AUSTRALIA AND NEW ZEALAND EDITION

Nursing and Midwifery RESEARCH

AUSTRALIA AND NEW ZEALAND EDITION

Nursing and Midwifery RESEARCH

methods and appraisal for evidence-based practice

7th edition

Dean Whitehead, PhD, MSc/MPH, BEd, FCNA (NZ)
Federation University Australia, Institute of Health and Wellbeing, Berwick, Victoria, Australia

Daniel Terry, PhD, MIntlHlth, MBA, Grad Cert UniTeach, BN, RN
University of Southern Queensland, School of Nursing and Midwifery, Ipswich, Queensland, Australia

Geri LoBiondo-Wood, PhD, RN, FAAN
Professor and Coordinator, PhD in Nursing Program, University of Texas Health Science Center at Houston, School of Nursing, Houston, Texas, USA

Judith Haber, PhD, RN, FAAN
Ursula Springer Leadership Professor in Nursing, New York University, Rory Meyers College of Nursing, New York, New York, USA

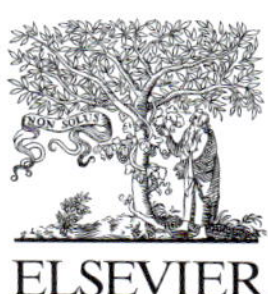

ELSEVIER

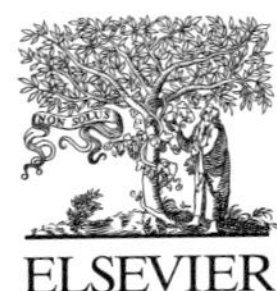

ELSEVIER

Elsevier Australia, ACN 001 002 357
(a division of Reed International Books Australia Pty Ltd)
Tower 1, 475 Victoria Avenue, Chatswood, NSW 2067

ISBN: 978-0-323-76291-5

This adaptation of Nursing Research: Methods and Critical Appraisal for Evidence-based Practice, tenth edition, by Geri LoBiondo-Wood and Judith Haber, was undertaken by Elsevier Australia and is published by arrangement with Elsevier Inc.

Nursing and Midwifery Research: methods and appraisal for evidence-based practice; Seventh Australia and New Zealand Edition

ISBN: 978-0-7295-4466-5

National Library of Australia Cataloguing-in-Publication Data

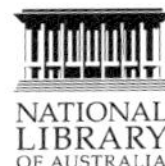

A catalogue record for this book is available from the National Library of Australia

Senior Content Strategist: Elizabeth Coady
Content Project Manager: Shruti Raj
Edited by Chris Wyard
Proofread by Tim Learner
Cover by Georgette Hall
Internal design: Standard
Index by Innodata Indexing
Typeset by GW Tech
Printed in Singapore by Markono Print Media Pte Ltd

Last digit is the print number: 9 8 7 6 5 4 3 2 1

TABLE OF CONTENTS

FOREWORD

The COVID-19 pandemic has been a clarion call for the importance of nurses and midwives in ensuring the health and wellbeing of our world. The pandemic has also underscored the importance of data-driven decision making and evidence-based practice. The ageing of the world's population, increasing geopolitical instability, soaring costs, widening inequities and the threats of global pandemics challenge existing models of care and generate many questions about what we can do better to address the needs of the populations we serve. A contemporary research agenda is not just about investigator-driven research but is also about considering the needs of individuals, families and communities in the context of contemporary social, political and economic dynamics. Co-design and co-production of research are critically important. The volume and speed of the introduction of new data require nurses and midwives to interpret, synthesise and apply research at an increasing rate. The burgeoning phenomenon of misinformation and disinformation increases the priority of these skills as a health professional.

In the framework of evolving and dynamic healthcare priorities, this seventh edition of *Nursing and Midwifery Research: methods and appraisal for evidence-based practice* comes at exactly the right time. In many ways, the world is at an inflection point emerging from the pandemic. Increasing digitalisation and the introduction of artificial intelligence are just two of the factors that signal a new era. To meet this challenge generations of committed, competent and credentialled nurses and midwives working across the healthcare ecosystem will be required.

Nursing and Midwifery Research: methods and appraisal for evidence-based practice builds upon the existing strengths of previous editions but is also adapted to the opportunities and challenges facing our world. The text provides a roadmap of the research journey from the conception of the big idea through planning, execution, evaluation and dissemination. Chapters tackle both methodological issues and pragmatic aspects of implementation, such as working in teams. Each chapter is structured on focused learning objectives and integrates tutorial and reflective exercises. Individually and collectively, these chapters provide an excellent resource for the nurse and midwife.

This impressive seventh edition is written by expert researchers who generously share their experience and wisdom to prepare the next generations of nurses and midwives. This text also marks another phase in the maturation of the research journey for nurses and midwives. Whether working in policy, practice, education or research, this text will remain a valuable resource beyond the classroom. The authors and editors are to be congratulated on this impressive contribution to the field and I hope it will inspire the current and next generation of researchers—the world needs you.

Patricia M. Davidson RN, PhD, FAAN
Dean Emerita
Johns Hopkins School of Nursing
United States of America;
Vice Chancellor & President
University of Wollongong
Australia

PREFACE

In the years since the first Australia–New Zealand edition of this book, nurses and midwives and allied healthcare professionals have continued to champion the need for critical appraisal and evaluation of research studies and reports. The ever-increasing acknowledgement behind basing practice on research evidence continues unchallenged—as does the importance of including nurses and midwives in the research process, either through conducting primary research and/or by implementing existing findings into practice. Effective knowledge regarding research methodology, process and design is mandatory in all healthcare settings today. All nurses and midwives need to understand what research findings mean and to realise its importance in defending, challenging and changing practice in complex healthcare environments. This seventh edition is dedicated, as were our previous editions, to all health professionals, research consumers and those conducting research. We, the Australasian editors/authors, have considerably revised previous content and pedagogy for this edition. As usual, we have updated supporting citation and the research sources and examples we use to illustrate the latest developments in the field. We gratefully acknowledge the contribution of our Australasian-based students, colleagues and reviewers of this text in making this edition more inclusive and broader in scope—while promoting a detailed account of the ever-changing nature and variety of the commonest research approaches in our disciplines.

This seventh edition is divided into three sections and 19 chapters.

Section 1: What you need to know about research to appreciate it and get started: This section sets the scene for the importance of nursing and midwifery research and provides an overview of research theory and its underpinning processes. It also includes chapters on critically searching for and reviewing the research literature and identifying research ideas, questions, statements and hypotheses.

Section 2: What you need to know about research to understand how it is applied: This section provides a detailed discussion of qualitative, quantitative and mixed-methods research approaches, with many useful examples from various settings. Chapters are devoted to implementation, sampling, collecting and analysing data in qualitative and quantitative approaches, assessing measuring instruments and applying research knowledge through evidence-based practice and knowledge translation. In addition, it also examines the ethical and legal issues to consider in research, along with a dedicated chapter examining Indigenous peoples and research.

Section 3: What you need to know about research if you want to conduct research: This section is designed to enhance the previous two sections through supporting both undergraduate and postgraduate students in their 'physical' research activities. Writing research proposals may be a requirement for undergraduates in their research program (especially at Honours level) and postgraduates will find the information useful for developing an ethics proposal or for applying for university and/or external funding. Research project management is included in this section—as well as presenting research findings, especially through the process of publication and other dissemination sources. The final chapter is designed to bring the 'whole' research process together by describing the beginning-to-end processes of a recently completed 'mixed-methods' research project. It should be of interest and advantage to both those new to the research process and those who are considering initial stages of conducting research in the field—as a 'live' example of research process.

We hope that you enjoy using the seventh edition of this text and that it stimulates and encourages you to read and think about research and its place in your professional practice and your wider 'world'. We also hope it assists in the development of your skills and confidence in critically searching for and appraising the research literature. Most importantly, we hope that you will share any new-found information about research with your colleagues and use research findings to inform the quality care that you deliver to your patients and clients. The delivery of quality nursing and midwifery evidence-based care is a challenge in our dynamic and complex healthcare environments and settings. Used appropriately, this text will be a valuable tool to assist you in that rewarding challenge.

Dean Whitehead and Daniel Terry
April 2024

EDITORS

Dean Whitehead, PhD, MSc/MPH, BEd, FCNA (NZ)
Federation University Australia, Institute of Health and Wellbeing, Berwick, Victoria, Australia

Daniel Terry, PhD, MIntlHlth, MBA, Grad Cert UniTeach, BN, RN
University of Southern Queensland, School of Nursing and Midwifery, Ipswich, Queensland, Australia

Geri LoBiondo-Wood, PhD, RN, FAAN
Professor and Coordinator, PhD in Nursing Program, University of Texas Health Science Center at Houston, School of Nursing, Houston, Texas, USA

Judith Haber, PhD, RN, FAAN
Ursula Springer Leadership Professor in Nursing, New York University, Rory Meyers College of Nursing, New York, New York, USA

ANZ CONTRIBUTORS

Elizabeth Brogan, PhD, MN, Grad Dip NURS, Grad Cert Perioperative, BN
Lecturer, School of Nursing and Midwifery, University of Technology Sydney, Ultimo, New South Wales, Australia

Raymond Chan, PhD, RN, FAAN, FACN
Deputy Vice-Chancellor (Research), Flinders University, Adelaide, South Australia, Australia

Deborah Davis, PhD, MNS, BN
Clinical Chair, Professor of Midwifery, Discipline of Midwifery, University of Canberra, Canberra, ACT, Australia

Jenny D'Antonio, MPET, BAppSc(Nursing)
Lecturer, Institute of Health and Wellbeing, Federation University Australia, Mt Helen, Victoria, Australia

Rebecca Feo, PhD, BPsych(Hons)
Senior Research Fellow, College of Nursing and Health Sciences, Flinders University, Adelaide, South Australia, Australia

Lynore Geia, PhD, MPH&TM, BNurse(Clinical), RM, RN
Professor of Nursing and Midwifery, School of Nursing and Midwifery, Edith Cowan University, Joondalup, Perth, Western Australia, Australia;
Adjunct Associate Professor,College of Health Care Sciences, James Cook University, Townsville, Queensland, Australia

Julia Gilbert, PhD
Lecturer, Institute of Health and Wellbeing, Federation University Australia, Ballarat, Victoria, Australia

Nicolas H. Hart, PhD, AES, CSCS, FESSA
Associate Professor, Human Performance Research Centre, University of Technology Sydney (UTS), Sydney, New South Wales, Australia

Darren Haywood, PhD, BPsych
Postdoctoral Research Fellow, School of Sport, Exercise, and Rehabilitation, University of Technology Sydney, Sydney, New South Wales, Australia

Danny Hills, PhD, MN Hons, Grad Cert Mgt, Grad Cert Ter Teach, BN
Monitoring and Evaluation Manager, Healthcare Solutions, Australian Primary Health Care Nurses Association, Melbourne, Victoria, Australia

Ha Hoang, PhD
Senior Lecturer in Rural Health, Centre for Rural Health, School of Health Sciences, University of Tasmania, Launceston, Tasmania, Australia

Alison Margaret Hutchinson, PhD, MBioeth, BAppSci (AdvNsg), RN
Professor, School of Nursing and Midwifery,Centre for Quality and Patient Safety, Institute for Health Transformation, Deakin University, Geelong, Victoria, Australia;
Chair in Nursing, Barwon Health, Geelong, Victoria, Australia

Sharon James, PhD, MPH, GradOHSN, BN, RN
Research Fellow/Project Manager AusCAPPS, SPHERE CRE, Department of General Practice, Monash University, Melbourne, Victoria, Australia

Jane Maguire, PhD, Grad Cert CFH, BA, BNurs(Hons)
Professor of Nursing, Deputy Head of School-Research, School of Nursing and Midwifery, University of Technology Sydney, Blaxland, New South Wales, Australia

Deb Massey, PhD, RN
Professor, Nursing and Midwifery, Edith Cowan University, Perth, Western Australia, Australia

Stephen Neville, PhD, RN, FCNA(NZ)
Professor, Nursing, Te Pūkenga, Hamilton, New Zealand

Hoang Nguyen, PhD
Lecturer, Wicking Dementia Research and Education Centre, College of Health and Medicine, University of Tasmania, Hobart, Tasmania, Australia

Rebecca O'Reilly, PhD
Professor of Nursing, Deputy Head of School, Nursing, Midwifery and Paramedicine, Australian Catholic University, New South Wales, Australia

Christopher Patterson, PhD, MN (MH), BN, RN
Associate Professor, Nursing, University of Wollongong, Wollongong, New South Wales, Australia

Hoang Phan, PhD, MD
Postdoctoral Research Fellow, Menzies Institute for Medical Research, University of Tasmania, Hobart, Tasmania, Australia

Tracy Robinson, PhD, BA(Hons)
Senior Lecturer, Nursing Innovation, School of Rural Health, Faculty of Medicine and Susan Wakil School of Nursing and Midwifery, University of Sydney, Sydney, New South Wales, Australia

Nicolette Sheridan, PhD, MPH, DipOHP, DipTT, RN
Head of School, School of Nursing
Professor, Nursing, Massey University, Auckland, New Zealand

Susan Stacpoole, PhD, BAppSc(Pod)
Adjunct Associate Professor, Institute of Health and Wellbeing, Federation University Australia, Victoria, Australia;
Research and Ethics Officer, School of Medicine, Rural Clinical School, University of Notre Dame Australia, Ballarat, Victoria, Australia

Linda Sweet, PhD, MNgS, GCHigherEd, BNg, RM, RN
Chair in Midwifery, School of Nursing and Midwifery, Deakin University, Burwood, Victoria, Australia;
Chair in Midwifery, Centre for Quality and Patient Safety, Western Health Partnership, St Albans, Victoria, Australia

Daniel Terry, PhD, MIntlHlth, MBA, BN
Associate Professor, School of Nursing and Midwifery, University of Southern Queensland, Ipswich, Queensland, Australia

Dean Whitehead, PhD, MSc, MPH, BEd, RN
Institute of Health and Wellbeing, Federation University Australia, Victoria, Australia

Nathan John Wilson, PhD, MSc, Grad Cert Sc (Applied Statistics), BSocSc, Dip Health Sc (Nursing)
Professor, School of Nursing and Midwifery, Western Sydney University, Richmond, New South Wales, Australia

ANZ REVIEWERS

Ashleigh E. Butler, PhD, MNurs, Grad Cert (Crit Care), Grad Cert Curriculum, Teaching and Learning in Higher Education, BNurs
Senior Research Fellow, School of Nursing and Midwifery, La Trobe University, Bundoora, Victoria, Australia

Carey Mather, PhD, MPH, GCert ULT, GCert Creative Media Technology, GCert Research PGrad Dip Health Promotion, BSc, RN, MACN, FAIDH, FHEA
Senior Lecturer, School of Nursing, College of Health and Medicine, University of Tasmania, Launceston, Australia

US CONTRIBUTORS

Karla M. Abela, PhD, RN, CCRN-K, CPN
Assistant Professor
University of Texas Health Science Center
Cizik School of Nursing
Houston, Texas, USA

Dian P. Baker, PhD, RN, APRN-BC
Professor
Nursing
California State University, Sacramento
Sacramento, California, USA

Julie Barroso, PhD, RN, FNAP, FAAN
Blair Chenault Professor of Nursing
Vanderbilt University School of Nursing
Nashville, Tennessee, USA

Carol Bova, PhD, RN, ANP
Professor
Graduate School of Nursing
University of Massachusetts Medical School
Worcester, Massachusetts, USA

Abraham A. Brody, PhD, RN, FAAN
Associate Professor of Nursing and Medicine
Associate Director, Hartford Institute for Geriatric Nursing
New York University
Rory Meyers College of Nursing
New York, New York, USA

Carolynn Spera Bruno, PhD, RN, APRN, CNS, FNP-C
Clinical Associate Professor
New York University
Rory Meyers College of Nursing
New York, New York, USA

Brynne A. Campbell, BA, MS
Health Sciences Reference Associate
Coles Science Center
New York University
Rory Meyers College of Nursing
New York, New York, USA

Dona M. Rinaldi, EdD, RN
Professor and Chairperson
Nursing
University of Scranton
Scranton, Pennsylvania, USA

Maja Djukic, PhD, RN, FAAN
John P. McGovern Distinguished Professor in Nursing
Associate Professor
University of Texas Health Science Center
Cizik School of Nursing
Houston, Texas, USA

Dalmacio Dennis Flores III, PhD, ACRN
Assistant Professor
Family and Community Health
University of Pennsylvania
School of Nursing
Pennsylvania, Philadelphia, USA

Mattia J. Gilmartin, PhD, RN, FAAN
Executive Director
Nurses Improving Care for Healthsystem Elders
New York University
Rory Meyers College of Nursing
New York, New York, USA

Judith Haber, PhD, RN, APRN, FAAN
Ursula Springer Leadership Professor in Nursing
New York University
Rory Meyers College of Nursing
New York, New York, USA

Tonda L. Hughes, PhD, RN, FAAN
Henik H. Bendixen Professor of International Nursing
Associate Dean, Global Health Nursing
Columbia University School of Nursing
New York, New York;
Professor of Psychiatry
Columbia University School of Medicine
New York, New York, USA

Susan Kaplan Jacobs, BSN, MLS, MA
Retired Curator, Health Sciences Librarian
Elmer Holmes Bobst Library
New York University Libraries
New York, New York, USA

Carl A. Kirton, DNP, RN, MBA
Chief Nursing Officer
Patient Care Services
University Hospital
Newark, New Jersey;
Adjunct Faculty-Nursing
New York University
Rory Meyers College of Nursing
New York, New York;
Adjunct Faculty
Business Administration
St. Peter's University
Jersey City, New Jersey, USA

Melanie McEwen, PhD, RN, CNE, ANEF, FAAN
Professor
University of Texas Health Science Center
Cizik School of Nursing
Houston, Texas, USA

Shannon Munro, PhD, APRN, NP
Researcher
Diffusion of Excellence Initiative
Veterans Health Administration
Salem, Virginia, USA

Brennan Parmelee Streck, PhD, RN
Cancer Prevention Fellow
Division of Cancer Prevention
National Cancer Institute, National Institutes of Health
Bethesda, Maryland, USA

Susan Sullivan-Bolyai, DNSc, CNS, RN, FAAN
Associate Dean for Research & Innovation
Graduate School of Nursing
University of Massachusetts Medical School
Worcester, Massachusetts, USA

Marita Titler, PhD, RN, FAAN
Professor Emerita
University of Michigan School of Nursing
Ann Arbor, Michigan, USA

Geri LoBiondo-Wood, PhD, RN, FAAN
Bette P. Thomas Distinguished Professor for Innovative Healthcare Delivery
Director, PhD in Nursing Program
University of Texas Health Science Center
Cizik School of Nursing
Houston, Texas, USA

ACKNOWLEDGEMENTS

Welcome to the seventh edition of this nursing and midwifery research text. Our deep appreciation is extended to all our Australasian-based contributors for their collegiality, in creating a friendly, supportive and cooperative environment in which to achieve our aims of producing a market-leading text in the important field of nursing and midwifery research and evidence-based practice. We, the Australasian editors, and authors, have considerably revised the previous edition content and pedagogy for this edition. As usual, we have also updated supporting citations and the primary research sources and examples that we use to illustrate the latest and seminal developments in the field.

The production of this edition was facilitated by the Elsevier (Australasia) publishing team with their assistance and support throughout the writing and production process: We would like to express our appreciation to Shruti Raj, Content Project Manager, and Elizabeth Coady, Senior Content Strategist, for their patience, guidance and unfailing assistance throughout the development of this book. We also thank the Australasian manuscript reviewers, colleagues and students who collectively provided feedback, suggestions and ideas to make this text even more relevant, useful and meaningful than previous editions. This is to the direct benefit of nurses, midwives and other related health professionals. Lastly, but by no means least, we are indebted to our families, who were enthusiastically with us all the way through this edition 'journey'. Dean would like to express his heartfelt gratitude to Katie, Thomas, James and Joshua for their unstinting love and support and their tolerance of re-locating from place to place. 'Chasing research' often means never standing still. Daniel would like to express his gratitude to his family, Melissa, Hannah, David, Rachel and Esther, for their sacrifice of time, their patience as plans changed and their sense of adventure in dad's pursuit of knowledge.

Dean Whitehead and Daniel Terry

SECTION 1

What You Need to Know About Research to Appreciate It and Get Started

1

The Significance of Nursing and Midwifery Research and Evidence-Based Practice

Dean Whitehead and Daniel Terry

LEARNING OUTCOMES

After reading this chapter, you should be able to:

- understand the value of research and evidence-based practice in relation to nursing- and midwifery-based practice
- identify Australasian perspectives of the relationships between research, education, policy and practice
- investigate the need for consumer engagement in nursing and midwifery research
- identify contemporary trends in terms of nursing and midwifery research and evidence-based practice.

KEY TERMS

evidence-based practice, p. 2
nursing- and midwifery-based research, p. 3
research awareness, p. 7
research consumers, p. 3
research utilisation, p. 7
translation science, p. 8

HOW THIS BOOK WORKS

The main aims of this book are to support nurses, midwives and other health professionals in developing research awareness and critical appraisal skills and research consumer expertise—as well as to provide foundational skills in conducting primary research. There are three 'logical' sections. Section 1 *What you need to know about research to appreciate it and get started* (for understanding the early reasons and processes for conducting research) examines the key aspects of research awareness, research theory and process, searching and reviewing the research literature, and formulating research ideas and questions. Section 2 *What you need to know about research to understand how it is applied* (for understanding how existing research is and can be used to influence practice) incorporates chapters on common qualitative and quantitative approaches/processes, mixed-methods (multi-methods) research, ethical and legal issues, Indigenous research approaches, and the application of evidence-based practice and knowledge translation. Section 3 *What you need to know about research if you want to conduct research* (for understanding of the full processes required for undertaking research projects) provides practical information about writing research proposals and grant applications, managing a research project, and presenting and publishing conducted research. It has a final chapter providing a detailed 'live' account of the progress from research idea through to publication and further dissemination of an actual clinical mixed-methods project.

INTRODUCTION

We intentionally want this introductory chapter to be briefer than others in this book. Many books start off with an over-long and over-complex lead-in and this can distract readers from the beginning. Research and **evidence-based practice** (EBP) can appear over-complex and so we want to leave more specific 'detail' until later chapters. This chapter, instead, is designed to offer a more gradual lead-in. For now, the early aim is to identify what research is, its important place in clinical (and non-clinical) practice, education and policy, and its close relationship with EBP. The purpose of this opening chapter, then, is to introduce the reader to the topics of this book and, overall, to clarify the significance of research and the implementation of evidence-based findings into nursing and midwifery (and all healthcare) practice. It is intended that this chapter and text, overall, will make a valuable contribution towards broadening the reader's understanding of research and EBP and further extending the knowledge base of those already familiar with aspects of it. As stated some time ago, 'Take nothing on its looks; take everything on evidence. There's no better rule.' (Charles Dickens).

WHY DO WE NEED RESEARCH?

TUTORIAL TRIGGER 1.1

Most nurses and midwives will understand the relevance of research and basing our practice on the 'best' available evidence—even if they don't always see or witness it in practice. Make a list of the main reasons why research and best evidence-based practice is core to nursing and midwifery practice.

Hopefully, most of us will acknowledge that research is an important aspect of nursing and midwifery practice—over a variety of settings and disciplines (i.e. clinical practice, education, management, policy setting, etc.). It is assumed that it is far better to be a research-based profession than not. It is vital to ensure credibility within and outside our professions—especially with the members of the public/communities that we serve. So why is it then that **nursing- and midwifery-based research** is often viewed as 'something that others do'—and far from a universal and widespread activity at the international, national, regional and local level? While many nurses and midwives are 'research aware', how many are highly knowledgeable '**research consumers**' and/or implement and practise research—especially outside of the Higher Degree Research (HDR) educational setting—where undertaking research projects is required to achieve certain degree qualifications?

In the healthcare/health service setting, a key objective is the delivery of safe and effective quality-driven patient care. To meet this objective, nurses and midwives are required to have at least a good understanding of the importance of the place of research—both as consumers and as conductors of research. This can be challenging given the continual change and complexities brought about in health and social care environments—in both acute and community settings. These challenges include an ageing and multicultural population as they relate to multimorbidity issues affecting children through to older adults—for instance, lifestyle-related chronic diseases (e.g. diabetes, respiratory and cardiovascular disease), new endemics and epidemics (we've recently got over the COVID-19 epidemic—but its legacy lingers in various forms) and evolving social issues such as low health literacy rates. Both acute and community-based healthcare settings are notably highly complex settings and they are ever changing and 'fluid'. That means our practices are ever changing and evolving, and we cannot stand still in such an environment. We must keep abreast of what the current evidence base is and what it is not—and what is predicted for the near future.

Interestingly, when one searches the nursing and midwifery 'current state of research' literature, there is little that discusses general issues around research across the professions in Australasia. The exception is Eckert et al (2022 p. 515) in their critical opinion piece article, in *The Medical Journal of Australia*, as authored by senior nurses and midwives across Australia and New Zealand. Their article is a rallying call for the nursing and midwifery workforce to boost Australia's clinical research impact. They argue that the largest health workforce has the greatest research potential, but that this workforce is underrepresented as recipients of research funding and that employment structures affect nursing and midwifery clinicians'/researchers' ability to lead research that improves the healthcare system overall. They state:

> *Nurses and midwives are the frontline workers in hospitals and communities and thus are well positioned to lead research addressing efficacy of clinical and health system interventions. Nurses and midwives work across all aspects of healthcare delivery, across all age groups, and from metropolitan to rural and remote areas, making their reach and potential impact substantial. To achieve meaningful and sustained impacts on health care outcomes, greater engagement with, and investment in, nursing- and midwifery-led research is needed.*

The authors suggest that, moving forward, strategies are needed to:

- **develop research skills:**
  - by further improving the teaching of undergraduate level research skills and enabling conversion to honours programs;

  - by improving doctoral and postdoctoral research training opportunities and ensuring suitability of programs for nurses and midwives, including those who remain clinically active; and
  - by improving the quality of nursing and midwifery research outputs; and
- **increase resources:**
  - by funding career frameworks for nurses and midwives to undertake research that is clinically embedded, whether or not they undertake direct clinical work; and
  - by creating nursing and midwifery roles that are part clinical and part research, and providing clinicians with dedicated time alongside their care duties to undertake clinical research and translation work—similar to medical colleagues.

To assist such called-for reform, authors such as Janerka et al (2023) have attempted to investigate research priorities in healthcare settings. Their study aimed to determine nursing and midwifery research priorities for a metropolitan health service (across five hospital sites) in Australia using a priority-setting partnership approach. They adopted a mixed-methods, multiphase study (see Chapter 12). This involved (i) formation of a steering group (consumers, clinicians); (ii) a cross-sectional survey of nurses, midwives, patients, carers and community members to identify research topics; (iii–iv) summarising and checking of research topics; (v) interim priority setting; (vi) a consensus workshop for final priority setting using a modified nominal group technique; and (vii) reporting. They concluded that priorities reflected a strong desire for research focus on clinical care, as well as education and systems to support nurses and midwives in providing care. Involving clinicians and consumers in research can help identify priorities that are of direct relevance to health service users and staff.

WHAT ARE THE BARRIERS AND ENABLERS FOR NURSING AND MIDWIFERY RESEARCH?

What we do know, despite our agreement that research is vital to our practice and that it should be a universal practice, is that there remain many barriers (negative influences) and enablers (positive influences) to nursing and midwifery research. Research requires time, effort and comprehensive understanding. The barriers and enablers, taken from existing research evidence, tend to relate to resourcing, funding, educational, cultural, professional and organisational factors. These are summarised in Table 1.1. The table contents are enablers. If they are absent, then they become the barriers.

RESEARCH IN BRIEF 1.1

Morrison et al's (2022) study examined factors influencing research activity among nurses in clinical practice. The commonly cited barriers included a lack of research knowledge, confidence and access to resources (particularly protected time), while enablers were reported as educational partnerships, research-motivated clinical nurses and access to research role models.

TUTORIAL TRIGGER 1.2

Referring back to Tutorial Trigger 1.1 and comparing with it, list the main reasons why you think that many nurses and midwives do not routinely use and/or conduct research in their practice. Is this a problem—and, if so, why?

HOW DOES RESEARCH AND EVIDENCE PROTECT US AND THE PUBLIC WE SERVE?

All healthcare professionals have a professional duty to acknowledge and draw upon a readily available knowledge base to protect the health-related interests of the public at large—and to protect health professionals themselves (Lehane et al 2019). Let's take a common clinical scenario. Imagine that you (or a colleague) have made an unintentional clinical/practice error and the consequence is that you are formally required to explain your (or their) actions to a clinical Line Manager. Most questioning from a Line Manager would probably centre on 'what was the knowledge and evidence base at the time to justify the actions taken—leading to the error?' (see Chapter 13). How would you go about justifying yourself/your colleague's practice? For many, if they could not clearly and specifically provide a clearly defined and proven research EBP rationale for the action, the type of responses typically might be 'we've always done it this way', 'nobody has questioned it before', 'I was told to do it', 'I didn't realise that there were alternatives', 'I *assumed* that this was best practice', etc. Although these types of responses in such circumstances might be commonplace, they are not viewed as a 'strong case' for justifying practice actions. There would be likely consequences if this were the case. Good-quality research and evidence exist to protect practitioners and the public at large.

It is a large part of our professional scope of practice and personal accountability to ensure that we are up to date with our research and evidence knowledge and understand

TABLE 1.1 Barriers and Enablers to Nursing and Midwifery Research

Resourcing	Funding	Cultural	Professional	Organisational
Research infrastructure—desk, computer, space, software Educational and development program (training and education) Peer and mentoring framework Access to library, IT systems and research findings	Financial support (open access publication, conference and travel support) Dedicated research positions Protected time (workforce and staffing) Research grant funding (internal and external)	Supportive research culture Access to mentors Access to research support activities Journal clubs In-service education Symposia and research showcases Continuing professional development Motivation Enthusiasm and passion Encouraging new and novel research methods Time Support from colleagues (communities of practice)	Dedicated research positions Strong local research teams focused on priorities Inter-professional/ disciplinary research opportunities Conference attendance Research skills, capabilities and attributes Teamwork Continuing professional development Networking and peer support Access to academic support Knowledge, skills, confidence, training	Access to research teams Protected time (workforce and staffing) Local, national and international research leadership Academic–clinical collaborations Workforce models Institutional and managerial support Organisational support Research frameworks and procedures Access to data Research translation and implementation

what best practice is—and, equally, what is not best practice. All registered health professionals are accountable and responsible for providing the best possible quality standard of patient care at all times—and ensuring that these standards are research defined and evidence based (Australian Nursing and Midwifery Council (ANMC) *Code of Professional Conduct for Nurses in Australia* 2018 https://www.nursingmidwiferyboard.gov.au/Codes-Guidelines-Statements/Professional-standards.aspx; *Nursing Council of New Zealand Code of Conduct and Scope of Practice* 2012 https://www.nursingcouncil.org.nz/Public/Nursing/Code_of_Conduct/NCNZ/nursing-section/Code_of_Conduct.aspx).

It is important to note that if you are an undergraduate student nurse you are not accountable to the ANMC or NCNZ; however, an ability to demonstrate compliance with their codes of conduct throughout your course is essential and is closely assessed in the clinical and higher education setting.

Experiential (hands-on) learning is important in the clinical setting where nurses and midwives see practice firsthand. Research studies provide information with examples which connect and relate to the theoretical aspects of the research and, hopefully, provide evidence-based information to impact real-life clinical situations. For instance, it is commonly reported that many students, especially early on in their training (both undergraduate and postgraduate), struggle with the demands of clinical placements. Often that experience seems to be related to the working relationship that students enjoy (or do not enjoy) with their clinical facilitators. How would we know what 'best practice' for clinical facilitators (and best practice for students working with them) looks like if we don't investigate such social phenomena? For instance, Ryan and McAllister (2019) conducted a qualitative, descriptive, interpretative study (see Chapter 5) on the experiences of clinical facilitators working with Australian nursing students. They uncovered four themes revealing participants' (clinical facilitators') different mindsets, actions and skills to provide insights into the complexity of the role. These four themes included *preparing to work with students, facilitating successful clinical experiences, facing unique challenges* and *encountering rewards along the way*. These themes alone offer valuable insight into common experiences between students and facilitators—and what we can further learn from such findings. Furthermore, Bradley et al (2023) explored how final year graduating students perceive themselves and are prepared for RN roles as 'work ready' in Australia. This included the role of the clinical preceptor in facilitating their role transition.

Hopefully, these related examples help the reader to understand the importance of exploring and acknowledging complex healthcare issues using a range of different research approaches and representing different participants and their worldviews. There is no single research study that can determine practice—nor any single perspective that can represent the only solution or 'truth'. Good-quality practice outcomes and effective knowledge can come only from asking and critically examining multiple research/evidence perspectives—and representing all approaches to research.

WHAT DO NURSES AND MIDWIVES GENERALLY RESEARCH?

Nursing and midwifery are diverse disciplines that can be explored in many different ways—from studying an '*nth* of one' (i.e. an in-depth study of one participant, i.e. case study, meta-ethnography) through to large epidemiological and census-based studies (large-scale population-based surveys), and from an in-depth understanding of unique personal experiences (usually qualitative) through to broad survey and clinical trial findings (usually quantitative). Healthcare and health service environments are highly complex and ever changing. Research agendas are often dictated by the most current topics—clinical and social. Whatever the topic/issue, a consistency is that the research agendas are often focused on patient care quality, efficacy, efficiency and safety. If we look, broadly, to the current nursing and midwifery research literature, common themes are noted. Box 1.1 lists some of the current research priorities seen in the nursing and midwifery research literature.

RESEARCH IN BRIEF 1.2

Becoming a competent midwife is a complex process. The aim of midwifery education is to support the development of competence in midwifery skills and knowledge and to prepare graduates to meet the responsibilities inherent in the midwifery role. In Patterson et al's (2019) New Zealand online survey-based study, it was asked how well newly graduated midwifery practitioners perceived their midwifery program had prepared them for beginning midwifery practice. The findings highlighted that those respondents viewed becoming a midwife as a blend/combination of: (1) *gaining the knowledge and practical skills required for the profession*; (2) *management skills in areas of running a business, working with other people, navigating local procedures and processes effectively and balancing work with personal life*; (3) *gaining confidence in one's competence*; and (4) *having support along the way*. The study concluded that content that facilitates these four finding requirements should be included in midwifery programs to support the transition from student to practitioner—and paves the way for approaching transition to practice while being mindful of these factors.

HOW DO WE KNOW WHAT GOOD RESEARCH LOOKS LIKE?

Although many nurses and midwives may not actually physically conduct research, most will recognise the need to possess the skills to critically find, read, review and appraise published research—particularly in the age of 'predatory journals' (see Chapter 3 for more detail).

BOX 1.1 Nursing and Midwifery Research Priorities

The following list, while not exhaustive, highlights common research priorities that are notable in the current nursing and midwifery literature.

- Patient safety and quality care
- Workforce, professional issues and advanced practice (see Research in brief 1.2—Patterson et al (2019))
- Health services research—acute and primary healthcare
- Ageing, chronic and palliative care
- Cancer, oncology and recovery care
- Patient experience and compassionate care
- Quality of life (i.e. symptom management and self-management)
- Vulnerable populations
- Integrated, community and transitional care
- Models of care (e.g. nurse-led care)
- Maternal, child and family health
- Mental health (see Research in brief 1.3—De Cieri et al (2019))
- Digital health
- Patient-centred and family-centred care
- Health economics and policy
- Knowledge transfer, implementation science and research translation
- Interdisciplinary/agency research

RESEARCH IN BRIEF 1.3

It is well known that healthcare service workplaces are often demanding and stressful workplaces in which to live. The impact of work-related stress on mental and physical health is particularly notable within nurses and midwives, who have been found to face exposure to a wide range of work-related stressors. The introduction of mental health 'mindfulness' has been gaining popularity in recent years to counter workplace stress and encourage and maintain positive mental wellbeing. De Cieri et al (2019) identify that mindfulness is defined as 'the awareness that emerges through paying attention on purpose, in the present moment and non-judgmentally to the unfolding of experience moment by moment'. This finding emerged from their Victoria-based cross-sectional survey reporting the findings of 702 nursing and healthcare worker participants. Their findings were that participants reported higher levels of work-related stress and poorer mental health compared with available norms, whereas their levels of physical health were within the normal range. Analysis showed that work-related stressors were important predictors of employee mental health, but that mindfulness was the stronger predictor. There was a slightly stronger relationship between employee physical health and work-related stress compared with mindfulness. Furthermore, being younger and being employed in a non-nursing role were associated with better physical health. Such findings add to the evidence base supporting mindfulness in the workplace and assist in informing further research in this important area.

Oermann et al (2017) conducted a study into predatory journals in nursing in 2016. At the time, 70,000 predatory journal articles within biomedicine (including nursing and midwifery) were published by 2014. Their finding that most of the articles reviewed were rated as of poor or average quality supports the fact that consumers of the nursing literature cannot rely on articles published in these journals for credible, sound evidence on which to base nursing practice or build nursing knowledge. Therefore, nurses and midwives need to acquire the critical appraisal skills to understand good-quality research findings and separate them out from those of poor quality. A mistaken assumption, by many, is that 'if something is published then it must be of good quality'. That simply is not the case.

Within this context, it is vital to develop an understanding of published research, not only of the findings that may impact practice, but also that the quality of the research is sufficiently robust to 'trust' or have confidence in the findings; thus critical decisions about practice change can be made. This is commonly the first step that health professionals take in their journey to become familiar with research and the processes of research—that is, the critical searching for and the reviewing/appraisal of gathered research literature (see Chapter 3). It is also one of the first steps towards 'research awareness'—which is the emphasis of the first section of this book.

TRANSLATING AND IMPLEMENTING RESEARCH KNOWLEDGE TO PRACTICE

Evidence-based nursing (EBN) and evidence-based midwifery (EBM) have their roots in the evidence-based medicine movement that grew from clinicians' concerns about the growing mass of clinical trials conducted that did not make their findings into medical practice. Evidence-based medicine was focused initially on appraising the best-available medical research and incorporating it into practice. As EBP has evolved, there is a need for high-quality and up-to-date research that is able to be understood, which supports clinicians to improve their own practice and to provide patients with relevant and current information (Schaefer & Welton 2018).

EBP encompasses three key elements, which include clinical expertise, patient preferences and high-quality research, and it is these three elements that contribute to good clinical decision making. EBP has been instrumental in improving the quality of nursing practice and care, minimising potential healthcare complications and reducing healthcare costs. It is considered the highest standard in supporting clinicians with making healthcare decisions (D'Souza et al 2021).

Overall, EBN and EBM have brought about a change in emphasis from **doing** research to **understanding** research, which reflects a move from 'research generation' towards '**research utilisation**' in practice (Lehane et al 2019). An accompanying strong policy and legislation emphasis on clinical effectiveness and quality (clinical governance) means that nurses and midwives are routinely called upon to justify their clinical decisions and outcomes to clients, peers, colleagues, commissioners and all consumers of healthcare (Fowler 2014).

Research awareness is an important stage of beginning the process of learning research and EBP. It allows us to identify what research is and where it is located, and to recognise it when we see it. It also allows us to discuss research in an informed manner with other health professional colleagues and clients. Watanabe et al (2013 p. 232) state that 'research awareness is an important consideration necessary for providing superior nursing care'. However, we also understand that superior nursing care is often not the norm of clinical practice.

Being research aware does not always 'translate to practice'. Being a research consumer, however, moves us forwards, which means that this translation process must occur. To help illustrate, Curtis et al (2017 p. 862) have stated:

> *There is universal acknowledgement that the clinical care provided to individuals should be informed on the best available evidence. Knowledge and evidence derived from robust scholarly methods should drive our clinical practice, decisions and change to improve the way we deliver care. Translating research evidence to clinical practice is essential to safe, transparent, effective and efficient healthcare provision and meeting the expectations of patients, families and society. Despite its importance, translating research into clinical practice is challenging. There are more nurses in the frontline of healthcare than any other healthcare profession. As such, nurse-led [and midwifery-led] research is increasingly recognised as a critical pathway to practical and effective ways of improving patient outcomes.*

Being a research consumer also encourages a more critical 'lens' to view practice and question and challenge gaps and inconsistencies in the existing knowledge base. For instance, see 'Research in brief 1.4' by Hungerford et al (2019) related to differences in mandated undergraduate nursing student practice hours between four different countries. The study essentially asks: 'Why are there differences and is any one system better?' Such questions are important to ask in terms of critically evaluating practice as we compare and contrast different 'systems'.

RESEARCH IN BRIEF 1.4

Hungerford et al (2019) have identified that there is a global acceptance of the need for undergraduate nursing students to complete practice experience hours during their program of education—yet questions remain about these practice experiences, including those related to duration. They report a scoping review (see Chapter 3) that compared the number of practice experience hours mandated for students undertaking courses that led to Registered Nurse (RN) licensure in Australia, New Zealand, the United Kingdom and the United States. They found that substantial differences were evident between the four countries regarding the number of mandated practice experience hours and identified that there is no clearly linked research evidence to justify the decision made in relation to the mandated number of hours. They conclude that, internationally, there is a need to re-examine the rationale for mandating a minimum number of practice experience hours for students in programs of education that lead to qualifying as an RN.

RESEARCH TO EVIDENCE-BASED PRACTICE TO TRANSLATIONAL SCIENCE/KNOWLEDGE TRANSLATION

The Joanna Briggs Institute (JBI, based in South Australia), alongside other organisations such as the Cochrane Library (see Additional Resources), seeks to facilitate and support EBP in all healthcare settings across the world. Based on the updated JBI model of evidence-based healthcare (see Chapter 15), healthcare practitioners, policy makers and others involved in the management or delivery of care can draw on a number of key steps in getting evidence into practice which best suits the organisational context (JBI: https://jbi.global/jbi-model-of-EBHC). The steps and processes to get evidence into practice within the JBI model are well documented (Jordan et al 2019), with the five 'As' of EBP, which include Ask, Acquire, Appraise, Apply and Audit. The JBI model provides a greater understanding of the EBP process as:

1. searching for the best available international evidence
2. appraising the evidence
3. summarising and disseminating usable and valid evidence
4. embedding appraised and rated evidence in practice and organisational systems
5. utilising the evidence
6. evaluating the use and impact of evidence-based practices and policies on outcomes.

Closely related to EBP, the concept of **translation science** (knowledge translation, knowledge transfer, implementation science, etc.) is a relatively new discipline of investigation that is rapidly growing in the healthcare sciences. Its premise is based on the notable gap between the availability of EBP recommendations and the actual subsequent application of evidence to improve patient care and population health. Translation science is designed to test and measure implementation interventions to improve the uptake and use of evidence in the healthcare arena. This field has emerged to investigate which implementation strategies work to promote use of tried and tested EBPs. Advancements in translation science can sustain the successful integration of evidence in practice to improve care delivery, population health and health outcomes. Helpfully, Titler (2018) offers an introductory overview of translation science and addresses issues in this field of science such as variations in terminology, theories and models, implementation strategies, and context and implementation related to EBPs.

TUTORIAL TRIGGER 1.3

You have been employed by a large hospital as a clinical nurse researcher. Very little research has so far been undertaken by the nursing and midwifery staff at the hospital. Your role involves promoting nursing and midwifery research and creating a stimulating, friendly and supportive environment for this purpose.

How might you best go about your role?

AN UNEXPECTED HURDLE

Sarah is a recently graduated registered health professional. From her undergraduate training, she has a good awareness of the contribution of good-quality research to influence clinical practice. She is keen to establish a research career. Faced with a specific clinical issue at work associated with wound care, she searched for a more recent and 'robust' research study that seemed to offer alternative and safer care to current practice. Sarah presented the study findings to the wound care team but was disheartened when encountering resistance to her proposal. Usual practice remained in place.

Could Sarah have approached this differently to meet the unexpected resistance—and what early steps could she take to begin her research career interest?

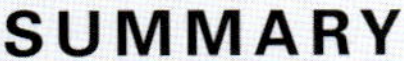

SUMMARY

The future of nursing and midwifery research in the Australasian region looks to be an exciting one. At the present time, Australian and New Zealand nurses and midwives continue to develop a strong research base as evidenced in the many research publications. Research continues to grow and flourish despite the difficulties experienced by the professions within the evolving healthcare environment. This chapter has aimed to identify the nature and place of nursing and midwifery research in building efficient and effective quality-based practice. It is intended that readers are beginning to appreciate the vital place of nursing and midwifery research and EBP and to understand their place as a current/future research consumer. The following chapter is intended to lead readers to a beginning understanding of the actual process and design of research in relation to its theoretical and philosophical underpinnings.

KEY POINTS

- Nursing and midwifery research is primarily concerned with determining and evaluating quality patient outcomes and improving practice. Research provides the basis for expanding the body of scientific knowledge that forms the foundation of nursing and midwifery practice. Thus research links education, theory, practice, management and policy.
- Nurses and midwives, at all levels, have a responsibility to understand and participate in the research process. We are all encouraged to move beyond being activity and task focused and to move towards a focus on solving clinical problems, cultivating better practices and improving patient care and outcomes. Therefore, as consumers of research, we must have a basic understanding of the research process and critical appraisal skills that provide a standard for evaluating the strengths and weaknesses of research studies before considering applying them in clinical practice.

TIME TO REFLECT

Happell B, Waks S, Bocking J, et al., 2019. 'I felt some prejudice in the back of my head': nursing students' perspectives on learning about mental health from 'Experts by Experience'. J. Psychiatr. Ment. Health Nurs. 26 (7–8), 233–243. doi:10.1111/jpm.12540

Aim: Even though mental health is an important component of undergraduate and postgraduate nursing and midwifery education, and though many of our clients suffer issues of mental health at any time on the lifespan and in different healthcare settings, negative attitudes and stereotypes persist with health professionals. Evidence suggests that the use of mental health service consumers (Experts by Experience) can influence positive attitudes in nursing students. Research in this area to date is limited and primarily from Australia and New Zealand. Happell et al (2019) sought to identify nursing students' perspectives and experiences of being taught mental health by an 'Expert by Experience'.

Design: A qualitative exploratory approach was used. Focus groups were conducted with nursing students from seven universities in Australia and Europe. Data were analysed thematically.

Reflect on the following as reported in the study: Student participants described how exposure to Experts by Experience challenged their views and attitudes and provided a mechanism for reflection, critique and change.

Continued

TIME TO REFLECT—cont'd

The main theme 'changing mindset' includes two subthemes: *exposing stereotypes* and *reflection*. This unique international study demonstrates the capacity for Experts by Experience to contribute to positive attitudinal change towards mental illness in nursing students. This changed mindset must occur for policy goals to be realised. Nurses in all areas of practice will work with people labelled with mental illness and experiencing mental distress. Overcoming stereotypes and adopting more positive attitudes is essential to delivering quality mental health care.

Questions

Reflect on the information given and answer the following questions:

a. Can you identify the research design? Do you know of other research designs that could have been used?
b. Do you think that the chosen design is appropriate for this study?
c. What information did the researchers want and did they get it?
d. Do you think that the objectives are achievable using this design?

All healthcare professionals have a professional duty to acknowledge and draw upon a readily available knowledge base to protect the health-related interests of the public at large—and to protect health professionals themselves.

Does this study fulfil that duty?

LEARNING ACTIVITIES

1. A research consumer is one who:
   a. wants to join a research team to participate in the conduct of research
   b. wants to change practice in the clinical area
   c. wants to read critically and evaluate research findings for implementation into nursing practice
   d. wants to conduct research in the clinical area.
2. Nurses and midwives do not always conduct research because:
   a. they find it difficult to translate findings into practice
   b. they think that research findings are irrelevant and that their practice is good enough
   c. they do not have the time to change their practice
   d. they find it difficult to conduct research in the clinical area.
3. The Australian College of Nursing and the New Zealand Nurses Organisation:
   a. want all nurses to conduct research
   b. do not think that all research is important
   c. think that all nurses should undertake higher degrees in nursing
   d. want to promote research as an integral part of nursing practice.
4. Nurses and midwives, whether consumers or producers of research or both:
   a. need to recognise the research process as contributing to the professionalism of their discipline
   b. need to understand that only senior nurses should be involved in research
   c. want all research findings to be implemented in practice
   d. want every nurse and midwife to be involved in writing research proposals.
5. The primary objective of EBP is:
   a to reduce healthcare costs
   b to improve patient outcomes
   c to increase healthcare provider job satisfaction
   d to attract new patients to a healthcare facility.
6. Translation science is an emerging and important discipline that seeks:
   a. to make nursing and midwifery practice more scientific
   b. to improve the uptake and use of evidence in the healthcare setting
   c. to allow us to be more critical of existing practice
   d. to identify which research approaches are the best.

For further content associated with this chapter visit: https://evolve.elsevier.com/cs/product/9780729596794?role=student 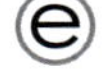

ADDITIONAL RESOURCES

Cochrane Library. https://www.cochrane.org/evidence.

Joanna Briggs Institute approach to evidence-based healthcare. https://jbi.global/.

National Health and Medical Research Council. 2016. Guidance for Guidelines Development. https://www.nhmrc.gov.au/guidelines.

REFERENCES

Bradley, L., Barr, J.A., Finn J., 2023. Work readiness of graduating nursing students: case study research. Teach. Learn. Nurs. 18 (3), 383–388. doi:10.1016/j.teln.2023.03.012

Curtis, K., Fry, M., Shaban, R.Z., et al., 2017. Translating research findings to clinical nursing practice. J. Clin. Nurs. 26, 862–872. doi:10.1111/jocn.13586

De Cieri, H., Shea, T., Cooper, B., et al., 2019. Effects of work-related stressors and mindfulness on mental and physical health among Australian nurses and healthcare workers. J. Nurs. Scholarsh. 51 (5), 580–589. doi:10.1111/jnu.12502

D'Souza, P., George, A., Nair, S., et al., 2021. Effectiveness of an evidence- based practice training program for nurse educators: a cluster- randomized controlled trail. Worldviews Evid.-based Nurs. 18 (4) 261–271. doi:10.1111/wvn.12521

Eckert, M., Rickard, C. M., Forsythe, D., et al., 2022. Harnessing the nursing and midwifery workforce to boost Australia's clinical research impact. Med. J. Aust. 217(10), 514.

Fowler, F.J. Jr., 2014. The problem with survey research. Contemp. Sociol. 43 (5), 660. doi:10.1177/0094306114545742f

Happell, B., Waks, S., Bocking, J., et al., 2019. 'I felt some prejudice in the back of my head': nursing students' perspectives on learning about mental health from 'Experts by Experience'. J. Psychiatr. Ment. Health Nurs. 26 (7–8), 233–243. doi:10.1111/jpm.12540

Hungerford, C., Blanchard, D., Bragg, S., et al., 2019. An international scoping exercise examining practice experience hours completed by nursing students. J. Nurs. Educ. 58 (1), 33–41. doi:10.3928/01484834-20190103-06

Janerka, C., Mellan, M., Wright, R., et al., 2023. Nursing and midwifery research priorities for an Australian health service: a priority-setting partnership approach. Collegian 30, 693–700. doi:10.1016/j.colegn.2023.08.004

Jordan, Z., Lockwood, C., Munn, Z., et al., 2019. The updated Joanna Briggs Institute model of evidence-based healthcare. JBI Evid. Implement. 17(1), 58–71.

Lehane, E., Leahy-Warren, P., O'Riordan, C., et al., 2019. Evidence-based practice education for healthcare professions: an expert view. BMJ Evid. Based Med. 24, 103–108.

Morrison, L., Johnston, B., Cooper, M., 2022. Mixed methods systematic review: factors influencing research activity among nurses in clinical practice. J. Clin. Nurs. 31, 2450–2464. doi:10.1111/jocn.16133

Oermann, M.H., Nicoll, L.H., Chinn, P.L., et al., 2017. Quality of articles published in predatory nursing journals. Nurs. Outlook 66 (1), 4–10. doi:10.1016/j.outlook.2017.05.005

Patterson, J., Macznik, A.K., Miller, S., et al., 2019. Becoming a midwife: a survey study of midwifery alumni. Women Birth 32 (3), e399–e408. doi:10.1016/j.wombi.2018.07.022

Ryan, C., McAllister, M., 2019. The experiences of clinical facilitators working with nursing students in Australia: an interpretive description. Collegian 26 (2), 281–287. doi:10.1016/j.colegn.2018.07.005

Schaefer, J. D., Welton, J.M., 2018. Evidence based practice readiness: a concept analysis. J. Nurs. Manage. 26 (6), 621–629. doi:10.1111/jonm.12599

Titler, M.G., 2018. Translation research in practice: an introduction. Online J. Iss. Nurs. 23 (2), 1. doi:10.3912/OJIN.Vol-23No02Man01

Watanabe, Y., Oe, M., Takemura, Y., et al., 2013. Four factor Research Awareness Scale for nurses in Japan: instrument development study. Jpn. J. Nurs. Sci. 10, 232–241. doi:10.1111/jjns.12009

2

An Overview of Research Theory, Process and Design

Linda Sweet and Deborah Davis

LEARNING OUTCOMES

After reading this chapter, you should be able to:

- discuss the theoretical and philosophical positions that underpin different research approaches
- examine the relationships between paradigms, methodologies and frameworks
- describe broad commonalities and differences between qualitative and quantitative research approaches
- list the sequential elements that form the research process and research design.

KEY TERMS

constructionism, p. 14
critical social theory, p. 16
epistemology, p. 13
interpretivism, p. 16
ontology, p. 13
paradigm tension, p. 18
paradigms, p. 13
philosophy, p. 13
positivism, p. 15
post-positivism, p. 15
qualitative, p. 16
quantitative, p. 15
research design, p. 20
research frameworks, p. 19
research process, p. 20
research theory, p. 19

INTRODUCTION

The field of research can be confusing, with many different concepts and processes to understand. As midwives and nurses, we must grapple with these to use evidence to inform our practice or contribute to the body of knowledge that constitutes our profession and practice. The former positions us as 'consumers of research' and the latter as 'producers' of knowledge. In either case, a robust understanding of research is required.

Healthcare services and service users are demanding high-quality care from their healthcare professionals, which means providing care informed by the best available evidence. Applying the best evidence to clinical practice is known as evidence-based practice (EBP; see Chapter 15), and while there are challenges in implementing EBP it remains the goal of all modern healthcare services. Consider for a moment a newspaper article that sensationally reports on the benefits of a new wound care technology for venous leg ulcers. As a nurse, do you begin recommending this to your patients? It is more likely that you will try to locate the research that initiated the newspaper article. Once you have located the research article, you will need to appraise the research to determine whether it should change your practice in relation to the management of venous leg ulcers. To appraise the research in this way requires an understanding of the **research process**.

While all nurses and midwives require an understanding of research to use research to inform their practice, many will also become involved in the conduct of research. The later chapters of this book focus on those who are engaged or ready to engage in 'primary' research. Nurses and midwives make excellent researchers and have contributed significantly to the body of research evidence shaping healthcare practices in a variety of fields. Midwifery researchers, for example, are largely responsible for the body of evidence that demonstrates the benefits of midwifery-led continuity of care for childbearing women (Sandall et al 2016), which is now considered the gold standard of maternity care. Due to the nature of nurses' and midwives' work and their close connection to the recipients of healthcare and their family members, they often ask different kinds of research questions to other healthcare professionals. It is important that the body of evidence informing our practice addresses a full range of research questions to be most useful overall to healthcare recipients and healthcare providers (Kennedy et al 2016).

Although a firm understanding of the foundations of research is important, this can be challenging for a range of reasons. A notable barrier is a lack of agreement in the literature on definitions and relationships between the key concepts in research; hence the need for a beginning chapter, like this one, to clarify research concepts and contexts. For example, concepts such as theory, framework, paradigm, philosophy, methodology, method and design are often defined differently by various authors. In many cases, terms are used incorrectly and/or interchangeably. Therefore, midwives and nurses are encouraged to read widely around these concepts to build understanding. This chapter presents the foundational theoretical and philosophical knowledge necessary for understanding research, as well as mapping out the frameworks and processes that emerge from these positions. The intention is to produce a solid foundation from which beginning consumers of research or novice researchers can proceed in a safe and informed manner.

TUTORIAL TRIGGER 2.1

1. Why do you think nurses and midwives should study research theory and philosophy?
2. How might the absence of knowledge of the underpinning theories and philosophies of research affect nursing and midwifery research?

BEHIND THE METHODOLOGY AND METHOD: ONTOLOGY AND EPISTEMOLOGY

When we think 'research', we often think about the 'doing' bits of research, for example, doing interviews or analysing data. We often instinctively do the same with nursing and midwifery practice, where we may be drawn to the practical application of skills without necessarily being drawn to the theoretical underpinnings. Yet behind the 'doing' lie assumptions about the nature of reality and life and the nature of knowledge. These positions dictate what can be known, what type of knowledge is valuable and how knowledge can be acquired. These positions and questions are addressed by the branches of **philosophy** known as **ontology** and **epistemology**. Ontology is 'the study of the nature of being', and epistemology is 'the study of the nature of knowledge' (Al-Ababneh 2020, Reed 2018). Related **paradigms** reflect an agreed set of beliefs and assumptions about how problems in certain areas should be understood and researched. All research paradigms are underpinned by an ontological and epistemological position that shapes all aspects of the research process, including the research aims or questions, data collection techniques, ways of analysing or interpreting data and the meaning or implications of the results or findings.

It is important for those consuming or performing research to understand what lies behind the practical research method because it is here that certain assumptions are made that are integral to the way we interpret, understand and potentially use the research (Davies & Fisher 2018). In addition, researchers need to be clear about the underpinnings of any paradigm or methodology adopted for a study to ensure the researcher agrees with its assumptions and that there is congruence between the study aims, data collection, analysis and interpretation—in essence, that the study is robust. Let us now examine the role of ontology and epistemology in a little more detail.

Ontology

Ontology is the philosophical study of *being*; it is about the nature of being, existence and reality (Al-Ababneh 2020). It is a branch of philosophy that is concerned with what constitutes reality or, put simply, explores the assumptions we make in order to believe something is real or makes sense (Al-Ababneh 2020). Ontological assumptions consider *what is*—that is, what entities exist or may be said to exist and, as such, researchers take a position regarding their perceptions of how things really are and how things really work (Al-Ababneh 2020). This ontological position may be explicit and declared, or may be assumed in the research methods chosen for a study. What is clear is that research methods can be traced back, through methodology and epistemology, to an ontological position (Al-Ababneh 2020).

Epistemology

There are three main epistemological positions underpinning all research approaches, although they are usually implicitly rather than explicitly stated in a research report; these are *objectivism*, *constructionism* and *subjectivism* (Gray 2018). Objectivism holds that there is one objective truth or reality and that this exists apart from any human perception of it. Subjectivism is at the other end of the spectrum, positing that there is no objective truth but that we wholly impose meaning on an object or phenomenon. Within this position, there can be multiple truths and realities. Furthermore, there can also be multiple truths and realities in **constructionism**, which holds that meaning comes into existence through our engagement with the world, where meaning is thus constructed. To illustrate the differences between these epistemological positions, let us examine the phenomenon of insomnia. If we were researching this from an objectivist position, we would be working with an explicit diagnostic criterion for the disorder, and we would be able to use this to verify whether someone did or did not have the condition. The fact that insomnia exists and many people experience it would, therefore, be an objective truth. From a constructionist position, we would appreciate that insomnia may be experienced differently by different people, and that while a certain number of hours or quality of sleep may be non-debilitating for one person it might have serious consequences for another. From a constructionist perspective, the true meaning of insomnia arises from the interplay of the phenomenon and those engaging with it. A subjectivist position might see us questioning the phenomenon of insomnia altogether, noting that, as a social phenomenon, the concept is a human construct with no essential meaning.

RESEARCH PARADIGMS

A research paradigm is a belief system shared amongst certain groups (e.g. climate scientists, child development psychologists) that includes how certain phenomena should be understood and addressed by research (Davies & Fisher 2018). The research paradigm, therefore, shapes the type of research questions asked, the research methods used and the ways the findings or results are understood. Inherent in the paradigm are certain assumptions, including the nature of being (ontology) and knowledge (epistemology) as already highlighted. This next section outlines the three main research paradigms: *positivist*, *interpretivist* and *critical*, although there are others.

Do note that, while many research terms at first appear unfamiliar, there are often 'clues' in the term to assist: that is, positivist (to be 'positive' of a certain outcome), reductionist (to 'reduce' down to), constructionist (to be 'constructed' from), interpretative (to 'interpret'), critical (to be 'critical' of), deductive (to 'deduce' something—think Sherlock Holmes), etc. When considering the difference between terms such as positivist and positivism, we refer to the etymology of words. The suffix '-ism' means adherence to or the following of an ideology, while the suffix '-ist' is an agent noun, indicating a person is involved in a certain activity, field or mindset. At the same time we can use tables to compare, contrast and simplify terms. For instance, Table 2.1 presents a simplified comparison between positivist, interpretive and critical research paradigms for this chapter section.

The Positivist Paradigm

The positivist or 'scientific' paradigm emerged from the 'Enlightenment' and is often associated with the 'Age of Reason'. This is the historical period (17th and early 18th century) in which a blind faith in God (or other entity) began to give way to scientific reasoning. Consider, for example, the scientific discoveries of Galileo Galilei (1564–1642), who used the telescope to chart the heavens. With the laws and principles governing the movement of celestial bodies understood, humankind could predict their movement, and the heavens were no longer a mysterious reflection of God's will (Park et al 2020). An objectivist epistemological position underpins the scientific paradigm. Here, there is one objective truth that can be identified with a robust method of scientific inquiry. Robust scientific inquiry refers to the development of hypotheses, the use of objective measures and the prediction and testing of causal relationships (see Chapter 8).

TABLE 2.1 A Simplified Comparison of Positivist, Interpretive and Critical Research Paradigms

	Positivist	Interpretive	Critical
Position	Empirico-analytical, reductionist	Post-positive, postmodern, naturalistic	Post-positive, postmodern, post-structural, emancipatory
Methodology	Experimental, quasi-experimental, correlational, etc.	Phenomenology, grounded theory, ethnography, exploratory/ descriptive, case study, historical, Delphi	Feminist research, action research, critical ethnography, etc.
Data collection	Experiments, closed surveys and interviews	Open observation or interviews, focus groups	Open observation or interviews, focus groups
Researcher position	Distant	Close	Close

Within this paradigm, authentic knowledge can be gained only from the senses (something must be seen to be believed; *empirical evidence*) or extensions of the senses (measurement tools such as psychometric testing, for example—see Chapter 11) (Durepos et al 2018). This is also where the term '**positivism**' comes from. 'Posited' knowledge is that derived from the senses rather than from speculation. 'Empirical-analytical' or 'logical positivism' are also terms used to describe this research paradigm. Another related concept in this research paradigm is that of 'deductive reasoning'. This describes a logical thought process whereby research hypotheses are derived from theory and where reasoning moves from the general (what is already known) to the particular (what is being tested/measured). This is often conceptualised as a top-down approach. This contrasts with 'inductive reasoning', which moves from the particular to the general, as in the case of developing themes from interview data, which is a bottom-up approach (think inductive cooker top). Although the research landscape has changed considerably over the last decade or so, we often 'assume' that most 'medical' research adopts the positivist paradigm (i.e. clinical trials).

While the scientific method was first used to understand the natural world better, it was soon extended to the social world. Critics, however, began to realise the limitations of the positivist paradigm for researching social issues as the approach necessarily reduces human experience to measurable variables under controlled conditions (*reductionism*). Durepos et al (2018 p. 2293), however, make a case for the importance of empirics in the development of nursing knowledge, commenting '... using methods of measurement and reductionism is essential to developing empiric evidence, advancing nursing knowledge and supporting nurses' collaboration with natural sciences like medicine'.

The Post-Positivist Paradigm

Post-positivism emerged in response to the positivist movement and represents a softening of some of the positivist assertions concerning truth and objectivity. Post-positivism acknowledges the fallibility of the research process (or human beings) in achieving 'true/absolute' objectivity—hence we note terms like 'error' in research (Durepos et al 2018). While true objectivity remains an ideal, research questions underpinning our quest for truth are reframed as conjecture (hypotheses), and these hypotheses become the central point in the research endeavour, to be accepted or rejected after rigorous testing (see Chapter 4). Post-positivism brings us the *null hypothesis* (the framing of the research hypothesis in the null or negative) and probability (*p* values, for instance), which reflects a more tentative (predictive) rather than a certain approach to truth. Corry et al (2019) argue that post-positivism has superseded positivism as the guiding paradigm of the scientific method.

Research within the positivist paradigm will most often use **quantitative** data and statistical analysis. Chapters 8 through to 11 offer a detailed account of quantitative research approaches and methods. Perhaps the most well-known research method within this paradigm (in healthcare research especially) is the randomised controlled trial (RCT). It is often, perhaps misleadingly, referred to as the 'gold standard' in medicine.

RESEARCH IN BRIEF 2.1

Goldfeld et al (2022) undertook an RCT to investigate the benefits of an Australian nurse home-visiting program in promoting children's language and learning, general and mental health, maternal mental health and wellbeing, and parenting and family relationships. At the child's age of between 4 and 5 years, outcomes were assessed via parent interviews and direct assessment of children's language and learning. Outcomes were compared between the intervention and usual care arms. They demonstrated that the nurse-led intervention of home visiting showed statistically significant benefits for child and maternal mental health and wellbeing, and parenting and family relationships.

The Interpretive Paradigm

The *interpretive* paradigm emerged in response to positivism, especially regarding the application of the scientific method to social situations. It is one thing to use the scientific method to predict how atoms, molecules or cells might behave in each situation, but another to use it to predict human behaviour. Shunning many of the principles of the scientific method, research within the interpretive paradigm does not aim to predict, measure and control but, instead, to describe, explore and generate meaning within a social context. The interpretive paradigm is underpinned by a *constructionist epistemology*, which holds that there can be multiple truths and realities and that meaning is constructed by individuals and their engagement with the world. This means that meaning and truth are subjective and context dependent. This also means that researchers are not considered objective but rather involved in 'meaning making' as they engage with the processes and phenomena under study. For the interpretive researcher, reality is a flexible position whereby the phenomenon being investigated exists within many different possibilities and meanings (Cuthbertson et al 2020). Meanings are therefore located in a particular context or situation and time and, generally, meanings emerge from the study process. Interpretive methods ensure dialogue between the researcher and the participants to construct a meaningful reality collaboratively. The rationality of this perspective is that the researcher is not, and cannot be, separated from the people and the processes involved. The goal is a deep and self-reflexive engagement with the phenomenon being studied (Crowther & Thomson 2020).

Research within the interpretive paradigm will most often use **qualitative** data and thematic or other methodologically driven modes of analysis. Chapters 5 through to 7 offer a detailed account of qualitative research methods. The most well-known 'traditional' research methods within this paradigm include phenomenology, grounded theory and ethnography (see Chapter 5).

RESEARCH IN BRIEF 2.2

Prussing et al (2023) examined the implementation of midwifery continuity models within regional settings in Australia. The study used a grounded theory methodology. Grounded theory studies lead to the articulation of theory developed from the data; this is an inductive process. The analysis identified three concepts: 'engaging the gatekeepers', 'midwives lacking confidence' and 'women rallying together'. These concepts led to the substantive theory: 'A partnership between midwives and women is required to build confidence and enable the promotion of current evidence; this is essential for engaging key hospital stakeholders to invest in the implementation of midwifery continuity of care models' (Prussing et al 2023 p. 99). This research provides new evidence of the importance of midwives educating and partnering with women to enable regional Australia to transition to midwifery continuity of care models.

TUTORIAL TRIGGER 2.2

Grounded theory methodology is an interpretivist research approach that generates theory that is 'grounded' in the data. These types of studies do not usually result in 'generalisable' findings—in other words, findings that may apply to a wider population (often a main purpose of positivism/post-positivism approaches).

- How then can the outcomes of studies, such as Prussing et al's (2023), 'widely' inform the disciplines of nursing and midwifery and other health professions?

The Critical Paradigm

The *critical* paradigm developed in response to both positivism and **interpretivism**. For critical researchers, it is not enough to work within the given social structures to predict, describe or even better understand various phenomena. Research within the critical paradigm seeks emancipation, empowerment and social change—especially for those who are known to be oppressed and disadvantaged members of communities where 'inequity' between groups is a known phenomenon. These approaches generally raise the issue of power and question the *status quo* of social institutions (Koopmans & Schiller 2022). The researcher adopts a position that is free from the limitations of tradition and seeks to minimise the 'distance' between the researcher and the study participants. Critical approaches usually look to encourage empowerment and equality for research participants and to challenge and change oppressive social structures (Kailemia et al 2023).

Research within the critical paradigm can be underpinned by subjectivist or constructionist epistemologies. *Post-structural* research approaches (informed, for instance, by popular theorists such as Foucault) are most often associated with *subjectivist epistemology* as they encourage us to rethink all accepted truths, categories and norms—through highlighting their social, rather than their essential, nature. Within this approach, things or phenomena do not have an essential nature where they exist on their own but, instead, meaning is wholly imposed by the actions/inactions of human beings. What makes this approach 'critical' is that the meaning imposed on these things reflects our society's social structures, values and beliefs. Take, for example, what it means to be a woman in our society. Women are not inherently less capable of leadership than men, although often an inherent 'understanding' has been imposed on the category of 'woman' and exacerbated by deeply embedded, traditional (and cultural) social structures.

Critical approaches are also referred to as 'emancipatory'. In nursing, emancipation has emerged from a long-standing history of social oppression addressed through **critical social theory** and, in particular, through *feminist* theory and research (Kiguwa 2019). Feminist research aims to explore issues that are known to cause discrepancies and inequities in women's lives (Dupius et al 2022, Parry 2020). Women's activities are not disregarded in the process—they are instead emancipated (Parry 2020). Although it is a useful approach for investigating issues in nursing, midwifery and women's healthcare generally, overall feminist research represents a small body of research work in these disciplines. Therefore, we acknowledge the place of feminist research here, but do not include an in-depth discussion. Readers who wish to know more about feminist theory and research are directed to the above references as well as actual research examples (Gauci et al 2022, Morley et al 2020, Paynter et al 2022, Westergren et al 2019).

Action research is another common example of a research approach within the critical paradigm (see Chapter 12). It is a critical inquiry that describes and interprets social situations and, in doing so, aims to improve social division/inequality through participant/co-researcher involvement. It is essentially a critique of existing social organisational/community situations, via collaboration and partnership, to generate social change in those environments. Action research is an example that is underpinned by constructionist epistemologies.

Research within the critical paradigm will most often use qualitative data and a variety of analytical approaches. Chapters 5 to 7 offer a detailed account of qualitative research methods.

RESEARCH IN BRIEF 2.3

Woods et al (2022) used participatory action research to explore whether, and how, professional nurse educator identity is co-constructed by a community of practice. This approach enabled purposeful and sustainable social change that recognises participants as researchers and generators of knowledge. Following three distinct phases, participation in the research resulted in collective meaning making, praxis, knowledge generation and the co-construction of the nurse educator's professional identities (Woods et al 2022).

METHODOLOGY: LINKING PARADIGMS, APPROACHES AND METHODS

Methodology is not a fancy word for methods. They are two different things. 'Method' refers to the data collection tools used in a study (questionnaire or interview, for example), whereas 'methodology' provides the lens through which data are analysed and understood. Examples of methodologies include phenomenology, ethnography, quasi-experimental studies and feminist research (see Table 2.1). Inherent in the methodology is a certain epistemological position and research paradigm, and, very often, methodologies also draw on the work of particular theorists. In a robust study there is congruence and clear linking between the key elements of research: epistemology → research paradigm → methodology → methods. One would not expect a research study that aims for an in-depth understanding of an experience (implying constructionist epistemology and interpretive research paradigm) to use a survey (methodology) with structured questionnaires (method) that had a drop-down menu of choices and the results presented as descriptive (summary) proportions or frequencies of participants responding in a certain way. Agreement of the key elements of research design is vital to ensure rigour in research. Rigour is a concept that refers to the trustworthiness of the study and is managed in different ways depending on the research approaches used. The implication of not understanding the requisite alignment of methodology and methods is that it will probably result in research lacking rigour. 'Research in brief 2.4' illustrates these points related to paradigms, methodology, methods and alignment.

RESEARCH IN BRIEF 2.4

Nurse researchers Ryan et al (2022) wanted to understand 'what it means to care for older patients dying from traumatic injuries in the emergency department' (p. 562). They used a phenomenological methodology and, because there are a few different theorists informing phenomenology, they chose two theorists, Heidegger and van Manen (see Chapter 5). The choice of Heidegger and van Manen meant that the research process did not include a practice called 'bracketing' (identifying and putting aside pre-existing researcher presumptions), common to other types of phenomenology. Phenomenology aims for a deep understanding of human experience (Wertz 2023), so the researchers chose in-depth interviews as their data collection method. Hopefully, the reader can appreciate why something like a survey would not necessarily be appropriate for this methodology. The researchers state: 'the phenomenological "facts" of lived experience are meaningfully (hermeneutically) captured in language as an interpretive process' (p. 563), which implies a constructionist epistemology and interpretive research paradigm. Driven by the methodology, the analytical lens is focused on the meaning of the experience from the perspectives of those with the phenomenon (nurses caring for older people dying from traumatic injuries in the emergency department). The analysis is not focused on cause-and-effect relationships, as it might be if the research were underpinned by an objectivist epistemology within a scientific research paradigm. The analysis describes the existential dimensions of temporality and spatiality, revealing new insights into what it means to care for elderly patients dying from traumatic injuries.

Research Approaches

At the most simplistic level, research approaches are often thought of as belonging to two main 'camps': qualitative or quantitative. At the same time, though, there is a rapidly growing interest in and place for mixed-methods approaches that incorporate both 'camps' (see Chapter 12). The reasons for selecting a qualitative approach rather than a quantitative one, or vice versa, are based on the research question and the purpose of the study. Formulating the research problem (research question, problem statement or hypothesis) is an initial and key step in the research process, regardless of the method used (see Chapter 4). As a research consumer, you should examine the consistency between the research problem and the methodology and methods used to address that problem. Critical appraisal/evaluation skills are required to review research studies effectively and judge whether the findings could be applied to practice. Recognition of the similarities and differences between the characteristics of qualitative research and quantitative research means that the nurse or midwife is better equipped to interpret research findings and identify ways they might be applied to practice. Writers such as Mehrad and Zangeneh (2019) offer simplified explanations of the relationships, similarities and differences between quantitative and qualitative research approaches. The origins and belief systems for the qualitative and quantitative approaches are described and compared in Table 2.2.

Researchers may sometimes be under the impression that the differences between qualitative and quantitative approaches are so wide that one position is incompatible with the other (Adu et al 2022). Sometimes the terms '**paradigm tension**/war', or similar, are seen to describe this unhelpful viewpoint (Adu et al 2022). Although not intended, the information in Table 2.2 may exaggerate the apparent division between them. Instead, it is important to acknowledge their obvious 'connectedness' and interrelationships. Both approaches are complementary—not competitive. They are both equally important and play

TABLE 2.2 A Comparison of Qualitative and Quantitative Approaches

Concepts	Qualitative	Quantitative
Origins	Search for meaning; interactive approach	Search for truth in an objective, controlled manner
Beliefs	Human beings are complex beings who attribute unique meanings to situations.	Human beings are biopsychosocial beings with measurable components.
Truth	Subjective with multiple realities	Objective reality
Basis of knowing	Meaning, discovery	Cause-and-effect relationships
Focus	Complex and broad	Concise and narrow
Level	Holistic	Reductionist
Reasoning	Dialectic (conversational), inductive	Logical, deductive
Setting	Occurs in uncontrolled naturalistic (social or human) settings.	Investigator seeks experimental control of the setting.
Purpose	Develops theory by exploring meaning and describing relationships.	Tests hypotheses, theories by control and observation.
Sample	People in the sample are referred to as participants or, in ethnographic studies, informants.	People in a group are termed the sample, and are referred to as subjects, cases or respondents.
Researcher position	An active and interactive participant, immersed in the setting	Uses measuring instruments or tools (e.g. questionnaires)
Data elements	Written form (words), art, artefacts	Numerical form (numbers)
Analyses	Interpretive analysis usually undertaken manually—although data can be loaded into software such as NVivo that facilitates review and management of data.	Statistical analysis using software (e.g. SAS, SPSS, Minitab, Statview, R)
Outcomes	Are often thematic or conceptual, but not quantifiable and are expressed in words.	Must be measurable and are reported in numerical terms.
Clinical application	Exploration of unique experiences of individuals or groups.	Findings able to be generalised to similar groups.

their part according to the nature and intention of the research objectives. Broadly speaking, both approaches are scientific and rigorous and follow similar process, design and methodology structures. Neither quantitative nor qualitative research can occur by chance; both are governed by systematic attention to the method and design of the research process (explained later in this chapter).

In the late 1970s, 'hierarchies of research evidence' were developed and popularised, which has contributed (intentionally or not) to a paradigm tension. The 'hidden' suggestion of these hierarchies is that some methods of research (especially positivist approaches) are better (or more important) than others. This led to much debate about the quality and reliability of evidence, and multiple hierarchies have ensued. However, the more recent perspective is that different research methods are needed to answer different clinical questions. Therefore effectiveness, appropriateness and feasibility of methodology are more important indicators than hierarchy. Table 2.3 highlights the frequently cited National Health & Medical Research Council (NHMRC) hierarchy of research evidence, although it is important to note that it represents a quantitative hierarchy only.

Most researchers are now realising the limitations of championing or rejecting one research approach at the expense of another. It is now accepted by many to be both naive and simplistic to suggest either that one research approach is better than another or that they are so different that researchers can adopt only one or the other. It is also acknowledged that, in many instances, adopting a single research approach or methodology might prove inadequate when it comes to answering research questions/hypotheses. The key issue is that the researcher chooses the most appropriate methodology for the task at hand.

A mixed-methods approach to answering clinical questions has grown in popularity (see Chapter 12). This approach is one which employs both qualitative and quantitative approaches to answer the research question.

TABLE 2.3 Designations of Levels of Evidence According to Type of Research Question

Level	Intervention
1	Systematic reviews of level 2 studies
2	Randomised controlled trials (RCTs)
3a	Pseudo RCTs
3b	Comparative studies with concurrent controls
3c	Comparative studies without concurrent controls
4	Case series

(Source: National Health & Medical Research Council, 2009. NHMRC additional levels of evidence and grades for recommendations for developers of guidelines. Retrieved from https://www.mja.com.au/sites/default/files/NHMRC.levels.of.evidence.2008-09.pdf.)

RESEARCH IN BRIEF 2.5

Cameron et al (2023) undertook a mixed-methods study to evaluate a statewide smoking cessation initiative for Aboriginal mothers called Quit for New Life (QFNL). They aimed to assess (1) models of implementation of QFNL, (2) the uptake of QFNL, (3) the impact of QFNL on smoking behaviours and (4) stakeholder perceptions of the initiative. They conducted semistructured interviews with clients and health service stakeholders and sourced routinely collected clinical outcome data. Stakeholders shared stories of success; however, the quantitative analysis found no statistically significant impact of QFNL on smoking cessation rates. They did find that the QFNL was acceptable to both clients and stakeholders, increased awareness about smoking cessation and gave staff resources to support clients (Cameron et al 2023).

TUTORIAL TRIGGER 2.3

From what you have read so far, do you believe there is a 'best' method to use for conducting nursing or midwifery research? Justify your decision.

THEORETICAL AND CONCEPTUAL FRAMEWORKS

Research theory and *theoretical* and *conceptual frameworks* are often used in the language of research to represent similar things but have subtle differences in meaning (Varpio et al 2020). Theories (theoretical approaches, frameworks, perspectives) are often implicit (and sometimes explicit) in the research process and can be understood as a system of ideas or a set of relationships between certain concepts that are offered as an explanation for something. Theories provide a lens through which a phenomenon is viewed. Varpio et al (2020) provide a useful discussion on the use of theoretical and conceptual frameworks in research and offer a robust critique of the divergence of definitions. **Research frameworks** that are embedded in the methodology or are additional to the stated design provide the knowledge and theory basis for conducting research studies. Theoretical research frameworks represent known and tested theories. There are many 'tried and tested' theories in nursing and midwifery that researchers can cross-reference. Therefore this foundational knowledge serves as a 'frame of reference' from which researchers can either predict or explain their study outcomes. For instance, Oruc et al (2023) explored the experiences of women diagnosed with gynaecological cancers from the theoretical perspective of 'salutogenesis'. Salutogenesis is a theory developed by social anthropologist Aaron Antonovsky that focuses on factors that contribute to health, rather than those that contribute to disease. Among other important findings, Oruc et al (2023) identified that, even if the women did not have resilience initially, it developed over time with supportive interventions and inner resources. This is described in their core category of 'Formation of resilience: power of the resources' (Oruc et al 2023 p. 3).

Where studies are unique and explore either unknown or previously unexplored issues, it may be that there is no theoretical framework to guide the researcher. In this case, conceptual frameworks can identify single or multiple concepts that are related—but remain untested.

Research Process

If we look at a series of 'typical' research studies, regardless of which paradigm and approach is used, they all follow essentially the same **research process**. By paying attention to this methodological process, critical research consumers can appreciate the logical nature of research methods and the relevance of certain guiding forces on the outcomes of research. To clarify the forces, drivers and process of research, this book is designed to take the reader step by step through a sequential process-driven research journey—chapter by chapter. The structure of the chapters in this book is designed to follow the sequence of the research process. The research process typically follows the following structure:

1. identifying the (clinical) problem/issue
2. critically searching and appraising the available primary (research-based) and conceptual (theory-based) literature
3. refining research ideas, questions, statements or hypotheses
4. identifying and minimising ethical issues and procedures
5. identifying and justifying an appropriate research methodology and method
6. sampling (choosing) appropriate research populations (participants/elements)
7. collecting or generating research data from participants/elements
8. analysing collected research data
9. interpreting and making sense of research results/findings
10. disseminating (sharing) research findings to wider audiences.

We can note from the research process list that several factors determine the nature and extent of the conducted research, which, in turn, influences the choice of research methodology or approach. Regardless of the research approach, however, the process remains constant. This can also be seen by looking at the decision path for selecting a research approach, as outlined in Fig. 2.1.

AN UNEXPECTED HURDLE

A study was undertaken to investigate mothers' and care providers' experiences of Assumption of Care, which is the forcible removal of a baby by the State immediately after birth. 'Assumption of Care most often involves some of society's most vulnerable women, including those experiencing drug and alcohol dependencies, mental health issues, domestic violence, poverty, homelessness and personal histories of child abuse and neglect' (Marsh et al 2017 p. 64). This study involved participants who were considered vulnerable by research ethics, and the topic was a sensitive topic, which caused several research hurdles. Issues such as trust, power imbalance, discrimination, confidentiality and exploitation were of concern. To overcome these, efforts were made to give power to the participants, establish a trusting relationship and use narrative inquiry methods. As a result, only three mothers were recruited (Marsh et al 2019).

1. How could the researchers have modified their research design to encourage the recruitment of women?
2. What may be the consequence of the small sample size?

Research Design

Research design refers to the planning of the research, the selection of methodology or design, and associated methods for identifying and recruiting the sample/participants, and collecting and analysing data. The following is useful as a guide for designing research:

1. selecting the specific methodology and method/methods to be used (i.e. qualitative–phenomenology or quantitative–experimental, or potentially both in the case of mixed-methods research—see Chapters 5, 8 and 12)
2. determining ethical issues and obtaining ethical consent and approval (see Chapter 13)

If your beliefs are:

Researcher beliefs	Humans are biopsychosocial beings, known by their biological, psychological and social characteristics. Truth is objective reality that can be experienced with the senses and measured by the researcher.	or	Humans are complex beings who attribute unique meaning to their life situations. They are known by their personal expressions. Truth is the subjective expression of reality as perceived by the participant and shared with the researcher. Truth is context-laden.

then you'll ask questions, such as:

Example questions	What is the difference in blood pressure and heart rate for adolescents who are angry compared to those who are not angry?	or	What is the structure of the lived experience of anger for adolescents?

and select approaches:

Approaches	**Quantitative/deductive**	or	**Qualitative/inductive**

leading to research activities

Research activities	Researcher selects a representative (of population) sample and determines size before collecting data. Researcher uses an extensive approach to collect data. Questionnaires and measurement devices are, according to a standard protocol, administered to control for extraneous (unexpected) variables. Primarily deductive analysis is used, generating a numerical summary that allows the researcher to reject or accept the null hypothesis.	or	Researcher selects participants who are experiencing the phenomenon of interest and collects data until saturation is reached. Researcher uses an intensive approach to collect data. Researcher conducts interviews and participant or non-participant observation in environments where participants usually spend their time. Researcher bias is acknowledged and set aside. Primarily inductive analysis is used, leading to a narrative summary which synthesises participant information, creating a description of human experience.

Fig. 2.1 Decision path for selecting a research approach

3. developing a sampling framework and technique (i.e. the rationale for choosing an appropriate population of research participants, subjects or elements to study), such as a random sample of first-year nursing or midwifery students (see Chapters 6 and 9)
4. for quantitative research, operationally defining variables (see Chapter 9)
5. in the case of many quantitative research studies, developing, selecting and evaluating measuring instruments through a pilot study before using in the larger study (see Chapter 10)
6. employing data collection techniques (see Chapters 6 and 9)
7. analysing collected data (see Chapters 7 and 11)
8. evaluating results/findings (see Chapters 7 and 11)
9. discussing results and their applicability to practice if a clinical study is undertaken (see Chapter 15)
10. disseminating study outcomes through publication/presentations/seminars/workshops (see Chapter 18).

Published research in academic journals closely follows this process in disseminating published research findings. The research then is usually reported in a logical fashion. There are many considerations when publishing research, such as who can be named as an author (ICMJE 2022) and avoiding plagiarism (breaches in academic integrity). McClunie-Trust (2018) points out the importance of writing about how the research was conducted and not just the findings of the research. Nursing- and midwifery-related academic journal articles are usually presented in the following systematic manner (with likely headings highlighted in brackets):

1. the identification of a research problem, idea or issue (introduction)
2. a review of previous research and conceptual work on the identified topic (literature review/background)
3. specification of the research question, statement or hypothesis (aim)
4. a description of how the study was conducted (design, method or approach—to include the possible subheadings of sampling, ethical considerations, data collection and data analysis)
5. discussion on the results of the research (results/findings)
6. the interpretation of the research findings (discussion—including limitations, recommendations and conclusion/summary).

SUMMARY

Understanding how research works and what methods and processes it adopts is a vital part of becoming a knowledgeable research consumer. This knowledge base ensures that our practice is more likely to be evidence based and that we are well placed to understand and communicate the 'language' of research with our immediate and wider healthcare colleagues. Although some theoretical and philosophical terms might initially appear somewhat confusing, they need to be understood to grasp the whys and wherefores of conducting and/or consuming research. A good understanding serves as a solid platform to advance novices towards the first steps of the research process—where they are more likely to 'not just consume research findings but engage in and conduct primary research themselves'. Much of the available research literature routinely uses the terminology and concepts highlighted in this chapter and expects the reader to be readily familiar with this material. Chapter 3 is devoted to the initial, yet vital, research process steps of critically searching for, retrieving and appraising existing research literature, while Chapter 4 looks at identifying research ideas, questions, statements and hypotheses. In Section 2, Chapter 13 looks at ethical and legal issues in research,

KEY POINTS

- Research originates from and is underpinned by several theoretical and philosophical positions. These positions inform the 'worldview' of the researcher, which in turn enables the researcher to select the most appropriate methodology to answer the research question/s asked.
- The two major categories (camps) of research are qualitative and quantitative (although some now refer to the third category of 'mixed-methods' research; see Chapter 12). All research paradigms and methodologies have their differences and similarities, but, ultimately, the paradigm chosen (if not all of them) by researchers should be determined based on which is the most appropriate and will result in answering the research question/s.
- Research is necessarily conducted according to established scientific, systematic and structured processes. These must be understood before the research consumer can start to apply/translate research findings or conduct research, particularly practice-focused research that potentially has implications for other healthcare professionals and the broader population.

TIME TO REFLECT

Feltrin, C., Newton, J..M, Willetts, G., 2019. How graduate nurses adapt to individual ward culture: A grounded theory study. J. Adv. Nurs. 75(3), 616–627. doi:10.1111/jan.13884

Aim: to explore how graduate nurses adapt to individual ward culture.

TIME TO REFLECT—cont'd

Objective: to increase understanding of strategies that graduate nurses use on a day-to-day basis to integrate themselves into pre-existing social frameworks.
Design: qualitative—grounded theory.

Questions

1. Is the research design appropriate? Why or why not?
2. Reflect on the information given and answer these questions:
   a. What were the reasons for the researchers wanting to understand adaptation strategies used by nurses?
   b. Are there any issues that you could foresee relating to researching new graduate nurses in clinical settings?

LEARNING ACTIVITIES

1. The first step in becoming a knowledgeable research consumer involves:
   a. understanding how to conduct research
   b. understanding the 'language' of research
   c. understanding how research works, its underpinning theories and what methods and processes it adopts
   d. understanding how research impacts on nursing practice.
2. Research is guided by the following concepts (and related questions):
   a. ontology, epistemology and methodology
   b. ontology, epistemology and oncology
   c. ontology, pedagogy and methodology
   d. ontology, pedagogy and dermatology.
3. Further delineation of qualitative and quantitative research is outlined in a common classification of research paradigms. These are:
   a. deductive, inductive and productive
   b. positivist, critical and interpretive
   c. negativist, uncritical and interpretive
   d. positivist, critical and productive.
4. The term *positivism* refers to the:
   a. philosophical position reflecting the traditional scientific approach of subjective observation and causal relationships
   b. philosophical position reflecting the traditional scientific approach of objective observation and nursing relationships
   c. philosophical position reflecting the traditional scientific approach of objective observation and causal relationships
   d. philosophical position reflecting the traditional scientific approach of subjective observation and nursing relationships.
5. Critical and interpretive research paradigms generally use:
   a. qualitative methods to examine phenomena of interest
   b. quantitative methods to examine phenomena of interest
   c. qualitative methods to examine hypotheses
   d. quantitative methods to examine hypotheses.
6. Mixed-methods research is used when:
   a. a researcher is feeling anxious about a particular research approach
   b. one research paradigm is superior to another
   c. two different paradigms are used in one study
   d. only one paradigm is used.
7. Research frameworks serve as a frame of reference from which researchers can either predict or explain their:
   a. study methods
   b. study designs
   c. study inputs
   d. study outcomes.
8. The first part of the research process involves:
   a. identifying the problem/issue
   b. critically searching and reviewing the available primary (research-based) and conceptual (theory-based) literature
   c. identifying research ideas, questions, statements or hypotheses
   d. all of the above.
9. The last part of the research process involves:
   a. analysing collected research data
   b. determining research results/findings
   c. disseminating research findings
   d. all of the above.
10. The research design (plan) is dependent upon the following starting points:
    a. the purpose and the question/s being asked
    b. the nature of the issue or problem being investigated
    c. what is likely to offer the 'best fit' and potential outcomes
    d. all of the above.

For further content associated with this chapter visit: https://evolve.elsevier.com/cs/product/9780729596794?role=student 

ADDITIONAL RESOURCES

Joanna Briggs Institute. https://jbi.global/.
National Institute of Nursing Research. https://www.ninr.nih.gov/.
Nursing Education Expert. https://nursingeducationexpert.com/theoretical-frameworks/.
Nursing theories. https://www.currentnursing.com/nursing_theory/research_and_nursing_theories.html.
Philosophy of research. https://conjointly.com/kb/philosophy-of-research/.

REFERENCES

Adu J, Owusu MF, Martin-Yeboah E, et al., 2022. A discussion of some controversies in mixed methods research for emerging researchers. Methodol. Innov. 15 (3), 321-330. doi:10.1177/20597991221123398

Al-Ababneh, M. 2020. Linking ontology, epistemology and research methodology. Sci. Philos. 8 (1), 75–91.

Cameron, E., Bryant, J., Cashmore, A., et al. 2023 A mixed methods evaluation of Quit for new life, a smoking cessation initiative for women having an Aboriginal baby. BMC Health Services Res. 23 (1), 532.

Corry, M., Porter, S., McKenna, H., 2019. The redundancy of positivism as a paradigm for nursing research. Nurs. Philos. 20 (1), e12230. doi:10.1111/nup.12230

Crowther, S., Thomson, G., 2020. From description to interpretive leap: using philosophical notions to unpack and surface meaning in hermeneutic phenomenology research. International J. Qual. Method. 19, 1609406920969264. doi:10.1177/1609406920969264

Cuthbertson, L. M., Robb, Y. A., Blair, S., 2020. Theory and application of research principles and philosophical underpinning for a study utilising interpretative phenomenological analysis. Radiography 26 (2), e94–e102.

Davies, C., Fisher, M., 2018. Understanding research paradigms. J. Australas. Rehab. Nurses Assoc., 21 (3), 21–25. doi:10.3316/informit.160174725752074

Dupuis C, Harcourt W, Gaybor J, et al., 2022. Introduction: feminism as method—navigating theory and practice. In: Harcourt, W., van den Berg, K., Dupuis, C., et al. (Eds.), Feminist Methodologies: Experiments, Collaborations and Reflections.Springer International Publishing, Champaign, IL, pp. 1–20. doi:10.1007/978-3-030-82654-3_1

Durepos, P., Orr, E., Ploeg, J., et al., 2018. The value of measurement for development of nursing knowledge: underlying philosophy, contributions and critiques. J. Adv. Nurs. 74 (10), 2290–2300. doi:10.1111/jan.13778.

Gauci, P., Peters, K., O'Reilly, K., et al., 2022. The experience of workplace gender discrimination for women registered nurses: a qualitative study. J. Adv. Nurs. 78 (6), 1743–1754. doi:10.1111/jan.15137

Goldfeld, S., Bryson, H., Mensah, F., et al. 2022. Nurse home visiting to improve child and maternal outcomes:5-year follow-up of an Australian randomised controlled trial. PLoSONE 17(11), e0277773. doi:10.1371/journal.pone.0277773

Gray, D.E., 2018. Doing Research in the Real World, fourth ed. SAGE Publications, London.

International Committee of Medical Journal Editors (ICMJE), 2022. ICMJE Recommendations: defining the role of authors and contributors. Retrieved 28 September 2023 from https://www.ICMJE.org/recommendations/browse/roles-and-responsibilities/defining-the-role-of-authors-and-contributors.html.

Kailemia, P.N., Lee, E.C., Renfrew, M.J., 2023. Intersection of social determinants of symptomatic breast cancer presentation in a rural setting: a critical ethnographic study. J Adv. Nurs. 79 (5), 1882-897.

Kennedy, H.P., Yoshida, S., Costello, A., et al., 2016. Asking different questions: research priorities to improve the quality of care for every woman, every child. Lancet Glob. Health 4 (11), e777–e779. doi:10.1016/S2214-109X(16)30183-8

Kiguwa, P., 2019. Feminist approaches: an exploration of women's gendered experiences. In: Laher, S., Fynn, A., Kramer, S. (Eds.), Transforming Research Methods in the Social Sciences: Case Studies from South Africa. Wits University Press, Johannesburg, pp. 220–235. Retrieved from https://www.jstor.org/stable/10.18772/22019032750.19.

Koopmans, E., Schiller, D.C., 2022. Understanding causation in healthcare: an introduction to critical realism. Qual. Health Res. 32 (8/9), 1207–1214.

Marsh, C. A., Browne, J., Taylor, J., et al., 2017. A researcher's journey: exploring a sensitive topic with vulnerable women. Women Birth 30 (1), 63-69. doi:10.1016/j.wombi.2016.07.003

Marsh, C. A., Browne, J., Taylor, J., et al., 2019. Making the hidden seen: a narrative analysis of the experiences of Assumption of Care at birth. Women Birth 32 (1), e1-e11. doi:10.1016/j.wombi.2018.04.009

McClunie-Trust, P., 2018. Writing about the 'how' of research. Kai Tiaki: Nurs. N. Z. 24 (2), 34–35.

Mehrad, A., Zangeneh, M.H.T., 2019. Comparison between qualitative and quantitative research approaches: social sciences. Int. J. Res. Educ. Stud. 5 (7), 1–7. doi:10.53555/es.v5i7.998

Morley, G., Bradbury-Jones, C., Ives, J. 2022 What is 'moral distress' in nursing? A feminist empirical bioethics study. Nurs. Ethics 27 (5), 1297–1314. doi:10.1177/0969733019874492

National Health & Medical Research Council (NHMRC), 2009. NHMRC additional levels of evidence and grades for recommendations for developers of guidelines. Retrieved from https://www.mja.com.au/sites/default/files/NHMRC.levels.of.evidence.2008-09.pdf.

Oruc, M., Deliktas Demirci, A., Kabukcuoglu, K., 2023. A grounded theory of resilience experiences of women with gynecological cancer. Eur. J. Oncol. Nurs. 2023, 64. doi:10.1016/j.ejon.2023.102323

Park, Y., Konge, L., Artino, A. R., 2020. The positivism paradigm of research. Acad. Med. 95 (5), 690–694. doi:10.1097/ACM.0000000000003093

Parry B. 2020 Feminist research principles and practices. In: Kramer, S., Laher, S., Fynn, A., et al. (Eds.), Online Readings in Research Methods. Psychological Society of South Africa, Johannesburg, Ch. 5. doi:10.17605/OSF.IO/BNPFS

Paynter, M., Jefferies, K., Carrier, L., et al., 2022. Feminist abolitionist nursing. ANS Adv. Nurs. Sci. 45 (1), 53–68. doi:10.1097/ANS.0000000000000385

Prussing E, Browne G, Dowse E, et al., 2023. Implementing midwifery continuity of care models in regional Australia: a constructivist grounded theory study. Women Birth 36 (1), 99–107.

Reed, P.G., 2018. Philosophical issues and nursing science. Nurs. Sci. Q. 31 (1), 31–35. doi:10.1177/089431841774110

Ryan, K., Windsor, C., Jack, L. 2022. The phenomenon of caring for older patients who are dying from traumatic injuries in the emergency department: an interpretive phenomenological study. J. Nurs. Scholarship 54 (5), 562–568. doi:10.1111/jnu.12764

Sandall, J., Soltani, H., Gates, S., et al., 2016. Midwife-led continuity models versus other models of care for childbearing women. Cochrane Database Syst. Rev. 4, CD004667, doi:10.1002/14651858.CD004667.pub5

Varpio, L., Paradis, E., Uijtdehaage, S., et al., 2020. The distinctions between theory, theoretical framework, and conceptual framework. Acad. Med. 95 (7), 989–994. doi:10.1097/ACM.0000000000003075

Wertz, F.J., 2023. Phenomenological methodology, methods, and procedures for research in psychology. APA handbook of research methods in psychology: research designs: quantitative, qualitative, neuropsychological, and biological, vol. 2, second ed. American Psychological Association, Washington DC, pp. 83–105. doi:10.1037/0000319-005

Westergren, A., Edin, K., Walsh, D., et al., 2019. Autonomous and dependent—the dichotomy of birth: a feminist analysis of birth plans in Sweden. Midwifery 68, 56–64. doi:10.1016/j.midw.2018.10.008

Woods, A., Cashin, A., Horstmanshof, L. 2022. The social construction of nurse educator professional identities: exploring the impact of a community of practice through participatory action research. J. Adv. Nurs. 78 (8), 2522–2536.

3

Critically Searching and Reviewing the Research Literature

Dean Whitehead and Debbie Massey

LEARNING OUTCOMES

After reading this chapter, you should be able to:

- identify a variety of different research literature sources
- outline the main components of a literature review and understand different types of literature reviews
- conduct a detailed and focused search of the literature using an effective search strategy
- discuss searched literature in relation to specific research designs and methodologies
- begin to apply criteria to evaluate (summarise and critique/critically appraise) research articles and broader research literature on a specific topic.

KEY TERMS

artificial intelligence, p. 38
bibliographical databases, p. 30
critical appraisal/evaluation/review, p. 38
grey literature, p. 36
literature review, p. 27
literature searches, p. 27
open access, p. 29
primary source, p. 27
refereed (peer-reviewed) journals, p. 27
secondary source, p. 27

INTRODUCTION

A competent research consumer is expected to demonstrate skills and knowledge about how to conduct a literature search, select relevant research articles or other resources for review, critically evaluate the selected research literature and then report it in a progressively sophisticated manner. The ability to critically synthesise and analyse a defined body of research literature is a skill commonly developed and assessed in both undergraduate and postgraduate coursework and research degree programs. It is also increasingly required by clinicians for quality improvement and to promote evidence-based practice (EBP) with the aim of improving patient care and outcomes (see Chapter 15). For those who conduct research and then share their research findings (see Chapter 18), the requirement is the same. The clinical environment is complex and often overwhelming. Through promoting access to quality, evidenced-based information at the point of care, improvements have been demonstrated in safer patient care and increased students' knowledge base and confidence (Wilson et al 2022).

Conducting research literature searches and then critiquing the gathered research literature is a vital part of successful primary 'research process' (see Chapter 2). It is equally important for those who don't currently conduct research but consume its findings for clinical practice, education, professional development and reflective practice. While in the higher education setting, nursing and midwifery students are expected to craft academic assignments that demonstrate effective abilities to find, critically appraise and relate research findings to practice issues, at the same time, it is widely acknowledged that this is a core skill that many students (both undergraduate and postgraduate) fail to appreciate the value of (Carter et al 2023, Gimenez 2019, Riley 2019). The term 'academic literacy' is now being applied to the skill development that most nursing and midwifery students now require—such as Jefferies et al's (2018) systematic review titled 'The importance of academic literacy for undergraduate nursing students'. Learning effective literature search and review/appraisal skills greatly assists academic literacy (Garvey et al 2023).

A systematic approach to searching scholarly and professional literature is the first step in a **literature review** on a particular topic of interest. Information and communications technology (ICT) has revolutionised the contemporary process of searching the research literature. It is by far the most convenient and expansive resource at hand—assuming one has access to reliable internet connections and institutional subscription to a range of ICT-type databases. A range of online resources is now available to anyone with internet access, including websites, electronic books (e-books), literature databases of published journal articles, full-text journal repositories and e-journals. At the 'local' level, nursing and midwifery students are commonly using 'learning portals' developed through course management software systems (such as Moodle—*Modular Object-Oriented Dynamic Learning Environment*) that create environments where students can access a whole range of learning resources—including library and bibliographical database resources for searching and accessing the research literature. The proliferation of social media and related media, such as podcasting, wikis, Facebook, X (Twitter), Flickr, Reddit, etc., adds to this armoury of resources—or at least adds to the way that nursing and midwifery research is accessed and understood. As well as 'academic literacy', another related required skill is 'digital literacy'. Ross and Cross (2019) state 'the internet and social media have changed the way society communicates, requiring the nursing workforce to develop effective digital literacy skills and attain levels of e-professionalism'. As well as social media, there is also 'academic social media' to consider—that is, ResearchGate, Academia.Edu, Kudos, LinkedIn, etc. (Manca 2018).

This chapter examines sources of academic literature and describes search strategies before moving on to the critical review of gathered literature. The logical steps of the **literature search** and review process are:

1. formulating a review question (or it could be an academic assignment question)—see Chapter 4
2. conducting a comprehensive and systematic search of the available literature
3. assessing studies for inclusion in the review
4. critically appraising the selected studies
5. synthesising findings from individual studies and a wider 'body' of studies
6. reporting results, discussing the impact of the results and making recommendations for practice.

Steps 1–3 represent the research literature *search* phase, while steps 4–6 represent the critical *review* of the research literature phase. Both phases are logical, sequential and interrelated. Knowledge and skills for both searching the literature and critically reviewing the literature are essential and complementary for both research consumers and primary researchers conducting research 'in the field' (Usher et al 2023). In practical terms, searching for and critically reviewing the research literature should be a complementary, continuous and seamless process.

Before this chapter begins to describe the process of critically searching the research literature, it first needs to identify the nature and scope of the different types of literature that are available.

TYPES OF RESEARCH LITERATURE SOURCES

Primary and Secondary Literature Sources

Broadly speaking, academic and clinical literature is divided into two source classifications: **primary source** and **secondary source**. Both types of sources are accessible through **refereed (peer-reviewed) journals**, electronic or print databases and websites. Experience in working with these sources is a requirement for nursing graduates in clinical, educational, research and professional settings. A credible literature review reflects the use of mainly primary sources of information—that is, original research or original development of theory (see Chapter 2). Most primary research sources are found in the published literature as refereed journal articles, mostly online (see 'Refereed journals' later in this chapter). Academic theses (at the Honours', Master's and Doctoral level) are also primary sources.

A secondary source is commonly a summary and critique of a range of primary studies on a specific topic (O'Connor 2020) (e.g. a literature review, integrative review, systematic review or narrative review paper—see later in this chapter), a conceptual paper (concept or discourse analysis) or an in-depth analysis of an issue or problem (e.g. critical editorials). Four common reasons for using secondary sources are:

- *full-text primary sources are unavailable*—this may occur with early classic papers or those written in publications with a limited distribution;
- *a secondary source provides a different interpretation of an issue or problem*—secondary sources help students develop the ability to see things from another point of view, which is an essential aspect of critically reading a wide range of literature;
- *when an issue or topic is not yet well established and has not, yet, been applied to nursing or midwifery practice*—so

there is currently little or no primary research in that field of knowledge.

Another common form of secondary sources is 'general topic' nursing and midwifery texts (such as this one you are reading now). The advantages of secondary sources are that they review the state of the science and form an important component in the application of knowledge to practice (O'Connor 2020). In turn, they may include recommendations for practice and/or contributions to the development of the science of nursing. Research consumers do, however, need to consider potential limitations of biases with secondary sources. For example, reviews may not fully cover the existing knowledge, or purposely 'promote' a particular approach or opinion. The authors do not always have to demonstrate a rigour/audit trail commonly associated with primary sources (i.e. measures of validity, reliability and trustworthiness—see Section 2 chapters). It should be noted, as well, that there are certain exceptions. In terms of 'hierarchy of research evidence', systematic reviews and meta-analyses (see later in this chapter) are secondary sources, but (hopefully) rigorously applied and often considered 'best' evidence for practice development. However, this is a contested assumption and not always the case (see Chapter 15).

Several resources focus purely on facilitating secondary research and resulting publications, including systematic reviews, meta-analyses, meta-syntheses and clinical practice guidelines designed to support EBP (see Box 3.1).

Publishers now also produce a range of secondary texts as e-books on the internet for organisational subscribers such as universities and health departments (e.g. *Elsevier's ClinicalKey for Nursing*: https://www.clinicalkey.com.au/nursing/#!/). This format enables regular web-based updates rather than waiting for the next edition of a book to be revised on a routine 3- to 5-year publication cycle. Accompanying the notable new-generation of affordable and reliable e-readers, many publishers are automatically converting new 'hard copy' texts to this format. From a clinical practice perspective, there are notable advantages in having access to large portable libraries of clinical information. Many Australasian university libraries are now moving towards 'e-book/resource preferred' purchasing models that are available on the 'aggregator' platforms such as EBL, EBrary and EBSCOhost. Part of the advantage of this approach is that students can purchase parts of books rather than the whole. Some publishing houses (e.g. Wolters Kluwer) enable purchasers to take a 'cook-book' approach to developing their own custom texts that combine different chapters from different related texts contained in their own catalogue.

Refereed Journals

Until quite recently, 'hard copy' print journals were the most popular form for publishing the latest primary research studies, reviews of literature and/or theoretical/conceptual papers. Today, it is far more common to encounter 'online-focused' academic journals—which have the option of hard copy for paid subscribers. A main advantage of online-focused journals is that they are supported by internet resources with pre-print (in press/advance access) publication and current and archived full-text articles available on publisher or journal websites.

BOX 3.1 Examples of Resources Using Secondary Sources That Directly Influence Evidence-Based Clinical Practice

Journals

Evidence-Based Nursing—https://ebn.bmj.com

International Journal of Evidence-Based Healthcare—https://onlinelibrary.wiley.com/journal/17441609

Worldviews on Evidence-Based Nursing—https://sigmapubs.onlinelibrary.wiley.com/journal/17416787

Organisations

Australian and New Zealand Guidelines Network—https://anz-guideline-network.webnode.page

Campbell Collaboration—https://www.campbellcollaboration.org/ (US)

Cochrane Collaboration—https://www.cochrane.org/ (UK), https://australia.cochrane.org/ (Australia), https://nz.cochrane.org/ (New Zealand)

Institute for Healthcare Improvement—https://www.ihi.org/ (US)

Joanna Briggs Institute—https://joannabriggs.org/ (Australasia)

National Institute of Clinical Studies—https://www.clinicalguidelines.gov.au (Australia)

Clearinghouses/Literature Repositories

National Guideline Clearinghouse—https://www.ahrq.gov/gam/index.html (US)

National Quality Measures Clearinghouse—https://www.ahrq.gov/gam/index.html (US)

National Institute for Health and Clinical Excellence—https://www.nice.org.uk/ (UK)

Some journals (mainly Open Access—see later) are published only in electronic form on the internet (e.g. Bentham Open's *The Open Nursing Journal*—for which one of this chapter authors is the current Editor-in-Chief).

TUTORIAL TRIGGER 3.1

Journal articles that are available 'in advance' and/or 'in press' and/or 'early view' are assigned a Digital Object Identifier (DOI) number for direct reference—but have not yet been assigned volume/issue numbers or page numbers. Those details are reserved for when the article becomes available as a 'hard copy' of 'full online' version. Consider how these two versions of the same document differ and would be cited differently as part of an end-text reference list or bibliography. Identify the correct format for both and make a note for future reference.

For a research consumer, refereed (peer-reviewed) journals are the first source for accessing scholarly literature—primary and secondary. A refereed journal usually has an editor-in-chief/editor and co-editors and an editorial board of experts in the discipline, and uses peer review as a means to critically review submitted manuscripts for possible publication (Trotter 2021). Two or three peer reviewers are commonly assigned to critique and review a submitted manuscript. The aim is to evaluate whether the quality, clarity and rigour of the research study process, content and writing are suitable for publication in the selected journal. For those wanting to publish or know more of the publication process, Chapter 18 provides a detailed account of the many procedures and processes involved in journal (or otherwise) manuscript preparation, submission and review.

Especially with the more recent development of internet-only journals, there exist a number of nursing and midwifery journals competing in an increasingly crowded and competitive market. Most of these disciplinary and professional journals publish primary research and review papers on the state of current knowledge, including articles on practice, theory, policy and education. In previous editions of this text, a list of 'established' scholarly and professional nursing and midwifery journals was presented. However, especially with the more recent advance of 'open access' (see following section), it would be difficult to present a representative list that covers all that is now available.

Open Access Journals

As already stated, the notable increase of national and international journals on the back of ever-increasing competitiveness and competition for researchers to publish (the 'publish or perish' phenomenon—see Chapter 18) has witnessed the nature of journals continuously adapting over recent times. Fifteen years ago, journal articles were available only in hard copy format or online via personal/institutional subscription. If a reader didn't have a subscription, then they could pay a 'one-off' fee to access one or more articles. That model still exists, but that tradition has rapidly changed towards 'open access' formats—either online only or more traditional formats. The main change has been from 'subscription-only' access (where subscription fees provided the revenue and income for publishing companies) towards open access (where 'up-front' production/publication fees are generated, instead, from the authors themselves)—which means that readers can access them free of charge instead of having pay to subscription or one-off fees. This is seen by many to be a 'greener' and fairer way of disseminating research—especially for consumers in poorer/developing countries (de Jong 2017).

Inevitably, as with any 'competitive' industry, there are those who see the opportunity to exploit the current situation. Such companies have rightfully earned the title *predatory journals* and they tend to prey on the most vulnerable researchers (i.e. new researchers/authors 'desperate to publish' and/or researchers from developing countries). Legitimate **open access** journals commonly offer a publication process discount for authors from developing parts of the world—although predatory journals are also known to mimic this. Oermann et al (2018) conducted a study into predatory journals in nursing in 2016. Oermann et al (2022) have examined predatory journals and how to identify them.

At the time of the Oermann et al (2018) article, 70,000 predatory journal articles within biomedicine (including nursing and midwifery) were published. They identified that the initial number of articles for selection for their study was over 4000, published within just a few years. The finding that most of the articles reviewed were rated as poor or average supports the fact that consumers of the nursing literature cannot rely on articles published in such journals for credible, sound evidence on which to base nursing practice or build nursing knowledge. For instance, the nursing credentials of most authors (75.4%) could not be identified For each article reviewed, the research team rated its overall quality. From this assessment, 96.3% of the articles were rated as poor (n = 171) or average (n = 169). Only 13 articles (3.7%) were rated as excellent. They also identify that there are no current legal remedies to intervene in the practices of predatory publishers. The only reasonable intervention is to develop a well-informed community of scholars and practitioners who can determine that which is credible from that which is not. Midwifery is perhaps more immune to widespread predatory journals—but they do still exist.

A major area of concern is the lack of or questionable peer review processes with predatory journals (Oermann et al 2020, 2022). A useful scoping review (see later), titled 'What is a predatory journal?' identifying characteristics of predatory journals grouped them into six areas, one of which was having a poor or an incomplete peer review process on which to base decisions about articles to publish (Cobey et al 2018). The aim of peer review is to identify weaknesses in methodology, ethical concerns and other issues related to the quality of the paper, and importantly the manuscript's contribution to knowledge. As Oermann et al (2018) state, predatory journals lack the safeguards of traditional publishing practices. They appear legitimate 'on the surface' by conforming to an expected structure—but they are often not. That is where critical review/appraisal skills (see later in this chapter) are required to identify, eliminate and ignore low-quality predatory publications. A lack of quality is usually evident, representing inadequate peer review and editorial processes, in an attempt by predatory journals to publish quickly and receive up-front paid fees as quickly as possible.

Readers of this chapter may ask (especially if they are interested in publishing themselves), 'how do authors avoid getting "tricked" into publishing in predatory journals?' (it's a bit like avoiding common general online 'scams' overall) and 'how can I avoid the same mistake?' There are certain 'red flags' (warnings) that make it reasonably easy to identify predatory journals, or at least raise awareness so that further investigation is required. Perhaps the number one red flag with predatory journals is always to be very wary when any publishing company/journal approaches you directly. There are some established open access journal corporations (e.g. SAGE, BMC Central) that will contact you—but these are mostly general invitations—more based on 'do you know this journal/suite of journals exists—related to your topic area?'. If you are not sure, then the Directory of Open Access Journals (DOAJ)—https://doaj.org/—is a good site to check first. If the journal targeting you is not on their list, it's another red flag. Then there are many other red flags, such as:

- poor-quality online interface
- minimal and/or very broad journal scope (e.g. 'we publish almost anything related to nursing, midwifery or healthcare')
- poor English quality and grammatical errors
- the country of origin—many predatory journals are based in certain countries (usually sub-continent); some, however, will try to give the impression that they are based elsewhere with false addresses (e.g. US, Europe)
- unknown editors
- unknown or no editorial board and/or all based in the country of origin
- unsophisticated online manuscript submission processes (e.g. request to send a Word document by email)
- up-front publishing charges—legitimate journals will mostly ask for payment only once the article is in press/published
- not registered or associated with any reputable professional bodies and/or citation agencies—nor are credible *Impact Factor* sources stated (see later in this chapter 'Assessing the Quality of Journals')
- articles may not have been assigned a *Digital Object Identifier* (DOI) number
- the quality of existing articles in the journal—they are usually a very 'mixed bag' and often poor quality.

Literature Databases

Literature databases are repositories of published literature. They generally contain journal articles but some link to other sources, such as books or theses. This section discusses the common **bibliographical databases** used by nurses, midwives and other health professionals to examine the research literature. A 'portal' such as *PubMed* or *EBSCOhost* provides user-friendly access and search functions for a range of user-selected databases. Databases are developed by various companies or government agencies and access is commonly via a password-protected university or health service server restricted to enrolled students or employees—but such sources are also free to access generally. PubMed, a service of the US National Library of Medicine, is a particularly useful resource as it provides free public access through the internet for Medline searches—https://pubmed.ncbi.nlm.nih.gov/. The provided information in PubMed always includes at least the article abstract with access and, in many cases, access to free full-text article versions—for instance, Whitehead's (2021) editorial titled 'Preventative health improvement in orthopaedic and trauma practice: 20 years on—Are we there yet?' at: https://www.sciencedirect.com/science/article/pii/S1878124121000046?via%3Dihub.

Each database sources a range of journals particularly relevant to the related discipline/s of the database. Box 3.2 lists the common databases relevant for nursing and midwifery. There is overlap when a journal article is indexed to several different databases, while other journals will be indexed in one database but not another. Increasingly, international publishers are developing online literature databases for their own suite of journals such as 'publisher-based databases'—also highlighted in Box 3.2. The availability of full-text article access to a journal is usually determined by your organisation's subscription or if you have a personal subscription or are willing to pay a 'one-off' fee for individual articles. Open access journal articles are usually 'free to view'.

BOX 3.2 Common Literature Databases

Cochrane Collaboration: prepares, maintains and promotes the accessibility of systematic reviews of the effects of healthcare through a variety of documents and facilities, e.g. systematic reviews, clinical guidelines, databases—https://www.cochrane.org/

CINAHL (Cumulative Index to Nursing and Allied Health Literature): first published in 1956 as print-based *Cumulative Index to Nursing Literature*; CD-ROM database from 1982; online from 1995; indexes over 1600 journals. Contains the most comprehensive nursing information for reviewing the literature for research and research consumer purposes. Since 2003 it has been run through the EBSCOhost platform. The latest version is CINAHL complete https://www.ebsco.com/products/research-databases/cinahl-complete

Medline (Index Medicus): the oldest health-related literature index, first published in 1879; spans medicine, allied health, biophysical sciences, humanities, veterinary and nursing literature; primarily English-language or with English-translation abstracts; managed by the US National Library of Medicine (https://www.nlm.nih.gov/). Also provides free public access to PubMed for currently 21 million Medline citations—https://pubmed.ncbi.nlm.nih.gov/

MIDIRS: the Midwives Information and Resource Service is a subscriber information resource for maternity healthcare professionals. Resources include an online database, forums and *Midwifery Digest*—https://www.midirs.org/

OVID: a portal to scientific literature databases under the umbrella of Wolters Kluwer Health covering over 1200 journals (and includes Nursing@Ovid). Provides abstracts or full-text articles for a selection of nursing and midwifery journals sourced mainly from publishers and professional societies—https://www.wolterskluwer.com/en/solutions/ovid

EMBASE: provides coverage of international biomedical and pharmacological literature, with over 24 million indexed records and more than 7500 current, mostly peer-reviewed, biomedical journals—https://www.elsevier.com/products/embase

Psyclit: (online PsycINFO) database of psychology journals; managed by the American Psychological Association (APA). The APA has a widely used reference format which is a variant of the Harvard (author/date) style—https://www.apa.org/index.aspx

Educational Resources Information Center (ERIC): first published in 1969 in cooperation with Current Index to Journals in Education (CIJE). Claims to be the world's largest digital library of education-based literature—https://eric.ed.gov/

Australia/New Zealand Reference Centre: run by EBSCOhost, combines Australasian magazines, newspapers, newswires and reference books to create the largest collection of regional full-text content available to libraries in Oceania—https://www.ebsco.com/products/research-databases/australia-new-zealand-reference-centre

Sociofile: from Sociological Abstracts, Inc. of San Diego, California, provides over 445,000 citations and abstracts from the sociological abstracts and Social Planning/Policy and Development Abstracts (SOPODA) databases.

Scopus: from Elsevier, a large abstract and citation database of peer-reviewed literature: scientific journals, books and conference proceedings in the fields of science, technology, medicine, social sciences and arts and humanities—https://www.elsevier.com/products/scopus

Publisher-based databases: most multinational publishers maintain a website providing a database and repository of full-text articles for the journals they publish. Commonly accessed as a subscription service by university libraries for access to the full-text articles (as PDF documents). Examples include:

Wiley-Blackwell—https://www.wiley.com/en-au

Elsevier 'Science Direct'—https://www.sciencedirect.com/

Lippincott Williams & Wilkins (Wolters Kluwer Health)—https://lww.com/pages/default.aspx

Sage—https://us.sagepub.com/en-us/nam/home

Springer—https://www.springer.com/gp

Note: Website addresses in this box and throughout the book were functional and accurate at the time of writing. As addresses do change, if the site address does not work and there is no automatic redirection, use a generic search engine (e.g. Google) to locate the new site.

Databases that were established prior to digital storage (e.g. CINAHL, ERIC, Index Medicus, PsycINFO) all provided their information on journal articles as print-based sources to university and hospital libraries. These databases have been progressively adding early articles to their online versions (for those who wish to access early seminal research for historical reasons—and to compare with current studies in relation to similarities and differences), although there are some limitations. The online CINAHL database does not provide any information on articles published before 1982, while Medline goes back to 1966.

Email alerts containing information on current or forthcoming issues of specific journals are available for many journals and/or publishing house databases, either directly from the publisher or via portals such as Scopus (https://www.scopus.com) and Google Scholar (http://scholar.google.com.au). These portals are often free to access—or accessed through a university or health service institution library home page.

Websites

Today, there are literally many hundreds of nursing and midwifery-related academic journal websites. Most established and reputable journals, university schools or faculties and professional and regulatory organisations (Australasian councils, colleges and unions) have established websites. Many are likely to be quality assured and reliable, but caution is advised. It is especially important that the quality and accuracy of information available from the internet is assessed in a systematic manner. Compared with established journal articles and textbooks, there may have been no peer review process undertaken prior to the publication of internet material. Take, for instance, the popular Wikipedia site, which is difficult to officially verify as the text can be edited by anybody. As with many encyclopedias, Wikipedia is a tertiary source which is mostly considered inappropriate as an academic citation source. Therefore, consider the source of the website when judging the merits of any information. Web pages may be sponsored, or they may endorse a non-evidence-based position. Helpfully, *the National Library of Medicine* offers useful links on their page titled 'How do I evaluate health information that I find online?'—see https://support.nlm.nih.gov/knowledgebase/article/KA-04677/en-us.

With the volume of online resources increasing at a staggering rate, some may feel overwhelmed about what to access or not online—and what represents a good-quality online site about lay health and health professional consumers. Authors such as Hibbard (2017) seek to offer solutions. The following listed points may assist you to determine whether to use a particular website or not:

- Is the source a well-known, reputable organisation?
- What is the purpose of the information disseminated?
- Is the information substantiated by references/evidence?
- How does this information relate to other published material?
- Is there any inherent bias in the content?

> **TUTORIAL TRIGGER 3.2**
>
> Most healthcare professionals and consumers now use the internet to search for healthcare information. Think of a specific clinical topic that you are interested in and then use a generic search tool (e.g. Google Scholar) to locate written health-related material. How much information does this generic search yield? Look at the first page of results (as this is the most likely to be accessed by those performing an initial search). How much of it looks credible? Generate a set of questions that would be useful to assess the scientific merit of the healthcare information you see via a general web-based search. Work in a group to discuss proposed questions and gain consensus of which information could be used as evidence, and which would be questionable.

ASSESSING THE QUALITY OF LISTED JOURNALS

As already stated, while the nursing and midwifery journal industry grows at a rapid rate, there is an increasing need for research consumers to be able to judge the quality and credibility of the research information presented. There are several ways to 'rate' the quality of a journal or an individual article. The most common process is the use of *bibliometrics* (altmetrics) to calculate a journal's *impact factor* (IF) and an individual article's and overall journal's *citation rate*. These bibliometrics/altmetrics are contested but it also best noted that, in the absence of a current credible alternative, they are widely accepted by the 'academic' industry as the main mode of assessing journal and research article quality and impact (Smith & Watson 2016). Smith and Watson (2016), helpfully, unpack these metrics in their self-explanatory article titled 'Career development tips for today's nursing academic: bibliometrics, altmetrics and social media'.

An impact factor is calculated by identifying the number of articles in a journal that were subsequently cited by other articles (in their journal or different journals); that is:

$$\text{IF} = \frac{\text{number of articles in a journal cited by other articles}}{\text{total number of articles in the journal}}$$

A citation rate reflects the number of times an individual article is cited by other authors in more recent articles. It is influenced by what databases are used, the range of journals indexed in the database, the time lag between an article being published and it being cited by a more recent article, and inflation of citations by *self-citation* (an author referencing their own previous work). Some journal editors encourage the dubious practice of insisting that authors cite other studies from their own journal before they will allow publication. This helps to 'inflate' the impact factor of that journal, particularly if they are a low-ranking journal.

In terms of bibliometrics/altmetrics, there are two clear and established leaders that dominate. One is the US-based corporation Thomson Reuters' Institute of Scientific Information (ISI) and its Web of Science 'Core Collection' database (Clarivate Analytics)—see https://clarivate.com/products/web-of-science/. The other is European-based Elsevier's Scopus database—SCImago journal rank (SJR) indicator—see https://www.scimagojr.com/. SCImago is credited with bringing an 'alternative' ranking to the table: the Q ranking. The Q (Quartile) ranking is given as either Q1, Q2, Q3 or Q4, where Q1 indicates that the journal is in the top 25% of its subject category while Q4 indicates it is in the bottom 25% of the journals in that category. This ranking tends to report a similar outcome list to Impact Factor. SCImago uses both rankings in its database. These two databases and ranking metrics are discussed in more detail from a research author's perspective in Chapter 18.

CONDUCTING A SEARCH OF THE RESEARCH LITERATURE—THE 'LITERATURE REVIEW'

To conduct a literature search, the researcher/reviewer needs to know why, what and where to access the literature. It is also important to be able to clearly convey to the reader, reviewer or marker the approach and methods used during the literature search. The process must be clear, transparent and replicable. This will assist the reader to assess the extent to which all possible literature has been accessed and critically reviewed/appraised (see 'An unexpected hurdle'). This search should be detailed and comprehensive enough that readers would be confident to repeat the search themselves and come up with similar results. It should be noted here, and is covered in more detail later in this chapter, that there are many different types of 'literature review' (i.e. systematic, narrative, integrative, scoping, etc.). Until a later section in this chapter gets to the 'specifics' of these different types of reviews, we use the term 'literature review' to cover all these different approaches.

Formulation of a research question or topic is an important initial stage in the research process (Kumar 2019). Chapter 4 discusses the development of a research question or hypothesis for the purpose of a primary study. Once the question is constructed and refined, several subsequent steps guide the search process: selecting a database; refining the search strategy using keywords and filters; and examining and managing the search results.

Authors report their efforts to incorporate systematic database searches into nursing and midwifery education programs to assist students' understanding of the research process. Often, they work collaboratively with librarians who come highly recommended for those students new to database searching (Dhakal 2018). For instance, Nagle et al (2019) report that two experienced librarians were part of the literature search team/authors of their article titled 'Informing the development midwifery standards for practice: a literature review for policy development'.

Scope and Size of Search

In preparing a literature search, research consumers frequently ask themselves, 'How many articles do I need?' or 'How far back in the literature do I need to go?' The answers depend on the purpose of the search and the topic being investigated. The aim is to address the selected topic in a comprehensive and transparent way (Usher et al 2023). If the search is a student assignment/assessment task then students would be expected to demonstrate to the marker that they had accessed a broad, relevant and contemporary body of literature (both primary and secondary sources). The general 'rule of thumb' is that research literature that is less than 5 years old (especially for providing evidence for practice) is preferable, unless a particular period was known for *seminal* (strongly influencing later developments) articles, or a historical context is required. A review that explores a broad policy or clinical context issue may first seek literature less than 10 years old and then seek to include earlier original seminal work—especially as it is commonly seen that theory/policy development is 'cyclical' (i.e. it builds on the successful components of previously established practices).

To save 're-inventing the wheel', it can be useful to search for any existing recently conducted literature reviews (such as within Google Scholar) on a particular topic, as the availability of existing reviews could mean that much of the search work has already been done. If it appears that a credible and rigorous search has been conducted, you could draw on that material in your own work, while, of course, noting that you should never directly copy (plagiarise) such material for the purpose of your own articles or assessments. One would also still need to perform a new search of the literature published after the stated year range in the already published review.

Selecting a Database

A range of literature databases exists that lists nursing, midwifery and related health and medical literature, as described earlier in this chapter. Selection of an appropriate database/s relates to the purpose and topic of the search. Some portals enable searching of multiple databases simultaneously (e.g. EBSCO Nursing Resources: https://www.ebsco.com/health-care/for-nursing-allied-health). Alternatively, a search strategy can be saved and/or re-executed with another database if the initial results of the database/s were not satisfactory and/or one wishes to compare results against other databases—as they often produce differing results. Authors of published literature reviews should clearly outline the databases used. Nasrawi et al (2022) clearly identify the databases used in their integrative review.

Using Keywords

The abstraction and indexing process for each literature database relies on the use of keywords. This process has some limitations, and the accurate issue of keywords needs to be considered carefully. Each bibliographical database has a specific online search guide that provides information on the organisation of the entries and the keyword terms. For example:

- 'Medical Subject Headings' (MeSH) were developed by the US National Library of Medicine and are used particularly in Medline and PubMed and other important repositories such as the Cochrane databases.
- CINAHL uses nursing-specific terms that may differ from those used in Medline or other databases that use MeSH indicators.

Finding the correct keywords (or variables/concepts/terms) to include in a search is therefore an important element of the search process. The keyword functions of a database contain 'explode' or 'focus' features for terms where user-entered terms are mapped to the nearest keyword (e.g. 'mental health nursing' maps to 'psychiatric nursing' in CINAHL). The use of truncation is another useful tool. Truncation retrieves all variations of a root word in a single search by using a special symbol to replace the word endings. This broadens the search and is useful where limited information is available. The truncation symbol is often a question mark (?) (wildcard) or an asterisk (*). So, for instance, gyn* would reveal all literature title variants, such as gynaecology (European) or gynecology (American), gynaecological, gynecological etc. Caution is advised, though. A term like cerv* (for cervix or cervical) would also reveal literature related to the cervical spinal column.

Inclusion/exclusion Criteria for Keywords

Stated criteria for included keywords may be determined prior to a search strategy. *Inclusion criteria* are specific characteristics that the searched-for topic must possess to be eligible for inclusion in the final key studies. They are likely to range from quite broad requirements (e.g. age and/or gender) through to more specific criteria (e.g. have an existing disorder, such as osteoporosis). *Exclusion criteria* identify related characteristics and keywords but are considered 'just outside' what is the focus of the topic area—to avoid 'accidental' inclusion. It allows the reader further insight into the process—and to ask questions such as 'if I included the excluded keywords in another search, what would be the outcome?' Sometimes, the inclusion/exclusion criteria keywords are summarised in accompanying tables. Authors should identify their inclusion and exclusion criteria and provide sound justification for applying these criteria. See, for example, Chen et al's (2022) article investigating nurses' competency in electrocardiogram interpretation in acute care settings.

Using PICO/T to Develop Keywords

PICO/T is an acronym that describes the elements of a well-formed clinical question (Schiavenato & Chu 2021). Chapter 4 describes this process related to clinical question-setting in more detail. The acronym stands for:

P—for the 'patient' or 'problem'
I—for the 'intervention' of interest
C—for 'comparison'
O—for 'outcome'
T—for 'timeframe' (not always used)

Use of a PICO framework should help with search strategies, reducing noise and improving the precision of retrieval in the context of the clinician–librarian interaction (Booth et al 2000). PICO/T's primary purpose is to create clinical questions for research studies but, in literature searches, it can be used in a reverse manner. Essentially, it can be used to break down research questions into the specific keywords that were used to construct them. For example, you might want to know the effects of massage therapy on patients with cancer. The clinical question in PICO/T format would be something like: 'What are the effects of massage therapy for symptom relief on patients who have cancer compared with those who do not receive massage therapy?' The 'patients' are cancer sufferers, the 'intervention' is massage therapy, the 'comparison' is against cancer patients who do not receive the intervention, the 'outcome' is symptom relief and there is no 'timeframe'. The general keywords in the question would be 'cancer patients', 'massage therapy' and 'symptom relief'. Using these keywords, depending on the database/s you use, will lead you to a range of relevant studies such as Wyatt et al's (2019) review of the prevalence and types of complementary and integrative health therapies used by caregivers of patients with cancer.

 **TUTORIAL TRIGGER 3.3**

You have noticed an increased incidence of cannula infection rates on your ward and decide to search the literature for the latest information on prevention and treatment. Identify at least three keywords/phrases that you could use to begin the search. Use an appropriate literature database and identify: (1) how much literature is there?, (2) what type of literature is it (i.e. nursing/midwifery or medical or both; primary or secondary or both)? and (3) is there a dominant methodology/method reported?

Using Search Filters

In addition to keywords, other important search 'steps' narrow the focus of a search strategy. Numerous filters (database limits) are available as 'check boxes' to include only publications most relevant to your keyword search, especially if there are unmanageable amounts of research literature on a particular topic. Commonly used filters include:

- selecting a range of publication years (e.g. 2019–24)
- English-language publications only
- human research studies only (as opposed to including animal-research studies—see Chapter 13)
- available as full-text papers (the entire paper is available for reading) or just the title/abstract.

Searches can also be conducted for specific author, keyword, title and journal, using a range of search filters to further refine a search. Individual databases have different search filter features. The use of too many and/or 'random' use of filters will of course exclude papers, some of which may be useful to you. It is therefore advisable to take a stepwise approach where the focus becomes progressively narrower as more filters are added. Box 3.3 provides an example of such a process.

BOX 3.3 Conducting a Literature Search

Access the preferred database (e.g. 'CINAHL') on the computer search menu (library systems enable searching of multiple databases simultaneously) and you will be routed to the EBSCOhost platform. CINAHL generally limits the amount of institution users that can be online at any one time, which will vary between institutions, so you may have to try more than once to gain access. Imagine that you wanted to know what the current 'state of play' was in relation to clinical nurses and health promotion in terms of current EBP.

Before you start, note the main terms used. These are:

Explode

When you *Explode* a term, you create a search query that 'explodes' the subject heading. The headings are exploded to retrieve all references indexed to that term as well as all references indexed to any narrower subject terms.

In a database with a tree, such as *MeSH* or *CINAHL Headings*, exploding retrieves all documents containing any of the subject terms below the term you selected. In other databases, exploding retrieves all documents containing the selected term, as well as any of its first level of narrower terms. If a plus sign (+) appears next to a narrower or related term, there are narrower terms below it.

Major Concept

When you select *Major Concept* for a term, you create a search query that finds only those records for which the subject heading is a major point of the article. Searches are limited with specific qualifiers (subheadings) to improve the precision of the search and limited to major subject headings to indicate the main concept of an article.

Combining Explode and Major Concept

If you select both *Explode* and *Major Concept*, you retrieve all references indexed to your term (and its narrower terms) and all articles for which the subject heading is a major point of the article.

In this example, we will just use the major concept tick boxes and tick all their available tick boxes to illustrate.

- In the CINAHL Complete (EBSCOhost) database, type in the first search words/term. In this case it is 'nursing simulation'. Note that the term will prompt a drop-box of related terms. This may prompt you to click a different term—such as 'nursing simulation in nursing education'. In this case, we will stick with 'nursing simulation'. Then click the 'search' radio button. The result, at the time this search was conducted (late 2023), was 2770 'hits'.
- Repeat the search strategy for 'simulation training'—the result is 3835 hits. Now you will see both searches separately identified as S1 and S2. Then click on the 'select' box which will highlight S1 and S2 and then click on the 'search with AND' Boolean button (see footnote to this box regarding the use of Boolean terms). This creates S3—and the result is now 314 hits.
- Go to the left-hand column to view the limiters in 'Limit To'. Limit the search from 2013 to 2023—for S4 and 274 hits. Now go to the 'Subject: Major Heading' limiter list. Choose 'students, nursing'. This results in 94 hits. This will now give more narrow options—related to students and nursing. Click on education, nursing for S6. This results in 34 hits. Note that there are quite a few other limiters, e.g. 'Geography'. Here you will see

Continued

BOX 3.3 Conducting a Literature Search—cont'd

that you could limit to various parts of the world if you just wanted to review regional/national literature. Overall, this search has resulted in 34 hits and an output like:

#	Search History	Results
1	Nursing simulation	2770
2	Simulation training	3835
3	S1 AND S2 – S3	314
4	Limit to years 2013–2023 – S4	274
5	Limit to Students, nursing – S5	94
6	Limit to Education, nursing – S6	34

- The search resulted in 34 articles abstracted to CINAHL with 'nursing simulation' and 'simulation training' for the years 2013–23. That would generally, for most people's purposes, represent a manageable amount of literature to browse through and see whether the search provided the information needed, or would need to be repeated using an alternative strategy or perhaps an alternative database.
- Examine the 'display' (view results) of the results, reading the title and abstract to decide whether to keep the article in a folder and later access a full-text copy for further review. Results are displayed in reverse chronological order (most recent first) and have a relevancy score for each article to assist further.
- There are numerous facilities available—bibliographical details and abstracts can be emailed, RSS, imported into a bibliographical database or printed, and full-text articles can be printed in a variety of formats. Use a bibliographical database to manage your references and reference format (e.g. EndNote; see later in this chapter—reference managers).

Note: Boolean operators are words (such as 'AND', 'OR', 'NOT') used to combine and refine the results of searches. The term 'AND' was used as a Boolean in the above example to find articles related to both 'nursing simulation' and 'simulation training'. If 'OR' was used, then the sum of the two individual searches would be combined (i.e. resulting in 3835 articles).

Literature searches using computerised databases are limited by the range of journals indexed and a potential lack of precision in abstracting of keywords. Researchers may therefore conduct 'hand' or 'manual' searches of the table of contents of collected journals to identify other relevant publications that may have been missed during journal indexing in the databases and other sources such as thesis collections and conference proceedings. Alternatively, they may hand-search the reference lists of recent published articles for literature not identified in the electronic search process—particularly national, non-English, official or 'obscure' journal citations.

Searching the 'Grey' Literature

Grey literature is a term used to refer to evidence that may exist in a format that is often hard to find using a bibliographical index such as CINAHL or PubMed. For instance, research may be published in conference proceedings in an abridged version earlier than it is released into a refereed journal. ProQuest (https://www.proquest.com/) is a useful tool to find grey literature in their extensive product resources—such as conference proceedings and theses repositories. Paez (2017) provides a detailed description of the role and purpose of grey sources in literature reviews. OpenGrey (https://opengrey.eu/) is a resource that allows access to over 700,000 European grey literature sources and is expanding further. *Grey Literature Report* (https://www.nyam.org/library/collections-and-resources/grey-literature-report/) is a bimonthly update from the New York Academy of Medicine on health services and public health research.

RESEARCH IN BRIEF 3.1

Jaques et al (2018) report their literature review process related to 'Understanding the contemporary role of the intellectual disability nurse'. Adhering to the 'Preferred Reporting Items for Systematic Reviews and Meta-Analyses: The "PRISMA" Statement', six electronic databases were systematically searched: CINAHL, PubMed, Science Direct, Medline, ERIC and Scopus. The following search terms were used in conjunction with various medical subject headings: intellectual disability; developmental disability; nursing practice; advanced nursing practice; nursing practice, evidence-based; nursing practice, theory-based; nursing practice, research-based; differentiated nursing practice; intellectual disabilit* OR developmental disabilit* OR mental* retard* OR learning disabil* OR cognitive disabil* OR intellectual impairment OR mental deficiency OR mentally defective OR psychosocial retard* AND nursing practice OR advanced nursing practice OR evidence-based medicine OR nurs* rol*. The search initially included articles published in English language between the years 2000 and 2017. In total, 1040 articles were initially identified from the combined databases. After their critical review 'screening' process, a total of 27 key articles were eventually selected.

Overall, literature research search results should list the bibliographical details and abstracts (and possibly reference lists) of published articles from a specified list of journals. and may link to full-text versions of the journal

RESEARCH IN BRIEF 3.1—cont'd

article. Bibliographical details of a journal article will generally include author/s, publication year, article title, journal name, journal volume number, journal issue number and page numbers. Reading at least the offered abstract, in the first instance, is an important step as this provides a summary overview of the whole process undertaken (Wakefield 2014). The abstract enables you to decide whether to include the paper in your list of references and seek to retrieve the full-text article, or discard it as being outside the scope of your search topic.

There are many aspects related to learning effective search strategies. The search in Box 3.3 is a simplified illustration of an often-complex task that requires good instruction and experiential learning. Note that such a process may involve 'narrowing down' from a large corpus of literature to a much smaller body of literature. For instance, in Zhu et al's (2019) study, they narrowed from an initial 3397 'hits' down to six key studies.

REPORTING THE SEARCH STRATEGY

All the relevant elements of a search strategy should be reported in a secondary research paper (i.e. literature review, integrative review, systematic review or scoping review). This will include databases accessed; keywords used; publication year range; inclusion and/or exclusion criteria for papers; use of MeSH, Boolean and truncation terms; and search filters incorporated. Ideally, this process should be replicated (as much as possible) across several different databases—and each one reported, as well as all of them collectively. This enables the reader to critique the rigour and comprehensiveness of the search process. Sometimes, depending on the nature and depth of academic assignments, students may be called upon to do a similar exercise (see 'An unexpected hurdle').

AN UNEXPECTED HURDLE

Joshua conducted a 'critical' research literature review for one of his undergraduate assignments and it was marked as A+ (higher distinction). His lecturer encouraged him to submit his assignment for publication in a national nursing journal (see Chapter 18)—which he did. For the assignment, he used several different bibliographical databases and searched the relevant topic literature over the last 10 years. The submitted paper was rejected by the reviewers of the journal (see Chapter 18) mainly because the review was not 'critical enough' in

AN UNEXPECTED HURDLE—CONT'D

terms of reporting, in detail, the overall process and methods undertaken.

1. What could Joshua have done to make his research literature review as critical as possible—in terms of moving from an assignment format to a publication format? How do you think that the formats might differ?
2. Why is it important, when conducting 'critical' literature reviews, that a clear 'rigour trail' is indicated?

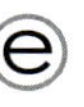

MANAGING THE COLLECTED RESEARCH LITERATURE

Bibliographical databases are software packages designed to create your own reference library. They form a useful tool in managing the literature search and review processes, as they store bibliographical details of journal articles, reports and other print materials. Examples of these databases include EndNote, Reference Manager, Pro-Cite, Papyrus, CiteULike, RefWorks, etc. (Francavilla 2018). Some universities provide research students with access to these types of bibliographical databases as part of a site-licence agreement, or they can be purchased individually.

Most literature databases provide an export function to common bibliographical databases, or the search results can be saved in a format that allows importing by a bibliographical database. This function eliminates re-keying of bibliographical information into the database fields. However, details should be checked to correct any errors during the import process. These databases also interface with word-processing software. Linkage of the two programs allows insertion of references into the body of a word-processed document (such as a literature review). The in-text citation and list of references can then be formatted automatically to a selected reference style—for example, AMA, APA, Chicago, Harvard and Vancouver (Gimenez 2019). Some journals will use a variation of one of these style manuals to reduce word count. EndNote possesses a clever self-explanatory tool known as 'cite while you write'. Elsevier's 'Mendeley' does similar. You can automatically cite references in your manuscript and automatically format bibliographies (reference lists) by moving between later EndNote versions and your word processor program.

Software Tools to Support Screening the Literature

The methods used in literature reviews often create large datasets that results in the need to 'screen' many numbers of articles to assess whether the literature meets the overall aim of the review. The first round of screening, usually the title and abstract screening, is time consuming and often requires more than one round of screening. To promote rigour and ensure reliability, this stage is often shared between different members of the review team—and is part of the overall **critical appraisal/evaluation/review** process (see later). As the number of published literature reviews grows and methods of searching the literature become more sophisticated, there has been a growing need to support more transparent, rigorous and pragmatic screening techniques. Software tools have been developed to facilitate this stage of the literature review process.

The two most common software tools used in healthcare to screen literature are *Covidence* https://www.covidence.org/ and *Rayyan* https://www.rayyan.ai/. Both tools were designed to expedite the review screening process by easing citation sharing and allowing comparisons by the review team in relation to include or exclude the literature. Harrison et al (2020), in their evaluation of software screening tools, state that Covidence and Rayyan provide a useful user experience for carrying out initial screening.

Writing Tools

Scrivener is one of many writing tools that helps to manage, tag, edit and organise collections of information including rich text files. Developed originally by a PhD student, but adapted for creative writing, it has also been adapted for business reports and thesis writing. Some useful tools assist you to keep and compare older versions of your document and to colour-code versions with a simple method for developing separate documents (such as chapters) and merging them. Desktop note-taking tools such as *Tomboy* can also assist in planning your document and aid chapter and heading structure for thesis development (https://wiki.gnome.org/Apps/Tomboy).

ChatGPT

ChatGPT, which stands for Chat Generative Pretrained Transformer, is an advanced, pretrained, deep-learning language model developed by OpenAI, an **artificial intelligence** (AI) research laboratory based in San Francisco, California. ChatGPT can process vast amounts of information and generate large amounts of coherent and informative text. ChatGPT produces high-quality written responses to queries or questions, it can paraphrase text, generate ideas, expand and contrast concepts and create a detailed logical structure to organise ideas and develop coherent arguments as well as powerful and compelling introductions and conclusions (Sun & Hoelscher 2023). However, it should be noted that, although generated text might sound convincing, the information produced is often not underpinned by evidence and is therefore unreliable. This should be particularly noted when using this resource for student assessments. ChatGPT is also a useful proofreading and editing tool. In addition, it can assist with word choice, suggest alternative phrasing and help maintain a consistent tone and style.

CRITICALLY REVIEWING AND APPRAISING THE RESEARCH LITERATURE

Readers who have searched and reviewed the research literature on a clinical topic previously (or intend to) will be able to relate to the need to explore a critical 'mass' (corpus or body) of research literature studies—and not just evaluate a single study. Practice should not be changed based on a single critically reviewed study, and good grades for academic assignments will not be achieved if a wide range of appropriate research studies is not included.

For those who wish to critically evaluate single or a small number of 'key' research articles, appraisal checklists are contained in Box 3.4 (qualitative) and Box 3.5 (quantitative). They are not recommended for a large body of collected studies as they are too detailed, and the process would be too time consuming—although one could adapt them and create one's own 'summary' form of them to assist. Other more simplified checklist tools—for example, the Critical Appraisal Skills Programme (CASP) https://casp-uk.net/casp-tools-checklists/—exist for that purpose.

Once an effective literature search has been completed, the next logical step is to review that gathered critical mass of research literature. In practice, it is best to view the search and review processes as seamless and continuous. A review of the research literature is a systematic and, hopefully, critical review of published papers on a particular topic of interest in a discipline (Hutchinson & Frazer 2023). Two contemporary issues have highlighted the importance for high-quality reviews of original research: first, the recent proliferation of nursing and midwifery knowledge through print, online publications and other sources and, second, the emphasis of clinical practice based on the best available evidence (see Chapter 15). This section presents the critical review of research literature as a process essential to the development of our disciplines, a thread that runs across practice, research, education and theory (see Fig. 3.1).

In relation to the four concepts in Fig. 3.1, a critical review of the literature presents:

- new knowledge that can lead to the development, testing or refinement of theories (see Chapter 2)
- gaps or limitations in the literature that can lead to new directions in original research
- the existing knowledge about a particular topic, concept or problem of clinical interest, and

BOX 3.4 Critical Review Guidelines for Qualitative Studies

Title and Abstract

1. Is the title of the research paper concise, clear and congruent with the text?
2. Were the aims and/or objectives stated? What are they?
3. Did the abstract contain sufficient information about the stages of the research process (e.g. aims, research approach, participants, data collection, data analysis, findings)?

Identifying the Phenomenon/Phenomena of Interest

1. Is the phenomenon focused on human experience within a natural setting?
2. Is the phenomenon relevant to nursing, midwifery and/or health?

Structuring the Study

1. Is it clear that the selected participants are living the phenomenon of interest?
2. How is published literature used in the study?
3. Does the question identify the context (participant/group/place) of the method to be followed?
4. Is the theoretical framework clearly stated?
5. Does the theoretical framework fit the research question?
6. Is the method of data collection and analysis clearly specified?
7. Does the qualitative method of data collection that has been chosen fit the research question (e.g. grounded theory, ethnography)?
8. Are the limitations of the study stated?

Research Question and Design

1. Was the research question determined by the need for the study? How was this determination made?
2. Are the data collection strategies appropriate for the research question?
3. Do the data collection strategies reflect the purpose and theoretical framework of the study (e.g. in-depth interviewing, focus groups)?
4. Can the data analysis strategy be identified and logically followed?

Participants

1. How were the participants and setting selected (e.g. sampling strategies)?
2. How was confidentiality of the participants assured?
3. How was the anonymity of participants assured?
4. What ethical issues were identified in the study?
5. How were the ethical issues addressed?

Data Analyses

1. How were the data analysed?
2. Is the analysis technique congruent with the research question?
3. Is there evidence that the researcher's interpretation captured the participants' meaning?
4. Did the researcher say how the criteria for judging the scientific rigour of the study were maintained in terms of credibility auditability, fittingness and confirmability?

Describing the Findings

1. Does the researcher demonstrate to the reader the method (e.g. audit trail) by which the data were analysed?
2. Does the researcher indicate how the findings are related to theory?
3. Is there a link between the findings to existing theory or literature, or is a new theory generated?

Researcher's Perspective

1. Are the biases of the researcher reported (e.g. researcher/participant expectations, researcher bias and power imbalance)?
2. Are the limitations of the study acknowledged?
3. Are recommendations suggested for further research?
4. Are implications for healthcare mentioned?

- research findings that inform EBP activities (development of clinical practice guidelines, practice development projects).

The focus of this chapter is primarily from the perspective of a research consumer in conducting a literature review and preparing a written report or perhaps an assignment. Some types of review are complex and require significant expertise and experience to complete. This being the case, this section will just touch on these principles and highlight where they are covered in more detail in other chapters.

Purposes of a Literature Review Related to Research

The overall purpose of a review of the literature is to examine the knowledge base to inform a defined area of clinical practice or theoretical perspective, or guide original research (Aveyard & Bradbury-Jones 2019). The common forms of a review include:

- a systematic summary of a series of original research papers—for example, a systematic review

BOX 3.5 Critical Review Guidelines for Quantitative Studies

The Title and Abstract

1. Is the title of the research paper congruent with the text?
2. Were the aims and/or objectives stated? What are they?
3. Did the abstract contain sufficient information about the stages of the research process (e.g. aims, hypothesis, research approach, sample, instruments and findings)?

Structuring the Study

1. Is the motivation for the study demonstrated through the literature review?
2. Is the literature cited current, relevant and comprehensive? Are the references recent?
3. Are the stated limitations and gaps in the reviewed literature appropriate and convincing?
4. How was the investigation carried out?
5. Is the hypothesis stated?
6. Which hypothesis is stated: the scientific hypothesis or the null hypothesis?
7. Does the hypothesis indicate that the researcher is interested in testing for differences between groups or in testing for relationships?

The Sample

1. Is the sample described?
2. Is the sample size large enough to prevent an extreme score from affecting the summary statistics used?
3. How was the sample size determined?
4. Was the sample size appropriate for the analyses used?

Data Collection

1. How were the data collected (questionnaires or other data collection tools)?
2. Who collected the data?
3. Are the data adequately described?
4. What is the origin of the measurement instruments?
5. Are the instruments adequately described?
6. How were the data collection instruments validated?
7. How was the reliability of the measurement instruments assessed?
8. Were ethical issues discussed?

Data Analysis

1. Are descriptive or inferential statistics reported?
2. What tests were used to analyse the data: parametric or non-parametric?
3. Were the descriptive statistics/inferential statistics appropriate to the level of measurement for each variable?
4. Were the appropriate tests used to analyse the data?
5. What is the level of measurement chosen for the independent and dependent variables?
6. Were the statistics appropriate for the research question and design?
7. Are there appropriate summary statistics for each major variable?
8. Were the statistics primarily descriptive, correlational or inferential?
9. Identify the outcome of each statistical analysis.
10. Explain the meaning of each outcome.

Findings

1. Were the findings expected? Which findings were not expected?
2. Is there enough information present to judge the results?
3. Are the results clearly and completely stated?
4. Describe the researcher's report of the findings.
5. Identify any limitations or gaps in the study.
6. Were suggestions for further research made?
7. Did the researcher mention the implications of the study for healthcare?
8. Was there sufficient information in the report to permit replication of the study?

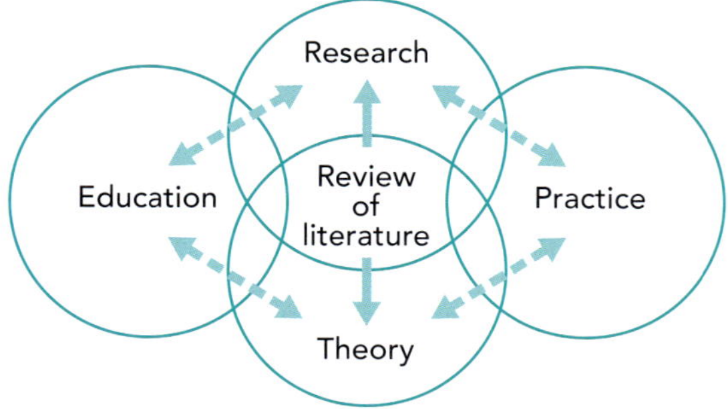

Fig. 3.1 Relationship of the review of literature to theory, research, education and practice

- a supporting background section for a clinical practice guideline or evidence-based recommendation
- the background section of an original research proposal, grant application or published field research paper.

A literature review therefore serves a purpose for both research consumers and primary researchers (see Sections 2 and 3 of this book). Primary researchers will usually conduct a detailed and rigorous literature search process to inform their research from beginning to end (Kumar 2019). Literature reviews are also, of course, undertaken by undergraduate and graduate coursework and research students for various learning purposes.

TUTORIAL TRIGGER 3.4

The review of literature is usually easy to find in a primary research paper. Most frequently, it is one of the early sections of the paper and is labelled 'Review of literature' or 'Background' or some other comparable term. Review any recent primary research article and notice the way in which the review of the literature is presented. Summarise its main points and decide whether you think that it is an effective review or not. Then repeat the process with another article. Compare and contrast the review sections of each article with one another.

RESEARCH IN BRIEF 3.2

Graj et al (2019) identify clinical placement as a fundamental aspect of student learning and skill development across healthcare disciplines. They also believe that participation in clinical placements can also present significant risk to students. Their systematic literature review sought to examine the range of risks and hazards encountered by students across healthcare disciplines during their clinical placements. The CINAHL Complete, Medline Complete and PsycINFO databases were searched. Search terms, searched within abstracts, included: (AB(health OR health care OR healthcare)) AND (AB(student* OR trainee*)) AND (AB(clinical placement* OR clinical practical* OR clinical practicum OR clinical practice placement* OR clinical fieldwork OR clinical rotation)) AND (AB(risk* OR occupational health and safety OR occupational risk* OR adverse health event* OR occupational safety OR hazard OR expos* OR problem* OR challenge*)). An English language limiter was used.

Studies investigating an element of risk faced by students during clinical placement were eligible for inclusion. Key study eligibility criteria included:

1. an investigation of risk to students
2. a focus on students undertaking training in a healthcare discipline, and
3. a clinical placement context.

All disciplines in which healthcare students were required to complete clinical placements as a part of their professional training were eligible. Studies published between 2013 and 2018 inclusive were eligible for inclusion. Research conducted in the context of all comparative international health systems, including Australia, New Zealand, the United States, Canada and the United Kingdom, were the focus of this study. Following removal of duplicates, abstracts were screened. The full texts of potentially relevant studies were located and

RESEARCH IN BRIEF 3.2—Cont'd

assessed against the eligibility criteria listed above. The reference lists of resulting articles were visually appraised; potentially relevant papers were screened for inclusion. After the initial 'hit' of 272 studies, the search eventually yielded a total of 50 records for inclusion in the review.

The review concludes that, as risks in unpredictable clinical environments cannot be eradicated, there is a critical need for educative action to enable students to manage risks competently and confidently, and to reduce occurrence of adverse health events.

Characteristics of a Critical Literature Review

A review usually includes a critical evaluation of both primary and secondary literature related to the clinical practice question or proposed study, as well as a summary of the overall strengths or weaknesses of the reviewed studies' conflicts and gaps in the literature (Hutchinson & Frazer 2023). From a student perspective, a critical review of the literature is essential to acquiring knowledge for the development of academic assignments, presentations and debates. Academic staff will expect students to include cited literature in support of their rationale for each clinical practice or theory activity (Gimenez 2019). Novice students, at first, may just be required to read and critique small numbers of primary studies to familiarise themselves with the terminology and processes of research overall. Students may be asked to critically appraise a single research study (see Boxes 3.4 and 3.5) to get an in-depth appreciation of certain paradigms and methodologies (see Chapter 2). However, especially in terms of practice change, students are often asked to draw on much broader collections of literature. This can be achieved by either searching for themselves or referring to 'prepacked' literature such as existing different types/styles of published literature reviews (see later in this chapter).

A student assignment might involve retrieving and critically reviewing the primary sources listed for a particular clinical practice guideline to determine the degree of support found for the interventions outlined in the guidelines (Hunker et al 2014). An effective literature review will reflect characteristics listed in Table 3.1. The development of skills in writing a literature review is experiential—more exposure to literature and more practice in writing will improve the quality and depth of a review. As a reviewer's experience grows, the style of review will usually transform from a descriptive summary of individual studies to a more integrated synthesis and analysis of collections of studies—such as Nagle et al's (2019) policy development literature

TABLE 3.1 Characteristics of a Written Review of Literature

Levels of Review	Criteria
Description	• Enough sources are identified, based on the clinical question, related keywords and appropriate range of publication years. • Review mainly consists of primary sources. • Summary of studies is presented in a logical flow using themes or categories. • Summary is succinct and adequately represents the reviewed literature/knowledge base of a specific topic • Summaries/paraphrasing of material (direct quotes of content used only for specific purposes and referenced appropriately).
Analysis	• Critical review of study methods, outcomes and applicability to clinical practice. • Assessment of study quality, using accepted review 'criteria' to analyse strengths, weaknesses or limitations and conflicts or gaps in information.
Synthesis	• Linking studies together to form a new whole. • Use of summary tables to facilitate critique of articles in sections or themes.

review 'Informing the development midwifery standards for practice'.

Steps in the Critical Review/Appraisal Process

Once the relevant studies have been selected from the literature search, a stepwise process for **critical reviewing/appraising** the literature is recommended. It includes:

- preliminary reading of available abstracts, which allows articles to be selected or discarded;
- obtaining a full-text print or electronic copy of all included articles (meeting eligibility/inclusion criteria) to enable organisation for priority critical reading and eventual sorting/analysing/synthesising into themes or categories;
- an initial read/skim/scan of all sources that identifies a set of core/key articles, as well as others that are useful and peripheral to your questions, and perhaps some that are not as useful as first thought and which may then be discarded from the review. This includes 'grey' literature sources—and the scanning of selected key article reference lists;
- describing the justification for discarding/excluding studies based on a clear rationale;
- organising findings into themes, allowing comparison and links between coherent studies during the review—often using summary tables as a guiding and organisational tool;
- potential citation/reference management using appropriate software (e.g. EndNote, Mendeley, etc.);
- critical reading/review/appraisal, which requires several readings, a certain level of knowledge across a broad range of methodological approaches and the use of a set of criteria/tools to evaluate the studies.

Once this process has been fully undertaken, the research consumer should have moved from the critical appraisal of individual studies to the appraisal of an overall collection or corpus of related studies. This collection must be organised into the sum of all its parts. It is from this point that we start to see how the main findings are related to the whole—such as with Foster et al's (2023) integrative review related to children and young people's participation in decision-making within healthcare organisations in New Zealand.

Summary Tables

For most styles of literature review, after an initial review of papers, it may be useful to construct some working summary tables to provide key characteristics of individual studies and how they relate to or differ from each other. For instance, Peberdy et al's (2022) review of knowledge, attitudes and practices of maternity healthcare professionals concerning umbilical cord clamping uses a data extraction table with the following headings: 'authors' aim, country, sample, design, finding's strengths and limitations'. Use of a data extraction table promotes the effective critique of studies in sections or themes and identifies questions and gaps in the literature. Initially, column headers are selected to allow analysis of the various papers under specific themes (see Table 3.2). The development and sophistication of the table then progresses as the review of papers continues. A table then allows summary information to be noted for each study (description) and enables identification of similarities and differences between the studies (synthesis) and limitations (analysis).

TABLE 3.2 Example of Summary Table Column Headers

Author/Date	Participants	Method/procedure	Outcome Variables	Findings
Paper A				
Paper B				
Paper C				

Schematic Tools

Many research consumers benefit from 'visual' representations and breakdown of research information. The same is true for literature reviews. Many nursing and midwifery-based literature 'systematic' literature reviews (see later) routinely incorporate such schematics. The most common ones are the likes of the previously mentioned PRISMA and CASP tools. A Word and PDF PRISMA template can be found at http://prisma-statement.org/PRISMAStatement/FlowDiagram.aspx. It should be noted that the PRISMA framework guideline and schematic were originally (and still are) developed for medical Cochrane-based systematic reviews (meta-analysis—see later) but have been 'adopted' by many for literature-based systematic reviews (Stovold et al 2014).

Types of Literature Review

The 'landscape' and popularity of literature reviews in nursing and midwifery has increased significantly over the last decade (Aveyard 2022). Literature reviews are valuable tools for EBP-conscious practitioners. Good-quality reviews usually demonstrate that the researchers have undertaken a systematic and effective process to search and appraise the available literature. To evaluate the quality of a review and determine whether the author/s have adhered to a systematic and transparent process, Box 3.6 identifies the main components that should have been followed. These can then be a potential supporting source of 'preappraised' clinical/educational evidence. For this reason, it's important to be clear about what a literature review is.

Aveyard and Bradbury-Jones (2019) conducted a 'mapping review' of literature reviews; essentially it is a critical literature review focused on literature review types and styles (a review of reviews). They report the recent emergence of many different methods for now performing a literature review. They refer to the 'early days' when there were essentially two types of review: a Cochrane systematic review and a narrative review. They correctly identify how the term 'systematic review' is now widely used to describe a variety of review types—different to the original medically defined Cochrane-based systematic review (meta-analysis). This recent phenomenon has resulted in what often happens with new nursing and midwifery terms: they are often used 'interchangeably'. What would have been called in the past (and is still used today) a 'literature review' is now more likely to be termed 'systematic', 'narrative', 'integrative', 'scoping', 'critical' and, sometimes, just 'review'. This presents a potential problem. Although there are similarities between the terms, they do not always mean the same thing. That said, for now, it appears that the best way to present the current situation is to go with the 'strong flow'—that is, call them all 'systematic' reviews. The reason we argue this is that the overall intention and process of any 'robust' literature review is that it should be 'systematic' and follow a certain rigour-trail process. However, given the growth in literature reviews and the confusion that surrounds them, it is

BOX 3.6 Critical Review of a Literature Review

1. Are all the relevant concepts and variables included in the review?
2. Are primary sources mainly used?
3. Does the literature review uncover gaps or inconsistencies in knowledge?
4. Does the summary of each reviewed study reflect the essential components of the study design, research process and analysis techniques?
5. Does the critique of each reviewed study include: strengths, weaknesses or limitations of the design; conflicts; and gaps or inconsistencies in information in relation to the area of interest?
6. What overall conclusions can be drawn from the synthesis of the literature?
7. Does the organisation and synthesis of the reviewed studies follow a logical sequence that justifies why there is a need for a particular study?
8. How does the review reflect critical thinking and EBP?

still important to identify the different types of literature reviews, as follows.

Narrative Review

A traditional narrative review was the original type of literature review. Narrative reviews are 'evidence round-ups' on specific healthcare topics. The topic is usually broad and may not include a focused clinical question or, in some cases, a defined search strategy. Analysis of the primary studies is classified as 'narrative' or 'thematic'—a narrative is purely descriptive, while a thematic analysis produces a basic synthesis of findings by identifying important and recurring themes (Polkki et al 2014). Such reviews are useful for informing readers about the context of topics but their potential for being less systematic than other reviews means that they are less likely to provide compelling evidence for practice change alone. Authors may have expert opinions (and biases) and find studies to support their preferred positions (selection bias). The approaches of concept and discourse analysis are, to some, 'purer' forms of narrative interpretive inquiry—for example, Connor et al (2023) and their concept analysis of clinical judgement in nursing.

Systematic Review (Meta-analysis)

As already highlighted by Aveyard and Bradbury-Jones (2019), historically a systematic review is a common strategy for examining an explicit issue in clinical practice, particularly for 'cause-and-effect' experimental studies where the effect of an intervention or treatment is tested (see Chapter 8). Commonly, but not always, this style of 'medical' systematic reviews also uses meta-analytical techniques. Meta-analyses should be based on systematic reviews but not all systematic reviews include a meta-analysis. When the data from studies in a systematic review are sufficiently equivalent, a meta-analysis of the pooled data can be examined using common quantitative analysis procedures. A meta-analysis combines the results of several studies that address a set of related research hypotheses. In its simplest form, this is normally by identification of a common measure of effect size (i.e. sample size), for which a weighted average might be the output of meta-analyses. Meta-analyses are covered in more detail in Chapter 12. The Cochrane Collaboration (Library) is the oldest and largest repository of medical systematic reviews. See their website for examples of study protocols and reports of systematic reviews—https://www.cochrane.org.

Systematic reviews and meta-analysis are far less 'popular' in nursing and midwifery research than 'literature systematic reviews' because of their statistical complexity. Driscoll et al (2018) offer an example. These authors sought to undertake a systematic review and meta-analysis examining the association between nurse staffing levels and nurse-sensitive patient outcomes in acute specialist units. Nine electronic databases were searched for English articles published between 2006 and 2017. The primary outcomes were nurse-sensitive patient outcomes. Of 3429 unique articles identified, only 35 met the inclusion criteria. All were quantitative cross-sectional studies (see Chapter 9) and the majority utilised large administrative databases. Higher staffing levels were associated with reduced mortality, medication errors, ulcers, restraint use, infections, pneumonia, higher aspirin use and a greater number of patients receiving percutaneous coronary intervention within 90 minutes. A meta-analysis involving 175,755 patients, from six studies, admitted to the intensive care unit and/or cardiac/cardiothoracic units showed that a higher nurse staffing level decreased the risk of in-hospital mortality by 14% (0.86, 95% confidence interval 0.79–0.94). However, the meta-analysis also showed high heterogeneity ($I^2 = 86\%$). They conclude that nurse-to-patient ratios influence many patient outcomes, most markedly in-hospital mortality. They identify that more studies need to be conducted on the association of nurse-to-patient ratios with nurse-sensitive patient outcomes to offset the paucity and weaknesses of research in this area. This would provide further evidence for recommendations of optimal nurse-to-patient ratios in acute specialist units.

Meta-synthesis

Systematic reviews and other quantitative reviews have been established for some time now. More recently, there is a demand for methods of synthesising the findings of qualitative research studies, especially in health-related research. This is particularly relevant for nursing and midwifery. The term 'meta-synthesis' is used to distinguish this from quantitative 'meta-analysis'. Meta-synthesis may also be used to integrate the findings from both quantitative and qualitative studies. For such reasons, there has been disagreement over whether a meta-synthesis is a form of systematic review (meta-analysis) (Sandelowski et al 2007). There are several different approaches to meta-synthesis, and a review of meta-synthesis methods for qualitative research lists about 10 methods (Barnett-Page & Thomas 2009). For nursing and midwifery, some examples of differing approaches are meta-summary (Kelly et al 2023) and meta-ethnography (Fernández-Basanta et al 2023), where collective qualitative study findings are designed to provide a more substantive and informative position than findings from separate qualitative studies alone. Zhu et al (2019) report their meta-synthesis (meta-aggregation) review into nursing students' experiences with faculty incivility in the clinical education context.

Scoping Reviews

Scoping reviews (sometimes called mapping reviews) may appear different to other literature reviews in that they are more useful where there are fewer primary research (qualitative, quantitative and mixed-methods) studies to draw on than there is 'other' literature (i.e. theoretical/conceptual, opinion-based, grey literature, literature reviews, etc.). This is most likely in 'developing' and evolving healthcare topics and/or topics that are not well researched for a variety of reasons to clarify concepts. They essentially draw on any existing and available literature to appraise. The appraisal may or may not be 'critical' in terms of synthesising existing qualitative, quantitative and mixed-methods-based studies. An 'initial' scoping review may be performed to facilitate a decision on whether to then proceed with a systematic review or not. That said, remember that nursing and midwifery are 'famous' for taking terms and using them interchangeably. It may well be that what is called a 'scoping review' is a 'standard' systematic review.

An example of a 'true' scoping review is Campbell et al's (2019) scoping review investigating factors influencing clinical decision making used by mental health nurses to provide provisional diagnosis. The authors identify that medical diagnosis has traditionally been the role of medical officers. However, mental health nurses working in crisis/emergency settings within Australia are expected to provide a provisional diagnosis post-assessment of a consumer. The researchers identify that there is 'limited literature and understanding' of how mental health nurses develop a provisional diagnosis, and aimed to first identify and describe the clinical decision-making processes used by mental health nurses across a variety of clinical settings. Second, they sought to explore the factors influencing mental health nurses' diagnostic practice in a variety of settings. Literature was searched using CINAHL (EBSCOhost), PubMed and ProQuest, and peer-reviewed literature published between 2007 and 2017 was used for this scoping review. They conclude that little is known about the use of diagnostic practice in mental health nursing in Australia; however, the limited literature revealed an overlap between the factors which influence clinical decision making and diagnostic practice, respectively, and the authors suggest that further research is required to expand on this context.

Integrative Reviews

An increasingly used literature review in nursing and midwifery is the integrative review (Whittemore & Knafl 2005). The integrative review method supports the use of diverse data sources, thereby developing a holistic understanding of the topic of interest by presenting the state of the science and contributing to theory development. An integrative review is a specific review method that summarises past empirical or theoretical literature to provide a more comprehensive understanding of a particular phenomenon or healthcare problem. Integrative reviews thus have the potential to build nursing science, informing research, practice and policy initiatives. Well-done integrative reviews present the state of the science, contribute to theory development and have direct applicability to practice and policy (Whittemore & Knafl 2005). Anderson et al's (2018) integrative review aimed to examine, thematically group and critically evaluate published literature around the impact of MAGNET designation on organisational culture within designated hospitals. Crevacore et al's (2023) integrative review examined factors impacting effective delegation practices by Registered Nurses to Nursing Assistants.

> **TUTORIAL TRIGGER 3.5**
>
> Summarise the main points that reflect the purposes of a literature review from a research consumer's perspective.

SUMMARY

Being able to both critically search for and then perform a critical review/appraisal of collected research literature is an acquired skill. The main objectives for a research consumer in relation to searching and reviewing the research literature are to acquire the ability to: conduct a critical database computer search, efficiently retrieve enough scholarly material for a literature review and critically evaluate the selected literature using accepted reviewing/appraisal criteria and tools. This chapter provides the instruction needed to enable effective retrieval of research literature and the beginning critical evaluation, analysis and synthesis of published studies on a specific topic of interest for a variety of purposes (e.g. student assignments, research theses and primary and secondary research projects).

KEY POINTS

- Primary sources are published articles reporting an original piece of research. Secondary sources are reviews of a series of primary studies on a specific topic.
- Primary sources are essential for literature reviews while secondary sources may provide important synthesised information on a topic of interest and are useful for developing clinical practice guidelines and modelling critical evaluation skills.
- Strategies for efficiently retrieving scholarly literature include experiential learning, seeking advice from

reference librarians and using a literature (bibliographical) database/s to collect and manage research literature.
- A critical review of the literature is a comprehensive, in-depth and systematic review of a variety of sources—such as scholarly publications, unpublished scholarly print materials, internet materials, audiovisual materials, personal communications and other written material.
- A literature review provides valuable information for both research consumers and researchers.
- The ability to critically review/appraise database literature is necessary for implementing research-based practice in nursing and midwifery.

TIME TO REFLECT

Jarden, R.J., Sandham, M., Siegert, R.J., et al., 2020. Intensive care nurses' well-being: a systematic review. Aust. Crit. Care 33 (1), 106–111. doi:10.1016/j.aucc.2018.11.068

Aim: Jarden et al (2020) state that the unique work challenges of intensive care nurses can cause both stress and distress to nurses, evident in the available literature. The objective of their review was to systematically identify, appraise and synthesise primary research reporting intensive care nurses' wellbeing regarding burnout, compassion, fatigue and moral distress.

Design: The search strategy included (1) bibliographical databases for published work and (2) forward and backward citation searches. Key search terms included [critical OR intensive] AND [nurs*] AND [well*]. Inclusion criteria were as follows: (1) population: critical or intensive care nurses working with adult or mixed adult and paediatric patients, (2) study type: primary research studies, (3) outcome: intensive care unit nurses' wellbeing; and (4) publication available in the English language. Studies were excluded if the group of intensive care nurses was not independently reported. Included studies were critically appraised, and results were synthesised and presented descriptively. Semantics of the included studies were explored to identify frequently used terms.

Reflect on the following: Database searches identified 1652 documents, with three additional records from citation searches. After removal of duplicates and title and abstract screening for potential inclusion, four full-text articles were assessed and met the inclusion criteria. The primary reason for exclusion was studies not reporting ICU nurses' wellbeing as an outcome.

Questions

1. What other designs could have been used in this study?
2. Reflect on the information given and answer the following:
   a. What was the research design?
   b. Is the design appropriate for this study?
   c. Is an eventual narrative sample of four key publications an appropriate amount of evidence?

LEARNING ACTIVITIES

1. You find that most of the articles retrieved during an electronic search of the literature are not useful. Which of the following is the next best step to follow?
   a. Use the articles obtained, knowing that there has been little research in this area.
   b. Change the keywords and do another search.
   c. Change the study and focus of the literature review.
   d. Use a print index to retrieve older papers.
2. The following words or phrases describe either primary or secondary sources. Place a P next to those describing primary sources and an S next to those describing secondary sources.
   a. Summaries of research studies
   b. First-hand accounts of participant interviews
   c. Biographies
   d. Textbooks
   e. Patient records
   f. Reports written by the researcher
   g. Doctoral or master's theses
3. A refereed journal:
   a. publishes both articles and critiques of studies
   b. is indexed in a bibliographical database
   c. uses a panel of reviewers to review submitted papers for possible publication
   d. is retrievable online
   e. all of the above.
4. How many years is it necessary to go back in the literature for an evidence-based project?
   a. 1 year is sufficient
   b. 5 years is preferred
   c. 10 years is expected
   d. all literature is to be included.
5. CINAHL stands for:
   a. Cumulative Indicators to Nursing and Allied Health Literature
   b. Comparative Indicators to Nursing and Aligned Health Literature
   c. Comparative Index to Nursing and Allied Health Literature

   d. Cumulative Index to Nursing and Allied Health Literature.
6. Impact factors (IF) are:
   a. bibliometric measurements of citation rates
   b. bibliometric measurements of factor rates
   c. bibliometric measurements of article rates
   d. bibliometric measurements of standard rates.
7. A summary table assists in:
   a. collecting a broad range of literature
   b. summarising the weaknesses of studies
   c. tracking the generalisability of studies
   d. synthesising key characteristics from studies.
8. A systematic (meta-analysis) review is the most appropriate type of review to examine:
   a. descriptive and exploratory studies
   b. cause-and-effect experimental studies
   c. studies in a meta-synthesis
   d. level III studies.
9. Which of the following is an example of 'grey literature'?
   a. Abstracts from an online bibliographical database
   b. Abstracts in printed proceedings from a conference
   c. Full-text papers in a published journal
   d. An abstract of a primary study in a textbook.
10. The characteristics of a literature review include:
   a. evidence of a comprehensive search of the literature
   b. a review of mainly secondary sources of literature
   c. summaries of overall strengths and weaknesses
   d. a logical flow using themes or categories.
      i. a, b and c
      ii. a, c and d
      iii. b, c and d
      iv. all of the above

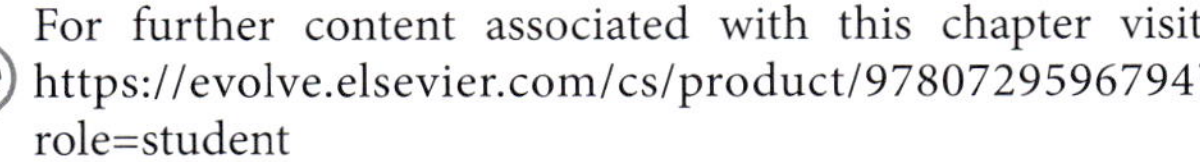
For further content associated with this chapter visit: https://evolve.elsevier.com/cs/product/9780729596794?role=student

ADDITIONAL RESOURCES

MIDIRS: Student support hub *(website)*. https://www.midirs.org/learning/student-support-hub/.

Vicky, R.N., 2019. Allnurses—how to conduct a literature review using CINAHL *(website)*. http://allnurses.com/nursing-student-assistance/how-conduct-literature-751831.html.

REFERENCES

Anderson, V. L., Johnston, A. N., Massey, D., et al., 2018. Impact of MAGNET hospital designation on nursing culture: an integrative review. Contemp. Nurse 54 (4–5), 483–510.

Aveyard, H., 2022. The future direction for the publication of literature reviews in the Journal of Advanced Nursing. J. Adv. Nurs. 78 (6), e82–e83. doi:10.1111/jan.15206

Aveyard, H., Bradbury-Jones, C., 2019. An analysis of current practices in undertaking literature reviews in nursing: findings from a focused mapping review and synthesis. BMC Med. Res. Methodol. 19, 105. doi:10.1186/s12874-019-0751-7

Barnett-Page, E., Thomas, J., 2009. Methods for the synthesis of qualitative research: a critical review. BMC Med. Res. Methodol. 9, 59–67.

Booth, A., O'Rourke, A. J., Ford, N. J. 2000. Structuring the presearch reference interview: a useful technique for handling clinical questions. Bull. Med. Library Assoc. 88 (3), 239.

Campbell, K., Massey, D., Broadbent, M., et al., 2019. Factors influencing clinical decision making used by mental health nurses to provide provisional diagnosis: a scoping review. Int. J. Ment. Health Nurs. 28, 407–424. doi:10.1111/inm.12553

Carter, R., Ramjan, L.M., Wilson, N.J., et al., 2023. "It keeps me on track": Undergraduate nursing students' experiences of using annotated exemplars—a qualitative study. Teach. Learn. Nurs. 18 (2), 286–292. doi:10.1016/j.teln.2023.01.003

Chen, Y., Kunst, E., Nasrawi, D., et al., 2022. Nurses' competency in electrocardiogram interpretation in acute care settings: a systematic review. J. Adv. Nurs. 78 (5), 1245–1266.

Cobey, K.D., Lalu, M.M., Skidmore, B., et al., 2018. What is a predatory journal? A scoping review. F1000Res. 7 (1001), 1–29. doi:10.12688/f1000research.15256.2

Connor, J., Flenady, T., Massey, D., et al., 2023. Clinical judgement in nursing – an evolutionary concept analysis. J. Clin. Nurs. 32, 3328–3340. doi:10.1111/jocn.16469

Crevacore, C., Jacob, E., Coventry, L. L., et al., 2023. Integrative review: Factors impacting effective delegation practices by registered nurses to assistants in nursing. J. Adv. Nurs. 79, 885–895. doi:10.1111/jan.15430

de Jong, G., 2017. Reasons to temper enthusiasm about open access nursing journals. Contemp. Nurse 53 (2), 262–266. doi:10.1080/10376178.2016.1257922

Dhakal, K., 2018. Librarians collaborating to teach evidence-based practice: exploring partnerships with professional organizations. J. Med. Libr. Assoc. 106 (3), 311–319. doi:10.5195/jmla.2018.341

Driscoll, A., Grant, M.J., Carroll, D., et al., 2018. The effect of nurse-to-patient ratios on nurse-sensitive patient outcomes in acute specialist units: a systematic review and meta-analysis. Eur. J. Cardiovasc. Nurs. 17 (1), 6–22. doi:10.1177/1474515117721561

Fernández-Basanta, S., Picallo-García, L., Movilla-Fernández, M.-J., 2023. Cultivating learning in vitro: a meta-ethnography of learning experiences of nursing students regarding high-fidelity simulation. J. Clin. Nurs. 32, 2056–2072. doi:10.1111/jocn.16269

Foster M, Blamires J, Moir C, et al., 2023 Children and young people's participation in decision-making within healthcare organisations in New Zealand: an integrative review. J. Child Health Care Feb 21, 13674935231153430 doi:10.1177/13674935231153430. Online ahead of print.

Francavilla, M.L., 2018. Learning, teaching and writing with reference managers. Pediatr. Radiol. 48, 1393–1398. doi:10.1007/s00247-018-4175-z

Garvey, L., Willetts, G., Herrmann, A., et al., 2023. A multi-layered approach to developing academic written communication skills for nursing students. Int. J. Nurs. Educ. Scholar. 20 (1), 20220107. doi:10.1515/ijnes-2022-0107

Gimenez, J., 2019. Writing for Nursing and Midwifery Students. Red Globe Press, London, UK.

Graj, E., Sheen, J., Dudley, A., et al., 2019. Adverse health events associated with clinical placement: a systematic review. Nurse Educ. Today 76, 178–190.

Harrison, H., Griffin, S.J., Kuhn, I., et al., 2020. Software tools to support title and abstract screening for systematic reviews in healthcare: an evaluation. BMC Med Res Methodol. 20 (7), 1—12. doi:10.1186/s12874-020-0897-3

Hibbard, J.H. 2017. Patient activation and the use of information to support informed health decisions. Patient Educ. Couns. 100 (1), 5–7. doi:10.1016/j.pec.2016.07.006

Hunker, D.F., Gazza, E.A., Shellenbarger, T., 2014. Evidence-based knowledge, skills, and attitudes for scholarly writing development across all levels of nursing education. J. Prof. Nurs. 30, 341–346.

Hutchinson, M., Frazer, K. 2023. Reading and appraising research. In: Jackson, D., Power, T., Walthall, H. (Eds.), Navigating the Maze of Research: enhancing nursing and midwifery practice. Elsevier Health Sciences, Chatswood, NSW, pp. 56–69.

Jaques, H., Lewis, P., O'Reilly, K., et al., 2018. Understanding the contemporary role of the intellectual disability nurse: a review of the literature. J. Clin. Nurs. 27, 3858–3871. doi:10.1111/jocn.14555

Jarden, R.J., Sandham, M., Siegert, R.J., et al., 2020. Intensive care nurses' well-being: a systematic review. Aust. Crit. Care, 33 (1), 106–111. doi:10.1016/j.aucc.2018.11.068

Jefferies, D., McNally, S., Roberts, K., et al., 2018. The importance of academic literacy for undergraduate nursing students and its relationship to future professional clinical practice: a systematic review. Nurse Educ. Today 60, 84–91. doi:10.1016/j.nedt.2017.09.020

Kelly, Y., O'Rourke, N., Flynn, R., et al., 2023. Factors that influence the implementation of (inter)nationally endorsed health and social care standards: a systematic review and meta-summary. BMJ Qual. Saf. 32 (12), 750–762. doi:10.1136/bmjqs-2022-015287

Kumar, R., 2019. Research Methodology: a step-by-step guide for beginners. SAGE Publications, London, UK.

Manca, S., 2018. ResearchGate and Academia.edu as networked socio-technical systems for scholarly communication: a literature review. Res. Learn. Technol. 26, 1–16. doi:10.25304/rlt.v26.2008

Nagle, C., McDonald, S., Morrow, J., et al., 2019. Informing the development midwifery standards for practice: a literature review for policy development. Midwifery 76, 8–20. doi:10.1016/j.midw.2019.05.007

Nasrawi, D., Reid, C., Megan Lee, M., et al., 2022. Nursing assessment and management of nutrition in older people with cancer: an integrative review. Collegian 29 (6), 924-930. doi:10.1016/j.colegn.2022.06.012

O'Connor, S. 2020. Secondary data analysis in nursing research: a contemporary discussion. Clin. Nurs Res. 29 (5), 279–284.

Oermann, M.H., Nicoll, L.H., Chinn, P.L., et al. 2018. Quality of articles published in predatory nursing journals. Nurs. Outlook 66 (1), 4–10. doi:10.1016/j.outlook.2017.05.005

Oermann, M.H., Nicoll, L.H., Ashton, K.S., et al., 2020. Analysis of citation patterns and impact of predatory sources in the nursing literature. J. Nurs. Scholarsh. 52 (3), 311–319.

Oermann, M.H., Nicoll, L.H., Carter-Templeton, H., et al., 2022. How to identify predatory journals in a search: Precautions for nurses. Nursing 52 (4), 41–45. doi:10.1097/01.NURSE.0000823280.93554.1a

Paez, A. (2017). Gray literature: an important resource in systematic reviews. J. Evid. Based Med. 10 (3), 233–240.

Peberdy, L., Young, J., Massey, D., et al., 2022. Integrated review of the knowledge, attitudes, and practices of maternity health care professionals concerning umbilical cord clamping. Birth, 49 (4), 595–615.

Polkki, T., Kanste, O., Kaariainen, M., et al., 2014. The methodological quality of systematic reviews published in high-impact nursing journals: a review of the literature. J. Clin. Nurs. 23, 315–332. doi:10.1111/jocn.12132

Riley, E., 2019. Exploring strategies to enhance scholarly writing for RN-BSN students using an online tutorial. Teach. Learn. Nurs. 14 (2), 128–134. doi:10.1016/j.teln.2018.12.011

Ross, P., Cross, R., 2019. Rise of the e-Nurse: the power of social media in nursing. Contemp. Nurse 55 (2–3), 211–220. doi:10.1080/10376178.2019.1641419

Sandelowski, M., Barroso, J., Voils, C., 2007. Using qualitative meta-summary to synthesize qualitative and quantitative descriptive findings. Res. Nurs. Health 30 (1), 99–111. doi:10.1002/nur.20176

Schiavenato, M., Chu, F. 2021. PICO: What it is and what it is not. Nurse Educ. Pract. 56, 103194.

Smith, D.R., Watson, R., 2016. Career development tips for today's nursing academic: bibliometrics, altmetrics and social media. J. Adv. Nurs. 72 (11), 2654–2661. doi:10.1111/jan.13067

Stovold, E., Beecher, D., Foxlee, R., et al., 2014. Study flow diagrams in Cochrane systematic review updates: an adapted PRISMA flow diagram. Syst. Rev. 3, 54. doi:10.1186/2046-4053-3-54

Sun, G.H., Hoelscher, S.H. 2023. The ChatGPT storm and what Faculty can do. Nurse Educ. 48 (3), 119–124. doi:10.1097/NNE.0000000000001390

Torres, C.G., 2022. Editorial misconduct: the case of online predatory journals. Heliyon 8 (3), e08999. doi:10.1016/j.heliyon.2022.e08999

Trotter, T. L. 2021. Using the peer review process to educate and empower emerging nurse scholars. J. Prof. Nurs. 37 (2), 488–492.

Usher, K., Aveyar, H., Bradbury-Jones, C., et al., 2023. Conducing and writing a literature review. In: Jackson, D., Power, T., Walthall, H. (Eds.), Navigating the Maze of Research: enhancing nursing and midwifery practice. Elsevier Health Sciences, Chatswood, NSW, pp. 28–44.

Wakefield, A., 2014. Searching and critiquing the research literature. Nurs. Stand. 28 (39), 49–57.

Whitehead D. 2021. Preventative health improvement in orthopaedic and trauma practice: 20 years on – are we there yet? Int. J. Orthop. Trauma Nurs. 40, 100847. doi:10.1016/j.ijotn.2021.100847

Whittemore, R., Knafl, K. 2005. The integrative review: updated methodology. J. Adv. Nurs. 52 (5), 546–553. doi:10.1111/j.1365-2648.2005.03621.x

Wilson, D., Aggar, C., Massey, D., et al., 2022. The use of mobile technology to support work integrated learning in undergraduate nursing programs: an integrative review. Nurse Educ. Today. 116, 105451. doi:10.1016/j.nedt.2022.105451

Wyatt, G.K., Lehto, R.H., Sender, J., 2019. The prevalence and types of complementary and integrative health therapies used by caregivers of patients with cancer. Semin. Oncol. Nurs. 35 (4), 342–347. doi 10.1016/j.soncn.2019.06.005

Zhu, Z., Xing, W., Lizarondo, L., et al., 2019. Nursing students' experiences with faculty incivility in the clinical education context: a qualitative systematic review and meta-synthesis. BMJ Open 9, e024383. doi:10.1136/bmjopen-2018-024383

4

Identifying Research Ideas, Questions, Statements and Hypotheses

Dean Whitehead

LEARNING OUTCOMES

After reading this chapter, you should be able to:

- describe the process of identifying and refining a research idea, question, problem, statement or hypothesis
- identify the process in matching research questions to appropriate research approaches
- identify the criteria for determining the significance of a research problem.

KEY TERMS

dependent variable, p. 58
hypothesis, p. 58
independent variable, p. 58
keywords, p. 53
null hypothesis, p. 58
research hypothesis, p. 58
research idea, p. 50
research problem, p. 50
research question, p. 51
research statement, p. 51

INTRODUCTION

To begin research the researcher needs to identify a research idea, question or statement closely aligned to the area of interest. The process involves adopting a **research idea**, developing a **research problem**, reviewing the research literature and following up with a clear and comprehensive statement of the purpose of the research. Deciding on the purpose and direction of a research project is essential because there are many issues to consider during this early stage that determine the direction and outcomes of the research undertaken—for instance, 'Why are you doing this research?', 'What is the motivation; what are you trying to achieve?', 'Who will benefit and how?' There are many reasons for undertaking research. For example, is the research to fulfil a research higher degree (RHD) qualification and/or is it part of an application for a research grant (see Chapter 16)? Is it needed for career progression and/or personal development? Perhaps, most importantly, is it required to change or defend current practice?

Many beginning researchers will be 'in a hurry' to start their research. Subsequently, 'corner cutting' may be expected. It is often this initial question-setting phase of the research process where this occurs despite it being a highly important phase. There may be a misleading belief that developing a research question or statement is relatively easy and possibly occurs naturally and/or as the research progresses. This is never the case. In addition, many may have already decided what methodology they want to use, the type of data they wish to collect or what they wish to find—without having considered a fully formed research question/s in the first place. However, think of the process used when we critically appraise/evaluate a research study (see Chapter 3). A key requirement in critical appraisal is to examine the consistency and relationship between the research problem, question or statement and the methods used to address it and then the extent to which the research problem has eventually been addressed (Boswell & Cannon 2020). Therefore, the early development of the research idea, issue, problem, question or statement (or hypothesis in some cases) is a vital step in the research process overall (see Chapter 2 for the research process).

WHY IS THIS QUITE A SHORT CHAPTER COMPARED WITH OTHERS?

This chapter is one of the shorter chapters in this book—not because it is less important than any other aspect of the research process and research design, but more the nature of the task. For instance, when writing/reading a higher degree dissertation/thesis, the questions, statements and hypotheses are developed and defined early in the process. The broad idea and 'overarching' question will be seen as part of the introductory first chapter. More specific questions will be seen in the methodology/method (design) chapter and then they are addressed again in the concluding recommendations/conclusion chapter—in terms of whether they have been met by the process and findings of the study process. When conducting research, therefore, researchers must bear in mind that they should be continually referring to the original aims, objectives and questions to 'cross-check' and remind themselves that they are keeping 'on track' according to the original aims and objectives (Mullaney & Rea 2022). Research questions, statements and hypotheses reflect a study's aims and objectives. Think of a degree/diploma course assessment. How is the marker/reader supposed to know what you intend to do or if you have achieved it if you do not clearly state the assessment's intentions (i.e. aims and objectives)? With research, this is demonstrated though clear questions, statements and hypotheses.

DEVELOPING AND REFINING A RESEARCH IDEA

As already mentioned, many nurses and midwives will have a reasonable idea of the topics they would like to research, usually focused on a specialty discipline issue or a problem to address. With research problems the general idea is to try to solve that problem (or at least parts of it) and/or contribute to further understanding and possible solutions. When thinking about a research problem or question, it is important to consider the ways in which a study will enhance understanding and knowledge of the topic (Ellis 2018). For example, will it lead to improved patient care, better clinical performance, tool development, theory development or the further development of nursing and midwifery education, management and administration?

TUTORIAL TRIGGER 4.1

Think of a research idea or problem that you would be interested in exploring further for a possible research study. At this moment, before you were to do a further literature review, what would that topic be? What do you already know about it? Do you already know/suspect that there might be knowledge gaps that require further research?

THE SIGNIFICANCE OF RESEARCH PROBLEMS TO NURSING AND MIDWIFERY

Once you have decided on a research idea or problem, it is important to consider the problem's potential significance to nursing or midwifery. The research problem should have the potential to contribute to and extend nursing or midwifery knowledge to professionals and to the public at large. The significance would be in relation to:

- the potential for patients, nurses, midwives, the healthcare community in general and society to benefit from the study
- the results being appropriate for extending the knowledge base of nursing and midwifery practice, education, policy or management
- the results providing theoretical relevance and clarity
- the findings supporting previously untested theoretical assumptions, extending or challenging an existing theory and clarifying conflicts and tensions in the theory
- the findings informing the formation or revision of nursing or midwifery practices or policies.

DEVELOPING AND REFINING A RESEARCH IDEA INTO A RESEARCH QUESTION

It takes considerable time to refine a research idea into an appropriate **research question**, **research statement** or hypothesis that will confirm or generate nursing and midwifery knowledge and practice (Kumar 2019). Much of that time will be spent critically searching, reviewing and appraising the existing research literature to assess the current 'state of affairs' and look for potential knowledge gaps to explore and address (see Table 4.1). That is why Chapter 3 (covering the literature search and appraisal process) comes before this chapter. One should 'naturally' lead to the other. An effective literature search and appraisal will inevitably 'pose' questions to be answered (White 2017).

TABLE 4.1 Factors Influencing the Development of a Research Idea

Factors	Influence	Example
Practical experience	Clinical practice provides a wealth of experience from which research problems can be derived. The nurse may observe the occurrence of a particular event or pattern and become curious about why it occurs, as well as its relationship to other factors in the patient's environment.	The effect of educational intervention on prevention of postpartum depression led to empowerment and increased awareness and internalisation of health control beliefs and less tendency towards external health control beliefs (Moshki et al 2013).
Critical appraisal of the scientific literature	A review of studies appearing in journals may indirectly suggest a problem area by stimulating the reader's thinking. A nurse may observe different approaches and suggestions in several related research studies and wonder which findings are most valid.	Children's negative emotional responses during or following hospitalisation are concerning for health professionals. A survey and psychometric approach were used to test initial reliability and validity of the Emotional Reactions Instrument—English (Kim et al 2012).
Gaps in the literature	A review may identify gaps in the literature and suggest areas for future study. Research ideas can also be generated by research reports that suggest the value of further studies to extend or refine the existing scientific knowledge base.	Previous studies on the effect of sociodemographic variables on burnout have shown various results. Neonatal intensive care units (NICUs) are very different working environments for nurses. A significant negative relationship was found between level of burnout and the quality of life of the nurses (Aytekin et al 2014).
Interest in untested theory or model	Verification of an untested nursing theory or model provides a relatively uncharted area from which research ideas/problems can be derived. Although theories or models themselves may not be tested, a researcher may investigate a particular concept related to a specific theory or model. Questions such as, 'If this theory/model is correct, what kind of behaviour would I expect to observe in particular patients and under which conditions?' or 'If this theory/model is valid, what kind of supporting evidence would I find?' are examples.	A structural model of study demands and resources, student burnout, engagement, health and satisfaction with life was tested. Burnout was positively associated with demands, lack of student resources, relationships with lecturers and social support of peers (Mokgele & Rothmann 2014). An instrument to measure hope in people with schizophrenia (the Schizophrenia Hope Scale, SHS-9) was developed. Reliability and validity of the Scale has been established (Choe 2014).

The research problem/idea should reflect a refinement of the researcher's thinking and should include:

- a defined or specific problem area to be further explored as indicated by a preliminary investigation of the related, existing research literature
- the topic and population under study, and
- the context and setting in which the study will take place (child health, aged care, acute or primary healthcare, etc.).

Often, researchers do not spend enough time on this stage of the research process. Hegde and Salvatore (2019) are critical of the fact that many clinical researchers experience problems in answering their research questions because they do not formulate/construct them properly in the first place. Tools are available (see later in this chapter) to assist researchers to craft specific questions and statements (Baker 2022). Such is the level of detail required at this stage that whole texts (e.g. White 2017) have been published that are devoted to this part of the research process.

Reviewing and Appraising the Relevant Literature

Related to developing a research problem, the preceding critical literature searching and appraisal process is a systematic and rigorous exploration of the existing literature related to the concept(s) of interest (this process is described in detail in Chapter 3). **Keywords** and concepts from an idea/problem statement are best used to determine the inclusion and exclusion criteria for searching the literature. The more structured, thorough and systematic the literature review is, the more likely the 'exact' question/s needed is achieved —in order to guide the methodology and lead to a higher likelihood of successful outcomes (Mullaney & Rea 2022).

Literature reviews are also important as they provide syntheses of findings from studies and analysis of themes and methods identified from the literature, when written in a clear and concise form (Boswell & Cannon 2020). There are numerous styles and steps to a literature review, which are discussed in detail in the previous chapter.

TUTORIAL TRIGGER 4.2

Referring back to Tutorial Trigger 4.1, relate back to your already chosen topic of interest. Conduct a very quick Google Scholar search on the topic. Has that topic and potential knowledge gap you chose clearly been filled, or is there scope to explore it further or in a different way?

RESEARCH IN BRIEF 4.1

Let us consider Barr et al's (2019) study as an example of addressing a national mental health 'problem'. They identify that reducing and eliminating the use of restrictive practices, such as seclusion and restraint, is a national priority for Australia's (and it would be the same for New Zealand's) mental health services. They do acknowledge that attempts have been made for legislation, organisation and practice changes to bring about a reduction in these practices. However, they also note that forensic mental health services continue to report high rates of restrictive practices in place. Forensic mental health care is complex, highly specialised and often delivered in an unpredictable environment. Viable alternatives to seclusion and restriction need to be considered for the benefit of clients and the wider community. Barr et al's (2019) qualitative study details their findings that examined the experiences of 32 nurses recruited from an Australian forensic mental health service. They found that, while high rates of restrictive practices may be linked to the unique characteristics of forensic patients, effective training, teamwork and leadership are critical factors influencing their use in this setting. They urge that nurses working in this area need to be further educated and supported to work confidently and safely with this high-risk patient cohort—which would lead to a reduction in the use of restrictive practices.

THE SIGNIFICANCE OF RESEARCH PROBLEMS TO NURSING OR MIDWIFERY

Once the researcher has decided on the research question or problem, it is important to consider the problem's significance to nursing or midwifery practice—and its potential impact on healthcare practice overall. The research problem/idea should have the capacity to contribute to and extend nursing or midwifery knowledge. The significance could be in relation to:

- the potential for patients, nurses, midwives, the healthcare community in general and society to benefit from the study
- the results extending the knowledge base of nursing and midwifery practice, education or management
- the results providing theoretical relevance and clarity
- the findings supporting previously untested theoretical/conceptual assumptions, extending or challenging an existing theory/concept or clarifying a conflict in the current literature
- the findings informing the introduction of or revision of nursing or midwifery practices and/or policies.

Defining a Specific Problem Area

As stated earlier, researchers begin with an idea and an interest in a broad topic area, such as pain management, family communication patterns, self-care activities of the aged, management of urinary incontinence, etc. When nurses and midwives ask questions such as 'Why are things done this way?', 'What would happen if ...?' or 'Is this the best way to ...?', they are already potentially developing a researchable question. Using qualitative methods, researchers are likely to be exploring individuals' personal responses to treatments, or experiences of a clinical condition or health/illness state—and the personal meanings attached to these (Baker 2022) (see Chapter 5). With quantitative methods, the researcher may, instead, focus on 'variables' of interest and their relationship to each other (Schneel et al 2021) (see Chapter 8). Regardless of the approach used, the researcher engages in a process linked usually to their topic choice and personal experience. This process guides the research question under consideration. For instance, Usher et al (2023), mindful of the general mental health impact of the recent COVID-19 epidemic, wondered about the mental health impact on preregistration students across Australia, especially in the university setting. They conducted a national cross-sectional study to answer their questions. Of the 516 students who completed the cross-sectional survey, over half (n = 300, 58.1%) reported mental health concerns and most students (n = 469, 90.9%) reported being impacted by COVID-19. Close to half of students (n = 255, 49.4%) reported signs of posttraumatic stress disorder. These findings allowed the researchers to suggest strategies to support nursing students manage their mental health and to safeguard the recruitment and retention of the future nursing workforce.

Fig. 4.1 illustrates how the development of a clinical research idea is influenced by practical experience and the scientific research literature.

Problem Questions and Statements

Problem questions or statements may be written in two main ways: either as a declaration (declarative) or as a problem statement that asks a question (interrogative), as illustrated in Table 4.2. Declarative statements are positive, explicit statements, whereas interrogative statements convey (ask) a question. The style chosen is largely related to the researcher's preference, experience and 'worldview' (see Chapter 2). An effective problem statement usually:

1. provides clear identification of the concepts of interest, phenomena or variables under investigation
2. specifies the population being studied
3. demonstrates the focus of the study (i.e. examination of experiences, exploration of variables and relationships and/or empirical testing).

Beginning to Structure Clinical Research Questions/Statements

So how do we go about developing and refining a research question/statement/hypothesis? There are common tools that can be used to assist. PICO/T is an acronym that describes the elements of a well-formed clinical question which is often the essence of a clinical topic. It signposts exactly what should happen in the topic study. Many journal article titles adopt a PICO-style format so that the reader is able to quickly understand what the study is about and it aids readers/researchers to easily find them through a 'keyword' search (see Chapter 3). Generally, PICO works best with quantitative experimental-type studies that use hypotheses (see Chapter 8), but that is not always the case. For instance, Mackie et al (2019) used the PICO format in their scoping review of the effect of interrupting prolonged sitting with frequent bouts of physical activity or standing on first or recurrent stroke risk factors.

The acronym PICO stands for and includes:

P—for the 'population'
I—for the 'intervention' of interest
C—for 'comparison'
O—for 'outcome'
T—for 'timeframe' (not always used).

An effective PICO question guides clinical research. For example, you might want to know if there is a difference in outcome between patients with a diagnosis of symptomatic heart failure (LVSD) receiving a self-management book manual program delivered and supported by a specialist cardiac nurse versus the same book manual program followed by the patient on their own. The area of interest would most likely be: which group, intervention or control had the better outcome of the two different approaches? Using a PICO/T format, the *patients* are individuals with a definitive diagnosis of symptomatic heart failure; the *intervention* is the self-management book manual program; the *comparison* is between those patients following a self-management plan delivered and supported by a specialist cardiac nurse and those patients who followed the same program on their own. The *outcome* refers to which group had the better/worse results overall.

Qualitative research questions also follow a logical format but are formulated differently to perform the task that is required (Green & Thorogood 2018). Below is a list of the common characteristics that 'typical' qualitative sentences will contain; either some or all of them.

- Use single sentences if possible.
- Include the purpose of the study.
- Include the central phenomenon.
- Use qualitative verbs (e.g. explore, understand, discover, uncover, etc.).
- Common qualitative terms are also words based on experience, attitudes, beliefs, opinions, perceptions, etc.
- Note the participants.
- State the research site.

Qualitative questions are 'open' questions—so they will commonly start with 'how', 'why', 'when', 'where', 'what', etc. (Baker 2022). For instance, Winnington et al (2023) ask their qualitative case study question as 'What are the learning experiences of first year graduate entry nursing students in New Zealand and Australia?' Note that it contains the majority of the already-stated criteria.

Idea emerges

Recovery processes of patients following hospital discharge with a diagnosis of myocardial infarction

Brainstorming

How do survivors from a recent myocardial infarction deal with their illness and recovery?

What factors impact on this recovery process?

How do these factors interrelate?

Review of the literature

The period after discharge following a myocardial infarction is noted as a vulnerable period with psychological morbidity a common phenomenon. The literature suggests that little is known about the process of adjustment for these survivors. Stress and coping are personal experiences, with factors such as age, personality traits and situational factors affecting appraisal and coping. Thus, an examination of issues that influence patients' recovery and compliance with lifestyle changes is necessary in the immediate post-hospitalisation period.

Identify variables

Potential variables:

- age
- disease morbidity
- health status
- health behaviours/risk factors
- coping
- social support
- health support needs

Research problem is formulated

To explore the health status, perceptions of coping and social support among survivors of a recent myocardial infarction in the first three weeks after discharge from hospitals

Fig. 4.1 Process of formulating a research problem.

TABLE 4.2 Problem Statements in Declarative and Interrogative Forms

Research Focus	Problem Statement
Declarative	
A randomised controlled trial of two antenatal education programs in Sydney, Australia.	A randomised controlled trial of two antenatal education programs for first-time parents was conducted. Three self-report surveys were completed by 170 women in both groups (Svensson et al 2009).
Evaluation of the psychometric properties of a Chinese version of the Diabetes Coping Measure scale (DCM-C).	A self-administered questionnaire was completed by 205 people with type 2 diabetes from three hospitals in Taiwan. Confirmatory factor analysis, criterion validity and internal consistency reliability were conducted to evaluate the psychometric properties of the tool (Huang et al 2009).
An exploration of differences in the general factor saturation of the Maslach Inventory-Student Survey with respect to: (a) when efficacy or inefficacy terms are included, (b) the strength of the correlations of the efficacy versus inefficacy scale with emotional exhaustion and depersonalisation and (c) the reliabilities of the different subscales.	Convenience sampling was used to obtain 512 university students in Johannesburg: 149 men and 363 women aged between 18 and 62 years. Participants were enrolled in a variety of faculties; factor analysis with bifactor rotations and polychoric correlations were performed. The findings have implications for research/theory and practice. It is recommended that the psychometric properties and loading of these two scales on the general burnout factor be explored (Morgan et al 2014).
Interrogative	
Competency standards for critical care nurses; do they measure up?	How effective and valid is the tool for assessing clinical practice of specialist level critical care nurses (Fisher et al 2005)?
A comparison of three groups: 1-hour single music session, 30 minutes of guided verbal relaxation and a control group. A randomised controlled trial.	How effective is music therapy and verbal relaxation on chemotherapy-induced anxiety (Lin et al 2011)?
An investigation across eight mental health services in Queensland of nurses' attitudes to the use of seclusion, which is a legally regulated practice in Australia.	Is there a relationship between burnout, job satisfaction and therapeutic optimism and justification and the use of seclusion (Happell & Koehn 2011)?

RESEARCH IN BRIEF 4.2

Cummins et al (2023) identify that perinatal mental health (PMH) conditions are associated with an increased risk of adverse perinatal outcomes including preterm birth. They conducted a retrospective cohort study (see Chapter 8) to compare perinatal outcomes in women with a mental health history between midwifery caseload practice (MCP) and standard models of maternity care. The cohort included 3028 women with PMH; 352 (11.6 %) received MCP. Their findings support MCP for women with PMH. The PICO/T components are readily notable within this study.

TUTORIAL TRIGGER 4.3

Think of a topic and write both a qualitative question and a quantitative question/statement. Compare and contrast them. Can you think of a methodology that would best suit each question?

MATCHING RESEARCH QUESTIONS/ STATEMENTS TO AN APPROPRIATE RESEARCH APPROACH

A research question/statement/hypothesis (please note that this chapter uses the term question more often to save the repetition of repeating all the terms—although note that there are differences between each of them) does not exist only to state the topic idea/problem/issue. It also serves to guide the whole research process—and especially the methodology and method (Hegde & Salvatore 2019). If the question uses terms like 'What are the experiences, opinions, attitudes of ... ?' then the likelihood is that a qualitative methodology/approach will be adopted. Furthermore 'lived experience' is often associated with phenomenology (see Chapter 5). If the question (more likely a statement/hypothesis) states 'What is the difference between ... ?' the likelihood leans more towards a quantitative methodology/approach.

Concept of Interest

The concepts of major interest in research studies are called phenomena (qualitative) or variables (quantitative). From a quantitative perspective, **variables** exhibit different values (i.e. the properties of the variable can vary, e.g. pain, anxiety) and they are 'measurable'. Properties that differ from each other, such as age, weight, height and blood pressure, are common examples of variables. Quantitative research attempts to understand how and why differences in one variable are related to differences in another variable—that is, how a change in one variable might affect the other. In experimental studies this phenomenon is often referred to as 'cause and effect'. For instance, if you 'cause' a wound product to be applied to a wound the researcher wants to observe what will be the 'effect', especially if it is then compared with the effects of other wound care products. Omura et al (2019) conducted a quasi-experimental study of two parallel groups (intervention and control) evaluating the impact of an assertiveness communication training program for 150 Japanese nursing students. Students in the intervention group participated in a 90-minute assertiveness communication workshop conducted by the researchers. A multimethod approach was used consisting of prereading, a PowerPoint presentation, videos, group discussion and role-plays. The control group did not receive the training program. The findings showed that, following the assertiveness communication training program, a higher percentage of students from the intervention group demonstrated the intention to speak up. The intervention group also displayed higher levels of assertiveness. This highlights that the 'cause' (the assertiveness program) had a positive 'effect' on those that received it compared with those that did not receive the program.

In qualitative studies, the concept (phenomenon) of interest is explored within a social context. Relationships or experiences of study participants are explored within a natural setting that is unique to them. To demonstrate, for example, Adams et al (2023) undertook a thematic review of qualitative research exploring home-visiting nurses' roles and identifying the challenges for nurses working with women experiencing family violence. The thematic synthesis identified two themes: (1) relationship building—with the client, with services and with colleagues/self, and (2) family violence practice—ask/screen, validate/name, assess risk/safety plan and safeguard children. The thematic synthesis confirmed the multiple roles fulfilled by home-visiting nurses and offered insight into the challenges they face as they undertake complex and demanding work. The roles of the home-visiting nurse evolved, with the initial focus on safeguarding children leading to broader family violence nursing practice roles, including the identification of family violence and safety planning discussions with vulnerable women.

Population of Interest

The terms **population** and **sample** are commonly used in research studies to identify the societal group of interest. The people or elements being studied need to be specified in the problem statement. If the scope of the problem has been narrowed to a specific focus and the variables have been clearly identified, the nature of the population will be evident to the reader of a research report. For example, Uhm et al (2019) identify their 'Implementation of an SBAR communication program based on experiential learning theory in a pediatric nursing practicum' study. The reader here can immediately identify that the population of interest is paediatric nurses in the clinical setting. The concepts of interest are SBAR communication and experiential learning theory.

AN UNEXPECTED HURDLE

Tahghighi et al (2019) utilised a comparative quantitative descriptive design to compare the psychological functioning and resilience of nurse shift workers and nursing non-shift workers. Many, including perhaps the researchers, might reasonably assume that shift workers (including night shifts) would have lower psychological functioning and resilience compared with non-shift workers working 'regular' daytime hours. Data were collected from employed Registered and Enrolled Nurses (n = 1369) who were members of the Queensland Nurses and Midwives Union (QNMU). The survey included standardised measures of resilience depression, anxiety, compassion satisfaction, compassion fatigue and intention to leave the profession. Generalised Linear Mixed Model analysis revealed shift workers had significantly lower levels of compassion satisfaction. However, there were no significant differences between the groups on resilience, depression,

Continued

AN UNEXPECTED HURDLE—cont'd

anxiety, stress, compassion fatigue or intention to leave nursing. The researchers suggest that their study requires replication using a longitudinal design to confirm these findings—perhaps because the results were unexpected.

Think of ways in which a similar study might be conducted differently to potentially identify significant differences in the areas where no significant difference was found.

Hypotheses and Hypothesis Testing

A **hypothesis** is a quantitative prediction/statement about the potential relationship between two or more 'variables' or phenomena that suggests an answer to the research question. Hypotheses provide the source from where many quantitative studies originate, and effective effort should be applied to testing them. They are not always clearly stated in published research articles. That represents a flaw in the research when it comes to critical appraisal if they are not clearly stated. Hypotheses flow from the problem statement, literature review and theoretical framework. Hypothesis testing is the most common purpose of *inferential statistics*. Inferential statistics are a set of statistical analytical procedures that allow inferences to be made about a population using existing data findings from a representative sample, thus enabling 'generalisability' of findings (see Chapter 9). What this means is that, if the chosen study sample population has the same characteristics of a much larger population, then it is 'reasonable' to expect that the study findings would be the same for the wider population had they been chosen as a population sample (Kumar 2019). Hypothesis testing is used to answer such questions as 'Is there a difference between the two groups?', 'What is the relationship between the two variables?' or 'What are the changes over time?'. Regardless of the specific format used to state the hypothesis, the statement should be worded in clear, simple and concise terms. The three main points to include in the statement are:

1. the *variables* of the hypothesis
2. the *population* being studied
3. the *predicted outcome/direction* (see later in this chapter) of the hypothesis.

RELATIONSHIPS BETWEEN HYPOTHESES, VARIABLES AND STUDY DESIGN—STATISTICAL VERSUS RESEARCH HYPOTHESES

The researcher may use one of two hypotheses. For example, they may use a 'statistical' hypothesis (also commonly called a **null hypothesis** (sometimes seen as H_0 in text) which states that there is no relationship between the *independent* and *dependent* variables), or they may use a **research hypothesis** (also called a *scientific hypothesis*—sometimes seen in text as H_1, H_2, etc.), which is a statement about the expected relationship between the variables. Regardless of the hypothesis used, there is a suggested relationship between the hypothesis and the research design of the study.

When we are exploring the relationship between variables there are always 'independent' and 'dependent' variable/s. The **independent variable** (also sometimes termed an 'explanatory' variable) is the 'property' that is being observed for any change to it. The **dependent variable** (also sometimes termed an 'outcome' variable) is the 'property' that is being applied to the independent variable to see whether it causes a change (remember 'cause and effect' mentioned earlier). For instance, a wound is an independent variable (i.e. a wound is a wound). A dependent variable would be the application of a 'wound-healing' application/product (Scheel et al 2021).

For example, when an experimental design (see Chapter 8) is used, we would expect to see hypotheses that reflect relationship *statements*, such as the following:

- X_1 is more effective than X_2 on Y (dressing A is more effective than dressing B on decubitus ulcers).
- The effect of X_1 on Y is greater than that of X_2 on Y (the effect of dressing A on decubitus ulcers is greater than the effect of dressing B).
- The incidence of Y will not differ between participants receiving X_1 or X_2 treatments (the incidence/occurrence of decubitus ulcers will be the same for participants receiving dressing A as for those receiving dressing B).
- The incidence of Y will be greater in participants after X_1 than after X_2 (the incidence/occurrence of decubitus ulcers will increase more in participants receiving dressing A than in those receiving dressing B).

Such hypotheses indicate that an experimental treatment will be used and that two groups of subjects—*experimental* and *control* groups—are being used to test whether the difference predicted by the hypothesis exists (Boswell & Cannon 2020). In contrast, non-experimental designs reflect 'associative' relationship statements, such as the following:

- X will be negatively related to Y (excessive pain will be negatively related to wound healing).
- X will be positively related to Y (a good nutritional diet will be positively related to wound healing).

If the researcher obtains statistically significant findings for a research hypothesis (i.e. their 'prediction' is strongly supported) then the hypothesis is supported. The examples in Table 4.3 are examples of statistical hypotheses.

TABLE 4.3 Examples of Statistical Hypotheses

Hypothesis	Variables[a]	Type of Hypothesis	Type of Design Suggested
Oxygen inhalation by nasal cannula of up to 6 L/min does not affect oral temperature measurement taken with an electronic thermometer.	IV: oxygen inhalation by nasal cannula DV: oral temperature	Statistical	Experimental
The incidence of pregnancy in adolescent girls attending birth control education classes will not differ from that of girls who do not attend birth control education classes.	IV: birth control education classes DV: adolescent pregnancy	Statistical	Experimental

[a] *IV*, independent variable; *DV*, dependent variable.

Types of Hypotheses

Directional Versus Non-directional Hypotheses

Hypotheses can be directional or non-directional. A *directional* hypothesis is one that specifies the expected direction of the relationship between the independent and dependent variables. An *independent variable* has a presumed effect on the *dependent variable*. In this case the existence of a relationship is proposed as well as the nature or direction of that relationship. An example of a directional hypothesis is: 'Hospitalised children will feel less anxious if their parents are permitted to remain with them'. The suggested direction is 'less' or 'least'. Alternatively, the 'opposite' directional hypothesis would be: 'Hospitalised children will feel more anxious if their parents are not permitted to remain with them'. Then the direction is 'more' or 'most'.

A *non-directional* hypothesis indicates the existence of a relationship between the variables but does not specify the anticipated direction of the relationship. An example of a non-directional hypothesis is: 'There will be a difference in anxiety levels in children if their parent is permitted to remain with them'. This would be used if it is anticipated that parents influence levels of anxiety in children—but it is not known exactly whether this may have a negative or a positive effect. Other examples of such hypotheses can be found in Table 4.4. In any study that involves statistical analysis, the underlying null hypothesis is usually assumed without being stated. Fig. 4.2 illustrates the decision path for determining the type of hypothesis presented in a study, as well as the study's readiness for a hypothesis testing design.

Shacklock et al (2014) used social exchange theory to examine associations between nurses' perceived organisational support and supervisor–nurse relationships with their job satisfaction, organisational commitment, engagement and intentions to quit. The researchers aimed to examine the strength and direction of the relationships. Eleven directional hypotheses were tested. Descriptive statistical analysis and exploratory factor analysis were used. Partial least squares modelling was used to test hypotheses 1–9, and mediation analysis was conducted using the Sobel test to analyse the path model. All 11 hypotheses were supported. Results showed that the higher the satisfaction with supervisor–nurse relationships and organisation support, the greater was nurses' engagement. In addition, job satisfaction predicted both affective commitment and quitting intentions.

In addition to directional and non-directional hypotheses, there is a *causal* hypothesis. As the name implies, a causal hypothesis suggests a cause for any change. For instance, Zhou et al (2022) examined the psychological distress of nursing students affected by COVID-19 and the pathway(s) between perceived social support and psychological wellbeing. One of their hypotheses was 'self-compassion and professional self-concept, in sequence, would mediate the association between perceived social support and psychological wellbeing among nursing students'. The researchers use the terms 'mediate' and 'sequence' to illustrate causality.

TUTORIAL TRIGGER 4.4

You are a student midwife attending an antenatal education class in the hospital. During the meeting the couples tell the midwife that they do not think that they are getting enough information about infant care and behaviours. They feel they are inadequately prepared for parenthood. You have heard the questions they are asking, and you think they are correct. You would like to investigate the reasons why the pregnant couples feel they are inadequately prepared for parenthood and if a type of intervention/program might improve their anxieties. You would like to test your hypothesis. Write (a) a directional hypothesis and (b) a non-directional hypothesis for the research study.

TABLE 4.4 Examples of Wording of Hypotheses

Hypothesis	Variables[a]	Type of Hypothesis	Type of Design Suggested
1. There will be a relationship between self-concept and suicidal behaviour.	IV: self-concept DV: suicidal behaviour	Non-directional research	Non-experimental
2. Synchrony of maternal and newborn sleep rhythms will be negatively related to postpartum blues.	IV: synchrony of maternal and newborn sleep rhythms DV: postpartum blues	Directional research	Non-experimental
3. Structured preoperative education is more effective than structured postoperative education in reducing the patient's perception of pain.	IV: preoperative education IV: postoperative education DV: perception of pain	Directional research	Experimental
4. The incidence and degree of severity of subject discomfort will be less after administration of medications by the Z-track intramuscular injection technique than after administration of medications by the standard intramuscular injection technique.	IV: Z-track intramuscular injection technique IV: standard intramuscular injection technique DV: subject discomfort	Directional research	Experimental
5. Progressive relaxation will be more effective in reducing indices of physiological arousal than hypnotic relaxation or self-relaxation in patients undergoing cardiac rehabilitation.	IV: progressive relaxation IV: hypnotic relaxation IV: self-relaxation DV: physiological arousal indices	Directional research	Experimental
6. There will be a relationship between years of nursing experience and attitude towards patients with human immunodeficiency virus (HIV) disease.	IV: years of experience DV: attitude towards HIV patients	Non-directional research	Non-experimental
7. There will be a positive relationship between trust and self-disclosure in marital relationships.	IV: trust DV: self-disclosure	Directional research	Non-experimental
8. There will be a greater decrease in post-test state anxiety scores in subjects treated with non-contact therapeutic touch than in subjects treated with contact therapeutic touch.	IV: non-contact therapeutic touch IV: contact therapeutic touch DV: state anxiety	Directional research	Experimental

[a] *IV*, independent variable; *DV*, dependent variable.

RESEARCH IN BRIEF 4.3

In Ng et al's (2023) study, drawing on self-determination theory, they investigated the combined relationship between abusive supervision (i.e. vertical mistreatment) and workplace bullying (i.e. horizontal mistreatment) on job satisfaction and public service motivation among Australian nurses. They proposed three hypotheses to test:

Hypothesis 1: Workplace bullying will moderate the negative relationship between abusive supervision and job satisfaction. Specifically, the relationship will be stronger when participants experience greater workplace bullying.

Hypothesis 2: Abusive supervision will have a negative indirect effect on public service motivation via job satisfaction.

Hypothesis 3: The indirect relationship of abusive supervision on public service motivation, via job satisfaction, will be moderated by the extent to which employees experience bullying, such that the indirect effects will be stronger for employees who experience high bullying.

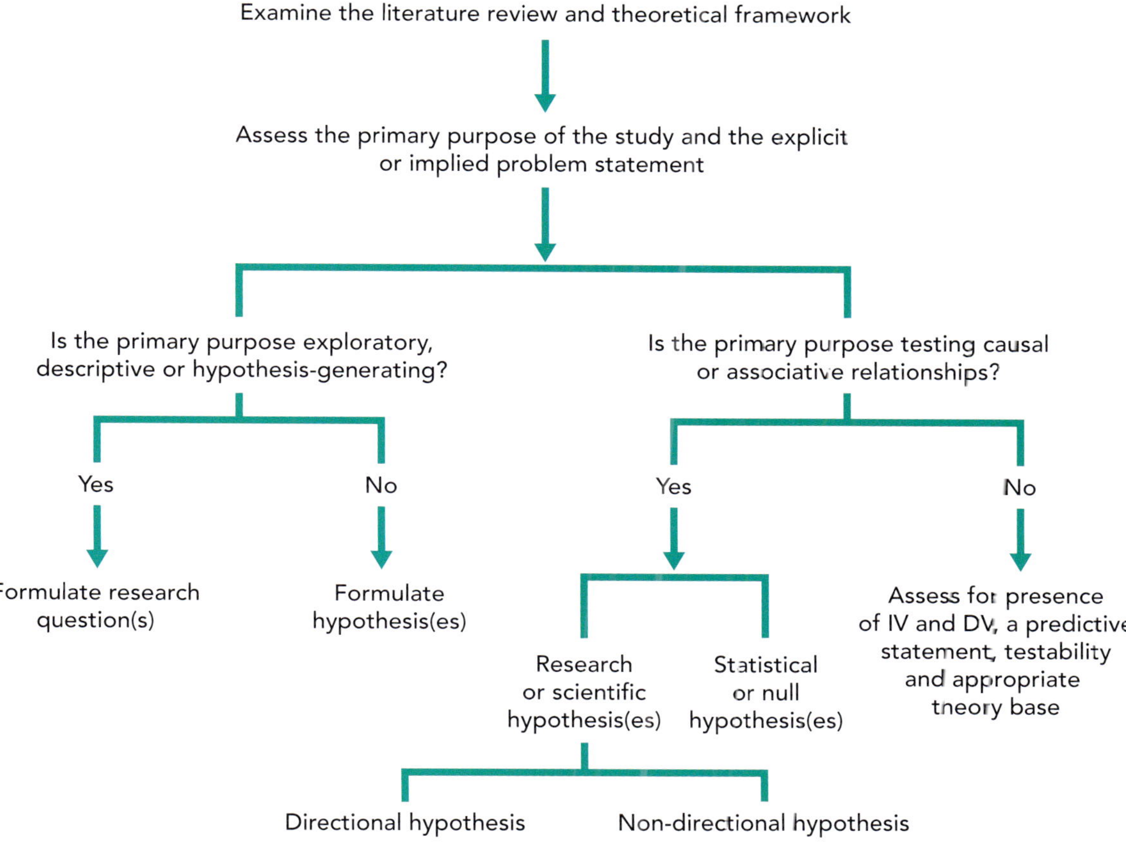

Fig. 4.2 Hypothesis testing decision path

SUMMARY

Identifying the most appropriate research idea, problem, question, statement or hypothesis is an integral part of successful research. It is vital in determining the nature and design of a research project. Researchers undertaking this part of the research process are advised to ask key questions of their research, to determine whether the right idea, problem, question, statement or hypothesis has been considered. These would include:

- the results being applicable for extending the knowledge base of nursing or midwifery practice, education or management
- the results providing theoretical relevance
- the findings supporting previously untested theoretical assumptions
- the findings informing the formulation or revision of nursing or midwifery practices or policies.

If the research idea, problem, question, statement or hypothesis has not met most of the stated types of criteria, then the relevance and significance of the research (qualitative and quantitative) is questionable. This chapter brings a close to the first section of this book. The next section goes on to explore how research methodology and methods are applied.

KEY POINTS

- Identification of the research question, statement or problem is an important key preliminary step in the research process. The extent to which this is properly structured often determines the accuracy and appropriateness of the research.
- Refinement of the research problem includes examination of the previous research literature and discussion of the potential significance of the problem to nursing or midwifery practice, education or theory.
- The research problem should have the potential for contributing to the body of nursing and midwifery knowledge.

TIME TO REFLECT

Begley, C., Guilliland, K., Dixon, L., et al., 2019. A qualitative exploration of techniques used by expert midwives to preserve the perineum intact. Women Birth 32 (1), 87–97.

Aim: To explore expert Irish and New Zealand midwives' views of the skills that they employ in preserving the perineum intact during spontaneous vaginal birth.

Design: A qualitative, descriptive study was undertaken. Semistructured, recorded interviews were transcribed and analysed using the constant comparative method. Expert midwives employed in New Zealand and one setting in Ireland were invited to join the study. 'Expert' was defined as achieving, in the preceding 3.5 years, an episiotomy rate for nulliparous women of <11.8%, a 'no suture' rate of 40% or greater and a severe perineal tear rate of <3.2%. Twenty-one midwives consented to join the study.

Reflect on the following: Four main themes emerged from the study: 'calm, controlled birth', 'position and techniques in early second stage', 'hands on or off?' and 'slow, blow and breathe the baby out'. Using the techniques described enabled these midwives to achieve rates, in nulliparous women, of 3.91% for episiotomy, 59.24% for 'no sutures' and 1.08% for serious lacerations.

Questions

1. What might be a good research question that would fit this study?
2. Think of other ways that this study might have been conducted.
3. Reflect on the information given:
   a. What are the benefits of conducting studies that compare and contrast practice in different countries?
   b. What are the main overall benefits of this study for practice?

LEARNING ACTIVITIES

1. In a higher degree research thesis/dissertation, the research questions are mostly likely to be noted in which chapters?
   a. The introduction chapter, the literature review chapter and the final chapter
   b. The introduction chapter, the method chapter and the final chapter
   c. The introduction chapter, the results chapter and the final chapter
   d. The introduction chapter, the theoretical chapter and the final chapter
2. The first part of developing research questions is:
   a. developing the research aim
   b. developing the research plan
   c. developing the research objective
   d. developing the research idea.
3. What is the main activity that 'narrows' a research idea into a research question?
   a. Conducting the literature review
   b. Developing the research method
   c. Deciding what variables are involved
   d. Knowing whether the question is answerable.
4. The acronym PICO stands for:
   a. predicter, intervention, comparison, operator
   b. population, intervention, comparison, outcome
   c. population, interest, content, outcome
   d. predictor, interest, content, operator.
5. The PICO acronym sometimes has a 'T' added, i.e. PICO/T. The 'T' stands for:
   a. tabulation
   b. traits
   c. timeframe
   d. total.
6. In qualitative studies the phenomena of interest are explored:
   a. within a holistic and humanistic context
   b. only in a community context
   c. only in the clinical area
   d. with a single focus group of people.
7. The 'null' hypothesis is also known as:
   a. the causal hypothesis
   b. the statistical hypothesis
   c. the non-scientific hypothesis
   d. the directional hypothesis.
8. The 'research' hypothesis is also known as:
   a. the statistical hypothesis
   b. the non-directional hypothesis
   c. the scientific hypothesis
   d. the negative hypothesis.
9. The variable that causes the change/effect is known as:
   a. the obvious variable
   b. the dependent variable
   c. the independent variable
   d. the context variable.

10. The term 'cause and effect' tends to refer to:
    a. experimental studies
    b. surveys
    c. non-experimental studies
    d. case studies.

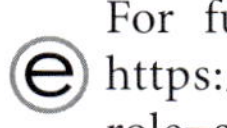

For further content associated with this chapter visit: https://evolve.elsevier.com/cs/product/9780729596794?role=student

ADDITIONAL RESOURCES

The Writing Centre—how to write a research question. https://writingcenter.gmu.edu/guides/how-to-write-a-research-question.

REFERENCES

Adams, C., Hooker, L. Taft, A., 2023. A systematic review and qualitative meta-synthesis of the roles of home-visiting nurses working with women experiencing family violence. J. Adv. Nurs. 79, 1189–1210. doi:10.1111/jan.15224

Aytekin, A., Yilmaz, F., Kuguolu, S., 2014. Burnout levels in neonatal intensive care nurses and its effects on their quality of life. Aust. J. Adv. Nurs. 31 (2), 39–47.

Baker, E. 2022. Crafting Qualitative Research Questions: a prequel to design. Sage Publications, Thousand Oaks, CA.

Barr, L., Wynaden, D., Heslop, K., 2019. Promoting positive and safe care in forensic mental health inpatient settings: evaluating critical factors that assist nurses to reduce the use of restrictive practices. Int. J. Ment. Health Nurs. 28, (4), 888–898. doi:10.1111/inm.12588

Begley C, Guilliland K, Dixon L, et al., 2019 A qualitative exploration of techniques used by expert midwives to preserve the perineum intact. Women Birth 32 (1), 87–97.

Boswell, C., Cannon, S., 2020. Introduction to Nursing Research: incorporating evidence-based practice. Jones & Bartlett Learning, Burlington, MA.

Choe, K., 2014. Development and preliminary testing of the Schizophrenia Hope Scale, a brief scale to measure hope in people with schizophrenia. Int. J. Nurs. Stud. 51, 927–933.

Cummins, C., Baird, C., Melov, S.J., et al., 2023. Does midwifery continuity of care make a difference to women with perinatal mental health conditions: a cohort study from Australia. Women Birth. 36 (2), e270–e275. doi:10.1016/j.wombi.2022.08.002

Ellis, P., 2018. Understanding Research for Nursing Students. Sage Publications, London, UK.

Fisher, M.J., Marshall, A.P., Kendrick, T.S., 2005. Competency standards for critical care nurses: do they measure up? Aust. J. Adv. Nurs. 22 (4), 32–40.

Green, J., Thorogood, N., 2018. Qualitative Methods for Health Research, fourth ed. Sage Publications, London.

Happell, B., Koehn, S., 2011. Seclusion as a necessary intervention: the relationship between burnout, job satisfaction and therapeutic optimism and justification for the use of seclusion. J. Adv. Nurs. 67 (6), 1222–1231.

Hegde, M.N., Salvatore, A.P. 2020. Clinical Research in Communication Disorders, principles and strategies. fourth ed. Plural Publishing, San Diego, CA.

Huang, M.F., Courtney, M., Edwards, H., et al., 2009. Psychometric evaluation of the Chinese version of the diabetes coping measure scale. J. Nurs. Scholarsh. 41 (4), 385–390.

Kim, J.S., Park, J.H., Foster, R.L., et al., 2012 Psychometric validation of Emotional Reaction Instrument–English to measure American children's emotional responses to hospitalisation. J. Clin. Nurs. 23, 1541–1551.

Kumar, R., 2019. Research Methodology—Step by Step for Beginners, fourth ed. Sage Publications, London.

Lin, M.F., Hsieh, Y.J., Hsu, Y.Y., et al., 2011. A randomized controlled trial of the effect of music therapy and verbal relaxation on chemotherapy-induced anxiety. J. Clin. Nurs 20, 988–999.

Mackie, P., Weerasekara, I., Crowfoot, G., et al., 2019. What is the effect of interrupting prolonged sitting with frequent bouts of physical activity or standing on first or recurrent stroke risk factors? A scoping review. PLoS One 14 (6), e0217981.

Mokgele, K.R.F., Rothmann, S., 2014. A structural model of student well-being. South Africa J. Psychol. 44 (4), 514–527.

Morgan, B., de Bruin, G.P., de Bruin, K., 2014. Operationalizing burnout in the Maslach Burnout Inventory—Student Survey: personal efficacy versus personal inefficacy. South Africa J. Psychol. 44 (2), 216–227

Moshki, M., Beydokhti, T.B., Cheravi, K., 2013. The effect of educational intervention on prevention of postpartum depression: an application of health locus of control. J. Clin. Nurs. 23 (15–16), 2256–2263.

Mullaney, T.S., Rea, C. 2022. Where Research Begins: choosing a research project that matters to you (and the world). University of Chicago Press, Chicago, IL.

Ng, N., Franken, E., Nguyen, D., et al., 2023. Job satisfaction and public service motivation in Australian nurses: the effects of abusive supervision and workplace bullying. Int. J. Hum. Res. Manag. 34(11), 2235–2264, doi:10.1080/09585192.2022.2070715

Omura, M., Levett-Jones, T., Stone, T.E., 2019. Evaluating the impact of an assertiveness communication training programme for Japanese nursing students: a quasi-experimental study. Nurs Open 6, 453–472.

Shacklock, K., Brunetto, Y., Teo, S., et al., 2014. The role of support antecedents in nurses' intentions to quit: the case of Australia. J. Adv. Nurs. 70 (4), 811–822.

Scheel, A.M., Tiokhin, L., Isager, P.M., et al., 2021. Why hypothesis testers should spend less time testing hypotheses. Perspect. Psychol. Sci. 16(4), 744–755. doi:10.1177/1745691620966795

Svensson, J., Barclay, L., Cooke, M., 2009. Randomised-controlled trial of two antenatal education programmes. Midwifery 25, 114–125.

Tahghighi, M., Brown, J.A., Breen, L.J., et al., 2019. A comparison of nurse shift workers' and non-shift workers' psychological functioning and resilience. J. Adv. Nurs. 75 (11), 2570–2578. doi:10.1111/jan.14023

Uhm, J.Y., Ko, Y., Kim, S., 2019. Implementation of an SBAR communication program based on experiential learning theory in a pediatric nursing practicum: a quasi-experimental study. Nurse Educ. Today 80, 78–84.

Usher Am, K., Jackson, D., Massey, D., et al., 2023. The mental health impact of COVID-19 on pre-registration nursing students in Australia: findings from a national cross-sectional study. J. Adv. Nurs. 79, 581–592. doi:10.1111/jan.15478

White, P., 2017. Developing Research Questions, second ed. Bloomsbury Publishing, London, UK.

Winnington, R., Shannon, K., Turner, R., et al., 2023. Learning experiences of first year graduate entry nursing students in New Zealand and Australia: a qualitative case study. BMC Nurs. 22 (1), 74-85. doi:10.1186/s12912-023-01233-9

Zhou, L., Sukpasjaroen, K., Wu, Y., et al., 2022. Perceived social support promotes nursing students' psychological wellbeing: explained with self-compassion and professional self-concept. Front. Psychol. 13, 835134. doi:10.3389/fpsyg.2022.835134

SECTION 2

What You Need to Know About Research to Understand How it Is Applied

5

Common Qualitative Methods

Dean Whitehead

LEARNING OUTCOMES

After reading this chapter, you should be able to:

- identify the general features of qualitative research
- describe the common range of qualitative research methodologies and approaches that may be used in the conduct of nursing and midwifery and health-related research
- appreciate the value of the knowledge gained from qualitative research for practice
- identify health-related experiences that might be explored using qualitative research approaches.

KEY TERMS

critical (approach), p. 67
descriptive (approach), p. 67
ethnography, p. 73
grounded theory, p. 71
interpretive (approach), p. 67
naturalistic (approach), p. 67
phenomenology, p. 67
qualitative methodologies, p. 66
qualitative meta-synthesis, p. 76

INTRODUCTION

Qualitative research refers to a range of methodologies and approaches to research that cluster under a 'paradigmatic umbrella' known as post-positivism or interpretivism (see Chapter 2). It is used by most disciplines including nursing and midwifery. Qualitative research helps us to make sense of human reality and the social world. Qualitative research is used when the understanding of human phenomena is needed and why such phenomena may occur. The main purpose of qualitative research is to develop rich description and meaning that makes sense of the social world that we live in (Lune & Berg 2016). Qualitative researchers seek knowledge and understanding through social science theories and a range of related research approaches available to them to explore phenomena in a meaningful way (Green & Thorogood 2018). A qualitative researcher's choice of methodological approach depends on the research question (see Chapter 4), which is obtained from exploring the literature and reflecting upon the research problem or concern, the nature of the study and the type of knowledge the researcher wishes to uncover. The range of **qualitative methodologies** include, but are not limited to, various schools of phenomenology, grounded theory, case study, narrative inquiry, naturalistic inquiry, historical research, concept/discourse analysis and feminist research. Each of these approaches holds a set of related but differing *ontological* (being-related), *epistemological* (knowledge-related) and methodological beliefs, principles or theories (see Chapter 2). It is these beliefs that shape the researcher's approach—that is, their research knowledge and beliefs, the methods used for data collection and analysis, and the product or results/outcomes of the research.

One of the main qualities of qualitative research is that it involves the exploration of subjective human experience with the aim of generating understanding, meaning and theory. In nursing, midwifery and healthcare, qualitative research provides rich descriptions of what it is like to be healthy or ill and why people behave or engage with healthcare in the way that they do. Qualitative research requires the researcher to often distinguish between another's world experience and their own, exploring these different 'worldviews' (Lune & Berg 2016). The qualitative research process involves close partnership between the researcher and participant. Research participants in qualitative research are viewed as 'knowers and participators'. They are regarded as having the knowledge that the researcher seeks to explore and uncover—whether or not the participant is aware of this.

The participants in qualitative research are always part of the phenomenon of interest. They are part of and have experienced the social environment or culture that the researcher is examining and exploring. It is for this reason that researchers should always 'choose' the most appropriate participants to gain the best possible insights and outcomes. This process is called 'sampling' and is explained in detail in Chapters 6 and 9: one from the qualitative perspective and the other quantitatively.

This chapter takes the reader through some of the most common qualitative methodologies in nursing-, midwifery- and health-related research. The following Chapters, 6 and 7, deal more with the specifics of qualitative research process and design—such as data collection, sampling techniques and data analysis.

WHY IS QUALITATIVE RESEARCH IMPORTANT?

Qualitative researchers aim to understand human experiences through personal perceptions, interpretations, opinions, values and beliefs of the chosen research participants. Qualitative research has proven invaluable in the disciplines of nursing and midwifery. Both disciplines seek insight and understanding of ways in which the people we care for experience and engage with healthcare delivery and services. Qualitative researchers, guided by research questions and the appropriate methodological approach, generally adopt a **descriptive**, **interpretive**, **naturalistic** or **critical approach** to viewing human phenomena (see Chapter 2). This means that nursing and midwifery qualitative research is designed to help us understand naturally occurring events through exploring experiences, social interactions, meanings, attitudes, beliefs and values of research participants within the context of health, disability and illness experiences. It has the potential, through such inquiry with its participants, to highlight the need for practice or intervention change, to inform theory development, to influence health policy and to highlight the need for further research. For these reasons, publication rates for qualitative research have increased over many years, with highly regarded nursing, midwifery and healthcare journals now publishing high-quality qualitative research (Merriam & Grenier 2019).

Qualitative approaches are governed by their methodology—the philosophical or theoretical knowledge and/or conceptual frameworks that guide and underpin the research approach. Taking a methodological stance, or 'lens', when conducting qualitative research requires the researcher to closely understand the relevant methodology: its philosophy, theory and concepts, and how they might be applied throughout the study process. Focusing on the main principles of the chosen methodology often requires a great deal of self-monitoring and reflection (Merriam & Grenier 2019). For example, **phenomenology** is the study of human phenomena. Phenomenologists ask: 'What is the nature and meaning of human experience?' and 'What is the essence of human experience?' They are interested in 'lived-through' experience and the quality of personal experiences. Ethnography, on the other hand, studies the culturally shared perceptions of everyday experiences. Ethnographers explore experience within the context of culture and social situations. They ask: 'What do people do here and why?' Grounded theory is underpinned by the theory of 'symbolic interactionism', taken from social psychology, which studies the network of people who interpret the world through social interactions. Grounded theorists ask: 'What is occurring here during social interactions?' They study relationships between how we see ourselves, how we see others and how we think others see us to provide a perspective on social behaviour. Grounded theorists seek to develop theory based on those social interactions and perspectives.

These noted qualitative methodologies share many similar properties. However, they explore experiences and phenomena in different ways and, therefore, produce different types of research outcomes. For this reason, much of this chapter is devoted to exploring selected research traditions, the detailing of how they are structured, and how they influence nursing and midwifery practice.

TUTORIAL TRIGGER 5.1

Identify healthcare experiences that you think would benefit from deeper personal understanding and insight. Propose ideas to explore possible research questions and approaches with your tutor. Consider lived experience, the impact of culture on human experiences and situations of human interaction to guide your thinking

A COMMON TREND IN QUALITATIVE RESEARCH

'Qualitative descriptive', 'interpretive descriptive' and 'descriptive exploratory' are all labels for qualitative research that rely on pure description rather than theory. This is distinct from some of the 'traditional' methodologies mentioned previously such as phenomenology, ethnography and grounded theory. The goal of qualitative descriptive research is to provide a 'comprehensive summary of the events in the everyday terms of those events ... and the task of the researcher is to stay close to the data and to the surface of words and events' (Sandelowski 2000 p. 334).

All research inquiry, both qualitative and quantitative, requires varying levels of description and all description requires interpretation. Levels of description always depend on the research participants' perspective or perception. For example, when describing an event, situation or experience, participants select what they will describe and in the process they have often already interpreted and transformed the experience or event (Sandelowski 2000). While descriptive exploratory research does describe the facts of the event, situation or experience, no attempt is made to place this within a methodological, philosophical, theoretical, conceptual or abstract framework. For example, phenomenology requires the researcher to use a 'phenomenological lens'. The phenomenological researcher interprets the data in terms of the 'life world' (Mohammadi et al 2018, van Manen 2017) to reveal essence, nature and meaning so that interpretation moves beyond description.

Qualitative descriptive methodology, then, is more an approach that adopts common aspects of all qualitative approaches. Qualitative descriptive researchers often collect rich narrative data from small sample populations and the analyses of that data thematically using broad 'free-form' methods.

Many authors do not specify their qualitative research methodology or approach. For example, Jarden at al (2023), in their qualitative descriptive study, explored 39 Australian nurses from two metropolitan healthcare organisations in Victoria. They examined perceptions and experiences of work wellbeing extending from what inspired participants to join the healthcare organisation, what created a 'great day' at work for them, through to what may have supported them to stay. Four themes were constructed for each of the key research questions. Inspiration to join the organisations transpired through organisational reputation, recruitment experiences, right position and right time, fit and feel. A great day at work was created through relationships with colleagues, experiences with managers, adequate resourcing and delivering quality care. Factors contributing to nurses resigning included COVID-19, uncertainty of role, workload and rostering, and, finally, not feeling supported, respected and valued. Factors that may have supported the nurses to stay included flexible work patterns and opportunities, improved workplace relationships, workload management and support, and supportive systems and environments. Cutting across these themes were five threads: (1) relationships, (2) communication, (3) a desire to learn and develop, (4) work–life balance and (5) providing quality patient care.

We therefore need to critically ask: 'What methodology, philosophy, theory, frameworks, knowledge, or concepts have guided interpretation and understanding of the data in these studies?' Of importance, when using qualitative descriptive methodology, the researcher should provide a justification as to why and how the chosen approach specifically addresses the aims of the study. Thomas et al (2023) adopted their qualitative descriptive approach specifically for its ability to represent undergraduate midwifery student participants' experiences with novice and expert midwifery preceptors, and to identify the benefits and challenges of working with novice and expert preceptors, from the perspective of undergraduate student midwives. The researchers highlight that this approach provided them with the flexibility to explore the issue without being restricted by a predetermined theory. They viewed 'qualitative description' as an appropriate method to answer their specific practice-based questions (see 'Research in brief 5.1').

RESEARCH IN BRIEF 5.1

The objective of Thomas et al's (2023) descriptive qualitative study was to examine the recent trend of increased midwifery university places in Australia offered to address midwifery workforce shortages. As a result, more graduate midwives entered the workforce, in turn leading to more midwifery students precepted by novice midwives when on professional placement. It is not known whether this more junior midwifery workforce impacts the student experience. Nineteen third/fourth-year Bachelor of Nursing/Bachelor of Midwifery (Honours) students attended six focus groups (ranging from two to five participants). Data were analysed thematically. Three overarching themes were identified: '*building relationships*', '*teaching and learning*' and '*improvements to professional placement*'. Benefits and challenges existed with both novice and expert preceptors. Importantly, feeling welcomed and receiving critical feedback were identified. The researchers concluded that the student/preceptor relationship is based upon feeling welcomed and relatability, and is developed more easily with novice preceptors. Expert preceptors provide insightful and valuable feedback and are more able to actively teach. Novice preceptors' consolidation of practice can impact student-learning opportunities. Including students in decision making aids development of critical thinking. Allocation practices which address student-learning needs will improve the student professional practice experience.

'TRADITIONAL' APPROACHES TO QUALITATIVE RESEARCH

As has already been stated, the more traditional approaches to qualitative research are often more complex and in-depth than the popular descriptive exploratory approaches just mentioned. Traditional approaches are governed by longstanding philosophical or theoretical positions that have evolved over many years—alongside enduring critical debate and comparison. Phenomenology is a key example of this, which questions the meaning of our/others' lived experience and the way in which we live it (Mohammadi et al 2018, van Manen 2017).

Phenomenology

Origins and Philosophical Underpinnings

Many researchers agree that there are significant distinctions between the natural and human sciences. These distinctions centre on the idea of holism and that the natural sciences cannot account for the human aspects that create science (van Manen 2014, 2017). The human sciences specifically aim to uncover the 'humanness' of science, and phenomenology is one such human science research approach. Phenomenology is widely accepted as appropriate when assisting health researchers in exploring and understanding the meaning of health, illness, disability and disease as it is witnessed and experienced (Green & Thorogood 2018).

Phenomenology is a methodology that uncovers thoughts, perspectives, understandings, feelings and behaviours from the perspective of the individual. It does not offer causal explanations or theories. Instead, it provides an account of the experience of 'being in the world' of everyday life, of living in and through the world. The main purpose of conducting phenomenological research, in healthcare, is to be focused on the lived experience of people during health and illness and how this might influence their engagement with health. By listening to the stories of those who live with and witness health-related issues, phenomenological researchers aim to bring understanding to aspects of lived experience that often seem elusive—or we just simply accept as 'normal'. In this sense, phenomenological research captures the 'pathic' knowledge needed by health carers to understand the illness experience. The term 'pathic' derives from the Latin word *pathos*, meaning 'suffering' and 'passion and disease' (van Manen 1999 p. 30).

It is the everyday language of people who live with disease, disability and illness (and health) that provides the 'richest' insights into what the experience really means to them. As van Manen (1990 p. 61) notes, everyday language is like a 'reservoir of human experience'. The goal of phenomenology is to develop an understanding of human experience as it is lived in the 'life-world', the real world. The phenomenological researcher is committed to understanding the experience of the whole phenomenon, rather than parts of that experience (Green & Thorogood 2018).

Ranse et al (2018), for example, used a hermeneutic phenomenological approach to explore the lived experiences of final year nursing students caring for a dying patient. The study involved in-depth interviews with six students. Analysis and interpretation of the data revealed the students' experiences of being caring, experiencing family-centred care, 'but recounted unexpectedness of both the dying trajectory and the physical changes in the dying patient' and, when reflecting on loss, students questioned their own actions and identified supportive relationships and ways to cope (see 'Research in brief 5.2').

RESEARCH IN BRIEF 5.2

Ranse et al's (2018) hermeneutic phenomenological study of the lived experiences of final year nursing students in caring for a dying patient in Queensland was guided by existential phenomenology, informed by the philosophies of Heidegger (1953/2010), Husserl (1900/2001) and Merleau-Ponty (1945/2002). Using phenomenology in this study meant using a phenomenological 'lens' to explore and understand the human experiences of the six final year nursing students who participated. First-hand experiential descriptions were collected through in-depth interviews and recorded reflections. Contextual understandings were enhanced with reflections of clinical experiences where the participants had cared for someone who had died, with questions like 'Can you tell me about the day that you cared for a patient at the end of their life?' The use of the hermeneutic circle approach was used to acknowledge the researchers as active participants in the research process 'whereby a co-authored understanding of the experience is produced'. The authors employed a modified Ranse and Arbon (2008) approach, using phenomenological validation criteria in an iterative manner, to ensure that 'the phenomenological texts produced were in-depth, orientated to the phenomenon and were a recognisable anecdote of the singularity of an experience'. The essence of the students' experiences was captured in three emerging themes and several subthemes: 'being caring' included 'caring for the patient and family', 'being present' and 'after-death care'. 'Unexpectedness in witnessing an expected death' included 'the death trajectory' and 'physical changes in the dying patient'. 'Experiencing loss'

Continued

 **RESEARCH IN BRIEF 5.2—cont'd**

included 'questioning one's actions', 'valued and being valued' and 'cope, cope, cope ... cry'. The findings of this study provide valuable insight into the impact for final year nursing students of caring for a patient who is dying—even when the death is expected.

There are many different philosophical *schools of thought* and subsequent interpretations of phenomenology. During the twentieth century it was Edmund Husserl and Martin Heidegger who notably launched the movement, with others such as Gadamer and van Manen following. For an overview of many of those who influenced the movement, see van Manen (2014—particularly Chapter 4, 'Beginnings'). There is scope in this chapter to describe only the most adopted phenomenological schools of philosophy: those of Husserl and Heidegger (summarised in Table 5.1). Wider reading will help to unearth important other schools, of which there are many. For example, articles such as those by Barkway (2001), Dowling (2007), McConnell-Henry et al (2009) and Earle (2010) offer detailed and insightful accounts of various phenomenological schools.

Husserlian Phenomenology

Phenomenology, as a philosophical movement, has its origins in Ancient Greek philosophy. It is, however, the German philosopher Edmund Husserl (1859–1938) who is

TABLE 5.1 A Summary of Husserl's and Heidegger's Philosophical 'Positioning'

Descriptive/realist phenomenology	• Developed by German philosopher Husserl (1859–1938) as an alternative to positivism (see Chapter 2). • Views human beings as subjects in a world of objects. • Aims to study the consciousness of those objects, which Husserl called 'phenomenology'. • Aims to explore the intentional structures of mental acts as they are directed at both real and ideal objects. • Primarily interested in 'What do we know ...?' • Aims to separate out (*bracket*) mood, thoughts, memories and emotions to focus on conscious awareness of objects. • *Epistemological* in nature (see Chapter 2)—asks questions of knowledge about objects gained through conscious awareness.
Transcendental phenomenology	• Husserl's later work takes the intuitive experience of phenomena as its starting point, and aims to extract the essential features of experiences and the essence of what we experience.
Interpretive phenomenology	• Developed by Heidegger (1889–1976), who was a pupil and colleague of Husserl. • Questions the relationship between consciousness and objects. • Most important claim is the practical 'situatedness' of human experience. • Aims to understand a person's 'position' related to their human experience and the necessary conditions for people being or existing in their world. • Ontological in nature (see Chapter 2)—hopes to understand the nature and the meaning of 'being'. • The notion of being or 'being-in-this-world' is fundamental. • Central aspects to this notion are the relationships between self, being, meaning, existence and temporality.
Hermeneutic phenomenology	• Provides a framework that defines a view of persons and their being-in-the-world. • Examines the collected data (text) by moving from parts to the whole. • Analysis informed by 'the hermeneutic circle' (see Chapter 7). • Generates knowledge about humans and their world; is subjective, temporal (of time and worldly) and historical. • Makes background assumptions visible. In language, the testing of assumptions is possible. For example, Whitehead (2002) refers to the 'phenomenological nod' that he experienced when investigating the academic assignment-writing experiences of a group of student nurses. This nod confirmed that the students' experiences were very similar to his past experiences and describes how they relate to the current and future experiences of both parties.

credited as the founder of the 20-century phenomenological movement. Husserl's desire was to seek an alternative to positivism (see Chapter 2) that would integrate the world of science alongside the real 'life-world' (*Lebenswelt*) experienced by people (Sadala & Adorno 2002). For Husserl, human beings were subjects in a world of objects and it was the study of the consciousness of those objects that he called phenomenology. From this focus, he developed one of the two main schools of phenomenology (*descriptive phenomenology*) and was primarily interested in the question: 'What do we know ...?' (Koivisto et al 2002). Husserl moved philosophical discussion from the question of whether objects in our 'conscious awareness' had a separate existence to the systematic analysis of consciousness together with its objects. To focus on conscious awareness of objects, he aimed to separate out (*bracket*) mood, thoughts, memories and emotions. He believed that understanding about intuition and judgement (therefore, logic and truth also) emerged because of reflecting upon experiences of life (Dahlberg et al 2001). Husserl's phenomenology, *epistemological* in nature (see Chapter 2), is thus concerned with asking questions of knowledge about objects gained through conscious awareness. Husserl concluded that 'essences', as the things that define experience, exist within the conscious experiences of people and that this consciousness (and its intention) is presented by people to the world (Sadala & Adorno 2002).

Heideggerian Phenomenology

Martin Heidegger (1889–1976), a pupil and colleague of Husserl, questioned the relationship between consciousness and objects and consequently moved significantly from Husserl's interpretations. Heidegger's views helped to form the other main school of phenomenological philosophy: *interpretive phenomenology*. For Heidegger, the practical 'situatedness' of human experience was his most important claim. Heidegger focused his efforts on the study of a person's 'position' related to their human experience and towards the understanding of the necessary conditions for people existing or being in their world. As such, Heideggerian phenomenology is *ontological* (see Chapter 2). This means that it hopes to understand the conditions whereby human beings can understand their existence and therefore the nature and the meaning of 'being'.

The notion of being or 'being-in-this-world' is central to Heidegger's interpretations and is referred to by Heidegger in the commonly used context of *dasein* (Heidegger 1962 p. 67). The German verb *dasein* means 'to exist', although there are other variations in interpretation. It is a contraction of the correct form of *das* and *sein* (*das* meaning 'the' and *sein* meaning 'being'). In this sense, Heidegger suggested that people are aware of their own existence and question what it means to be themselves in or outside their own world. This relates to the concept of 'self', which is linked to the wider position of the person's place in their community, the world and the cosmos. Therefore, Heidegger suggested that people can question the meaning of their experiences of being and that they interpret their different worlds through comparison with those around them. People can reflect on the meaning of their experience and can look forward to other possibilities of 'being'.

Heidegger also described *dasein* as something that exists in a world that is familiar to and understood by people. Worlds contain preunderstandings that people use to make sense of their situations. This notion lends itself to the commonly used term 'hermeneutics'. *Hermeneutic phenomenology* provides a framework by which to define the view of a person's world and their being in that world. It also defines how meaning and language are understood, and therefore how knowledge about humans and their world is subjective, temporal (of time and worldly) and historical. This 'hermeneutic circle' (Heidegger 1962 p. 119) describes the historical, cultural and personal interpretations through which human understanding is developed.

Also important to Heidegger (1962 p. 386) was the notion that 'being in the world' is always understood in terms of *temporality*. Temporality refers to the fact that life, as it is lived now, cannot be separated from the historical experience of living a life and the potential for that life in the future. Temporality is therefore directly related to 'the meaning of life'. In summary, Heideggerian philosophy has at its core the relationships between self, being, meaning, existence and temporality. For those who require a deeper understanding of Heidegger's interpretive phenomenology, Mackey (2005) provides a comprehensive description and analysis. Table 5.1 compares the two main philosophical schools of Husserl and Heidegger.

There are many different phenomenological approaches. The ones discussed so far are the most 'traditional' and most used—but there are many others (too many to cover in part of a single chapter like this). The more recent approaches are van Manen's latest work and interpretative phenomenological analysis (IPA). Refer to van Manen (2014) for his last text. Wilson et al's (2023) study on trauma-informed care in acute mental health units through the life-world of mental health nurses adopts van Manen's approach. For IPA, Kagi et al (2023) explored the experiences of primary healthcare nurses advancing their careers in a remote Western Australian location.

Grounded Theory

Origins and Theoretical Underpinnings

Grounded theory refers to the method initially developed and introduced by Glaser and Strauss (1967), and further discussed and developed in collaboration with other colleagues (Corbin & Strauss 1990, Glaser 1999, Strauss & Corbin 1998). Another notable name is Kathy Charmaz, a student of Glaser and Strauss, who 'progressed' grounded theory into the social constructivist paradigm (Hoare et al 2013). Glaser and Strauss, two non-health professional sociologists working in a US-based department of nursing doctoral studies in the 1960s, devised techniques for generating theory about social processes so that the theory became 'grounded'. Grounding is because the theories began and emerged through analysis of collected data. The data are collected from human actions and interactions as they occurred over time, collected by speaking with and listening to those who are engaged in the action and interaction—and sometimes from documents relating to that action and interaction.

Essentially, grounded theory is designed to develop theoretical explanations of socially constructed events. Its main strength lies in enabling researchers to use data to develop theory—rather than test it. However, it also ideally generates hypotheses for further research (see Chapter 4). Theory grounded in this way is often thought to produce more useful outcomes than those emerging from 'pure' theorising alone. Knowledge may increase through generating new theories rather than analysing data within existing theories. Grounded theory is a widely used qualitative methodology in nursing and midwifery research, especially to identify clinical issues of importance inductively by creating meaning about those issues through the analysis and modelling of theory (McCann et al 2018).

Grounded theory is associated by many with the concept of *symbolic interactionism*—a term coined by Blumer in 1937 (Chamberlain-Salaun et al 2013). This process aligns an *interactionist* approach alongside *naturalistic* inquiry to develop theory. People are seen as being both 'self-aware' and 'aware of others', and therefore can adapt their social interactions and situational behaviour to shape meaning and society (de Chesney 2014a). This is linked to the fact that many grounded theory research questions start with the intention of asking 'How do people ...?' For example, Smith et al (2018 p. 176) broadly ask, in their grounded theory study, 'How do nursing students determine satisfaction with learning?' Sudarsan et al (2023) ask 'how do beliefs, practices and experiences of asthma impact Indian immigrant children in New Zealand and their family caregivers?' Their 'constructivist' (see later) grounded theory study examines the Indian and the host New Zealand culture to highlight 'tensions' related to family carers' and children's preferences.

The Purpose and Process of Grounded Theory

Grounded theory remains popular among nursing and midwifery researchers. This is because it is not just focused on social processes but also has evolved to explain human action and interaction in clinically related issues of social, psychosocial or spiritual dimensions of life. The classic grounded theory methodology, as originally formulated and published by Glaser and Strauss (1967), has been modified so that there are now multiple versions (e.g. Charmaz 2000, Corbin & Strauss 1996, Strauss & Corbin 1998). The views of the four main authors—Glaser, Strauss, Corbin and Charmaz—have, over time, evolved and adapted to the point that they often appear to be in direct conflict with each other. The discipline of grounded theory, and its evolution over time, can resemble something of a 'battleground'. Take, for instance, Glaser's (2002) critique of Charmaz's constructivist grounded theory. He states that grounded theory cannot be constructivist—therefore seeking to challenge Charmaz's main contribution. In turn, Strauss has expressed concern about Glaser's version of grounded theory—that it places too much emphasis on its inductive nature and that there are distinct differences between approaches to coding data and developing categories (Bulawa 2014).

There are, on the other hand, also broad agreements—regarding, for example, theoretical sensitivity, sampling, constant comparative analysis and theoretical memoing (see Chapter 7). Different versions of grounded theory generally reflect different ideas about how data are analysed and theory is developed. That is why it is important to understand the differences and similarities between different grounded theory approaches before a researcher decides which methodology to adopt. Like different phenomenological approaches, many grounded theory approaches may appear to all 'do the same thing'—but the different approaches produce different findings and outcomes. In nursing and midwifery research, either classic grounded theory or the more recent version Strauss and Corbin (1990, 1998) are most used. Reference to Heath and Cowley's (2004) seminal paper, on comparing Glaser and Strauss's versions of grounded theory, will give the reader additional insight and understanding. Chen and Boore (2009) do similar, with the added benefit of including wider works by both Corbin and Charmaz. De Chesney's (2014a) text on grounded theory and its application to nursing research is also useful. Whole research texts are also devoted entirely to the works of single contemporary grounded theorists. For instance, Artinian et al's (2009) text titled *Glaserian Grounded Theory in Nursing Research* is a good example.

It is generally agreed that the framework for a grounded theory is that which is developed from data analysed to form and support the grounded theory. Here, the theoretical framework 'evolves during the research itself' (Strauss & Corbin 1990 p. 49). Grounded theory research can be conducted according to a variety of perspectives, with the primary ones being *objectivism* and *constructivism*. Objectivism considers that, as in the natural sciences, there are realities/truths/facts (an object) to be revealed. Objectivist grounded theory aims to find and uncover what is believed to be 'there' (to be real) about human action and interaction (Glaser 2002). In contrast, constructivism considers that, in human social science, there are multiple constructed realities that are determined according to the opinion of the person experiencing the situation and the person theorising (Charmaz 2000). Constructivist grounded theorists view their theory as representing one of multiple realities about what may be happening in relation to human action and interaction. The researchers' theorising 'lens' is shaped by factors such as culture, political ideology and moral stance.

Although the variety of grounded theory versions can appear overwhelming for some planning a grounded theory research project, this situation does provide choice, and adaptation of methods is also common (Glaser 1999). It is also important to understand that, although grounded theory analyses mostly qualitative data, quantitative-'type' data can also be collected and analysed. Grounded theory, therefore, is commonly viewed as the methodology that most closely bridges the 'gap' between quantitative and qualitative research.

RESEARCH IN BRIEF 5.3

Prussing et al (2023) identify that international evidence demonstrates significantly improved outcomes for women and their babies when supported by midwifery continuity of care models. They argue that, despite this, widespread implementation has not been achieved in Australia, especially in regional settings. They adopted a constructivist grounded theory approach to develop a theoretical understanding of the factors that facilitate or inhibit the implementation of midwifery continuity models within regional settings. They interviewed 34 participants from which three concepts of theory emerged: '*engaging the gatekeepers*', '*midwives lacking confidence*' and '*women rallying together*'. A substantive theory also emerged: *A partnership between midwives and women is required to build confidence and enable the promotion of current evidence; this is essential for engaging key hospital stakeholders to invest in the implementation of midwifery continuity of care models.* The study concluded that the implementation of midwifery continuity of care needs a coordinated ground-up approach in which midwives partner with women and

RESEARCH IN BRIEF 5.3—cont'd

promote widespread dissemination of evidence for this model, directed towards consumers, midwives and hospital management to increase awareness of the benefits.

TUTORIAL TRIGGER 5.2

Referring back to Tutorial trigger 5.1, could you use a grounded theory methodology to investigate your chosen clinical issue? Would you have to adjust your initial research question?

Ethnography

Origins and Theoretical Underpinnings

The term '**ethnography**' originates from the Greek *ethnos* (custom, culture, group) and the Latin *graphia* (drawing, writing or description). Therefore it is concerned with describing a custom, group or culture. Ethnography, as the descriptive study of cultures, has emerged as a subset of anthropological research (the study of humankind). It is an approach to research that aims to understand the activities and meanings of a social group with an emphasis on understanding its culture.

Different cultural groups (human societies) view relationships and meanings differently, with culture emerging from knowledge learned and shared. Consequently, interactions and behaviours within a group are interpreted and understood in a particular way by its group members. Ethnography is considered to be holistic in this sense, as it aims to understand the behaviour of a group of people within the context of their own culture. For instance, the aim of Molloy et al's (2019) ethnography was to explore the culture of mental health nursing as it related to the care of Aboriginal and Torres Strait Islander service users in public mental health services. The researchers describe the cultural context in terms of 'the dynamic and evolving socially constructed reality that exists in the minds of social group members'. They state that undertaking an ethnographic study of this area enabled research on beliefs within the group and how they were expressed in specialist nursing care. Studies of this nature are usually interested in forming a picture of the social whole in that behaviours and events are studied in relation to other factors that may influence or generate these events and behaviours. One of the main strengths of ethnographic research, in this sense, is in the *emic* (insider reality/perspective) and *etic* (outsider reality/perspective) interpretations of phenomena (see Table 5.2). An ethnographic researcher may have access to both *emic* and *etic* perspectives depending on their level of involvement within the culture.

TABLE 5.2 Common Ethnographic Approaches

Approach	Characteristics
Realist ethnography	• Aims to be objective. • Withholds personal judgements. • Involves long periods in the field. • Involves participant observation. • Aims to understand history, culture and worldviews. • Has anthropological origins. • Gives outsider/etic perspective. • Is generally narrated in third person. • Uses quotes of 'informants', but researcher has final interpretation.
Critical ethnography	• Embraces subjectivities and personal biases. • Advocates for the emancipation of marginalised groups. • Has critical social origins. • Is politically motivated. • Aims to create change. • Gives outsider/*etic* perspective. • Aims to understand power, inequity and dominance. • Entails researcher collaboration with participants to negotiate final report.
Case studies	• Generates understanding of a bounded system (individual or group). • Researcher locates the 'case' or 'cases' within their larger context. • Aims to link theory with practice. • Can be mixed-methods (see Chapter 12).
Autoethnography	• Aims to describe personal experience. • Aims to understand cultural experience. • Combines autobiographical and ethnographic approaches. • Has postmodernist social science origins. • Embraces personal subjectivity and emotionality. • Gives insider/emic perspective.
Ethnomethodology	• Focuses on micro levels of social life on a day-to-day basis. • Interprets interpersonal and social interaction. • Was developed by Harold Garfinkel. • Has sociological and phenomenological origins. • Is descriptive only—does not attempt to critique, explain or evaluate. • May use non-participant observations.

AN UNEXPECTED HURDLE

The purpose of Havery's (2019) study was to investigate how clinical facilitators' pedagogic practices in hospital settings enabled or constrained the learning of students for whom English was an additional/second language. The study used an ethnographic design to observe the interactions of 21 first-year students for whom English was an additional language and the relationship with their three facilitators. Observations occurred during three 2-week clinical placement blocks in three large metropolitan hospitals in Australia. The study found that there were multiple learning spaces in the hospitals, each of which was associated with learning activities between facilitators and students. These activities provided access to opportunities for learning core nursing skills, as well as for socialisation into the language of nursing. It was identified that data were collected from a range of sources owing to the complexity of the setting and sample population. Subsequently, the data collection did not follow a predetermined framework and the number of cases studied overall was small.

How might the study be approached differently to counter the hurdle of not being able to follow a predetermined data collection framework and resulting in small case numbers?

Critical ethnography is a type of ethnographic research that is underpinned by critical social theory (see Chapter 2). Through application of a critical lens, critical ethnographers explore marginalised groups from an *etic* (outsider) perspective. As with other critical approaches to research, it is politically motivated and aims to create change. Critical ethnographers aim to understand power, inequity and dominance. An example is Kaldal et al's (2023) ethnography investigating factors influencing newly graduated nurses' delivery of direct care in acute care hospital settings (see 'Research in brief 5.4'). The study identified the tension between a commitment to care and compromised care delivery that was born out of tensions between newly graduated nurses' professional beliefs and nursing values, a desire to integrate patients' needs and preferences, and organisational constraints on everyday practices where newly graduated nurses often worked alone without the support of a more experienced nurse.

Table 5.2 serves to highlight the nature of some of the main approaches to ethnography.

RESEARCH IN BRIEF 5.4

Kaldal et al (2023) sought to explore factors influencing newly graduated nurses' delivery of direct care in acute care hospital settings using an ethnographical approach. A total of 10 newly graduated nurses were purposively sampled, and data were collected through 96 hours of participant observation as well as 10 semistructured interviews. Three main structures emerged from the data: 'contrasting intentions and actions for care delivery', 'organisational constraints block interpersonal aspects of nursing care' and 'newly graduated nurses' suppressed need for support constitutes delay in care actions'. The study concluded that newly graduated nurses were committed to delivering high-quality care but were aware they sometimes provided compromised care. The paradox between a commitment to care and compromised care delivery was born out of tensions between newly graduated nurses' professional beliefs and nursing values, a desire to integrate patients' needs and preferences, and organisational constraints on everyday practices where newly graduated nurses often worked alone without the support of a more experienced nurse. Critical reflection on cultural, social and political forces that influence direct care delivery may support newly graduated nurses to deliver direct patient care more intentionally.

The Purpose and Process of Ethnography

A central belief related to ethnographic process is that individuals' experiences are socially organised. As such, the researcher examines these experiences and then proceeds to explore how these have been shaped by broader social relationships. To do this, all ethnographers must enter a research site to conduct their study, be it a community setting, a hospital unit, etc. The research setting is the '*conceptual field*' and the conduct of research in the field is known as *fieldwork*. The selection of the field depends on the research topic. In many nursing and midwifery examples the site is chosen based on convenience and/or familiarity. Ottrey et al's (2019) study on staff relationships at mealtimes provides a typical example. They chose ward environments familiar to them. Each ward contained 32 beds and was staffed by a healthcare team that included a wide range of clinical and support service personnel. Meals were plated in the kitchen and delivered to patients on the ward by food service staff. Mealtime assistance was provided to patients by nursing staff and/or volunteers. Therapy unrelated to eating was not scheduled at mealtimes, although a protected mealtime program was not in place. Additionally, nutrition in-services (i.e. malnutrition, therapeutic diets) were conducted by the dietitian as part of staff education.

TUTORIAL TRIGGER 5.3

Referring again to Tutorial trigger 5.1 and Tutorial trigger 5.2, could you use an ethnography methodology to investigate your chosen clinical issue/s? Would you have to adjust your initial research question?

OTHER QUALITATIVE METHODOLOGIES

The methodologies described so far are all categorised in the *interpretive* tradition of qualitative research (see Chapter 2). There are other research methodologies that are relevant to nursing and midwifery research. Two of these are categorised under the heading of '*critical research*' (or 'emancipatory research'). The first, *feminist research*, was briefly discussed in Chapter 2. The second, *action research*, is covered in Chapter 12, where the common argument is made that approaches such as action research and the *Delphi technique* do not come under the umbrella of qualitative research and that they are part of a separate paradigm—that of 'mixed methods'. They are briefly mentioned here, however, because many nursing and midwifery researchers continue to classify them as qualitative.

Historical Research

Historical research has a variety of uses and takes several different forms, but is most useful in the study of long-term societal change and connections between divergent social factors and social systems (Yuginovich 2000). For many, historical research simply provides the lens by which the past can be viewed in relation to current and future events and cycles. Nursing and midwifery practice has long been influenced by ongoing, repetitive trends that alter with each new generation (de Chesney 2014b). Many health professionals will appreciate the benefit of reflecting on past events in healthcare history. A historical perspective provides a frame of reference to consider past practices and potential mistakes and use this reflective learning to inform future practice.

In historical research, data are collected and analysed from a variety of sources. Most commonly, data are sought from archived written sources, such as letters, diaries, journals, reports, documents and meeting minutes. For example, Meehan (2012) drew on historical sources (dating from the 1820s) to investigate spirituality and spiritual care from a 'careful nursing' perspective—and sought to align findings with more contemporary contexts such as current professional practice models. More recently historical data has been sourced from outside traditional sources, with data now commonly collected through interviews from those involved in past events, or from descendants or relatives of those who have passed on.

As with feminist research, historical research has not been commonly adopted by nurses and midwives for some time now—but is still considered important. Beedholm et al (2013) provide an example of a historical approach in drawing on the philosopher Foucault's epistemological tradition in their work to uncover the meaning of 'ruptured thought' as it applies to a critical attitude to nursing research—and Smith (2018) explores American psychiatric nursing after World War II in the context of rapidly changing education, policy and practice around mental health and mental health nursing, and the passing of the National Mental Health Act in 1946.

As with history itself, research trends change and often repeat themselves over time, and thus historical approaches will be likely to come back into 'vogue' in health research in the future. For current writing on historical research, readers can find whole texts on the subject, such as Mason et al's (2011) text on the history of the nursing profession and de Chesney's (2014b) text on using life history to research nursing, as well as articles in the annual *Nursing History Review* through the American Association of the History of Nursing.

Qualitative Meta-synthesis

A relatively recent phenomenon in qualitative research has been the development of **qualitative meta-synthesis**. The term *meta-synthesis* is used to distinguish this approach from quantitative *meta-analysis* (see Chapter 3). Meta-synthesis may be used to integrate the data and findings of solely qualitative studies in a review of studies, or it may be used to integrate the findings from both quantitative and qualitative studies. Qualitative meta-synthesis applies systematic methods of searching, selecting and appraising existing qualitative research. Data is then analysed together and interpreted to explore and construct greater meaning than is possible from the individual studies alone (Erwin et al 2011). Meta-syntheses thereby also have potential to support change in clinical practice and health policy. There are many approaches to meta-synthesis and a review of meta-synthesis methods for qualitative research lists approximately 10 different methods (Barnett-Page & Thomas 2009), resulting in different terms associated with it, such as *meta-summary*. *Meta-ethnography* is a related approach—such as with Pangas et al's (2018) meta-ethnography of 25 qualitative studies on refugee women's experiences of negotiating motherhood and care in a new country. Whatever the approach, researchers essentially follow a method where all qualitative studies that exist on a particular topic are searched and reviewed and then matrices (tables) are used to compare studies and create a new interpretation of the collected data. Recent examples include Adams et al's (2023) Australian-based qualitative meta-synthesis of the roles of home-visiting nurses working with women experiencing family violence.

SUMMARY

The qualitative methodologies of qualitative description, phenomenology, grounded theory and ethnography have been explored in this chapter. Other less common, but important, qualitative methodologies have also been outlined. Each is an important approach in its own right and allows for different aspects to be explored. An appreciation of all these approaches will assist the beginning researcher to decide which methodology is appropriate to answer any chosen research question. Qualitative research represents a historically important part of nursing and midwifery research and theory development. It has an enduring place within health disciplinary research and is increasingly recognised as providing perspectives unable to be explored by any other approach. The popularity of qualitative research is especially assured with the emergence of the 'third paradigm' for research: mixed-methods research (see Chapter 12). Nurses, midwives and health researchers have an interest in maintaining this qualitative tradition and to continue to further explore understandings about the ways in which patients and clients in our care experience and engage with health and illness. Qualitative methods allow practitioners and researchers to seek and develop ways to improve healthcare experiences and outcomes. The following two chapters explore and describe design processes and methods as they apply to conducting qualitative research.

KEY POINTS

- Qualitative research is the search for understanding and meaning about human experience. It is used to gain deep understanding and insight and construct valid theory to guide disciplinary knowledge development. It can be used when little is known or when theory needs revising.
- Qualitative methodology helps us understand subjective human experience in the context of naturally occurring social phenomena. Qualitative methodologies guide researchers in their exploration of lived experience: the perceptions, attitudes, beliefs and values of people in a range of healthcare contexts and settings.
- There are a wide range of qualitative methodologies available—both traditional and emerging. The chosen methodology depends on the nature of the clinical topic under investigation and the guiding research question.
- Qualitative methods offer researchers the opportunity to gather rich information from research participants.
- The qualitative research perspective is holistic, inductive and uses interpretive processes.

TIME TO REFLECT

Hosie, A., Agar, M., Lobb, E., et al., 2014. Palliative care nurses' recognition and assessment of patients with delirium symptoms: a qualitative study using critical incident technique. Int. J. Nurs. Stud. 51, 1353–1365.

Aim: To explore the experiences, views and practices of inpatient palliative care nurses in delirium recognition and assessment.

Objective: Palliative care nurses may often recognise patients' delirium symptoms but there is variability in their capacity to comprehensively assess patients, situate the observed neurocognitive changes within a delirium framework and consistently apply accurate delirium terminology. The objective of this study is to understand more closely why this variability exists.

Design: Critical incident technique (CIT) was used to guide a series of semistructured interviews. Prior to interviews, participants were given a vignette of a palliative care inpatient with an unrecognised hypoactive delirium to prompt their recollection of a similar clinical incident. Clearly recalled and described incidents were analysed using thematic content analysis.

Reflect on the following:

- Nurses' intimate patient interactions over their first 24-hour assessment period make them ideally placed to recognise early delirium symptoms, assess the patient and apply appropriate treatment and supportive interventions. Yet nurses' capacity to effectively care for patients with delirium is limited by underrecognition of delirium, knowledge and practice gaps, and the distress and strain of caring for a patient with delirium.
- Routine use of delirium risk, screening and assessment tools is absent from practice. Adoption of available tools may assist palliative care nurses to shape their thinking about this complex syndrome and to enable them to respond to clinical changes in a more timely and appropriate way.
- How might we understand the experiences and/or interactions of people who present with delirium? What methodologies might you choose to use, and why?

Questions

1. What research questions might you pose if you were undertaking this study?
2. Think of other methodologies that could have been used.
3. Reflect on the information given and answer the following questions:
   a. Identify the research methodology.
   b. Is the design appropriate for this study?
   c. Might interviewing patients with delirium be an alternative approach?

LEARNING ACTIVITIES

1. Qualitative research's main aim is to:
   a. investigate issues that quantitative research is unable to reveal
   b. understand naturally occurring social phenomena
   c. include participants in the research
   d. determine what patients think about nurses and/or midwives
   e. all of the above.
2. Qualitative research, by its nature, is usually: (*emic* = insider; *etic* = outsider)

a. deductive, emic, naturalistic and holistic
b. deductive, etic, naturalistic and holistic
c. interpretive, emic, naturalistic and holistic
d. interpretive, etic, naturalistic and holistic
e. all of the above.

3. According to many researchers, the main advantage of qualitative descriptive exploratory approaches to research is:
   a. they can be easier to manage
   b. they don't use complicated terminology
   c. they do not limit the researcher to a particular philosophical worldview
   d. they can incorporate a variety of different perspectives
   e. all of the above.
4. Husserlian phenomenology is associated with:
   a. *lebenswelt*, epistemology, bracketing, descriptive phenomenology
   b. *lebenswelt*, ontology, bracketing, interpretive phenomenology
   c. *dasein*, epistemology, bracketing, descriptive phenomenology
   d. *dasein*, ontology, bracketing, interpretive phenomenology.
5. Heideggerian phenomenology is associated with:
   a. *lebenswelt*, epistemology, descriptive phenomenology
   b. *lebenswelt*, ontology, interpretive phenomenology
   c. *dasein*, epistemology, descriptive phenomenology
   d. *dasein*, ontology, interpretive phenomenology.
6. The hermeneutic circle describes:
   a. the fact that life experiences go around and around
   b. the fact that life cycles go around and around
   c. the historical, cultural and personal preconceptions from which understanding is developed
   d. the process by which all life is understood.
7. Grounded theory aims to:
   a. develop a well-rounded theory for use in later research
   b. develop a theoretical explanation for socially constructed events and ideally generate a hypothesis for further research
   c. develop a rationale for linking qualitative findings to quantitative findings
   d. develop a theoretical explanation for experimentally constructed events and ideally generate a hypothesis for further research.
8. Grounded theory originates from and has been further developed by:
   a. Strauss and Corbin
   b. Strauss and Chopin
   c. Glaser and Corbin
   d. Glaser and Strauss.
9. Ethnography has its origins in:
   a. quantitative research
   b. feminist research
   c. historical research
   d. anthropology.
10. Ethnography typically includes:
   a. the study of cultures, fieldwork, surveys, insider/outsider reality
   b. the study of cultures, fieldwork, observation, insider/outsider reality
   c. the study of individuals, fieldwork, observation, insider/outsider reality
   d. the study of individuals, laboratory work, observation, insider/outsider reality.

For further content associated with this chapter visit:  https://evolve.elsevier.com/cs/product/9780729596794?role=student

ADDITIONAL RESOURCES

Global Qualitative Nursing Research. https://journals.sagepub.com/home/gqn.

Grounded Theory Institute (with a focus on facilitating classic grounded theory method). https://www.groundedtheory.com.

Grounded Theory Online. https://www.groundedtheoryonline.com/what-is-grounded-theory/.

Norlyk, A., Harder, I., 2010. What makes phenomenological research phenomenological? An analysis of peer-reviewed empirical nursing studies. Qual. Health Res. 20, 420–431.

REFERENCES

Adams, C., Hooker, L., Taft, A., 2023. A systematic review and qualitative meta-synthesis of the roles of home-visiting nurses working with women experiencing family violence. J. Adv. Nurs. 79, 1189–1210. doi:10.1111/jan.15224

Artinian, B., Giske, T., Cone, P. (Eds.), 2009. Glaserian Grounded Theory in Nursing Research: trusting emergence. Springer, New York.

Barkway, P., 2001. Michael Crotty and nursing phenomenology: criticism or critique? Nurs. Inq. 8, 191–195.

Barnett-Page, E., Thomas, J., 2009. Methods for the synthesis of qualitative research: a critical review. BMC Med. Res. Methodol. 9, 59–67.

Beedholm, K., Lomborg, K., Frederiksen, K., 2013. Ruptured thought: rupture as a critical attitude to nursing research. Nurs. Philos. 15, 102–111.

Bulawa, P., 2014. Adapting grounded theory in qualitative research: reflections from personal experience. Int. Res. Educ. 2, 145–160.

Chamberlain-Salaun, J., Mills, J., Usher, K., 2013. Linking symbolic interactionism and grounded theory methods in a research design: from Corbin and Strauss' Assumptions to Action. Sage Open 3(3). doi:10.1177/2158244013505757

Charmaz, K., 2000. Grounded theory: objectivist and constructivist methods. In: Denzin, N., Lincoln, Y. (Eds.), Handbook of Qualitative Research, second ed. Sage Publications, Thousand Oaks, CA, pp. 509–535.
Chen, H.Y., Boore, J.R.P., 2009. Using a synthesized technique for grounded theory in nursing research. J. Clin. Nurs. 18, 2251–2260.
Corbin, J., Strauss, A., 1990. Grounded theory research: procedures, canons, and evaluative criteria. Qual. Sociol. 13 (1), 3–21.
Corbin, J., Strauss, A., 1996. Analytic ordering for theoretical purposes. Qual. Inq. 2 (2), 139–150.
Dahlberg, K., Drew, N., Nyström, M., 2001. Reflective Life World Research. Lund, Sweden.
De Chesney, M., 2014a. Nursing Research Using Grounded Theory: qualitative designs and methods in nursing. Springer, New York.
De Chesney, M., 2014b. Nursing Research Using Life History: qualitative designs and methods in nursing. Springer, New York.
Dowling, M., 2007. From Husserl to van Manen: a review of different phenomenological approaches. Int. J. Nurs. Stud. 44, 131–142.
Earle, V., 2010. Phenomenology as research method or substantive metaphysics? An overview of phenomenology uses in nursing. Nurs. Philos. 11, 286–296.
Erwin, E.J., Brotherson, M.J., Summers, J.A., 2011. Understanding qualitative metasynthesis. J Early Interv. 33 (3), 186–200.
Glaser, B., 1999. The future of grounded theory. Qual. Health Res. 9 (6), 836–845.
Glaser, B.G., 2002. Constructivist grounded theory? Forum Qual. Soc. Res. 3, (3). doi:10.17169/fqs-3.3.825
Glaser, B., Strauss, A., 1967. The Discovery of Grounded Theory: strategies for qualitative research. Aldine, New York.
Green, J., Thorogood, N., 2018. Qualitative Methods for Health Research. Sage Publications, London, UK.
Havery, C., 2019. The effects of clinical facilitators' pedagogic practices on learning opportunities for students who speak English as an additional language: an ethnographic study. Nurse Educ. Today 74, 1–6.
Heath, H., Cowley, S., 2004. Developing a grounded theory approach: a comparison of Glaser and Strauss. Int. J. Nurs. Stud. 41, 141–150.
Heidegger, M., 1962 (original work published 1927). Being and Time (Macquarie, J., Robinson, E., Trans.). Blackwell, Oxford.
Hoare, K.J., Mills, J., Francis, K., 2013. New graduate nurses as knowledge brokers in general practice in New Zealand: a constructivist grounded theory. Health Soc. Care Community 21, 423–431.
Hosie, A., Agar, M., Lobb, E., et al., 2014. Palliative care nurses' recognition and assessment of patients with delirium symptoms: a qualitative study using critical incident technique. Int. J. Nurs. Stud. 51, 1353–1365.
Husserl, E., 2001 (original work published 1900). Logical Investigations (Findlay, J., Trans.), vol. 1. Routledge, London.
Jarden, R J., Scott, S., Rickard, N., et al., 2023. Factors contributing to nurse resignation during COVID-19: a qualitative descriptive study. J. Adv. Nurs. 79, 2484–2501. doi:10.1111/jan.15596
Kagi, E, Rasiah, R, Moran, M., 2023. Experiences of primary health care nurses advancing their careers in a remote Western Australian location. Aust. J. Rural Health 31, 41–51. doi:10.1111/ajr.12904
Kaldal, M. H., Feo, R., Conroy, T., et al., 2023. New graduate nurses' delivery of patient care: A focused ethnography. J. Clin. Nurs. 32, 7454–7466. doi:10.1111/jocn.16804
Koivisto, K., Janhonen, S., Väisänen, L., 2002. Applying a phenomenological method of analysis derived from Giorgi to a psychiatric nursing study. J. Adv. Nurs. 39 (3), 258–265. doi:10.1046/j.1365-2648.2002.02272.x
Lune, H., Berg, B.L., 2016. Qualitative Research Methods for the Social Sciences, ninth ed. Pearson, Harlow, Essex.
McCann, T., Polacsek, M., 2018. Understanding, choosing and applying grounded theory: part 1. Nurse Res. 26 (3), doi:10.7748/nr.2018.e1592.
McConnell-Henry, T., Chapman, Y., Francis, K., 2009. Husserl and Heidegger: exploring the disparity. Int. J. Nurs. Pract. 15, 7–15.
Mackey, S., 2005. Phenomenological nursing research: methodological insights derived from Heidegger's interpretive phenomenology. Int. J. Nurs. Stud. 42, 179–186.
Mason, D.J., Isaacs, S.L., Colby, D.C., 2011. The Nursing Profession: development, challenges and opportunities. Jossey-Bass, San Francisco, CA.
Meehan, T.C., 2012. Spirituality and spiritual care from a Careful Nursing perspective. J. Nurs. Manag. 20 (8), 990–1001.
Merriam, S.B., Grenier, R.S., 2019. Qualitative Research in Practice: examples for discussion and analysis. Jossey-Bass, San Francisco, CA.
Mohammadi, N., Dianati, M., Omidi, A., et al., 2018. Lived experience of Male-to-Female transsexual people after sex reassignment surgery. Int. J. Med. Res. Health Sci. 5, 102–110.
Molloy L., Walker, K., Lakeman, R., et al., 2019. Encounters with difference: mental health nurses and Indigenous Australian users of mental health services. Int J Mental Health Nurs 28 (4), 922–929. doi:10.1111/inm.12592
Ottrey, E., Porter, J., Huggins, C.E., et al., 2019. Ward culture and staff relationships at hospital mealtimes in Australia: an ethnographic account. Nurs. Health Sci. 21, 78–84. doi:10.1111/nhs.12559
Pangas, J., Ogunsiji, O., Elmir, R., et al., 2018. Refugee women's experiences negotiating motherhood and maternity care in a new country: a meta-ethnographic review. Int. J. Nurs. Stud. 90, 31–45. doi:10.1016/j.ijnurstu.2018.10.005
Prussing, E., Browne, G., Eileen Dowse, E., et al., 2023. Implementing midwifery continuity of care models in regional Australia: a constructivist grounded theory study, Women Birth 36 (1), 99–107. doi:10.1016/j.wombi.2022.03.006
Ranse, J., Arbon, P., 2008. Graduate nurses' lived experience of in-hospital resuscitation: a hermeneutic phenomenological approach. Aust. Crit. Care 21 (1), 38–47. doi:10.1016/j.aucc.2007.12.001
Ranse, K., Ranse, J., Pelkowitz, M., 2018. Third-year nursing students' lived experience of caring for the dying: a hermeneutic

phenomenological approach. Contemp. Nurse 54 (2), 160–170. doi:10.1080/10376178.2018.1461572
Sadala, M.L.A., Adorno, R.C.F., 2002. Phenomenology as a method to investigate the experience lived: a perspective from Husserl and Merleau Ponty's thought. J. Adv. Nurs. 37, 282–293. doi:10.1046/j.1365-2648.2002.02071.x
Sandelowski, M., 2000. Focus on research methods. What ever happened to qualitative description? Res. Nurs. Health 23, 334–340.
Smith, K.M., 2018. Different places, different ideas: reimagining practice in American psychiatric nursing after World War II. Nurs. Hist. Rev. 26 (1), 17–47. doi:10.1891/1062-8061.26.17
Smith, M.R., Grealish, L., Henderson, S., 2018. Shaping a valued learning journey: student satisfaction with learning in undergraduate nursing programs, a grounded theory study. Nurse Educ. Today 64, 175–179. doi:10.1016/j.nedt.2018.02.020
Strauss, A., Corbin, J., 1990. Basics of Qualitative Research: grounded theory procedures and techniques. Sage Publications, Newbury Park, CA.
Strauss, A., Corbin, J., 1998. Basics of Qualitative Research: techniques and procedures for developing grounded theory, second ed. Sage Publications, Thousand Oaks, CA.
Sudarsan, I., Hoare, K., Sheridan, N., et al., 2023. Navigating asthma—the immigrant child in a tug-of-war: A constructivist grounded theory. J. Clin. Nurs. 32, 4009–4023. doi:10.1111/jocn.16521
Thomas, K.J., Yeganeh, L., Joanne VlahovichJ., et al., 2023. Midwifery professional placement: Undergraduate students' experiences with novice and expert preceptors, Nurse Educ. Today 131, 105976. doi:10.1016/j.nedt.2023.105976
van Manen, M., 1990. Researching Lived Experience: human science for an action sensitive pedagogy. State University of New York Press, London, Ontario.
van Manen, M., 1999. The pathic nature of inquiry and nursing. In: Madjar, I., Walton, J. (Eds.), Nursing and the Experience of Illness: phenomenology in practice. Allen & Unwin, St Leonards, NSW, pp. 17–35.
van Manen, M., 2014. Phenomenology of Practice: meaning-giving methods in phenomenological research and writing. Left Coast Press, Walnut Creek, CA.
van Manen, M., 2017. Phenomenology and meaning attribution. IPJP. 17 (1), 1–12.
Whitehead, D., 2002. The academic writing experiences of a group of student nurses: a phenomenological study. J. Adv. Nurs. 38, 498–506.
Wilson, A., Hurley, J., Hutchinson, M., et al., 2023. Trauma-informed care in acute mental health units through the life-world of mental health nurses: a phenomenological study. Int. J. Ment. Health Nurs. 32, 829–838. doi:10.1111/inm.13120
Yuginovich, T., 2000. More than time and place: using historical comparative research as a tool for nursing. Int. J. Nurs. Pract. 6, 70–75.

6

Data Collection and Sampling in Qualitative Research

Dean Whitehead and Sharon James

LEARNING OUTCOMES

After reading this chapter, you should be able to:

- understand the reasoning for qualitative data collection and sampling approaches
- discuss the benefits and limitations of qualitative data collection and sampling techniques
- describe different qualitative data collection and sampling approaches and appreciate research study examples for different approaches

KEY TERMS

INTRODUCTION

A key stage in all research process is determining the nature of the study population and then sampling from this population so that representative/appropriate data can then be collected. If something is missed in this process, it may be difficult to go back and collect more data, potentially impacting data quality for analysis and the study's duration. In qualitative research, the study population is nearly always human—although there are some exceptions that are discussed later in this chapter. Individuals taking part in a qualitative study are most commonly referred to as 'participants'. This chapter will focus on sampling and data collection techniques used in qualitative research—leading to the following chapter, which details the complementary process of analysing the collected data from the sample population.

SAMPLING TECHNIQUES AND PROCEDURES IN QUALITATIVE RESEARCH

The primary purpose of sampling is the selection of suitable participants (population) to enable the focus of the study to be researched. As with all types of research, effective sample selection is a vital part of the research design process (see Chapter 2). The choice of sampling method and subsequent data collection process is based on the chosen study methodology, aims and objectives and the research question/s.

TYPES OF SAMPLING

Sampling in qualitative research is termed *non-probability* sampling. Unlike *probability* sampling, used in quantitative research, non-probability sampling does not involve 'randomisation'. This means that members of a potential qualitative study population do not have an equal chance of being selected. Instead, they are often intentionally recruited by researchers as possessing the best characteristics related to the research topic's inclusion/exclusion criteria (see later) and/or are the most readily available. There are four main types of qualitative non-probability sampling most used in nursing and midwifery research:

1. convenience sampling
2. purposive sampling
3. snowball sampling
4. theoretical sampling.

Convenience Sampling

This is the most common form of **qualitative sampling** and occurs when people are invited to participate in the study because they are conveniently (opportunistic—sometimes called 'availability' or 'volunteer' sampling) available with regard to access, location, time and willingness. Convenience sampling is often described as a relatively fast and easy way to achieve the sample size needed for a study, particularly if participants are not readily identifiable. For example, in East et al's (2021) study about the experiences of individuals discussing sexual health in the context of cardiac illness with healthcare professionals, 13 participants were recruited using convenience sampling methods such as media releases as well as community and health professional advertisements. Given the potentially sensitive topic area and difficulty in identifying potential participants, convenience sampling was a useful method to collect data. Although it may be the most common form of sampling in qualitative research, the main limitation of using convenience sampling is that it may not provide the most data-rich method of data collection owing to either underrepresentation or overrepresentation of groups within the overall study population. For example, recruiting nursing students from a university library setting may result in representing only those students who are not currently on a clinical placement, those groups with imminent exams or assignments, or those who favour physical library environments over off-campus virtual resources. If a sample is not representative of the 'overall' population, it potentially limits the researchers' ability to socially generalise the findings to a wider similar population (Flick 2018). Some would argue that achieving a representative sample is not always important in qualitative studies. However, a considered sampling approach that aims to obtain a diverse group of participants (but who fit the inclusion criteria) representing the phenomena being studied is often an important factor.

Purposive (Purposeful) Sampling

Purposive sampling is a popular approach in qualitative research (Campbell et al 2020). It is also commonly called 'judgemental' (sometimes 'authoritative') sampling. Participants are recruited according to preselected criteria relevant to the research aims/questions of a given qualitative study. Purposive sampling is designed to recruit those who have the required status, experience or knowledge of interest to the researcher. An example of such a sampling approach is Adcock et al's (2022) study, which explored midwifery leaders' needs to effectively contribute to maternity services reform. Purposive sampling was used to recruit a total of 13 participants representing midwifery leaders across Australia. The inclusion criteria (see later in the chapter) were: midwives working in a range of midwifery leadership roles across every state and territory in Australia.

Two further types of sampling sit under the 'umbrella' of purposive sampling. These are quota sampling and maximum phenomena variation sampling. In *quota sampling*, the researcher decides on both the number of participants required and the characteristics of interest. These may be age, gender, profession, diagnosis, ethnicity and so forth. The population is divided into the groups of interest (e.g. men under the age of 45 years and men over 45 years). The researcher would then select men from each group to represent the proportion of each group in the wider population. If the desired sample size was 20 men and the proportion of men over 45 years in the desired population was 75%, then the sample would consist of 5 men under 45 years and 15 men older than 45 years. Quota sampling is thus considered more specific with respect to representing proportions of the sub-samples of interest in a given qualitative research study. An example of quota sampling is evident in Addo et al's (2019) study investigating the main factors driving changes in dietary and physical activity behaviours among Australian residents who were born in sub-Saharan Africa and the extent to which these factors are related to immigration. They describe their recruitment of 24 participants using a quota criterion to minimise selection bias based on ethnicity and demographic factors. These factors included sub-Saharan Africa subregion origin, state of residence, gender and living arrangement.

Maximum phenomena variation sampling is an approach used to ensure that the full range and extent of the investigated qualitative phenomena are represented—such as ensuring people experiencing milder to severe symptoms across a spectrum, in relation to a particular condition, are included, or perhaps ensuring a breadth of demographic factors are captured (e.g. across different age ranges) during data collection. An example is Calma et al's (2021) study, which explored final-year nursing students' perceptions of general practice nursing. Semistructured **interviews** were conducted with 16 participants with 'variation' based across the range of low, mid and high intention to work in general practice.

Snowball Sampling

Also known as 'chain referral' or 'networking' sampling, *snowball sampling* occurs when the researcher begins gathering information from one or a small number of participants and then requests they identify/suggest others who may be friends, relatives, colleagues or other significant contacts who they know have also experienced the phenomena of interest. This type of sampling can be a cost-effective way of recruiting participants and is especially useful in recruiting 'hidden populations'. This may be, for example, marginalised or stigmatised individuals who are not easily accessible to researchers, such as drug users, sex industry workers or members of cults/sects or other 'underground' subcultures. One example is Fauk et al's (2021) study, investigating the influences of cultural practices and religious beliefs on sexual relationships and behaviours of participants as contributors for HIV transmission in Indonesia. Given the interplay between culture, religion and HIV across the eventual sample size of 52 women and 40 men, this was achieved using snowball sampling over a 6-month period. While snowball sampling has traditionally been used with hard-to-reach/vulnerable participants, it is also worth noting that it has become more popular in relation to recruiting sample populations via social media—for instance, Bennetts et al's (2019) report that they used 'passive' snowball sampling via Facebook where users liked, shared or circulated the link to others.

The limitations of snowball sampling include a reliance on referrals from a small network of initial contacts to generate additional participants, or the process may not reveal the number or diversity of participants hoped for. The participants, therefore, may not be representative of the overall population being studied.

Theoretical Sampling

Theoretical (or *theory-based*) *sampling* is mostly used in grounded theory studies but is increasingly being used to gather data for the purpose of theory generation (see Chapter 2). The sampling starts from identifying a small (homogeneous) group of cases and moves to compare it with other larger (heterogeneous) groups (Campbell et al 2020). Sampling, in this case, occurs sequentially and alongside data analysis. Analysed data guide the relevant areas to be explored further in the next round of data collection and the sample focus to achieve this. The initial participants are usually purposively chosen or conveniently available. For example, McCullough et al (2021) described the perspectives of nurses about the actions and interactions involved in primary healthcare delivery in remote communities using a constructivist grounded theory perspective. Those nurses working in Australian community health centres or Aboriginal Medical Services located in areas classified as 'remote' or 'very remote' were invited to take part in the study. Participants were initially recruited from a remote nurse practitioner interest group and further participants were recruited using theoretical sampling and a snowball approach. This resulted in nurse practitioners (n = 13), remote area nurses (n = 7) and nursing academics with experience in remote area nursing (n = 4) participating in the study. Participants who demonstrated characteristics associated with developing categories (see Chapter 7) were invited to participate in telephone interviews and an expert reference group.

USING MORE THAN ONE SAMPLING TECHNIQUE IN A QUALITATIVE STUDY

As indicated for theoretical sampling, it is possible to use more than one form of sampling in other types of qualitative studies. For example, in a study by Huang et al (2021) investigating the attitudes and experiences of family caregivers and their shared decision-making involvement regarding people diagnosed with schizophrenia, the researchers used both convenience and purposive maximum variation sampling to ensure sample diversity. This was done by recruiting through a tertiary hospital facility and then the study sought nurses in psychiatry wards based on differing relationships to the patient, years of caregiving experience and educational attainment. Depending on context, studies that use more than one sampling technique may be classified as 'multi-method' studies (see Chapter 12).

SAMPLING CRITERIA

In qualitative research, targeted participants are viewed as individuals able to reflect upon and express their experiences, values, beliefs and opinions. Different qualitative approaches have varying sampling intentions regarding the targeted participants. The selection depends upon the **sampling criteria**. Sampling criteria identify the nature and characteristics of the **sample population** and their eligibility to be part of the study based on predetermined *inclusion* and *exclusion* requirements.

Inclusion Criteria

Inclusion criteria are specific characteristics that the person, population or 'elements' must possess in order to be eligible for a study. They are likely to range from quite broad requirements (e.g. age and/or gender) through to more specific criteria—that is, have an existing disorder (e.g. osteoporosis) and have experienced a hip fracture in the last 6 months. For example, in Ho et al's (2021) qualitative study on the older person's lived experience and adaptations to sensory impairment, the 13 community-dwelling adult participants were over 65 years of age, living independently, able to understand written and spoken English and had at least one sensory change (e.g. sight or hearing impairment). Inclusion criteria were based on the research questions: '1. To what extent is sensory change apparent to older people? 2. Which of the senses is the most important to older people? 3. What is the older person's experience of living with sensory change? 4. How do older people respond to and manage sensory change?'

The chosen qualitative methodology will also strongly guide the focus for inclusion criteria (Holloway & Galvin 2023). For instance, participants in phenomenological studies are mostly chosen because of their experience of the phenomenon being studied and because of their ability to express that experience. With ethnographic research, the researcher is usually 'in the field' and observing and recording the events and behaviours of participants as they occur. In this case, participants need to be present in the observable location.

Exclusion Criteria

Exclusion criteria are 'potential' characteristics that have been identified as not relevant to the study and lead to the exclusion of a potential participant from the study. For example, a study on young adults would normally exclude those under 18 years of age and may have a cap on those over 25 years of age. Of course, it is not always necessary to state exclusion criteria. For instance, a study involving 'giving birth' does not have to exclude men. Exclusion criteria may often be stated as the 'opposite' of the inclusion criteria—for example, if 'included' persons are registered nurses/midwives then 'excluded' would be non-registered nurses/midwives. This information is often not needed but is still commonly seen. In Hibberson et al's (2023) study, exploring multidisciplinary simulation training for perioperative teams in Australia, the inclusion criteria were: being currently employed in an Australian hospital, currently a nurse, surgeon or anaesthetist and currently registered with the Australian Health Practitioner Regulation Agency (AHPRA), and having undertaken simulation training within the last 5-years. It is worth noting that, often, inclusion and/or exclusion criteria are sometimes presented as a table or tables in an article.

Qualitative studies do not always report inclusion/exclusion criteria. However, this does not mean that anyone can be included in the study sample. The criteria may be assumed as the target individuals have common shared characteristics—for example, they are all new graduates in a specific university course.

TUTORIAL TRIGGER 6.1

You intend to research the perceptions of people living in the community setting with indwelling urinary catheters. What might you consider as inclusion/exclusion criteria?

SAMPLE SIZE IN QUALITATIVE RESEARCH

Unlike quantitative approaches, which aim to establish *statistical significance* by sampling a predetermined number of subjects or elements, qualitative researchers do not always begin a study with a predetermined sample size. In qualitative research, sample size can be determined by the aims of the study, the sampling technique and strategy, and the data quality as well as researcher judgement and experience (Mthuli et al 2022). Other factors include budget, time, population access, resource availability and selection criteria (Mthuli et al 2022). Predetermining an adequate sample size can be problematic. These decisions are based on context as well as iterative process during analysis (see Chapter 7). Essentially, the 'richness' of data collected is far more important than the number of participants. A useful guide to sampling in qualitative studies proposed by Mthuli et al (2022) is 'DEJA', which involves firstly reviewing the literature to **Define** the sampling strategy (e.g. non-probability), then **Explain** the techniques to be used (e.g. purposive, snowball), then **Justify** the sampling decisions based on the research intent, and lastly **Apply** these decisions to the research process overall.

Commonly, a sample size of between 8 and 20 participants is reported in qualitative studies but this can vary considerably; on average, it is between 2 and 60 participants (Mthuli et al 2022). Researchers, over time, have provided sample size guidelines for qualitative research designs. Isaacs (2014 p. 320) states that a 'rule of thumb' is 12–26 participants. Other authors are more specific in relation to different methodologies. For instance, Creswell and Poth (2018) recommend 3–5 participants for a case study, 10 for a phenomenological study and 15–20 for a grounded theory study, whereas Morse (1995) suggests a sample size ranging from 6 participants for a phenomenological study to 30–50 for an ethnographic study. For focus groups (see later in this chapter), Krueger and Casey (2015) suggest 5–10 participants in each focus group. However, in Guthrie et al's (2020) study of midwives, student midwives and Indigenous health workers—exploring woman-centred weight gain support across models of care—four focus groups were conducted ranging from 4 to 31 participants in each (n = 68). Occasionally, many participants may be involved; for example, Jenkins et al (2021) analysed open-ended qualitative survey responses from 1175 open-text responses in their New Zealand-based study investigating 'silver linings' from COVID-19 lock downs.

DATA COLLECTION IN QUALITATIVE RESEARCH

The process of data collection follows the identification and targeting of the sample population. Data collection can take the form of 'direct data' or 'indirect data'. *Direct data* include recordable spoken or written words and observable body language, actions and interactions. Here, the interactions may be human to human or human responses to inanimate objects—such as a haemodialysis machine. Whatever objects can be observed or communicated are potential or actual data (Merriam & Grenier 2019). The collection of direct data is relevant when considering the thoughts, feelings, experiences, meaning of experience, responses, actions, interactions, language and processes of individuals and groups within their social and/or cultural setting (Flick 2018). It is this type of data that mostly sets the 'context' of qualitative research. Direct data are, by far, the most common form of data in qualitative research.

Indirect data are generated, in the first instance, by someone or something else—such as through documents or media reporting an event, or an artistic rendition of an event or experience (e.g. novels, songs, paintings, poems, photographs and, more recently, social media representations). For instance, Foster and Whitehead (2018) highlight the value of using drawings as both a form of data collection and a medium to prompt discussion with children hospitalised in a paediatric high-dependency unit in New Zealand. The children were asked to draw a picture of a person in hospital. The drawing was then referred to in the interview to explore their experience of their hospital stay and their needs, for example by asking the child to describe what the significance of people, place and items included in the drawing meant to them. The drawings were analysed post-interview using an assessment tool that assessed the child's level of anxiety. Where indirect data need to be collected, these are sought through a variety of methods. These may include systematically searching archives or browsing the internet. The data collected may be in either hard-copy or electronic form.

Depending on the types of data required for a qualitative study, various methods of collecting data can be used singularly or in combination (multi-method—see Chapter 12) to obtain direct data. For direct data, these methods may include interview, observation, open-ended questionnaire, journalling (diary accounts) or 'think aloud' sessions. Direct data can be collected by the study participant at the request of the researcher (e.g. through writing a personal journal or diary) and then provided back to the researcher. Or, for topics where the population is geographically dispersed or diverse, sensitive in nature, a range of perspectives are sought or the focus is specific, an open-ended **questionnaire** may be more appropriate (Braun et al 2021). Most commonly, however, qualitative approaches gather data through interpersonal contact with participants (usually an interview) or through the presence of the researcher in proximity to events (usually observation) (Flick 2018). This is unlike quantitative research, where, frequently, interpersonal contact is deliberately limited with participants or events.

IS THERE MORE THAN ONE DATA COLLECTION METHOD IN A QUALITATIVE STUDY?

As with qualitative sampling techniques, it is also possible to use more than one **qualitative data collection** method in a single study (multi-method). This can be achieved in two different ways—that is, two different methods are employed at the same 'sitting' (with the same participants) or at different 'sittings'—usually with different participants. For instance, in Rees et al's (2018) 'same sitting' study on understanding Australian students' and clinicians' experiences of informal interprofessional workplace learning, 'general' interviews began by exploring students' and clinicians' understandings of workplace interprofessional student–clinician (IPSC) interactions. Following directly on, the same participants were asked to narrate (narrative interviewing) their workplace experiences of IPSC interactions. In a 'different sitting' example, Doughty et al (2018) in their Auckland-based study, separately used focus groups and semistructured interviews to explore the experiences and perceptions of new graduate nurses undertaking a new postgraduate program and the Directors of Nursing supporting them to complete the program.

Interviews

Interviews are regarded as the main method for qualitative data collection, used in many nursing- and midwifery-related research studies. Spoken 'narrative' is the basis of most qualitative data, where that narrative is mostly gathered through direct encounters between the researcher and the participant (or several participants) using in-depth interviews and/or focus group interviews. Interviews can be conducted by telephone, web-based conferencing or email, and through social communication and media conversations (e.g. micro-blogging—X (Twitter), Facebook, Tumblr).

Interviews in qualitative research may be unstructured, semistructured or occasionally structured. With *unstructured* interviews, neither the specific questions to be asked nor the range or type of possible answers are predetermined. The interviews are designed to be informal and conversational, with the aim of encouraging participants to express themselves in a natural manner. Unstructured interviews tend to start with single broad questions, such as 'What is your experience of ... ?' The researcher, however, has an idea in mind of the general issues to be covered and may use a topic list as a reminder. Quinney et al (2018) used unstructured interviews in their Queensland-based phenomenological study on professional insights from nurses who are carers for their own family supporting their chronic illness.

Semistructured interviews use an interview guide to provide a predetermined set of questions for discussion. The questions are set to ensure the research aims/questions are directly covered. However, there is flexibility to ask any questions in any order, follow 'tangents' or seek further clarification of previous answers or elaboration of responses. Therefore semistructured interviews steer the interview, yet are flexible enough to allow the interviewer to follow other leads and areas of interest. James et al (2021) used semistructured, one-on-one telephone interviews to examine Australian primary healthcare nurse participants' experiences in using telehealth during COVID-19. Interviews ranged from 19 to 59 minutes in duration and were audio recorded. Interviews were conducted by one of two investigators independently, using a semistructured interview guide to assist in directing the conversation.

Structured interviews are not commonly conducted in qualitative research. They follow a list of set questions, usually asked in a certain order—but these questions are still open ended—that is, usually commencing with words like 'how', 'why', 'where' or 'when'. This distinguishes them from structured *quantitative* interviews, which usually ask only closed-ended questions—such as 'how many'—to gather numerical data. Brunton and Cook (2018) identify their structured qualitative interview schedule in their 'Dis/integrating cultural difference in practice and communication' study of host and migrant registered nurse perspectives from New Zealand.

Common to all types of interview format is the need to avoid 'leading' questions at all times—ranging from structured to unstructured interview guides. The researcher should not lead or influence a participant down a particular line of thinking. This is a form of data bias. Questions should be neutral, balanced, objective and for general guidance only. There are several guides to formulating effective and unbiased interview question guides—such as Kross and Giust's (2019) article.

TUTORIAL TRIGGER 6.2

Prepare an interview schedule for investigating the experiences of clients who have an indwelling urinary catheter. What sort of questions might you ask of your participants?

Conducting Interviews

The structure and conduct of interviews are important; both factors will impact on the quality of the data generated. Many researchers perform 'dry/dummy runs' with peers and/or colleagues as a form of 'testing' the interview schedule and interview techniques. This is a valuable opportunity to gain evaluative feedback on the nature and structure of the question format and potentially make suggested changes.

There are several considerations for all researchers conducting any type of interview to enhance the experience and the quality of data collected. At the start of the interview it is important that the 'rules of engagement' are established and communicated—such as generating and maintaining a warm and non-judgemental manner towards the participant/s, asking questions in a balanced, unbiased, non-threatening, sensitive and clear way, and choosing a setting and time for the interview that is appropriate for both the interviewer and interviewee to explore the area of study (e.g. private setting if personal questions will be asked). Most interviews conducted in qualitative research are audio recorded and/or, less commonly, video recorded. Video recording, while useful for recording non-verbal data, is considered more 'intrusive'. Video conferencing audio (e.g. Zoom, Teams) or telephone interviews can be used for audio recording. Stevens et al (2019) used both audio and video recording for interviews and observation in their ethnographic study (see Chapter 5) of skin-to-skin contact and what women prefer in the first hours after a caesarean section. Both formats have an advantage over handwritten notes because it is often impossible to manually record everything the interviewer hears or observes.

During the interview it is important that the participant feels as comfortable as possible. Privacy and comfort are essential, and the researcher should minimise the likelihood of disruption as much as possible by, for example, ensuring that all items required are available (recording equipment, tapes, consent forms, participant information sheets, drinks, tissues, etc.). Researchers should take active steps to ensure privacy such as posting 'do not disturb' signs and disabling mobile telephone or pager devices. The issues of confidentiality and anonymity should be discussed with the participant before the interview is conducted. Any 'concern' questions are encouraged and answered. Potential issues are usually set out in the study information, and the participant, when undertaking consent (see Chapter 13), acknowledges that they understand the issues and have had the opportunity to discuss these with the researcher prior to interviews/observation. In most cases, it is made clear to the participant that they can request to discontinue/withdraw from the interview at any time during it. To promote informed consent, it is important to check participant understanding of all issues before consenting.

Appropriate time should be allowed for each interview. Giving the participant an approximate guide of likely interview duration at the time of recruitment is helpful, though interviews should not be hurried or terminated before they have naturally completed. If, however, the participant wishes to stop the interview, or the researcher senses that the participant is becoming tired or distressed, then the interview can be stopped or paused at any time. This may mean setting up a new appointment for another time. It is, however, preferable to resume as soon as possible so that flow and recall of previous discussion is not lost. It is recommended that no single interview last more than 1–2 hours, as otherwise 'interview fatigue' is likely to occur (Holloway & Galvin 2023).

The use of videoconferencing/virtual platforms (e.g. Zoom, FaceTime, Teams) to conduct qualitative interviews has significantly increased over recent years. Irani (2019) reports on the increasing use of this media option in their article titled 'The use of videoconferencing for qualitative interviewing: opportunities, challenges and considerations'. Carlson et al (2019) in their study explore the perception of nursing students—across three international universities in Australia, Hong Kong and Sweden—of peer learning during cross-cultural learning activities through student-led webinars via Zoom. Younas et al's (2023) qualitative study, exploring behavioural indicators of compassionate nursing care from the perspectives of individuals with multimorbidities and complex needs, utilises virtual interviewing.

 **TUTORIAL TRIGGER 6.3**

What might be the most important features of a 'desirable' environment for the conduct of qualitative interviews?

Vital to the process during an interview are the interviewer's presence and engagement (including how they listen and attend to, and end, responses—as well as bring the session to an end, i.e. summarise/debrief). It should be remembered, however, that the purpose is always to gain information from the participant; it is not for the researcher to express their own thoughts and feelings. In a structured or semistructured interview, an appropriate range of questions is asked. The purpose of the interview schedule in semistructured interviews is to support the interviewer to stay relatively focused. Questions may also be used to prompt expansion and elaboration with participants if further detail is required. An active listening position is adopted by the researcher, concentrating on what is being said as well as being alert to other cues—particularly participant non-verbal cues indicating distress or disengagement. During the interview, some researchers find it useful to record non-verbal aspects of the interview (memoing)—for example, if the participant laughs or cries and at what point this occurs. The memo notes can be later used to guide the data collected from the audio/videotaped interviews. Alongside this, the interviewer may document a reflective written account written immediately or soon after the interview session as a review of their own thoughts and feelings about the interview. These reflective memos may then also assist later data analysis.

Qualitative interviews should allow the participant to speak freely and offer in-depth and lengthy responses through techniques used singularly or in combination. Possible techniques include the following:

- *Funnelling*—beginning the interview with general and broad (non-probing) opening questions and then narrowing down to topic specifics as the interview progresses—once a degree of rapport and relationship has been established—and the participant feels more 'comfortable'.
- *Probing or prompting*—seeking further details or seeking clarification. Gauci et al (2022) used prompts as part of their interview guide to ensure the research aims were addressed in their study exploring women's experiences of workplace gender discrimination as registered nurses.
- *Paraphrasing*—repeating what the participant has said, without changing the meaning of what has been said, assists understanding and clarity and acts as a further prompt.

Cultural and Language Considerations

When conducting interviews, it is also important to consider the use of language and cultural context, especially in cross-cultural settings. In qualitative research, participants are often interviewed in a language that is not their first/native language. Where this occurs, it is important that the interviewer attends to language considerations and a culturally appropriate approach. In multicultural societies, such as Australia and New Zealand, research is often conducted involving participants from culturally and linguistically diverse (CALD) backgrounds for the purpose of describing, understanding and clarifying cultural 'worldviews'. It is important that researchers are aware of the need to create and maintain cultural competency and cultural safety, and consider their positionality (see Chapter 14) (Brion & Rogers-Shaw 2022). It is well known, for instance, that many remote-living Aboriginal and Torres Strait Islander Australian families lack access to consistent, culturally safe healthcare services. Campbell et al's (2018) Baby One Programme (BOP) presents their family-centred, Indigenous health worker-led, home-visiting model of care focused on promoting family health to give Indigenous children the best start in life. The program was developed by Aboriginal community-controlled Apunipima Cape York Health Council and delivered in Queensland's Cape York remote communities. The qualitative study used semistructured interviews with four family members enrolled in the BOP and 24 Apunipima staff members. In addition, 20 community members, including two program users, participated in a men's community focus group. Their findings showed that health worker education and training, and knowledge exchange between health workers, midwives and nurses, was critical to program effectiveness. The program is reported as growing despite substantial logistic, financial and practical challenges.

When data are collected in two or more languages, it is important to consider strategies to ensure data collection is completed in the same way as far as possible across language groups. Examples include employing bilingual researchers or professional interpreters. Internet searches for local and national language translation services will yield a variety of available resources and services.

Similar subcultural 'competency and safety' considerations are needed when dealing with 'vulnerable' participants. For instance, in Younas et al's (2023) qualitative study exploring behavioural indicators of compassionate nursing care from the perspectives of individuals with multiple morbidities and complex needs, face-to-face and virtual semistructured interviews were conducted with 23 individuals having experiences as complex patients. Among them were 19 homeless participants living in a shelter.

RESEARCH IN BRIEF 6.1

Staps et al (2019), in their study, identify that Māori have disproportionately high rates of bipolar disorder (BD) and subsequent mental health service use. Their qualitative study combining individual interviews and focus groups was conducted with the aim to explore mental health clinicians' and Māori mental health workers' perspectives of effective treatment for Māori with BD. Sixteen participants

 **RESEARCH IN BRIEF 6.1—cont'd**

took part in either individual interviews or focus groups, or both. The study found the importance of a Māori worldview; tikanga Māori (rituals), understanding the whānau (context), whakawhanaungatanga (connection), the powhiri (introduction) process and whakarongo (listening) were key to working effectively with Māori who had BD. The participants in this study identified the person and their culture rather than the psychiatric diagnosis as crucial to providing effective care to Māori with BD. Without a foundation in whakawhanaungatanga, engagement, diagnosis, treatment adherence, and the process of recovery was unlikely to be as effective for Māori with BD. It was stated from the findings that it was the person, not the diagnosis, that was central to therapeutic engagement.

Benefits of Interviews

Interviews provide the researcher with a valuable opportunity to enter the world of the participant and reflect on a particular event. Rapport and trust can be developed and are desirable to collect the extensive and detailed data that are needed. Interviews should develop as 'conversational encounters' that offer opportunities to clarify issues—as well as probe for ever-deeper insight and meaning. Interviews also offer an opportunity to collect unique data, as every participant can use their own words and draw on their own experiences. If emotive issues arise during the interview session, the interviewer can offer support appropriate to their role as a researcher, such as information on sources of counselling if the need exists or arises. Overall, qualitative interviews offer an opportunity to create productive, meaningful and supportive engagement that benefits both researchers and participants.

Limitations of Interviews

There is a range of challenges when conducting interviews. These challenges include securing access to and securing an adequate sample of participants, securing informed consent, the impact of discussing difficult or traumatic experiences on the interviewee and interviewer, developing an informed interview schedule, interview scheduling, capturing data in an acceptable and reliable way, establishing the interviewer–interviewee relationship and developing effective interviewer skills (Coleman 2019). Interviews are not so much limited by the techniques and methods used, as by how these are applied by the researcher. These are influenced by the researcher's background, preparation and experience as well as the approach (Coleman 2019). There is always a potential for an imbalance in the power relationship between interviewer and interviewee. This should be minimised as much as possible. An effective interview should be more of a discussion, focused on the participant, than a question-and-answer session.

Interviews can be time consuming and resource intensive to set up and conduct. Several factors will determine the extent of this—such as multiple venues and travel time, multiple interviewers, videoconferencing availability (if used), participant reliability, etc. To this extent, there may also be cost implications associated with interviews—for both participants and researchers.

Another consideration is that the interviewer, despite efforts to 'bracket' out their own experiences, ideas, prejudices and opinions prior to an interview session, will sometimes, inevitably, bring their own 'agenda' to interviews. The resulting data may, in part, be influenced by the interviewer, whether this is through body language and/or the nature of questions asked. There is the potential for degrees of 'subjectivity/influence' with many qualitative interviews.

Focus Group Interviews

Focus group interviews are conducted in a group setting and they can be used in several ways to generate data. Focus groups can be conducted to explore, develop and refine initial research questions and interview schedules as a form of data collection, or as a way of exploring the impact of findings generated through interviews (or another form of data collection) (Holloway & Galvin 2023). Focus groups use interview schedules but these differ in scope, nature and intention from other types of individual participant interviews. This is because of the unique nature of 'group dynamics' and insights gained from interaction between participants. Focus groups offer a collective set of values, experiences and observations of participants that are later interpreted in context. O'Neill et al (2023) explored the impact of the COVID-19 environment on nursing delivery of family-centred care (FCC) in an Australian paediatric hospital using focus groups. Nineteen nurses participated across seven focus groups. The focus groups were semistructured, with a flexible interview guide organising questions related to existing FCC framework tenets. Discussion included nurses' experiences providing FCC to inpatients and families during the COVID-19 pandemic in general. Other questions explored the impact of involving families in decision making, the quality of FCC provision and what might have been approached differently to deliver FCC during this time. Each focus group was up to 60 minutes in duration and was facilitated by two of the research team. The resulting four themes—*advocating with empathy*, *enabling communication*, *responding with flexibility* and *balancing competing considerations*—and the eight subthemes that were generated, outlined how nurses delivered FCC, and how these FCC actions were impacted by the COVID-19 environment and related hospital restrictions.

If a series of focus groups are scheduled, initial interviews usually identify broad issues and perspectives related to the focus of the study, while subsequent interviews seek to prioritise and narrow down issues.

Benefits of Focus Group Interviews

The main benefit of this method of data collection is the generation of data from multiple participants, which often allow a larger sample size compared with individual interview studies. Another advantage is that, for those who may find one-to-one interviews intimidating (both participants and researchers), the group setting may be more appealing and provide access to participants who may not participate otherwise. Focus groups offer supportive group interactions as each member is encouraged to identify, describe, analyse and resolve issues and are particularly valuable in obtaining different perspectives on the same topic. Focus group interviews are usually a more cost-effective way of collecting data when a larger sample size is required than individual interviews.

Limitations of Focus Group Interviews

There are several potential limitations to consider. Focus groups may not allow for the exploration of issues as deeply as one-on-one interviews. At the same time, as they may not be as intimate and private as individual interviews, sensitive or potentially emotive issues may not be discussed. Researchers require expertise to effectively conduct and 'control' focus group interviews in different ways. For instance, avoiding 'group think' outcomes (where members generally agree with each other—even if this is not the reality), preventing any individual from dominating conversations, as well as drawing out contributions from quieter members. Where focus groups do not present any of these dilemmas, the researchers should be mostly inconspicuous—often needing only to contribute to commence, prompt occasionally and finalise the session. For researchers who prefer to directly influence proceedings, this may be seen as an individual limitation.

RESEARCH IN BRIEF 6.2

In a study by Rogan et al (2022), they explore nursing and medical perceptions of factors that impact sepsis management in an emergency department. In this qualitative study, nurses and doctors were purposively recruited from a major referral hospital in New Zealand. The researchers identified that face-to-face focus groups were used to understand the views of the group as a collective,

Continued

RESEARCH IN BRIEF 6.2—cont'd

as well as allowing diversity of participant opinion. Six focus groups, three with nurses and three with doctors, were undertaken where participants were matched where possible with others of similar experience. Prior to interview, participants completed a form detailing their emergency department (ED) work experience. Three focus group facilitators were used: an ED registrar, an ED research nurse and a moderator to support facilitator development of the first two facilitators as well as ensuring interviews covered similar questions and were of similar format. All focus groups were transcribed and loaded into NVivo (Version 12, QSR International—see Chapter 7).

Observation

Observational methods are commonly used in qualitative research designs and vary between methods. **Observation** is the process of observing the daily life and behaviours of participants in their natural setting to record aspects such as their social position, role and function, and actions and interactions. Qualitative observation is traditionally adopted by ethnographers (Balcom et al 2021) but it can be used in other qualitative approaches. This is especially so with studies using an interpretive/constructivist approach (see Chapter 2), where exploring observed events is often used to interpret and understand behaviour.

In qualitative research, observation methods are mostly unstructured. In unstructured observation, researchers enter the observed 'field' with no predetermined schedule as to what they may or may not see or hear. However, some studies will use more structured observation and a template to record data—looking for specific events. A structured approach requires an 'observation protocol' to record the same information collected during observations by the data collectors across the site field/s. For instance, observers in a ward or clinic may focus observation on a certain clinical phenomenon of interest. Ottrey et al (2019) undertook an observational ethnographic study on two subacute wards to explore the relationships, roles and responsibilities of nurses involved at mealtimes and the influence on meal provision. Overall, 67 hours of observational fieldwork were conducted over 3 months. Observers moved throughout the wards, watching and listening to participants, and recording these data as handwritten field notes. Observation continued until patterns/themes were realised. Such an approach was designed to gain an enriched understanding of ward culture and staff relationships at hospital mealtimes, helping to uncover new knowledge on how the healthcare team engaged in and worked together to deliver nutrition care to patients.

Process of Observation

Methods of observation range from participation to observation where four distinct roles of participation and observation can be identified: *complete participant*, *participant-as-observer*, *observer-as-participant* and *complete observer*. These roles can also be adopted in quantitative research and are further discussed in Chapter 9. Differences in observer roles depend on the degree of researcher involvement (intervention) or detachment (concealment) with participants (see Fig. 6.1).

With *complete participation*, the researcher is an accepted and established member of the community (or group or subgroup) under observation. Complete participation gives the researcher the best opportunity to observe behaviours as the researcher is part of the community. Most anthropological studies use this technique, as the researcher is already a member of the community or attempts to be invited into and accepted by the community.

Complete Participant
- Researcher is immersed in group/community (complete intervention)
- Research is usually concealed (covert)

Participant as Observer
- Researcher steps into and out of groups/community (intervention)
- Research is known (open)

Observer as Participant
- Researcher mainly observes but occasionally enters field (brief intervention)
- Research is known (open)

Complete Observer
- Researcher does not participate
- Research is either known (open) or concealed (covert)

Fig. 6.1 Different roles of the observer in observational research.

Sometimes it is not known by the community that the participant observer is a researcher (a form of concealment) to avoid disruption of normal activity. In a *participant-as-observer* role, the researcher is acting as both participant and observer, with this openness allowing productive relationships to develop with other participants and the researcher to step in and out of the research environment when they think it is best. With *observer-as-participant*, the researcher's role is made public/known, and the researcher is first an observer, with participation a secondary role—such as with Ottrey et al's (2019) previously mentioned study. As a *complete observer*, a researcher is confined to observations only and has no interaction with participants. In this role, the research study itself may or may not be revealed to the participants. There are major ethical implications for not revealing to people that they are being observed for research purposes and so examples, not just in nursing and midwifery, are rare. Sometimes, it may be planned that participants are informed after the research has finished. However, this is still considered an ethical challenge (see Chapter 13).

A further aspect of observation is in the 'positioning approach' that the observer adopts. These are classified as *single*, *multiple* or *mobile*. In *single* positioning the observer occupies one location only, so is less likely to distract participants or to be distracted. *Multiple* positioning allows the observer to move to different locations and view events from different angles/perspectives. *Mobile* positioning is needed in situations where the observer must follow participants wherever they go as they go about daily activities.

Another method of conducting observational study is using video recording. Decisions on how to record observational data depend on the focus of the research question and the analytical approach proposed. A main advantage of this approach is that the researcher can play the video over and over, aiding the data analysis process and reducing personal observational bias. This method can be used to observe behaviour in a naturalistic setting. For example, James et al (2020a, 2020b) used non-participatory video recordings to analyse lifestyle risk communication during consultations between nurses and patients in general practice. Non-verbal communication was analysed quantitatively, and qualitative content analysis (see Chapter 7) of communication techniques was undertaken using the audio data. Using non-participatory video observation allowed for specific behaviours to be observed, and context-driven issues such as spatial constraints and perceptions of intrusion by having a researcher present were largely avoided (James et al 2019).

Benefits of Observation

Observational/field research produces a wealth of different data in different contexts and in different ways—and uses a range of available techniques, especially in relation to positioning and role. With some techniques, such as video observation, James et al (2019) suggest that using video provides rich data where the volume of data can be overwhelming for the researcher. However, good dynamics between the practitioner, patient, technology or other members of the team are needed in order to support contextual understanding of dynamics and communication, as well as needs in skills development and reflective practice. Where researchers are also participants, observation allows them to reflect on and evaluate their own feelings about their experiences in the field. In this case, researchers can choose to either 'step back from' or 'be immersed in' situations.

Limitations of Observation

Given the visual/situational aspects of data collection in observation, which cannot always be anticipated or controlled, there may be concerns about privacy and confidentiality of participants. If researching from an 'objective/distant' stance, it is necessary to be aware that observation is more susceptible to 'subjective' interpretation by the researcher than is usually the case with interview data. The data are directly interpreted by the observer. Field notes are often likely to be written up following the observation event—potentially adding to the subjectivity of data. A further consideration is the *Hawthorne effect* (participant reactivity) in observational research methods. This effect is a well-known phenomenon whereby people who know that they are being researched (particularly when observed) tend to behave in different ways than they would normally—either to please the researcher or to present themselves in a different and possibly more positive way (see Chapter 9 for a more detailed account of this phenomenon).

Table 6.1 highlights some of the overall benefits and limitations of the main qualitative data collection methods.

RESEARCH IN BRIEF 6.3

Belle and Cook's (2023) Tasmanian ethnography study is titled 'I've got no idea': an ethnography of Critical Care Nurses' (CCN) observed nuanced and ambiguous professional identities in regional Australia. They explored how CCNs construct professional identity and subjectively experience nursing practice. Observations were conducted over 8 months with thirteen CNNs, which resulted in 45 fieldwork visits and a total of 92 hours of observation. During observations, fieldwork notes included detailing the interactions between CCNs and physicians, allied health professionals, patients and patient visitors, as well as actions, symbols, rituals and artefacts

Continued

RESEARCH IN BRIEF 6.3—cont'd

of the CCN's work environment. All CCNs participated in informal conversations during the fieldwork, with eight also participating in semistructured interviews, which were guided by findings from observations. The researchers describe their 'positioning themselves in the centre of action, focusing on details, and bringing theoretical questions into participant discussions'.

TUTORIAL TRIGGER 6.4

Devise a plan for observing chronically ill children in a paediatric ward. What type of observer/participant role/s would you employ? What might you expect to observe?

WHEN HAVE ENOUGH DATA BEEN COLLECTED?

Qualitative researchers often experience uncertainty when not being able to socially generalise their findings to wider populations owing to the small sample sizes often used. They will often state a limitation of their study as the 'small' sample size. This can be overcome when researchers 'feel' that they have enough information at hand or, alternatively, the emerging data becomes repetitive or uncovers nothing new. Where this is the case, researchers are collecting data until data 'saturation' (redundancy of data) is achieved (see Chapter 7). This may occur even with smaller sample sizes. Data saturation is not dependent on the amount of data collected but rather is based on the richness of the emerging data set. Controversy exists, though, over whether it is possible to achieve true data 'redundancy' or saturation (Mthuli et al 2022). Therefore the point at which this situation seems to occur will vary with each study and cannot be predicted. Once the researchers are reasonably satisfied that they have reached the point that no further data is required, data collection can cease and they can move on to the next stage in the qualitative research process—*data analysis*. In Hall et al's (2023) study, they recruited women who had a positive experience and had given birth in Australia in the previous 12 months for individual semistructured interviews. The study aimed to understand the

TABLE 6.1 Summary of Benefits and Limitations of Main Qualitative Data Collection Methods

Data Collection Methods	Benefits	Limitations
Individual interview	• Allows participants to express their own ideas. • Allows interviewer to be responsive to individual differences and situational circumstances.	• Minimal control over the order in which the topics are covered. • Usually small sample size limited due to cost and time.
Focus group interview	• Allows organised discussion structured in a flexible way. • Provides opportunity for all to participate and give their opinions. • Dominant and submissive participants can be directed and controlled. • Discussion generated between participants. • Large quantity of information collected in a short amount of time.	• Researcher has less control over the flow of discussion. • Facilitating focus group interviews requires considerable skill. • Difficult to distinguish between individual view and group view. • More difficult to organise and order data for analysis.
Involved observation	• Allows researcher immersion and prolonged involvement with participants. • Encourages free and open conversation with the participants.	• Altered behaviours of observed groups by the presence of the researcher. • Takes time to build trust with participants.
Detached observation	• Reveals descriptions of behaviours by stepping outside the group. • Allows identification of recurring patterns of behaviours that participants may be unable to recognise or reveal themselves.	• Potential researcher bias in the design of a study. • Sources or participants may not be equally credible. • Analysis of observation can be biased.

health system factors that promoted a positive childbearing experience. They conducted 36 interviews, at which point they concluded that data saturation had been reached.

SUMMARY

With qualitative research, sampling methods and methods of collecting data are a vital and integral component of study design. A number of different options are available, which, in turn, will determine the nature and approach of the research to be conducted—and the direction it takes. Attention to detail is required with both sampling and data collection processes. Errors in either are likely to affect overall study outcomes. The effectiveness of these processes greatly impacts on the next stage of qualitative design process: that of data analysis. Qualitative data analysis is the focus of the following chapter.

KEY POINTS

- A wide range of methods and techniques is used for both sampling and collecting data from the population sample of interest in qualitative research.
- The four main types of sampling used in qualitative research are *convenience* sampling, *purposive* sampling, *snowball* sampling and *theoretical* sampling.
- Choosing a sample size and sampling scheme and collecting data from the chosen sample should be an active process of reflection, which is central to qualitative research.
- Qualitative research mostly employs interviews (including focus groups) and/or observation to collect data from sample populations. Each has strengths and limitations.

TIME TO REFLECT

Tourangeau, A.E., Cummings, G., Cranley, L.A., et al., 2010. Determinants of hospital nurse intention to remain employed: broadening our understanding. J. Adv. Nurs. 66 (1), 22–32.

Aim: Tourangeau et al (2010) conducted a study to identify nurse-reported determinants of intention to remain employed and to develop a model explaining determinants of hospital nurse intention to remain employed.

Design: A descriptive qualitative study using focus group methodology was implemented.

Reflect on the following: Thirteen focus groups including 78 nurses were carried out in two Canadian provinces. Each focus group was led by two moderators consisting of a researcher and a research assistant. One moderator led the group and the other attended to participant needs, functioning and location of digital recorders and ensuring a comfortable environment. Focus groups were digitally recorded. A semistructured question guide was prepared that included one main question and several probing questions. Focus groups were opened with one question reflecting the study research question: 'What circumstances in your work or life influence your decision to remain in or leave employment in your job at this hospital?' Probing questions were developed based on current knowledge of determinants of intention to remain employed from the literature, but were not required. Moderators sought clarification intermittently.

Questions

1. What aspects of good focus group conduct are evident in the above description?
2. What further information would be helpful in assessing the quality of the process and impact on data collection?
3. What are the limitations of using focus groups for this particular research question?

LEARNING ACTIVITIES

1. In sampling, the inclusion criteria indicate:
   a. characteristics or properties of the chosen sample that the researcher would not want them to possess
   b. characteristics or properties of the chosen sample that the researcher would most want them to possess
   c. characteristics or properties of the sample that the researcher would find most attractive
   d. characteristics or properties of the chosen sample that the researcher would find least attractive.
2. Which group of participants below would represent a purposive sample?
   a. All the people working in a hospital
   b. Specialist nurses recommending other specialist nurses
   c. Specialist nurses working in intensive care
   d. All inpatients in a hospital
3. When sampling methods are applied to data already collected, this is called:
   a. data sampling
   b. information sampling
   c. theoretical sampling
   d. non-theoretical sampling.

4. What is the most common method used for collecting qualitative data?
   a. Questionnaire
   b. Interview
   c. Observation
   d. Survey
5. When interviewing, starting off with simple and broad questions to help ease the participant into the process is referred to as:
   a. nurturing
   b. channelling
   c. funnelling
   d. easing.
6. Observational methods can employ which of the following approaches?
   a. In-place participant; participant-as-observer; observer-as-participant; and absolute observer
   b. Complete participant; participant-as-observer; observer-as-participant; and complete observer
   c. Absolute participant; participant-as-observer; observer-as-participant; and in-place observer
   d. Complete participant; in-place observer; in-place participant; and complete observer.
7. Observation techniques are most commonly used in:
   a. phenomenology
   b. grounded theory
   c. historical research
   d. ethnography.
8. A qualitative researcher knows that it is not useful to collect any further data:
   a. when they sense that this is the case
   b. when the participants say that they have nothing more to say
   c. when data saturation/redundancy of data is reached
   d. when data overload is reached.
9. A form of methodological triangulation applies when:
   a. participants are mixed up
   b. different methods for collecting data are employed in the same study
   c. different methods for collecting data are employed in different studies
   d. the data collection methods are mixed up.
10. The Hawthorne effect, in observational research, is when:
    a. participants behave in different ways than they would normally
    b. participants are observed when the research is concealed from them
    c. the researcher becomes totally integrated into the community being researched
    d. there is more than one observer and observations are integrated for objectivity.

For further content associated with this chapter visit: https://evolve.elsevier.com/cs/product/9780729596794?role=student 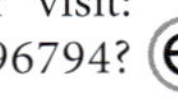

ADDITIONAL RESOURCES

Interviews and focus groups in qualitative research. www.qualres.org/HomeInte-3595.html.

Observation in qualitative research. https://www.qualitative-research.net/index.php/fqs/article/view/466/996.

Sampling in qualitative research. https://saylordotorg.github.io/text_principles-of-sociological-inquiry-qualitative-and-quantitative-methods/s10-02-sampling-in-qualitative-resear.html.

REFERENCES

Adcock, J.E., Sidebotham, M., Gamble, J., 2022. What do midwifery leaders need in order to be effective in contributing to the reform of maternity services? Women Birth 35 (2), e142–e152.

Addo, I.Y., Brener, L., Asante, A.D., et al., 2019. Determinants of post-migration changes in dietary and physical activity behaviours and implications for health promotion: evidence from Australian residents of sub-Saharan African ancestry. Health Promot. J. Austr. 30 (S1), 62–71.

Balcom, S., Doucet, S., Dubé, A., 2021. Observation and institutional ethnography: helping us to see better. Qual Health Res, 31(8), 1534–1541.

Belle, M.-J., Cook, P.S., 2023. 'I've got no idea': an ethnography of Critical Care Nurses' nuanced and ambiguous professional identities in regional Australia. Health Sociol. Rev. 32 (2), 129–144. doi:10.1080/14461242.2022.2091947

Bennetts, S.K., Hokke, S., Crawford, S., et al., 2019. Using paid and free Facebook methods to recruit Australian parents to an online survey: an evaluation. J. Med. Internet Res. 21 (3), e11206. doi:10.2196/11206

Braun, V., Clarke, V., Boulton, E., et al., 2021. The online survey as a qualitative research tool. Int. J. Soc. Res. Methodol. 24 (6), 641–654.

Brion, C., Rogers-Shaw, C., 2022. Becoming culturally proficient qualitative researchers by crossing geographic and methodological borders. Qual. Rep. 27 (10), 2091–2112.

Brunton, M., Cook, C., 2018. Dis/Integrating cultural difference in practice and communication: a qualitative study of host and migrant Registered Nurse perspectives from New Zealand. Int. J. Nurs. Stud. 83, 18–24.

Calma, K. R. B., Halcomb, E., Williams, A., et al., 2021. Final-year undergraduate nursing students' perceptions of general practice nursing: a qualitative study. J. Clin. Nurs. 30 (7–8), 1144–1153.

Campbell, S., McCalman, J., Redman-MacLaren, M., et al., 2018. Implementing the Baby One Program: a qualitative evaluation of family-centred child health promotion in remote Australian Aboriginal communities. BMC Pregnancy Childbirth 18, 73. doi:10.1186/s12884-018-1711-7

Campbell, S., Greenwood, M., Prior, S., et al., 2020. Purposive sampling: complex or simple? Research case examples. J. Res. Nurs. 25 (8), 652–661.

Carlson, E., Stenberg, M., Lai, T., et al., 2019. Nursing students' perceptions of peer learning through cross-cultural student-led webinars: a qualitative study. J. Adv. Nurs. 75, 1518–1526. doi:10.1111/jan.13983

Coleman, P. 2019. In-depth interviewing as a research method in healthcare practice and education: value, limitations and considerations. Int. J. Caring Sci. 12 (3), 1879–1885.

Creswell, J.W., Poth, C., 2018. Qualitative Inquiry and Research Design: choosing among five approaches, forty-second ed. Sage Publications, London, UK.

Doughty, L., McKillop, A., Dixon, R., et al., 2018. Educating new graduate nurses in their first year of practice: the perspective and experiences of the new graduate nurses and the director of nursing. Nurse Educ. Pract. 30, 101–105.

East, L., Jackson, D., Manias, E., et al., 2021. Patient perspectives and experiences of sexual health conversations and cardiovascular disease: a qualitative study. J. Clin. Nurs. 30 (21–22), 3194–3204.

Fauk, N. K., Ward, P. R., Hawke, K., et al., 2021. Cultural and religious determinants of HIV transmission: A qualitative study with people living with HIV in Belu and Yogyakarta, Indonesia. PLoS One 16 (11), e0257906–e0257906.

Flick, U., 2018. An Introduction to Qualitative Research, sixth ed. Sage Publications, London, UK.

Foster, M., Whitehead, L., 2018. Using drawings to understand the child's experience of child-centred care on admission to a pediatric high dependency unit. J. Child. Health Care 23 (1), 102–117. doi:10.1177/1367493518778389

Gauci, P., Peters, K., O'Reilly, K., et al., 2022. The experience of workplace gender discrimination for women registered nurses: a qualitative study. J. Adv. Nurs. 78 (6), 1743–1754.

Guthrie, T. M., de Jersey, S. J., New, K., 2020. Midwife readiness to provide woman-centred weight gain support: exploring perspectives across models of care. Women Birth 33 (6), e567–e573.

Hall, H., Fooladi, E., Kloester, J., et al., 2023. Factors that promote a positive childbearing experience: a qualitative study. J. Midwifery Womens Health. 68, 44–51. doi:10.1111/jmwh.13402

Hibberson, M., Lawton, J., Whitehead, D., 2023. Multidisciplinary simulation training for perioperative teams: a qualitative descriptive exploratory study. J. Periop. Nurs. in press.

Ho, I. C., Chenoweth, L., Williams, A., 2021. Older people's experiences of living with, responding to and managing sensory loss. Healthcare 9 (3), 329.

Holloway, I., Galvin, K. 2023. Qualitative Research in Nursing and Healthcare, fifth ed. Wiley-Blackwell, London, UK.

Huang, C., Lam, L., Plummer, V., et al., 2021. Feeling responsible: family caregivers' attitudes and experiences of shared decision-making regarding people diagnosed with schizophrenia: a qualitative study. Patient Educ. Counsel.104 (7), 1553–1559.

Irani, E., 2019. The use of videoconferencing for qualitative interviewing: opportunities, challenges, and considerations. Clin. Nurs. Res. 28 (1), 3–8. doi:10.1177/1054773818803170

Isaacs, A.N., 2014. An overview of qualitative research methodology for public health researchers. Int. J. Med. Public Health 4, 318–323.

James, S , Desborough, J., McInnes, S., et al., 2019. Strategies for using non-participatory video research methods in general practice. Nurse Res. 27(2), 32–37.

James, S., Desborough, J., McInnes, S., et al., 2020a. Nonverbal communication between registered nurses and patients during chronic disease management consultations: Observations from general practice. J. Clin. Nurs. 29 (13–14), 2378–2387.

James, S., McInnes, S., Halcomb, E., et al., 2020b. Lifestyle risk factor communication by nurses in general practice: understanding the interactional elements. J. Adv. Nurs. 76 (1), 234–242.

James, S., Ashley, C., Williams, A., et al., 2021. Experiences of Australian primary healthcare nurses in using telehealth during COVID-19: a qualitative study. BMJ Open 11 (8), e049095.

Jenkins, M., Hoek, J., Jenkin, G., et al., 2021. Silver linings of the COVID-19 lockdown in New Zealand. PLoS One 16 (4), e0249678.

Kross, J , Giust, A., 2019. Elements of research questions in relation to qualitative inquiry. Qual. Rep. 24 (1), 24–30.

Krueger, R.A., Casey, M.A., 2015. Focus Groups: a practical guide for applied research, fourth ed. Sage Publications, London, UK.

McCullough, K., Whitehead, L ., Bayes, S ., et al., 2021. Remote area nursing: best practice or paternalism in action? The importance of consumer perspectives on primary health care nursing practice in remote communities. Aust. J. Primary Health 27, 62–66.

Merriam, S.B., Grenier, R.S., 2019. Qualitative Research in Practice: examples for discussion and analysis. Jossey-Bass, San Francisco, CA.

Morse, J.M., 1995. The significance of saturation. Qual. Health Res. 5, 147–149.

Mthuli S.A., Ruffin, F., Singh, N. (2022). 'Define, Explain, Justify, Apply' (DEJA): an analytic tool for guiding qualitative research sample size. Int. J. Soc. Res. Methodol. 25 (6), 809–821.

O'Neill, J., Devsam, B., Kinney, S., et al., 2023. Exploring the impact of the COVID-19 environment on nursing delivery of family-centred care in a paediatric hospital. J. Adv. Nurs.79, 320–331. doi:10.1111/jan.15469

Ottrey, E., Porter, J., Huggins, C.E., et al., 2019. Ward culture and staff relationships at hospital mealtimes in Australia: an ethnographic account. Nurs. Health Sci. 21, 78–84. doi:10.1111/nhs.12559

Quinney, L., Dwyer, T., Chapman, Y., 2018. Professional insights from nurses who are carers for family with chronic illness: a phenomenological approach. Collegian 25 (3), 263–269.

Rees, C.E., Crampton, P., Kent, F., et al., 2018. Understanding students' and clinicians' experiences of informal interprofessional workplace learning: an Australian qualitative study. BMJ Open 8, e021238. doi:10.1136/bmjopen-2017-02123

Rogan, A., Lockett, J., Peckler, B., et al., 2022. Exploring nursing and medical perceptions of sepsis management in a New

Zealand emergency department: a qualitative study. Emerg. Med. Australas, 34 (3), 417–427.

Staps, C., Crowe, M., Lacey, C., 2019. Effective care for Māori with bipolar disorder: a qualitative study. Int. J. Ment. Health Nurs. 28, 776–783. doi:10.1111/inm.12582

Stevens, J., Schmeid, V., Burns, E., et al., 2018. Who owns the baby? A video ethnography of skin-to-skin contact after a caesarean section. Women Birth 31 (6), 453–462.

Tourangeau, A.E., Cummings, G., Cranley, L.A., et al., 2010. Determinants of hospital nurse intention to remain employed: broadening our understanding. J. Adv. Nurs. 66 (1), 22–32.

Younas, A., Porr, C., Maddigan, J., et al., 2023. Behavioural indicators of compassionate nursing care of individuals with complex needs: a naturalistic inquiry. J. Clin. Nurs. 32, 4024–4036. doi:10.1111/jocn.16542

7

Analysing Data in Qualitative Research

Stephen Neville and Dean Whitehead

LEARNING OUTCOMES

After reading this chapter, you should be able to:

- recognise the major styles of qualitative data analysis
- describe common processes involved with coding, categorising and comparing qualitative data
- identify strategies used for analysis in narrative research and discourse analyses
- consider options for organising qualitative data and managing qualitative data analysis
- identify strategies that enhance trustworthiness of a qualitative study
- describe qualitative meta-synthesis
- consider options for presentation and dissemination of qualitative results.

KEY TERMS

categorising, p. 103
coding, p. 103
concept analysis, p. 106
conceptual ordering, p. 102
content analysis, p. 105
discourse analysis, p. 106
explanatory schema, p. 98
inductive reasoning, p. 98
narrative analysis, p. 106
qualitative data analysis, p. 97
thematic analysis, p. 105
trustworthiness, p. 108

INTRODUCTION

Qualitative data analysis is the formal interpretation of collected qualitative data to create order, elicit meaning and communicate findings. It can be challenging because it involves large amounts of data and requires considerable time for ordering and interpreting the data. As Lester et al (2020 p. 94) state, 'Part of this challenge is due to the seemingly limitless approaches that a qualitative researcher might leverage, as well as simply learning to *think* like a qualitative researcher when analyzing data'. There is no 'one size fits all' method for analysis and therefore the researcher is required to be deliberate, considered and systematic while applying abstract and conceptual thinking. As there is no single approach, the process requires careful planning and reflection before implementation. Despite these challenges, it is well worth the effort, as results add richness to the unique nursing and midwifery body of knowledge directed at improving clinical outcomes.

This chapter discusses the key issues relevant to analysing qualitative data. Initially, three major aspects of **qualitative data analysis** are presented: *coding and categorising, constant comparison* and *thematic analysis*. In addition, the chapter clarifies the data analysis process for those using narrative and discursive methodologies which collect qualitative data from existing material (e.g. journal texts). This is then followed by discussion of a relatively recent approach to using qualitative research within a systematic review process: *meta-synthesis*. Finally, there is consideration of trustworthiness (research rigour) and ways of reporting and disseminating qualitative results.

KEY ISSUES IN THE ANALYSIS OF QUALITATIVE DATA

Defining Qualitative Data Analysis

There are a number of different strategies that can be applied to qualitative data analysis where the chosen method is a result of the researcher's philosophical/theoretical approach and research design (see Chapter 2). Whatever approach is used requires active engagement with initial and emerging data through analytical processes to find new meanings. What is important to note is that most qualitative data analysis approaches are matched to the research methodology that underpins them—that is, interpretative phenomenological analysis (IPA) (see later in this chapter).

Table 7.1 presents an overview of some common qualitative methodologies (see Chapter 5 also) and the analytical processes generally associated with them. Qualitative researchers can choose to use set processes related to particular methods. However, sometimes the research context is not well suited to limiting the data analysis to only one strategy or a single way of undertaking the data analytical process. This is a distinct advantage of qualitative research in that there exist different interpretations and the flexibility to adapt to different 'social' circumstances (Bettez 2015). However, this does not suggest that 'any' methodology or method can be used. Instead, the researcher always chooses the most appropriate data analytical strategy that best suits the methodology used and is closely aligned to the way the qualitative data has been collected.

What can be challenging for the novice/early career qualitative researcher is understanding the terminology used. This is the same for research language overall. There can be many words or terms used for similar (or dissimilar) concepts or processes—such as different types of coding, labelling, categorisation and memoing. Table 7.2 provides a list of commonly used words and terms in qualitative data analysis (and their definitions) to assist.

Reasoning Processes in Qualitative Data Analysis

A key feature of qualitative data analysis is the application of **inductive reasoning**, which generates ideas from the collected data. This type of reasoning is the counter logic to *deductive reasoning* used in quantitative data analysis (see Chapter 11). The qualitative researcher works with the data to develop insightful interpretations (explanations and interpretations) and requires the skills of comprehension, synthesis, theorising, reflection and recontextualising. The researcher is involved in developing an understanding of the phenomenon being investigated through creating a schematic picture (**explanatory schema**) that accounts for relationships between related concepts, explaining why these relationships occur and then relating this new knowledge back to previously developed knowledge (Merriam & Grenier 2019).

TABLE 7.1 Comparison of Approaches to Data Analysis of Popular Qualitative Methodologies

Research Approach	Research Focus	Type of Data	Analysis Strategies
Grounded theory	Human action and interaction	Anything relevant to the study can be data: • interviews • observations • field notes	Coding (open, axial, selective) • Categorisation • Constant comparison
Phenomenology	The experience and meaning of phenomena	Texts, e.g. interview transcripts	Coding • Categorisation • Thematising • Interpreting
Ethnography	The social organisation of experience	Anything relevant to the study: • interviews • observations • field notes	Coding • Categorising • Interpreting
Narrative	How individuals construct understanding of an event	Individuals' stories (usually interviews)	Coding • Thematising • Restorying
Descriptive exploratory	Explanation of phenomena	Anything relevant to the study: • interviews • observations • objects and artefacts • documents	Coding • Content analysis • Summarising

TABLE 7.2 Commonly Used Terms in Qualitative Data Analysis

Term	Definition
Categorisation	The logical grouping of concepts emerging from the data.
Core category	The central category that is used to integrate all the categories identified during analysis in grounded theory research.
Coding	Transforming the raw data into a standardised layout for analysis, through identifying and labelling recurrent words, themes or concepts.
Axial coding	In grounded theory, following open coding, the data are reassembled as categories are developed.
Open coding	In grounded theory, the process of identifying and labelling concepts.
Selective	Selection of the core category, which integrates all the other major categories.
Theoretical	Conceptualisation of how the substantive codes in grounded theory may be related to one another as hypotheses to be integrated into the theory.
Conceptual ordering	The process of organising data into discrete categories according to the identified underlying meanings.
Constant comparison	A process fundamental to grounded theory analysis where the data are collected and coded, and simultaneously analysed by comparing with other pieces of data, then more data are collected and analysed in the same manner and so on.
Content analysis	A type of analysis where the researcher counts and reports the frequency of concepts/words/behaviours found in the data.
Diagramming	Making visual representation of the linkages emerging from the data.
Explanatory schema	A framework or concept that organises and interprets data.
Field notes	Notes or memos made during or after observation of a specific phenomenon. They help the researcher remember the behaviours, activities and events observed. They can become data for the analysis.
Inductive analysis	A process of logical thought in which generalisations are developed from specific observations.
Iterative process	Repeatedly returning to the data, e.g. undertaking a preliminary analysis, using that to guide the next phase of data collection, and continuing in this manner until data collection is complete.
Memoing	Making notes during data collection and analysis. The notes track the researcher's thinking and can guide the final conceptualisation. These can also become data.
Coding memos	Recording why a concept label was applied to a section of the data.
Theoretical memos	Thoughts about possible connections between concepts.
Saturation	A point of 'diminishing returns', i.e. analysis of new data only serves to confirm the conclusions already reached.

Methodological Assumptions Underpinning Qualitative Data Analysis

The choices that researchers make with respect to relevant data collection and analysis are influenced by their methodological assumptions—that is, their theoretical stance and/or philosophical perspective. Researchers might have a prechosen *theoretical framework* (e.g. symbolic interactionism) or a theoretical stance related to the study's purpose (e.g. in feminist research—see Chapter 5 for both). They may also adopt a philosophical stance—as with various phenomenological approaches (again see Chapter 5). In either situation, the data will most likely be collected, viewed and analysed through a 'theoretical lens', where aspects of the theory/philosophy guide the researcher as to what is most important in the data (Nguyen et al 2022). For example, Neville et al (2018) used an environmental gerontological theoretical framework to demonstrate how the physical environment influences older people's ability to engage in their local community. In addition to *theoretical frameworks*, the reader may come across the related term of *conceptual frameworks*. The two terms are often used interchangeably. However, there are notable differences—for example, theoretical frameworks are 'established' and may have been 'tested'. In contrast, conceptual frameworks are often newly developed and/or evolving before they become established. For instance, Lukewich et al (2022) adopt the Organization for Economic Cooperation and Development (OECD) Patient Reported Indicator Surveys (PaRIS) conceptual framework to investigate the effectiveness of Registered Nurses on patient outcomes in primary care.

When Is Qualitative Data Analysis Performed?

In quantitative research, data are analysed following data collection. However, with qualitative research there are potentially three different strategies for the timing of analysis. These are:

1. *Analysis is a separate step following data collection*—here the focus is on the complete data set that has been collected or already exists. This is common, for example, in phenomenology, discourse analysis and narrative research (see Chapter 5).
2. *Analysis occurs simultaneously with data collection*—in this method some data are collected then analysed, then more data are collected and analysed and so on. This approach is a distinctive feature of grounded theory. The amount of data collected before and between analyses varies.
3. *Phased data collection and analysis*—in this scenario one type of data collection, such as interviews or focus groups, is completed and analysed before proceeding to the next type of data collection—such as a quantitative survey questionnaire. This approach is commonly found in mixed-method/method triangulation research designs which use both qualitative and quantitative approaches in a single study (see Chapter 12). It can also be found in 'multimethod' approaches which use a single-paradigm approach—that is, two different qualitative approaches/data collection methods in the same study (again see Chapter 12).

> **TUTORIAL TRIGGER 7.1**
>
> 1. What factors make qualitative research challenging and need consideration before/when undertaking it?
> 2. The terms 'analysis' and 'interpretation' are often used interchangeably. What is the difference between them? Why has 'interpretive description' become an increasingly popular approach to qualitative data analysis?

CONDUCTING QUALITATIVE DATA ANALYSIS: GENERAL PRINCIPLES

Conducted properly, qualitative data are subject to intense scrutiny. It is as though the researcher were using a microscope during analysis to look for different aspects, which may or may not be related to one another, to address the study research question/s. Here, the researcher's 'theoretical lens' about the human experience is shaped and ultimately understood using spoken or written language.

With most specific approaches there are guidelines for data analysis that can be selected and followed. For instance, when using grounded theory methods there are established, contemporary analysis guidelines as well as more recent variations and modifications. The fundamental feature of grounded theory, as noted in Table 7.2, is the *constant comparative method* (Belgrave & Seide 2019). With this method, concepts are developed from the data through coding and analysing at the same time using multiple stages of collecting while refining and categorising the data (see later). In contrast, with phenomenological data analysis for instance, rather than using set processes for data analysis, frameworks can be used as 'guides'—for example, Colaizzi's (Wirihana et al 2018) and van Manen's (van Manen 2023) analytical frameworks. Sheikhnezhad et al (2023) report their study on the blaming experiences of women with breast cancer who have been subjected to intimate partner violence, which is informed by using van Manen's analytical approach.

When undertaking descriptive, exploratory qualitative research (see Chapter 5), it is recommended that researchers use an approach that best suits answering the research question or addressing the research aim. The researcher is not 'tied' to a specific analytical framework or technique. When using this approach, data analysis is referred to as being data driven, and mainly inductive, and the findings should be easily understood by consumers of the research (Doyle et al 2020). However, in most cases this requires using either a content or thematic analytical approach. As noted previously, the chosen data analytical framework is at the discretion of the researcher, but it must be congruent with the methodological framework used in the research.

If the purpose of a study is to increase our understanding of a participant's experience of a phenomenon, then this type of research usually provides 'themes' that are explained fully and often written in a narrative form—like a story. Macdiarmid et al (2020) used this approach to gain insights into the health professional's experience of facilitating debriefing following a simulated experience in New Zealand. In this hermeneutic phenomenological study, 10 health professionals participated in face-to-face interviews and were asked to describe their experiences using a conversational style approach to data collection. Hermeneutic phenomenology requires data collection and data analysis to occur at the same time. Data analysis used an iterative process that required in-depth engagement with the interview material. Following this, findings were developed and presented as stories. These stories were presented as 'Getting started', 'Supporting the debrief to unfold' and 'Knowing when to end'.

Most approaches to conducting research will position the literature review (see Chapter 2) as being undertaken before data collection; however, this is not always the case. For example, with grounded theory there is some debate about the timing of the literature review. In classic grounded theory, it is recommended that the literature review not be undertaken before data analysis or even until codes and categories are beginning to emerge. It is argued that this prevents researcher bias in predetermining the emerging theory. An alternative perspective recommends that a preliminary review of the literature is taken before commencing the study, which is later expanded on, or a secondary review is written while undertaking data collection and analysis (Soa-Diaz & Valverde-Berrocoso 2022).

TEAM APPROACH OR WORKING ALONE?

Qualitative data analysis can be performed by one researcher. For instance, Nowell et al (2017) report their single-author study related to mentorship in nursing academia.

It should be noted, however, this is becoming far less common. Qualitative studies are far more likely to involve more than one researcher, as in Jedwab et al's (2022) study on understanding nurses' perceptions of barriers and enablers to use of a new electronic medical record system in Australia. That study's data were analysed by five team members adopting a deductive content analysis approach aligned to the 14-domain Theoretical Domains Framework.

There is a common agreement that analysis by several people is preferable. This assumes that multiple viewpoints will produce results that are more accurate or a richer description of the phenomenon under investigation, as well as lessen the chance of individual bias. It is also argued that group analysis produces results that are more consistent and reliable. This is not always the case, though. Sometimes, a singular subjectivity is more likely to produce a single-reality outcome that may be preferred by the researcher.

When a group/team conducts qualitative data analysis, several potential strategies exist, including the following:

- One researcher (or more) will do all or part of the analysis, then provide the results to the other team members who view those results prior to or during their analysis of data. This might be done separately or collectively, with further communication and negotiation until agreement is achieved—for example, Irani et al's (2018) study on how home health nurses plan their workday.
- The researchers conduct the analysis separately then, afterwards, discuss until agreement is reached—for example, in Salamonson et al's (2018) exploration of the experiences of first-year undergraduate students trying to work and study at the same time. Each of the researchers independently analysed the interview transcripts then compared and discussed their individual findings until consensus was reached. Overall, consensus related to the classification and naming of the themes.

ANALYSING QUALITATIVE DATA ACCORDING TO THE WAY DATA WERE COLLECTED

Qualitative research data can be collected in various ways, such as audio or video recording, observation, field notes, documents, letters and photographs. Audio recordings are usually transcribed into a written form for closer investigation and coding; this may occur with video recordings as well. Data such as works of art, photographs or documents/reports may not be recorded and are often directly interpreted. For example, underpinned by a qualitative participatory research design, Dixon et al (2022) used a 'photo-voice' technique combined with semistructured interviews to explore women's experiences of participating in a women-only mental health prevention and recovery program in Australia. In this study, participants were asked to take pictures that represented their experiences of engaging in the program.

In all cases, the process of data analysis needs to be appropriate and aligned to the style of data collection and recording. For instance, a line-by-line analysis may be sufficient in transcribing an audio recording but would not be appropriate for a transcribed video recording as non-verbal body language data would be lost. Ethnographical fieldwork and observational data will often fall into this category of 'non-verbal' data. For instance, Stevens et al (2018) used a video ethnography in their Australian midwifery study exploring skin-to-skin contact between mother and baby following caesarean section. No matter what the method chosen for the collection and translation of audible or visual data into the written form, it remains an interpretive process requiring the researcher to justify decisions about the level of detail and how to represent the data (Holloway & Galvin 2017).

COMPLEMENTARY PROCESSES THAT AID DATA ANALYSIS

Depending on the research approach used, there may be complementary processes that assist overall analysis—such as writing different types of memos (i e. coding memos, theoretical memos, operational or 'field' notes; see Table 7.2).

An example of a complementary process may be using diagrams/maps to convey understanding about the research focus or phenomenon. This can be helpful when working out possible links between concepts while thinking about them and placing them in order (**conceptual ordering**). Williams et al (2018) provide an example of 'situational maps' that helped make sense of online narratives about people who live with an eating disorder. These situational maps resulted from a creative process utilising data collected, prior knowledge and literature related to the topic. This mapping approach allowed the complexities of living with an eating disorder—including the fear associated with disclosure, the challenges of having an eating disorder and the stigmatisation experienced—to be explored. Situational maps illustrate who and what are involved in the phenomenon of interest, why they are and how they became involved, and what would make a difference to the situation under investigation (Williams et al 2018). These are often presented diagrammatically and commonly featured alongside the written results of a study. Kimmerle et al (2023) use situational analysis and mapping to illustrate the emergence of a new early childhood intervention with paediatric nurses. They highlight that the mapping strategies were harnessed to structure discourse material to show the positioning of different elements in the professional 'arena'.

MANAGING DATA ANALYSIS

Manual Analysis

Qualitative research can generate vast amounts of 'raw' data. Transcribing an interview is time consuming and can take up to 10 hours per hour of talk/narrative. It is likely to produce many pages of physical text, which is the beginning of the manual data analytical process. Manual analysis can be undertaken when data is produced either as paper copies of the text or saved as a 'Word' file or other computer-based documents—but some 'traditionalists' prefer paper-based methods. Using paper-based methods can be problematic in relation to recording the analysis process, reanalysis, linkages between analyses and sorting of analyses for conceptual ordering. Manual analysis, while designed to be thorough and immersive, is also time consuming and labour intensive.

The researcher can choose a range of visual paper-based strategies when sorting and connecting different data-related interpretations and outcomes. For instance, different coloured cards, index files or labelling stickers can have concepts or memos written onto them and then sorted into different patterns or hierarchies and placed visually on large noticeboards, tabletops, etc. Online 'whiteboard' software, such as Miro, can potentially be used (https://miro.com/).

Single or multiple manual systems can be used throughout qualitative data analysis, although a key message is to keep things as simple and accessible as is possible, noting that access may be required over long periods of time—especially if using larger sample sizes and/or collecting qualitative data over time.

Software Analysis

An increasing number of qualitative researchers are now using *computer-assisted qualitative data analysis software* (CAQDAS) packages. CAQDAS are now accepted tools for data analysis as they reduce the time involved in managing data and allow the researcher to spend more time immersed in the actual analysis. However, computer software cannot replace the human intuitive and reflective processes needed to analyse qualitative data, and there are those who caution that there is a danger that the 'tool' replaces the thought processes that are essential to conceptualising and mapping qualitative data analysis (Rodik & Primorac 2015). A wide range of CAQDAS packages are now available such as NVivo, ATLAS.ti and MAXQDA. Whole texts, such as those written by Jackson and Bazeley (2019), are devoted to using and applying such software. These software programs assist with condensing, organising and managing the vast amounts of qualitative research data generated through the storage of data in multiple recorded forms (including aural, visual, video and word forms) within a large-capacity project file and subfiles where:

- labels for concepts interpreted from data can be recorded next to data
- linkages are recorded with relationships able to be created and displayed visually and flexibly
- hierarchies of conceptual ordering can be developed, diagrammed, recorded and reformed; reanalyses are facilitated
- memos can be recorded and linked to data or analyses
- tables, pictures and images can be imported
- data security is maintained
- quantitative data analyses can be connected to qualitative data analyses (see Chapter 12, 'Mixed-methods research')
- analyses by different people or different projects can be merged
- navigation around the project file and subfiles is relatively easy.

Although CAQDAS programs perform similar functions, there are some differences, and some may be better suited to specific methodologies. For example, the *Ethnograph* package was designed specifically for ethnographic analysis and assists in the management and analysis of text-based data such as transcripts of interviews, field notes and diaries. Sometimes the decision on which CAQDAS to use is purely pragmatic (e.g. a particular program is already available or there is previous experience). This was the case with Rogan et al's (2021) qualitative descriptive study exploring nursing and medical perceptions of sepsis management in a New Zealand emergency department. Thematic analysis was performed with the aid of NVivo 12 software.

TUTORIAL TRIGGER 7.2

What might be the disadvantages for a novice qualitative researcher using a CAQDAS program to organise data and manage data collection?

WRITING UP DATA ANALYSIS

In quantitative research, data analysis is completed before writing the results into a report. In qualitative research studies, by contrast, data analysis typically continues as the findings are being written into a report. With some qualitative research approaches, such as phenomenology, writing and rewriting are considered an essential part of the reading and reflection needed for thematic analysis. During the writing phase, the need for further refinement of categories, conceptualisations or interpretive work may need to be undertaken. In most cases, writing is a mechanism that assists with providing clarity and meaning about what the data are saying. This process also assists the researcher with determining when *data saturation* (the point where no new information is noted) is reached and analysis is viewed as complete. In Mayes et al's (2018) Australian exploration of midwives' and doctors' views on STan analysis monitoring (ST-Analysis (STan) is a technology that adds information to conventional fetal monitoring (cardiotocography) during labour), interviews were conducted until data saturation was deemed reached at the 15th participant—but continued until the 18th participant to ensure that all clinical roles were represented.

METHODS OF DATA ANALYSIS

The research methodology that underpins the research project will determine the data analytical process to be undertaken. Consequently, there are a variety of approaches to qualitative data analysis. Rather than attempt to provide a 'recipe' or formula for qualitative data analysis, the following section provides an overview of key steps undertaken in the overall processes.

Getting to Know the Data

Following 'verbatim' (as it is) transcription of the collected narrative/documentation, the researcher is often left with a voluminous amount of data to make sense of. The first step in the data analytical process is to begin to make sense of the data (sense-meaning), or to develop what can be referred to as 'first impressions' of the data. This is an important component as it requires researchers to immerse themselves in the data (Borkan 2021). Reading and rereading are key tasks associated with data immersion. This process can be at the level of each word, each line (line-by-line analysis), each sentence, each paragraph, etc.—or all levels—and sets the researcher up for the following stages of coding. It depends on the adopted strategy (and can be dictated by the methodology) as to whether this process occurs separately with each transcript and/or across all the interview/observation transcripts.

Coding and Categorising

The second stage in the data analytical process, and one that is common to many qualitative methodologies, is **coding** and **categorising**. The first step is to divide the data into abstract 'bits' called 'codes'. This requires close reading, understanding and then interrogation of the data—which should have already occurred in the initial 'getting to know your data' phase. If using written data, such as transcripts, this would mean once again reading and rereading them to identify and label recurrent words, ideas and concepts. With written forms of data, usually after having read the whole transcript at least once, there are two fundamental methods for coding:

1. *line-by-line code*—carefully examining words, phrases, or sentences for data relevant to the overall research question.
2. *scanning paragraphs for units of meaning relevant to answering the research question, which are then denoted (or abstracted) into descriptive codes*—there may be several such denotations per paragraph or perhaps none.

When found, the 'bit' of data is denoted into codes—that is, another word, or words (terms), that is an interpretation of emerging insights. Sometimes the words in the data are abstract enough and cannot be improved upon (i.e. represented in another form). The codes are then marked onto the transcripts or field notes and a separate list of the codes is created with a short definition; this is sometimes termed the 'attributes' of the code (Miles et al 2019).

After line-by-line coding the abstracted codes are then grouped logically—'like with like'—and a tentative 'label' is allocated. This process is called **categorisation**. This may commence quite early on or might only be done after all data are coded. The categories are labelled to signify the interpretation represented by the grouping of the codes. The categories may be temporary as there might be revision in the light of further analysis and the labels may be changed to enhance clarity, or abandoned as the codes are recategorised, and some might be 'collapsed' together—that is, two or three similar and related codes become one overall representative code (Lester et al 2020).

The final step is to establish relationships conceptually by establishing a hierarchy of categories and subcategories. A category will tend to have multiple subcategories; sometimes there may be more than two levels in the hierarchy, with the third level sometimes referred to as 'properties' of the subcategory. Thus, there may be categories, subcategories and properties of subcategories. It is possible that the processes of coding, categorising and conceptual 'ordering' (establishing hierarchies) will be cyclical, with the researcher moving back and forth from one to the other—rather than there being discrete linear steps (Locke et al 2022). Overall, the relationships identified are extensively explored and reduced to the least number of categories possible for overall sense making and manageability. When the researcher's carefully considered opinion is that data have been coded, categorised and conceptually ordered satisfactorily, data analysis will stop. Jarden et al (2019) used a six-phase content-driven inductive approach to their analysis related to workplace wellbeing perceptions of Australasian intensive care nurses. After initial coding, categorised codes were developed at three levels consistent with the initial probe questions.

Some research approaches specify what type of coding should be conducted and how this is to be done. For instance, in the classic grounded theory method (see Chapter 5), two forms of coding, 'open' and 'theoretical', are required (see Table 7.2). *Open coding* (involving some coding and categorisation) is the process of looking for underlying meaning and uniform patterns in and across data. *Theoretical coding*—a type of conceptual ordering—involves connecting concepts that have arisen from open coding. The connections between concepts are related to the overarching 'core' category as relationships between categories, subcategories and their properties are analysed.

With grounded theory, other sets of guidelines might direct a different way to code. For instance, following open coding, *axial coding* may take place, where relationships between the 'open codes' are identified. It is termed 'axial' because coding occurs around the axis of a category, with categories and subcategories being linked (Youn-Joo & Yun-Jung 2022). Additionally, a form of theoretical coding is possible, termed *selective coding*. Here a central, organising category is identified and data are selectively coded to this core variable.

It is also possible to start qualitative data analysis with a predetermined list of codes and then search for examples of data that fit into these codes, referred to as *deductive coding* (Reynolds et al 2022). This process is a bit like using a 'pigeonhole' in a mailroom: the pigeonhole is the pre-existing code into which relevant bits of data are slotted (counted and coded). With some forms of 'content analysis' this style may be required, especially when there are many data sources, and several people are needed to do the analysis (multiple coders). Usually, the codes are developed from a range of opinions, previously reported research or as suggested by experts. Potentially, in this instance, the interview questions (or observation guidelines) are designed to focus on each separate code. The codes may also already be grouped into categories that predate analysis.

TUTORIAL TRIGGER 7.3—GROUP EXERCISE

Each person in the tutorial writes a paragraph about their first clinical placement (either as an undergraduate or as a new graduate): what were the challenges? Leave a large margin on the right-hand side of the paragraph and then exchange that paragraph with another person's paragraph. It is then exchanged with another person's paragraph and so on. Analysis of these data is done solo—keeping the descriptive exploratory research question in mind: 'What were the challenges encountered in the first clinical placement?' Perform line-by-line coding of relevant data, placing the labelled codes in the wide margin. Collectively as a group, share the codes generated and then list on a whiteboard. Next, collectively categorise the codes (i.e. place like-codes into groups, giving each category an appropriate label). From here, observe whether 'naturally occurring' themes arise (see next section).

RESEARCH IN BRIEF 7.1

Gautam et al (2022) used a grounded theory approach to provide a theoretical explanation of how older adults seek and maintain connections when living in residential aged care. Data were collected through undertaking digitally recorded face-to-face interviews with 17 older people residing in a residential aged care facility in Nepal. The writing of memos that captured the researchers' ideas and reflections occurred alongside the interviews. Data collection and data analysis occurred simultaneously. Analysis of the interviews and memos involved line-by-line analysis to develop codes and constant comparison of these codes to establish categories. An ongoing and iterative process involving open, axial and selective

RESEARCH IN BRIEF 7.1—cont'd

coding processes resulted in the emergence of one core category supported by the meanings inherent in the data. This core category formed the foundation for the naming of the emergent theory entitled 'seeking connections'. This research found that older adults living in residential aged care 'seek connections' through the subcategories of 'identifying sources', 'developing connections' and 'appraising responses'. In their article, findings were depicted diagrammatically and through the use of data excerpts.

TYPES OF QUALITATIVE ANALYSIS

Thematic Analysis

Thematic analysis is widely utilised in qualitative research as a process for condensing, organising, analysing, describing and reporting themes (patterns) identified in a data set (Braun et al 2019). This style of analysis treats the data set as a 'corpus' of information that can be best understood as a whole, rather than by breaking it up into small abstracted sections. The analysis process is about understanding the overall themes evident in the data set. These themes, then, can be uncovered only by 'having a feel' for the overall meaning of the whole set of data. A theme is broader than a category because it appears consistently throughout the data set as a central idea/s.

Thematic analysis requires becoming familiar with the data through a method appropriate to the data (e.g. reading and rereading if working with written or spoken narrative/words). The researcher then goes back to the data for further analysis and reflection and so on, until 'meaning making' occurs—that is, the data becomes less abstract and the overall picture emerges. Data analysis, in this sense, is termed *iterative*. This means that the researcher is moving back and forth over the data rather than in linear steps (Locke et al 2022). This style of data analysis is useful for both specific and general approaches to undertaking qualitative data analysis, including phenomenology, as well as qualitative descriptive and interpretive methodologies. It is worth noting that Braun et al (2019) identify thematic analysis as an umbrella term that is distinguished by distinct conceptualisations of what a theme is as well as, sometimes, radically different methods for theme identification and development—alongside coding.

Content Analysis

Content analysis is the other main approach to analysing qualitative data after thematic analysis. Historically, content analysis has its origins within the quantitative paradigm and was used exclusively as a means of 'counting' the occurrence of phenomena. Graneheim et al (2017 p. 29), however, state 'content analysis has changed from a counting game to a more interpretative approach'. Modifications to how content analysis can be used have been expanded to include the analysis of qualitative data and it is now widely used (Kleinheksel et al 2020). This method means that qualitative data can be analysed either inductively or deductively (as well as *abductively*—generating theory from qualitative observation). This is the same type of approach that can be incorporated into grounded theory.

Like thematic analysis, content analysis uses a set of techniques to analyse textual/narrative data that brings together similarities evident across data sets (Vears & Gillam 2022). However, content analysis differs from thematic analysis in that it creates meaningful units, subcategories and categories to explain the phenomena, which can then be presented as a theme. Bengtsson (2016) helpfully identifies four main steps to be followed when undertaking content analysis. These are *decontextualisation*, *recontextualisation*, *categorisation* and *compilation* of the data. A main aim, therefore, is to uncover the logic of how themes and categories are interpreted, abstracted and connected to the main aim and outcomes. As with thematic analysis, content analysis can be used for specific as well as general approaches to undertaking qualitative data analysis. It also includes qualitative descriptive and interpretive methodologies but, more specifically, can be used in case study research (Jackson et al 2019).

It should be carefully noted that, often, the two terms 'thematic analysis' and 'content analysis' are mistakenly reported interchangeably. They are different things and different processes. The reader/appraiser should caution against this fact when exploring the qualitative literature.

RESEARCH IN BRIEF 7.2

This 'Research in brief' provides two examples of studies that have respectively utilised thematic and content data analytical techniques. First, taking a qualitative descriptive approach, Zhao et al (2022) interviewed 23 older Chinese migrants to explore their perceptions of loneliness and social isolation. Using a data-driven thematic analytical process involving identifying repeated patterns from the transcripts, these researchers identified three key themes. These themes were named as 'high value placed on meeting family obligations', 'feeling a deep sense of imbalanced reciprocity' and 'moving away from filial obligations'. Second, Hoedl et al (2022) used a content analytical method of data analysis, with a combined inductive and deductive coding framework. The aim of this qualitative study was to assess burdens placed on and consequences of the COVID-19 pandemic on nursing

Continued

RESEARCH IN BRIEF 7.2—cont'd

home staff. Digitally recorded individual semistructured interviews were undertaken with eight registered nurses, eight healthcare assistants and two care aids (n = 18). Findings from undertaking this content analysis resulted in addressing the research aim through the creation of six categories: 'quantitative work load', 'qualitative workload', 'work organisation', 'social working environment', 'physical consequences' and 'psychological consequences'.

What do you see as some of the challenges you might face when undertaking either a thematic or a content analysis when engaging with qualitative data?

Narrative Analysis, Discourse Analysis and Concept Analysis—Qualitative 'Language' Analysis

Unlike 'primary' (collecting new data from research participants) analysis with certain qualitative research approaches, the collected data is 'shaped' into a written form for analysis or already exists in the form of existing written narrative. Therefore, speech or written texts are not the *experience* itself, but they are, instead, linguistic representations of it. Three popular styles of analysis that focus on language and how it is used to create understanding are *narrative analysis*, *discourse analysis* and *concept analysis*. Their contexts are often defined through the discipline of 'linguistics' and linguistic research.

Narrative analysis can take several forms and use a range of analytical styles. However, the essential feature is the *life-story method*, where people express their life experiences through storytelling. This is 'restorying', where the researcher reorganises the stories into a framework and, where necessary, places them in a chronological and/or hierarchical order (i.e. main theme first). As the restorying occurs the researcher highlights and links the ideas and themes that exist in the stories. The analysis may consist of a description of the story and themes, or it can be taken to a deeper level of analysis, with a 'deconstruction' of the stories to expose and explore inconsistencies and contradictions (Sandberg 2022).

Carson et al (2017) used narrative analysis to tell the birth experiences of 81 young mothers aged 15 to 24 years. The data analysis process consisted of four steps: (1) listening to the entire interview, (2) transcribing the interview verbatim, (3) organising the data into key categories, (4) comparing data from one transcript to the next to identify commonly occurring stories and (5) placing events in chronological order, with subheadings signposting the narrative content. The findings revealed that these young women's identities as mothers were significantly shaped by their birth experiences.

There are a variety of theoretical perspectives with respect to **discourse analysis**, which means that there are also a variety of ways in which the data for this approach can be analysed. For some researchers, the focus may be as narrow as the study of a single statement or a conversation between two people, while for others it could constitute all forms of talk or writing, or the way the talk is 'meshed' together. Although the term 'discourse' has been described in a variety of ways, it can be essentially understood as the way in which language (and visual and spatial arrangements) is used to construct our understanding of experiences. Therefore, discourse analysis aims to reveal the meaning of the way ideas are communicated through language, and to uncover the ideological influences underlying human behaviour and thought (Johnstone 2018). In contrast to other qualitative methodologies, which seek to understand or interpret social reality as it exists, discourse analysis seeks to uncover 'reality' as it is produced. For example, in one approach to discourse analysis, Joergensen and Praestegaard (2018) used critical discourse analysis to better understand the influences driving patient participation as consumers of mental health services. In this article the concept of discourse was applied to textual data in three ways. First, the texts were interrogated linguistically, looking at the type of language that was used to describe ways patient participation was represented. Second, the main discourses evident in texts that enable people to talk about patient participation were identified. Finally, the social contexts within which patient participation occurs were illuminated. Findings from this study identify that patient participation in mental health services is limited and that biomedical and management discourses dominate patients' participation in their care. These contradictory discourses also serve and support the stigmatisation of people living with mental illness (Joergensen & Praestegaard 2018).

Concept analysis is a popular linguistic approach used in nursing- and midwifery-related qualitative research, with the main methodologies originally constructed by nurses and midwives. They include different, but related, approaches by seminal authors such as Rogers, Walker and Avant and Morse. The process is used when terms and concepts are new, ill defined or used incorrectly—that is, when common terms are used interchangeably such as, for instance (as earlier highlighted in this chapter), the concepts of thematic analysis and content analysis. They often share common characteristics (i.e. definitions, attributes, antecedents, 'case-study/vignettes')—all designed to illustrate and 'pinpoint' a clearer understanding of the concept at hand as analysed and interpreted through common themes in the existing literature. For instance, Pueyo-Garrigues et al (2019) conducted a Rogerian evolutionary concept analysis on health education to clarify the concept, to enable translation of its theory into practice.

Other Styles of Analysing Qualitative Data

A number of 'other' methods exist to approach qualitative data analysis. This chapter has, so far, identified several of the key approaches such as thematic and content analysis. There are too many others to cover them all in a single chapter. Other approaches, *transactional analysis* (TA) and *interpretative phenomenological analysis* (IPA), are two commonly used in nursing/midwifery research. TA is an inductive approach that overarches constant comparative methods. It draws on elements of qualitative thematic and narrative analysis underpinned by the theoretical notions of Bakhtin and Rosenblatt (Stewart 2011). Stewart goes on to state that TA provides a mechanism that transcends thematic analysis in that it goes beyond the overall identification of themes to focus on the moments of 'shaping' as themes are constructed. Burns and Peacock (2019) helpfully analyse and compare different interpretative phenomenological methodologies as a lead-in to IPA. IPA is a phenomenological approach that operates within the iterative hermeneutical circle process (see Chapter 5—Heidegger) of lived experience. Moustakas (1994) is credited with the original structured analysis process that often underpins the IPA methodology. Anderson et al (2019) report their New Zealand-based study using IPA to explore clinical decision making aligned to clinical intuition and expertise. Knight-Agarwal et al (2023) used IPA to explore the knowledge, practices and beliefs of Australian health professionals and pregnant women regarding physical activity and weight management during the antenatal period. Three major themes emerged: (1) women rely on multiple sources of pregnancy-related healthy lifestyle information, (2) discussions around healthy lifestyle behaviours are low priority and often inconsistent and (3) lifestyle-related topics perceived as sensitive make some conversations and actions difficult.

QUALITATIVE META-SYNTHESIS

The findings from qualitative research can enrich healthcare practice as they provide a deeper, more insightful understanding of the healthcare experience. There has been concern, however, that qualitative research tends to be conducted in isolation, lacks links with previous research and is often not used to inform nursing and midwifery practice. An analytical strategy to counter this is the use of qualitative *meta-synthesis*, which pulls together the findings from qualitative studies relevant to a specific research question and situates them in a wider interpretive context, therefore providing a greater understanding of the phenomenon (Achterbergh et al 2020). Qualitative meta-synthesis is neither a meta-summary (i.e. a quantitatively oriented aggregation of qualitative findings) nor a systematic or integrated literature review. Instead, it combines and integrates qualitative research to describe and explain findings from primary studies to create insights (Rene et al 2022). As such, new knowledge is generated through comparison and analysis of the selected studies. It is now a relatively common qualitative research approach and several authors have provided procedures for undertaking qualitative meta-synthesis (e.g. Paterson et al 2001, Sandelowski et al 2007).

Meta-synthesis has been used to generate knowledge across a diverse range of healthcare experience, such as the experience of chronic pain across a number of long-term conditions (Crowe et al 2017), Public Health Nurses' perceptions and experiences of identifying and managing women with perinatal mental health problems (Noonan et al 2017), exploring diabetic people's perceptions and experiences of diabetic foot ulcer in order to identify how they could be better supported to prevent ulceration or manage its impact (Coffey et al 2019) and Zheng et al's (2018) systematic review and qualitative meta-synthesis of nurses' coping strategies when dealing with a patient's death. Thorne (2017) argues that meta-syntheses ably contribute to evidence-based practice where, often, quantitative studies are viewed as the most appropriate form of evidence for practice change. Attempts have been made to make the process as robust as possible for nursing and midwifery—such as with the Adelaide Joanna Briggs Institute-based ConQual synthesis approach of Munn et al (2014).

RESEARCH IN BRIEF 7.3

Kim and Chang (2022) undertook their meta-synthesis in accordance with the ENTREQ (enhancing transparency in reporting the synthesis of qualitative research) statement (Tong et al 2012). The focus of this meta-synthesis was to understand nurse resilience by integrating qualitative research findings on nurses' resilience-related experiences. They used 16 studies published between January 2011 and September 2021 from five databases (PubMed, EMBASE, Web of Science, CINAHL and PsychINFO). Data synthesis identified four themes: 'self-development based on one's inner self', 'fostering a positive attitude toward life', 'developing personal strategies for overcoming adversity' and 'building professionalism to become a better nurse'. They concluded that nurses who were resilient demonstrated increased problem-solving abilities leading to improved quality of care provided to consumers of healthcare services. Other recommendations included opportunities for all nurses to participate in professional development programs focused on increasing resilience.

QUALITATIVE DATA ANALYSIS RIGOUR—TRUSTWORTHINESS

In quantitative research, the basic principle for assessing the quality of the research is that of 'rigour' through the concepts of 'reliability' and 'validity'. Central to determining rigour in quantitative research is the ability for findings to be generalised or be identified in other sample groups. Discussion related to the generalisability of findings in qualitative research is both complex and contested (Smith 2018). Some qualitative researchers cite a lack of generalisability, as it relates to quantitative research, as a weakness or limitation of qualitative studies. In contrast, others claim that generalisability can be demonstrated in qualitative studies. For example, Darnell et al (2018) claim qualitative findings can drive the construction of concepts and theories that can be applied across different settings or contexts, also referred to as analytical generalisations. Some see qualitative meta-synthesis (see previous section) as a 'veiled' attempt to generalise.

For many years now, reliability and validity are generally not seen as appropriate methods to evaluate the findings of qualitative research. Throughout this time, and even recently, there remains considerable debate among qualitative researchers about how best to determine rigour in qualitative research. A common and unified approach to describing the criteria for quality is not evident. It may be that there is no one method that can be identified, as the nature of qualitative research makes it difficult to reach agreement on criteria for assessing its quality. Due to its complexity, authors such as Tong et al (2007) have developed the *consolidated criteria for reporting qualitative research* (COREQ) guidelines to assist with the critical assessment and appraisal of published qualitative research. Many journals now require authors to state that they have referred to the COREQ guidelines when preparing their manuscript for publication (see Chapter 18).

It is often accepted that rigour in qualitative research is determined by *trustworthiness*. **Trustworthiness** can be defined as the extent to which qualitative data that has been collected represents participants' perceptions and experiences (Guba 1981). Currently, there are six broad positions that can be adopted with respect to the criteria for trustworthiness. A researcher will generally select from one or more of these positions in making the claim of trustworthiness and therefore demonstrating qualitative rigour:

Position 1—Using the Criteria of Quantitative Research

This position argues that the process of quantitative reliability and validity remain appropriate concepts for ensuring rigour in qualitative research. From a qualitative perspective the concepts of reliability and validity are broadly concerned with addressing trustworthiness in a study (Coleman 2021). To ensure rigour the use of verification strategies, procedural precision and documenting an auditable trail of key decisions made during the data analytical process are vital. To a certain extent, meta-synthesis (just discussed) suits this position.

Position 2—Parallel Methodological Criteria

This position argues that qualitative research requires a different set of criteria for evaluating trustworthiness. Commonly cited are those of Guba and Lincoln (1989), who developed criteria that have a parallel relationship to those used in quantitative research. These are: 'credibility with internal validity', 'auditability (dependability) with reliability', 'fittingness (transferability) with external validity' and 'confirmability with objectivity'. The four criteria are listed with explanations in Table 7.3.

Position 3—Multiple Criteria

This position argues one list of criteria per qualitative research approach. For example, it has been proposed that the trustworthiness of an ethnographic report can be

TABLE 7.3 Criteria for Judging Trustworthiness: Credibility, Auditability, Fittingness and Confirmability

Criteria	Criteria Characteristic
Credibility	Truth of findings as judged by participants and others within the discipline.
Auditability	Accountability as judged by the adequacy of information leading the reader from the research question and raw data through various steps of analysis to the interpretation of findings.
Fittingness	Faithfulness to everyday reality of the participants, described in enough detail so that others in the discipline can evaluate importance for their own practice, research and theory development.
Confirmability	Findings that reflect implementation of credibility, auditability and fittingness standards.

evaluated by the application of three criteria: veracity, objectivity and perspicacity (Stewart 1998). In grounded theory, various forms have been suggested. Khademi et al (2017), in their grounded theory study on humanistic nursing in acute care environments, used the terms of 'fit', 'work', 'relevance' and 'modifiability' to demonstrate rigour. Other grounded theorists, such as Strauss and Corbin (2014), advocate for criteria more closely aligned with quantitative research: 'validity', 'reliability', 'efficiency' and 'sensitivity'.

Position 4—Each Study Develops Suitable, Justifiable Criteria

Growing in popularity is the flexibility for researchers to develop their own list of criteria to assess rigour of a study. Some common criteria selected are described below.

- *An audit (decision trail)*, where care is taken to record the decisions made, particularly regarding design planning, sampling, data collection methods and analysis decisions. Dyar (2021) asserts that a systematic approach to outlining the research procedures undertaken needs to be documented. This gives assurance that a rigorous research process has been undertaken by the researcher, which can be externally assessed by the reader. Doing so promotes transparency associated with all aspects of the research process.
- *Member (participant) checking*, where researchers seek to determine rigour by checking the descriptions, categories, concepts or theory produced with the participants for their approval and acceptance (Erdmann & Potthoff 2023). This may be problematic, as participants may not agree with the analysis or change their mind. However, the use of member checking may be methodologically determined and therefore needs to occur where this is the case. However, not all researchers agree, particularly those undertaking critical qualitative studies, who argue that doing so raises significant epistemological concerns (see Chapter 2) highlighting the impartiality of knowledge (Motulsky 2021).
- *Reflexivity*, where a process of critical questioning related to all aspects of the research process by the researcher or research team occurs. In their study, Rettke et al (2018) described the key decisions made while designing their project. They then reflected on each of the decisions made as to how it went and what could have been done better, and used these reflections to guide the ongoing conceptualisation, execution and evaluation of the project.

Position 5—No Criteria Are Necessary

There is also a postmodern position (see Chapter 2) that rejects the need for criteria to be selected or stated by a researcher regarding trustworthiness of a qualitative research study or its product. Part of the reasoning for this position is that the findings in qualitative research, particularly those findings derived from postmodern or post-structural studies, are frequently contradictory, messy and complex (Holtz 2020). The findings are therefore a subjective construction in which the knowledge, beliefs and activities of the researchers play a significant role. The findings are 'unique social interactions' and, for this reason, qualitative research can never be truly 'generalisable'. The research and its reported product are accepted or rejected by the reader of the report or user of the product according to their own subjective criteria.

> **TUTORIAL TRIGGER 7.4**
>
> In groups of two or three, find a qualitative research article relevant to your area of practice or that relates to patient care. Answer the following questions:
>
> - Is there a clear statement of the aims of the research?
> - Was the research design appropriate to address the research aims?
> - Were the data collected in a way that addressed the research issue?
> - Was the method of data analysis appropriate?
> - How is the trustworthiness of the research established?
> - Are the findings clearly stated?
> - How valuable is the research?

REPORTING AND DISSEMINATING QUALITATIVE DATA FINDINGS

Writing and publishing qualitative research data findings generally require the same principal skills as quantitative research. However, there may be specific challenges for the qualitative researcher. Unlike quantitative research and depending on the methodology employed, in some cases it is acceptable for qualitative findings and discussion about the findings to be integrated. Usually segments of data (e.g. direct quotes from participants or parts of field notes) are integrated into reported results. As with any research report, limitations, implications and recommendations need to be offered and the trustworthiness criteria applied should be listed and justified. The essential element is to write the findings so that they capture and sustain the reader's interest and provide the best representation of the narrative data possible. To accommodate this required process, some journals might allow an additional word count over the usual maximum for any other type of manuscript.

However, it is important that the journal author guidelines for presenting qualitative work is adhered to.

The style of presenting the results of qualitative data analysis is often governed by the research approach that has been applied. Different options may include the following.

Sequential presentation of concepts. This either may be done completely by descriptive and explanatory narrative following an ordered sequence of concepts or may be supplemented by a list or lists of categories and subcategories, perhaps presented as tables or within an appendix. In the narrative, at appropriate points, there are usually embedded samples of illustrative data (e.g. quotes from participants).

A flow of themes. Thematic analysis results tend to be written as a flowing narrative. A list of the themes may be provided prior to the narrative commencing. Headings may or may not be used in the narrative when a different theme is being written about. Quotes from the participants are also included.

Multiple forms of presentation. With some research approaches, such as grounded theory, the results can be presented in multiple forms that may include combinations of diagramming, tables of hierarchical concepts, a succinct 'storyline' and a necessarily detailed narrative text (also with embedded illustrative data).

A creative synthesis or representation. Becoming more acceptable are types of creative synthesis or representation of results. Possible choices include poems, 'fictionalised' or 'semifictionalised' novels or short stories, performance (e.g. plays, monologues, movies, dance), visual art (e.g. painting, montage, sculpture, photographs, series of cartoons) or auditory art (e.g. song, orchestral arrangement).

SUMMARY

Qualitative data analysis is a field which is dynamic and evolving. Qualitative research throughout healthcare settings offers a wealth of understanding that enhances care delivery. Data analysis styles are numerous, although some are more common than others. A degree of flexibility exists, but formal directions are encouraged for the purpose of research rigour to ensure or evaluate the trustworthiness of qualitative research studies and results, plus offering varying ways in which to report findings. Continuing growth of qualitative meta-synthesis and mixed-methods research (see Chapter 12) further cements the contribution to knowledge development. The next decade or so should ensure a maturing of a whole range of alternative or further-refined qualitative forms of healthcare research across all healthcare disciplines.

KEY POINTS

- Qualitative data analysis is a formal, systematic process of interpretation where the most common style of qualitative data analysis involves associated abstractions of data via 'coding' that incorporates description, categorisation and conceptualisation.
- There are a variety of qualitative data analysis styles, sometimes linked to specific research approaches like content analysis, discourse analysis and ethnography.
- It is possible to follow specific directions regarding styles of qualitative data analysis, as is often offered by methodologists regarding qualitative research approaches, or to have flexibility by using the style free form (descriptive exploratory).
- The reporting and dissemination of qualitative research results can be presented in various forms.

TIME TO REFLECT

Ranse, K., Ranse, J., Pelkowitz, M., 2018. Third-year nursing students' lived experience of caring for the dying: a hermeneutic phenomenological approach. Contemp. Nurse 54 (2), 160–170.

Aim: Ranse et al's (2018) study looked to explore nursing students' lived experience of caring for a dying patient and their family within an Australian context.

Design: A hermeneutic phenomenological methodology.

Reflect on the following:

- The provision of palliative care services is integral to nursing practice. As students prepare to become registered nurses, it is essential that they are adequately equipped to provide care to people who are dying and their significant others. Previous studies have acknowledged that upon registration many nurses have had limited theoretical and clinical preparation related to working with someone who is dying. Consequently, newly registered nurses are confronted with the expectation to care for a patient who is dying with often no prior experience. Integrating end-of-life theory and practice opportunities during nurses' undergraduate preparation will assist in them being able to provide quality holistic care to this group of people. The researchers identify the knowledge gained from this study will improve nurse preparation to ensure a skilled approach to the provision of palliative care services and identify any additional support that student nurses may require.

TIME TO REFLECT—cont'd

- Data were collected from a group of students studying nursing in an Australian university. Following ethical approval, researchers invited nursing students to participate. Six female nursing students participated in an individual interview. The types of questions asked at interview included 'Can you tell me about the day you cared for a patient at the end of their life?' Following transcription data were analysed thematically and included a hermeneutic circle approach. Phenomenological validation criteria were used to ensure the analytical process was orientated to the phenomenon being investigated. In-depth verbatim quotations were presented in the article to highlight examples of student nurses' experiences of caring for a person who is dying and their significant others.

Questions

1. Are there other designs that could have been used in this study? If so, what are they?
2. Reflect on the information given and answer the questions:
   a. Identify the research design.
   b. Is the design appropriate for this study?
   c. Is the data analytical process congruent with the methodology deployed?

LEARNING ACTIVITIES

1. The purpose of qualitative data analysis is to:
   a. establish cause-and-effect relationships
   b. order the data to enhance understanding
   c. manipulate the data to answer the research question
   d. all of the above.
2. Coding is the process of 'interrogating' the data for:
   a. themes and topics
   b. ideas and concepts
   c. terms, phrases and keywords
   d. all of the above.
3. Constant comparative data analysis involves:
   a. collection of all data then analysis of that data
   b. sequential segments of data collection and data analysis
   c. analysis of data during the collection of data
   d. cyclical collection of data, with simultaneous coding and analysis by comparison with other data, followed by further data collection and analysis and so on.
4. CAQDAS is an acronym which stands for:
   a. computer-assisted qualitative data analysis systems
   b. computer-assisted qualitative data analysis software
   c. computer-assisted quantitative data analysis software
   d. computer-assisted qualitative data analytical systems.
5. The main advantage of conducting qualitative research by a single researcher is:
   a. it is easier to conduct
   b. a singular subjectivity is more likely to produce a single-reality outcome
   c. they are less 'shackled' by following a particular methodology
   d. the data analysis process is more likely to be accurate.
6. Which of the following methods of qualitative analysis require immersion in the data as the beginning of the analysis process?
   a. Grounded theory
   b. Thematic analysis
   c. Discourse analysis
   d. All of the above
7. Thematic analysis is normally associated with:
   a. breaking the data up into abstracted bits
   b. researcher objectivity
   c. line-by-line coding
   d. an inductive, iterative process.
8. The key feature of inductive analysis is:
   a. the use of predetermined codes
   b. hypothesis testing
   c. applying your values and assumptions to the data
   d. using reasoning to interpret and organise meanings from the data.
9. Methods to avoid an overly biased interpretation of the data may include:
   a. asking peers external to the study to review the analysis
   b. providing an audit trail that allows others to draw conclusions about the data
   c. providing examples from the original data to illustrate the identified themes when writing up
   d. all of the above.
10. The underlying assumption of 'member checking' is:
    a. it prevents researcher subjectivity
    b. participants are best positioned to evaluate an interpretation of their experience
    c. this allows researcher reflexivity
    d. all of the above.

For further content associated with this chapter visit: https://evolve.elsevier.com/cs/product/9780729596794?role=student 

ADDITIONAL RESOURCES

Association for Qualitative Research: An international organisation that aims to further the practice and study of qualitative research. www.aqr.org.au.

Janesick, V.J., 2016. 'Stretching' Exercises for Qualitative Researchers, ed. 4. Sage Publications, Thousand Oaks, CA.

Lester, J., Cho, Y., Lochmiller, C., 2020. Learning to do qualitative data analysis: A starting point. Hum. Resour. Dev. Rev. 19 (1), 94–106.

Lewins, A., Silver, C., 2014. Using Software for Qualitative Data Analysis: a step-by-step guide, ed. 2. Sage Publications, London, UK.

Qualitative Health Research: an interdisciplinary journal of qualitative health research. https://journals.sagepub.com/home/qhr.

The International Journal of Qualitative Methods: An interdisciplinary journal with a focus on methodological advances in qualitative or mixed methods studies. https://journals.sagepub.com/description/IJQ.

REFERENCES

Achterbergh, L., Pitman, A., Birken, M. et al., 2020. The experience of loneliness among young people with depression: a qualitative meta-synthesis of the literature. BMC Psychiatry 20, 415. doi:10.1186/s12888-020-02818-3

Anderson, N.E., Slark, J., Gott, M., 2019. Unlocking intuition and expertise: using interpretative phenomenological analysis to explore clinical decision making. J. Res. Nurs. 24 (1–2), 88–101. doi:10.1177/1744987118809528

Belgrave, L., Seide, K., 2019. Grounded theory methodology: principles and practices. In: Liamputtong, P. (Ed.), Handbook of Research Methods in Health Social Sciences. Springer, Singapore, pp. 299–316.

Bengtsson, M., 2016. How to plan and perform a qualitative study using content analysis. NursingPlus Open 2, 8–14.

Bettez, S.C., 2015. Navigating the complexity of qualitative research in postmodern contexts: assemblage, critical reflexivity, and communion as guides. Int. J. Qual. Stud. Educ. 28, 932–954.

Borkan, J., 2021. Immersion–crystallization: a valuable analytic tool for healthcare research. Family Pract. XX, 1–5.

Braun, V., Clarke, V., Hayfield, N., et al., 2019. Thematic analysis. In: Liamputtong, P. (Ed.) Handbook of Research Methods in Health Social Sciences. Springer, Singapore, pp. 843–860.

Burns, M., Peacock, S., 2019. Interpretative phenomenological methodologists in nursing: a critical analysis and comparison. Nurs. Inq. 26 (2), e12280. doi:10.1111/nin.12280

Carson, A., Chabot, C., Greyson, D., et al., 2017. A narrative analysis of birth stories of early-age mothers. Sociol. Health Ill. 39 (6), 816–831.

Coffey, L., Mahon, C., Gallagher, P. 2019. Perceptions and experiences of diabetic foot ulceration and foot care in people with diabetes: a qualitative meta-synthesis. Int. Wound J. 16, 183–210.

Coleman, P., 2021. Validity and reliability within qualitative research in the caring sciences. Int. J. Caring Sci. 14 (3), 2041–2045.

Crowe, M., Whitehead, L., Seaton, P., et al., 2017. Qualitative meta-synthesis: the experience of chronic pain across conditions. J. Adv. Nurs. 73 (5), 1004–1016.

Darnell, S., Chawansky, M., Marchesseault, D., et al., 2018. The state of play: critical sociological insights into recent 'Sport for Development and Peace' research. Int. Rev. Sociol. Sport 53 (2), 133–151.

Dixon, K., Fossey, E., Petrakis, M., 2022. Using photovoice to explore women's experiences of a women-only prevention and recovery care service in Australia. Health Soc. Care Community 30, e5839–e5847.

Doyle, l., McCabe, C., Keogh, B., et al., 2020. An overview of the qualitative descriptive design within nursing research. J. Nurs. Res. 25 (5), 443–455.

Dyar, K., 2021. Qualitative inquiry in nursing: creating rigor. Nurs. Forum 57 (1), 187–200. doi:10.1111/nuf.12661

Erdmann, A., Potthoff, S., 2023. Decision criteria for the ethically reflected choice of a member check method in qualitative research: a proposal for discussion. Int. J. Qual. Methods 22, 1–11.

Gautam, S., Montayre, J., Neville, S., 2022. Seeking and maintaining connections: a grounded theory study of maintaining spirituality in residential aged care facilities. Int. J. Older People Nurs. 17, e12435.

Graneheim, U.H., Lindgren, B.M., Lundman, B., 2017. Methodological challenges in qualitative content analysis: a discussion paper. Nurse Educ. Today 56, 29–34.

Guba, E.G., 1981. Criteria for assessing the trustworthiness of naturalistic inquiries. Educ. Commun. Technol. 29, 75–91.

Guba, E. G., Lincoln, Y., 1989. Fourth Generation Evaluation. Sage Publications, London, UK.

Hoedl, M., Thonhofer, N., Schoberer, D., 2022. COVID-19 pandemic: burdens on and consequences for nursing home staff. J. Adv. Nurs. 78, 2495–2506.

Holloway, I., Galvin, K., 2017. Qualitative Research in Nursing and Healthcare, fourth ed. Wiley Blackwell, Chichester, West Sussex.

Holtz, P., 2020. Does postmodernism really entail a disregard for the truth? Similarities and differences in postmodern and critical rationalist conceptualizations of truth, progress, and empirical research methods. Front. Psychol. 11, 545959.

Irani, E., Hirschman, K., Cacchione, P., et al., 2018. How home health nurses plan their work schedules: a qualitative descriptive study. J. Clin. Nurs. 27, 4066–4076.

Jackson, D., Borbasi, S., Power, T., 2019. Qualitative research. In: Borbasi, S., Jackson, D. (Eds.), Navigating the Maze of Research: enhancing nursing and midwifery practice, fifth ed. Elsevier Australia, Chatswood, NSW, Australia, pp. 143–170.

Jackson, K., Bazeley, P., 2019. Qualitative Data Analysis with NVivo, third ed. Sage Publications, Los Angeles, CA.

Jarden, R.J., Sandham, M., Siegert, R.J., et al., 2019. Strengthening workplace well-being: perceptions of intensive care nurses. Nurs. Crit. Care 24 (1), 15–23.

Jedwab, R.M., Manias, E., Hutchinson, A.M., et al., 2022. Understanding nurses' perceptions of barriers and enablers to use of a new electronic medical record system in Australia: a qualitative study. Int. J. Med. Inform. 158, 104654. doi:10.1016/j.ijmedinf.2021.104654

Joergensen, K., Praestegaard, J., 2018. Patient participation as discursive practice: a critical discourse analysis of Danish mental healthcare. Nurs. Inq. 25, e12218. doi:10.1111/nin.12218

Johnstone, B., 2018. Discourse Analysis, third ed. John Wiley & Sons, New York.

Khademi, M., Mohammadi, E., Vanaki, Z., 2017. A grounded theory of humanistic nursing in acute care work environments. Nurs. Ethics 24 (8), 908–921.

Kim, E.Y., Chang, S.O., 2022. Exploring nurse perceptions and experiences of resilience: a meta-synthesis study. BMC Nurs. 21 (1), 26. doi:10.1186/s12912-021-00803-z. Erratum in: BMC Nurs. 2022, 21 (1), 44.

Kimmerle, B., zu Sayn-Wittgenstein Hohenstein, F., Offenberger, U., 2023. Pediatric nurses in early childhood intervention in Germany—emergence of a new professional role: situational analysis and mapping. Forum Qual. Soc. Res. 24 (2), 5. doi:10.17169/fqs-24.2.4036

Kleinheksel, A., Rockich-Winston, N., Tawfik, H., et al., 2020. Qualitative research in pharmacy education. Demystifying content analysis. Am. J. Pharm. Educ. 84 (1), 127–137.

Knight-Agarwal, C., Minehan, M., Cockburn, B., et al., 2023. Different experiences of weight management and physical activity during pregnancy – a qualitative study of women and healthcare professionals in Australia. Int. J. Qual. Stud. Health Well-being 18, 1. doi:10.1080/17482631.2023.2202973

Lester, J., Cho, Y., Lochmiller, C., 2020. Learning to do qualitative data analysis: a starting point. Hum. Resour. Dev. Rev. 19 (1), 94–106.

Locke, K., Feldman, M., Golden-Biddle, K., 2022. Coding practices and iterativity: beyond templates for analyzing qualitative data. Org. Res. Methods 25 (2), 262–284.

Lukewich, J., Martin-Misener, R., Norful, A.A., et al., 2022. Effectiveness of registered nurses on patient outcomes in primary care: a systematic review. BMC Health Serv. Res. 22, 740. doi:10.1186/s12913-022-07866-x

Macdiarmid, R., Neville, S., Zambas, S., 2020. The experience of facilitating debriefing after simulation: a qualitative study. Nurs. Praxis Aotearoa N. Z. 36 (3), 51–60.

Mayes, M.E., Wilkinson, C., Kuah, S., et al., 2018. Change in practice: a qualitative exploration of midwives' and doctors' views about the introduction of STan monitoring in an Australian hospital. BMC Health Serv. Res. 18, 119.

Merriam, S.B., Grenier, R.S., 2019. Qualitative Research in Practice: examples for discussion and analysis. John Wiley & Sons, New York..

Miles, M., Huberman, A., Saldana, J., 2019. Qualitative Data Analysis: a methods sourcebook, fourth ed. Sage Publications, Los Angeles, CA.

Motulsky, S., 2021. Is member checking the gold standard of quality in qualitative research? Qual. Psychol. 8 (3), 389–406.

Moustakas, C., 1994. Phenomenological Research Methods. Sage Publications, Thousand Oaks, CA.

Munn, Z., Porritt, K., Lockwood, C., et al., 2014. Establishing confidence in the output of qualitative research synthesis: the ConQual approach. BMC Med. Res. Methodol. 14, 108.

Neville, S., Adams, J., Napier, S., et al., 2018. "Engaging in my rural community": perceptions of people aged 85 years and over. Qual. Stud. Health Wellbeing 13 (1), 1503908.

Nguyen, T., Whitehead, L., Demody, G., et al., 2022. The use of theory in qualitative research: challenges, development of a framework and exemplar. J. Adv. Nurs. 78, e21–e28.

Noonan, M., Galvin, R., Doody, O., et al., 2017. A qualitative meta-analysis: public health nurses' role in the identification and management of perinatal mental health problems. J. Adv. Nurs. 73 (3), 545–557.

Nowell, L., Norris, J., White, D., et al., 2017. Thematic analysis: striving to meet the trustworthiness criteria. Int. J. Qual. Methods 16, 1–13.

Paterson, B., Thorne, S., Canam, C., et al., 2001. Meta-study of Qualitative Research. Sage Publications, Thousand Oaks, CA.

Pueyo-Garrigues, M., Whitehead, D., Pardavila-Belio, M., et al. 2019. Health education: a Rogerian concept analysis to translate theory into practice. Int. J. Nurs. Stud. 94, 131–138. doi:10.1016/j.ijnurstu.2019.03.005

Ranse, K., Ranse, J., Pelkowitz, M., 2018. Third-year nursing students' lived experience of caring for the dying: a hermeneutic phenomenological approach. Contemp. Nurse. 54 (2), 160–170.

Rene, C., Landry, I., de Montingny, F., 2022. Couples' experiences of pregnancy resulting from assisted reproductive technologies: a qualitative meta-synthesis. Int. J. Nurs. Stud. Adv. 4, 100059. doi:10.1016/j.ijnsa.2021.100059

Rettke, H., Pretto, M., Spichiger, E., et al., 2018. Using reflexive thinking to establish rigour in qualitative research. Nurs. Res. 67 (6), 490–497.

Reynolds, S., Woltz, P., Neff, J., 2022. Program evaluation of implementation science outcomes from an intervention to improve compliance with chorhexidine gluconate bathing. A qualitative study. Dimens. Crit. Care Nurs. 41 (4), 200–208. doi:10.1097/DCC.0000000000000530

Rodik, P., Primorac, J., 2015. To use or not to use: computer-assisted qualitative data analysis software usage among early-career sociologists in Croatia. Qual. Soc. Res. 16 (1), 12.

Rogan, A., Lockett, J., Peckler, B., et al., 2022. Exploring nursing and medical perceptions of sepsis management in a New Zealand emergency department: a qualitative study. Emerg. Med. Australas. 34, 417–427. doi:10.1111/1742-6723.13911

Salamonson, Y., Priddis, H., Woodmass, J., et al., 2018. The price of journeying towards the prize: commencing nursing students' experiences of working and studying: a qualitative study. J. Clin. Nurs. 27, 4141–4149.

Sandberg, S., 2022. Narrative analysis in criminology. J. Crim. Justice Educ. 33 (2), 212–229.

Sandelowski, M., Barroso, J., Voils, C., I, 2007. Using qualitative metasummary to synthesize qualitative and quantitative descriptive findings. Res. Nurs. Health 30 (1), 99–111.

Sheikhnezhad, L., Hassankhani, H., Sawin, E., et al., 2023. Blaming in women with breast cancer subjected to intimate partner violence: a hermeneutic phenomenological study. Asia-Pac. J. Oncol. Nurs. 10 (3), 100193.

Smith, B., 2018. Generalizability in qualitative research: misunderstandings, opportunities and recommendations for the sport and exercise sciences. Qual. Res. Sport Exerc. Health 10 (1), 137–149.

Soa-Diaz, M., Valverde-Berrocoso, J., 2022. Grounded theory as a research methodology in educational technology. Int. J. Qual. Methods 21, 1–13.

Stevens, J., Schmeid, V., Burns, E., et al., 2018. Who owns the baby? A video ethnography of skin-to-skin contact after a caesarean section. Women Birth 31 (6), 453–462.

Stewart, A., 1998. The Ethnographer's Method. Sage Publications, Thousand Oaks, CA.

Stewart, T.T., 2011. Transactional analysis: conceptualizing a framework for illuminating human experience. Int. J. Qual. Methods 10 (3), 282–295.

Strauss, A., Corbin, J., 2014. Basics of Qualitative Research: techniques and procedures for developing grounded theory, 4th ed. Sage Publications, Thousand Oaks, CA.

Thorne, S., 2017. Metasynthetic madness: what kind of monster have we created? Qual. Health Res. 27 (1), 3–12.

Tong, A., Sainsbury, P., Craig, J., 2007. Consolidated criteria for reporting qualitative research (COREQ): a 32-item checklist for interviews and focus groups. Int. J. Qual. Health Care 19, 349–357.

Tong, A., Flemming , K., McInnes, E., et al., 2012. Enhancing transparency in reporting the synthesis of qualitative research: ENTREQ. BMC Med Res Methodol. 12 (1), 181.

van Manen, M., 2023. Phenomenology of Practice: meaning-giving methods in phenomenological research and writing. Left Coast Press, Taylor & Francis Group, Walnut Creek, CA.

Vears, D., Gillam, L., 2022. Indictive content analysis: a guide for beginning qualitative researchers. Focus Health Prof. Educ. 23 (1), 111–127.

Williams, E., Russell-Mayhew, S., Ireland, A., 2018. Disclosing an eating disorder: a situational analysis of online accounts. Qual. Rep. 23 (4), 914–931.

Wirihana, L., Welch, A., Willamson, M., et al., 2018. Using Colaizzi's method of data analysis to explore the experiences of nurse academics teaching on satellite campuses. Nurs. Res. 25 (4), 30–34.

Youn-Joo, U., Yun-Jung, C,. 2022. A grounded theory on school nursing experiences with major pandemic diseases. Inquiry 59, 469580221090405. doi:10.1177/00469580221090405

Zhao, I., Holroyd, E., Wright-St Clair, V., et al., 2022. Feeling a deep sense of loneliness: Chinese late-life immigrants in New Zealand. Australas. J. Ageing 41, 448–456.

Zheng, R., Lee, S., Bloomer, M., 2018. How nurses cope with patient death: a systematic review and qualitative meta-synthesis. J. Clin. Nurs. 27, e39–e49.

8

Common Quantitative Methods

Daniel Terry and Ha Hoang

LEARNING OUTCOMES

After reading this chapter, you should be able to:

- describe the overall purpose of quantitative designs
- distinguish the difference between key research designs that use quantitative methods including randomised controlled trials, non-randomised studies and observational studies
- list the criteria necessary for inferring cause-and-effect relationships
- apply critical review criteria to evaluate the findings of selected quantitative studies.

KEY TERMS

control, p. 118
dependent (outcome) variables, p. 115
explanatory (independent) variable, p. 119
independent (predictor) variables, p. 115
manipulation, p. 119
non-randomised studies of interventions, p. 125
observational (non-experimental) designs, p. 120
randomisation, p. 118
randomised controlled trials, p. 116

INTRODUCTION

This chapter provides an overview of the meaning, purpose and issues related to quantitative research designs, while presenting the common approaches used to answer a variety of nursing and midwifery questions. Related factors such as sampling, data collection, assessment of measurement instruments and data analysis are discussed in Chapters 9–11. The focus here is on providing you, as a research consumer or budding researcher, with the information to evaluate quantitative studies critically.

When examining the fundamental building blocks of research, there is an easy method to recognise whether a research study is quantitative or qualitative. Quantitative research measures something and will include numbers. Qualitative research is word based rather than number based. A rudimentary method to identify quantitative research is to search for words such as 'measure', 'test' or 'calculate', whereas qualitative research uses words such as 'explore', 'describe', 'in-depth', 'examine' and so forth. It is important to note that any research which includes a social component is not always qualitative. For example, a survey can measure psychosocial aspects of health and, despite the study/survey having social aspects, by definition it is quantitative.

In nursing and midwifery, the methods of quantitative research fall into randomised and non-randomised studies, which may be interventional, as well as observational and correlational research. All research, whether quantitative or qualitative, starts with research questions. Those research questions will drive all aspects of the study, and indeed will determine which method is required. Quantitative research often has a hypothesis, which is a statement concerning a relationship between two or more variables and derived from the research question. The hypothesis is then tested by studying the effects of **independent ('predictor') variables** on **dependent ('outcome') variables** using inferential statistical methods (see Chapter 11 for more detail). However, the ability of any method to determine cause-and-effect relationships between variables will differ. There is a hierarchy in how this is achieved, as illustrated in Table 8.1.

QUALITY OF EVIDENCE

All research generates data or 'evidence'. However, not all evidence is the same. It is vital that the best evidence is used in nursing and midwifery practice. To that end, the National Health and Medical Research Council of Australia (NHMRC) (2019) recommends the Grading of Recommendations Assessment, Development and Evaluation (GRADE) system, an internationally recognised approach, as the standard in clinical guideline development. The GRADE system is also used in Cochrane Collaboration systematic reviews to grade the quality of evidence; however, there are other approaches to grading the quality of evidence (see Chapter 15). Nevertheless, this system of grading the quality of evidence updates earlier advice from the NHMRC, which indicated to use only the research design considerations for evidence grading. In contrast, the GRADE approach involves rating the quality of evidence for *each outcome* along a continuum of very low, low, moderate or high quality (Table 8.2). Evidence from **randomised controlled trials (RCTs)**

TABLE 8.1 Continuum of Quantitative Research Designs

Design Increasing Control and Ability to Assign Causality	Sub-types	Features
Observational	Descriptive	Describes variables.
	Correlational	Examines relationships between variables.
	Cross-sectional	Examines variables and relationships at one point in time.
	Retrospective	Retraces participants with a certain outcome backwards to find a possible exposure.
	Case-control	Cases matched to controls.
	Cohort	Follows participants from exposure to outcome.
	Longitudinal	Repeated measurements of participants over time.
Non-randomised studies of interventions	Time-series	Manipulation (intervention).
	Non-equivalent control group	Manipulation + control.
Randomised controlled trials	Parallel or crossover randomised controlled trial	Control & manipulation + random assignment to groups.
	Cluster-randomised controlled trial	Groups of participants (not individuals) are randomised.

TABLE 8.2 Explanations for Interpreting Level of Evidence

Evidence Grading	Explanation
High	Very confident that the true effect in the target population is close to the estimate of the effect observed from the participants included in prior research.
Moderate	Moderately confident that the true effect in the target population is close to the estimate of the effect observed from the participants included in prior research.
Low	Limited confidence that the true effect in the target population may be substantially close to the estimate of the effect observed from the participants included in prior research.
Very low	Little confidence that the true effect in the target population is likely to be substantially close to the estimate of the effect observed from the participants included in prior research.

(or meta-analysis where the results of multiple RCTs have been combined using a statistical approach) is automatically assigned a rating of *high* quality and non-randomised studies automatically assigned a *low* rating. However, the evidence rating is then modified downwards within GRADE if there are concerns about:

1. **limitations**: the risk of bias associated with the design of the study or studies that provided evidence for that outcome (assessed by risk of detection, performance, attrition);
2. **imprecision**: how precise the study results are;
3. **inconsistency**: the degree to which results from different similar studies (comparing the same interventions, for example) have varied;
4. **indirectness**: the evidence not being totally relevant to the research question at hand; and
5. **publication bias**: the completeness of reporting of research.

It is also possible to *upgrade* the quality of evidence assigned to an outcome from a non-randomised or observational study. Upgrading evidence quality for an observational study can be considered when a dose–response gradient is present and large effects are identified (i.e. 2–5-fold reductions or increases in risk) (Bezerra et al 2022).

The most suitable appropriate methods to test cause-and-effect relationships is the RCT (Rajasekar & Kumar 2019). Other designs allow for the effect of variables that will bring a degree of bias to the study, thus reducing the likelihood of the study to determine whether measured differences in a particular outcome were due to an intervention or some external factor. For example, if a less robust design is used, the outcome between a group of people who received a particular intervention/treatment could potentially be because of that intervention/treatment or due to some other external reason (Rajasekar & Kumar 2019). The RCT should be conducted with every effort possible to minimise the risk of bias. It is considered the 'gold standard' in quantitative research. However, conducting an RCT is often difficult. It may not be practical to allocate participants randomly. It may also not be feasible to blind participants or the researchers as to what arm (branch) of the study they have been allocated. There are many reasons why a RCT may not be possible or ethical; as such, the GRADE approach aids in classifying the quality of evidence from non-randomised and observational studies to guide decision making.

Concepts Underpinning Quantitative Research

The empirical paradigm that informs quantitative research designs emphasises 'objective' observation, accuracy and control. Not only medicine but also other disciplines such as nursing and midwifery have followed this tradition when conducting quantitative research. Fig. 8.1 illustrates the focus on variables and relationships for each type of quantitative design.

The term 'design' implies the organisation of research components into a coherent and systematic plan. It also represents the major distinctive approach selected for the specific purpose of answering an explicit research question. The research question or aims and objectives influence and guide the choice of design. A clear understanding of research design is important to make an informed choice about which design will best answer the research question, and for a consumer to understand the implications and the use of research. On this basis alone, clinicians can begin to determine whether a journal article describing a research study could be of value in informing their practice (Greenhalgh 2019). One of the most valuable places to find up-to-date information about quantitative

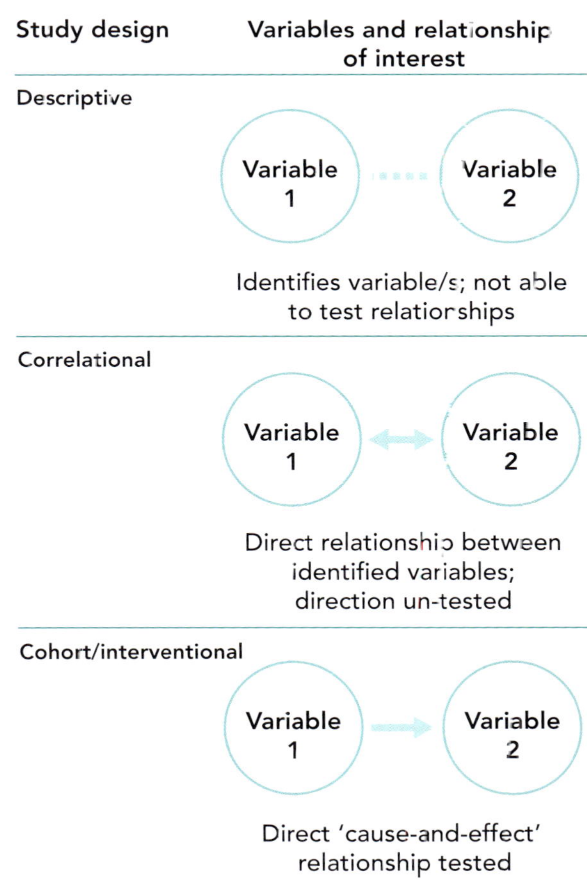

Fig. 8.1 Examining variables in quantitative designs.

research is the Cochrane Collaboration, a not-for-profit organisation focused on providing clinicians, researchers and communities with accessible and effective health information and healthcare interventions through its systematic review of best evidence.

Important aspects of quantitative research include objectivity in the conceptualisation of the problem, hypothesis testing, operational definition, feasibility, accuracy, control of intervention and control conditions, replication, internal validity and external validity. Selection of a particular design gives a researcher more or less control over these aspects, particularly three major concepts:

1. control
2. randomisation
3. manipulation.

RCTs (the strongest designs) contain aspects of all three of these concepts.

Control

Control is achieved in a study by comparing an outcome between one or more groups while ensuring that all participants involved in the research receive the same treatment, except for one key aspect that only an intervention group receives. In a **parallel group** RCT, the group of participants who receives the usual care or treatment is typically termed the 'control' group and the group of participants who receives the alternative treatment of interest is termed the 'intervention' group. In a **crossover** RCT design, participants act as their own controls—for example, two groups of participants in a recent study examined the impact of the immersive experience of nature through the use of virtual reality technology to assist those undergoing haemodialysis. Each group received either the intervention or no intervention for a period of 4 weeks and then 'crossed over' to receive the opposite for a similar period of time (Smyth et al 2022). The sequence in which each participant received the intervention was randomised (see next section).

The strength and rigour of a quantitative design relate to controlling the effects of any extraneous variables that may cause bias (threats to internal validity, such as selection, history and maturation) and influence the study findings. These variables can be either antecedent or intervening. An antecedent (preceding) variable occurs before the study commences but may affect the outcome variable of interest and influence findings. For example, age, gender, pre-existing health status or socioeconomic status could affect outcomes such as recovery time and ability to integrate healthcare behaviours. Similarly, an intervening (mediating) variable is not part of the study design but rather occurs during the course of the study and may affect the outcome variable—for instance, a change in the model of clinical care during a longitudinal study. Threats to 'internal validity' are discussed further in Chapter 9.

Randomisation

Randomisation (random assignment) to study groups is intended to ensure that groups or participants are similar with respect to the variables of interest, so that differences in the outcome variable can be attributed solely to the intervention. Efforts should be made to ensure that participants are assigned to either the experimental or control group purely by chance. Each participant therefore has an equal and known probability of being assigned to any group. If randomisation is not possible, the design should simply be described as 'non-randomised'. Sometimes, you may also see the term 'quasi-experimental' being used, which, unlike true experimental designs, does not rely on random assignment but is based on non-random conditions or criteria. This is sometimes seen in clinical settings where true randomisation cannot be achieved, such as the study by Hawkins et al (2023), which examined the experiences of negative workplace behaviours and coping among nursing staff in relation to educational workshops, where there may have been potential contamination due to participants communicating with each other during the intervention period. Nevertheless, when random assignment is possible, it may be achieved individually or by groups, with a variety of approaches available—from a very simple coin toss or 'draw from a hat' to more sophisticated techniques such as a table of random numbers (see Chapter 9) and computerised random number generation (see Box 8.1).

It is also important to note that the people who are measuring the outcomes of the study should not know how the randomisation falls, or who goes into which groups. This is termed 'allocation concealment'. In a study of the methodological quality of 250 controlled trials, empirical evidence of bias was discovered with larger effect sizes reported in studies that did not adequately report allocation concealment (Boutron et al 2023). There are many potential explanations for this finding—one being that researchers might inadvertently influence participant selection if inadequate methods are used to conceal allocation assignments. As allocation concealment is a known source of bias associated with RCTs, the Consolidated Standards of Reporting Trials (CONSORT) statement recommends that the method used to conceal the allocation sequence is always outlined explicitly in studies reporting results of RCTs (Schulz et al 2010). Studies should report a comparison between groups on demographic and

BOX 8.1 Excerpts from Randomised Controlled Trial With Random Assignment to Study Groups

The parallel pilot RCT was conducted between January 2018 and January 2019 at three long-term care facilities (LTCFs) in Australia. Participants were randomly assigned to either an intervention (PARO—an advanced interactive therapeutic robot with usual care) or a control group (usual care only) via a computer-generated randomisation list by an independent researcher who was not involved in the recruitment or data collection (Pu et al 2020 p. 1079).

In an RCT that examined the effects of different educational interventions on the rate of pneumococcal vaccination among patients with chronic disease, the unit of randomisation was the weeks of the intervention. In this study, 'each week of the 10-week study period was randomised to either intervention or control using random numbers generated by https://www.random.org/. For each location, five weeks were allocated to intervention and five to the control' (Chan et al 2015 p. 319). For each nurse clinic, a computer-generated (using IBM® SPSS Statistics v19), sequentially numbered randomisation list was developed in advance by the Chief Investigator. Block randomisation (block size 20) with stratification for established Type 2 Diabetes (T2D) was applied at a 1:1 ratio to allocate participants to either nurse intervention or standard care (Carrington & Zimmet 2022 pp. 27–28)

'[Alternate] allocation to each treatment group was determined based on the selection of a sealed [blank] envelope by the treating nurse. The envelopes were locked in a filing cabinet and accessed when a patient was recruited ... envelopes were shuffled each time a patient was recruited' (Goedemans et al 2014 p. 63).

clinical characteristics for each group to further highlight the presence or lack of biases (similarity or differences) between groups (Schulz et al 2010). In this case, the randomisation of groups would suggest the differences between groups should be minimal, otherwise if too dissimilar the risk of bias may impact the trustworthiness of results.

In addition to concealing the allocation sequence from the researchers enrolling patients into trials, efforts should be made to ensure that:

1. the participants enrolled in the study do not know to which group they have been assigned (to reduce risk of performance bias);
2. the clinicians delivering care to the participant do not know to which group they have been assigned (to reduce risk of performance bias); and
3. the researchers measuring outcomes do not know to which group the participants have been assigned (to reduce risk of detection bias).

Employing these safeguards will minimise the influence from those applying the intervention or treatment under investigation or measuring its effects. A crude (and imaginary) example is a study of an ointment for wound healing. The ointment containing the relevant medication is being compared with another ointment that does not contain the medication (a placebo). If the researchers and their assistants, or the nurses working with the patients, know which ointment is being applied to the wound, they may influence the results by perhaps (even unconsciously) cleaning the wound better prior to applying the medicated ointment rather than the non-medicated one. By blinding the ointment so no one knows which one is being applied, and then comparing the results, a true indication of the effectiveness of the ointment can be identified.

In addition, the patients on whom the ointment is being tested should not know what treatment they have received either. This is difficult to achieve in many areas of nursing and midwifery practice where a process (a particular method to deliver nursing or midwifery care) is being evaluated. Although this is difficult to achieve in some circumstances, efforts to implement blinding should always be considered in the planning stages of a RCT because, by ensuring that no one knows which patients receive the intervention and which ones receive the control or 'placebo' condition, a more accurate estimation of the effect of the intervention will be obtained (Webster et al 2021).

Manipulation

Both RCTs and non-randomised studies of interventions use **manipulation**. A researcher manipulates the causal or '**explanatory (independent) variable**' by introducing a 'treatment' or 'intervention'. The intervention (treatment) group receives manipulation of the explanatory variable, whereas the control group does not. The intervention might be, for example, a treatment, a teaching plan or a medication. For example, Slykerman et al (2022) conducted a large RCT among nurses to understand whether a daily probiotic supplement reduced perceived stress and symptoms of illness. In this case the intervention was the introduction of the probiotic while the control group received a placebo; the effect of this manipulation was measured to determine the effect of the intervention. A study protocol or procedure ensures that all participants in the intervention group will receive the same treatment, while also assisting a reader of the study to understand the nature of the experimental treatment and manipulation of variables.

There are three major categories of quantitative designs: observational, non-randomised studies of interventions and RCTs. Each category includes a range of design choices. Choice of a design relates to the research question or hypothesis, the amount of control a researcher can have and the study feasibility. Examples of these categories of design from nursing and midwifery research are discussed in the following sections.

OBSERVATIONAL DESIGNS

Observational (non-experimental) designs are used when a researcher wishes to construct a picture of a phenomenon or explore events, people or situations as they occur naturally in the environment. The aim is therefore to observe and identify variables of interest and explore relationships between those variables. These designs are used when:

- there is little information or research about the topic of interest, or
- the phenomena of interest are not amenable to experimental designs (e.g. when ethical considerations do not allow a 'treatment' to be denied to a control group).

Observational designs work from a clear, concise problem statement based within an appropriate theoretical framework. Although a researcher does not actively manipulate an intervention variable in this design, the concepts of control and rigour are still important and should be evident to the reader. Demographic data are collected to describe the sample of participants, such as age, gender, income level, ethnicity, occupation and educational level. Reporting this information assists readers in considering the generalisability of the study and the potential application of the findings to their own practice setting. The common types of observational designs are discussed below, noting their advantages and disadvantages, and using examples from published clinical research to illustrate features of specific designs.

RESEARCH IN BRIEF 8.1

After several reports in the local newspaper and ongoing debates across several rural Australian communities regarding the use of agricultural sprays impacting the incidence of asthma and hospitalisations, a group of

RESEARCH IN BRIEF 8.1—cont'd

researchers undertook a retrospective study. This was an observational study to examine hospital separation data between 2010 and 2015 across the whole state, where agricultural sprays were of concern, to understand the true drivers of hospital admissions. In rural settings, other than being male, there were no significant predictors of asthma hospital admissions among those aged 0–14 years and no predictors among individuals aged 15 and above (Terry et al 2017). A further follow-up retrospective study was necessary to confirm the findings, as not all hospital presentations led to hospital admissions and several limitations associated with the data were recognised. Using hierarchical multiple regression, it was noted in the follow-up study that key factors such as age, population density and private health insurance were associated with asthma emergency presentations among males and females aged 0–14 years, whereas socioeconomic status and rurality were not predictive (Terry et al 2022). The research team went on to suggest that agricultural sprays were not predictive of hospital presentations.

Descriptive/Exploratory Studies

Descriptive studies can be either quantitative or qualitative. In quantitative research, descriptive studies seek to describe the status of a variable or phenomenon with no attempt to manipulate the conditions or events. Data for these studies are gathered through several ways including direct observations, questionnaires and retrospective or prospective audit of available data. Descriptive studies can often be used as a precursor to other quantitative research. In a descriptive study, the researcher does not usually begin with a hypothesis, though one may be developed after the data is collected.

A survey is a common type of observational design that enables collection of information about the characteristics of particular individuals, groups, institutions or situations, or about the frequency of a phenomenon's occurrence, particularly when little is known about it. There are both advantages and disadvantages to consider when undertaking survey research (see Table 8.3). For example, surveys can be useful when investigating participants' knowledge, beliefs or attitudes about a particular topic or concept, and data collection can be relatively inexpensive. However, questions or items within the survey may have issues of reliability, while participant willingness to answer questions accurately or honestly may be problematic or be a limitation of the study design (Siedlecki 2020).

TABLE 8.3 Advantages and Disadvantages of Survey Studies

Advantages	Disadvantages
A lot of information can be obtained from a large population in an economical manner.	Large-scale surveys can be time consuming and costly.
Accurate if the sample is representative of the population of interest.	Information tends to be brief and superficial, with breadth rather than depth of data.
	Requires expertise in a variety of research areas (e.g. sampling techniques, questionnaire construction, interviewing, data analysis) to produce a reliable and valid study.

AN UNEXPECTED HURDLE

When testing the impact or efficacy of a new drug, treatment or procedure, RCTs remain the benchmark or gold standard as a high level of trustworthiness exists as to the item or procedure being tested or examined. As outlined earlier, the fictitious ointment treatment is one example of how this may be achieved. However, in some cases it may not be feasible or ethical to blind patients, clinicians or researchers to the control or placebo condition in an RCT. To address this issue, a placebo is administered within the study with the blinding or deception removed so that the patient is fully aware that they are receiving the placebo. This is what is termed an 'open trial' or 'open-label placebo' (OLP). Although this may be considered a more ethical approach for certain studies, where clinicians and researchers are fully transparent and patients are cognisant, it also does come with some limitations by introducing bias. Some examples where there has been moderate risk of bias, but with promising outcomes, include high-risk studies associated with treatments for allergic rhinitis, attention deficit hyperactivity disorder, back pain, cancer-related fatigue, irritable bowel syndrome, major depression and hot flushes associated with menopause (von Wernsdorff et al 2021).

If you were to undertake a high-risk study, how might you answer the following questions:

1. What ethical issues may exist if deception of the patient is evident when providing a medical or healthcare intervention?
2. If deceiving a patient regarding their treatment by using a placebo, how can they be accurately, completely and comprehensively informed concerning their care?
3. What are the implications to a study if OLP is used?
4. What alternatives may be available to the researchers?

Correlational Studies

An extension of descriptive research, correlational studies explore the relationships between variables to provide a deeper insight into the phenomenon of interest. These studies enable examination of the relationship between pairs of variables, as well as a comparison between groups. A researcher uses this design to quantify the strength of the relationship between variables (i.e. as one variable changes, does a related change occur in the other variable?). For example, using a correlational design, a study examining job satisfaction and career intention of Australian general practice nurses was able to identify that most of the 786 nurses who responded enjoyed the work they undertook. However, among those respondents (23%) who were not sure or were less satisfied in their current roles, a relationship existed between job dissatisfaction and intention to leave general practice employment (Halcomb & Bird 2020).

Correlational designs cannot test a 'cause-and-effect' relationship (i.e. whether a change in one variable causes a measurable change in another variable). A common misuse of a correlational design is a researcher's attempt to conclude that a causal relationship exists between the study variables; as such, keep in mind that correlation does not imply causation. When reading a correlational study, it is important to identify the variables and the relationship being tested and consider whether the implied relationship is consistent with the conceptual framework and research question being asked. The advantages and disadvantages of correlational studies are listed in Table 8.4.

Cross-sectional Studies

Studies that measure data at one point in time (i.e. data are collected on only one occasion with the same participants rather than on the same participants at several points in time) are called cross-sectional studies. These studies are

TABLE 8.4 Advantages and Disadvantages of Correlational Studies

Advantages	Disadvantages
Increased flexibility to investigate relationships among variables.	Unable to determine a causal relationship between variables because of the lack of manipulation, control and randomisation.
Efficient and effective method of collecting a large amount of data about an issue of interest.	No random sampling possible with pre-existing groups—the ability to generalise is therefore decreased.
Provides a framework for exploring the relationship between variables that are not able to be manipulated.	Unable to manipulate the variables of interest.
A foundation for potential, future interventional studies.	

categorised as either 'descriptive' or 'analytical' (Wang & Cheng 2020). Cross-sectional analytical studies vary from other descriptive studies because they use inferential statistics to infer a relationship between two or more variables. A limitation of the cross-sectional design is that the outcome of interest and the causal factor are measured simultaneously. The lack of time as a factor therefore provides only weak evidence of causality. In contrast, a longitudinal study, which follows a group of people for a period during a series of studies, provides greater evidence of causality.

Retrospective Studies

Observational studies can be either retrospective or prospective. In a retrospective design, data are collected and recorded from previously occurring events, whereas in a prospective or longitudinal design the data collection is planned and occurs after the study has begun.

Nurses and midwives often review patients' medical records retrospectively to answer their research questions. An example is a study retrospectively examining the dialysis attendance patterns of Aboriginal patients attending dialysis services throughout all Australian locations. It was found that among patients who missed two or more dialysis treatments a month were those attending urban services. As such, urban patients were twice as likely to have a hospital admission and three times as likely to have an emergency presentation. Rural patients experienced higher dialysis attendance and lower health service utilisation (Gorham et al 2022).

Case–Control Studies

A case–control study is an approach which examines participants on the basis of a study outcome (clinical characteristic, condition or disease) that is or is not present (e.g. delirium). The study direction is usually retrospective: from the study outcome backwards to the cause or the exposure. Individuals with the outcome of interest are the 'cases'. Cases are matched with 'controls', a sample of people who come from the same 'study base' (like the cases for characteristics such as age, gender or clinical procedure), but do not have the outcome of interest. Detailed past histories, particularly in relation to possible risk factors (exposure), are examined from both groups to see whether the cases have been more exposed to the suspected causative factor than the controls.

Selection bias may exist if the cases are not from a well-defined study base (in time and place). A critical reader therefore needs to cautiously evaluate the conclusions drawn in relation to measurement error. Advantages are like those of a correlational design, but a higher level of control is possible. Disadvantages include an inability to draw a causal linkage between the two variables (an alternative hypothesis may cause the relationship) and finding naturally occurring groups of participants who are similar in all respects except for their exposure to the variable of interest is very difficult.

RESEARCH IN BRIEF 8.2

A case–control study was used by a group of Australian nurse researchers to identify risk factors for incident delirium in patients admitted to hospital for acute medical care (Tomlinson et al 2017). An audit tool was used to review medical records of patients admitted to acute medical units for data regarding potential risk factors for delirium. Cases were 161 patients admitted to an acute medical ward and diagnosed with incident delirium. Controls were 321 patients sampled from the acute medical population admitted within the same time range, stratified for admission location but without a diagnosis of incident delirium during their admission. The researchers identified a selection of predisposing and precipitating risk factors. Predisposing risk factors included dementia, cognitive impairment, functional impairment, previous delirium and fracture on admission. Precipitating risk factors included the use of an indwelling catheter, adding more than three medications during admission and having an abnormal sodium level during admission.

Cohort Studies

A cohort study is an approach where the direction of study is prospective from the exposure to the outcome, or from the cause to the presumed effect. Commonly, a researcher studies the development of a particular health outcome or disease state (e.g. long-term cognitive impairment). Participants are selected from a population known to be free of the health outcome under study, and then classified according to whether they have one or more explanatory variables hypothetically related to the outcome. These participants (referred to as the cohort) are then studied over a time ranging from days to months to years, to determine who develops the outcome of interest. The incidence of the study outcome is observed in relation to exposure to possible causes/risk factors.

Cohort studies can be cross-sectional or longitudinal. Cross-sectional studies examine cohorts at one point in time, or perhaps sequences of time-points, whereas longitudinal cohort studies investigate cohorts over long time periods. A disadvantage of this design is the time and high costs involved, as there may be a considerable time lag between time of exposure and the subsequent study outcome. This may be partly overcome in an historical cohort study if some of the data of individuals exposed in the past are available for use.

A prospective cohort study design was used by nurse researchers to study long-term cognitive impairment in patients discharged from an Australian intensive care unit (ICU) (Mitchell et al 2018). The researchers hypothesised that a longer episode of delirium and a longer period of ventilation while in the ICU may be associated with long-term cognitive impairment once discharged. Of 148 study participants, 91 (61%) completed assessment at 3 and 6 months. The incidence of delirium was 19%, with 41% cognitively impaired at 3 months and 24% remaining impaired at 6 months. The researchers did not find an association between global cognitive function and ICU delirium, but there was a positive association with information-processing speed and executive functioning at 6 months post-discharge. In addition, there was a positive association between executive functioning speed and mechanical ventilation, although this was not statistically significant.

Longitudinal Studies

In contrast to a cross-sectional design, longitudinal studies collect data from the same group of participants at different points in time (repeated measures). By collecting data from each participant at certain intervals, a longitudinal perspective of the outcome variable is possible. An example of a longitudinal cohort study is the classic Nurses' Health Study, one of the largest cohort studies of risk factors for major chronic diseases in women. In 1976 over 120,000 married registered nurses aged 30–55 years were initially enrolled in the study (Belanger et al 1978) and the cohort continues to be followed, examining a wide range of issues including diet, menopause and breast cancer (Li et al 2020). Contemporary articles continue to be published from follow-up assessments (see the Nurses' Health Study website in 'Additional resources' at the end of this chapter).

There are three types of longitudinal design, each with their advantages and disadvantages:

1. longitudinal trend studies
2. longitudinal cohort studies
3. longitudinal panel studies.

Longitudinal Trend Studies

This type of design is good for looking at general trends in populations; however, it is not suitable for following individuals. Trend studies are used, for example, by newspapers in the run-up to a general election and are carried out by taking regular samples from the population to find out what voting patterns are likely to be. Therefore, trend studies use the same population but different samples from it over time. Trend studies are unique in longitudinal designs in being immune to attrition, or dropout, from the study as they make no effort to resample the same people (although they may do this incidentally) and sampling at each stage simply proceeds until sufficient participants have responded. For instance, Koch et al (2017) examined trends in sun-protection behaviour in Western Australia by conducting annual cross-sectional telephone surveys of a randomly selected sample. Over a 10-year period the researchers found that, despite slight fluctuations in the use of sunscreen and protective clothing, sun-protection behaviour among Western Australian adults remained relatively unchanged.

Longitudinal Cohort Studies

This type of design uses a sample—called a cohort—and runs a study over time at regular intervals by sampling from that cohort. For example, the cohort may be all the students graduating in one year in nursing from a large university nursing program. A university may be interested in following up this cohort over the years after graduation and they can do this by sending out questionnaires to students in the group. A random sample may be selected from the cohort or the whole cohort may be sampled. In this design the cohort, not the individual, is of interest. There is no effort to sample the same people, although many of the same people will respond; rather it is information about the whole group that is being sought through those sampled at each stage. Clearly, this design is more vulnerable to attrition than the trend design.

A good example of a longitudinal cohort study is the Australian Longitudinal Study on Women's Health (https://alswh.org.au/), which has been providing insights into Australian women's health for the past 20 years and which has been used to inform policy and clinical practice.

Longitudinal Panel Studies

This type of design is like the cohort design as it follows a defined group of people; however, unlike the cohort design, a panel study is designed to follow individuals over time and makes every effort to re-recruit and, thereby, resample precisely the same people at each stage in the study. This is a very powerful way of studying individual change and individual differences over time but it provides less information about a whole group than a cohort study and little information about the population. Because of the need to re-recruit specific individuals, panel studies are very vulnerable to attrition, as once someone is lost to the study they rarely reappear. While statistical methods exist to compensate, their data are essentially lost to the study. The advantages and disadvantages of a longitudinal design are listed in Table 8.5.

A longitudinal panel design was chosen to examine how undergraduate nursing students' career expectations relate to their career choices, particularly employment in care of older people (Abrahamsen 2019). Overall findings from the study were that the likelihood of moving into care of older people increase with time in nursing careers and relates to nurses' expectations of achieving leadership roles and working part-time. Box 8.2 includes examples of longitudinal data sets.

Causality in Observational Designs

As noted earlier, observational designs are often limited in their ability to determine 'causality'—where one variable influences another in a cause-and-effect relationship. Historically, only experimental research has been able to support the concept of causality. There are, however, many instances in clinical research where experimental studies cannot be conducted because of ethical or practical reasons. To overcome this limitation, several statistical analytical techniques are available to explain relationships among variables and establish causal links. These causal modelling analyses (also termed 'causal analysis', 'path analysis', 'linear

BOX 8.2 Some Examples of Longitudinal Data Sets

There are many longitudinal data sets available for study around the world, and the custodians of these are keen for other investigators to use them. Consider approaching authors if you are interested in doing this sort of work. It is an interesting approach to quantitative research that can yield not only worthwhile results but also publications in high-ranking journals. The following is a list of some such data sets:

- Australian Longitudinal Study on Women's Health: https://alswh.org.au/
- Avon Longitudinal Study of Parents and Children (ALSPAC): https://www.bristol.ac.uk/alspac/
- Footprints in Time – The Longitudinal Study of Indigenous Children (LSIC) https://www.dss.gov.au/about-the-department/longitudinal-studies/footprints-in-time-lsic-longitudinal-study-of-indigenous-children-overview
- Mater University Study of Pregnancy (MUSP): https://social-science.uq.edu.au/mater-university-queensland-study-pregnancy
- Medicine in Australia: Balancing Employment and Life (MABEL) Australia's national longitudinal survey of doctors: https://melbourneinstitute.unimelb.edu.au/mabel/home#mabel
- The Dunedin Multidisciplinary Health & Development Study: https://dunedinstudy.otago.ac.nz/studies/assessment-phases
- The Dutch Famine Birth Cohort Study: https://www.hongerwinter.nl/?lang=en
- The Raine Study: https://rainestudy.org.au/

TABLE 8.5 Advantages and Disadvantages of Longitudinal Studies

Advantages	Disadvantages
Participants are followed separately and therefore act as their own control.	Long duration of data collection—costly in terms of time, effort and resources.
Both relationships and differences can be explored between variables.	Threats to internal validity include 'testing' and 'mortality' (loss to follow-up), and the influence of confounding variables.
Changes in the variables of interest are assessed over time; early trends in data can be investigated at a subsequent measurement.	Social desirability bias is possible (participants respond in a way they believe is congruent with the researchers' expectations)—'Hawthorne effect'.

structural relation analysis (LISREL)' and 'structural equation modelling (SEM)') are introduced in Chapter 11.

Non-randomised Studies of Interventions

The gold standard for testing interventions is usually an experimental design such as an RCT, but for many reasons this type of design may be impractical to conduct. For example, suppose you were interested in the effects of a new cardiac education program that is being introduced into your service. You could randomly assign participants to receive either the new program or the usual program, but there may be several practical, ethical or administrative reasons why this is impossible. As an alternative, you may decide it is more feasible to compare the outcomes of your unit's patients (the intervention group) with those of a similar unit at a site yet to implement the program (the control group).

These types of **non-randomised studies of interventions** manipulate the treatment (intervention, explanatory variable) but lack at least one of the other characteristics of a 'true' experimental design—either a control or randomisation. This group of designs is able to test cause-and-effect relationships, but the lack of a control and/or randomisation threatens the study's internal validity and weakens any causal inference. Many different designs exist; the common types are discussed here (Fig. 8.2) (see Table 8.6 for advantages and disadvantages of non-randomised studies of interventions).

Non-equivalent Control Group Studies

This design is similar to a true experimental design, except participants are unable to be randomised to study groups owing to practicality or feasibility issues (Fig. 8.2A). Despite the lack of randomisation, this design is commonly used in clinical research as it is relatively robust to threats to internal validity. Collection of pre-intervention data allows for a comparison of the two groups before the intervention is introduced, which enables the researcher to control for

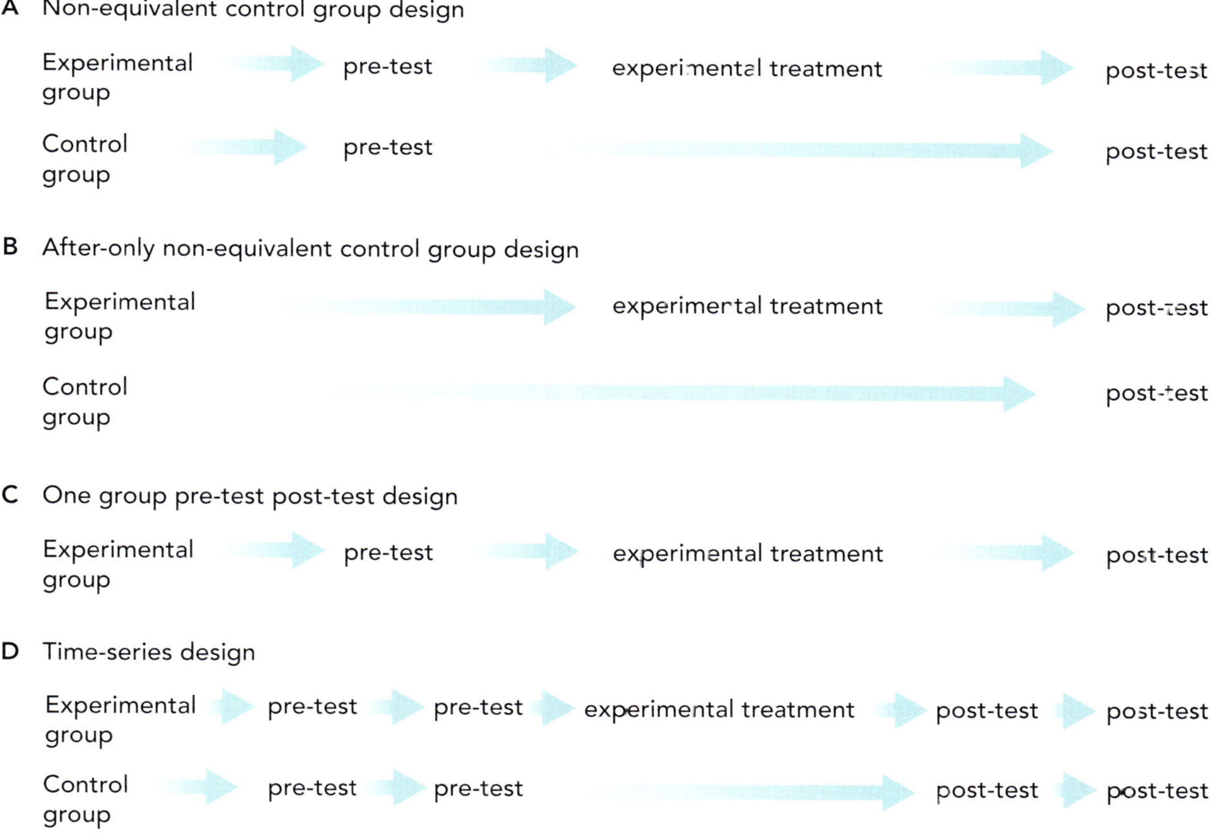

Fig. 8.2 Comparison of designs for non-randomised studies of interventions.

TABLE 8.6 Advantages and Disadvantages of Non-randomised Studies of Interventions

Advantages	Disadvantages
Practical, feasible and able to be generalised. May be the only design to evaluate some hypotheses, particularly in clinical settings. More adaptable to the real-world practice setting than controlled experimental designs.	Need to rule out any plausible alternative explanations for the findings—control by design or statistical analysis. Unable to make clear cause-and-effect inferences.

differences during data analysis. This feature strengthens the influence of the intervention and minimises any effects of extraneous variables.

RESEARCH IN BRIEF 8.3

Kozlowski et al (2018) used a non-equivalent control group design to test the effect of a brief Emotional Intelligence training program for registered nurses. A validated Emotional Intelligence self-assessment tool was administered to two groups of nurses (the intervention and a control group) at two time-points 3 months apart. The intervention group received an Emotional Intelligence training program which consisted of a 5-hour workshop, a 30-minute one-on-one feedback session with a trainer and an individualised follow-up reminder SMS. The study found that Emotional Intelligence scores significantly increased over baseline levels for the intervention group whereas scores for the control group remained unchanged.

After-only Non-equivalent Control Group Studies

In some circumstances a researcher may be unable to measure specific characteristics of the participants before the introduction of a new intervention, but still wishes to collect data demonstrating the efficacy of the program/intervention (shown in Fig. 8.2B). This type of opportunistic study can also be referred to as a 'natural experiment' because the participants (or groups of participants) are exposed to the intervention or control based on factors outside the control of the researchers. This design has the benefit of minimising 'testing effects' (whereby completing a pretest affects the post-test scores), but it is a weaker design because it assumes that the two groups are equivalent before the intervention is introduced.

A team of Australian nurse researchers used an after-only non-equivalent control group design to opportunistically evaluate the impact of an initiative to add unregulated nursing support workers to wards in acute care hospitals (Duffield et al 2018). A sample of five wards where the use of nursing support workers had been introduced were compared with a group of five wards where there were no nursing support workers. A cross-sectional survey was administered to staff and patients in both groups. The patient survey consisted of the Patient Evaluation of Emotional Care during Hospitalisation (PEECH) tool and the staff survey consisted of the Practice Environment Scale. The results showed that adding nursing support workers to ward staffing did not lead to improvements in patient care or practice environment. The researchers identified limitations with the study design and suggested the inclusion of baseline measurements and matching in future research to allow for more robust conclusions to be drawn.

One-group Pretest–Post-test Studies

A one-group pretest–post-test design is another approach used to determine the effect of a treatment or intervention on a given sample (Fig. 8.2C). However, the lack of randomisation and a control group means that confounding variables are not accounted for, which significantly limits the internal validity of the studies. The design is most frequently used to study the effectiveness of educational programs, or the restructuring of social groups and organisations or the implementation of behavioural interventions. In nursing research this design is most frequently used to evaluate education interventions.

As an example, Kol et al (2021) used a pretest–post-test design to determine the effect of using standardised patients in the simulated hospital environment on first-year nursing students' psychomotor skills. The research found that students developed psychomotor skills more fully in a learning environment designed in a similar way to a real hospital clinic setting. The researchers acknowledged that the generalisability of the findings was limited because the study was conducted at a single site with no control group.

Before–After Design

Sometimes researchers use a 'before–after' design to test the effects of an introduced intervention where the participants are different individuals before the intervention to those involved after the intervention. This design is particularly common in health service research and implementation studies where the focus of the intervention is at the service or facility level. Similar to all non-randomised designs, the lack of randomisation increases the risk of bias from systematic errors.

A before–after study design was used by Australian nurse researchers to determine the impact of an evidence-based intervention (a thermal care bundle) on the prevention, detection and treatment of perioperative inadvertent hypothermia (a temperature <36°C before, during or after surgery) (Duff et al 2018). The incidence of perioperative hypothermia and compliance with the evidence-based care bundle were collected at two time-points before and after the implementation of the intervention. The study found that the bundle improved the management of perioperative inadvertent hypothermia through increased risk assessment, temperature recording and active warming, but did not impact on the incidence of perioperative inadvertent hypothermia.

TUTORIAL TRIGGER 8.1

Given the information in the 'after-only non-equivalent control group' section, describe the reasons why a RCT design was not possible in the Australian study (Duffield et al 2018).

Interrupted Time Series Studies

Another approach when only one group is available is to study that group over a longer period using a time series design (illustrated in Fig. 8.2D). In this design, the variable of interest is measured at multiple time-points with the intervention introduced at a predetermined mid-point. If the intervention has a causal effect then the mean, or the slope of the trend, of the pre-intervention data should be different to that of the post-intervention data.

A team of UK nurse researchers used an interrupted time series design to evaluate whether the introduction of portable nursing stations into wards reduced inpatient falls (Ali et al 2018). Inpatient falls data were collected monthly across 17 wards for 24 months prior to and 12 months following the introduction of portable nursing stations. The study found that portable nursing stations were associated with lower monthly falls rates. The slope of the pre-intervention data trend was 0.119 (95% confidence interval (CI), 0.045 to 0.194) compared with −0.222 (95% CI −0.350 to −0.093) for the post-intervention data, which equated to a statistically significant change of 0.341 (95% CI, 0.159 to 0.524; $p = 0.001$).

RANDOMISED CONTROLLED TRIAL DESIGNS

RCT designs have all three identifying properties: randomisation, control and manipulation. These designs are used to test cause-and-effect relationships between an intervention (treatment) and an outcome, and minimise or control alternative explanations (threats to validity) for the study findings (Rajasekar & Kumar 2019). To infer causality, the study requires that:

- the explanatory (causal) and outcome (effect) variables must be associated with each other
- the cause precedes the effect, and
- the relationship is not able to be explained by another (extraneous) variable/s.

Conducting an RCT can be challenging, as all relevant variables need to be identified and then controlled, manipulated or measured. However, RCTs are an important way that nurses and midwives can generate research relevant to their knowledge and evidence requirements. One challenge is to design the study in such a way that minimises the potential that the treatment to which patients have been randomly assigned cannot be delivered as intended. Bias from this so-called 'contamination' can occur if a participant allocated to a specific study group receives the alternative intervention. Another challenge is implementing strategies to ensure that as many patients enrolled in the study as possible can complete it, otherwise there may be incomplete outcome data. Attrition bias can occur if there are systematic differences between groups in the number of patients who do not complete the study.

There are many different designs that can be used to conduct an RCT. The central design element is that participants are randomly assigned to the control or intervention condition(s).

When reading an RCT, the prime focus is on assessing the validity of the results. How certain is it that the intervention (explanatory variable) caused the effect on the outcome variable? The validity of the results and consequent interpretations depend on how well the researcher has controlled other variables that may also explain any change in the outcome variables. Although random assignment and control minimise the effects of threats to internal validity, it is not perfect in practice as some are difficult to control. Mortality effects (a threat to internal validity) may be a problem for studies with long follow-up periods, as participants tend to drop out because of the burden over an extended period of time (called 'loss to follow-up' or attrition bias). There may be important differences between participants who withdraw and those who complete the study; these differences, and not the intervention, may explain the study findings. Guidelines for reporting results of RCTs have been developed by the CONSORT (Consolidated

Standards of Reporting Trials) group for reporting these types of threats (Liampas et al 2019); see 'Additional resources' at the end of this chapter). Specifically, it is very important to examine and discuss any loss to follow-up in studies as these may influence a study's findings. Incomplete data at the end of a study may impact how confident we are that the results are demonstrating a relationship (internal validity) or whether some other factor has led to these results occurring. This issue is discussed in more detail in Chapter 9.

TUTORIAL TRIGGER 8.2

The group assignment for your research subject is to critique an assigned quantitative study. To proceed, you must first decide on the design to be used. You think it is a before-and-after design; the others in the group think it is an experimental design because it has several explicit hypotheses. How would you convince them that you are correct?

Types of Randomised Controlled Trials

An RCT is the gold standard for testing cause-and-effect relationships in clinical research (Rajasekar & Kumar 2019). As introduced above, there are numerous types of RCT designs. They can be broadly categorised by the unit of randomisation used (individual participant or cluster of participants) and as either parallel (outcomes compared between groups) or crossover (outcomes compared within groups at more than one time-point) designs. The number of participants required in a trial generally increases if more than two conditions (e.g. two different alternative interventions and control conditions) are being tested. The most common RCT design is a parallel group RCT comparing one intervention with a control condition. In the parallel group RCT, participants are randomly assigned to intervention and control conditions, so that any pre-intervention differences (antecedent variables) are measured and/or controlled. Pretest measures or observations can be measured to provide a baseline score for verifying similar characteristics between control and treatment groups, and therefore the effect of the intervention. The intervention is then introduced, and the outcome variable is again measured to see whether it has changed. Outcomes for the control group are also measured for comparison. The difference between the groups at post-test reflects whether a causal link exists between the explanatory and the outcome variables.

A recent example of a parallel group RCT comparing a control and an intervention that is relevant to nursing practice involved the testing of forced-air warming during procedures performed with sedation in a cardiac catheterisation laboratory (Conway et al 2018). In this study, 140 participants from two hospitals were randomised in a 1:1 ratio either to be warmed with a forced-air warming device during their procedure or to receive usual care, which consisted of passive warming with heated cotton blankets. Block randomisation (groups of two to five patients) was used to enhance the success of balancing the demographic and clinical characteristics between groups, which is generally recommended for RCTs with small sample sizes. Furthermore, the randomisation sequence was stratified into groups of patients at each site and according to whether or not the sedation was administered by an anaesthetist. Balanced randomisation using stratification involves incorporating baseline covariates into the randomisation scheme, which is an effective way to minimise the chance that groups will differ in important characteristics post-randomisation (Bruce et al 2022). The primary outcome was the proportion of participants who were hypothermic (defined as a temperature below 36°C) after procedures. Data were collected prior to and after procedures. Forced-air warming was found to decrease risk of hypothermia and increase post-procedural temperature as well as ratings of thermal comfort (Conway et al 2018).

Cluster-randomised Controlled Trials

A cluster-randomised controlled trial (c-RCT) uses coherent groups or clusters of individuals, such as outpatient clinics (Logan et al 2023), ICUs (Lynch et al 2020), hospital clinical work area (Haskell et al 2021) or aged care settings (Luliano et al 2021), as the random allocation unit, rather than individuals. All individuals in the group allocated to the intervention then receive the experimental treatment. This aspect of the cluster RCT is particularly suited to testing competing interventions that are common or routine in nursing and midwifery practice, because in this situation there is a high risk that clinicians may implement the control condition to patients randomised to the intervention condition (and vice versa). Such incorrect implementation of the randomised allocations is called 'contamination'. Randomising participants at the cluster level is one way to reduce risk of bias from contamination.

A disadvantage of cluster randomisation to consider is that the number of participants required to be enrolled in the trial heavily depends on the degree to which measurements of the outcome of interest are similar within each cluster (termed intracluster correlation (ICC)) (Hemming & Taljaard 2020). In trials with high ICCs (similar measurements within clusters) each measurement contributes less to the overall ability for the study to be able to detect a statistically significant difference between the intervention and the control conditions (Hemming & Taljaard 2020). In these situations, more clusters need to be added (instead of more participants within each cluster), which may not always be possible. To overcome this problem, a solution is to apply the crossover method to the cluster-level randomisation design by breaking it into a series of repeated measurements fluctuating (in random order) between intervention and control conditions.

Another type of cluster RCT design is the stepped wedge design. In this design, the intervention conditions are implemented in the clusters over time periods in a randomised order such that, at the end of the trial, all clusters will be using the intervention being tested. Although there are variations to the stepped wedge design that can be used, the most common implementation involves measuring outcomes in each cluster over the whole period (Hemming & Taljaard 2020). This type of clustered design is suited to situations where the intervention requires considerable resources to implement, necessitating that only a small number of sites receive the intervention at any one point in time. Another situation that particularly suits the stepped wedge design is a nursing or midwifery research study primarily aiming to implement evidence into practice. A systematic review of stepped wedge trials identified that most studies included in the review were used to evaluate interventions in routine care that have already been shown to be effective in more controlled research settings (Mdege et al 2011). In these situations where evidence of efficacy is already available, it is often more feasible to recruit and retain sites in a trial if the intervention will be implemented at all sites. This differs to a typical cluster RCT, where only intervention sites will receive the intervention.

BOX 8.3 Criteria for Evaluating Quantitative Designs

1. What design was used in the study (observational, non-randomised or randomised controlled trial)?
2. Which specific type of the above design was used in the study, and was it appropriate?
3. Was the design appropriate for the research problem and data collection methods?
4. Was the problem examining a cause-and-effect relationship?
5. Were the common threats to the validity of findings for this design addressed?
6. Was the design suited to the study setting?
7. Were the limitations of the design adequately discussed?
8. Were there other limitations related to the design that you identified but were not discussed?
9. For observational designs, did the report go beyond the parameters of this design, and infer cause-and-effect relationships between variables?
10. How were randomisation, control and manipulation applied?
11. What were the plausible alternative explanations for findings, and were they discussed and discounted?
12. Are the findings able to be generalised to other practice settings and the larger population of interest?

SUMMARY

Quantitative research methods use numerical data to answer specific research questions and draw inferences from their findings to estimate effects in the target population. Observational designs are used to construct a picture or description of events as they naturally occur but cannot establish cause-and-effect relationships between variables. Non-randomised studies of interventions are frequently used in clinical research to explore cause-and-effect relationships, as there are times when an RCT design, which can test this relationship, is impractical to conduct within that setting. RCTs are characterised by control of extraneous variables, manipulation of the explanatory variable and random assignment of participants to study groups.

Chapter 15 discusses the critical review process, which is directed towards evaluating the appropriateness of the study design in relation to factors such as the research problem, theoretical framework, hypothesis, methods of data analysis and interpretation. The overall purpose of reviewing studies is to assess the validity of findings and to determine whether these findings are worth incorporating into your professional practice and/or as the evidence base for current institutional clinical practices. Criteria for the review of quantitative designs relate to how well any potential biases in the methods have been addressed (see Box 8.3).

The most important question to ask as you read an RCT is, 'What else could have happened to explain the findings?' This question of potential alternative explanations will be addressed by a well-written report, which will systematically review potential threats to the validity of the findings. You must then decide whether the author's explanations are clear and logical.

KEY POINTS

- Three main strengths of quantitative approaches are objectivity, precision and control afforded through design, sampling strategies and analytical tests.

- Quantitative designs allow nurses and midwives to justify, in a scientific manner, the outcomes of their actions and provide the basis for effective high-quality and evidence-based clinical practice.
- Extraneous and confounding variables represent a major influence on the interpretation of any quantitative study. These types of variables limit the validity of the study and generalisability of the findings; this is particularly evident with observational designs.
- When reviewing quantitative studies, check that the author has addressed all of the relevant issues, such as evidence of a representative sample, and minimal and unbiased loss to follow-up.

TIME TO REFLECT

Hermanson, Å., Åstrand, L.L., 2020. The effects of early pacifier use on breastfeeding: a randomised controlled trial. Women Birth 33(5), e473–e482. doi: 10.1016/j.wombi.2019.10.001

Aim: To investigate whether a recommendation of early pacifier use affects the proportion of breastfeeding at 6 months compared with a recommendation to avoid pacifier use during the first 2 weeks.

Methods: An open RCT with parallel group design; 239 primiparous mothers and their term infants were randomly assigned to an intervention group or a control group. The primary outcome was the proportion of breastfeeding at 6 months. Secondary outcomes were the proportions of breastfeeding and breastfeeding problems at 2 and 4 months. To investigate factors which may influence breastfeeding, a multivariate logistic regressions analysis was performed.

Reflect on the following: When reflecting on this study, you may consider whether the design used was appropriate for the study considering the stated aim, the strengths and limitations of the design, and whether it would have been possible to use an alternative design to examine whether early pacifier use impacts the proportion of infants who are breastfeeding at 6 months.

Questions

1. Could this study be considered a non-randomised study of an intervention? If so, why?
2. Is the design appropriate for this study?
3. Why did the researchers collect information using an open RCT approach?
4. Are the aims achievable using this design?
5. Why was it important to report the differences between groups within this study?

LEARNING ACTIVITIES: QUIZ

1. The purpose of quantitative research is to explore, examine and describe.
   True
   False
2. A study which uses questionnaires with numerical scores to examine feelings, perceptions or social effects is a quantitative study.
   True
   False
3. Assigning an intervention to only one group of participants but not another is an RCT.
   True
   False
4. Bias happens when the participants know whether they are in the group that the intervention is being tested.
   True
   False
5. Non-randomised correlation studies are used frequently in nursing and midwifery because RCTs are not possible in that field.
   True
   False
6. RCTs are always the only way to conduct a study.
   True
   False
7. RCTs are best way to conduct a study, if possible.
   True
   False
8. A randomised controlled trial design includes four aspects—randomisation, blinding, control and manipulation.
   True
   False
9. Sometimes a control can be implemented by manipulating one variable and not another.
   True
   False
10. A case–control study is the most powerful type of design for examining cause-and-effect relationships.
    True
    False

11. When data are collected before and after the introduction of the intervention, the design is called a case–control study.
    True
    False
12. In non-randomised studies of interventions, blinding may be used.
    True
    False
13. Loss to follow-up is one of the potential disadvantages of longitudinal studies.
    True
    False

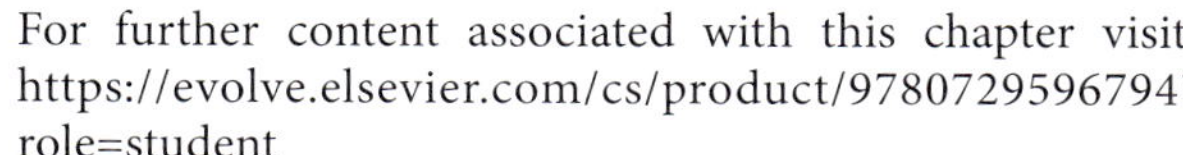
For further content associated with this chapter visit: https://evolve.elsevier.com/cs/product/9780729596794?role=student

ADDITIONAL RESOURCES

CASP International: Critical Appraisal Tools. http://caspinternational.org/?o=1012.
Cochrane Collaboration. https://www.cochrane.org/.
GRADE working group. https://www.gradeworkinggroup.org/.
National Health and Medical Research Council. 2023. Building a healthy Australia. Australian Government. Available from https://www.nhmrc.gov.au/.
Nurses' Health Study. https://nurseshealthstudy.org/.
The Dunedin Multidisciplinary Health and Development Study. https://dunedinstudy.otago.ac.nz/studies/assessment-phases.
The Raine Study. https://rainestudy.org.au/.

REFERENCES

Abrahamsen, B., 2019. A longitudinal study of nurses' career choices: The importance of career expectations on employment in care of older people. J. Adv. Nurs. 75 (2), 348–356.

Ali, U.M., Judge, A., Foster, C., et al., 2018. Do portable nursing stations within bays of hospital wards reduce the rate of inpatient falls? An interrupted time-series analysis. Age Ageing 47 (6), 818–824. doi:10.1093/ageing/afy097

Belanger, C.F., Hennekens, C.H., Rosner, B., et al., 1978. The nurses' health study. Am. J. Nurs. 78, 1039–1040.

Bezerra, C.T., Grande, A.J., Galvão, V.K., et al., 2022. Assessment of the strength of recommendation and quality of evidence: GRADE checklist. A descriptive study. Sao Paulo Med. J. 140, 829–836.

Boutron, I., Page, M.J., Higgins, J.P., et al.; Cochrane Bias Methods Group, 2023. Considering bias and conflicts of interest among the included studies. In: Higgins, J., Thomas, J. (Eds) Cochrane Handbook for Systematic Reviews of Interventions, Ch. 7, 177–204.

Bruce, C.L., Juszczak, E., Ogollah, R., et al., 2022. A systematic review of randomisation method use in RCTs and association of trial design characteristics with method selection. BMC Med. Res. Methodol. 22 (1), 314.

Carrington, M.J, Zimmet, P.Z., 2022. Nurse co-ordinated health and lifestyle modification for reducing multiple cardio-metabolic risk factors in regional adults: outcomes from the MODERN randomized controlled trial. Eur. J. Cardiovasc. Nurs. 21 (1), 26–35.

Chan, S.S.C., Leung, D.Y.P., Leung, A.Y.P., et al., 2015. A nurse-delivered brief health education intervention to improve pneumococcal vaccination rate among older patients with chronic disease: a cluster randomised trial. Int. J. Nurs. Stud. 52, 317–324.

Conway, A., Ersotelos, S., Sutherland, J., et al., 2018. Forced air warming during sedation in the cardiac catheterisation laboratory: a randomised controlled trial. Heart 104, 685–690.

Duff, J., Walker, K., Edward, K.L., et al., 2018. Effect of a thermal care bundle on the prevention, detection and treatment of perioperative inadvertent hypothermia. J. Clin. Nurs. 27 (5–6), 1239–1249.

Duffield, C., Roche, M., Twigg, D., et al., 2018. Adding unregulated nursing support workers to ward staffing: exploration of a natural experiment. J. Clin. Nurs. 27 (19–20), 3768–3779.

Goedemans, A., Liang, K., Cottell, B., et al., 2014. Topical Arnica and mucopolysaccharide polysulfate (Hirudoid) to decrease bruising and pain associated with haemodialysis cannulation-related infiltration: a pilot study. Ren. Soc. Australas J. 10 (2), 62–65.

Gorham, G., Howard, K., Cunningham, J., et al., 2022. Dialysis attendance patterns and health care utilisation of Aboriginal patients attending dialysis services in urban, rural and remote locations. BMC Health Serv. Res. 22 (1), 251.

Greenhalgh, T., 2019. How to Read a Paper: the basics of evidence-based medicine and healthcare. John Wiley & Sons, New York.

Halcomb, E., Bird, S., 2020. Job satisfaction and career intention of Australian general practice nurses: a cross-sectional survey. J. Nurs. Scholarsh. 52 (3), 270–280.

Haskell, L., Tavender, E.J., O'Brien, S., et al., 2021. Process evaluation of a cluster randomised controlled trial to improve bronchiolitis management – a PREDICT mixed-methods study. BMC Health Serv. Res. 21 (1), 1–13.

Hawkins, N., Jeong, S.Y.S., Smith, T., et al., 2023. Creating respectful workplaces for nurses in regional acute care settings: a quasi-experimental design. Nurs. Open, 10 (1), 78–89.

Hemming, K., Taljaard, M., 2020. Reflection on modern methods: when is a stepped-wedge cluster randomized trial a good study design choice?. Int. J. Epidemiol. 49 (3), 1043–1052.

Hermanson, Å., Åstrand, L.L., 2020. The effects of early pacifier use on breastfeeding: a randomised controlled trial. Women Birth 33 (5), e473–e482. doi:10.1016/j.wombi.2019.10.001

Koch, S., Pettigrew, S., Minto, C., et al., 2017. Trends in sun-protection behaviour in Australian adults 2007–2012. Australas. J. Dermatol. 58 (2), 111–116. doi:10.1111/ajd.12433

Kol, E., Ince, S., Işik, R.D., et al., 2021. The effect of using standardized patients in the Simulated Hospital Environment on first-year nursing students psychomotor skills learning. Nurse Educ. Today 107, 105147.

Kozlowski, D., Hutchinson, M., Hurley, J., et al., 2018. Increasing nurses' emotional intelligence with a brief intervention. Appl. Nurs. Res. 41, 59–61.

Li, Y., Schoufour, J., Wang, D.D., et al., 2020. Healthy lifestyle and life expectancy free of cancer, cardiovascular disease, and type 2 diabetes: prospective cohort study. BMJ, 368, 16669. doi:10.1136/bmj.l6669

Liampas, I., Chlinos, A., Siokas, V., et al., 2019. Assessment of the reporting quality of RCTs for novel oral anticoagulants in venous thromboembolic disease based on the CONSORT statement. J. Thromb. Thrombolysis, 48 (4), 542–553.

Logan, B., Viecelli, A.K., Johnson, D.W., et al., 2023. Study protocol for The GOAL Trial: comprehensive geriatric assessment for frail older people with chronic kidney disease to increase attainment of patient-identified goals—a cluster randomised controlled trial. Trials 24 (1), 365.

Luliano, S., Poon, S., Robbins, J., et al., 2021. Effect of dietary sources of calcium and protein on hip fractures and falls in older adults in residential care: cluster randomised controlled trial. BMJ, 375, n2364.

Lynch, J., Rolls, K., Hou, Y.C., et al., 2020. Delirium in intensive care: a stepped-wedge cluster randomised controlled trial for a nurse-led intervention to reduce the incidence and duration of delirium among adults admitted to the intensive care unit (protocol). Aust. Crit. Care 33 (5), 475–479.

Mdege, N.D., Man, M.S., Taylor, C.A., et al., 2011. Systematic review of stepped wedge cluster randomized trials shows that design is particularly used to evaluate interventions during routine implementation. J. Clin. Epidemiol. 64 (9), 936–948.

Mitchell, M.L., Shum, D.H., Mihala, G., et al., 2018. Long-term cognitive impairment and delirium in intensive care: a prospective cohort study. Aust. Crit. Care 31 (4), 204–211.

National Health and Medical Research Council (NHMRC), 2019. Guidelines for Guidelines. Assessing certainty of evidence. Retrieved from: https://www.nhmrc.gov.au/guidelines-forguidelines/develop/assessing-certainty-evidence.

Pu L, Moyle W, Jones C, et al., 2020. The effect of using PARO for people living with dementia and chronic pain: a pilot randomized controlled trial. J. Am. Med. Dir. Assoc. 21 (8), 1079–1085.

Rajasekar, A., Kumar, V., 2019. Randomized controlled trials: gold standard of evidence. Drug Invent. Today 12 (6), 1215–1217.

Schulz, K., Altman, D., Moher, D., 2010. CONSORT 2010 Statement: updated guidelines for reporting parallel group randomised trials. BMJ 340, c332. doi:10.1136/bmj.c332

Siedlecki, S.L., 2020. Understanding descriptive research designs and methods. Clin. Nurse Spec. 34 (1), 8–12.

Slykerman, R.F., Li, E., 2022. A randomized trial of probiotic supplementation in nurses to reduce stress and viral illness. Sci. Rep. 12 (1), 14742.

Smyth, W., McArdle, J., Body-Dempsey, J., et al., 2022. Immersive virtual reality in a northern Queensland haemodialysis unit: study protocol for a cross-over randomized controlled feasibility trial. Contemp. Clin. Trials Commun. 28, 100956.

Terry, D., Peck, B., Kloot, K., et al., 2022. Pediatric emergency asthma presentations in Southwest Victoria: a retrospective cross-sectional study 2017 to 2020. J. Asthma 59 (2), 264–272.

Terry, D., Robins, S., Gardiner, S., et al., 2017. Asthma hospitalisation trends from 2010 to 2015: variation among rural and metropolitan Australians. BMC Public Health 17 (1), 723.

Tomlinson, E.J., Phillips, N.M., Mohebbi, M., et al., 2017. Risk factors for incident delirium in an acute general medical setting: a retrospective case–control study. J. Clin. Nurs. 26 (5–6), 658–667.

Wang, X., Cheng, Z., 2020. Cross-sectional studies: strengths, weaknesses, and recommendations. Chest 158 (1), S65–S71.

Webster, R.K., Bishop, F., Collins, G.S., et al., 2021. Measuring the success of blinding in placebo-controlled trials: should we be so quick to dismiss it? J. Clin. Epidemiol. 135, 176–181.

von Wernsdorff M, Loef M, Tuschen-Caffier B, et al., 2021. Effects of open-label placebos in clinical trials: a systematic review and meta-analysis. Sci. Rep. 11 (1), 1–4.

9

Data Collection and Sampling in Quantitative Research

Daniel Terry and Hoang Phan

LEARNING OUTCOMES

After reading this chapter, you should be able to:

- describe the purpose of sampling
- define element, population and sample
- describe the protocols and procedures for drawing samples
- describe the types of probability and non-probability sampling
- discuss the factors that determine sample size
- discuss eligibility, inclusion and exclusion criteria for sample selection
- examine and categorise study variable/s
- describe appropriate methods of collecting data in quantitative research
- analyse key considerations for selecting the most appropriate quantitative research methods
- explore and clarify potential risks to internal validity
- describe external validity and key considerations
- critique published peer-reviewed articles and describe the study methods, data collection and study validity
- describe and apply key considerations for understanding different quantitative data collection methods.

KEY TERMS

external validity, p. 134
inclusion and/or exclusion criteria, p. 134
internal validity, p. 134
measurement, p. 133
non-probability sampling, p. 135
observation, p. 141
probability sampling, p. 135
questionnaires, p. 141
records, databases and other documentations, p. 142
study validity, p. 133
types of sampling strategies, p. 135
variables, p. 133

INTRODUCTION

It is critical that sampling, data collection tools and methods are cohesive to study design so as to ensure the credibility and validity of the study. Specifically, sampling in quantitative research design to promote selection of the most appropriate data collection method, while also ensuring cohesion with any applicable theoretical or conceptual frameworks. Quantitative studies use numerical data which are analysed via statistical methods to answer research questions. A logical flow and congruency exist between research questions, aims, objectives, outcomes and design, including sampling and data collection methods, should therefore be clear to a reader. The 'methods' of a research proposal, grant application, report or published journal article describe the researcher's operational plan, the procedure or simply the process of how the data were collected to answer the research question, objective or hypothesis.

This chapter introduces the basic concepts of sampling applicable to quantitative research studies, while also focusing on types of quantitative data collection methods and **study validity**. It is an assumption in quantitative research that the **variables** of interest can be quantified through a **measurement** process that is expressed in a numerical format. The common approaches to data collection in health research are varied but are often included within the domains of social determinants and psychosocial, physiological or biological measurements. Data collection measurements of these domains could include physiological data collection tools such as the Mini Mental State Examination Tool, fall assessment using a Timed Up and Go Test (TUGT); social determinants could include social economic index, economic analysis and demographic data (Batko-Szwaczka et al 2020). These approaches involving collection of data about participants are identifiable and repeatable steps that enable the major variables to be studied in a systematic, objective and rigorous manner. Quantitative data should be collected in a standardised method following a protocol which limits any influence by the sample, an observer or data collector.

Where appropriate there should also be a registered study protocol for any quantitative interventional study, which is published with the data collection methods and follows appropriate international guideline documents for the quantitative study design. Internal and external validity are used to reflect whether study findings are meaningful and trustworthy. **Internal validity** refers to the degree of confidence in a study to establish a trustworthy causal relationship between a treatment and an outcome. **External validity** refers to results from a study which can be generalised to larger groups.

SAMPLING CONCEPTS

The purpose of sampling from a quantitative perspective is to obtain a sample that has a minimum of bias and that represents the characteristics of interest of those in the target population. If an appropriate sampling strategy is used then a reasonably accurate understanding of the phenomena of interest in the target population is made possible by obtaining data from the study sample. A **target population** is the entire group of people in which the researcher is interested. Examples of bias are threats to internal validity, such as selection, history and maturation. The validity of generalising from a sample to the population depends on how representative the sample is of the population; thus the sampling approaches used remain vital, as an incorrect sampling approach may increase the level of bias in the data and render the outcomes poor or, in a clinical situation, hazardous.

As it is difficult and inefficient to access a population, a researcher employs sampling strategies and techniques that aim to reduce sampling bias. Samples should therefore be drawn to ensure that valid inferences or generalisations can be made from the sample to the population; a quality sample is one that is representative of the wider population from which it is drawn. A population is a set of all the cases of interest and can be composed of people, animals, objects or events. A population can be broadly defined and potentially involve thousands of people or narrowly specified to include only several hundred people.

Population criteria are a precise description of the population that enable generalisability of the findings from a quantitative study to similar populations. The population criteria are then reflected in the **eligibility criteria** of the sample, so that the important characteristics of the population and sample are congruent. Populations may be difficult or challenging to access (e.g. minority groups), so a specific list of available subjects with the characteristics relevant to the study must be developed. This list is called a **sampling frame** and it is from this list that potential participants will be drawn. Instead of a specific list, researchers can instead develop a rule for describing the sampling frame. A *sample* is a subset of the population drawn from the sampling frame and each person is called an *element*.

Inclusion and Exclusion Criteria

The population criteria establish the target population—the entire set of participants or cases that are the focus of the study. The study criteria identify the specific characteristics required for participants in the study sample and are commonly listed in proposals or published papers as **inclusion and/or exclusion criteria**. Eligibility criteria can be viewed as delimitations or those characteristics that restrict the population to a homogeneous group of participants, such as: gender, age, marital status, socioeconomic status, English-speaking status, religion, ethnicity, level of education, age of children, diagnosis, hospitalisation status, nursing specialty, sexuality and so on.

SAMPLE SIZE AND POWER ANALYSIS

For quantitative research, particularly interventional studies and clinical trials where an effect is being measured, sample size must be determined prior to study commencement. This should be calculated and written into the study protocol, prior to applying for ethical approval. Consultation with a biostatistician may be needed, so it is always good to ask a research mentor for assistance and guidance when calculating a sample size. Several factors influence the proposed sample size, including the design, the need for generalisability, the proposed size of the effect of any intervention, the level of statistical significance, the feasibility and the costs. Generally, a larger sample size has more chance of demonstrating an effect, although this may be costly and may not always be necessary, depending on the size of the effect being measured.

Power analysis is a statistical calculation used to determine the correct size of a sample so that accurate inferences can be made about the true relationship between the study variables. Power is the product of sample size, the effect of the study intervention and the chosen level of statistical significance. A study suitably 'powered' provides confidence in interpreting the findings (see 'An unexpected hurdle'). Power reflects the ability of a statistical test to reject a null hypothesis that is false (Cohen 1988). If the sample in a study is too small and power is not achieved, it is possible that a *type II error* may occur. A type II error occurs when a null hypothesis that is false is accepted (see Chapter 11 for a more detailed discussion of power analysis and type I and type II errors).

The study by Alananzeh et al (2019) in the following 'Research in brief 9.1' highlights the importance of a clearly defined target group, adequate sample size determined through power analysis, mechanisms to ensure representativeness of the sample through the provision of bilingual research, and a method to ensure maximum participation through recruitment through the Arab community and religious organisations. Convenience sampling was used.

RESEARCH IN BRIEF 9.1

Alananzeh et al (2019) explored the unmet supportive needs of Arab Australian and Arab Jordanian cancer survivors living in Sydney, Australia and Amman, Jordan. Arab people living in Sydney and Amman with a diagnosis of cancer within the last 5 years were invited to participate. Participants completed a questionnaire that measured unmet supportive care needs, depression and language acculturation. It was calculated that a total sample of 124 participants (ideally 62 from Jordan and 62 from Australia) were needed, allowing for 20% incomplete or missing data. Participants were recruited from oncology clinicians, where hospitals provided brochures written in English and Arabic. A bilingual researcher was employed to conduct the study. Arab-speaking persons diagnosed with any type of cancer, up to 5 years post-diagnosis, 18 years or older and able to read and/or speak English or Arabic were eligible for the study. A convenience sample was used. The final sample was 143 participants (66 from Australia and 77 from Jordan). Researchers concluded that Arab Australians had higher unmet needs compared with their Jordanian counterparts. This confirmed previous research that there are disparities in unmet needs for Arab immigrant cancer survivors.

TYPES OF SAMPLES

There are two **types of sampling strategies**: non-probability sampling and probability sampling (see Tables 9.1 and 9.2). In **non-probability sampling**, elements are chosen by non-random methods; there is no way of checking that each sampling element has been included in the sample. In contrast, **probability sampling** uses some form of *random selection* when choosing the sample units and therefore minimises bias and supports generalisability of the findings. This more rigorous sampling strategy is more likely to result in a representative sample, an important consideration in quantitative research.

Non-probability Sampling

As noted in Chapter 6, this sampling approach is most appropriate for qualitative research, as well as small exploratory quantitative studies, although it is also used in observational research and clinical trials. Non-probability samples are those in which the participants are chosen by the researcher or choose themselves so that the chance of being selected is not known. Non-probability samples are useful when information on the total population is unknown or unavailable. Non-probability sampling strategy is less rigorous for quantitative research approaches than probability as, in such cases, it tends to produce less accurate and less representative samples—thus limiting the ability of the researcher to make generalisations about the findings at a population level. In order to make generalisations, the sample must be representative of the population. If the sample characteristics are not typical of the population, then a sampling error has occurred, which threatens the external validity of the study. The three major types of non-probability sampling are convenience, quota and purposive sampling (see Table 9.1).

TUTORIAL TRIGGER 9.1

One thousand pregnant patients were seen by registered midwives in the perinatal clinic of hospital X. You have been asked by the Patient Experience Manager to send a patient satisfaction questionnaire to this group and have been advised that a sample of 330 patients is adequate.

How would you select a simple random sample from the group of 1000 patients?

Probability Sampling

The purpose of quantitative research is to make inferences about a population based on the findings of research conducted on a sample that has been drawn from that population. In order to make generalisations to the population the sample must be representative of the population; that is, the sample must have the same proportion of characteristics as found in the population.

TABLE 9.1 Non-Probability Sampling Strategies

Sample strategy	Description
Convenience sampling	*Ease of drawing:* Very easy although snowball may be more labour intensive. *Risk of bias:* Considerable. *Representative of the sample:* Because participants tend to volunteer, representativeness is questionable. *When to use:* When the researcher has ready access to participants. Note: Snowball samples usually require participants who are already recruited to identify others. *Things to consider:* It is the most readily accessible and has willing persons or objects as study participants. Clinical trials often involve convenience sampling as the researchers can access the patients from hospitals or clinics. Convenience sampling may be easier for the researcher to obtain participants. The only concern is obtaining enough participants who meet the criteria dictated by the study. The major disadvantage is that the risk of bias is greater than in any other type of sample. The problem of bias exists because convenience samples tend to be self-selecting, and the information obtained comes only from those people who volunteer to participate.
Quota sampling	*Ease of drawing:* Relatively easy. *Risk of bias:* Contains unknown source of bias that affects external validity. *Representative of the sample:* Builds in some representativeness by using knowledge about the population of interest. *When to use:* When the researcher needs to recruit participants to specific subgroups. *Things to consider:* It addresses the issue of appropriate representation for each segment of a population. This non-probability sampling approach uses prior knowledge about the population of interest to build some representativeness into the sample. A quota sample accounts for the proportion of various strata in a population. Characteristics chosen to form the strata are selected according to a researcher's judgement based on knowledge of the population and the literature, to reflect important differences in the variables of interest—for example, age, gender, religion, ethnicity, diagnosis, socioeconomic status, level of completed education or occupation. Participants who meet the eligibility criteria of the study would be recruited until the quota for each stratum was filled.
Purposive sampling	*Ease of drawing:* Relatively easy. *Risk of bias:* Bias increases with greater heterogeneity of the population; conscious bias is also a danger. *Representative of the sample:* Very limited ability to generalise because sample is hand picked. *When to use:* When the researchers choose the sample based on who they think would be appropriate for the study. Primarily used when there is a limited number of people with knowledge in the area being studied. *Things to consider:* It is the researchers' knowledge of the population, and its elements are used to hand-pick cases typical of the population to be included in the sample. A purposive sample can be used to study a highly unusual group, such as those individuals with a rare genetic disease. In another situation a researcher may wish to interview individuals who reflect different ends of the range of a particular characteristic. When using a purposive sample in a quantitative study, a researcher assumes that errors of judgement in overrepresenting and underrepresenting elements of the population in the sample will tend to balance out. However, there is no objective method for determining the validity of this assumption.

TABLE 9.2 Probability Sampling Strategies

Sample strategy	Description
Simple random sampling	*Ease of drawing:* Laborious. *Risk of bias:* Low. *Representative of the sample:* Maximised; probability of non-representativeness decreases with increased sample size. *When to use:* When a full list of all members of the population of interest is available, who are then selected using a method such as a random number generator. *Things to consider:* In simple random sampling, the population elements are identified and the sample is then selected, using some form of random number generation. The numbers corresponding with the sampling frame indicate units to be chosen for the sample. This process continues until a sample of the desired size is drawn. *Advantages:* The sample selection is not subject to the unconscious biases of the researcher; the representativeness of the sample in relation to the population characteristics is maximised; the differences in the characteristics of the sample and the population are purely a function of chance; and the probability of choosing a non-representative sample decreases as the size of the sample increases. *Disadvantages:* It can be time consuming and an inefficient method for obtaining a random sample. It can be costly, resource intensive and time consuming if potential participants are widely dispersed. In addition, although participants have been randomly selected, not all those selected may choose to participate in the study, resulting in a sample that is not always representative.
Stratified random sampling	*Ease of drawing:* Time consuming. *Risk of bias:* Low. *Representative of the sample:* Enhanced. *When to use:* When there are specific subgroups within the population of interest. Each subgroup is treated as a separate sampling frame. *Things to consider:* It divides the population into 'strata' or subgroups that are homogeneous (composed of similar or identical elements). An appropriate number of elements from each subset are randomly selected on the basis of their proportion in the population to maintain representativeness in the sample. The population is stratified according to any number of attributes (e.g. age, gender, sexuality, ethnicity, religion, socioeconomic status, level of education, diagnosis, type/stage of disease and so on). The variables selected to make up the strata should be adaptable to homogeneous subsets for the attributes being studied. This approach is equivalent to quota sampling (Fig. 9.1 provides an example that illustrates proportional stratified random sampling). *Advantages:* This method captures key population characteristics in the sample. *Disadvantages:* Can lack the ability to classify every member of the population into various subgroups, while developing a definitive and exhaustive list of the whole population can be problematic.
Cluster sampling	*Ease of drawing:* Less time consuming than simple or stratified. *Risk of bias:* Subject to more sampling errors than simple or stratified. *Representative of the sample:* Less representative than simple or stratified. *When to use:* When the target population can be organised into clusters, such as general practices, hospitals or local health districts and the unit of analysis is the cluster rather than the individuals within it.

Continued

TABLE 9.2 Probability Sampling Strategies—cont'd

Sample strategy	Description
	Things to consider: It is where clusters of individuals are selected rather than the individuals themselves. Clusters can take many forms: GP practices, patients attending particular GPs, wards within hospitals, hospitals within an area health district or state and so on. A one-stage cluster sample is where the researcher selects all participants within each of the clusters. Two-stage or multistage cluster sampling involves successive random sampling of units (clusters) that progress from large to small and meet sample eligibility criteria. The first-stage sampling unit consists of large units or clusters. The second-stage sampling unit consists of smaller units or clusters and so on. Sampling units or clusters can be selected by simple random or stratified random sampling methods. In both one-stage and two- or multistage cluster samples, the unit of analysis is the cluster. *Advantages:* It is more economical in terms of time and money than other types of probability sampling, particularly when the population is large and geographically dispersed or when a sampling frame of the elements is not available. *Disadvantages:* Greater sampling errors tend to occur than other random sampling methods, the sample size needs to be increased, and the statistical analysis is more complex.
Systematic sampling	*Ease of drawing:* More convenient and efficient than simple, stratified or cluster sampling. *Risk of bias:* Bias in the form of non-randomness can be inadvertently introduced. *Representative of the sample:* Less representative if bias occurs because of coincidental non-randomness. *When to use:* When a list of all members of the population of interest is available and participants are chosen from the list at a given uniform interval, using a randomly selected starting point. *Things to consider:* It maximises the efficiency of a research study, increases the accuracy and meaningfulness of the findings and enhances the generalisability of the findings from the sample to the population. Systematic sampling involves the selection of cases drawn from a population list at fixed intervals ('*k*'). Systematic sampling may sometimes represent a non-probability strategy. Systematic and simple random samplings are essentially the same procedure. *Advantages:* The results are obtained in a more convenient and efficient manner. *Disadvantages:* Bias in the form of non-randomness can be introduced inadvertently. This may occur if the population list is arranged so that a certain type of element is listed at intervals that coincide with the sampling interval.

The primary characteristic of probability sampling is the random selection of elements from the target population. Each participant in the population therefore has an equal, known and independent chance (probability) of being selected in the sample. As noted in Table 9.2, four commonly used probability sampling strategies are: simple random, stratified random, cluster and systematic.

The degree of difference between the sample and the population is what is referred to as *sampling error*. The sampling strategy, sample size and participant attrition rate will affect the degree of sampling error in a study and therefore the extent of external validity of a study. The use of probability sampling, coupled with a sufficient sample size and good response rate, will limit sampling error, therefore limiting the threat to external validity.

It is important to be aware that there can be overlap in some of the sampling techniques. It is possible to obtain a convenience quota sample or a stratified convenience

40	23	0	29	10	94	17	58	12	85	13	25	80	84	72	74	54	63	55	31
32	98	49	23	74	97	51	42	21	87	48	64	54	38	84	68	14	17	35	48
84	34	84	14	53	65	67	37	2	45	84	21	71	34	10	80	72	27	11	13
86	37	24	89	23	4	44	40	72	81	44	69	25	44	34	34	34	75	50	50
50	58	85	8	22	24	73	20	63	35	60	87	91	92	96	80	19	22	87	24
1	87	43	82	9	31	40	88	33	28	82	73	18	6	48	64	59	45	34	3
21	19	42	76	84	67	29	68	8	66	93	89	96	28	12	14	38	47	52	65
32	66	33	21	81	97	39	76	67	27	97	22	76	89	41	11	91	29	6	66
16	82	42	75	35	42	92	90	77	24	21	8	36	16	5	54	89	51	57	85
74	32	63	65	93	96	18	36	82	72	39	69	37	97	51	17	36	71	38	30
50	94	4	66	17	37	10	53	8	29	67	74	88	38	11	59	60	91	56	17
71	47	81	18	53	98	7	87	29	37	22	93	13	6	95	7	95	71	14	6
71	93	48	16	33	19	46	21	60	44	52	91	52	58	10	9	41	31	35	18
20	94	13	99	45	6	53	54	1	25	79	28	1	48	36	26	68	37	59	7
75	22	69	56	62	40	64	45	40	99	94	14	98	84	22	38	24	87	43	71
16	87	41	0	88	83	11	37	71	78	22	39	43	37	75	84	84	11	55	58
92	90	80	2	30	37	85	55	56	50	3	71	24	13	62	74	82	44	90	32
96	89	31	32	37	45	70	67	80	55	58	9	55	60	61	55	86	44	27	77
38	29	36	94	65	39	56	29	29	65	88	13	71	38	71	8	81	66	31	44
20	6	61	66	90	13	70	60	92	53	87	49	34	42	14	47	75	33	26	9
63	44	94	21	14	13	41	80	39	72	29	3	25	89	44	88	13	49	18	58
13	32	93	90	31	75	86	95	18	51	61	59	84	95	67	54	40	30	29	63
26	35	48	81	19	24	36	36	76	16	46	5	93	41	97	46	79	54	95	49
89	74	96	95	94	69	31	60	16	69	76	42	28	71	69	34	46	55	20	42
50	39	28	64	20	68	60	33	92	82	61	70	5	68	95	88	12	85	18	94
55	86	5	96	87	69	75	93	54	79	0	57	45	8	86	59	25	21	9	29
75	35	1	2	86	62	70	83	85	13	97	37	13	73	16	38	36	23	54	11
74	50	1	77	87	92	68	87	57	36	17	47	0	97	78	72	72	45	54	51
34	24	35	13	26	42	22	75	47	2	34	87	15	50	65	27	5	72	28	68
73	33	42	65	91	24	44	84	71	55	70	1	27	30	8	61	65	61	18	92
7	55	12	6	61	17	23	95	91	58	60	30	35	61	34	27	75	44	35	64
10	94	18	4	3	19	21	37	28	55	76	25	10	29	80	64	8	81	20	32
20	48	92	87	95	58	57	73	42	1	12	81	94	85	63	97	24	19	93	51
81	10	92	49	70	15	76	4	36	92	62	99	78	32	86	74	43	22	98	46
66	67	82	94	67	75	16	88	84	98	0	52	37	0	43	9	0	51	2	62
64	92	36	11	3	52	44	65	45	67	97	86	92	2	50	5	93	66	73	40
36	29	98	46	88	23	28	44	8	71	69	43	53	16	87	21	56	23	37	24
15	11	82	30	59	94	23	30	40	25	87	26	24	30	44	53	33	65	72	55
89	57	49	79	83	88	42	45	41	93	38	24	15	80	97	18	61	12	13	42
23	36	65	9	64	26	93	37	26	44	42	17	45	68	27	77	74	56	49	34
9	93	90	61	45	40	75	85	64	66	36	89	72	43	99	90	92	10	10	85
53	94	30	31	62	92	82	30	94	56	40	4	50	53	9	74	87	2	36	36
18	69	77	38	89	78	30	68	71	92	22	93	91	74	52	1	97	69	71	42
50	20	76	36	6	20	75	56	36	5	14	70	9	78	23	33	91	33	25	72
30	46	1	10	16	72	69	26	94	39	80	36	36	68	92	74	22	74	41	42
59	47	7	92	77	55	2	12	5	24	0	30	25	62	83	36	92	96	36	75
93	22	3	20	82	44	16	69	98	72	30	57	77	15	90	29	32	38	3	48
9	55	27	41	40	94	77	14	54	10	25	75	1	74	72	15	69	80	33	58
70	8	3	5	46	89	28	86	40	6	25	40	81	26	63	97	87	48	26	41
19	6	89	31	80	60	13	89	17	69	38	93	58	55	54	69	74	33	8	55

Fig. 9.1 Table of random numbers

sample. For example, a convenience sample of women with breast cancer can be stratified by age and/or stage of cancer (Gordon et al 2019). Nevertheless, the type of sampling strategy used depends on a number of factors including the research question(s) or hypotheses underpinning the study, the research design (e.g. exploratory, descriptive, observational, randomised controlled trial), the accessibility of participants, and time and resource constraints, as well as ethical and governance requirements. Once a sample has been established, the researcher needs to move towards considering what data are being collected and how they will be measured, along with the validity of the measures and processes.

RESEARCH IN BRIEF 9.2

A cross-sectional study funded by the Australian Centre for Behavioural Research in Diabetes by Diabetes Victoria and Deakin University aimed to examine the association of diabetes stigma with psychological, behavioural and haemoglobin A_{1c} (HbA_{1c}) outcomes and to investigate moderation effects of self-esteem, self-efficacy and/or social support. This study, which was conducted in 2015, used data from a national online survey of English-speaking Australians aged 15–75 with diabetes. Researchers surveyed a stratified random sample of 20,000 National Diabetes Services Scheme (NDSS) registrants, stratified by diabetes types and state of residents, using postal invitation directly by the NDSS (which directed them to the online survey website and provided researcher contact details). In addition, all participants of a previous study conducted in 2011, including 2065 NDSS registrants who agreed to being contacted about future surveys, were mailed/emailed study invitations directly by the researchers. In total, 2342 eligible participants took part in the study, comprising 1838 respondents to the self-report postal survey (2015 new cohort) and 504 respondents who were participants of the previous study (2011 cohort). The sample represented registrants having type 1 diabetes or type 2 diabetes, from six states and two territories of Australia. The response rate of the study was generally low, including 9% of the 20,000 NDSS registrants via the postal survey and 24% participants of the previous cohort study (Holmes-Truscott et al 2020). The sample representation of geographical location was maintained with minor differences, despite a relatively low response rate.

TUTORIAL TRIGGER 9.2

Your research group wants to obtain a sample of New Zealand practice nurses to determine their perceptions of research utilisation and the degree to which it informs their clinical practice in primary care.

Which sampling strategies would you employ to recruit the participants?

What might the inclusion/exclusion criteria be for your study?

GETTING THE OPERATIONAL DEFINITIONS RIGHT

Clinical practice issues that require research often focus on clinical variables that are of interest and measurable. Providing an internationally recognised definition of the variable of interest is essential to improve translations of outcomes and the ability to replicate study results. Biological and physiological indicators of health, such as blood pressure and heart rate, are generally easy to operationally define and amenable to measurement using standard and accepted units—for example, mmHg or beats per minute. In contrast, psychosocial variables, such as distress, anxiety, hope, wellness, social support, self-efficacy or health-related quality of life, have a number of validated established data collection tools that research teams can choose from to include in their study to measure the primary or secondary outcomes of interest.

DATA COLLECTION METHODS

Psychosocial, Physiological and Social Determinants of Biological Measurements

In clinical practice, nurses and midwives collect and document a range of quantitative measurements numerous times during a day. These data collection points often use specialised equipment. Measurements can be physiological (e.g. weight, blood pressure, temperature, pulse oximetry), biochemical (e.g. urinalysis, blood glucose level), microbiological (e.g. bacterial cultures) or anatomical (e.g. radiological examinations). Physiological or biological measurement is particularly suited to the study of several types of clinical issues, including investigation of the effectiveness of specific clinical or nursing practice activities.

The advantages of using physiological data collection methods include their objectivity, precision and sensitivity (ability to detect subtle variations in the measured variable of interest), assuming that calibration and instrument error has been addressed and the study protocol has been followed. These methods are considered more reliable because, unless there is a technical malfunction, two readings of the same instrument taken at the same time are likely to yield similar results. (See Chapter 10 for detailed discussion on measuring instruments.)

The limitations of physiological or biological measurements include the cost involved in obtaining specialised knowledge and training of personnel to collect the data reliably, environmental influences and/or the effect of instrumentation and testing on collection of data (see 'Internal validity' later in this chapter). For example, the presence of a heart rate monitor may elicit a stress response and make some patients anxious and may increase their heart rate, unless suitable information is provided to allay their concerns.

Observation

Observation can be suitable as a data collection method in complex research situations that are best viewed as total entities or difficult to measure in parts, such as studies dealing with patients who are unable to tell you their response. This approach may also be the best way to develop an operational definition for some variables of interest, particularly individual characteristics and conditions, such as traits and symptoms, verbal and non-verbal communication behaviours, activities, skill attainment or environmental characteristics. Observation may be structured or relatively unstructured. Structured observation uses tools, checklists or rating scales to document observed activities or behaviours. The behaviours or events to be observed are specified in advance, and data collection forms are prepared for documentation.

RESEARCH IN BRIEF 9.3

Xu et al (2017) conducted a cross-sectional study to examine the association between dietary patterns and anaemia, and to assess whether biomarkers of serum magnesium, C-reactive protein (CRP) and serum ferritin can mediate these associations for older Chinese people (n = 2401). The results inform the strategy for anaemia prevention. A questionnaire provided data on each participant's background information (e.g. age, gender and education), health history and health-related behaviours (e.g. smoking and alcohol consumption). Dietary data assessment is based on each participant's 24-hour recall, with information being collected over three consecutive days. Biomarker and anthropometric data were also collected. Blood was collected by venepuncture and tested immediately for glucose and HbA_{1c} after an overnight fast. Plasma and serum samples were then frozen and stored at −86°C for later laboratory analysis. Height and body weight were measured by trained health workers based on a standard protocol recommended by the World Health Organization. Ethical approval was obtained

Descriptive analyses (e.g. mean, standard deviation) were undertaken to present the dietary consumption, CRP and serum ferritin. Exploratory factor analysis was used to identify dietary patterns. Poisson regressions were used to examine the associations between anaemia and dietary patterns, and the interaction between dietary patterns and serum magnesium. In summary, a traditional dietary pattern (high intake of rice, pork and vegetables) was positively associated with anaemia; a modern dietary pattern (high intake of fruit and fast food) was inversely associated with anaemia. The association between dietary patterns and anaemia is mediated by serum magnesium. Understanding the association between diet in relation to the key biomarkers and anaemia can provide appropriate preventive measures against anaemia for the older Chinese population.

Questionnaires

Questionnaires are instruments designed to collect data from participants in a quantitative study. Questionnaires are generally self-administered, or participants are asked the questions by a researcher or clinician. They consist of a set of purposefully constructed questions (or items) that will be used to measure the study variable/s of interest. Numerous questionnaires are available to measure variables that are of interest to nursing and midwifery researchers (see 'Additional resources' at the end of this chapter for examples of books and websites that list health research instruments). A set of items on a questionnaire can be created and assembled into a variety of instrument forms (see Table 9.3).

Question items should:

- be written so that the intent of the question and the nature of the information sought are clear and unambiguous to the respondent
- relate to only one construct and ask only one question at a time
- not be open to alternative interpretations but allow for respondents with different opinions to provide different answers
- flow logically from one question item to the next

TABLE 9.3 Forms of Measuring Instruments

Instrument Form	Description
Scale	Individual item scores are combined to obtain an overall score.
Profile	A comprehensive instrument that assesses different components of a concept within one measurement approach.
Battery	Comparable to a profile with assessment of multiple components but derived from different original sources.
Index	A single number (usually total score) derived from various sources and/or list of items.

- be grammatically correct and free of jargon and value-laden terms
- be written at a level of language understandable to respondents.

The researcher must not assume the validity and reliability of established or existing questionnaires. This is particularly important if the questionnaire was designed for a specific group in a specific country.

Questionnaires identified during a literature search may be used in original form or may be adapted for use in a new study. When used in a different cultural context from that originally used, this adaptation takes the form of ensuring that the questions are not culturally biased. If adapted, it is important to be aware that any modification may alter the instrument's accuracy and validity. If instruments are already available, a researcher should obtain permission for their use from the original author or copyright holder (often the publisher of the journal where the instrument or article was first published) and there may or may not be a fee for its use.

Questionnaires can be administered in a paper-based format or an electronic format (e.g. delivered via a smartphone or tablet device). Items used in questionnaires can also include open ended or closed ended. Open-ended items enable participants to respond in their own words and can be used when the researcher does not know all possible alternative responses. Closed-ended items use a fixed number of alternative responses, although the format can vary (e.g. fixed response, multiple-choice formats or lists of responses where participants rank-order the responses) (Chin et al 2021). Fixed-response items can be used for questions requiring a dichotomous 'yes' or 'no' response, or when there are categories such as languages spoken at home, highest educational level or employment status. Structured, fixed-response items are best used when the question has a limited number of responses; the participant is asked to choose the response closest to their preferred answer. Although fixed-response items have the advantage of simplifying the respondent's task and the researcher's analysis, they may miss some important information about participants' views regarding the variable/s of interest.

A rating scale, such as a Likert scale or Likert-type scale, is an example of a fixed-response format used to determine a participant's attitude or opinion. For example, lists of statements are provided for the respondents to indicate whether they 'strongly agree', 'agree', 'disagree' or 'strongly disagree'. Likert-type scales are commonly constructed as 4-, 5-, 7- or 10-point scales (Box 9.1 illustrates a 5-point scale). By including a neutral response such as 'neither agree nor disagree', an odd-point scale is created, although a neutral category may limit analysis and be difficult to interpret.

Questionnaires are most useful when there is a finite set of questions to be asked and the researcher can be assured of the clarity and specificity of the items. If questionnaires are too long or complicated, they are less likely to be completed; this relates to 'respondent burden' and may result in missing data.

TUTORIAL TRIGGER 9.3

Imagine you are working as a registered nurse in a community palliative care team. You have noticed that it is always similar populations being referred to your services. You suspect there are certain population groups in your community who do not access the services.

Describe three different quantitative data collection methods that could assist you to explore this concern.

Records, Databases and Other Documentations

All data collection methods previously discussed illustrate the approaches researchers use to gather new or 'primary' data of interest to study. **Records, databases and other documentations** are termed 'secondary' sources, and include hospital records, care plans, clinical databases and census or population data (see 'Additional resources' at the end of this chapter). These existing data sources can also be used to answer specific primary research questions.

With the exponential increase in clinical data collection and storage, the use of 'data mining' approaches now enables examination of clinical practice issues (Mallappallil et al 2020).

BOX 9.1 Examples of Closed-ended and Open-ended Questions

Closed-Ended: Likert-Type Scale

How satisfied are you with your learning in this current research subject?

1. Very satisfied
2. Moderately satisfied
3. Undecided
4. Moderately dissatisfied
5. Very dissatisfied

To what extent do the following factors contribute to your current level of satisfaction?

	Not at All	Very Little	Somewhat	Moderate Amount	A Great Deal
Subject content	1	2	3	4	5
Learning process	1	2	3	4	5
Related readings	1	2	3	4	5
Student activities	1	2	3	4	5
Assessments	1	2	3	4	5

Closed-Ended

On average, how many clients do you see in the community health centre in a day?

1. 1–4
2. 5–9
3. 10–14
4. 15–19
5. 20 or more

How would you characterise the pace of your intensive care department?

1. Too slow
2. Slow
3. About right
4. Busy
5. Too busy

Closed-ended: Analogue Scale (Linear Analogue Anxiety Scale—LAAS)

Mark an 'X' on the scale below to indicate the amount of anxiety you are experiencing now.

1 2 3 4 5 6 7 8 9 10

No anxiety — Extreme anxiety

Open-Ended

Are there incentives for members that the Australian College of Critical Care Nurses ought to provide that are currently not being offered?

Contemporary data mining involves specific approaches and steps as one element in an emerging discipline called 'knowledge discovery in databases'. Data mining uses specific software to undertake automated processes utilising algorithms for interrogating the dataset. Either a hypothetic–deductive (hypothesise and test) or an inductive (test and hypothesise) approach can be used (Mallappallil et al 2020).

Using available data has distinct advantages. As the data collection step of the research process is sometimes a challenging and time-consuming task, the use of available records enables significant timesaving. If records have been kept in a similar manner over time, as with clinical databases, analysis of these records allows for the examination of trends over time. However, potential major challenges from using existing data also exist. For example, administrative data include valuable sources of information that are collected primarily for day-to-day operations of an agency (e.g. hospital) and are not always captured for research purposes. As such, there are some disadvantages associated with the reliability of administrative data for research purposes and also due to the lack of adequate control variables (Johnson et al 2013).

In addition to these challenges, various government privacy acts protect the rights of individuals who may be identified in records. As a result, healthcare institutions may be reluctant to allow researchers access to medical records unless the information is provided in a format that is de-identified, thus preserving anonymity (Altman et al 2018). Current policies on storage of research data in Australia are governed by the National Health and Medical Research Council (NHMRC) (see 'Additional resources' at the end of this chapter).

Data quality is particularly important as a potential bias with existing datasets (Mallappallil et al 2020), and it may be difficult for a research consumer or primary researcher to uncover these types of subtle biases. Despite these potential limitations, health records and other available data constitute a rich source for study.

TUTORIAL TRIGGER 9.4

You want to increase nursing engagement with evidence-based practice and enhance their knowledge utilisation and translation capabilities. You have been reading some literature on the experiences of nursing students across Australia and New Zealand and have a fair idea about some of the issues impacting on their clinical placement. Design a Likert-type questionnaire to obtain quantitative data from the same cohort of students about their perceptions of these issues.

STUDY VALIDITY

For a study to form the basis of further research, practice and theory development, the findings must be both believable and dependable. Two important criteria for evaluating the credibility and dependability of findings are internal validity and external validity. Internal validity (credibility) must be established before considering external validity (generalisability). The aim of a researcher is to select a design, sampling approach and data collection method that maximises both internal and external validity. A threat to internal validity can also be a threat to external validity (see Fig. 9.2).

Internal Validity

Internal validity relates to whether the intervention (explanatory or independent variable) had a real measurable effect on the outcome (dependent) variable, or whether some 'confounding' variable influenced and jeopardised the results. Confounding of findings occurs when extraneous variables are not controlled in the experimental design. A study, therefore, has internal validity when all confounding variables have been controlled or minimised (Sterne et al 2023). These threats are considered when planning the design and methods of a study, and before implementing results into practice. Threats to internal validity are most clearly applicable to experimental designs, but these factors should be considered in all quantitative designs (see Table 9.4).

Researchers should report any aspects of participant recruitment and retention that may influence a study's

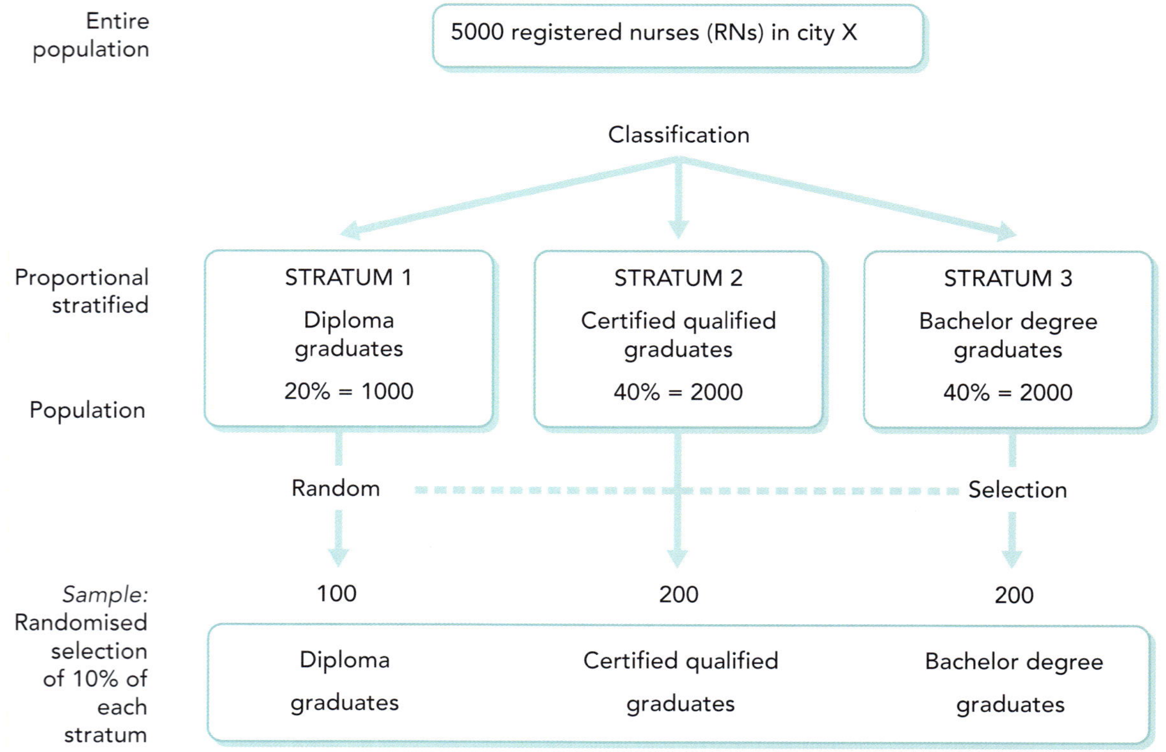

Fig. 9.2 Participant selection using a proportional stratified random sampling strategy

TABLE 9.4 Description of Threats to Internal Validity

Threat	Description
Selection bias	Study participants need to be a representative sample of the population of interest; problematic where individuals self-select for participation in a study. *Things to consider:* Selection effects are an issue where actual study participants do not constitute a representative sample (e.g. participants self-select for a study). In situations where a random sample cannot be obtained, bias becomes a concern as the study findings may not be generalised to other samples or population of interest. This becomes an external validity issue.
Mortality (dropout; loss to follow-up)	Non-response of enrolled participants from the first data collection point (pretest) to the final data collection point (post-test). *Things to consider:* When, for various reasons, participants withdraw from a study. This 'study mortality' or 'loss to follow-up' may affect the study findings if participants who withdraw are significantly different on the important study variables from those who remain. The final sample may not be representative of the original sample of the population of interest. This is also an external validity issue.
Maturation	Developmental, biological or psychological processes of an individual that change over time and may influence the study variable. *Things to consider:* The natural process of 'maturation' by participants (particularly in a longitudinal study) may also influence their responses to study variables—for example, a study may investigate the relationship between two methods of teaching on the knowledge of self-care for children with a chronic illness. Post-tests of student learning would need to be conducted in a relatively short timeframe after the teaching intervention is completed. This is to ensure that the findings are not influenced by the maturation of children who are learning new skills rapidly.
Instrumentation	Changes in measurement or observational techniques of the variables that may influence measurement; includes consistency for multiple observers (inter-rater reliability). *Things to consider:* Instrumentation threats are changes in the measurement of variables or observational techniques that may account for changes in the obtained measurement. For example, if an investigator has several research assistants collecting observational data, all must be trained in a similar manner. If they are not similarly trained, a lack of consistency may occur in their ratings and, therefore, a major threat to internal validity will occur.
Testing	The effect (experience) of taking a pretest on the score of a post-test. *Things to consider:* When a study uses a pretest, exposure to the test may prime participants and affect their responses at post-test. The differences between post-test and pretest scores may, therefore, not be a direct result of the intervention, but rather of the experience gained through testing.
History	A specific event that may affect the study variable, either within or external to the study setting. *Things to consider:* History refers to an event external to the intervention that occurs between the measurement points. For example, in a study of the effects of a quit smoking program, an event such as the graphic pictures of lip cancer and decayed teeth in external government-sponsored media advertisements may threaten internal validity. In this instance, the researcher would be in some doubt as to which event had a greater influence on participants' responses.

findings, as outlined in the CONSORT statement (see 'Additional resources' at the end of this chapter). More than one threat may exist in a study depending on the type of study design. Threats to internal validity in a study are usually acknowledged by the investigator in the results or discussion section of the study. Identifying a threat to internal validity does not invalidate the results but calls causality into question.

External Validity

External validity refers to the generalisability of a study's findings to other populations or settings. Factors that may affect external validity are related to the selection of participants, study conditions and types of observations. These factors are termed:

- interaction effect of selection
- reactive effects of being studied
- reactive or interaction effect of testing.

As noted in Fig. 9.2, there are inherent links between the factors of selection and testing, and those of threats to internal validity. When considered as internal threats, the focus is on how they influence the variables within the study. When assessing them as external threats the focus is in terms of generalisability, or applicability outside the study to other populations and settings. It is important to remember that this path is not exhaustive in describing the type of threats and their interactions.

AN UNEXPECTED HURDLE

A prospective, multicentre, randomised controlled trial was designed to compare outcomes of emergency versus delayed coronary angiogram (CAG) in survivors of out-of-hospital cardiac arrest with no obvious non-cardiac cause of arrest. The main aim of the study was to assess the 180-day survival rate with no or minimal neurological sequelae in patients who were resuscitated from an out-of-hospital cardiac arrest without ST segment elevation and who will be managed with either emergency or delayed CAG. The trial is a prospective national randomised open parallel group trial, in which survivors of out-of-hospital cardiac arrest were randomly assigned (1:1) into either emergency CAG (control group) or 48–96-hour delayed CAG (comparison group). In order to establish power at 0.8 for an alpha level of 0.01 and account for a 10% lost-to-follow-up rate and a crossover rate of 30%, the sample size for each group (immediate versus delayed CAG) was calculated to be $n = 485$ (total sample size: 970) (Hauw-Berlemont et al 2020, 2022).

During participant recruitment, the researchers encountered unanticipated hurdles. There were 338 eligible patients recruited and randomised. After 59 participants were excluded for various reasons (i.e. lack of informed consent, did not meet inclusion criteria, and others), a total of 279 patients were enrolled, including 141 in the emergency CAG group and 138 in the delayed CAG group. There was no difference in the 180-day survival rate between these two groups (emergency CAG 34.1% versus delayed CAG 30.7%). However, with approximately only one-quarter of the planned number of participants enrolled, this study was well below the sample size threshold for power analysis and could result in a type II error (Hauw-Berlemont et al 2022).

Effect of Selection

Selection relates to the generalisability of study results to other populations, and is influenced by the 'selection bias', 'mortality' and 'maturation' of internal validity threats. An example is when the sampling strategy used has not resulted in a representative sample/group. At times, the numbers of available participants may be low or not accessible to a researcher, who may then need to choose a non-probability method of sampling over a probability method, where a probability sample is one in which every possible eligible participant in the population has an equal chance of being selected into the sample. This may be difficult to achieve if a listing of all eligible participants (sampling frame) is not readily available.

Reactive Effect of Testing

Administration of a pretest in an intervention study may also affect external validity, influencing the generalisability of findings to other clinical situations or populations. Reactivity is influenced by the internal validity effects of 'maturation', 'instrumentation' and 'testing'. Suppose a researcher wants to assess changing knowledge of nurses on anticoagulant medications. To accomplish this, an education program on anticoagulation is implemented as an intervention. To evaluate whether the education program changes knowledge related to anticoagulation, knowledge tests are administered before and after the education intervention. The pretest on knowledge, however, may prompt participants to reflect on their knowledge and practice regarding anticoagulation medications. The participants' responses on follow-up testing may, therefore, differ from those of individuals who were given the education program but did not undertake the pretest.

Reactive Effects of Being Studied

Reactivity reflects participants' responses to being studied and is influenced by the internal validity threats 'testing' and 'history'. Participants may respond to a researcher as an extraneous response to being studied, not because of the actual study procedures. This is known as the 'Hawthorne effect', named after Western Electric Corporation's Hawthorne plant (in the United States), where a study of working conditions was conducted in the early 1900s. In this classic study, the researchers implemented several different working conditions (e.g. turning up the lights, piping in music loudly or softly and changing work hours). The researchers noted, however, that no matter what intervention was introduced the workers' productivity increased. It was therefore concluded that production increased as a result of the workers knowing that they were being studied rather than because of the actual experimental conditions. The

Hawthorne effect continues to be identified as a threat to internal validity.

All studies should have clearly identified data collection methods. The conceptual and particularly the operational definitions of all important variables should be presented. The researcher may provide a rationale for the method chosen; however, the published study should adequately describe the methods and data collection procedures for the reader. Several questions can be considered when examining the study procedure (see Box 9.2).

Questionnaires should be clearly described to allow a reader to decide whether the variables were adequately operationalised to allow measurement. Evaluating the adequacy of measuring instruments is often challenging for research consumers, as the actual instrument used is not always provided in the published study for inspection, and the reader may not feel confident about judging the adequacy of the method without reviewing it. Therefore, readers may need to check the reference list of the published study and obtain any other published studies that describe or evaluate the instrument(s). Once the reader has decided that the data collection method was appropriate to the problem and the procedures were appropriate for the sample studied, the reliability and validity of the instruments themselves need to be considered. These issues are discussed in the following chapter.

SUMMARY

Sampling is a process through which a researcher selects participants from the population for study. The purpose of sampling from a quantitative perspective is to obtain a sample which is representative of the population guided by various criteria to control for bias. Non-probability sampling is less rigorous and accurate, whereas probability sampling refers to the random selection of participants from the target population and aims to ensure that each participant in the population has an equal chance of being selected; nevertheless, there is still no guarantee of a representative sample of the population. Factors such as sample heterogeneity, sample size, the characteristics of those who consent to be in the study, response rate and participant dropout may affect representativeness. Overall, quantitative designs guide the choice of sampling techniques and data collection methods. Data collection methods include physiological or biological measurements, observation, interviews, questionnaires and records, databases and other documentations. Internal validity and external validity are

BOX 9.2 Criteria for Evaluating Data Collection Methods

In General

1. Are all data collection instruments clearly identified and described?
2. Is the rationale for their selection given?
3. Is the method used appropriate to the problem being studied?
4. Is the method used appropriate to the clinical situation?
5. Are the data collection procedures similar for all subjects?

Physiological or Biological Measurement

1. Is the instrument used appropriate and consistent with the research problem?
2. Is a rationale given for why a particular instrument was selected?
3. Is there a provision for evaluating the reliability, validity and responsiveness of the instrument and those who use it?

Observational Methods

1. Were the observations performed using the principles of informed consent?
2. How were any observers trained to minimise any bias?
3. Was there an observers' guide?
4. Were the observers required to make inferences about what they observed?
5. Is there any reason to believe that the presence of the observers affected the behaviour of the subjects?

Interview Questions/Questionnaires

1. Is the instrument (interview question/questionnaire) adequately described to assess whether it addresses the concept of interest?
2. Is there evidence that participants were able to complete the responses?
3. Is there a clear indication that the participants understood the interview questions/questionnaire?
4. Are the majority of the items appropriately closed-ended or open-ended?

Records Databases and Other Documentations

1. Are the records used appropriate to the problem being studied?
2. Are the data examined in such a way as to provide new information rather than summarising current information?
3. Is there any indication of selection bias in the available records?

important criteria for determining the credibility, dependability and generalisability of research findings.

KEY POINTS

- Sampling is a process that selects representative units of a population for study. Researchers sample representative segments of the population because it is rarely feasible or necessary to sample entire populations of interest to obtain accurate and meaningful information.
- Types of non-probability sampling are convenience, quota and purposive sampling.
- Criteria for drawing a sample vary according to the sampling strategy; systematic organisation of the sampling procedure minimises bias.
- A representative sample is one whose key characteristics closely approximate those of the population.
- An appropriate sampling plan will maximise the efficiency of a research study; it will increase the accuracy and meaningfulness of the findings and enhance the generalisability of the findings from the sample to the population.
- Simple random sampling is the basic technique of probability sampling; other probability sampling techniques include stratified, cluster and systematic methods.
- Probability sampling ensures that all elements have an equal chance of being selected in the sample, thereby minimising bias and enabling generalisability of the findings, and should be used as it reduces the probability of sampling error.
- Convenience sampling is the weakest form of sampling in terms of generalisability, as it produces a degree of sampling error and should be avoided if the intent of the research is to make inferences about the population. When critically analysing a study that employed this sampling strategy, the external validity of the findings should be examined.
- Non-probability samples are useful when the total population is unknown or unavailable.
- Power analysis is a statistical calculation used to determine the correct size of a sample so that accurate inferences can be made about the true relationship between the study variables.
- Clinical research is often based on non-probability sampling, with additional rigour introduced by randomisation of participants into treatment or control groups.
- Data collection methods are both objective (data are not influenced by the data collector) and systematic (data are collected in the same way for each study participant).
- Physiological or biological measurements use technical instruments to collect data about patients' physiological or biological status; the advantages of physiological or biological measurements are objectivity, precision and sensitivity.
- Observational methods are used when the variables of interest are events or behaviours; quantitative observation requires preplanning, systematic recording and controlling observations.
- Interviews and questionnaires are commonly used in nursing and midwifery research; participants report information about themselves, responding to open-ended or closed-ended items (questions or statements); the item should be clear to the respondent, free of bias and grammatically correct.
- Records, databases and other documentations are important sources for research, and can save considerable time and money when conducting a study. However, data are subject to problems of availability, authenticity and accuracy.
- Internal validity and external validity must be considered within the sampling design and data collection procedures.

TIME TO REFLECT

The following is based on a hypothetical study.

Aim: To explore whether a nurse-delivered educational intervention for adults with atrial fibrillation reduced unplanned hospital presentations during the 12 months following a first presentation to an emergency department.

Objective: Following a first presentation to emergency and subsequent hospital admission, adults were randomised to receive either standard care or a targeted educational intervention involving standard education plus a home visit by a cardiovascular specialist nurse after each subsequent emergency presentation. Each patient received a total of six home visits. The researchers proposed that the intervention would reduce hospital presentations by 40%. A total sample size of 220 (110 in the intervention group and 110 in the control group) was required, with an additional 20% required owing to loss to follow-up.

Design: The research was a randomised controlled trial. The sampling type was convenience, with every prospective, consecutive adult presenting with a subsequent hospital admission being invited into the study. Participants were recruited from seven major teaching

TIME TO REFLECT—cont'd

hospitals in Australia. The primary outcome was the number of hospitalisations, including emergency department visits, obtained via the hospital electronic medical record.

Questions

Reflect on the information given and answer these questions:

1. What type of sampling procedure was used for this study?
2. Was this an appropriate sampling procedure?
3. Why did the researchers want to collect information on medication adherence and confidence in managing atrial fibrillation symptoms?
4. What are the variables of interest?
5. What research instruments could be used?
6. What internal and external validity factors need to be considered?
7. Is the design appropriate for this study?
8. What issues will influence the generalisability of the results to the wider, global population living outside of Australia?

LEARNING ACTIVITIES

1. The purpose of sampling is to:
   a. make predictions about the study
   b. obtain a sample that is representative of the population
   c. increase the efficiency of a research study
   d. recruit as many participants as possible.
2. Which of the following is a probability sampling technique?
   a. Convenience sampling
   b. Quota sampling
   c. Snowball sampling
   d. Simple random sampling
3. The population criteria establish the:
   a. way a sample is drawn
   b. representativeness of a sample
   c. number of participants in a study
   d. target population.
4. A convenience sample:
   a. allows generalisability of the findings to the population
   b. gives everyone an opportunity to participate in a study
   c. is made up of the most readily available and accessible persons
   d. is made up of people who enjoy being part of a research study.
5. Which of the following is an example of a non-probability sampling technique?
   a. Stratified random sampling
   b. Cluster sampling
   c. Convenience sampling
   d. Systematic sampling
6. The primary characteristic of probability sampling is:
   a. the random selection of elements from the population
   b. the opportunity to generalise the findings of the study to the population
   c. to select participants who meet the study criteria
   d. to ensure the findings will be credible.
7. Stratified random sampling divides the population into strata that are:
   a. heterogeneous
   b. homogeneous
   c. purposefully chosen for the study
   d. different for each conceptual category.
8. What is the main advantage of using a self-administered questionnaire as a data collection method in quantitative research?
   a. It allows for more in-depth responses from participants.
   b. It eliminates bias in the selection of participants.
   c. It is less expensive and can be administered to large groups of people.
   d. It provides the opportunity for the researcher to clarify responses.
9. Criteria for inclusion/exclusion in a study are designed to:
   a. control for any bias or extraneous variability
   b. keep the wrong participants out of the study
   c. get the best participants into the study
   d. make it difficult for researchers to exclude participants.
10. What is the main advantage of using a random sampling technique?
    a. It is easy to implement and does not require a lot of resources.
    b. It allows researchers to ensure that certain subgroups of the population are represented in the sample.
    c. It eliminates bias in the selection of participants.
    d. It ensures that every member of the population has an equal chance of being selected.

For further content associated with this chapter visit: https://evolve.elsevier.com/cs/product/9780729596794?role=student 

ADDITIONAL RESOURCES

Bannigan, K., Watson, R., 2009. Reliability and validity in a nutshell. J. Clin. Nurs. 18, 3237–3243.

CONSORT Group statement. http://www.consort-statement.org/.

Faul, F., Erdfelder, E., Buchner, A., et al., 2009. Statistical power analyses using G*Power 3.1: tests for correlation and regression analyses. Behav. Res. Methods 41, 1149–1160. doi:10.3758/BRM.41.4.1149

National Health & Medical Research Council (NHMRC): policies on research data storage and protection. https://nhmrc.gov.au/research-policy.

Younas, A., Porr, C., 2018. A step-by-step approach to developing scales for survey research. Nurse Res. 26 (3), 14–19. doi:10.7748/nr.2018.e1585

REFERENCES

Alananzeh Alananzeh, I.M., Levesque, J.V., Kwok, C., et al., 2019. The unmet supportive care needs of Arab Australian and Arab Jordanian cancer survivors: an international comparative survey. Cancer Nurs. 42 (3), E51–E60; doi:10.1097/NCC.0000000000000609

Altman, M., Wood, A., O'Brien, D.R., et al., 2018. Practical approaches to big data privacy over time. Int. Data Priv. Law 8, 29–51.

Batko-Szwaczka, A., Wilczyński, K., Hornik, B., et al., 2020. Predicting adverse outcomes in healthy aging community-dwelling early-old adults with the timed up and go test. Clin. Interv. Aging, 5, 1263–1270. doi:10.2147/CIA.S256312

Chin, H., Chew, C.M., Lim, H.L., 2021. Development and validation of online cognitive diagnostic assessment with ordered multiple-choice items for 'Multiplication of Time'. Int. J. Sci. Math. Educ. 20, 1–21. doi:10.1007/s10763-021-10170-5

Cohen, J., 1988. Statistical Power Analysis for the Behavioral Sciences, second ed. Lawrence Erlbaum Associates, Hillsdale, NJ.

Gordon, J.R., Baik, S.H., Schwartz, K.T., et al., 2019. Comparing the mental health of sexual minority and heterosexual cancer survivors: a systematic review. LGBT Health 6 (6), 271–288.

Hauw-Berlemont, C., Lamhaut, L., Diehl, J.L., et al., 2022. Emergency vs delayed coronary angiogram in survivors of out-of-hospital cardiac arrest: results of the randomized, multicentric EMERGE trial. JAMA Cardiol. 7 (7), 700–707.

Hauw-Berlemont, C., Lamhaut, L., Diehl, J.L., et al., 2020. EMERGEncy versus delayed coronary angiogram in survivors of out-of-hospital cardiac arrest with no obvious non-cardiac cause of arrest: design of the EMERGE trial. Am. Heart J. 222, 131–138.

Holmes-Truscott, E., Ventura, A.D., Thuraisingam, S., et al., 2020. Psychosocial moderators of the impact of diabetes stigma: results from the second diabetes MILES–Australia (MILES-2) study. Diabetes Care 43 (11), 2651–2659.

Johnson, E.K., Nelson, C.P., 2013. Utility and pitfalls in the use of administrative databases for outcomes assessment. J. Urol. 190 (1), 17–18.

Mallappallil, M., Sabu, J., Gruessner, A., et al., 2020. A review of big data and medical research. SAGE Open Med. 8, 2050312120934839.

Sterne, J.A., Hernán, M.A., McAleenan, A., et al., 2023. Assessing risk of bias in a non-randomized study. In: Higgins, J., Thomas, J. (Eds) Cochrane handbook for systematic reviews of interventions, Ch 25, pp. 621–641. Retrieved from: https://training.cochrane.org/handbook/current/chapter-25.

Xu, X., Hall, J.J., Byles, J.E., et al., 2017. Dietary pattern, serum magnesium, ferritin, C-reactive protein (CRP) and anaemia among older people. Clin. Nutr. 36 (2), 444–451. doi:10.1016/j.clnu.2015.12.015

10

Assessing Measuring Instruments

Daniel Terry and Hoang Nguyen

LEARNING OUTCOMES

After reading this chapter, you should be able to:

- describe how measurement error can affect study findings
- discuss the reasons for testing reliability, validity and responsiveness
- describe the tests of stability, equivalence and internal consistency as they relate to the concept of reliability
- define validity in relation to a measuring instrument
- discuss the approaches used to examine content, construct and criterion-related validity
- outline the issues related to the measurement of responsiveness
- identify the criteria for evaluating the reliability and validity of measuring instruments
- evaluate the reliability and validity of measuring instruments.

KEY TERMS

consistency, p. 152
equivalence, p. 156
homogeneity, p. 156
internal consistency, p. 154
minimal important difference, p. 162
random errors, p. 152
reliability, p. 152
responsiveness, p. 162
stability, p. 154
systematic (constant) error, p. 153
validity, p. 152

INTRODUCTION

Many topic areas in nursing and midwifery research involve concepts that are easily observable, such as age or gender, and there is little misunderstanding about their meaning. However, other more abstract concepts, such as quality of life or fatigue, have different meanings to different people. Even experts may disagree about the meanings of such frequently used concepts. As end-users of research, it is important for nurses to understand how the concepts and measures used in the research are defined and measured. It is only when valid and reliable measures are used in a study that research users can have some confidence that its conclusions are trustworthy and valid. This chapter focuses on assessing the quality of tools or instruments used to measure concepts in a research study.

This chapter also examines issues related to the assessment of measuring instruments, also called *psychometrics*. Instrument evaluation in clinical research focuses on the major concepts of 'reliability' and 'validity' but should also consider the related concept 'responsiveness', where responsiveness, or sensitivity to change, refers to the instrument's ability to detect significant or important changes when they occur over time (Mokkink et al 2021).

The common approaches for assessing instrument reliability and validity are explored in relation to how these concepts inform the development, selection and evaluation of measurement tools used in nursing or midwifery research. Demonstrating acceptable levels of reliability and validity in a quantitative study is critical when: (1) using a previously developed instrument with different study participants, (2) comparing similar instruments that are supposed to measure the same study variable or concept and (3) developing a new assessment instrument.

KEY CONCEPTS AND BUILDING BLOCKS

Before getting into the more complex elements of the assessment of measuring instruments, we should take a step back for a moment and define some of the terms that are used. At times, learning these key concepts are a little unexciting; however, understanding what things mean and how they may work is important, particularly when there are many new terms at the very beginning. You may find that you are returning to this chapter from time to time or even often to recall a definition, term or meaning. Please use this chapter as a resource to develop and maintain your understanding of these core concepts.

Within this context and as a beginning step in measurement, we must define the concept of *measure* itself. In this case, measure or measurement is centred on an item or set of items that enables the quantity or nature of the phenomenon under study to be indicated (American Psychological Association 2023). It must be noted that 'measure' and 'instrument' can and are often used interchangeably, which you may notice within this text. Nevertheless, the next step associated with measurement is to define the concept(s) of interest or variable. An abstract *concept* is a mental image, and when it is defined in a way that it can be observed, it can be measured. The term *variable* refers to some aspect of a concept that varies and for which there is a concrete set of indicators that can be measured. This process of measurement of variables involves assigning numbers to observations to quantify concepts. The term *construct* describes concepts used by researchers that are based on theoretical premises that cannot be seen either directly or indirectly but can be measured (e.g. anxiety, distress or quality of life). The term *operationalise* means to turn an abstract concept into something that is measurable, such as creativity, confidence or even customer loyalty, while an *attribute* is the quality of an object or thing being measured.

A *measuring instrument* is a research tool that enables measurement of the individual study variables. An instrument can be a questionnaire, survey, observational case report form, physiological equipment or laboratory test. The ability to measure variables of interest accurately and consistently is a major focus for nurse and midwife researchers who use quantitative research methods. The term *scale* is used in two ways. First, it is used to denote a measurement instrument that incorporates a collection of items combined to make a composite score and is intended to reveal some underlying construct such as fatigue, quality of life or caregiver burden (DeVellis & Thorpe 2021). In the second definition, a scale is the potential numeric values when a rating or score is assigned to each response, such as when 0 denotes 'strongly disagree', 1 denotes 'disagree', 2 denotes 'unsure', etc.

There are two key considerations when approaching variables: **reliability**, the **consistency** with which an instrument measures the construct of interest, and **validity**, the degree to which an instrument accurately measures what it is supposed to measure. Any instrument must exhibit acceptable reliability and validity when measuring the construct of interest—that is, consistency and accuracy. A lack of reliability and validity in measurement means the findings or results may not reflect reality. If this is the case, it would limit the ability to draw an inference (a conclusion drawn from the evidence) that the independent variable is truly causing or influencing the dependent variable (i.e. internal validity). Therefore, any conclusions drawn may be invalid and fail to advance our understanding of that construct.

Measurement Error

Before discussing reliability, validity and responsiveness in more detail, the theory of 'measurement error' warrants examination. An important issue to consider initially is to what extent a measuring instrument displays errors when measuring the concept of interest. Ideally, the instrument scores obtained from a sample of participants are consistent and true measures of the construct for that population of interest, and therefore an accurate reflection of the real differences between individuals. No instrument is completely accurate; all measures contain some error. An observed test score actually consists of the true score ('signal') plus the error ('noise') (see Fig. 10.1). The extent of variability in test scores attributed to error, rather than the true score, is the *error variance*. The error component may be either chance (or random) error, or it may be systematic (or constant) error.

Nurse and midwife researchers usually work with instruments that are subject to errors. For example, instruments that measure psychological variables such as anxiety and physiological variables such as blood pressure will never be 100% accurate in measurement every time they are used. Differences between the 'true' value (signal) and the 'measured' value may be due to random error or systematic error (noise). The aim for researchers working in psychometrics and instrument development is to produce instruments that most closely measure the 'true' score and limit both systematic and random error.

Random Error

Chance or **random errors** are unsystematic in nature, difficult to control and it is unknown how they influence (or bias) the study results. These errors reflect a transient state in a participant or measuring instrument, within the context of a study. For example, a participant may be anxious about being tested, which may then

Observed scores	=	True variance	+	Error variance	
Actual score obtained		Consistent, hypothetical stable or true score		*Chance/random error* • Transient participant factors • Instrumentation variations • Transient environmental factors	*Systematic error* • Consistent instrument, participant or environmental factors

Fig. 10.1 Components of observed scores

influence their response to questions on the instrument. These perceptions or behaviours that occur at a specific point in time are transient and are often beyond the awareness or control of a researcher. Random error can also occur because of the instrument itself—for example, different clinicians assessing blood pressure on the same patient but obtaining different measurements (inter-rater error), or the same clinician obtaining different blood pressure values on repeated assessment on the same patient when no real change has occurred (intra-rater error).

Systematic Error

Systematic (constant) error occurs from relatively stable characteristics of the study population, which may also bias participants' behaviour and/or cause incorrect instrument calibration. This error has a systematic bias influencing their responses, and therefore influences instrument validity. Level of education, socioeconomic status, social desirability or other characteristics may influence the validity of an instrument by altering measurement of the 'true' responses in a systematic way (DeVellis & Thorpe 2021). For example, a participant who wants to please a researcher may consistently answer items in a socially desirable way—that is, they want to be seen in a good light, making the measurement inaccurate. This is also known as social desirability bias.

Systematic error also occurs when an instrument is improperly calibrated, such as a set of scales for weighing infants. If the scales were incorrectly calibrated and consistently weighed each infant at 500 grams less than their actual body weight, the scale would be reliable (capable of reproducing a stable repeatable measurement), but the results would be incorrect and therefore invalid. When appraising research, it is important to consider how systematic or random measurement errors may occur with different types of instruments. For example, inter-observer variation may occur when assessing nurse hand hygiene performance, where nurses who may be doing the same task judge or record the observations differently (Bredin et al 2022).

Performance Characteristics of an Instrument

The psychometric properties of an instrument consist of the major characteristics of reliability, validity and responsiveness. When reading and appraising research, it is important to independently assess the reliability and the validity of the instruments, to determine the soundness of instrument selection relative to the constructs being investigated and the likelihood that the results reflect reality. Reliable and valid measures produce consistent estimates of the measures of variables in the sample, thereby affecting internal validity, where internal validity is the level of confidence that the relationship between items is not being influenced by other factors, as discussed in Chapter 9.

Further, if the sampling strategy is based on probability methods (i.e. each member of a population has a known probability of being selected in the sample), reliable and valid measures allow accurate generalisations to the populations being studied, enabling external validity and the ability to apply research findings in clinical practice. Assessment of the reliability and validity of an instrument is therefore an important skill for a critical reader of nursing and midwifery research to develop. Instrument assessment can be a challenging process, and a range of resources are available to assist nurses and midwives when evaluating these properties for instruments commonly used in studies (see 'Additional resources' at the end of this chapter). The specific purpose of instrument testing guides the type of analytical test used to establish reliability and validity. The reader needs to be familiar with these purposes and the

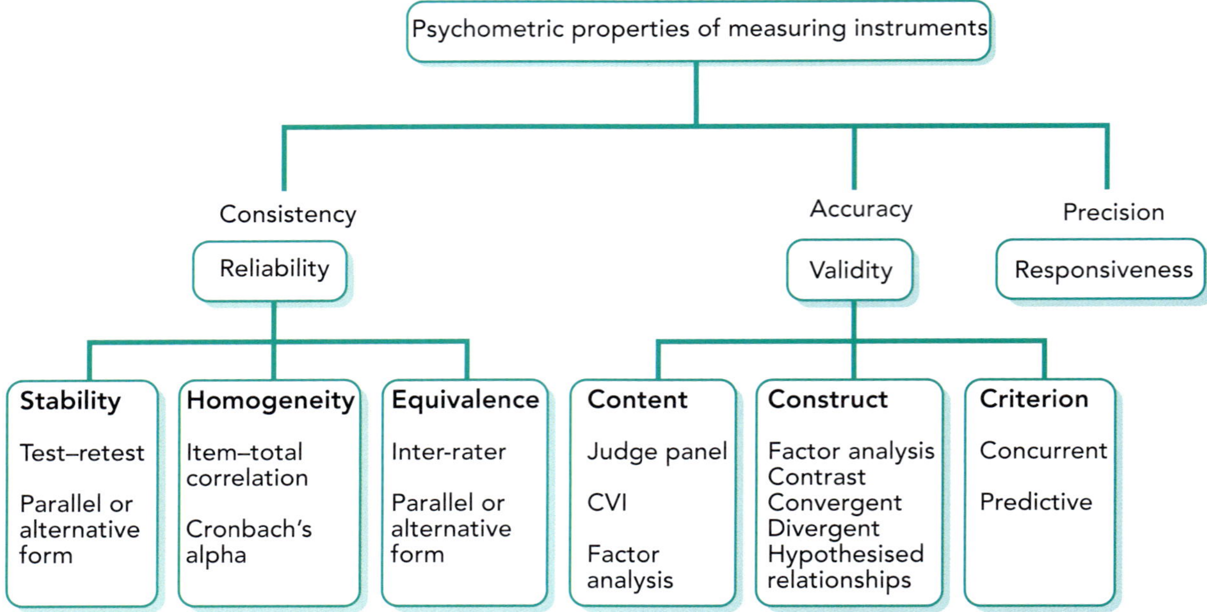

Fig. 10.2 Performance characteristics of a measuring instrument

results obtained from the analyses (Fig. 10.2). The following subsections examine each property separately.

Reliability

The reliability of an instrument is the consistency with which it measures the target attribute (quantity of a thing or object), such as frailty or quality of life, and produces the same results on repeated measures when the attribute has not changed. As a basic example, if an uncalibrated sphygmomanometer was used to measure adult blood pressure at the baseline of a study and then measured at a later point using the same tool, this time calibrated prior to the follow-up measure, any differences between the before and after results might reflect difference in the measuring tool itself rather than changes in blood pressure. A question to consider always when reading a report of a quantitative study is, 'How reliable is the instrument?' Thus, reliability can be equated with a measure's stability, **internal consistency** and equivalence (each of these will be explored in more detail later in this chapter). Attributes of reliability are concerned with the degree of consistency between scores:

- obtained at two or more independent times of testing (i.e. stability)
- within a scale, where a number of items are used to measure a construct (i.e. internal consistency)
- between different observers or between different forms of the instrument (i.e. equivalence).

The test of association between items and/or instruments is commonly expressed as a 'correlation coefficient', and ranges from 0 to 1. This value reflects the relationship between the error variance, true variance (differences among research participants in the measured attributes) and the observed score (American Psychological Association 2023). The closer the coefficient is to 1, the more reliable is the measure. A correlation closer to zero indicates that there is no significant relationship between two or more scores. A reliability coefficient of 0.90 indicates that an instrument has little measurement error (the error is small). In contrast, a reliability coefficient of 0.50 reflects high error (the measurement error is of concern).

When appraising a study, assess whether the method of reliability testing is consistent with the study's aim and the type of measure used. Reliability analysis essentially tests three different attributes—stability, internal consistency and equivalence—using five major tests of reliability, depending on the purpose and format of the instruments (see Table 10.1).

Stability

An instrument exhibits **stability** when the same results are obtained on repeated administration of the instrument.

TABLE 10.1 Measures to Test Different Attributes of Reliability

Psychometric Property	Test	Purpose
Stability Produces the same result on repeated testing.	Test–retest reliability	Tests the consistency of an instrument on repeated measures.
Internal consistency (i.e. homogeneity) All items measure the same concept or construct.	Cronbach's alpha[a]	Tests the internal consistency of an instrument with Likert-type response levels.
	Item–total correlation	Tests individual items against the total instrument.
Equivalence Same results are obtained with different observers, or similar equivalent instruments.	Inter-rater reliability	Tests the consistency between two or more observers.
	Parallel (alternative form)[b]	Tests the consistency between alternative forms of an instrument.

[a] The use of Cronbach's alpha on ordinal data should be used with caution as it will underestimate the true value. Alternatives may include polychoric correlation or McDonald's omega.

[b] This test can examine both the 'stability' and the 'equivalence' of an instrument.

The stability of an instrument to measure a construct consistently over a period is an important issue for researchers. It is expected that personality traits or other characteristics remain relatively constant or stable over time. This stability is important when an instrument is used in a repeated-measures longitudinal study.

For example, 'trait anxiety' is a relatively stable variable, and so if we measured it 2 weeks apart we would expect to get a similar result both times. However, 'state' anxiety fluctuates relative to the situation it is measured in, so if we measured state anxiety 2 weeks apart we should expect that we would get different results. Thus, stability should be used only to demonstrate reliability of a measure if that measure is not expected to vary between the two time periods (whatever the time period is). The two most common tests to assess stability are test–retest (described in the next paragraph) and parallel form (which is described in the section 'Equivalence', later in the chapter; the procedures for assessing stability using parallel forms are the same as those for equivalence).

Test–Retest Reliability

Test–retest reliability is the administration of the same instrument to the same participants under similar conditions on two or more occasions when true stability of the observed behaviour or characteristic is expected. Scores on repeated testing are compared and expressed as a correlation coefficient, usually Pearson's *r*, which determines the strength of association between the two sets of scores. However, it must be noted that Spearman's rho is a more suitable test for ordinal variables or when non-normally distributed data exists (see Chapter 11 for information about correlation coefficients). The interval between repeated administrations is critical, and ideally should be long enough that values obtained from the second administration will not be affected by the previous measurement (e.g. the respondent's memory of responses to the first administration). Therefore, the timeframe should be sufficient to minimise the risk of bias related to 'testing' (a threat to 'internal validity'; previously discussed in Chapter 9).

In a small-scale study of patients with dementia, the test–retest reliability of functional magnetic resonance imaging (fMRI) to detect neural changes (during word retrieval measures) was evaluated (Paek et al 2019). This study included seven patients with dementia and nine age- and education-matched healthy controls; fMRI was repeated three times over a 2-month span. Test–retest reliability was measured using the intraclass correlation coefficient (ICC). The magnitude of test–retest reliability was also assessed by calculating single-measure ICCs in six predefined regions of interest related to word retrieval processing. The researchers concluded that there was an unacceptable degree of variation across brain regions at each of the three fMRI measures, especially for patients with dementia, suggesting that one-time fMRI scanning may inadequately represent an individual's typical brain activation pattern. Thus, due to the poor test–retest reliability, multiple imaging baselines were recommended.

Internal Consistency

Internal consistency, also known as '**homogeneity**', is a measure of the extent to which items within a scale are correlated, therefore measuring the same concept. A unidimensional scale is one that measures one construct, whereas a multidimensional scale measures different but related constructs. For instance, the Faces Anxiety Scale is a unidimensional scale (Cao et al 2017, Prasad et al 2020). In contrast, the Hospital Anxiety and Depression Scale (HADS) (Eriksen et al 2019, Zigmond & Snaith 1983) is bidimensional, and the Depression Anxiety and Stress Scale (DASS) (Lovibond & Lovibond 1995, Nashwan 2021) is multidimensional. While there are numerous methods to assess internal consistency reliability, the two methods most used are item-to-total correlations and Cronbach's alpha (α).

Cronbach's alpha. The most widely used test of internal consistency for an instrument that has several items measuring the same underlying construct is Cronbach's alpha (α), where each item in the scale is compared simultaneously with all other items. A low Cronbach's alpha (<0.80) suggests a lack of correlation between items within a scale, and therefore is an unreliable measure of the underlying construct. Conversely, a high Cronbach's alpha (>0.95) indicates a high correlation between scale items and redundancy of one or more items, which may be removed without affecting the reliability of the scale.

Item-to-total correlations. Item-to-total correlations measure the relationship between each of the items and the total scale, reflected as a correlation coefficient (i.e. the degree of association between two or more variables). When item-to-total correlations are calculated, a correlation for each item on the scale is generated. Items that do not achieve a high correlation may be deleted from the instrument. Usually in a study not all the item-to-total correlations are reported unless the study is a report of how the researcher developed the tool (i.e. a methodological study reporting on psychometric properties of a new instrument). Typically, the lowest and highest correlations are reported, or a table may present analysis of all items tested. Correlation coefficients can range in value from −1.0 to +1.0 and can also be zero.

One aim of this test when developing a new or short-form version of an instrument is to eliminate items that have correlations that are too low (e.g. <0.30) and accept other items that measure the same concept without being redundant. In addition, if item-to-total correlations are found to be too high (e.g. >0.80), there is redundancy, as a specific item is measuring the same dimension as the total instrument. That is, they overlap rather than complement each other. This is unlike the other measures of reliability in which a higher correlation is generally desirable. It must be noted that there are differing schools of thought among some researchers who may examine the corrected item–total correlations to see whether removing any of the items could improve internal reliability. Although the approach is slightly different, the premise to improve the internal consistency remains the same.

RESEARCH IN BRIEF 10.1

While there are accepted gold standard measures, any deviation from or adaptation of the gold standard needs to undergo further assessment for tool validity and reliability. For example, the King's Parkinson's Disease Pain Scale (KPPS) was originally developed and validated by Chaudhuri et al in their multicentre European field study in 2015. It has since been proven to be a reliable and valid tool in different studies. Taghizadeh et al (2021) examined the psychometric properties of a Persian version of the KPPS (KPPS-P) among 480 people with Parkinson's disease. Cronbach alpha (α = 0.88) indicated good internal consistency, and ICC (0.97–0.99) values of test–retest reliability suggested sufficient stability of the KPPS-P over time. These findings confirmed the comparability of the Persian version of the KPPS to its original version.

RESEARCH IN BRIEF 10.2

A study examined sleep problems using the Insomnia Severity Index (ISI) among a sample of 96 people with chronic obstructive pulmonary disease (COPD). The ISI contains seven items with item–total correlations that ranged from 0.51 to 0.80 (mean = 0.67), indicating that all items contribute to the ISI total score. The overall findings, including the item–total correlation of all items, indicate that the ISI is a valid instrument for assessing insomnia severity in the COPD population (Jun et al 2022).

Equivalence

In the context of reliability assessment, **equivalence** is the consistency or agreement among different observers using the same or alternative forms of a measuring instrument. The two methods to test equivalence are inter-rater reliability and alternative or parallel form. An instrument demonstrates equivalence when there is a high percentage of agreement of an observed behaviour.

Inter-rater reliability. Measurement instruments that use direct observations and systematic recording of variables from more than one observer need to be tested for inter-rater reliability. For example, assessing the presence of an intravenous cannula (IVC) site infection may require the assessment of two independent raters to establish the severity of infection. Two main ways that inter-rater reliability is used are: (a) testing to see how similarly people *categorise* items (e.g. events, behaviours) and (b) how similarly people *score* items.

To achieve inter-rater reliability, two or more individuals observe the same behaviour or event to ensure that there is consistency of observations between observers. Observers are trained to observe and record the behaviour in a standard, consistent manner. When establishing inter-rater reliability, it is the reliability of the observers rather than the reliability of the instrument that is being tested. However, it must be noted that sometimes it may be the ambiguous wording of an instrument, a poorly designed scale or response options that may possibly contribute to the variability in a rater's interpretation and recording of a variable.

Inter-rater reliability is expressed as a percentage of agreement between scorers, kappa (κ is used for categorical level data) or as an intraclass correlation coefficient (for interval-level data) between scores assigned to the observed behaviours. The strength of agreement for kappa and intraclass coefficients has been interpreted as 0.0–0.20: no agreement; 0.21–0.39: minimal agreement; 0.40–0.59: weak agreement; 0.60–0.79: moderate agreement; 0.80–0.90: strong agreement; above.90: almost perfect agreement. Overall, 'any kappa below 0.60 indicates inadequate agreement among the raters' (McHugh 2012 p. 279).

AN UNEXPECTED HURDLE

Inter-rater reliability evaluates consistency in how observers categorise items, and how similarly observers score items.

The aim of a (hypothetical) Australian multisite randomised controlled trial was to test the relationship between different methods used by nurses when completing regular IVC site assessment on the rates of IVC site infections in hospitalised patients receiving daily antibiotics. The main study outcome was the detection of a localised IVC site infection during their hospital admission. As part of the data collection, multiple observers (i.e. data collectors) at each hospital site had to perform IVC site inspections on the enrolled patients for signs of infection and record their findings on a specially devised data collection tool. The data collection tool used to measure inter-rater reliability included questions with accompanying descriptions asking outcome assessors to identify the severity of the IVC site infection. With the study underway the early inter-rater checks indicated that there was variation (i.e. observer bias) among data collectors' IVC site assessments. In this study, the researchers were challenged to ensure that data collectors were able to assess IVC site infection in relation to presence (absent/present) and, when an IVC site infection was present, to grade the severity using the objective descriptors provided.

1. ***How might the researchers have dealt with this hurdle?***
2. ***What are some of the considerations when developing the IVC site assessment tool used to establish inter-rater reliability between outcome assessors?***
3. ***What strategies could the researchers have used to minimise observer bias in the data collectors' assessment of IVC site infection and severity?***

RESEARCH IN BRIEF 10.3

Katijjahbe et al (2020) examined the psychometric properties of the shortened version of the Functional Difficulties Questionnaire (FDQ), which is used to measure physical function of the thoracic region following cardiac surgery. The study involved a total of 225 participants across four tertiary care hospitals in Australia. The original 13-item FDQ was shortened to a 10-item scale (FDQ-s) after item reduction analysis. The authors also reported excellent internal consistency (Cronbach's α >0.90) and test–retest reliability (ICC = 0.89–0.92). The overall results indicated that the FDQ-s exhibits robust psychometric properties in this setting.

Parallel form reliability. Parallel (or alternative) form reliability is applicable if two comparable forms of the same instrument measuring the same construct exist. Parallel form instruments contain the same types of items that are based on the same domain or construct but the wording of the items is different. It is like test–retest reliability in that the same individuals are tested simultaneously using both measures. The scores from the two versions of the measure are then correlated to assess the consistency of results across alternative versions.

Development of parallel forms is important if the instrument is intended to measure a variable for which a researcher believes that 'testing' bias will influence a study's internal validity. If alternative forms of an instrument yield a high correlation then stability is demonstrated. This approach is also used to examine the equivalence between two instruments measuring the same construct. In practice, it is difficult to develop alternative forms of an instrument when considering the many issues required for instrument validity. For example, a nurse researcher develops a large set of questions that are split into two halves. Each set of questions is administered to a randomly selected half of the target sample so that each person is given both versions of the instrument to complete. The test that gives the most consistent results (i.e. highest correlation) is used.

TUTORIAL TRIGGER 10.1

Clinical trial nurses that are engaged in data collection and participant recruitment for clinical trials are required to undertake training. Why is this a critical step in research?

What other strategies may be employed by researchers to improve intra-rater and inter-rater reliability?

Validity

Validity examines the accuracy of a measuring instrument in reflecting all aspects of the construct of interest. The quality and rigour of any quantitative study are judged in part by the ability of the instruments used to measure what they were designed to measure. Importantly, assessment of the validity of an instrument is based on the way the measure is constructed, its relationship to measures of other constructs and its ability to predict specific events (DeVellis & Thorpe 2021). As with reliability, the validity of an instrument is not a dichotomous state (present or absent) but rather is supported on a continuum by evidence developed for the validity of an instrument as more studies use and examine the instrument. Therefore, nursing and midwifery researchers do not validate an instrument, but rather an application of it. For instance, a measure of anxiety may be valid for preoperative patients on the day of surgery but not necessarily for nursing students on the day of an exam. Establishment of construct validity is a complex process, involving numerous studies and different approaches over time. There are three types of validity: content validity, construct validity and criterion-related validity. Table 10.2 outlines the distinctions between the three types of validity.

A measure can, however, be reliable but not valid. A valid instrument that is supposed to measure anxiety does so; it does not measure some other construct, such as stress. Consider an illogical hypothesis where a researcher wanted to measure anxiety in patients by measuring their body temperatures. The researcher could obtain highly accurate, consistent and precise temperature recordings, but such a measure could not be a valid indicator of anxiety. The high reliability of an instrument (in this case, a thermometer) is not necessarily congruent with evidence of validity. Conversely, for an instrument to be considered valid, it must also demonstrate acceptable reliability. An instrument cannot validly measure the attribute of interest if it is erratic, inconsistent and imprecise—that is, if it demonstrates poor reliability.

A research consumer evaluates whether sufficient evidence of validity is present and whether the type of validity is appropriate to the design and the instruments used in the study. Instrument (measurement) validity is examined in relation to content, structure and establishing evidence of relationships between the measure and other variables. Table 10.2 summarises the validity-related psychometric properties of measuring instruments. One example of validity is when a new instrument was developed to measure nurses' perceptions of their responsibilities related to healthcare quality (Oldland et al 2021). Once developed and tested, the Nurses Responsibilities in Healthcare Quality Questionnaire was then shown to be acceptable in terms of validity and reliability. It now assists education providers and health service managers to identify gaps between nurses' beliefs and professional role expectations and helps in developing the knowledge, skills and attitudes of healthcare quality among nurses.

RESEARCH IN BRIEF 10.4

The Consumer Access, Appraisal and Application of Services and Information for Dementia (CAAASI-Dem) scale was developed over three phrases (Doherty et al 2020). In Phase 1, systematic review, expert reviews and respondent debriefing resulted in a 65-item CAAASI-Dem. In Phase 2, the scale was assessed and modified via a pilot test among 1412 participants, which led to the removal of 34 items. The revised 31-item CAAASI-Dem was then further refined and validated using exploratory factor analysis (EFA) in Phase 3, involving a sample of 3146 participants. This multistage process resulted in the final 26-item 5-factor CAAASI-Dem which showed good psychometric properties. In a follow-up study by Nguyen et al (2022) among 3277 participants, the structural validity and reliability of the CAAASI-Dem was evaluated using different statistical methods, including confirmatory factor analysis (CFA). The results indicated that the 24-item 5-factor CAAASI-Dem was a valid and reliable scale to examine individuals' self-assessed confidence in their ability to access, appraise and use dementia services and information.

TABLE 10.2 The Different Types of Validity Used to Assess Measuring Instruments

Type of Validity	Test	Purpose
Content		
Degree to which a measure includes every single element of the construct.	Face	Assesses the extent to which measurement items are subjectively considered to cover the concept the measure is supposed to be measuring—that is, how representative the measure is at 'face value' of the concept it is measuring.
	Judge panel Content Validity Index (CVI)	Assesses the 'relevancy' of each individual scale item on a measure. Removes redundant or unclear items.
Construct		
Factor analysis Degree to which a set of scale items measures an underlying construct or dimensions of a construct.	Exploratory factor analysis Confirmatory factor analysis	Identifies dimensions of an underlying construct, and enables identification of redundant scale items to create a more concise version of a scale.
Contrasted groups Degree to which groups are expected to differ on some construct of interest.	Analysis of variance (ANOVA) *t*-test	Identifies two or more groups of individuals who are expected to score extremely high or low on the characteristic being measured.
Divergent Degree to which two constructs are expected to differ.	Correlation coefficient	Assesses the differences in two measures that theoretically measure the same construct.
Convergent Degree to which two constructs are expected to be related.	Correlation coefficient	Assesses the similarities in two measures that theoretically measure the same construct.
Hypothesis-testing approach Testing hypothesised relationships on the basis of theory or prior research.	Correlation coefficient	Identifies differences in individuals' scores on a measure that enables inferences to be drawn about the construct validity of the instrument to measure the underlying constructs of interest.
Criterion		
Concurrent Degree of correlation between two measures of the same concept administered simultaneously.	Correlation coefficient	Assesses the performance of a new instrument against an established measure.
Predictive Degree to which a measure predicts performance on some future criterion.	Correlation coefficient	Assesses a measure's ability to predict something it should be able to predict.

Content validity. In the early stages of instrument development, the sampling adequacy or completeness of a set of items to reflect a content domain (i.e. construct) is assessed by the research team to have face validity, which is the extent to which the items seem to measure the construct. There are no formal tests for this, as it is a simple judgement that the researchers make. The next step in this 'judging' involves the use of an expert panel to assess more formally the extent to which the items measure the construct. The most widely used method of quantifying content validity for multi-item scales among nurse researchers is the Content Validity Index (CVI) (Yusoff 2019). The CVI is based on expert ratings of the relevance of each item and ranges from 1 'not relevant', through 2 'somewhat relevant' and 3 'quite relevant' to 4 'highly relevant'. CVI values may be computed for each item as well as for the overall scale and indicates either the proportion of items given a rating of 3 or 4 or the proportion of the raters giving a rating of 3 or 4.

Savage et al (2022) developed a new tool called KAnt Fall for assessing newborn fall risk in the acute care setting. The content validity of KAnt Fall was evaluated among 27 intensive care unit nurses. Item-level content validity indices (I-CVIs) and an average scale content validity index (S-CVI/Ave) were calculated, resulting in the removal of 14 items with low I-CVI scores from the initial 28-item scale. The modified 14-item scale (S-CVI/Ave = 0.92) was then tested for inter-rater reliability among 130 nurses. The intraclass correlation coefficient (ICC = 0.99) indicated excellent interrater reliability.

Construct validity. Construct validity (see Table 10.2) comprises a range of approaches used to assess the similarities or differences in performance between an instrument and other similar measures. Construct validity is an essential component when judging the quality of a study and concerns aspects about the measures used to operationalise the variables. The key question a research consumer needs to ask is: 'What is this instrument really measuring?' The different types of tests to establish construct validity (factor analysis, contrast, convergent/divergent, hypothesised relationships) are discussed in the following sections.

Factor analysis. Factor analysis is one of the methods used to assess construct validity and it provides quantitative assessment about the extent to which a set of items measure the same underlying construct or dimension of a construct, and whether the items in the instrument reflect a single construct or several constructs. Factor analysis assesses the degree to which the individual items on a scale truly cluster together around one or more dimensions (Black & Babin 2019). The correlation or relationship between an item or variable and their underlying factor is known as *factor loading*. Those items designed to measure different dimensions should be less correlated with some of the items and should load on different factors, which is discussed in more detail in Chapter 11. Montazeri et al (2020) developed the Hospital Nurse Interpersonal Empathy Questionnaire (HNIEQ) and examined its psychometric properties among 250 hospital nurses in Iran. The construct validity of the HNIEQ was assessed using exploratory factor analysis, which revealed six factors explaining 52.7% of the total variance. These include empathetic and ethical attention, perspective adoption, emotional affectability, altruism, emotion identification and responsivity, and reflection forecasting. Along with high internal consistency (Cronbach's α = 0.953) and test–retest reliability (ICC = 0.97), the HNIEQ is demonstrated to be a valid and reliable instrument for empathy assessment among nurses in this setting.

Contrasted-groups approach. Another approach often used to assess construct validity is the 'known-groups' method. This approach is generally acceptable when two or more groups have characteristics that are clearly different to one another. In this case, you are anticipating that one group will score higher while the other group is anticipated to score lower (Portney 2020). The instrument is administered to both the high-scoring and the low-scoring groups and the differences in scores are examined. If the instrument is sensitive to individual differences in the trait being measured, the groups will differ significantly, and evidence of construct validity is supported.

RESEARCH IN BRIEF 10.5

A study by Allen et al (2022) reported on the development and preliminary evaluation of the Everyday Ageism Scale (EAS) among 2048 older adults in the US. Exploratory factor analysis identified three factors, which explained 62.66% of the variance, including exposure to ageist messages, ageism in interpersonal interactions and internalised ageism. The tool demonstrated sufficient internal consistency (Cronbach's α = 0.768) and known-group validity between the older age group and their younger counterparts. The study provides evidence for EAS as having strong psychometric properties which can be used to explore the multidimensional nature of everyday ageism and its relationship with health.

Convergent and divergent approaches. Convergent validity is another approach used to assess construct validity and test measures of a construct when no gold standard (i.e. established measure) exists. Two or more instruments that theoretically measure the same construct are identified and administered to the same participants. A correlation analysis is performed to assess whether each participant's scores for both instruments change in the same way—that is, when one increases so does the other. If the measures are positively correlated, convergent validity is supported.

In contrast, divergent (discriminant) validity assesses the differentiation from one construct to another that may be potentially equivalent. A researcher may sometimes want to use instruments that measure the opposites of a construct. If the divergent measure is negatively related to other measures, validity for the measure is strengthened. Data from a factor analysis can also be used to determine divergent validity.

CASE STUDY

The convergent and discriminant validity of three frailty instruments (the frailty phenotype, the St Vincent's frailty instrument and the SHARE frailty instrument) were evaluated in an Australian study of 131 adults with heart failure (McDonagh et al 2020). All three frailty instruments measure five physical frailty domains to give an overall classification of frail, pre-frail or non-frail. Convergent validity was tested by reporting the correlations between the frailty instruments and heart failure-related subconstructs, such as depression, low quality of life and poor physical performance. Discriminant validity was assessed by evaluating the ability of each frailty instrument to discriminate between normal and abnormal scores of other physical and psychosocial scales specific to heart failure. The St Vincent's frailty instrument showed the highest correlations to the relevant subconstructs tested, displaying good convergent validity. The SHARE frailty instrument and the St Vincent's frailty instrument both detected significant group differences between the three frailty classifications (frail, pre-frail and non-frail) and they were both able to discriminate between normal and abnormal scores in three out of five of the heart failure-related subconstructs tested, providing evidence of discriminant validity. The study results concluded that the St Vincent's frailty instrument and the SHARE frailty instrument displayed the strongest convergent and discriminant validity, but these results need to be confirmed in a larger cohort.

A specific method of assessing convergent and divergent validity is the multitrait–multimethod approach. Similar to the approaches previously described, this method involves examining the relationship between indicators that should measure the same construct and those that should measure different constructs (Portney 2020). Anxiety, for example, can be measured by a variety of strategies, such as:

- a questionnaire—for example, the State-Trait Anxiety Inventory heart rate and blood pressure readings
- asking a participant directly about their anxious feelings
- observing a participant's behaviour
- measuring urinary or serum catecholamines.

The results of one of these measures can be correlated with results of each of the others in a multitrait–multimethod matrix (Portney 2020). The use of multiple measures such as self-report, observation, interview and collection of physiological data will also decrease the effect of systematic error, improving instrument validity.

Hypothesis-testing approach. This approach to construct validity uses an underlying theory of the instrument's design to develop and test hypotheses regarding the behaviour of individuals with varying scores on the measure. Empirical testing supports or rejects the relationships predicted among concepts and provides support for the construct validity of the instrument measuring those concepts. Data collected test the hypotheses and enable inferences about whether the rationale underlying the instrument's construction is adequate to explain the findings.

In an international study that measured the criteria-led discharge checklist to determine postoperative recovery, a hypothesis-testing approach was used to assess the checklist's capacity to measure physiological recovery after surgery (Boden et al 2021). The researchers used pair-wise chi-square with Bonferroni adjustments to assess between-group differences. The results showed that the criteria-led discharge checklist was like current discharge planning approaches and was particularly accurate in more complex cases ($p < 0.001$). The researchers concluded that measuring physiological recovery using the criteria-led discharge following emergency and elective abdominal surgery was akin to current practice, and the new checklist has the potential to reduce hospital length of stay.

Criterion validity. An instrument is said to have criterion validity if scores on a scale correlate highly with scores on an external criterion. This approach can be used only when there is an established, reliable and valid measure for a construct, or if there is a reliable and valid outcome that will occur in the future if the construct is present.

Concurrent validity

Criterion validity can be tested using a concurrent approach which examines the degree of correlation between two measures of the same concept administered at the same time. The instrument is valid if its scores correlate highly (i.e. 0.70) on the criterion (DeVellis & Thorpe 2021). This process is used to assess the performance of a new instrument compared with an established instrument—the 'gold standard'. The gold standard label is given to an instrument or test that is the best available measurement of a concept, attitude, behaviour or physical state. Sometimes the established gold standard may be a long or complicated measurement process, and a researcher may decide to construct a shorter instrument with less respondent burden (i.e. the amount of effort and time required from the participants).

For example, a multimethod and multiphase study was conducted by Dellafiore et al (2021) to develop and validate a self-efficacy scale for nurses to assess the nutritional care of older adults (SE-NNC). Confirmatory factor analysis was performed on data collected from 160 nurses who also completed the nursing profession self-efficacy scale (NPSES) as the 'gold standard' for concurrent validity. The final 27-item three-factor scale demonstrated good internal consistency (Cronbach's $\alpha = 0.979$) and adequate concurrent validity (ICC = 0.763).

Predictive validity. Predictive validity is another type of criterion validity and explores the degree of correlation between the measure of the construct of interest and some future measure or outcome of the same construct. Consider the following examples: blood sugar level testing may predict future diabetes, and academic achievement at high school predicts students' university grade point average. With the passage of time, correlation coefficients are likely to be lower for predictive validity studies.

A study by Abbass-Dick et al (2020) developed and examined the psychometric properties of the 28-item Comprehensive Breastfeeding Knowledge Scale (CBKS) among 217 Canadian expectant parents. The predictive validity of the CBKS was examined in relation to breastfeeding exclusivity outcomes. CBKS scores were demonstrated to be predictive of exclusive breastfeeding at 4 and 12 weeks postpartum.

Responsiveness

Reliability and validity are the two most important criteria for evaluating measuring instruments; however, sometimes nursing and midwifery researchers need to consider other qualities such as **responsiveness**. Responsiveness is the ability of an instrument to detect clinically important changes in a patient's status even when these differences are small (DeVellis & Thorpe 2021). Responsive instruments demonstrate:

- maximum change when clinically important changes in status occur
- minimal change on repeated applications to stable patients.

Responsiveness is therefore the magnitude of change in a participant's score on an instrument that corresponds to a **minimal important difference** (DeVellis & Thorpe 2021, Mokkink et al 2021). Responsiveness is measured by comparing instrument scores before and after a treatment of known effect. Effect size (change in scores due to treatment effect) can also be used to examine responsiveness as it relates to changes in the mean score compared with the standard deviation of baseline scores or score changes among stable patients (Mokkink et al 2021). The responsiveness or precision of an instrument is limited by 'floor and ceiling' effects—that is, the range of responses possible. The end-points (extremes) of the scale limit the responses that truly reflect a participant's status for that dimension. Floor and ceiling effects are considered present if more than 15% of respondents achieved the lowest or highest possible scores, respectively (Mokkink et al 2021).

Smith et al (2022) examined the responsiveness of the Patient-Reported Outcomes Measurement Information System (PROMIS) Cancer Function Brief 3D Profile among 209 patients across five tertiary care centres. The results indicated sufficient responsiveness in that PROMIS scores responded well to changes in scores of the Karnofsky Performance Scale (KPS) and numeric pain rating scale (NRS).

Knowledge of previous responsiveness characteristics of instruments aids in instrument selection and allows for more accurate sample size and statistical power estimations. However, assessment and reporting of responsiveness has been minimal when compared with the evaluation of reliability and validity. It is therefore often difficult to select an instrument based on its comparative responsiveness against other measures. Responsiveness can be improved by:

- increasing the number of response categories
- arranging scores into subgroups (e.g. gender, level of education, ethnicity) to allow the identification of emerging patterns
- including transition questions
- using individualised questions.

DEVELOPING A MEASURING INSTRUMENT

An abundance of instruments exists for measuring a wide range of clinical, psychological and educational constructs that are relevant to nursing and midwifery researchers. Reliable, valid and responsive instruments require substantial development and testing, involving a suite of testing processes and related studies, often over a number of years. Despite a plethora of available instruments, a researcher sometimes cannot locate an instrument or method with acceptable reliability and validity that measures their variable of interest. This may be the case when examining an element of a theory or when evaluating the effect of a clinical intervention. When deciding to develop a new instrument, a researcher needs to balance the disciplinary and academic need against the complex and time-consuming processes required. The development process includes:

- defining the construct of interest; a concept developed for a specific research purpose
- constructing items that reflect elements of the construct
- validation of the items
- pilot testing
- formal testing for reliability and validity of the entire instrument.

Defining the Construct

A construct is a concept used by researchers. Examples of constructs are pain, distress, fatigue or health-related quality of life. Defining a construct requires an extensive review of the theoretical literature as well as the existing knowledge base for all instruments developed to measure the concept. This background information enables the construct to be operationalised into a variable (i.e. defined in a way it can be measured). A well-constructed instrument consists of an objective, standardised measure of a clearly defined variable (e.g. a behaviour or characteristic).

Item Construction

Once the construct is defined, individual items (questions) can be developed. The collection of items should be comprehensive in covering all aspects of the construct. More items are initially developed than needed to address each aspect of the construct or subconstruct. In general, there should be a minimum four to six items for each independent aspect of the construct—more is not always better. There remains a debate regarding the minimum number of items possible; however, ideally a smaller number of items may be used when a larger sample size exists or is anticipated (Koran 2020). Nevertheless, items need to:

- reflect the operational definition of the construct (the extent items appear to accomplish this reflects the validity of the instrument)
- be unambiguous, concise, exact statements with only one idea per item (negative stems or items with negatively phrased response possibilities that result in a double negative may cause ambiguity)
- use a limited number of formats (errors may occur if respondents are confused by shifting from one format to another)
- be neutral in style so as to not influence a respondent (unless carefully constructed, an item may indicate an expected response, or an expected response to a subsequent item)
- be not unnecessarily complex or require exact operations
- be appropriate to the educational level of participants.

Item Validation

Newly constructed items are then evaluated by a panel of experts in the field to ensure that the items reflect what they are intended to measure. During the process of item validation, the Content Validity Index is calculated and based on this the number of items will be reduced as some items will not fit as intended and will be discarded. In this phase the researcher needs to ensure consistency among the items, as well as consistency in testing and scoring procedures.

Pilot Test

The developing instrument is then commonly tested on a small, carefully chosen representative sample of participants who display the behaviour of interest. This process assesses the quality of the instrument as a whole (reliability and validity), as well as the ability of each individual item to discriminate between respondents (variance in item response). Instrument administration is standardised using a set of uniform items and response possibilities that are consistently administered and scored. After pilot testing, modifications may be required prior to using the instrument in a larger study.

It is important that researchers who invest significant amounts of time in instrument development disseminate their findings. This type of research serves not only to introduce other researchers to the instrument but also to ultimately enhance the discipline, as our ability to conduct meaningful research is supported by our ability to measure important variables in a reliable and valid way.

RESEARCH IN BRIEF 10.6

Depression is common in patients with coronary heart disease. This may be undetected and undertreated by clinicians. The PHQ-9 is a validated instrument commonly used to assess depression in clinical trials. Gholizadeh et al (2019) aimed to develop and validate a Persian version of the PHQ-9. Researchers developed and administered a Persian version of the PHQ-9 to 150 patients with coronary artery disease in Tehran, Iran. The new Persian version of the PHQ-9 showed acceptable internal consistency, researchers reported a Cronbach's alpha coefficient of 0.80. The optimal cut-off score of ≥7 demonstrated a sensitivity of 76, specificity of 78 and the area under curve of 0.82. Researchers concluded that the Persian PHQ-9 had acceptable psychometric properties to screen and detect depression in patients with coronary artery disease, with a recommended cut-off score of ≥7.

Assessing Instruments

Reliability and validity are critical factors when assessing a measurement instrument (see Fig. 10.2). An effective critique includes establishing the instrument's level of reliability and validity and comparing the setting to the context under investigation. In a research report the reliability and validity for each measure should be presented. If these are not reported, a reviewer should question the merit and use of the instrument and the study's results. If appropriate, responsiveness of the instrument should also be reported.

Appropriate reliability tests should be reported in the original and subsequent reports of the instrument. If the initial testing sample and the current sample have different characteristics, a reader would expect that:

- a pilot study for the present sample was conducted to confirm that the reliability was maintained
- a reliability estimate was calculated on the current sample.

Satisfactory evidence of validity is probably the most difficult aspect for a reviewer to determine, but it is this that is most likely to fail to meet the required criteria. Validity studies are time consuming, as well as complex, and researchers may present only minimal validity data in a published paper. A reader should therefore closely examine the item content of an instrument when evaluating its strengths and weaknesses and try to find evidence of its validity. Articles may, however, not include the instrument, or provide only a few sample items available for review. In this case, a reviewer will need to appraise other articles that examine the instrument more fully.

A reader would expect to see reliability and validity discussed in relation to other instruments created to measure the same variable/construct. The relationship of the findings to strengths and weaknesses in instrument reliability and validity would be another important discussion point. Finally, recommendations for improving future studies in relation to instrument reliability, validity and responsiveness should be proposed. Refer to Box 10.1 for criteria for evaluating psychometric properties of instruments.

BOX 10.1 Criteria for Evaluating Psychometric Properties of Instruments

1. Was an appropriate method used to test the reliability of the instrument?
2. Is the reliability of the instrument adequate?
3. Was an appropriate method used to test the validity of the instrument?
4. Is the validity of the instrument adequate?
5. If the sample from the developmental stage of the instrument is different from the current sample, was the reliability and validity recalculated to determine if the tool remains consistent?
6. Are strengths and weaknesses of instrument reliability and validity appropriately addressed in the Discussion, Strengths, Limitations or Recommendations sections of the paper?
7. Is the precision or responsiveness of the instrument discussed in relation to clinically important differences?

TUTORIAL TRIGGER 10.2

You are working as an RN in the community health centre. You are asked to lead a journal club as part of your research and education program. The study that you have selected to critique is a randomised controlled trial of a new approach to wound care for patients with diabetic foot ulcers, which also examines their levels of depression. The study reports using three measures for depression including a modified, 17-item, Hamilton rating scale for depression, the Beck Depression Inventory and the Zung self-rating anxiety scale. You are not familiar with these scales; however, you would like to appraise the validity and reliability of each of the instruments to determine their acceptability.

How would you appraise validity and reliability of these instruments?

SUMMARY

The concepts of reliability and validity can often be challenging for a beginning researcher to appraise with confidence. This chapter described the systematic assessment of the psychometric aspects of an instrument. Discussing these issues with colleagues or research mentors is also a useful approach to assist in developing your skills to critically appraise the hallmarks and shortcomings of existing, as well as newly developed, instruments that are reported in the nursing or midwifery literature. These exchanges promote understanding of the basic concepts of psychometrics as well as the exploration of alternative methods of observation and the use of reliable and valid tools in clinical practice.

KEY POINTS

- Reliability examines the consistency of a measuring instrument—stability, homogeneity and equivalence—using tests such as test–retest, parallel or alternative form, split-half, item-to-total correlation, Cronbach's alpha and inter-rater reliability.
- Validity refers to whether an instrument measures what it is purported to measure (i.e. its accuracy) and is a crucial aspect of evaluating a tool.
- Testing of instrument responsiveness is an under-researched area but is an important issue for determining appropriate sample size and power calculations.
- The selection of a method for establishing reliability and validity depends on the purpose of the study, the characteristics of the construct and instrument and the testing method used for collecting data from the representative sample.

TIME TO REFLECT

Leahy-Warren, P., Mulcahy, H., Lehane, E., 2019. The development and psychometric testing of the Perinatal Infant Care Social Support (PICSS) instrument. J. Psychosom. Res. 126, 109813.

Aim: To develop a reliable and valid instrument to measure social support for new mothers in the perinatal period.

Design: Cohort survey.

Questions

1. Reflect on the information given and answer these questions:
   a. What was the research design?
   b. Is the design appropriate for this study?
   c. What constructs were the researchers interested in measuring?
   d. How did the researchers assess the construct validity of the scales?
   e. How was reliability (internal consistency) of the instrument items assessed?
   f. Was the instrument considered to be reliable? Please give a rationale.
   g. What methods did the researchers use to establish content validity?
2. Think of other methods that could have been used in this study to assess reliability and validity. Why do you think these methods were not used?
3. What are some of the strengths and limitations of the validity and reliability methods used in the study?
4. Could the PICSS scales be easily adapted and used in other settings and samples? Please give a rationale.

LEARNING ACTIVITIES

1. Which type of validity refers to the degree to which a research instrument measures the same construct as a previously established instrument?
   a. Content validity
   b. Criterion-related validity
   c. Concurrent validity
   d. Construct validity
2. Which of the following is an example of a construct?
   a. Height
   b. Weight
   c. Intelligence
   d. Age
3. Which of the following statements are true? An instrument can be:
   a. valid but not reliable
   b. reliable but not valid
   c. neither reliable nor valid
   d. both reliable and valid.
      i. a, b and c
      ii. b, c and d
      iii. a, c and d
      iv. a, b, c and d
4. A test score or measurement consists of:
   a. random errors plus constant errors
   b. random errors plus the true score
   c. constant errors plus error variance
   d. error variance plus the true score.
5. What is the most common way to establish content validity?
   a. Through statistical analysis
   b. Through expert judgement
   c. Through test-retest reliability
   d. Through internal consistency
6. A Cronbach's alpha coefficient of 0.80 indicates that:
   a. the frequency in each category is different from what would be expected by chance
   b. the instrument actually measures the concepts it was intended to measure
   c. the instrument is consistent—that is, data are collected consistently.
   d. none of the above.
7. Which type of reliability refers to the degree to which different items on a research instrument measure the same construct?
   a. Internal consistency reliability
   b. Test–retest reliability
   c. Parallel form's reliability
   d. Inter-rater reliability
8. Which type of validity refers to the degree to which a research instrument measures a theoretical construct that has not been previously established?
   a. Content validity
   b. Criterion-related validity
   c. Concurrent validity
   d. Construct validity
9. Tests that are used to estimate the stability of an instrument include:
   a. test–retest reliability
   b. parallel reliability
   c. Cronbach's alpha.
      i. a and b
      ii. a and c
      iii. b and c

10. When a variety of measurement strategies is used to examine the relationships between instruments that purport to measure the same construct and between those that should measure different constructs, this approach is called a:
    a. contrasted groups approach
    b. convergent approach
    c. multitrait–multimethod approach
    d. divergent approach.

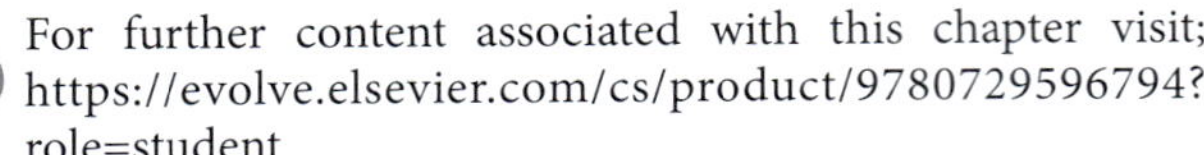

For further content associated with this chapter visit; https://evolve.elsevier.com/cs/product/9780729596794?role=student

ADDITIONAL RESOURCES

Abramson, J., Abramson, Z.H., 2011. Research Methods in Community Medicine: surveys, epidemiological research, programme evaluation, clinical trials. John Wiley & Sons, New York.

Mikkonen, K., Tomietto, M., Watson, R., 2022. Instrument development and psychometric testing in nursing education research. Nurse Educ. Today, 119, 105603.

Taherdoost, H., 2016. Validity and reliability of the research instrument; how to test the validation of a questionnaire/survey in a research: how to test the validation of a questionnaire/survey in a research. Int. J. Acad. Res. Manage. 5, 28–36. doi:10.2139/ssrn.3205040

REFERENCES

Abbass-Dick, J., Newport, A., Pattison, D., et al., 2020. Development, psychometric assessment, and predictive validity of the comprehensive breastfeeding knowledge scale, Midwifery 83, 102642. doi:10.1016/j.midw.2020.102642

Allen, J.O., Solway, E., Kirch, M., et al., 2022. The Everyday Ageism Scale: development and evaluation. J. Aging Health 34 (2), 147–157. doi:10.1177/08982643211036131

American Psychological Association. 2023. APA Dictionary of Psychology. American Psychological Association, Washington DC. Retrieved from: https://dictionary.apa.org/.

Black, W., Babin, B.J., 2019. Multivariate data analysis: its approach, evolution, and impact. In: Babin, B.J., Sarstedt, M. (Eds.), The Great Facilitator: reflections on the contributions of Joseph F. Hair, Jr. to marketing and business research. Springer International, Cham, Germany, pp. 121–130.

Boden, I., Peng, C., Lockstone, J., et al., 2021. Validity and utility testing of a criteria-led discharge checklist to determine post-operative recovery after abdominal surgery: an international multicentre prospective cohort trial. World J. Surg. 45, 719–729. doi:10.1007/s00268-020-05873-9

Bredin, D., O'Doherty, D., Hannigan, A., et al., 2022. Hand hygiene compliance by direct observation in physicians and nurses: a systematic review and meta-analysis. J. Hosp. Infect. 130, 20–33.

Cao, X., Yumul, R., Elvir Lazo, O.L., et al., 2017. A novel visual facial anxiety scale for assessing preoperative anxiety. PloS One, 12 (2), e0171233.

Chaudhuri, K.R., Rizos, A., Trenkwalder, C., et al., 2015. King's Parkinson's disease pain scale, the first scale for pain in PD: an international validation. Mov. Disord. 30 (12), 1623–1631.

Dellafiore,F., Caruso, R., Arrigoni, C. , et al., 2021. The development of a self-efficacy scale for nurses to assess the nutritional care of older adults: a multi-phase study, Clin. Nutrit. 40 (3), 1260–1267. doi:10.1016/j.clnu.2020.08.008

DeVellis, R.F., Thorpe, C.T., 2021. Scale Development: theory and applications, fifth ed. Sage Publications, Thousand Oaks, CA.

Doherty, K.V., Nguyen, H., Eccleston, C.E.A., et al., 2020. Measuring consumer access, appraisal and application of services and information for dementia (CAAASI-Dem): a key component of dementia literacy. BMC Geriatr. 20, 484. doi:10.1186/s12877-020-01891-3

Eriksen, S., Bjørkløf, G.H., Helvik, A.S., et al., 2019. The validity of the hospital anxiety and depression scale and the geriatric depression scale-5 in home-dwelling old adults in Norway*. J. Affect. Disord. 256, 380-385.

Gholizadeh, L., Shahmansouri, N., Heydari, M., et al., 2019. Assessment and detection of depression in patients with coronary artery disease: validation of the Persian version of the PHQ-9. Contemp. Nurse 55 (2–3), 185–194.

Jun, J., Park, C.G., Kapelle, M.C., 2022. Psychometric properties of the Insomnia Severity Index for people with chronic obstructive pulmonary disease, Sleep Med. 95, 120–125. doi:10.1016/j.sleep.2022.04.017

Katijjahbe M.A., Denehy, L., Granger, C.L., et al, 2020. Psychometric evaluation of the shortened version of the Functional Difficulties Questionnaire to assess thoracic physical function. Clin. Rehab. 34 (1), 132–140. doi:10.1177/0269215519879476

Koran, J., 2020. Indicators per factor in confirmatory factor analysis: more is not always better. Struct. Equ. Modeling 27 (5), 765–772.

Leahy-Warren, P., Mulcahy, H., Lehane, E., 2019. The development and psychometric testing of the Perinatal Infant Care Social Support (PICSS) instrument. J. Psychosom. Res. 126, 109813.

Lovibond, P., Lovibond, S., 1995. The structure of negative emotional states: comparison of the Depression Anxiety Stress Scale (DASS) with the Beck Depression and Anxiety Inventories. Behav. Res. Ther. 33, 335–343.

McDonagh, J., Salamonson, Y., Ferguson, C., et al., 2020. Evaluating the convergent and discriminant validity of three versions of the frailty phenotype in heart failure: results from the FRAME-HF study. Eur. J. Cardiovasc. Nurs. 19 (1), 55-63. doi:10.1177/1474515119865150

McHugh, M.I., 2012. Interrater reliability: the kappa statistic. Biochem. Med. 22 (3), 276–282.

Mokkink, L., Terwee, C., de Vet, H., 2021. Key concepts in clinical epidemiology: responsiveness, the longitudinal aspect of validity. J. Clin. Epidemiol. 140, 159–162. doi:10.1016/j.jclinepi.2021.06.002

Montazeri, M., Tagharrobi, Z., Sooki, Z., et al., 2020. Development and psychometric evaluation of the Hospital Nurse Interpersonal Empathy Questionnaire. Int. J. Nurs. Sci. 7 (3), 337–343. doi:10.1016/j.ijnss.2020.06.012

Nashwan, A.J., Villar, R.C., Al-Qudimat, A.R., et al., 2021. Quality of life, sleep quality, depression, anxiety, stress, eating habits, and social bounds in nurses during the coronavirus disease 2019 pandemic in Qatar (The PROTECTOR Study): a cross-sectional, comparative study. J. Pers. Med. 11 (9), 918.

Nguyen, H., Doherty, K. V., Eccleston, C. E. A, et al., 2022. Consumer Access, Appraisal, and Application of Services and Information for Dementia (CAAASI-Dem): a validation study, Aging Ment. Health 26 (12), 2489–2495. doi:10.1080/13607863.2021.1991277

Oldland, E., Hutchinson, A.M., Redley, B., et al., 2021. Evaluation of the validity and reliability of the Nurses' Responsibility in Healthcare Quality Questionnaire: an instrument design study. Nurs. Health Sci. 23 (2), 525–537.

Paek, E.J., Murray, L.L., Newman, S.D., et al., 2019. Test–retest reliability in an fMRI study of naming in dementia. Brain Lang. 191, 31–45.

Portney, L.G. 2020. Foundations of Clinical Research: applications to practice, fourth ed. Pearson, Upper Saddle River, NJ.

Prasad, M.G., Nasreen, A., Krishna, A.N.R., et al., 2020. Novel Animated Visual Facial Anxiety/Pain Rating Scale-Its reliability and validity in assessing dental pain/anxiety in children. Pediatr. Dent. J. 30 (2), 64–71.

Savage, K., Antista, H., Diamond, T., et al., 2023. Content validity and interrater reliability of a newborn fall risk assessment tool: KAnt Fall. Adv. Neonatal Care 23 (2), 167–172. doi:10.1097/ANC.0000000000001041

Smith, S.R., Vargo, M., Zucker, D.S., et al. 2022. Responsiveness and interpretation of the PROMIS Cancer Function Brief 3D Profile. Cancer 128 (17), 3217–3223. doi:10.1002/cncr.34376

Taghizadeh, E., Gheibihayat, S.M., Taheri, F., et al., 2021. LncRNAs as putative biomarkers and therapeutic targets for Parkinson's disease. Neurol. Sci. 42 (10), 4007–4015. doi:10.1007/s10072-021-05408-7

Yusoff, M.S.B., 2019. ABC of content validation and content validity index calculation. Educ. Med. J. 11 (2), 49–54.

Zigmond, A.S., Snaith, R.P., 1983. The hospital anxiety and depression scale. Acta Psychiatr. Scand. 67, 361–370.

11

Analysing Data in Quantitative Research

Daniel Terry and Danny Hills

LEARNING OUTCOMES

After reading this chapter, you should be able to:

- describe the differences between ratio, interval, ordinal and nominal levels of measurement
- describe the differences between, and state the purposes of, descriptive and inferential statistics
- identify the statistical procedures appropriate for each level of measurement
- describe the differences between parametric and non-parametric tests
- explain the concept of probability as it applies to the analysis of sample data
- explain type I and type II errors
- interpret 95% confidence intervals
- explain effect size, power and alpha levels and their relationship to sample size
- determine whether results of a study are objectively reported and include generalisations and limitations.

KEY TERMS

confidence intervals, p. 180
descriptive statistics, p. 168
effect size, p. 182
inferential statistics, p. 168
levels of measurement, p. 169
measures of central tendency, p. 169
null hypothesis, p. 178
power analysis, p. 181
standard deviation, p. 175

INTRODUCTION

This chapter outlines and describes common statistical procedures used in nursing and midwifery research, which encompass **descriptive statistics** (statistics used to describe a sample or population) and **inferential statistics** (statistics used to determine differences between samples or relationships of variables). An intricate knowledge of how to calculate these statistics is not always crucial; however, it is essential to understand what they mean, how they are used, how they are presented and their key limitations. In any case, spreadsheet and statistical computer applications greatly simplify data analysis such that, so long as the fundamentals of knowledge and understanding conveyed in this chapter can be applied and, with a little practice, relative novices may manage descriptive statistical analyses, at the very least (Grove & Cipher 2019).

Certainly, clinicians need to understand how to critically read and evaluate research studies to be able to translate clinically and administratively relevant research evidence into nursing and midwifery practice. Nurses and midwives are increasingly involved in higher-order clinical decision making. Consequently, there are greater expectations to use the best evidence to make effective and justifiable decisions in practice, even in the presence of periodic and persistent challenges and barriers (e.g. time constraints, insufficient support, insufficient knowledge of research and statistical analysis).

DESCRIPTIVE STATISTICS

Statistical methods are used to give organisation and meaning to numerical data. Data are analysed using two broad categories of analytical procedures. Procedures that enable researchers to describe, organise and summarise raw data are known as *descriptive statistics*. Procedures that enable researchers to estimate how reliably they can make predictions and generalise their findings based on the data are known as *inferential statistics* (Mishra et al 2019a, 2019b; Siedlecki 2020).

The primary purpose of descriptive statistics is to order and summarise quantitative data and facilitate the interpretation of the data. Descriptive statistics aid in summarising or representing the characteristics of the subject of investigation. Graphical and numerical techniques for organising and interpreting the data enable differences and trends to be identified. This can be achieved through simple statistical calculations, such as frequencies, percentages and proportions; the results are then organised into tables and graphical figures, such as pie charts, bar charts, line graphs and scatter plots. Descriptive statistics can also help in the identification of how data points are distributed and any data abnormalities, such as outliers at the extremes of data distributions, or missing or incomplete data (Amrhein et al 2019, Mishra et al 2019a).

Descriptive statistics also help to condense or summarise large quantities of numerical information into meaningful units. Data can be condensed and summarised using statistical **measures of central tendency** (i.e. mode, median and mean), measures of variability (e.g. range, interquartile range, standard deviation and confidence intervals) and some correlational techniques (these concepts are covered in detail later in the chapter). However, there is a need to clearly understand the use of a particular set of statistical techniques for data analysis. To evaluate the appropriateness of the statistical procedures used in a study, an individual should first develop an understanding of the levels of measurement that are appropriate for each statistical technique (Amrhein et al 2019, Mishra et al 2019a).

Levels of Measurement

Measurement is the assignment of numbers to objects or events according to certain rules and is determined by the nature of the subject of investigation being measured. **Levels of measurement** in ascending order are nominal, ordinal, interval and ratio (with the acronym NOIR). Nominal and ordinal measurements are also known as categorical data, and interval and ratio measurement are known as numerical data. The higher the level of measurement, the greater the flexibility a researcher has in choosing statistical procedures (Grove & Cipher 2019). Every attempt should be made to use the highest level of measurement possible so that the maximum amount of information can be obtained from the data. Table 11.1 shows levels of measurement and various examples.

Nominal Measurement

Nominal measurement refers to named categories and is used to classify objects or events into discrete groups (for example, a set of all whole numbers) and data are neither measured nor ordered. For example, male subjects may be assigned the number 1, female subjects the number 2 and non-binary subjects the number 3. The assignment of these numbers indicates that the categories of male and female are different and exclusive, and the object or event being examined either has a characteristic or does not. The numbers assigned to each category are nothing more than labels (names) and therefore cannot be arithmetically

TABLE 11.1 Levels of Measurement

Increasing level of measurement	Measurement	Description	Measures of Central Tendency	Measures of Variability	Example
	Nominal	Classification	Mode	Modal percentage, range, frequency distribution	Binary (yes/no)
	Ordinal	Relative rankings	Mode, median	Range, percentile, interquartile range, frequency distribution	Status (high, medium, low)
	Interval	Rank ordering with equal intervals	Mode, median, mean	Range, percentile, semi-quartile range, standard deviation	Temperature, height
	Ratio	Rank ordering with equal intervals and absolute zero	Mode, median, mean	All	Number of patients seen, age

manipulated. The numbers do not give the reader any more information about the nature of the difference. Nominal measurement can be used to categorise a sample of information such as gender, hair colour, eye colour, marital status or occupation (Amrhein et al 2019, Mishra et al 2019a).

Further, when measuring a phenomenon at the nominal level, the categories of response must be exclusive, can be assigned to only one category and are exhaustive (there are sufficient categories to enable all things or people being assigned to a category). For example, Terry and Peck (2020) examined how levels of consistency of interest and perseverance of effort (grit) among nursing students impacted their self-perceived academic and clinical performance. From a total sample of 435 students, they compared participant demographic characteristics (see Table 11.2).

TABLE 11.2 Comparison of Demographic Variables Among Student Sample

Demographic information	Frequency	Percentage (%)
Year of Program (*n* = 434)		
First year	149	34.3
Second year	164	37.8
Third year	121	27.9
Study Mode (*n* = 434)		
Flexible (online) students	199	45.9
Standard (face-to-face) students	235	54.1
Study Schedule (*n* = 434)		
Part time student	76	17.5
Full time student	358	82.5
Gender (*n* = 362)		
Female	329	90.8
Male	31	8.6
Other	2	0.6
Age (years) (*n* = 385)		
Under 20	32	8.3
20–30 years	147	38.2
30–39 years	118	30.6
40–49 years	61	15.8
50 years and over	27	7.0
Born in Australia (*n* = 362)		
Yes	257	70.9
No	105	29.1
Marital Status (*n* = 346)		
Single	123	35.5
Married/partnered	200	57.8
Divorced/separated	19	5.5
Other	4	1.2
Highest Level of Education (*n* = 349)		
Secondary school (year 12 or less)	108	30.9
Vocational education or trade training	198	56.7
Bachelor degree or above	39	11.1
Other	6	1.7
Employment Status (*n* = 399)		
Not in paid labour force	48	12.1
Casual employee (no guaranteed hours of work)	130	32.6
Part-time employee (less than 38 h/week)	167	41.9
Full-time employee (38 h/week)	54	13.5
Current After-Tax Income (AUD$) Per Week (*n* = 376)		
Less than $400	142	37.8
$400–$799	165	43.9
$800 –$1499	62	16.5
$1500–$3000	7	1.9
Healthcare (low income) card (*n* = 360)	137	35.8

(Source: Terry, D., Peck, B., 2020. Academic and clinical performance among nursing students: what's grit got to do with it? Nurs. Educ. Today 88, 104371.)

The variables in the table cover two types of measurements described in this text: nominal and ordinal. The nominal variables in this table include gender, study mode, study schedule, birthplace and marital status. They are all presented with associated frequencies (*n*) and percentages (%).

The nominal level of measurement allows the least amount of mathematical manipulation: only frequencies and proportions. Other than determining frequencies and proportions, the most frequently used statistical procedure for nominal data is the chi-square (χ^2) test. This test is covered in the later section on non-parametric tests.

Ordinal Measurement

Ordinal data are arranged in ordered categories and convey more information than nominal data, being arranged by relative ranking in a hierarchical order. For example, student grades are often represented as ordinal measures, typically being arranged as fail (<40%), marginal fail (40%–49%), pass (50%–59%), credit (60%–69%), distinction (70%–79%) and high distinction (80%–100%). Data or measures assigned to each category can be compared and those of a higher category can be said to have more of an attribute than one in a lower category. The intervals (spaces) between numbers on the scale are not necessarily equal, nor is there an absolute zero. For example, student nurses may be invited to nominate their clinical placement experience in order of preference on a Likert-type scale numbering 1 to 5, where number 1 is assigned to the 'least enjoyed placement' and number 5 to the 'most enjoyed placement'. However, the difference in actual score between students may differ widely (Grove & Cipher 2019). As with nominal level data, ordinal level categories are exclusive and exhaustive. In Table 11.2, the variable age group, level of education or income categories are measured on an ordinal scale, with higher numbers indicating older students, a higher level of education or higher income within the cohort. The limitation of ordinal measurement is that the intervals between the ranked categories cannot be treated as equal; ordinal scales add 'greater than' and 'less than', rather than 'greater than or equal to' and 'less than or equal to' to the measurement process. Mathematical manipulation of data is limited. However, in addition to what is possible with nominal data, medians, percentiles and rank order coefficients of correlation can also be calculated.

Interval Measurement

In an interval scale, the differences between scores or measures can be treated as equal, as there is a specific numerical distance between each of the levels. However, the zero point remains arbitrary. For example, in measuring temperatures on the Celsius scale, the distances between degrees are equal, but the zero point is arbitrary, reflecting the freezing point of water, which is not the same as having no heat.

In many areas of psychometric testing, including nursing, midwifery and the social sciences, there is much controversy over the classification of the level of measurement of intelligence, aptitude and personality tests, as well as quality of life and pain measures, with some regarding these measurements as ordinal and others as interval (Grove & Cipher 2019). The researcher needs to be aware of this controversy and to look at each study individually in terms of how the data are analysed (Reynolds et al 2021). Interval level data allow some manipulation such as addition and subtraction, but they do not necessarily allow multiplication and division. For example, 20°C on the Celsius scale is not half as hot as 40°C.

Ratio Measurement

Ratio measurement shows ranking of events or objects on scales with equal intervals and absolute zeros. The zero point makes the ratio of scale values meaningful. This is the highest level of measurement, but it is often achieved only in the physical sciences (Grove & Cipher 2019). Physical scales measuring height, weight, distance, pulse and blood pressure can usually be treated as ratio scales. Because there is a zero point in ratio scales, it is possible to state that 'a baby weighing four kilograms is twice as heavy as one weighing two kilograms'. In Table 11.2, although the 'age' variable was measured on an ordinal scale, the researchers could have, depending on their research question, measured age using a ratio scale, where a measure of central tendency and dispersion such as the median and interquartile range may have been reported.

Frequency Distribution

Frequency distribution is the most basic way of organising data. It is a statistical method for summarising the occurrences (frequencies) of events in a study. Although not always reported, it is usually the first step researchers undertake when exploring and summarising their data. For example, a lecturer reporting the results of an examination could report the number of students receiving each grade or could group the grades and report the number in each group. Table 11.3 illustrates the results of an examination given to a class of 51 students. The results of the examination are reported in several ways. The columns on the left show the raw data tally and the frequency for each grade, whereas the columns on the right show the grouped data tally and grouped frequencies (Grove & Cipher 2019).

When data are grouped, it is necessary to define the size of the group or the interval width so that no score will appear twice in the same group. The grouping of the data

TABLE 11.3 Frequency Distribution

INDIVIDUAL			GROUP		
Score	**Tally**	**Frequency**	**Score**	**Tally**	**Frequency**
90	|	1	>89	|	1
88	|	1			
86	|	1	80–89	|||| |||| ||||	15
84	|||| |	6			
82	||	2	70–79	|||| |||| |||| |||| |||	23
80	||||	5			
78	||||	5			
76	|	1	60–69	|||| ||||	10
74	|||| ||	7			
72	|||| ||||	9	<60	||	2
70	|	1			
68	|||	3			
66	||	2			
64	||||	4			
62	|	1			
60		0			
58	|	1			
56		0			
54	|	1			
52		0			
50		0			
Total		51			51

Mean, 74.5; standard deviation 7.8; median, 74; mode, 72; range, 36 (54–90)

in Table 11.3 prevents overlap. Each score falls into only one group, namely scores above 89, 80–89, 70–79, 60–69 and below 60. The interval widths should not be too large. Very large interval widths lead to loss of data information and may hide patterns in the data.

Fig. 11.1 shows an example of a histogram and a frequency polygon. The two examples are similar in that both plot scores against frequency. The greater the number of points plotted, the smoother is the resulting graph. The shape of the resulting graph allows for observations that

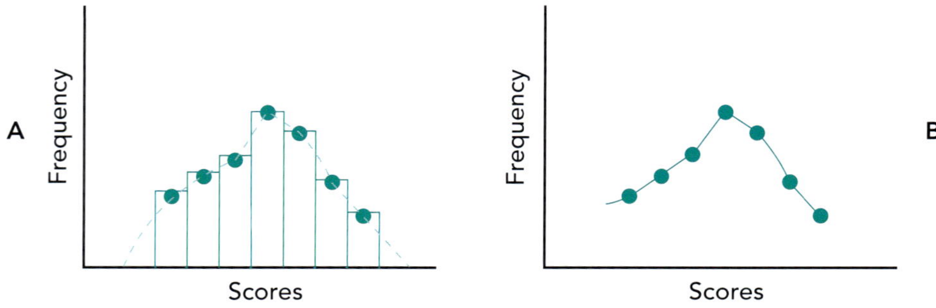

Fig. 11.1 Frequency distributions—A, histogram; B, frequency polygon

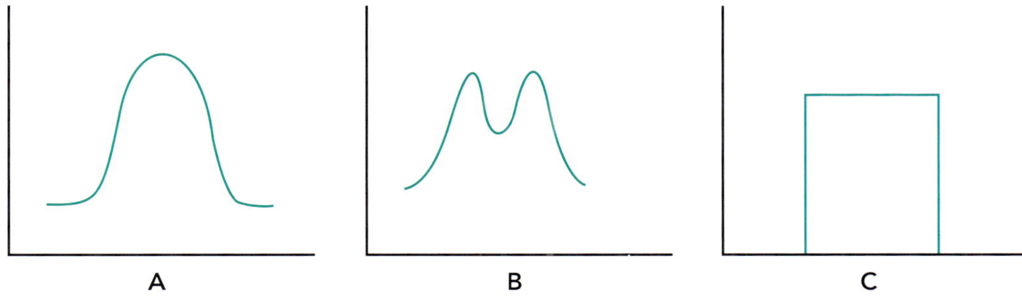

Fig. 11.2 Symmetrical distributions—A, unimoda ; B, bimodal; C, uniform

will further describe the data, particularly in terms of a normal or skewed distribution (described in more detail later in this chapter).

Measures of Central Tendency

A measure of central tendency is a single central score that enables a researcher to summarise the data set. Measures of central tendency describe the centre of a distribution of scores. These are the mode, the median and the mean. The mode refers to the numerical score that occurs with the greatest frequency in a distribution (i.e. most frequent) (Amrhein et al 2019, Mishra et al 2019a). The median is that point on a scale where half the scores fall above and half fall below (i.e. the middle score). The mean is the arithmetic average score. Measures of central tendency or summary statistics describe and give meaning to large amounts of numbers. As the measures of central tendency are sample specific, they will change with each sample (Mishra et al 2019a). The characteristics of a sample in a study are described in terms of summary statistics. The mean test score reported in Table 11.3 ($\bar{X} = 74.5$) is an example of such a statistic. If a different group of students were given the same test, it is likely that the mean would be different (Amrhein et al 2019). Measures of central tendency should be reported with one or more descriptions of dispersion appropriate for that measure of central tendency (described in more detail later in this chapter).

Mode

The mode is the most frequently occurring score in a frequency distribution and is the only measure of central tendency to be used with nominal data. It can, however, be used with all levels of measurement (see Table 11.1 above). A distribution can have more than one mode. The number of modes contained in a distribution is called the *modality of the distribution*. Fig. 11.2A and Fig. 11.3 illustrate unimodal or one-peak distributions. A multimodal distribution having two peaks is shown in Fig. 11.2B. Fig. 11.2C shows a uniform distribution, where all values are the same. Table 11.4 illustrates how the change in a few scores can change the modality of a distribution from unimodal to bimodal. Since the mode takes account of only the most frequently occurring scores, it is not always a very useful measure of central tendency (Amrhein et al 2019, Mishra et al 2019a).

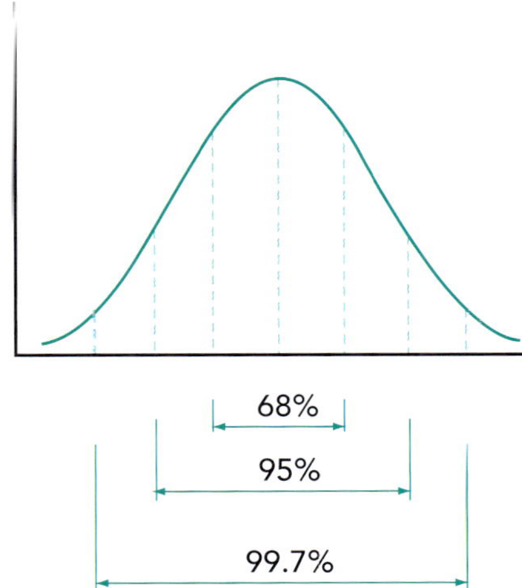

Fig. 11.3 Normal distribution (mesokurtosis) with associated standard deviations uniform

Median

The median is the middle score, or the score where 50% of the scores are above it and 50% of the scores are below it. The scores must first be ordered from lowest to highest in order to locate the median. In a set of an odd number of scores, the median is the middle score and in a set of an even number of scores, the median is the average of the two middle scores. For example, in the following set of odd-numbered scores 9 8 8 6 5 5 3, the median is 6, a value that is present in the data.

TABLE 11.4 Measures of Central Tendency

Score	Frequency	Measure
Unimodal		
35	||||	
36	|||| |||	Mode
37	|||	Median, mean
38	||||	
39	||||	
40	|||| |	
Bimodal		
35	||||	
36	|||| |||	Mode
37	|||	Mean
38	||||	Median
39	|||| |||	Mode
40	|||| |	

If there is one other score added so the data are now 10 9 8 8 6 5 5 3, the median is 7 ([8 + 6] ÷ 2), a value not actually present in the data. However, it is still meaningful to say that there are an equal number of scores above and below 7. For ordinal scale data, either the mode or the median can be used. The median presents more information about the distribution of scores by taking the rank order of the values into account. The median is not sensitive to extremes in high and low scores (Amrhein et al 2019, Mishra et al 2019a). As such, the median is best used if interval/ratio data are skewed (see below) and the researcher is interested in the 'typical' score. For example, if age is a variable and there is a wide range of ages that may affect the mean, it would be appropriate to also report the median. The median is easy to find by either inspection or calculation and can be used with ordinal or higher-level data, as shown in Table 11.1.

Mean

The mean is the most widely reported measure of central tendency. The mean is the mathematical average of all the scores and is most appropriately used with interval or ratio data (see Table 11.1), and is the only measure that reflects, and is affected by, all scores in the distribution. In a group of scores (e.g. age, income, height, test results), the mean is calculated by adding all the scores and dividing the total by the number of scores in the group (Amrhein et al 2019). Like the median, the mean can also take on a value not actually represented in the data. From the sample included above in relation to the median, the mean of the scores 9 8 8 6 5 5 3 is 6.29 and the median is 6. In small samples (where the number of participants or cases is <30) the mean can be affected by extreme values (also called outliers). Again, using the above example, if the values were 27 8 8 6 5 5 3, the mean is now 8.86; the mean has been dragged upwards by the extreme value of 27. Note that the median is still 6. However, the larger the sample size, the less affected the mean will be by a single extreme score.

Measures of Dispersion or Variability

Dispersion (or variability) is concerned with the spread of the data. Two or more samples with the same median or mean could differ in the distribution of values around those medians or means (Amrhein et al 2019, Mishra et al 2019a). Measures of dispersion answer the question, 'Is a sample homogeneous (similar) or heterogeneous (different)?' If a researcher measures oral temperatures in two samples, one sample drawn from a healthy population and one sample from a population hospitalised with an infectious illness, it is possible that the two samples will have a similar mean temperature (Amrhein et al 2019, Mishra et al 2019a). However, it is likely that there will be a wider range of temperatures in the hospitalised sample than in the healthy sample. Measures of dispersion describe the extent to which individuals or scores in the sample are spread out or vary. Many measures of variability exist. The modal frequency is the easiest to calculate. The most common measures used are the range, variance, standard deviation and interquartile range, which are unique for each sample of data.

Range

The range is the simplest and most unstable measure of dispersion. It is simply the difference between the highest and lowest scores. The range in Table 11.3 is 36, that is, 90 − 54 = 36. The disadvantage of the range is that it depends upon the two extreme scores only, which may be outliers (extreme scores) compared with the rest of the scores (Grove & Cipher 2019).

Quartiles and the Interquartile Range

The quartiles are values that cut the observations into four equal amounts/sections. There are three quartiles Q^1, Q^2 and Q^3. If you remember from the discussion of the median, the middle score, you may recognise that Q^2 is the median score. The distance between Q^1 (the 25th percentile) and Q^3 (the 75th percentile) is called the interquartile range. The interquartile range represents the middle 50% of the scores (Mishra et al 2019a); it is more stable than the range because it is less likely to be changed by a single extreme score. The middle 50% of the scores in Table 11.3 lies between 70 and 80 and the interquartile range is 10.

The middle 50% of the scores in Table 11.3 lies between 70 and 80 and the interquartile range is 10.

The formula to locate Q^1 is

$$\frac{(N+1)}{4}$$

where N = the number of data points. In the data shown in Table 11.3 there are 51 data points. Substituting 51 for N in the above equation to find Q^1 we count up 13 values, starting with the lowest value, and find that $Q^1 = 70$. The formula for Q^3 is

$$3 \times \frac{(N+1)}{4}$$

Again, starting with the lowest value, we count up 39 values and find that $Q^3 = 80$. The IQR is used in conjunction with the median to describe the centre and dispersion of ordinal level data or interval/ratio level data with a skewed distribution (see below).

Percentile

A percentile represents the percentage of cases a given score exceeds. The median is the 50% percentile and in Table 11.3 it is a score of 74. A score in the 90th percentile is exceeded by only 10% of the scores. The zero percentile and the 100th percentile are usually dropped.

Variance

A strategy commonly used to permit mathematical manipulation of different scores is to square them. Variance is a measure of variability that includes every score in the distribution. Some of the scores will be greater than the mean and some smaller. The deviation is the difference between the actual score and the mean. The deviation will be negative if the actual score is smaller than the mean. When negative deviations are squared, they become positive. To calculate the 'variance', the squared scores are summed and the mean of the summed scores is calculated. In short, the variance is the mean of the sum of squares. A small value for the variance (i.e. close to zero) indicates that the values are very close to the mean and therefore similar to each other; a large value for the variance indicates that the values are very spread out around the mean and from each other (Grove & Cipher 2019). Table 11.5 illustrates variance.

Sum of squares = 30

Number of values: 4

$$\text{Variance} = \frac{\text{Sum of squares}}{\text{Number of values}} = \frac{30}{4} = 7.5$$

TABLE 11.5 How Variance Is Calculated

Score	Mean	Deviation (Score – Mean)	Squared Deviation
2	6	−4	+16
4	6	−2	+4
7	6	+1	+1
9	6	+3	+9

Because the deviations from the mean are squared, it will be noted that the variance is expressed in units different from the scores. In order to convert back to the original units of measurement, it is necessary to find the square root of the variance. The value thus obtained is the standard deviation.

$$\begin{aligned}\text{Standard deviation} &= \text{square root of variance}\\ &= \sqrt{7.5}\\ &\approx 2.7\end{aligned}$$

Standard Deviation

The **standard deviation** (SD) is the most frequently used measure of dispersion/variability and it is based on the concept of the normal distribution or normal curve (see Fig. 11.3). It is a measure of average deviation or distance of each score from the group mean in a normal distribution (see below). When reporting the mean, the standard deviation should also be reported. It takes all scores into account and can be used to interpret individual scores (Mishra et al 2019a). Regardless of the mean and standard deviation, in a normal distribution of scores, **68% of the sample will fall within one standard deviation either side of the mean (34% on one side, 34% on the other),** two standard deviations encompass 95.2% of the scores and three standard deviations encompass 99.7% of scores. For example, the mean ($\bar{X}$) for the examination in Table 11.3 was 74.5 and the standard deviation (SD) was 7.8 (commonly reported as 74.5 ± 7.8 or ($\bar{X}$) 74.5, SD 7.8). This means that 68% of the grades were between 66.7 (i.e. 74.5 − 7.8 = 66.7) and 82.3 (i.e. 74.5 + 7.8 = 82.3). If a student received a grade of 88, they would know they did better than most of the class, whereas a grade of 58 would indicate they did not do as well as most of the class.

The smaller the SD in relation to the mean, the less variability within the sample and the more similar the scores are to the mean and to each other. One limitation of the SD is that it is expressed in terms of the units used in the measurement and cannot be used to compare means that have different units. If researchers were interested in the relationship between height measured in centimetres and weight measured in kilograms, it would be necessary for them to convert the height and weight measurements to standard units or z scores (see below). As noted above, the SD is the square root of the variance.

Z Scores

The z score is used to compare measurements/values in standard units. z scores take account of the mean and SD of the distribution. Each of the scores is converted to a z score and then the z scores are used to examine the relative distance of the scores from the mean. This process is called *standardising the score*. Any value in a distribution can be converted into a z score or value. The following formula will illustrate this concept:

$$\text{z score} = \frac{\text{Original value} - \text{mean}}{\text{Standard Deviation}}$$

As an example, the mean score on a drug calculation test was 70/100 and the standard deviation was 10. Mary's score on the test was 80. Using the above formula, from Mary's score (80), we subtract the mean (70) and divide it by the SD (10). We find then that Mary's score is 1 standard deviation above the mean. A z score of 1.5 means that the observation is +1.5 SD above the mean, whereas a score of −2 means that the observation is 2 SDs below the mean.

By using z scores, a researcher can compare results from scales that use different units, such as height and weight. For example, a participant in a research study may be 1.5 SDs above the mean for height, but 1.0 SD below the mean for weight. This tells us that the participant is taller than average for the sample, but also thinner than average.

Normal Distribution

The concept of the normal distribution is a theoretical one. It is based on the observation that data from repeated measures of some interval or ratio level data group themselves about a midpoint in a distribution that closely approximates the normal curve (also called the Gaussian distribution or bell curve), as illustrated in Fig. 11.3. The vertical line or Y-axis represents the frequency of occurrences of the values. The base line or X-axis shows the actual values of the scores increasing in number from left to right. In addition, if the means of many samples of the same interval or ratio data are calculated and plotted on a graph, that curve also approximates the normal curve (Mishra et al 2019a). This tendency of the means to approximate the normal curve is termed the sampling distribution of the means. The mean of the population is derived from the means of the sampling distribution (see Chapter 9).

A normal distribution is bell shaped, symmetrical about the mean and unimodal. The mean, median and mode are equal. Most of the values are clustered around the mean with smaller frequencies moving away from the mean or centre on either side. A characteristic of the normal curve is that a fixed percentage of the scores falls within a given distance of the mean (Mishra et al 2019a). As shown in Fig. 11.3, about 68% of the scores or means will fall within one standard deviation (SD) either side of the mean (±34%), 95.2% fall within two SDs of the mean (±47.6%) and 99.7% fall within three SDs of the mean (±49.85%). This is known as the empirical rule, put simply as the 68–95–99.7 rule. The mean and the standard deviation are known as the parameters (characteristics of a population) of a normal distribution. The mean provides the central point of the distribution and the standard deviation describes the spread.

TUTORIAL TRIGGER 11.1

You are undertaking a study that examines the length of hospital stay, in hours, among people who have been admitted to a maternity ward unit following a normal spontaneous vaginal delivery of their first child. You note the average length of stay is 23 hours (SD = 9.5 hours).

So, if a person has stayed for 33 hours, they are at the top of 34% of your study population, above the mean, and thus at the top of 84% of the study population (50 + 34 = 84) in terms of length of stay. If you have a person who stays 13 hours, what conclusions can be made?

Skewness

Skewness refers to the asymmetry of a distribution of interval or ratio scores. Not all samples of data approximate the normal curve. It is more common for samples to be non-symmetrical and have the peak of the curve off-centre. In these cases, where one tail is longer than the other, the distribution is described in terms of skew, with the skew relating to the direction (positive or negative) of the tail. In a positive skew, the bulk of the data are at the low end of the range and there is a longer tail pointing to the right or the positive end of the graph. Individual income has a positive skew, with most individuals in the low-to-medium range and very few in the upper range. The mean in a positive skew is to the right of the median. In a negative skew the bulk of the data are in the high range and there is a longer tail pointing to the left, or the negative end, of the graph, with the mean less than the median (Amrhein et al 2019). Fig. 11.4 illustrates positive and negative skews. In

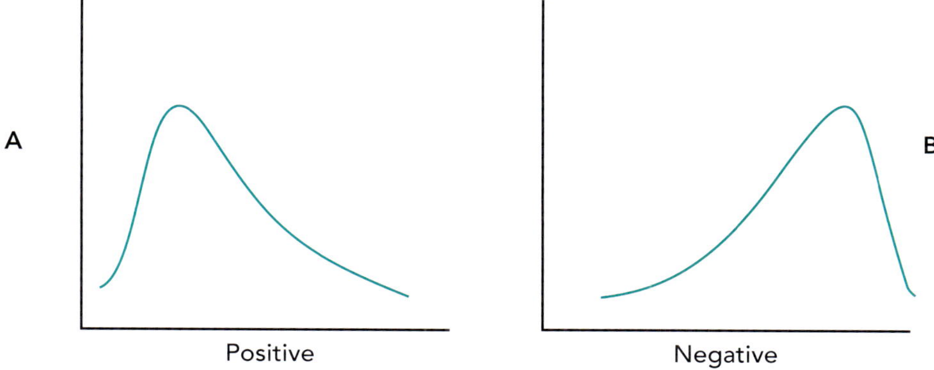

Fig. 11.4 Skewed distributions—**A**, positive skew; **B**, negative skew

each diagram the peak is off-centre and one tail is longer. Age at death in Australia has a negative skew because most deaths occur at older ages.

There are a number of ways in which skew can be detected. The simplest involves visual inspection of a frequency distribution of the data (as in Fig. 11.4). In practice, obtaining a completely normal distribution is rare and the researcher must determine whether the data can be considered approximately normal or whether the skew is of concern. One method for determining whether the skew is of concern that can be obtained in most statistical packages is the Kolmogorov–Smirnov test. With this test, however, even minor departures from normality can be detected as statistically significant in large sample sizes. Another method involves comparing the size of the skew statistic relative to its associated standard error (Dugard 2022). The skew statistic and its standard error can be generated in most statistical software packages. When the data are skewed, the mean and standard deviation do not describe the data accurately. Data transformation methods, such as using the logarithms of the data, can be employed to help enable data to achieve a near-normal distribution (Amrhein et al 2019). Logarithmic transformation must be done on a case-by-case basis and is not always successful. There is also a suite of statistics called non-parametric methods that are appropriate to use when data are skewed (described in more detail later in the chapter).

Kurtosis

Kurtosis is related to the peakness or flatness of a distribution. The peakness or flatness of a distribution is related to the spread of the data. The further the data are spread out on a scale, the flatter the peak. A distribution that peaks sharply is called leptokurtic, whereas a broad, flat distribution is called platykurtic (Amrhein et al 2019). Fig. 11.5 illustrates kurtosis. A normal distribution is described as mesokurtic (see Fig. 11.3).

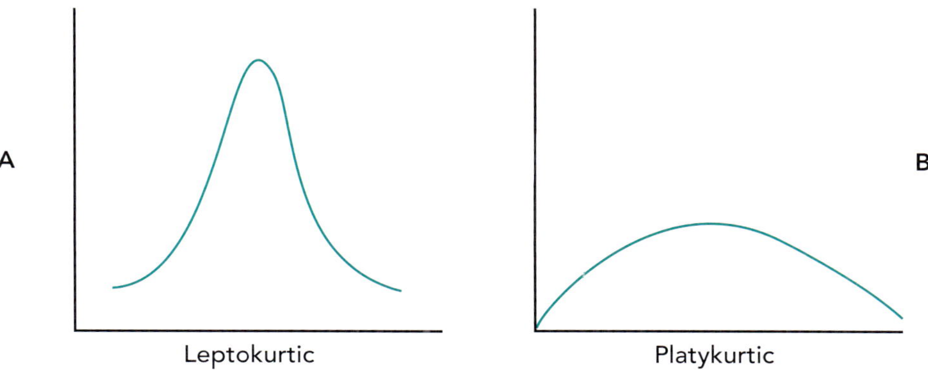

Fig. 11.5 Kurtosis—**A**, leptokurtosis; **B**, platykurtosis

TUTORIAL TRIGGER 11.2

You have collected data on the length of hospital stay in days for 18 mothers to be admitted to a maternity ward unit following the birth of their child. Calculate the mode, median and mean. What conclusions can be made from the distribution of scores?

Days	Frequency of Scores
2	2
3	5
4	5
5	3
6	2
7	1

INFERENTIAL STATISTICS

Descriptive statistics refer to various methods of summarising numerical data; however, at times the researcher seeks additional information. Inferential statistics seek to enable inferences (conclusions) to be drawn from those data. Statistical inference is based on probability theory and permits the generalisation from a specific sample, or samples, to the entire population. Statistical inference is generally used for two purposes, which include estimating the probability that statistics found in a random sample accurately reflect the population parameter (usually the median or mean) and testing hypotheses about a population. In the first instance, a parameter is a characteristic of a population, whereas a statistic is a characteristic of a sample. A researcher is rarely able to study an entire population, so inferential statistics allow statements about the larger population to be made from studying a random sample drawn from that population. Statistics are used to estimate population parameters (Mishra et al 2019c).

Statistical inference is inductive and indirect. General conclusions (inductive) are drawn about populations based on specific samples tested in an experiment. It is indirect because it begins by assuming a **null hypothesis** (H_0). The null hypothesis is that any differences are due to sampling variability (also sometimes in the literature referred to as 'chance'). The null hypothesis is used because statistical tests are designed to reject, rather than fail to reject, hypotheses. The null hypothesis states that there is no actual relationship or difference between the variables and that any observed relationship or difference is merely a function of chance fluctuations in sampling. The alternative hypothesis is that there is a relationship or difference (Mishra et al 2019c).

For example, if a research study is measuring nursing students' confidence in taking blood pressure readings before and then after instruction and practice, the null hypothesis would state that there will be no difference in confidence between the two time-points. The alternative hypothesis (also referred to as the research or scientific hypothesis) is the researcher's actual expectation about the outcome of a study, and what they are hoping to find when conducting the study and assessing the outcome through hypothesis testing. In the above example, the alternative hypothesis is that there will be an improvement in confidence scores following blood pressure instruction and practice (Mishra et al 2019c).

Hypothesis Testing

The most common use of inferential statistics in experimental studies is hypothesis testing. Hypothesis testing allows researchers to make objective decisions about the outcome of their interventional study, and answers the question, 'Is the difference between the two groups likely to be due to sampling variability or to the intervention?' Statistical hypothesis testing is a process of rejection or non-rejection of the null hypothesis, not proof. The decision to reject or not to reject a null hypothesis depends on the evidence presented, not on the actual 'truth' of the null hypothesis. Hypothesis testing is utilised routinely in intervention studies. The intervention may be an education program, a psychological treatment or a drug trial. At its most basic, a measurement is taken before the intervention and then after the intervention to see whether there is a change that is statistically significant (and, in terms of clinical interventions, if it is clinically significant) (Mishra et al 2019c).

Using the example of nursing students' confidence in taking blood pressure before and then after instruction and practice, the researchers may state the null hypothesis as 'There is no difference in nursing students' confidence in taking blood pressure before and after instruction and practice'. They will use a particular survey tool to measure confidence before any instruction and practice, deliver the appropriate teaching, allow the appropriate practice and then re-administer the confidence survey. Using a statistical test, if a difference in confidence is found the researchers will reject the null hypothesis. If no difference is found, they will not reject (but accept) the null hypothesis.

Probability and the Level of Significance

The concept of probability derives from probability theory and is central to our understanding of inferential statistics. Probability is given the symbol p and is expressed as a proportion between 0 (the event will not occur) and 1 (the event will occur). The probability of an event is the event's long-run relative frequency in repeated trials under similar conditions. It is the notion of repeated trials that allows researchers to use probability to test hypotheses. The statistician does not think of the probability of obtaining a single result from a single study, but rather of the chances of obtaining the same result from an idealised study that can be carried out many times under identical conditions (Mishra et al 2019c).

The term 'statistically significant' means that the result is unlikely to have occurred because of chance fluctuations in sampling. The probability that is chosen to indicate that an outcome is statistically significant is called the 'level of significance' or 'alpha level', denoted by the Greek symbol α. The level of significance for rejecting or failing to reject the null hypothesis must be chosen prior to the commencement of the study, and not after statistical analyses have been completed. The three most commonly reported alpha levels are: the 0.05 ($\alpha = 0.05$), the 0.01 ($\alpha = 0.01$) and the 0.001 levels of significance ($\alpha = 0.001$). They act as 'cut-off' values for determination of statistical significance. In scientific reports, this will be reported as, respectively, $p < 0.05$, $p < 0.01$ and $p < 0.001$. Values equal to or greater than the required alpha levels will consequently be reported as not statistically significant (Grove & Cipher 2019, Mishra et al 2019c).

The level of significance is the probability of making a type I error (the probability of rejecting a 'true' null hypothesis). If the researcher sets the alpha level or level of significance at 0.05, the researcher is willing to accept that, if the study were repeated 100 times, the decision to reject the null hypothesis would be wrong five times out of those 100 trials. An alpha level of 0.05 means that the researcher is prepared to accept a 5% risk that the results are an error. When hypothesis-testing life-or-death matters, researchers may set the alpha level at 0.01; this means the researcher is willing to accept that, if the study were repeated 100 times, the decision to reject the null hypothesis would be wrong only one time out of those 100 trials—there is, therefore, only a 1% risk of the results being in error (Mishra et al 2019c). The decision on how strictly the alpha level should be set depends on how important it is not to make an error. If the results of a study are to be used to determine whether a great deal of money should be spent in an area of nursing care, the researcher may decide that the accuracy of the results is so important that an alpha level of 0.01 is chosen. Usually, the minimum level of significance acceptable for all scientific disciplines, including nursing and midwifery, is 0.05.

Statistical probability is based on the concept of sampling error, and inferential statistics are based on random sampling. However, even when samples are randomly selected, there is always the possibility of some errors in sampling. Therefore, the characteristics of any given sample may be different from those of the entire population. Suppose a group of clinical nurses had access to a large number of patients with venous leg ulcers and wanted to find out the average length of time the ulcers take to heal with the usual nursing care. If the nurses studied the entire population, they might obtain an average healing time of 50 days, with a standard deviation (SD) of 10 days. This means that 68% of ulcers will be healed between 40 and 60 days. Suppose that there were insufficient funds to study all the patients and instead the nurses conducted several consecutive studies on the group of patients. They would first sample a group of 25 patients, calculate the mean and SD, and then return the sample to the main group before selecting the next sample. This process would be repeated many times and the nurses might end up with different means in healing time (Grove & Cipher 2019, Mishra et al 2019c). If they then placed the means in a frequency distribution, it might appear as in Fig. 11.6. As the number of samples drawn increases, the curve will approximate the normal curve. This frequency distribution is called the sampling distribution of the means. It shows that the nurses might find that one sample's mean is 50.5 days, the next sample is 47.5 days and the next sample is 52.5 days, and so on. The tendency for statistics to fluctuate from one sample to another is called the 'sampling error'.

In practice, researchers do not routinely draw on consecutive samples from the same population for many reasons, including but not limited to time, cost, feasibility and the ethical impact of delaying treatment. Usually, they compute statistics and make inferences based on one sample. However, the knowledge of the properties of the sampling distribution—if these repeated samples are hypothetically obtained—permits the researcher to draw a conclusion based on one sample. This is possible because the sampling distribution of the means follows a normal curve, and the

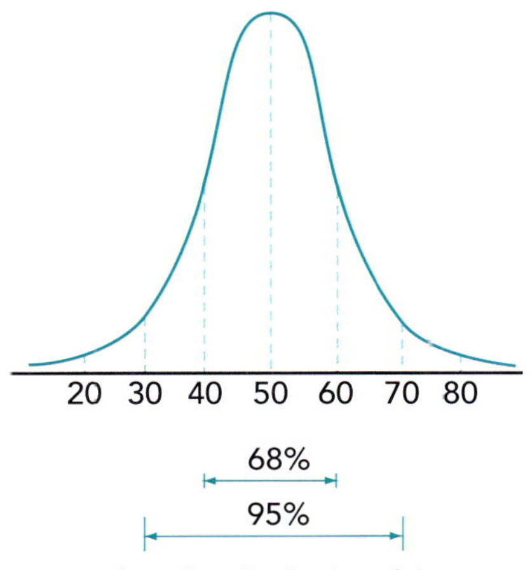

Fig. 11.6 Sampling distribution of the means

mean of the sampling distribution will be the mean of the population. The fact that the sampling distribution of the means is normal implies several important things. When scores are normally distributed, we know that 68% of the cases will fall between +1 SD and −1 SD (Mishra et al 2019c). The SD of a theoretical distribution of sample means is called the 'standard error of the mean', usually abbreviated to SE. The word 'error' is used because the various means that make up the distribution contain some error in their estimates of the population mean. The error is considered to be standard because it implies the magnitude of the average error, just as a standard deviation implies the average variation from one mean.

Although researchers rarely construct sampling distributions, the standard error can be estimated because it bears a systematic relationship to the sample SD and the size of the sample using the formula $SE = SD/\sqrt{n}$. **This tells us that increasing the size of the sample will increase the accuracy of our estimates of population parameters (smaller values for the SE indicate less error).** The other reason that the sampling distribution is so important is that there are sampling distributions for all statistics (Mishra et al 2019c). Researchers consult these distributions when making determinations about rejecting the null hypothesis.

95% Confidence Interval

As mentioned previously, researchers are usually limited by time, cost and other feasibility constraints to obtaining data from only one sample or a limited number of samples. The statistics obtained relate only to the sample(s) under study—these estimates do not tell us what the actual values might be in the wider population from which the sample was drawn. Researchers usually intend that their results should be generalised to the target population. To implement an intervention beyond the study setting, the researcher needs some level of confidence that the improvements seen in a particular group (the sample) due to a particular intervention are also likely to occur in the target population from which the sample came (Grove & Cipher 2019).

Confidence intervals (CIs) are one way to help a researcher assess what the values might be in the target population. They provide the plausible range of values bracketed by lower and upper limits that encompass the unknown population or 'true' value estimated by the sample value. These values of interest are commonly the means, differences between means, odds ratios, risk ratios or hazard ratios (Grove & Cipher 2019).

For example, the 95% confidence interval (95% CI) of a mean indicates that, if we took 100 similar samples and calculated their means, 95 of the CIs for those samples would contain the 'true' population mean and 5% would not.

The formula is:

$$95\%\ CI = \bar{X} \pm 1.96\,(SD/\sqrt{n})$$

Consider the example of the mean postnatal depression score and associated SD at 6 months after the birth of the baby for 72 women who received a depression intervention. The mean depression score was 6.12 ± 2.54 out of a possible maximum score of 30, with scores above 9 being of concern and scores of 12 or more indicating possible clinical depression. Using the above formula, the 95% CI for the mean intervention 6-month depression score is 5.53–6.70. This indicates that there is a 95% probability that, in the target population, the 6-month mean postnatal depression score of women who received the intervention would score between 5.53 and 6.70 out of a possible score of 30. Similar calculations were undertaken for a control group of women who did not receive the intervention. Table 11.6 shows how these results would be presented in the literature.

Note that the 95% CI for the intervention group (5.53–6.70) does not include the score that indicates scores of concern (9) while the 95% CI for the control group of women (8.73–12.49) does include this score as well as the score indicating potential clinical depression (12). This is important information for wider implementation of the intervention, as it implies that the intervention is successful in reducing postnatal depression.

As indicated above, CIs also apply to other statistics, and give an indication of the precision of the statistic under study. A wide CI indicates uncertainty, whereas a narrower CI indicates the statistic has been measured with more certainty or precision. CIs can also be associated with sample size. Smaller sample sizes tend to have wider CIs. It is preferable that research findings should present CIs in relation to the relevant statistic, in addition to *p*-values (American Psychological Association 2019, Grove & Cipher 2019).

Odds Ratio

Another way of presenting probabilities is the 'odds ratio' (OR) statistic. The OR is a summary statistic that estimates the odds of an event occurring in one group compared

TABLE 11.6 Differences in Postnatal Depression Scores Between Control and Intervention Groups

Group	*n*	Mean (SD)	95% CI	*p*-Value
Intervention	72	6.12 (2.54)	5.53–6.70	<0.001
Control	63	10.61 (7.63)	8.73–12.49	

with another. The odds ratio is a measure of strength of association (Grove & Cipher 2019). As an example, a study of a trial medication found that, of 982 patients who took the medication, 881 survived and 101 died, whereas of the 989 patients who did not take the medication 662 survived and 327 died. The odds of surviving if the medication was taken is 881/101 = 8.72, and if the medication was not taken it is 662/327 = 2.04. The OR is 8.72/2.04 = 4.27. The odds of surviving are therefore 4.27 times higher if the medication was taken than if it was not taken. ORs of 1 indicate that either event is likely, that there is no difference between the two groups. ORs greater than 1 indicate that the event is more likely to happen, whereas ORs less than 1 indicate that the event is less likely to happen. ORs can be obtained using chi-square analyses (for 2 × 2 tables), or logistic regression (where the outcome is dichotomous) and are also used as a way of presenting the results of a meta-analysis. A related concept, the hazard ratio (HR), is found in Cox regression, a type of survival analysis.

RESEARCH IN BRIEF 11.1

Margadant et al (2020) explored the relationship between nursing workload and mortality using the Nursing Activities Score. They found that a Nursing Activities Score per nurse ratio (NNR) greater than 61 at day 1 and mean for in-hospital mortality were associated with a higher mortality, with odds ratios of 1.26 (95% CI 1.12–1.50) and 1.43 (95% CI 1.20–1.70) respectively. The OR of 1.26 (which can also be interpreted as a 26% increase in risk) related to the NNR score of >61 at day 1 and the 95% CI around the OR indicates that the OR might be as low as 1.12 (only a 12% increase in risk) to 1.50 (a 50% increase in risk).

Note that, in this example, if the OR were still 1.26 (for day 1 values) but the 95% CI was 0.98–1.50, the interpretation would be that there was no relationship between an NNR score of >61 at day 1 and increased in-hospital mortality, as the CI passes through/includes 1, and ORs of 1 indicate that the outcome under study is equally likely in both groups. **If the 95% CI of the OR does not include 1, then the difference between the two groups is statistically significant (p <0.05).**

Errors in Statistical Inference: Type I and Type II Errors

The decision to reject or not reject the null hypothesis depends on the evidence presented, not whether the null hypothesis is 'true'. Because data on the entire population are not available, the researcher cannot categorically assert that the null hypothesis is or is not true, as he/she has only a sample from that population available. It is possible that statistical decision making may result in incorrect decisions (Grove & Cipher 2019).

There are two types of error in statistical inference: type I error and type II error. A *type I error* occurs when the null hypothesis is rejected when it is actually true for the population (the statistics say a treatment is effective when it is not). A type I error can be thought of as a false positive. A *type II error* is the failure to reject a null hypothesis that is actually false for the population (the statistics say the treatment is not effective when it is). A type II error is therefore a false negative. When conducting research on samples, it is impossible to eliminate these errors, but researchers will try and minimise them by conducting an appropriate power analysis (see below) (Grove & Cipher 2019).

Fig. 11.7 shows the relationship between the two types of error. Type I errors are usually considered more serious because if the researcher says that there are differences where there are none then the potential exists for patient care to be adversely affected. Type II errors (false negatives) occur because of a too-stringent level of α (e.g. 0.01 rather than 0.05), a small sample size or a small difference in measured effect.

Power Analysis

Researchers usually conduct a study in the expectation that they will find the relationship or effect that they are looking for (providing it really does exist). Statistical **power analysis** refers to procedures and formulas that help to identify the minimum number of subjects required to detect the relationship or effect at the appropriate level of statistical significance (Grove & Cipher 2019).

For example, consider that a researcher wants to assess the difference in mean scores of some measure between two groups (e.g. postnatal depression scores between women who did and those who did not receive an intervention). The null hypothesis is that there is no difference in postnatal depression scores between the two groups of women. The researcher will draw a sample of women from a wider population, randomly assign them to groups, administer the appropriate questionnaire, deliver the intervention to the intervention group only, then re-administer the questionnaire to both groups at the appropriate time, and then test whether there is a difference in mean scores between the two groups using a test such as the independent groups t-test (Grove & Cipher 2019). The power of the test is the probability that the test will find a statistically significant difference (p <0.05) in mean scores, should such a difference exist. For the test to have sufficient power, an adequate sample size is crucial (see 'An unexpected

Conclusion of test of significance	Reality	
	Null hypothesis is true	Null hypothesis is not true
Not statistically significant	Correct conclusion	Type II error
Statistically significant	Type I error	Correct conclusion

Fig. 11.7 Outcome of statistical decision making

hurdle'). Prior to collecting data, the researcher will need to conduct a power analysis to determine the appropriate sample size.

AN UNEXPECTED HURDLE

The aim of the study was to evaluate the effect of a multicomponent behavioural intervention for improving weight loss outcomes in obese patients with type 2 diabetes and depression. Patients were randomised to receive either the intervention or a usual care control condition. The multicomponent behavioural intervention involved 17 structured lifestyle sessions based on the Diabetes Prevention Program, targeting weight loss and depressive symptoms as well as diet and physical activity. Weight, glycaemic control and depression were assessed at baseline for participants in both the intervention and the control arms, with follow-up assessments being conducted at 6 and 12 months.

A power analysis was conducted and a medium (0.50) effect size was nominated as clinically relevant. With this effect size, alpha level of 0.05 and power of 0.80, a sample size of 64 in each group was required, with an additional 20% to allow for loss to follow-up.

The intervention was administered by two trained therapists within a clinical setting. Within the first 6 months of operation of the study, one of the trained therapists, who was in her third trimester, gave birth prematurely and was unable to continue running her remaining sessions. These issues resulted in only 39 patients recruited to the control group and 43 to the intervention. This meant the study was underpowered. It was not possible to have a third therapist finish the remaining sessions.

Think of possible ways in which the researchers might still be able to assess the effectiveness of the intervention for weight loss and depression among obese individuals with type 2 diabetes.

Power analysis and a related concept, sample size estimation, are important in experimental designs because the decision to reject or not reject the null hypothesis is dependent upon their correct computation. Broadly defined, *power* is the probability that a study will reject a false null hypothesis. Specifically, power is $1-\beta$ (the type II error rate) and ranges from 0 to 1; the minimal acceptable level for power to detect an effect is usually 0.80 (or 80%). This can be interpreted to mean that, if the experiment were repeated 100 times, the same result would be obtained 80% of the time. The significance level is usually $\alpha = 0.05$ (the type I error rate) (Grove & Cipher 2019). An adequate level of power strengthens the meaning of a study's findings. For further discussion on low power (too few subjects, too little data) and high power (too much data) and related software programs see the website: https://www.abs.gov.au/websitedbs/D3310114.nsf/home/Sample+Size+Calculator.

The required sample size depends on the following parameters, which must be relevant for the research being undertaken (Cohen 1988, Rudy 1991):

- α level (usually set at 0.05)
- power (usually set at 0.80)
- effect size (ES).

The alpha level, the power, the effect size and the associated sample size are all part of the 'evidence' required to reject or fail to reject the null hypothesis.

Effect Size

Effect size equates to the magnitude of the effect of an intervention or treatment. For example, in the study looking at postnatal depression, the mean depression scores and associated SDs were 6.12 ± 2.54 for the intervention group and 10.61 ± 7.63 for the control group. How 'big' a difference in mean scores is this? A significant *p*-value tells the researchers that there is an effect of the intervention but does not tell them whether or not that effect is clinically meaningful. Whereas statistical significance is determined by the *p*-value returned from a statistical test, clinical significance is determined by the effect size. Clinical significance relates to the practical importance of a treatment effect and can reflect the impact of change, in terms of it making a real difference to lives, how long the effects last, acceptability of a patient or consumer, cost effectiveness, or how easy something will be to implement (Bloom et al 2023).

Cohen (1988), in his seminal work, established three levels of standardised effect sizes: small, medium and large. A small effect size can be detected only statistically, a medium effect size is one where the difference or effect under study can be detected by a trained observer, and a large effect size is one that can be detected by an untrained observer. It is up to the clinicians involved in the study to determine what magnitude of effect size is clinically important. Unfortunately, many nursing and midwifery papers do not report effect sizes or the power of studies, making it difficult for researchers attempting to replicate studies to establish appropriate sample sizes. It also makes it difficult to interpret the effect of nursing interventions (Amrhein et al 2019, Grove & Cipher 2019). Effect sizes have been calculated for a variety of parametric tests (see Table 11.7).

Cohen's *d* is a measure of effect size and is derived from the results of a *t*-test. It is the difference in means between two groups divided by their combined (pooled) standard deviation. This indicates how many standard deviations of difference there are between the means of the intervention (treatment) and comparison conditions. A *d* value of 0.20 is considered small, 0.50 is medium and 0.80 is large. The effect size (Cohen's *d*) between the postnatal depression intervention group mean of 6.12 ± 2.54 and the control group mean of 10.61 ± 7.63 is -0.79.

This implies that a trained observer would detect a difference in depression behaviours between the two groups of women, and it might even be obvious to an untrained observer (Lovakov et al 2021). The negative effect size is due to the intervention group mean being smaller than the control group mean and does not affect interpretation. This effect size was determined using an online effect size calculator available at https://lbecker.uccs.edu/. There are many other effect size calculators available online.

As with the alpha level, researchers must propose the clinically significant effect size *before* conducting the research and will usually use the effect size found in previous relevant research or from pilot studies. If there is no previous research on which to draw, clinicians must make an informed decision based on their expertise as to a clinically relevant effect size in the area under study. Proposing an appropriate effect size is crucial when planning a study, as sample size depends on the proposed effect size (among other parameters—see above). Small effect sizes require large sample sizes as they are difficult to detect, whereas large effect sizes require smaller sample sizes as they are easier to detect (Cohen 1988, Lovakov et al 2021).

As well as Cohen's *d*, effect size can be expressed in terms of correlation units (Pearson's *r*), *f* values (Cohen's *f* in analysis of variance (ANOVA)) and linear regression coefficients, as well as ORs and their associated 95% CIs. It should be noted, however, that only Cohen's *d* and *f* and Pearson's *r* have standardised reference values (see Table 11.7). In addition to the reporting of CIs and *p*-values, effect sizes should also be reported (American Psychological Association 2019).

TABLE 11.7 Parametric Tests and Effect Size

Sample of Parametric Tests	EFFECT SIZE VALUES		
	Small	Medium	Large
t-test	0.20	0.50	0.80
ANOVA	0.10	0.25	0.40
Correlation	0.10	0.30	0.50

(Adapted from Cohen 1988 pp. 40, 79, 85–87.)

RESEARCH IN BRIEF 11.2

Deek et al (2017) evaluated the effect of involving family caregivers in the self-care of patients with heart failure on the risk of hospital re-admission through a randomised controlled trial. Based on re-admission rates published in previous studies, the researchers had calculated that 'to demonstrate a reduction from 30% to 15%', 130 patients in each group were needed 'given a 2-tailed significance level of 0.05, a power of 80% and an attrition rate of 10%' (p. 104). The researchers therefore had determined that a sample size involving 130 patients per control and intervention arm was required to show a clinically significant reduction in hospital re-admissions by 15%.

In this study, it was found that rate of re-admission at 30 days for the intervention group (9%) was approximately 52% lower than the rate of re-admission at 30 days for the control group (19%). This difference was statistically significant ($p = 0.02$) with an OR of 0.40 (95%, CI 0.02–0.10). In other words, the 'intervention' reduced the odds of re-admission at 30 days by 60% ($[1 - 0.4] \times 100$).

Tests of Statistical Significance

Tests of significance may be either parametric or nonparametric. Parametric tests are used to analyse interval or ratio scale data that are normally distributed, and non-parametric (so-called 'distribution free') tests are used for analysing nominal data, ordinal scale data or skewed interval/ratio data. In both types of tests, researchers aim to discover the probability of their findings assuming the null hypothesis to be 'true' for the population. There are many different statistical tests of significance that researchers use to test hypotheses. The procedure and the rationale for their use are similar from test to test (Grove & Cipher 2019, Mishra et al 2019b). Once the researcher has conducted a power analysis and collected the data, the data are used to compute the appropriate test statistic. These are available in statistical software packages such as SPSS, SAS, Stata and R. Based on the statistical results, the researcher either rejects or fails to reject the null hypothesis and then reports the statistical result and its probability, the relevant effect size and any relevant confidence intervals.

When conducting a statistical test, the outcome variable (the effect the researcher is measuring) is also called the dependent variable (DV) (see Chapter 8). Depending on that outcome, the DV can be: interval/ratio (e.g. systolic blood pressure, tumour size, time in weeks to healing of leg ulcer), ordinal (e.g. quality of life, levels of satisfaction/agreement, fatigue rating) or nominal (e.g. yes/no, died/survived, rehospitalised/not rehospitalised, healed/not healed). The variables that are the 'cause' of the outcome can be any level of measurement and are known as independent variables (IVs) (Amrhein et al 2019, Mishra et al 2019b). They are also known as predictor variables. The type of test to use is determined by the specific hypothesis or research question under study and the levels of measurement used for the DV and IVs.

There is a standardised format in which statistical results are presented and this format is commonly used in refereed journals. Once you become familiar with this format, it becomes easy to interpret reported findings from any statistical test. The test that is used depends on the level of the measurement of the variables (interval/ratio, ordinal or nominal) and the type of hypothesis being studied. Commonly used statistical tests are reported in Table 11.8 and Table 11.9. Basically, these statistics test two types of hypotheses: that there is a difference between groups or that there is a relationship (association) between two or more variables.

Degrees of Freedom

Any statistical significance testing involves the concept of degrees of freedom (usually abbreviated to df), which represent the number of data points in any given set of data that are free to vary (Grove & Cipher 2019). As an example, 10 nurses need medical ward placements. When nine nurses have been placed, the 10th nurse must take the 10th place; there is no choice. So, although there are 10 nurses (n), there are only nine ($n - 1$) degrees of freedom. Degrees of freedom can be thought of as the number of useful pieces of information available for analysis. In the above example, the 10th nurse is considered to provide no useful information as her placement is already known or fixed by the preceding nine placements. Statistical significance is based on the degrees of freedom—that is, the amount of useful information, which is a function of sample size and

TABLE 11.8 Common Tests of Differences

Level of Measurement	Type of Distribution	One Group	TWO GROUPS Related	TWO GROUPS Independent	MORE THAN TWO GROUPS Related	MORE THAN TWO GROUPS Independent
Nominal	Non-parametric	Chi-square goodness of fit	McNemar	Chi-square test of independence Fisher exact	Cochran's Q	Chi-square test of independence
Ordinal	Non-parametric	Chi-square goodness of fit	Wilcoxon signed-rank test	Mann–Whitney Wilcoxon rank sum	Friedman	Kruskal–Wallis
Interval/ratio	Parametric	One sample *t*-test ANOVA (repeated measures)	Paired *t*-test	Independent *t*-test ANOVA MANOVA ANCOVA		ANOVA MANOVA ANCOVA
Interval/ratio	Non-parametric (skewed data)		Wilcoxon signed-rank test	Mann–Whitney Wilcoxon rank sum	Friedman	Kruskal–Wallis

TABLE 11.9 Tests of Association

Level of Measurement	Two Variables	More Than Two Variables
Non-Parametric		
Nominal	Cramer's *V* Lambda Phi coefficient Point-biserial	Contingency coefficient Logistic regression
Ordinal	Kendall's tau Spearman's rho	Discriminant function analysis Principal components analysis Factor analysis
Parametric		
Interval or ratio	Pearson's *r* Simple linear regression	Multiple linear regression Path analysis Canonical correlation

the number of parameters (independent variables) in the analysis. It is important to note that how degrees of freedom are calculated depends on the type of statistical test (Grove & Cipher 2019).

Parametric Tests

Parametric tests make certain assumptions about the variables being studied, particularly that variances of scores (when two or more groups are being compared) are the same among the groups—that is, normally distributed in the population. This is called *homogeneity of variance*.

The advantages of using parametric tests are that the mathematical calculations are more sophisticated and robust than non-parametric tests. They permit analysis of interactions between two or more variables, and can be more powerful in identifying significant differences, providing the outcome variable is ratio or interval and normally distributed. For data that do not have these attributes—for example, ordinal data or skewed data—parametric tests are not appropriate to use and, in these instances, non-parametric tests are more appropriate. Many of the parametric tests are robust to some departures from normality, and there are options relevant to these tests to determine whether the departures are serious enough to warrant non-parametric tests to be employed, where available, instead (Mishra et al 2019b, Siedlecki 2020).

Non-parametric Tests

Non-parametric statistical tests are best used when the data cannot be assumed to be at the interval/ratio level of measurement, or when the sample is small and the normality of the underlying distribution cannot be established or inferred. Non-parametric tests are based on fewer assumptions than parametric tests but are less powerful and, therefore, less likely to identify significant differences; however, they are more appropriate when data do not meet the assumptions for parametric tests (Mishra et al 2019b, Siedlecki 2020).

The type of statistical analysis conducted (parametric or non-parametric) within a study is often stated within the paper methodology. For example, in a study by Jha et al (2016), two groups were compared (frail or not frail) for patients being assessed for heart transplantation. Within the statistical analysis section of the paper, it states that: 'Associations between the frailty category and age, sex, depression, cognitive impairment, markers of heart failure severity, haematological and biochemical parameters were made using independent *t*-tests or Mann–Whitney U test for continuous [interval/ratio] variables and chi-square (χ^2) test for categorical [nominal/ordinal] variables' (p. 431). You should be able to trace why each statistical test was chosen using Table 11.8.

TUTORIAL TRIGGER 11.3

A study by Lynch et al (2020) examined the factors that are associated with similarity index of undergraduate nursing students. Data in relation to the students and their similarity indexes were obtained from the university's administration database: Callista and the Grade centre of the subject online learning site (Blackboard learning platform).

Examine the 95% confidence intervals for the cumulative access (HITS) to the learning site over the semester. Based on these are there statistically significant differences between low, mid and high range users of the site and their relationship with similarity index?

Tests of Difference

Commonly used parametric tests of difference include *t*-tests and various ANOVA techniques. There are two types of *t*-test. The independent groups *t*-test tests for differences in mean outcome between two mutually exclusive groups (e.g. males or females, frail or not frail, surgery or non-surgery patients, etc.) at one time-point only. A paired *t*-test tests for differences in the one group at two separate time-points (e.g. a pre–post study on the same patients before and after surgery) (Grove & Cipher 2019). Non-parametric equivalents to the independent groups and paired *t*-tests are shown in Table 11.8.

ANOVA can also be used to explore differences between three or more groups at one time-point (cross-sectional), between three or more groups at two or more time-points or between two groups at three or more time-points (repeated measures). Analysis of covariance (ANCOVA) also measures differences among group means and uses a statistical technique to equate the groups on an important variable. Another expansion of the notion of analysis of variance is multiple analysis of variance (MANOVA), which is used to determine differences in group means when there is more than one dependent variable and those dependent variables are correlated with each other (Mishra et al 2019b).

When data are at the nominal level and the researcher wants to determine whether groups are proportionally different, the chi-square (χ^2) statistic is used. Chi-square is a non-parametric statistic that is used to determine whether the frequency in each category under study is different from what would be expected if there were no association between the categories (the null hypothesis). Chi-square can be used for 2 × 2 data, such as exploring whether or not there is a difference in the proportions between gender (male or female) and tertiary education (yes or no) or larger tables, such as 2 × 3, 3 × 3, 3 × 4 and so on. As with the *t*-test and ANOVA, if the calculated chi-square value is high enough and the *p*-value low enough (<0.05), the researcher would conclude that the frequencies found would not be expected if the null hypothesis were true (no association) and it would be rejected. This test cannot be used to compare frequencies when the sample size is small. In this instance, the Fisher's exact test is used, but only for 2 × 2 tables. The chi-square test of independence is used when the categories are mutually exclusive. The McNemar test is used if the categories are dependent, such as in a pre–post (before–after) design (Mishra et al 2019b).

Tests of Relationships

Correlations measure to what extent two variables are mathematically related or connected to each other. Correlations are used most commonly with ordinal or higher-level data. Correlation coefficients can range in value from −1.0 to +1.0, including zero. A zero coefficient means that there is no relationship between the variables. A positive correlation coefficient means that as one variable increases so does the other, and a negative correlation coefficient means that as one variable increases the other decreases (Grove & Cipher 2019). A perfect correlation implies that one variable is directly related to the other and all the data points fall along a straight, 45-degree line. Fig. 11.8 provides graphical illustrations, known as scatter plots, which show the strength and direction of the relationship between two variables.

As with other statistical tests of significance, the larger the sample, the greater is the likelihood of finding a significant correlation. There are parametric and non-parametric versions of correlation (see Table 11.9). It is important to note that correlations describe mathematical relationships (i.e. as one variable gets larger/smaller, so does the other one) and do not imply causality.

Linear regression is a popular technique for predicting a dependent variable (or outcome of interest under study) from one or more independent variables (or predictors).

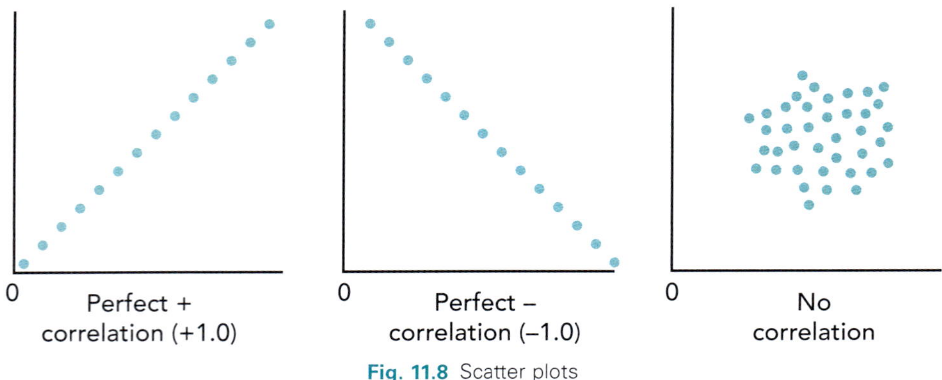

Fig. 11.8 Scatter plots

The DV must be a ratio or interval, while the IVs can be of any level of measurement. Simple linear regression is when there is only one IV. Multiple regression is when there are several different IVs. In either type, there can only be one DV (Grove & Cipher 2019). For example, a researcher working in an aged care facility is interested in identifying what variables are predictive of resident confidence in avoiding falls. Falls are of concern, and maximising confidence in avoiding falls is paramount to residents' safety and quality of life. The researcher has developed a questionnaire to measure confidence (the DV), and for the IVs has collected information on patients' age, gender, number and type of comorbidities, physical and cognitive function and length of stay in the facility. Multiple linear regression will identify which IVs are statistically significant predictors of confidence in avoiding falls, as well as how strongly predictive is each of those significant variables. Linear regression provides the unit change in the DV based on a unit change in an IV. For example, as the number of comorbidities increases, confidence in avoiding pressure injury might decrease and, as physical functioning increases, confidence might also increase.

Logistic regression is appropriate when the outcome is dichotomous (yes/no, pregnant/not pregnant, passed/failed and so on). As with linear regression, the predictors can be of any level of measurement. Logistic regression predicts the probability of an event occurring, expressed as an odds ratio.

Meta-analysis

As outlined earlier, it is not usually possible for researchers to repeatedly test the same hypothesis on different samples drawn from the same population. Meta-analysis, conducted as a secondary analysis in systematic literature reviews, is a series of statistical tests used for pooling the results of several empirical studies that assess the same hypothesis; meta-analyses aggregate data in order to have higher statistical power to assess the statistical and clinical importance of a particular effect (Grove & Cipher 2019).

Tests of Multivariate Relationships

Nursing and midwifery problems are rarely so simple that they can be explained by bivariate relationships—the relationship between two variables. For studying complex multivariate relationships—relationships among more than two variables—techniques other than those so far discussed are used. Examples of multivariate techniques include multiple regression, multiple discriminant analysis and logistic regression, principal component and exploratory factor analysis, multivariate analysis of variance and covariance, and structural equation modelling.

Structural Equation Modelling Techniques

Structural equation modelling (SEM) is an umbrella term for various methods (e.g. path analysis, confirmatory factor analysis and structure models) used to test theory expressed in the form of a systematic set of relationships between multiple observed or non-observed (latent), dependent or independent variables. SEM requires specific software such as LISREL (linear structural relations), AMOS or Stata. As many of the variables of interest to nursing are not easily defined and measured and because we are interested in causal models, SEM techniques are becoming more commonly used in nursing studies (Wang & Rhemtulla 2021). Many other statistical techniques are available to nurse and midwifery researchers, including those described in the *Electronic Statistics Textbook*, available at https://www.spotfire.com/products/data-science.

RESEARCH IN BRIEF 11.3

Terry et al (2023), using SEM, explored how a global crisis that permeated all aspects of life may have influenced the predictors of consistency of interest (passion) and perseverance of effort (persistence) to aid in the development of grit among nursing students. They found, using pathway models of grit, that within months of the global pandemic occurring, where all individuals' lives were disrupted, challenged and in some cases changed, the key predictors of consistency of interest and perseverance of effort were, on the most part, shown to fundamentally alter. Specifically, the model demonstrated that 1 standard deviation increase in the personality trait of conscientiousness was associated with a 0.33 standard deviation increase in consistency of interest, followed by openness (0.15), while hope (−0.15) and neuroticism (−0.16) had a negative impact on predicted consistency of interest. In addition, 1 standard deviation increase in the personality trait of conscientiousness was associated with a 0.39 standard deviation increase in perseverance of effort, while efficacy (0.30) also directly predicted perseverance of effort. These key predictors centred on key personality traits such as conscientiousness, openness and neuroticism were consistently present, while elements of psychological capital, particularly hope and efficacy, also influenced nursing students' capacity to persevere, while all other elements such as age, gender and income were unimportant in impacting student grit. Understanding these key drivers of grit, particularly those essential at or around the time of a crisis, guides our understanding how to better support nursing or healthcare students when times are tough, both as they study and as they enter the workforce.

SUMMARY

Descriptive statistics are statistical procedures used to organise and give meaning to data, and may be illustrated in a variety of visual ways (e.g. frequency distributions, skewed distributions and measures of variability). Inferential statistics allow researchers to estimate population parameters, test hypotheses and make objective decisions about the outcome of a study based on the rejection or non-rejection of the null hypothesis. Statistical inference permits a conclusion about a population to be made based upon a sample of that population. Statistical hypothesis testing is subject to two types of error: type I and type II. The results of tests are reported to be statistically significant or non-significant depending upon the α-level specified prior to any data collection. Tests of statistical significance may be parametric (when data meet certain assumptions) or non-parametric (used when the data cannot be assumed to be at the interval level of measurement or are skewed). These tests are used according to specific criteria. Effect size is an indicator of the clinical, as opposed to statistical, significance of an intervention or difference between two groups.

Alpha level, power and effect size are related to the required sample size, and the researcher must make an informed and appropriate decision in relation to these. Confidence intervals provide the plausible range of values for means, differences between means or odds ratios in the wider population from which the study samples have been drawn. More advanced statistical techniques, used to study complex multivariate relationships, were briefly described.

KEY POINTS

- Descriptive statistics refer to the measures used to describe raw data. Data can be presented in tables, histograms, bar charts, pie charts, polygons and scatter plots.
- The frequency distribution presents data in tabular or graphic form and allows for the calculation of observations of characteristics of the distribution of the data, including skewness, symmetry, modality and kurtosis.
- The standard deviation is the most stable and useful measure of variability for interval and ratio level data. It is derived from the concept of the normal distribution.
- Inferential statistics allow researchers to estimate population parameters, test hypotheses and make objective decisions about the outcome of a study based on sample data. Such decisions are based on the rejection or non-rejection of the null hypothesis.
- Failure to reject the null hypothesis indicates that the findings are likely to have occurred by sampling variation (chance). If the null hypothesis is rejected, the researcher finds in favour of the alternative hypothesis of a relationship being present between the variables.
- Statistical hypothesis testing is subject to two types of error: type I and type II. A type I error occurs when the researcher rejects a null hypothesis that is actually true. A type II error occurs when the researcher fails to reject a null hypothesis that is actually false. The risk of making a type I error is controlled by setting the alpha level or level of significance. Reducing the risk of a type I error by reducing the level of significance increases the risk of making a type II error. Type II errors can be minimised by an adequate sample size.
- The results of statistical tests are reported to be statistically significant or non-significant. Obtaining a probability value (p-value) of less than 0.05 or 0.01 (depending on the level of significance set by the researcher) can indicate a statistically significant result. This means the result is not likely to be due to sampling variation (chance).
- Commonly used parametric statistical tests include those that test for differences between means, such as the various t-tests and ANOVA techniques, with non-parametric equivalents being the Wilcoxon rank-sum test and Mann–Whitney U test and those that test for differences in proportions, such as the chi-square test.
- Tests that examine data for the presence of relationships (association) include Pearson's r and various regression techniques. Non-parametric equivalents are Spearman's rho and Kendall's tau. There is no non-parametric equivalent for regression.
- Any study involving inferential statistical analysis should also provide an appropriate power analysis, with the proposed effect size, alpha level and power used to determine sample size. Clues to the appropriate statistical test to use should stem from the researcher's hypotheses.
- To ascertain the precision of the reported statistics and what the plausible range of values are for those statistics in the wider population, confidence intervals should be reported where appropriate. To determine clinical as opposed to statistical significance, effect sizes should be reported where appropriate.

TIME TO REFLECT

Middleton, S., Dale, S., Wah Cheug, N., et al., 2019. Nurse-initiated acute stroke care in emergency departments: the triage, treatment, and transfer implementation cluster randomized controlled trial. Stroke 50 (6), 1346–1355. doi:10.1161/ STROKEAHA.118.020701

Aim: To evaluate the effectiveness of an intervention to improve triage, treatment and transfer for patients with acute stroke admitted to the emergency department (ED).

Design: A pragmatic, blinded, multicentre, parallel group, cluster randomised controlled trial was conducted in 26 Australian EDs with stroke units and tissue-type plasminogen activator (tPA) protocols. Eligible ED patients had acute stroke <48 hours from symptom onset and were admitted to the stroke unit via ED. The nurse-initiated intervention outcomes were assessed. The primary outcome was 90-day death or dependency (modified Rankin Scale score of ≥2); secondary outcomes were functional dependency (Barthel Index ≥95), health status (Short Form [36] Health Survey) and ED quality of care (Australasian Triage Scale; monitoring and management of tPA, fever, hyperglycaemia, swallowing, prompt transfer). Intention-to-treat analysis adjusted for preintervention outcomes and ED clustering. Patients, outcome assessors and statisticians were masked to group allocation.

Results: Twenty-six EDs (13 intervention and 13 control) recruited 2242 patients (645 preintervention and 1597 postintervention). There were no statistically significant differences at follow-up for 90-day modified Rankin Scale (intervention: $n = 400$ [53.5%]; control $n = 266$ [48.7%]; $p = 0.24$) or secondary outcomes.

Reflect on the following:

- What design was used for this study?
- Was this an appropriate design?
- At what level of measurement were the independent variables measured?
- What statistical procedures, descriptive and inferential, would be appropriate for each level of measurement?

Questions

Reflect on the information given and answer these questions:

1. What was the research design?
2. What is the difference between a single- and a double-blind RCT?
3. Is the design appropriate for this study?
4. What are the intervention and control arms in this study?
5. What was the sample size? Do you think it is sufficient for this study?
6. How would you know whether the effect of the intervention was statistically significant?

LEARNING ACTIVITIES

1. Which of the following is NOT a measure of central tendency?
   a. Mean
   b. Mode
   c. Range
   d. Median
2. Variance is a measure of variability that includes:
   a. every score in the distribution
   b. the highest scores in the distribution
   c. the lowest scores in the distribution
   d. most of the scores in the distribution.
3. A non-parametric test can operate:
   a. when measurements assume a normal curve
   b. without the assumptions about the normality of the distributions
   c. with any measurement of central tendency
   d. only when means and SDs are calculated.
4. A *p*-value of 0.05 indicates:
   a. there is a 5% chance of a type I error
   b. there is a 5% chance of a type II error
   c. the null hypothesis is likely to be true
   d. the alternative hypothesis is likely to be true.
5. If measurements were at the interval level and normally distributed, what test of difference would be used to analyse the data?
   a. Mann–Whitney U test
   b. Chi-square test
   c. *t*-test
   d. Pearson correlation.
6. Which of the following is a statistical test used to determine if there is a significant difference between the means of two groups?
   a. Chi-square test
   b. *t*-test
   c. ANOVA
   d. Regression analysis
7. If the power of a study is low, what could the researcher manipulate to improve power?
   a. increase the sample size
   b. decrease the effect size
   c. decrease the sample size
   d. alter the significance level from 0.05 to 0.01.
8. As effect size increases, sample size:
   a. stays the same
   b. increases

c. decreases
d. needs to be multiplied by 1.96.

9. What is the definition of standard deviation?
   a. A measure of the average deviation from the mean
   b. A measure of the spread of data around the median
   c. A measure of the spread of data around the mode
   d. A measure of the central tendency of the data
10. What is the definition of correlation coefficient?
   a. A measure of the average deviation from the mean
   b. A measure of the spread of data around the median
   c. A measure of the spread of data around the mode
   d. A measure of the strength of the linear relationship between two variables
11. A researcher reports a p value of <0.05 for a null hypothesis test. This means the researcher:
   a. has failed to reject the null hypothesis
   b. did not have enough power in the study
   c. has rejected the null hypothesis
   d. has reported a medium effect size.
12. What are the odds of tossing heads with a coin?
   a. 1:1
   b. 0.5
   c. 50:50
   d. a and c.

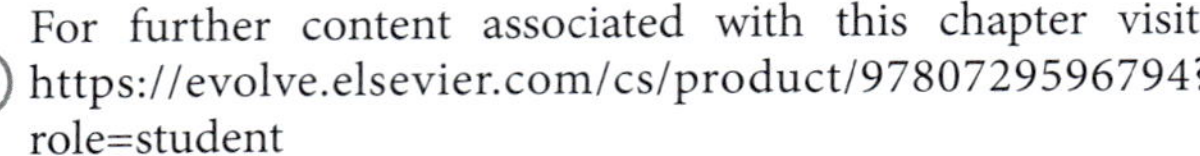
For further content associated with this chapter visit: https://evolve.elsevier.com/cs/product/9780729596794?role=student

ACKNOWLEDGEMENT

The 7th edition authors would like to thank and acknowledge Fahad Shaikh and Sunita R. Jha for their contribution to this chapter in previous editions of the text.

ADDITIONAL RESOURCES

Andrade, C., 2015. Understanding relative risk, odds ratio, and related terms: as simple as it can get. J. Clin. Psychiatry 76 (07), e857–e861.

Crichton, N., 2001. Information point: regression analysis. J. Clin. Nurs. 10 (4), 462.

Field, A., 2013. Discovering Statistics Using SPSS, fourth ed. Sage Publications, Thousand Oaks, CA.

G*Power. Free power analysis software for Windows or Macs from: https://gpower.software.informer.com/3.1/.

Gaskin, C.J., Happell, B., 2014. Power, effects, confidence, and significance: an investigation of statistical practices in nursing research. Int. J. Nurs. Stud. 51, 795–806.

Guo, P., East, L., Arthur, A., 2012. A preoperative education intervention to reduce anxiety and improve recovery among Chinese cardiac patients: a randomized controlled trial. Int. J. Nurs. Stud. 49, 129–137.

Leech, N.L., Barrett, K.C., Morgan, G.A., 2015. IBM SPSS for Intermediate Statistics: use and interpretation, fifth ed. New York, NY.

Mackridge, A., Rowe, P., 2018. A Practical Approach to Using Statistics in Health Research: from planning to reporting. John Wiley & Sons, New York.

Norton, E., Dowd, B., Maciejewski, M., 2018. Odds ratios—current best practice and use. JAMA. 320 (1), 84.

Pacquay, L., Verstraete, S., Wouters, R., et al., 2010. Implementation of a guideline for pressure ulcer prevention in home care: pre-test-post-test study. J. Clin. Nurs. 19, 1803–1811.

Ratcliffe, P., 1998. Using the 'new' statistics in nursing research. J. Adv. Nurs. 27, 132–139.

Virtual Statistics Textbook. https://onlinestatbook.com/.

REFERENCES

American Psychological Association (APA), 2019. Publication Manual of the American Psychological Association, seventh ed. APA, Washington DC.

Amrhein, V., Trafimow, D., Greenland, S., 2019. Inferential statistics as descriptive statistics: There is no replication crisis if we don't expect replication. Am. Stat. 73 (Suppl.), 262–270.

Bloom, D.A., Kaplan, D.J., Mojica, E., et al. 2023. The minimal clinically important difference: a review of clinical significance. Am. J. Sports Med. 51 (2), 520–524.

Cohen, J., 1988. Statistical Power Analysis for the Behavioral Sciences, 2nd ed. Lawrence Erlbaum Associates, Hillsdale, NJ.

Deek, H., Chang, S., Newton, P., et al., 2017. An evaluation of involving family caregivers in the self-care of heart failure patients on hospital readmission: randomised controlled trial (the FAMILY study). Int. J. Nurs. Stud. 75, 101–111.

Dugard, P., Todman, J., Staines, H., 2022. Approaching Multivariate Analysis: a practical introduction, second ed. Taylor & Francis, London.

Grove, S.K., Cipher, D.J., 2019. Statistics for Nursing Research-e-book: a workbook for evidence-based practice, third ed. Elsevier Health Sciences, Philadelphia.

Jha, S.R., Hannu, M.K., Chang, S., et al., 2016. The prevalence and prognostic significance of frailty in patients with advanced heart failure referred for heart transplantation. Transplantation 100 (2), 429–436.

Lovakov, A., Agadullina, E.R., 2021. Empirically derived guidelines for effect size interpretation in social psychology. Eur. J. Soc. Psychol. 51 (3), 485–504.

Lynch, J., Ramjan, L., Glew, P., et al., 2020. Factors associated with similarity index (SI) scores among a large cohort of undergraduate nursing students. Nurse Educ. Pract. 43, 102735.

Margadant, C., Wortel, S., Hoogendoorn, M., et al., 2020. The nursing activities score per nurse ratio is associated with in-hospital mortality, whereas the patients per nurse ratio is not. Crit. Care Med. 48 (1), 3–9.

Middleton, S., Dale, S., Wah Cheug, N., et al., 2019. Nurse-initiated acute stroke care in emergency departments: the

Triage, Treatment, and Transfer Implementation Cluster Randomized Controlled Trial. Stroke 50 (6), 1346–1355. doi:10.1161/STROKEAHA.118.020701

Mishra, P., Pandey, C.M., Singh, U., et al. 2019a. Descriptive statistics and normality tests for statistical data. Ann. Card. Anaesth. 22(1), 67–72.

Mishra, P., Singh, U., Pandey, C.M., et al. 2019b. Application of student's t-test, analysis of variance, and covariance. Ann. Card. Anaesth. 22 (4), 407–411.

Mishra, P., Pandey, C.M., Singh, U., et al. 2019c. Selection of appropriate statistical methods for data analysis. Ann. Card. Anaesth. 22 (3), 297–301.

Reynolds, C.R. Altmann, R.A., Livingston, R.A., 2021. Mastering Modern Psychological Testing: theories and methods, second ed. Springer International Publishing, New York. doi:10.1007/978-3-030-59455-8

Rudy, E.B., 1991. Unravelling the mystique of power analysis. Heart Lung 20 (5), 517–522.

Siedlecki, S.L., 2020. Understanding descriptive research designs and methods. Clin. Nurse Spec. 34 (1), 8–12. doi:10.1097/NUR.0000000000000493

Terry, D., Peck, B.. 2020. Academic and clinical performance among nursing students: what's grit go to do with it? Nurs. Educ. Today 88, 104371.

Terry, D., Peck, B., Biangone, M., 2023. Changes in grit and psychological capital at the time of major crisis: nursing students' perseverance, resources, and resilience. Int. J. Nurs. Educ. Scholarsh. 20 (1), 20220114.

Wang, Y.A., Rhemtulla, M., 2021. Power analysis for parameter estimation in structural equation modeling: a discussion and tutorial. Adv. Method. Pract. Psychol. Sci. 4 (1), 2515245920918253.

12

Mixed-Methods Research

Dean Whitehead

LEARNING OUTCOMES

After reading this chapter, you should be able to:

- understand the principles underpinning mixed-methods and multimethods research
- describe the value, benefits and dilemmas encountered when using qualitative and quantitative methods in a single study
- explain the purpose, process, value and constraints of action research
- explain the purpose, process, value and constraints of Delphi technique research
- describe the purpose, process, value and constraints of case studies and Q methodology.

KEY TERMS

action research, p. 198
case study, p. 203
Delphi technique, p. 202
mixed-methods research, p. 193
pragmatic paradigm, p. 194
Q methodology, p. 204
transformative paradigm, p. 194

INTRODUCTION

In the 1950s and 1960s, nursing and midwifery research was mostly undertaken within the quantitative paradigm. Then, during the 1970s and 1980s, a move towards research grounded in the qualitative paradigm became evident (Poth 2018). During these periods, there was general support for the separateness of quantitative and qualitative research approaches and most researchers chose one or the other approach—resulting in a noted and unhelpful 'paradigm tension'. However, soon after that, more and more researchers started to become concerned that neither approach, in isolation, could truly provide an 'overall' understanding of human beings and the complexity of their health-related needs, problems or care. This gradual realisation has brought about the development of what some refer to as the 'third paradigm': *mixed-methods* (also previously called method triangulation).

Mixed-methods research involves the integration of both quantitative and qualitative research approaches within the same study. This approach seeks to provide a deeper insight into the phenomenon of interest, by maximising the strengths of each approach and minimising their respective weaknesses. Halcomb (2018) highlights this shift, describing a notable increase in nursing- and midwifery-related mixed-methods research in recent years. This trend continues as multidisciplinary health research becomes more the norm and each discipline brings its own unique research 'worldview' to collaborative projects. The final chapter in this book reports a clinical multidisciplinary mixed-methods project which complements this chapter in illustrating the actual and potential wide-reaching impact of such approaches—as well as the challenges and complexity that all research approaches face.

In addition, current interest in *translational research*—that which strives to translate knowledge and render it operational so that it reaches the client—has strengthened interest in mixed-methods research (Brownson et al 2017). Stemming from the rising popularity of mixed-methods, journals (e.g. the *Journal of Mixed Methods Research*) and whole texts have become available to support the application of this approach and put into clearer context its place in health research, including research texts such as that by

Creswell and Plano Clark (2017), as well as texts specific to nursing and midwifery research such as that by Andrew and Halcomb (2009, 2012). Best practice for mixed-methods research in the health sciences overall is also described (see Creswell et al 2011).

WHAT IS MIXED-METHODS RESEARCH?

Tashakkori and Creswell (2007 p. 4), in their seminal work, clearly define **mixed-methods research** as 'research in which the investigator collects and analyses data, integrates the findings and draws inferences using both qualitative and quantitative approaches or methods in a single study or program of inquiry'. There are many benefits from not separating out quantitative and qualitative research but, instead, acknowledging and understanding their interrelated nature, assumptions and processes. Healthcare researchers, regardless of discipline, can and should choose from an increasingly wide and diverse range of research methods from both paradigms and within studies, to explore and understand increasingly complex clinical issues (Poth 2023, Sandelowski 2014). The available combinations (see later in this chapter) highlight the *pragmatic* approach often associated with mixed-methods research, an approach focused on practical applications of research and 'what works' (Creswell 2014, Tashakkori et al 2020). Each mixed-methods component can stand alone while also being linked to other parts and other studies. This is of great value when researchers want to understand how parts of clinical issues they are investigating relate to the whole picture—adding to the comprehensiveness of study findings (Poth 2020, 2023).

It is important to note, early on, that many healthcare researchers use the terms 'mixed-methods' and 'multiple/multi-methods' interchangeably—such as with Helliwell et al's (2018) managing polymyalgia rheumatica multimethods study in general practice. They are, however, different things. To illustrate further see Morse and Niehaus's (2009) study design list later in the chapter 'Rationale and designs for conducting mixed-methods research'.

Triangulation—the 'Emerging' Debate

A common but contested term in mixed-methods research is 'triangulation'. It generally refers to different mixed-methods design strategies (i.e. methodological, theory, investigative, data and multidisciplinary triangulation). The term, to a certain extent, is 'self-explanatory'. Mixed-method studies start, from the outset, to answer an overarching topic question that can only be answered through exploring different paradigms/worldviews (i.e. both qualitative and quantitative). To do so it 'should' compare one approach with the other throughout the study. In other words, it has to '*triangulate*' various aspects of the study to reach the overall findings. This chapter still uses the term but does so against the just-stated context Morgan (2019 p. 10) summarises well, in the *Journal of Mixed Methods Research*, the current dilemma surrounding triangulation:

> *In many ways, triangulation was a victim of its own success. From the 1970s into the 1990s, it was by far the best-known reason for doing mixed methods research (MMR). Hence, anyone doing MMR during that period might have been tempted to use triangulation as a justification, if only because there were few obvious alternatives. As a result, triangulation came to mean too many things. Yet that does not imply that the original purposes of triangulation have disappeared; instead, those purposes have been clarified and expanded. Today, we still have the goal of comparing the results of qualitative and quantitative studies on the same phenomena, but we have developed a better understanding of the alternative reasons for making such comparisons ... Building on these advances creates greater clarity about the differences between convergence, complementarity, and divergence.*

The 'takeaway' message here is that, while we will still see the term triangulation for some time to come it is advisable (especially for those conducting mixed-methods studies) to keep a close watch on the concepts of *convergence*, *complementarity* and *divergence*. It is not necessary, for now, to go into any further depth on this issue in this chapter.

Pragmatic and Transformative Paradigms in Mixed-Methods Research

It has already been highlighted in this chapter that a main benefit of mixed-methods research is its 'practical' outcomes, a better understanding of what works and a more heightened sense of 'completeness'. *Pragmatism* involves addressing positivist and post-positivist (see Chapter 2) 'rigid' worldviews and replacing them with the goal of problem solving through understanding wider experiences of various phenomena for better outcomes, with the belief that these goals can be achieved using various types of knowledge (Florczak 2014). Rorty's (1979) seminal work adds emphasis, with pragmatic approaches being '... a mixture of methods deployed on a problematic situation ... to appropriate the ideal possibilities of the current situation to aid action' (Maxcy 2003 pp. 79–80). To further illustrate the term 'action', see 'Action research' later in this chapter. For many, pragmatism is a philosophy—as well as an action. It is a means of 'uncovering truth'. Therefore, many will refer to pragmatism as a paradigm. It remains 'practical' though so, even as a paradigm, we shouldn't lose sight of its direct applicability to practice and knowledge. The key element in pragmatic research, therefore, is establishing that the research has been of direct clinical assistance and impact and answered the original overarching question while remembering that '... all knowledge is knowledge from some point of view ...' (Feilzer 2010 p. 8).

As well as its place as a **pragmatic paradigm**, mixed-methods research is also viewed as a potentially **transformative paradigm**. What is meant here is that mixed-method approaches, because they explore more than one worldview, have a higher likelihood of providing mechanisms and evidence for addressing the complexities of research in complex clinical settings and thus providing a basis for social change in those settings. As Mertens (2007 p. 212) articulately states:

> *The intersection of mixed methods and social justice has implications for the role of the researcher and choices of specific paradigmatic perspectives. The transformative paradigm with its associated philosophical assumptions provides a framework for addressing inequality and injustice in society using culturally competent, mixed methods strategies. The recognition that realities are constructed and shaped by social, political, cultural, economic, and racial/ethnic values indicates that power and privilege are important determinants of which reality will be privileged in a research context. Methodological inferences based on the underlying assumptions of the transformative paradigm reveal the potential strength of combining qualitative and quantitative methods.*

Poradzisz and Florczak (2018), in their article, ask the question 'Transformative research: a new frontier for nursing [and midwifery]?' Their definition of transformational research identifies mixed methods as the preferred process for those who conduct such studies. They highlight why transformational research is a useful and natural paradigm approach for many specific 'social justice' concerns of the healthcare professions. The reader can look to 'Action research' later in this chapter to add context. Participatory action research (PAR), a branch of action research, comes under the umbrella of critical social theory (emancipatory) research designed to address organisational and community 'inequality'.

Rationale and Designs for Conducting Mixed-Methods Research

The assumption underpinning mixed-methods approaches is that research which collects wider types of data provides a more comprehensive understanding of the research problem than would emerge from any single type of data considered in isolation (Creswell 2014, Poth 2023, Tashakkori et al 2020). The main rationales for conducting a mixed-methods study potentially are the complexity of the phenomena being studied, overlapping and different aspects of the phenomena in question, required triangulation of data (see later), completeness of multiple and complementary findings, off-setting weaknesses and providing stronger inferences, adding scope and depth to single studies, potential hypotheses development and testing, and possible instrument development and testing.

In research, there is always the consideration that there is more than one way to approach a research issue, with the research question, statement or hypothesis guiding the approach (see Chapter 4), and that we are not confined nor limited to having to use just a single methodology and method. This highlights the nature and place of mixed-methods research which 'integrates'. Two or more methods are integrated if: they both relate to the same topic area, they are both planned prior to the research program commencing, one informs the other and, as an outcome, they all expand the related field of inquiry (Poth 2023, Tashakkori et al 2020).

Careful and due attention is required in mixed-methods research to avoid mixed-methods errors. For instance, a common error in mixed-methods research is where the researcher has essentially conducted two separate studies—one quantitative and one qualitative—and then attempts to 'bolt them together' to form a mixed-methods study. It is usually quite notable where this occurs and should be part of the critical appraisal when reviewing mixed-methods studies. Pluye et al (2009) have, helpfully, developed a scoring system (Mixed Studies Reviews) for assessing mixed-methods studies. Such overall guides assist mixed-methods approach and design considerations—but they do vary and continue to adapt and update. For instance, there is Creswell's four characteristics of mixed methods (which can be part of a review/appraisal checklist) that include:

1. level of interaction between phases
2. sequence of data collection—simultaneous/sequential/concurrent
3. priority of data sets
4. timing of integration.

To help avoid mixed-methods errors, it is necessary to have a good understanding of different types and combinations of methods before commencing or reviewing/appraising this type of research. There are several different combinations in mixed-methods research with each influencing the type of mixed-methods design and eventual outcomes. This section of this chapter draws on Schoonenboom and Johnson's (2017) interpretation of the main 'current' designs. They commence with Creswell and Plano Clark's (2017) six 'major' mixed-methods designs:

- *Convergent parallel design*—the quantitative and qualitative phases are performed independently—and their results are brought together in the overall interpretation.
- *Explanatory sequential design*—a first phase of quantitative data collection and analysis is followed by the collection of qualitative data, which are used to explain the initial quantitative results.
- *Exploratory sequential design*—a first phase of qualitative data collection and analysis is followed by the collection of quantitative data to test or generalise the initial qualitative results.
- *Embedded design*—further to the 'classic' adoption of a single qualitative or quantitative phase, a further phase (qualitative or quantitative) is adopted.
- *Transformative design*—a transformative critical social theory (see Chapter 2) theoretical framework (emancipatory) (e.g. feminism) underpins and shapes the interaction, priority, timing and mixing of the qualitative and quantitative phases.
- *Multiphase design*—a complex design where more than two phases, or both sequential and concurrent processes, are combined over a period within a program of study addressing an overall program objective (overarching question).

Schoonenboom and Johnson (2017) identify their 'shorthand' adaptation of Morse and Niehaus's (2009) eight main design combinations—that is, qualitative is abbreviated to QUAL (qual) and quantitative to QUAN (quan). Upper-case terms denote the dominant phase and lower-case the less dominant phase. Morse and Niehaus (2009) refer to upper and lower-case as 'core' and 'supplemental':

- QUAL + quan—an inductive-simultaneous design where the core component is qualitative and the supplemental component is quantitative;
- QUAL → quan—an inductive-sequential design where the core component is qualitative and the supplemental component is quantitative;
- QUAN + qual—a deductive-simultaneous design where the core component is quantitative and the supplemental component is qualitative;
- QUAN → qual—a deductive-sequential design where the core component is quantitative and the supplemental component is qualitative;
- QUAL + qual—an inductive-simultaneous design where both components are qualitative; this is a multimethod design rather than a mixed-methods design;
- QUAL → qual—an inductive-sequential design where both components are qualitative; multimethod design;
- QUAN + quan—a deductive-simultaneous design where both components are quantitative; a multimethod design;
- QUAN → quan—a deductive-sequential design where both components are quantitative; a multimethod design.

We are reminded that the list is just for two-phase study designs. For, say, embedded designs the 'formulas' could be a combination of (QUAL + QUAN) → QUAN → QUAL, with any phase being core or supplemental and in any order. The choice cannot be 'random' though. The overall order and order of the core or supplemental phases will affect overall outcomes.

Confusion can arise when designing and interpreting mixed-methods research, so attempts need to be made to clarify the triangulation method and design used (Sandelowski 2014). It can appear that two or three discrete or independent studies have been conducted rather than a planned mixed-methods strategy. This is not to be confused with the earlier-mentioned mixed-methods error of 'bolting together' studies. One must remember that a research problem or question is determined by the aim of the study with a consequent design that follows in a 'seamless' manner. For instance, Lieschke et al (2022) wanted to explore the existing research capacity amongst nurses and midwives in a large Local Health District in New South Wales, Australia to inform the development of a nuanced capacity building program directed towards building a sustainable embedded research culture. A sequential mixed-methods study design was adopted. Phase one, the exploratory phase, involved an online survey of all nurses and midwives ($n = 8156$) working in metropolitan, rural and remote health services across the district. The survey measured research activity, skills, intention, value and relevance, organisational support, capability and culture, and research translation. Phase two, the explanatory phase, involved six focus groups with senior nursing and midwifery clinicians, educators and unit managers, with discussion centred on the results of Phase one.

Table 12.1 offers useful examples of the common types and combinations of mixed methods, while Table 12.2 offers an example of a mixed-methods approach used in a single study.

As clinical issues and environments become increasingly complex, researchers often attempt to push and extend the range and diversity of mixed-methods research. As an example, Searby et al (2023) aimed to examine the current alcohol and other drug (AOD) nurse practitioner workforce, and to explore barriers and facilitators to AOD nurse practitioner uptake in Australia. This is because the AOD nurse practitioner is a highly specialised provider of holistic care to people who use alcohol and other drugs,

TABLE 12.1 Simultaneous and Sequential Combinations of Quantitative and Qualitative Mixed-Methods Approaches

Combination	Rationale	Example
Simultaneous		
Qualitative + quantitative	There is a qualitative foundation and quantitative methods are used to provide additional complementary information.	The research is focused on the experiences of feeling depressed after miscarriage. Phenomenological methods could be used to address the question, and use of a depression scale would provide complementary information.
Quantitative + qualitative	There is a quantitative foundation and qualitative methods are used to provide additional information.	The research is testing hypotheses about depression after miscarriage. The phenomenological method is used to uncover the experience for a select group who acknowledge feelings of depression.
Qualitative + qualitative	There is a qualitative foundation and other qualitative methods used to provide additional information.	The phenomenological method is used to uncover the experience for a select group who acknowledge feelings of depression. Concurrent focus groups explore impacts of depression feelings on support-seeking behaviours.
Quantitative + quantitative	There is a quantitative foundation and other quantitative methods used to provide additional information.	Collection of physiological measures from women diagnosed with depression after miscarriage. Concurrent survey collecting social, health and depression scale information.
Sequential		
Qualitative → quantitative	Findings from qualitative investigation lead to use of the quantitative supplementary approach.	The research has described the experience of feeling depressed after miscarriage. The themes emerging from the data are then used to create a depression scale, which is tested for reliability and validity.
Quantitative → qualitative	Findings from quantitative investigation lead to use of the qualitative supplementary approach.	The research has tested hypotheses linking miscarriage with depression and found no significant relationships. A qualitative study is undertaken to uncover the experience of living through miscarriage, in an effort to let the data lead to common thoughts and feelings.
Qualitative → qualitative	Findings from qualitative investigation lead to use of the supplementary qualitative approach.	The research has described the experience of feeling depressed after miscarriage. The themes emerging from the data are then used during focus groups to explore impacts on family life.
Quantitative → quantitative	Findings from quantitative investigation lead to use of the supplementary quantitative approach.	The research has conducted a descriptive cross-sectional survey on those with depression after miscarriage. Those findings are then followed with an experimental clinical trial—where the treatment group receives a specific counselling intervention—and the other group receives 'standard' support.

(Adapted from Morse, J.M., Niehaus, L., 2009. Mixed Method Design: principles and procedures. Walnut Creek, CA: Left Coast Press, p. 25.)

TABLE 12.2 Use of a Triangulated Approach in One Study

Research Process Components	Qualitative Approach First Phase	Quantitative Approach Second Phase	Quantitative Approach Third Phase
Design	Descriptive, exploratory.	Correlational, Health Needs Instrument (HNI) tool development and testing.	Descriptive, correlational. Implementation of HNI tool.
Participants	Purposive sample of 34 older patients.	Purposive sample of 32 older patients.	Purposive sample of 54 older patients.
Data collection	Semistructured interviews.	Structured demographic data from HNI (35 nominal questions).	Structured interviews.
Analysis	Content/thematic analysis.	Internal consistency, content and concurrent validity.	Descriptive measures of variance and distribution.
Findings	Health needs included: help in managing tangible things, psychological support, health information, medical support and participation in decision making.	A significant negative correlation with patients' tangible needs for help with activities of daily life (ADL) during hospitalisation transition. Strong correlation between educational level and the need for health-related information.	A significant correlation between psychological needs with the need for medical support, informational needs and maintaining ADLs during period of hospitalisation.

(Source: Shih, S.-N., Gau, M.-L., Kao, C.-H., et al., 2005. Health needs instrument for hospitalised single-living Taiwanese elders with heart disease: triangulation research design. J. Clin. Nurs. 14, 1210–1222.)

with AOD nurse practitioners performing advanced roles such as prescribing and medication management.

TUTORIAL TRIGGER 12.1

When considering the notion of methodological 'best fit' for a research topic, what factors could affirm the 'fit' of a mixed-methods approach? For example, when would simultaneous methods be a better 'fit' than sequential methods?

Limitations Associated With Mixed-Methods Research

As with any area of research, accompanying the value and benefits of a research method, the limitations and challenges also need to be considered. The limitations associated with mixed-methods research include their time-consuming nature and resource intensiveness (i.e. generating more complex data for collection and analysis), the complexity of conducting both qualitative and quantitative phases, the complexity of a team approach (specialists in different methodology and methods) and the need for the principal researcher/s to have a sound working knowledge of both quantitative and qualitative paradigms including knowledge of how to combine them to ensure good outcomes (Halcomb & Andrew 2009; Tashakkori et al 2020). Undertaking mixed-methods research is usually a more complex undertaking than single-design studies.

SPECIFIC APPROACHES TO MIXED-METHODS RESEARCH

Over the last 10 years or so, mixed-methods research has 'exploded' in nursing and midwifery research and in general health services research. Its context, justification, place and importance across all health disciplines have become much clearer and far more widely accepted (Poth 2018). Prior to this shift, many health professionals felt the need to 'locate' their mixed-methods research to a specific approach. This was because mixed-methods research on its own was still often viewed as unclear and misunderstood. There has been a rapid swing from this position. It is a similar case to descriptive, exploratory qualitative methodology more recently becoming the most widely used qualitative approach in nursing and midwifery research (see Chapter 5). They are now the dominant approach. Chapter 5 starts with the 'general' descriptive exploratory dominant approach and then moves on to the most common 'traditional' specific methodologies. Similarly, here, there is still a need to highlight specific mixed-methods approaches because they remain important, and they perform functions and outcomes that 'generic' mixed-methods approaches cannot fully address. In terms of nursing and midwifery research, the following-mentioned four specific methodologies are explored and, currently, are addressed in terms of current 'popularity and commonality'.

Action Research

Action research is an important and established research approach in nursing and midwifery. The term '**action research**', informed by critical social theory (see Chapter 2), was coined in 1946 by the social psychologist Kurt Lewin to describe the research program he developed in response to post-World War II social problems in America (Lewin 1946). Lewin's interest was in narrowing the gap between research recommendation and action so that democratic inquiry could pave the way to group decisions and a commitment to organisational change and improvement (Lewin 1951). He wanted to develop a structured process for translating research evidence into action—rather than 'research for the sake of research'. The more recent emergence of 'practice development' (linked to research and knowledge translation—see Chapter 15) in health-related environments has reinforced the use of action research process to engage health professionals to collaboratively solve practice-based issues. For example, Hickey et al (2018) highlight the increasing demand for capacity building among the Aboriginal and Torres Strait Islander (Indigenous) maternal and infant health workforce to improve health outcomes for mothers. Their partnership project aimed at improving maternity services for Indigenous families in South-East Queensland. They report that their participatory action research study was a very effective method to actively mentor and engage all team members in reflective, collaborative research practice, resulting in positive changes for the maternity care service overall. The research assistants described learning to conduct interviews and infant assessments, as well as gaining confidence to build rapport with families. Reflecting on the stories shared by the women participating in the study opened 'a whole new world and interest' in studying midwifery and child health after learning the difficulties and strengths of families during pregnancy and beyond.

The Process of Action Research

In action research, group members are brought together to explore and address issues affecting them. While most forms of research are a series of linear steps, from question/hypothesis development (see Chapter 4) through to recommendations for action, action research is cyclical in design (Crozier et al 2012). It uses a cyclical research process that enables actions to be developed by the group, actioned, monitored, analysed and evaluated. The cyclic process forms the basis for reflection on the success of plans and the possibility of modifying them and starting another cycle of planning, action, data collection, analysis, evaluation and reflection. The spiral or cycle consists of several stages—some of which are repeated until the situation under examination improves or is abandoned. Fig. 12.1 describes each following and continuing cyclical stage, starting with initial diagnosis of the clinical problem/s, through to data collection and analysis, and resultant feedback to participants. Following on from this is the actioning of changes leading to the processes of reflection and program evaluation, before planning further action and starting the cycle again. It is worth noting that in action research many projects develop subprojects, with their own distinct spirals, that can become their own individual projects—with further co-researchers and funding involved.

Action research involves the use of social/organisational change 'experiments' with real people and their real problems in their own social systems. The function of action research is to focus on 'real-world' events, as opposed to controlled environments or generalisable outcomes—such as with experimental research (Coghlan 2019). Preliminary investigations involve a mix of methods (e.g. interviews, survey, audit, etc.) to explore the context and extent of the problems under consideration and assist the research team to develop specific research question/s. In action research, the change/action cycles emerge from the creation of new knowledge obtained from the processes of 'cycles of agreement' (consensus building or co-design/production). Employing both sequential and/or concurrent methods of data collection (see earlier in this chapter), these processes observe and reflect on immediate experiences, form concepts, and test and apply these experiences in new situations. Depending on the nature of the study, action research designs will be different—some resembling exploratory mixed-methods approaches and, at other times, transformative or multiphase mixed-methods research.

RESEARCH IN BRIEF 12.1

Kiser and Hulton's (2018) study adopted a unique approach to addressing the health needs of a rural homeless population using core principles relevant to community-based participatory research (CBPR)—an action research approach. The objective of the *Healthcare for the Homeless Suitcase Clinic* (HHSC) project was to create a community-based practice model of healthcare through unconventional portable, mobile 'Suitcase Clinics' staffed by

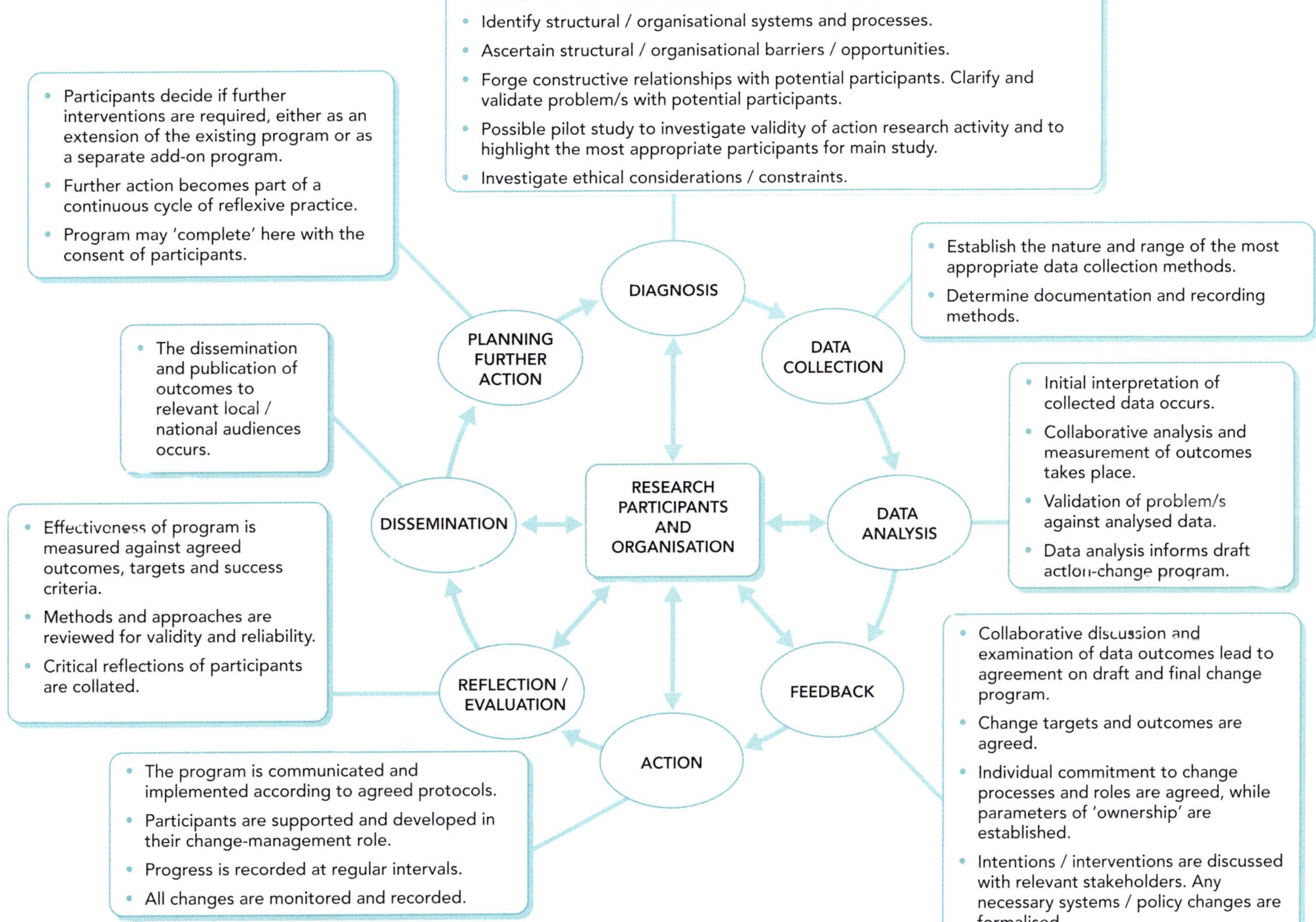

Fig. 12.1 An organisational-change action research cycle (Source: adapted from: Whitehead, D., Taket, A., Smith P., 2003. Action research in health promotion. Health Educ. J. 62, 5–22. Reprinted by permission of Sage.)

RESEARCH IN BRIEF 12.1—cont'd

volunteer providers and a Nurse Case Manager. These clinics addressed complex health concerns of the homeless in five unique shelter settings in a rural community. Using CBPR, community-academic partners worked systematically to explore the issues of homelessness in one community using action research data collection cycles, reflection and capacity building. In the most recent sampling of their Patient Satisfaction Survey (n = 47), 60% of the HHSC clients surveyed indicated that the HHSC kept them from going to the emergency department. Additional results from the Patient Satisfaction Survey demonstrated that 70% of the respondents listed the HHSC as their primary source of care. Moreover, 77% of those surveyed indicated satisfaction with the level of privacy and confidentiality provided by the HHSC, and 96% indicated a willingness to use the HHSC again. The HHSC demonstrated positive outcomes through community-wide collaborations, including several homeless clients acquiring health benefits including disability benefits. In addition, finding a medical home through other safety net providers has become a reality for homeless clients with the HHSC as a connecting link. Most importantly, they state, homeless clients have moved into housing, with demonstrated success in health outcomes.

Action research is necessarily 'insider' research in the sense that practitioners research their own professional actions and look for the best outcomes for their clients. There are several strategies that are used to facilitate the widest possible involvement of representative stakeholders—both clients and all those that influence. Box 12.1 highlights how various stakeholder groups might interact with the action research process. For instance, Neville et al's (2022) study sought to identify barriers to older Pacific people's participation in the healthcare system in Aotearoa New Zealand. A participatory action research design was used. In total, 104 Pacific co-researchers contributed to focus groups using *Talanoa*, a traditional method of conversational dialogue deeply rooted in Pacific Island culture. Data were collected in Pacific Island languages from storytelling and conversations shared within the focus groups. Data were translated into English and analysed using a collaborative approach. The findings captured older Pacific peoples' barriers to participation in the healthcare system: accessing healthcare, relationships with healthcare providers and understanding the healthcare system.

TUTORIAL TRIGGER 12.2

Who might the 'key' stakeholders be for an action research study on improving consumer direction/decision making for older people who access community-based health services? If you were conducting an action research project with this group and setting, what do you think would be the main priorities? What type of processes and research methods (for collecting research data) might you use?

The Value of Action Research

Perhaps the greatest value of action research is that it allows health professionals to learn about their local situation and facilitate the implementation and evaluation of research into this situation. Added to this is the obvious benefit that this type of research approach lends itself to ongoing evidence-based practice change and translation of change knowledge into practice (see Chapter 15). Action research also offers the flexibility for research projects to evolve naturally. As the study evolves and changes, the co-researchers

BOX 12.1 Action Research Project Structure

- Identify a health-related situation that needs improvement or a health concern for a group of people.
- Establish a collaborative research group concerned with addressing the situation (this group may include stakeholders).
- Establish a reference group composed of all key stakeholders to oversee and advise on the project.
- Conduct training action research workshops for researcher group members.
- Conduct a preliminary investigation to develop baseline data and understand the context and scope of the concern.
- Implement the first action plan, collect and analyse data.
- Research group reflection and replanning through the spiral or cycle.
- Meet with the reference group throughout the project to discuss/examine the evolving data and assess the proposed plans.
- Meet with the reference group to discuss project results.
- Disseminate the findings in accessible formats to all stakeholders (see Chapter 18).

can further develop and refine the process and provide a much fuller and more comprehensive picture of the problem at hand (Chevalier & Buckles 2019). Action research studies, therefore, have the potential to reach aims and outcomes that may not have been recognised or realised at project commencement. Many action research projects gain their own 'momentum' and researchers often want to keep working through more cycles to achieve better outcomes—usually until funding or support has discontinued and/or the project aims have been achieved. Although action research works best when the intention is to effect community-wide or overall organisational change, it can also be applied to a localised context—such as a single ward/unit and across subacute settings (e.g. Hills et al's (2022) nursing perspectives on reducing sedentary behaviour in subacute hospital settings across five Australian sites).

Limitations of Action Research

Action researchers will usually approach an action research-related study knowing the immense potential benefits that it can bring, especially in relation to measurable change in practice and community/organisational structures. At the same time, action researchers are also acutely aware of the limitations that can contradict its nature and intention. As one might already appreciate, action research is not easy to set up or initiate. Great effort, enthusiasm, equal participation, trust and prolonged engagement are necessary for effective process (Coghlan 2019). It can be noted, though, that the literature can be critical of action research's ability to offer genuine equality, empowerment and participation (Whitehead et al 2003). The nature and intention of action research is often quite broad as it relates to the whole situation under investigation. This means that process and outcomes are often difficult to predict. Action researchers face situations where they may not know exactly what to investigate, when and where to start or even when the research is likely to be complete. Therefore participants (co-researchers) are often unaware of exactly where their research 'journey' will take them (MacDonald 2012). This aspect of action research has implications for gaining funding and organisational support and for seeking human research ethics approval (see Chapter 13).

Action research can be viewed by some as an insensitive 'blunt tool', as it carefully examines and challenges organisations or communities. The suggestion, prior to the outset of the action research process, is that something is wrong and requires fixing/change—even though any criticism is intended to be constructive and improve practice. In addition, action research is often applied in situations where groups or communities are often perceived to be powerless, vulnerable, or oppressed by a dominant group, organisation or culture (Chevalier & Buckles 2019). Action research, therefore, can appear threatening to the research participants and the organisation/community/service being investigated. The aim of action research to bring about change can be challenging and difficult for participants and others within the study context, possibly because of prior experiences with change, differing perceptions about need, varying willingness to change, and organisational culture or conflict (Coghlan 2019). The need for many stakeholders to be involved at different levels can also provide challenges.

AN UNEXPECTED HURDLE

Nurses working in very remote areas of Australia (RANs) work in complex and isolated settings for which they are often inadequately prepared, and stress levels are notably high. Lenthall et al's (2018) study evaluated the development and implementation of an intervention to reduce and prevent the impact of occupational stress in the RAN workforce in the Northern Territory.

The study adopted a combined participatory action research/organisational development model, involving seven steps, to develop and implement system changes within the (then) Northern Territory Department of Health and Families (NTDH&F). The development, implementation and evaluation were informed via information from participants collected during workshops and interviews. Pre- and post-study surveys were undertaken to evaluate the study.

Findings demonstrated that occupational stress interventions, developed by the workgroups, were categorised into four main groups: (1) remote context, (2) workload and scope of practice, (3) poor management and (4) violence and safety concerns. The main interventions centred on promoting a well-educated, stable workforce. The authors state that there were very few measurable changes because of the interventions, as many were not able to be implemented in the period of the study—but they add that the project is 'continuing'.

1. Action research claims that actions are an outcome of the cyclic processes that govern this research method. What types of action might unfold from action research in a setting such as the one described in this study? Were any actions evident in the study described above?

2. The study honestly reports that there were very few 'measurable' changes. Should change always be measurable? Is some change, rather than no change, desirable? The time period is stated as a factor that prevented widespread action and change. What other factors may have been involved? What circumstances might have contributed to this?

Delphi Technique

The **Delphi technique** is named with reference to the Ancient Greek god Apollo. He 'connected with mortals' via the Temple of Apollo in Delphi (Greece). The 'Pythia', who was the high priestess of the temple, held the title 'Oracle of Delphi'. The Delphi Oracles were viewed as Apollo's most expert, truthful and trustworthy representative/informant on 'earth'. As a research approach, the Delphi technique is an effective method for collecting informed and trustworthy 'expert' opinion on a specific topic (Foth et al 2016). Information is collected from experts on the topic and usually responses remain anonymous. This prevents the personality, reputation or authority of any one participant from dominating others in the process. It is also argued that this anonymity frees participants from personal biases and encourages a more open disclosure and debate. The Delphi process is achieved by inviting the viewpoints of all parties, enabling individual viewpoints and ultimately achieving a degree of *consensus*. The Delphi technique is a useful strategy for examining an area with a limited empirical research base and/or for where there are questions for which there may be no known answers. The technique is particularly useful for determining best academic and practice standards and as a basis for forming policy-driven mechanisms where there is 'confusion' (Whitehead 2008).

The Delphi Process

A Delphi study involves a series of interviews/questionnaires (both qualitative and quantitative) with controlled feedback from usually anonymous participants or identified experts. Stages of the Delphi process include selection of the expert panel, formulation of the open question(s), generation of statements, reduction and categorisation of statements, rating of statements, and analysis and iteration (Bryar et al 2013). It is important to note that studies may state that they have adopted a 'modified' Delphi technique. Where this occurs, the authors should clearly identify what this means and its rationale (e.g. in Sim et al's (2018) four-round modified Delphi survey seeking indicators of quality nursing practice, resulting in eight overarching constructs, namely: care and caring, communication, coordination and collaboration, safety, patient characteristics, workload, nurses' work environment and organisational characteristics).

Typically, with Delphi studies, the first-round questionnaire collects qualitative data through unstructured questions seeking open responses. This type of data is needed initially to provide the richness of data necessary to formulate subsequent focused questions or statements. Qualitative content and thematic analysis processes of the collected first-round data are used as a basis to synthesise responses for each survey round (see Chapter 7). This analysis reveals several categories which are, in turn, grouped and listed. Generally, the data from the first round are specific and structured, but then require further quantification. Conventionally, they are formulated as a list of Likert scale statements/questions, or sometimes visual analogue/semantic differential scale-related items (see Chapter 9), and returned to the study participants for review and feedback. In many cases, the initial first-round analysis reveals several domains (categories) containing many statements (indicators) overall. For instance, Nkwanyana et al's (2019) study investigating a health system framework for perinatal care in South African district hospitals, for their second round, identified 36 domains containing 149 indicators.

The aim of a Delphi study is to identify an acceptably 'narrow' consensus on the investigated topic. Where this is the case, it usually requires several similarly structured Likert-style questionnaire rounds to help reduce the categories into a manageable number. The lowest-scoring questions are removed whereas the highest scores are kept for the following rounds. A predetermined consensus level or percentage is often set prior to commencing the study. For instance, Button et al's (2019) Queensland-based study sought to provide expert consensus on the clinical indicators that signal when a person with a haematological malignancy is at high risk of deteriorating and dying. Consensus was achieved if 70% of responses fell within two points on their seven-point Likert scales. Once the main points are manageable and/or cannot be broken down further, a degree of data 'saturation' or consensus is considered to have been met. In most cases it is by the second or third round that this is achieved, but there is always the option to continue with additional rounds. Sim et al's (2018) study used four rounds.

RESEARCH IN BRIEF 12.2

Dawson et al (2023), in their Delphi study, invited all midwifery staff within the maternity unit of a private hospital in Melbourne to identify their workplace change needs and priorities for research. In round one, participants joined face-to-face focus groups to put forward their ideas for workplace change and research ideas, and these data were developed into themes. In round two, participants ranked the themes in priority order. The top four ranked themes identified by this cohort of midwives were: 'ways of working—investigating alternative ways of working to enable greater flexibility and opportunities', 'understanding midwifery—working with the executive team to highlight the nuances of maternity care', 'education—increase in staff in the education

RESEARCH IN BRIEF 12.2—cont'd

team to provide a greater presence and opportunity for education' and 'postnatal specific—review ways of working in postnatal areas'. Several priority research and change areas were identified which, if implemented, would strengthen both midwifery practice and midwife retention in that workplace.

The Value of the Delphi Technique

The benefits of the Delphi technique include the ability to harness many opinions across geographical distance, the freedom of individuals to express their opinion without being influenced by others, and allowing individuals to participate at a convenient time and with relatively small cost and resources required. Delphi can also be performed over relatively short periods of time, especially if conducted using electronic mail/media. These benefits can overcome the potential limitations of other consensus methods such as focus groups, nominal group technique or consensus conferences. Potentially, small study groups can be used, and the range can be anywhere from a handful to hundreds of participants. For example, Button et al's (2019) study recruited 27 participants, while Al-Yateem et al's (2019) nurse-identified patient care and health services research priorities Delphi survey approached 1032 participants.

Limitations of the Delphi Technique

As well as several benefits, there are some methodological considerations to address with Delphi studies. These include inadequate descriptions of panelist characteristics (especially in terms of identifying who or what constitutes an expert), subjective researcher interpretation of definitions and measures of consensus, and high wastage of respondents due to 'response fatigue'—especially where there are more than two rounds. It is also important to remember that the findings of a Delphi study represent expert opinion but not indisputable fact (Whitehead 2008).

Case Study Approach

The term '**case study**' has different meanings in research and clinical contexts. For instance, case study research is often confused with the case study teaching method, 'case presentation' of a particular clinical case, or a 'case–control' study of an epidemiological design (see Chapter 8). A mixed-methods case study approach stems more from an approach that enables a detailed examination of a complex or simple single 'case' or 'unit' within a real-life and contemporary context using multiple data sources (e.g. Creswell 2013). The mixed-methods case study approach is an inquiry which is exploratory, observational and responsive to the social context and, therefore, both qualitative and quantitative in terms of its philosophical/theoretical position. The case (phenomenon of interest) is usually a group or community—but can also be an organisation. Regarding 'community', the community in Sami et al's (2018) mixed-methods case study is mothers and babies located in displaced camps in South Sudan. The researchers wanted to explore the factors that influenced the implementation of a package of facility- and community-based neonatal interventions in four displaced persons camps in South Sudan using a health systems framework—using focus groups, interviews, observation and existing documentation. A key solution was seen to be authorising the task-shifting of emergency newborn care to mid-level cadre, transitioning facility-based traditional birth attendants to community health workers and scaling up institutions to upgrade community midwives into professional midwives.

Whiteing et al (2022), in exploring the practice of rural and remote nurses in Australia, looked to do similar. The case study comprised three phases of data collection: first, a content analysis of 42 documents relating to the context of nursing, specifically rural and remote nursing; second, a content analysis of an online questionnaire ($n = 75$); and third, a thematic analysis of semistructured interviews ($n = 20$). COREQ reporting guidelines were used. Each phase of data collection informed subsequent data collection and analysis within the study. Following triangulation of data from each phase of the study, the major themes reported were '*a medley of preparation for rural and remote work*', '*being held accountable*', '*alone, with or without someone*' and '*spiralling wellbeing*'.

Triangulation of methods for mixed-methods case study (Yin 2018) enables use of a full range of data collection strategies—such as interviews, field notes, participant observation, audiovisual materials, survey tools, contemporary documents, etc.—both qualitatively and quantitatively (Creswell 2013). Data analysis can use a constant comparative approach (see Chapter 7) or be more structured. Data can be examined in their own right with no requirement for generalisability, or the study procedure may include steps to ensure reliability, validity and generalisability (Yin 2018).

RESEARCH IN BRIEF 12.3

Hayes et al (2019) explored the phenomenon of adolescent mental health in the inpatient setting using a prospective, longitudinal mixed-methods approach. They stated that little is known about the models of care (MoC)

Continued

RESEARCH IN BRIEF 12.3—cont'd

offered in inpatient units, or whether adolescents perceive these as helpful, and the perspectives of caregivers and clinicians. Accordingly, they were interested in developing a clinical protocol. The sample population consisted of adolescents, caregivers and clinicians at a single inpatient unit in Melbourne. Standardised outcome measures, including semistructured interviews, were administered to adolescents at three time-points: T1 (admission), T2 (discharge) and T3 (6 months post-discharge). Caregivers were also interviewed at T1, T2 and T3. Clinicians were interviewed once. The measures included the Life Problems Inventory, Quick Inventory of Depressive Symptomatology, Kessler Psychological Distress Scale and the Youth Self-Report. Health of the Nation Outcome Scales for Children and Adolescents were collected at the T1 and T2 points. Quantitative analysis included descriptive statistics and paired *t*-tests summarising adolescents admitted to the unit, clinical characteristics and longitudinal data on symptomatology. Qualitative data were analysed using both thematic and trajectory analysis. From this the Models of Community Hospital Activity (MoCHA) protocol has been developed.

Q Methodology

Q methodology uses a unique set of processes to reveal subjective attitudes and perspectives of participants about a particular topic. The technique reveals the structure of views and is useful for exploring values, beliefs and perceptions of life experiences. It is an alternative method for studying individual subjectivity (qualitative part) using factor analysis (see Chapter 10). Wolf and Peace (2018) identify the abductive nature of factor-analysed Q-methodology data and how this is aligned subjectively to the research topic. There is a misbelief that Q methodology is mainly about psychometric testing, but it is far more a systematic process of assessing qualitative data (Rhoads 2014). A set of stimulus material (i.e. textual statements, pictures, or recordings) is usually constructed. These are mostly obtained from prior interviews to form the Q sample. Statements in the Q sample are representative, but not exhaustive, of the diversity of attitudes and perceptions related to the topic. Once the set of statements has been verified and finalised, each statement or material is placed on an individual card to enable the cards to be sorted into some order. Participants are instructed on how to rank-order the set of Q-sample statements or materials. This is referred to as the Q-sort technique. Ranking commonly follows a Likert scale format (see Chapter 9)—for example, from strongly agree to strongly disagree using a quasi-normal distribution. That is, least cards can be assigned scores at the ends of the scale while proportionally more can be in the middle of the distribution. Q methodology, in this respect, applies quantitative analysis to qualitatively derived data. Fig. 12.2 illustrates a hypothetical example for a 36-item Q sample, with an 11-point Likert scale, from strongly disagree (−5) to strongly agree (+5). One card is placed per cell on the Q-sort diagram. In this example, only one card can be placed in the +5 location, while four statements can be located at −2. The

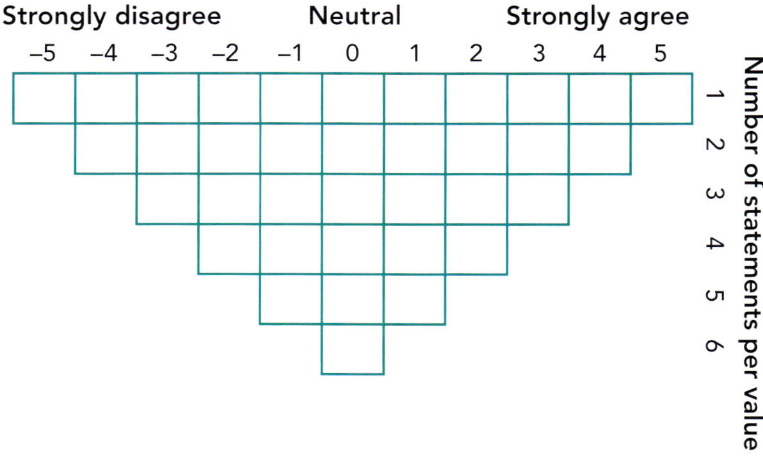

Fig. 12.2 Q-sort diagram (Modified from Denzin, N.K., 1978. The Research Act: a theoretical introduction to sociological methods, second ed. McGraw-Hill, New York; and Janesick V J 1994 The dance of qualitative research design: metaphor, methodolatory, and meaning. In: Denzin, N.K., Lincoln, Y.S. (Eds.) Handbook of Qualitative Research. Sage Publications, Thousand Oaks, CA.)

resulting order is then analysed using quantitative techniques to produce correlational matrices and factor analysis solutions (see Chapter 10). The use of factor analysis enabled the statements to be collated for clearer interpretation (Wolf & Peace 2018).

RESEARCH IN BRIEF 12.4

Younas et al (2023), in their exploratory sequential mixed methods study, performed a Q-sort survey as part of their study into implementing strategies to promote compassionate nursing care of complex patients. Phase 2 developed a Q-sort survey of implementation strategies for phase 3. Nurses, nurse managers, healthcare administrators, policymakers and compassionate care experts responded to the survey by ranking the 21 implementation strategies, out of which five met the Q-factor analysis criteria. Participant-perceived barriers to nurse compassion could be categorised under knowledge, intentions, skills, social influences, behavioural regulation, reinforcement, emotion, and environmental context and resources. The five highest-ranked strategies included facilitation, consultation with stress experts, involvement of patients and families, modelling compassion through shadowing and utilising implementation teams. The study concluded that enablement and modelling were the integration functions represented by the highest-ranked implementation strategies. Enabling nurses to provide compassionate care through emotional support and mental health counselling, and modelling compassion and compassionate care through shadowing, were recommended and rated as highly relevant by the majority of stakeholders.

TUTORIAL TRIGGER 12.3

You and your study group have been asked to present the steps involved in a Q-methodology study using a published paper to illustrate the concepts. Access two published Q-methodology papers and identify the common steps undertaken. Provide a one-paragraph general description with an accompanying example.

Mixing and Matching Mixed Methods

It is worth noting that mixed-methods approaches can adopt more than one 'specific' mixed-methods methodology. As with any 'newer' research paradigm, some researchers are naturally curious and inclined to test new, novel and creative approaches. For instance, Kirschbaum et al's (2019) study title should help to illustrate in their 'Q-sample construction: a novel approach incorporating a Delphi technique to explore opinions about codeine dependence' study. It 'mixes' Q methodology and Delphi.

SUMMARY

The value and contribution of mixed-methods research to and for nursing and midwifery practice is beyond question. Many researchers, with good understanding of mixed-methods approaches, will be able to appreciate the benefits of expanding research intentions and outcomes to accommodate a range of approaches and methods. While researchers need to be aware that mixed-methods research brings with it a unique set of challenges, compared with single-methodology studies, it is argued that the benefits outweigh this. This is particularly the case in relation to a higher likelihood of research comprehensiveness, completeness and notable/more likely changes in practice. In bringing together the paradigms of both qualitative and quantitative research (to create a third paradigm of mixed methods), this chapter and mixed-methods research brings together the 'paradigmatic circle' of quantitative and qualitative approaches.

KEY POINTS

- Mixed-methods research continues to rapidly gain recognition and approval in nursing and midwifery. Mixed-methods research combines methods, paradigms and the approaches of qualitative and quantitative research to enable a broader and more comprehensive picture of clinical research.
- Action research is a useful method to use when researchers want to understand and improve a situation, as it is action focused and context specific, and therefore can address problems of practical concern. Action research uses a cyclical process in which research, implementation, evaluation and theorising are linked to reduce the theory–practice gap.
- Delphi studies seek to gain expert consensus when there is confusion or a lack of 'general' understanding of a health-related issue, and typically combine qualitative and quantitative data from a series of open and closed questionnaire rounds.
- A case study approach enables a detailed examination of a single 'case' or 'unit' within a real-life setting. The 'case' can be an individual, social group, community, organisation or event.
- Q methodology combines interview (qualitative) data to form statements about the topic of interest, which are then rank-ordered to produce quantitative data.

TIME TO REFLECT

Palermo, C., King, O., Brock, T., et al., 2019. Setting priorities for health education research: a mixed methods study. Med. Teach. 41 (9), 1029–1038. doi: 10.1080/0142159X.2019.1612520

Aim: Palermo et al (2019) set about their mixed-methods study with a view to inform the development of a health education research strategy through addressing the following questions:

1. What are the health education research priorities over the next 3–5 years according to multiple stakeholders?
2. What is the rationale provided by multiple stakeholders for prioritising specific health education research topics?
3. What are the similarities and differences in health education research priorities across the range of stakeholders?

Design: A three-stage sequential mixed-methods study was conducted. Priorities for health education research were identified through a qualitative survey with 104 students, patients, academics and clinicians across five health sciences and 12 professions (stage 1). These findings were analysed using framework analysis and transposed into a quantitative survey whereby 780 stakeholders rated and ranked the identified priorities. Descriptive statistics identified priorities, exploratory factor analysis grouped priorities and differences between stakeholders were determined using Mann–Whitney U tests (stage 2). Six individual or group interviews with 16 participants (stage 3) further explicated the results from previous stages.

Reflect on the following: Through a sequential mixed-methods design engaging various stakeholders, their study identified the top three priorities as: understanding how to ensure students develop the required skills for work, how to promote resiliency and wellbeing in students and now to ensure the curriculum prepares students for work. Understanding how to develop communication skills, ensuring assessments led to fitness for practice and providing more useful feedback and the role of workplace-based learning as part of health-related curricula were also identified as high priorities through Likert ratings but not necessarily through rank (ranked 4th, 6th, 12th and 13th). The priorities were grouped under six factors: (i) culture of learning together in the workplace, (ii) preparation for work, (iii) meeting future Australian healthcare needs, (iv) pedagogical effectiveness, (v) workforce issues and (vi) curriculum integration. Priorities were typically similar across different types of participants; the study found only three significant differences in the perspectives of different stakeholder groups. The authors identify that the sequential mixed-methods approach to identifying priorities allowed for participants in Stage 1 to have genuine input into the list of priorities presented in Stage 2, meaning that the priorities ranked in Stage 2 were participant rather than researcher derived. They state that they thus remain unsure whether their findings reflect research gaps or participants' perceptions of these gaps.

Questions

1. Think of other designs that could have been used in this study.
2. Reflect on the information given and answer these questions:
   a. What was the research design?
   b. Is the design appropriate for this study?
   c. What could the researchers have done to avoid the uncertainty that their findings reflected actual research gaps or participants' perceptions of these gaps?

LEARNING ACTIVITIES

1. The main value of using mixed-methods research in nursing is that it:
   a. allows the researcher to understand a wider range of research methods
   b. helps researchers to champion particular research paradigms
   c. offers a higher probability that the conducted research will be viewed as complete and comprehensive
   d. assists in reducing research error.
2. Data triangulation involves:
   a. prioritising data into discrete groups in a single study
   b. using a variety of data sources in a single study
   c. differentiating between data sources in a single study
   d. using specific data sources in a single study.
3. A mixed-methods research study that sought to initially identify the lived health-related experiences of a group of patients and follow this up by using a tool to measure the extent of those health-related experiences would be using which of the following combinations?
   a. Simultaneous—qualitative and quantitative
   b. Simultaneous—quantitative and qualitative
   c. Sequential—quantitative leading to qualitative
   d. Sequential—qualitative leading to quantitative
4. Conventional Delphi studies have the following properties:
   a. use experts, quantitative first-round, qualitative second-round, consensus
   b. use clients, qualitative first-round, quantitative second-round, consensus

c. use experts, qualitative first-round, quantitative second-round, consensus
d. use clients, qualitative first-round, quantitative second-round, non-consensus.

5. With the Delphi technique, how many questionnaire rounds are most likely to occur?
   a. 1
   b. 2
   c. 3
   d. 4
6. The main features of action research are:
   a. mixed methods, participation, randomisation, change cycles
   b. mixed methods, change cycles, participation, empowerment
   c. participation, mixed methods, empowerment, organisational
   d. change cycles, socio-community, mixed methods, empowerment.
7. An action research cycle or spiral would typically contain the stages:
   a. diagnosis, data collection and analysis, feedback, actioning, reflection and evaluation, and further change cycles
   b. diagnosis, evaluation, feedback, actioning, and further change cycles
   c. diagnosis, data collection and analysis, feedback, actioning, reflection and evaluation
   d. diagnosis, data collection and analysis, feedback, reflection and evaluation, and further change cycles.
8. Action research studies mainly focus on one of two broad areas:
   a. organisational development/operational development
   b. organisational development/community development
   c. procedural development/community development
   d. organisational development/procedural development.
9. With a case study, the phenomenon of interest can be:
   a. an individual/s, a group or community, a conference, a process, an event
   b. an individual/s, a nation, an organisation, a process, an event
   c. an individual/s, a culture, an organisation, a process, an event
   d. an individual/s, a group or community, an organisation, a process, an event.
10. With Q methodology, participants are instructed how to rank-order the set of Q sample statements or materials. This process is called the:
    a. Q-filter technique
    b. Q-sort technique
    c. Q-sieve technique
    d. Q-sift technique.

For further content associated with this chapter visit:  https://evolve.elsevier.com/cs/product/9780729596794?role=student

ADDITIONAL RESOURCES

Creswell, J. 2013. What is mixed-methods research? https://www.youtube.com/watch?v=1OaNiTlpyX8.

What is triangulation? https://www.youtube.com/watch?v=DPOhrdBGsLc.

REFERENCES

Al-Yateem, N., Al-Tamimi, M., Brenner, M., et al., 2019. Nurse-identified patient care and health services research priorities in the United Arab Emirates: a Delphi study. BMC Health Serv. Res. 19, 77. doi:10.1186/s12913-019-3888-5

Andrew, S., Halcomb, E.J. (Eds.), 2009. Mixed Methods Research for Nursing and the Health Sciences. Wiley-Blackwell, London, UK.

Andrew, S., Halcomb, E.J., 2012. Mixed method research. In: Borbasi S., Jackson, D. (Eds.), Navigating the Maze of Research: enhancing nursing and midwifery practice. Elsevier Australia, Chatswood, NSW, pp. 147–155.

Brownson, R.C., Colditz, G., Proctor, E.K., 2017. Dissemination and Implementation Research in Health: translating science to practice, second ed. Oxford University Press, New York. doi:10.1093/oso/9780190683214.001.0001

Bryar, R., Anto-Awuakye, S., Christie, J., et al. 2013. Using the Delphi approach to identify priority areas for Health Visiting practice in an area of deprivation. Nurs. Res. Pract.—open access. doi:10.1155/2013/780315. Retrieved from: https://www.hindawi.com/journals/nrp/2013/780315/

Button, E., Gavin, N.C., Chan, R.J., et al., 2019. Harnessing the power of clinician judgement. Identifying risk of deteriorating and dying in people with a haematological malignancy: a Delphi study. J. Adv. Nurs. 75, 161–174. doi:10.1111/jan.13889

Chevalier, J., Buckles, D., 2019. Participatory Action Research. Routledge, London. doi:10.4324/9781351033268

Coghlan, D., 2019. Doing Action Research in Your Own Organization, fifth ed. Sage Publications, London.

Creswell, J.W., 2013. Qualitative Inquiry and Research Design: choosing among five approaches, third ed. Sage Publications, Thousand Oaks, CA.

Creswell, J.W., 2014. Research Design: qualitative, quantitative, and mixed-methods approaches, fourth ed. & international student edition. Sage Publications, Thousand Oaks, CA.

Creswell, J.W., Plano Clark, V.L., 2017. Designing and Conducting Mixed Methods Research, third ed. Sage Publications, Thousand Oaks, CA.

Creswell, J.W., Klassen, A.C., Plano Clark, V.L., et al., 2011. Best Practices for Mixed Methods Research in the Health Sciences. National Institutes of Health, Bethesda, MD.

Crozier, K., Moore, J., Kite, K., 2012. Innovations and action research to develop research skills for nursing and midwifery

practice: the Innovations in Nursing and Midwifery Practice Project study. J. Clin. Nurs. 21, 1716–1725.
Dawson, K., Bayes, S., Gilbert, S., et al., 2023. Working with private hospital midwives in Victoria, Australia to identify practice change priorities: outcomes of a Delphi study. Midwifery, 124, 103767.
Denzin, N.K., 1978. The Research Act: a theoretical introduction to sociological methods, second ed. McGraw-Hill, New York.
Feilzer, M., 2010. Doing mixed methods research pragmatically: implications for the rediscovery of pragmatism as a research paradigm. J. Mix. Methods Res. 4 (1), 6–16. doi:10.1177/1558689809349691
Florczak, K.L., 2014. Purists need not apply: the case for pragmatism in mixed methods research. Nurs. Sci. Q. 27 (4), 278–282. doi:10.1177/0894318414546419
Foth, T., Efstathiou, N., Vanderspank-Wright, B., et al., 2016. The use of Delphi and Nominal Group Technique in nursing education: a review. Int. J. Nurs. Stud. 60, 112–120.
Halcomb, E., 2018. Appraising mixed methods research. In: Liamputtong, P. (Ed.), Research Methods in Health Social Sciences. Springer Nature, Singapore, pp. 1051–1067.
Halcomb, E.J., Andrew, S., 2009. Practical considerations for higher degree research students undertaking mixed methods projects. Int. J. Mult. Res. Approaches 3 (2), 153–162.
Hayes, C., Palmer, V.J., Simmons, M., et al., 2019. Protocol for a prospective, longitudinal mixed-methods case study: supporting a Model of Care for Healthier Adolescents (The MoCHA study). BMJ Open 9, e025098. doi:10.1136/bmjopen-2018-025098
Helliwell, T., Muller, S., Hider, S.L., et al., 2018. Challenges of diagnosing and managing polymyalgia rheumatica: a multi-methods study in UK general practice. Br. J. Gen. Pract. 68 (676), e783–e793. doi:10.3399/bjgp18X699557
Hickey, S.D., Maidment, S.J., Heinemann, K.M., et al., 2018. Participatory action research opens doors: mentoring Indigenous researchers to improve midwifery in urban Australia. Women Birth 31 (4), 263–268.
Hills, D., Ekegren, C., Plummer, V., et al. 2022. Nursing perspectives on reducing sedentary behaviour in sub-acute hospital settings: a mixed methods study. J. Clin. Nurs. 31 (9–10), 1348–1361.
Janesick, V.J., 1994. The dance of qualitative research design: metaphor, methodolatory, and meaning. In: Denzin, N.K., Lincoln, Y.S. (Eds.), Handbook of Qualitative Research. Sage Publications, Thousand Oaks, CA, pp. 209–219.
Kirschbaum, M., Barnett, T., Cross, M., 2019. Q sample construction: a novel approach incorporating a Delphi technique to explore opinions about codeine dependence. BMC Med. Res. Methodol. 19, 101. doi:10.1186/s12874-019-0741-9
Kiser, T., Hulton, L., 2018. Addressing health care needs in the homeless population: a new approach using participatory action research. SAGE Open 2018 (7–9), 1–7. doi:10.1177/2158244018789750
Lenthall, S., Wakerman, J., Dollard, M., et al., 2018. Reducing occupational stress among registered nurses in very remote Australia: a participatory action research approach. Collegian 25 (2), 181–191.
Lewin, K., 1946. Action research and minority problems. J. Soc. Issues 2 (4), 34–46.
Lewin, K., 1951. Field Theory in Social Science. Harper, New York.
Lieschke, G., Giles, M., Ball, J., et al., 2022. Towards translational research participation for nurses and midwives: a mixed method study. BMC Nurs. 21 (1), 1–12.
MacDonald, C., 2012. Understanding participatory action research: a qualitative research methodology option. Can. J. Action Res. 13 (2), 34–50.
Maxcy, S.J., 2003. Pragmatic threads in mixed methods research in the social sciences: the search for multiple modes of enquiry and the end of the philosophy of formalism. In: Tashakkori, A., Teddlie, C. (Eds.), Handbook of Mixed Methods in Social and Behavioral Research. Sage Publications, Thousand Oaks, CA, pp. 51–90.
Mertens, D.M., 2007. Transformative paradigm: mixed methods and social justice. J. Mix. Methods Res. 1 (3), 212–225. doi:10.1177/1558689807302811
Morgan, D.L., 2019. Commentary—after triangulation, what next? J. Mix. Methods Res. 13 (1), 6–11. doi:10.1177/1558689818780596
Morse, J.M., Niehaus, L., 2009. Mixed Method Design: principles and procedures. Left Coast Press, Walnut Creek, CA.
Neville S., Wrapson, W., Savila, F., et al., 2022. Barriers to older Pacific peoples' participation in the health-care system in Aotearoa New Zealand. J. Prim. Health Care 14, 124–129. doi:10.1071/HC21146
Nkwanyana, N.M., Voce, A.S., Mnqayi, S.O., et al., 2019. A health system framework for perinatal care in South African district hospitals: a Delphi technique. BMC Health Serv. Res. 19, 402. doi:10.1186/s12913-019-4200-4
Palermo, C., King, O., Brock, T., et al., 2019. Setting priorities for health education research: a mixed methods study. Med. Teach. 41 (9), 1029–1038. doi:10.1080/0142159X.2019.1612520
Pluye, P., Gagon, M.P., Griffiths, F., et al., 2009. A scoring system for appraising mixed methods research, and concomitantly appraising qualitative, quantitative and mixed methods primary studies in Mixed Studies Reviews. Int. J. Nurs. Stud. 46, 529–546.
Poradzisz, M., Florczak, K.L., 2018. Transformative research: a new frontier for nursing? Nurs. Sci. Q. 31 (2), 117–120. doi:10.1177/0894318418755741
Poth, C.N., 2018. Innovation in Mixed Methods Research. Sage Publications, London, UK.
Poth, C.N., 2020. Confronting complex problems with adaptive mixed methods research practices. CJMMR. 1 (1), 29–46.
Poth, C.N., 2023. (Ed) The Sage Handbook of Mixed Method Research Design. Sage Publications, London.
Rhoads, J.C., 2014. Q Methodology. Sage Publications, London.
Rorty, R., 1979. Philosophy and the Mirror of Nature. Princeton University Press, Princeton, NJ.
Sami, S., Amsalu, R., Dimiti, A., et al., 2018. Understanding health systems to improve community and facility level newborn care among displaced populations in South Sudan: a mixed methods case study. BMC Pregnancy Childbirth 18, 325. doi:10.1186/s12884-018-1953-4

Sandelowski, M., 2014. Unmixing mixed-methods research. Res. Nurs. Health 37, 3–8.
Schoonenboom, J., Johnson, R.B., 2017. How to construct a mixed methods research design. Kolner Z. Soz. Sozialpsychol. (Aufl) 69 (Suppl. 2), 107–131. doi:10.1007/s11577-017-0454-1
Searby, A., Burr, D., Blums, C., et al., 2023. Barriers and facilitators to becoming an alcohol and other drug nurse practitioner in Australia: a mixed methods study. Int. J. Mental Health Nurs. 32, 839–853. doi:10.1111/inm.13125
Shih, S.-N., Gau, M.-L., Kao, C.-H., et al., 2005. Health needs instrument for hospitalised single-living Taiwanese elders with heart disease: triangulation research design. J. Clin. Nurs. 14, 1210–1222.
Sim, J., Crookes, P., Walsh, K., et al., 2018. Measuring the outcomes of nursing practice: a Delphi study. J. Clin. Nurs. 27, e368–e378. doi:10.1111/jocn.13971
Tashakkori, A., Creswell, J.W., 2007. Editorial: the new era of mixed methods. J. Mix. Methods Res. 1 (1), 3–7.
Tashakkori, A., Johnson, R.B., Teddlie, C., 2020. Foundations of mixed methods research: Integrating quantitative and qualitative approaches in the social and behavioral sciences. Sage Publications, Thousand Oaks, CA.
Whitehead, D., 2008. An international Delphi study examining health promotion and health education in nursing practice, education and policy. J. Clin. Nurs. 17, 891–900.
Whitehead, D., Taket, A., Smith, P., 2003. Action research in health promotion. Health Educ. J. 62, 5–22.
Whiteing, N., Barr, J., Rossi, D.M., 2022. The practice of rural and remote nurses in Australia: a case study. J. Clin. Nurs. 31, 1502–1518. doi:10.1111/jocn.16002
Wolf, A., Peace, R., 2018. Understanding Q Methodology Data Abductively: an ideal social science institution. Sage Publications, London, UK.
Yin, R.K., 2018. Case Study Research: design and method, sixth ed. Sage Publications, Thousand Oaks, CA.
Younas, A., Porr, C., Maddigan, J., et al., 2023. Implementation strategies to promote compassionate nursing care of complex patients: an exploratory sequential mixed methods study. J. Nurs. Scholarsh. 55, 805–824. doi:10.1111/jnu.12869

13

Ethical and Legal Issues in Research

Julia Gilbert, Susan Stacpoole and Jenny D'Antonio

LEARNING OUTCOMES

After reading this chapter, you should be able to:

- summarise the human rights violations that led to the development of international ethical codes and regulations to guide the conduct of research involving humans
- describe the ethical principles underpinning the conduct of research involving human participants
- identify the responsibilities of the researcher in relationship to research ethics and governance
- identify the laws, regulations and codes that apply to the conduct of research in Australia and/or New Zealand
- explain the essential elements for gaining informed consent from prospective research participants.

KEY TERMS

anonymity, p. 225
autonomy, p. 221
beneficence, p. 219
code of ethics, p. 215
confidentiality, p. 226
cultural diversity, p. 221
human research ethics committee (HREC), p. 215
human rights, p. 216
informed consent, p. 222
justice, p. 218
privacy, p. 225
respect for persons, p. 216
risk/benefit, p. 219
vulnerable participants, p. 210

INTRODUCTION

Ethical awareness and competence are critical to practice in all areas of healthcare. These skills are foundational to ensuring that all healthcare professionals uphold the values of their professions, respect the rights of all stakeholders and respond to the responsibilities and duties of their positions. Ethical principles and ethical competence also shape the way in which nurses and midwives interact with patients, their families, other health professionals, the community and issues arising from within the broader social agenda(s) of the public domain. Improving patient outcomes and reducing morbidity and mortality globally require the timely completion of high-quality research studies. However, these outcomes can be achieved only through the contribution of eligible, willing and informed participants. A number of fundamental ethical principles or imperatives apply to the conduct of research with these participants, many of whom will be **vulnerable participants**; to name a few principles, participants must be adequately protected, fully informed of the benefits and risks of the research and they must agree to participate freely. As nurses and midwives, you will be interacting with and caring for people who may be eligible research participants and/or current research participants; alternatively, you may be contributing to a global research agenda by conducting or leading a program of research as a nurse scientist. The likelihood that you will be exposed to some aspect of research within your professional life makes having a sound understanding of research ethics an essential prerequisite for the next generation of nurses.

This chapter provides an overview of the evolution of human research ethics and the current global efforts directed towards supporting and developing ethical competence among researchers, upholding and strengthening core ethical principles and ensuring awareness of and adherence to agreed international standards. Discussion of the nature of ethical and legal issues relating to human research is provided, followed by an in-depth examination of the moral principles that guide ethical decision making in research, with palliative populations as an example. The chapter emphasises rigorous and defensible research practices which adhere to accepted international and national standards of researcher integrity, respond to legal and regulatory requirements and recognise the central role of the oversight provided by committees such as the Human Research Ethics Committee (HREC) in Australia, or the Institutional Review Board (IRB) in many other countries. The chapter considers the role of these ethics committees as guardians and interpreters of national and international standards, and arbitrators of disagreement about standards. Finally, the chapter describes and examines the evaluation of a research project from an ethical viewpoint.

BACKGROUND

Both research and healthcare have significant and often complex moral and legal dimensions, largely explained by their great potential to either benefit or harm human beings. Human research involves research conducted on humans including their data or tissue. It includes humans: completing surveys, being interviewed or forming a focus group; agreeing to undergo testing or treatment including psychological, physiological or medical interventions; agreeing to be observed by researchers completing specific activities; agreeing to the collection and use of their body organs and tissues or fluids including exhaled breath; and granting access to their personal information, including anonymous and individually identifiable, as part of a researcher database (National Health and Medical Research Council (NHMRC) 2023).

Researchers and participants bring their own interests and unique perspectives to the research process, and these are shaped by their professional, academic, business, societal and cultural experiences. People often assume multiple roles, are bound by duties and responsibilities, and have their own individual and/or collective agendas and complex multifaceted relationships with each other. For example, cultural or religious imperatives might interfere with a participant's capacity or willingness to fully participate in one aspect of a study; or a political commitment might affect the nature of a participant's engagement in a study. These kinds of factors make research involving humans, and especially health-related research, not only deeply fascinating but also imbued with legal and ethical problems that differ from other forms of research.

This chapter highlights the essential roles of ethics in human research, that of achieving maximum benefit for society, containing scientific value, showing respect for human dignity, being subject to independent review and ensuring participants have provided informed consent. The detailed and relevant ethical principles of autonomy, beneficence, non-maleficence and justice form the basis of ethical conduct in contemporary human research (Artal & Rubenfeld 2017). The ethical principles protect research participants by ensuring the absence or minimisation of harm, trauma, pain, anxiety or discomfort during any research project involving human beings. Ethical codes and legal regulations are regularly updated and amended to try to ensure the protection of participants in research studies and the dissemination of research findings for the betterment of others.

What Are Ethical Principles?

Ethical principles are general standards of conduct that make up an ethical system. These principles are generally considered to be the main moral justification for the professional activities of all healthcare professionals. They provide a useful guide to moral decision making and action in research.

1. Principle 1: Non-maleficence—do no harm.
2. Principle 2: Beneficence—for the benefit of a person.
3. Principle 3: Respect for autonomy—allowing people to make their own choices.
4. Principle 4: Justice—being fair.

Non-maleficence is the principle that one should not deliberately inflict harm on another person. Beneficence is an ethical principle that addresses the idea that a person's actions should promote good. Doing good is thought of as doing what is best for another person. Beneficence should not be confused with the closely related ethical principle of non-maleficence, which states that one should not do harm to others. Beneficence involves actively contributing to the welfare of others.

Autonomy is a form of self-governance where individuals are allowed legally to make their own decisions about how they want to live. It refers to the ability of a person with legal capacity to make informed decisions about one's life in order to determine whether a course of action is in their best interests. A person's beliefs, values and commitments form the basis for autonomy as they constitute the person's reasons for making the choices and decisions they do. Respect for autonomy is inherent in research, as participants must be allowed to make their own decision to participate or not. Any actions by researchers that attempt to persuade or coerce the person into making a choice are violations of this principle.

Justice ensures fairness in the treatment of all persons; they have the right to be treated equally, regardless of their background or condition, and should not be discriminated against based on personal characteristics, beliefs or values (Barrow et al 2022).

As healthcare professionals, individual nurses and midwives need to be aware of their direct responsibilities in research governance and ethics. Research governance review ensures institution acceptability of legal and policy and compliance requirements (Kolstoe & Pugh 2023). Whether functioning as a researcher, research assistant or healthcare provider, nurses and midwives need to be cognisant of their legal and ethical responsibilities and competent to act in accordance with them. As both disciplines continue to be increasingly research based, it follows that nurses and midwives need to be familiar with exacting requirements of research governance, and alert to the potential ethical and legal problems inherent in the choice of: research questions, design and methodology; data collection and analysis; and the dissemination of research findings. By virtue of their training and experience, nurses and midwives are often highly attuned to the vulnerabilities of those with whom they are engaged; consequently, they are ideally positioned to advocate on behalf of others in terms of facilitating access to research opportunities and to ensuring that others are neither harmed nor subject to the violation of their rights during their research process.

What Is ethics?

Ethics, simply defined, describes what is expected in terms of right or correct and wrong or incorrect in terms of behaviour. When most people think of ethics (or morals), they think of rules for distinguishing between right and wrong, such as the Golden Rule ('Do unto others as you would have them do unto you'), a code of professional conduct like the Hippocratic Oath ('First of all, do no harm'), a religious creed like the Ten Commandments ('Thou Shalt not kill ...') or wise aphorisms like the sayings of Confucius. This is the most common way of defining 'ethics': norms for conduct that distinguish between acceptable and unacceptable behaviour.

THE EVOLUTION OF ETHICAL RESEARCH PRINCIPLES

Codes of conduct and systems of ethical review and oversight of health-related research evolved in the 20th century as a result of a series of serious human rights violations. Past unethical research studies, where uninformed and unaware individuals were exposed to disease or were subject to unproven and dangerous experiments, signalled the need for rules governing the design and conduct of human research. The Nuremberg Code was developed after WWII when evidence was discovered of gross research experiments conducted on prisoners in Nuremberg Nazi concentration camps (Barrow et al 2022). This landmark ethical code offered a set of ethical principles that were intended to apply to all future international research involving human participants. Despite wide promotion of this strong ethical guidance statement, in the decades since the establishment of the Nuremberg Code other highly unethical research involving humans has been conducted, including: the Vipeholm human experiments, sponsored by the sugar industry and conducted in a Swedish mental hospital during the mid 1940s with patients provided with excessive sugar to provoke dental caries (Gustafsson et al 1953); Milgram's (1963) experiments on obedience to authority involving members of the general public; Zimbardo's (1972) Stanford prison experiment on the effects of dehumanising social control; and the infamous 'Tuskegee Syphilis Trial' where members of a large community of African-American people in southern USA with syphilis were not informed of this infection so that its natural progression could be studied (Kampmeier 1974, Tuskegee Syphilis Study Legacy Committee 1996). From these much more recent travesties it is clear that the lessons and principles applied from the Nuremberg Code required considerable strengthening.

International efforts to reach agreement on what constitutes ethical conduct in health research culminated in the *Declaration of Helsinki*, which was adopted by the World Medical Association in 1964 and has been modified over ensuing decades. The declaration provides advice regarding the design and performance of a research study and mandates that research be clearly formulated in a protocol and then submitted to an *independent ethics committee* for review, comment, guidance and approval. The most recent version of the *Declaration of Helsinki* (World Medical Association 2013) contains the initial key ethical principles that were developed to expand the Nuremberg Code and also incorporates earlier versions of the *Declaration of Helsinki*. Among the ethical principles it stipulates are the medical researcher's duty to protect the life, health, privacy, autonomy and dignity of human participants (World Medical Association 2023).

However, even when countries are signatories to such high-level international agreements, unethical research practices can still occur. This is evidenced by the unethical experiments, referred to as the 'Green Experiments', which commenced in 1966 at the National Women's Hospital in Auckland, New Zealand, but which were not exposed and investigated until the 1980s (Cartwright 1988). The Cartwright Inquiry investigated a two-armed natural history study that aimed to determine the extent to which untreated carcinoma-in-situ progressed to become invasive carcinoma. Green (1969) hypothesised that carcinoma-in-situ did not lead to invasive cervical cancer, despite there being compelling evidence to the contrary. Unfortunately, the women with carcinoma-in-situ who were not treated after 2 years of follow-up had four times the risk of developing invasive cancer, causing many to die prematurely (McIndoe et al 1984). At the time this study was conducted, the National Women's Hospital in Auckland had the necessary institutional mechanisms in place to promote accountability on the part of clinical researchers. Green's research proposal was reviewed and approved by two committees (Jones 2017). Despite ethical concerns being raised about this natural history study of carcinoma-in-situ with senior hospital leaders, including the medical superintendent, hospital board and superintendent-in-chief, and concerns about this seriously unethical research being published in an international medical journal (McIndoe et al 1984), Green's research was allowed to continue (Batt 2017). It is unclear why the hospital leadership with the authority to intervene failed to act when it was clear that the health, wellbeing and survival of these women were in serious jeopardy (Jones 2017).

The Cartwright Inquiry found that the National Women's Hospital Board, senior clinicians and professors, particularly head of the Board, were all implicated, with this investigation leading to a number of human research ethics reforms (Cartwright 1988). The Inquiry noted the reluctance of other healthcare professionals to impinge upon the clinical freedom of their research colleagues as one explanation of the failure to address ethical concerns about the Green Experiments (Cartwright 1988). Such reluctance draws attention to the responsibilities of all professionals to be rigorous in assessing evidence and to defend and protect the instantiation of an ethical culture within the workplace.

In an effort to prevent further unethical biomedical research, the United Nations Educational, Scientific and Cultural Organisation (UNESCO) requires adherence to standards of integrity, responsibility and accountability in human research; the most recently adopted international declaration being the *Universal Declaration on Bioethics and Human Rights* (United Nations Educational 2005). This UNESCO Declaration provides a universal framework of principles and procedures to guide countries in developing relevant legislation, policies and ethical review committees. It also sets out the responsibilities of individuals, groups, communities, institutions and public and private corporations involved in bioethics, promotes respect for human dignity and upholds the protection of human rights and fundamental freedoms. Core principles of the UNESCO Declaration are: (1) respect for autonomy and individual responsibility (informed consent); (2) respect for privacy, anonymity and confidentiality; (3) respect for justice, beneficence; (4) respect for human vulnerability and personal integrity; and (5) respect for cultural diversity. These core principles are instantiated in relevant materials produced in many countries that support the UNESCO Declaration.

LEGAL AND ETHICAL REGULATORY MECHANISMS IN AUSTRALIA AND NEW ZEALAND

In both Australia and New Zealand, research-focused law reflects concerns about traditional areas, such as: informed consent, contractual obligation, negligent action and intellectual property rights (copyright). Other laws extend well beyond the domain of research, such as those concerned with privacy and human rights laws, but these also have important implications for the conduct of research and associated relationships. While there is international agreement about core ethical considerations applying to all research involving humans, adherence to the guidelines has not always been strict.

For instance, evidence emerged during the Cartwright Inquiry (Cartwright 1988) in New Zealand that the institutional committee overseeing the research failed to adequately review the scientific merit of the study and protect participants. The establishment of national ethical standards and review by independent human research ethical committees for all health research proposals and experimental treatments were two of the key recommendations to emerge from the Cartwright Inquiry. These recommendations have subsequently been reflected in the legislation and national policies of other countries, either because of unethical research practices and/or to strengthen human rights and health-related legislation that affords greater protection to research participants. Consequently, in accordance with the *Declaration of Helsinki*, a growing number of countries have specific laws governing the establishment and regulation of public research funding and/or monitoring agencies. This *Declaration of Helsinki* provided a template for the regulation of ethical conduct of research in Australia and New Zealand, which motivated the establishment of the Australian National Health and Medical Research Council (NHMRC), a statutory body operating in accordance with the *National Health and Medical Research Council Act 1992* (NHMRC Act 1992) and responsible for funding, monitoring and providing guidelines for ethical research (NHMRC 2018, 2023). Meanwhile, in New Zealand the Health Research Council (HRC) was established and charged with monitoring public research and providing ethical guidelines (Health Research Council of New Zealand 2010, 2021). The HRC operates under the *Health Research Council Act 1990* (Health Research Council Act 1990) and is responsible to the Minister of Health for, among other things, the maintenance of an ethical and safe health research environment.

The imperatives of the *Declaration of Helsinki* have been reflected in all versions of the Australian National Health and Medical Research Council's *Statement on Human*

Experimentation, since its initial publication in 1966, and are also reflected in the new *National Statement on Ethical Conduct in Human Research* (NHMRC 2023), which provides the blueprint for overall governance of ethical research in Australia, offering guidelines for researchers, HRECs and those engaged in the ethical review of research.

Ethical Review of Research Involving Indigenous Peoples

Australia and New Zealand are multicultural nations that people of many nations call home. The astute researcher will contemplate the valued perspective that Indigenous Peoples bring to the creation of new knowledge with and about our communities, whether incidentally or as a focus of research. Specifically designed for health researchers, the CONSIDER statement lends an eight-part checklist for reporting research but is also valuable for structure, evaluating the ethical integrity of research literature and designing new studies (Huria et al 2019). The first three checklist items show alignment with respectful diversity for contributions, and these are *Governance*, *Prioritisation* and *Relationships*. 'Indigenous' is not a description used by all cultures and in New Zealand Māori are recognised as *tangata whenua* (the original inhabitants) of New Zealand, and the Treaty of Waitangi provides principles that are the foundation for activities like research (Waitangi Tribunal 2020). Indigenous to Australia are two recognised Indigenous Peoples: Australian Aboriginal and Torres Strait Islanders. Within the Aboriginal peoples there are also more than 300 distinct nations, all with their own traditions, stories, symbols, art works and languages (Jackson-Barrett et al 2015). Historically, Australian and New Zealand research may have been intended to be to the benefit of all peoples, often planned for reducing the disproportionately negative representation of Indigenous Peoples and social determinants of health, but ultimately created Western knowledge about Indigenous Peoples for the benefit of the researcher, an institution, a university or a political agenda. This meant that research was predominantly a 'silencing of Indigenous ways of knowing', where Western scientific processes that compared and contrasted individual people as objects of study at that point in time were valued above precolonisation knowledge (Wilson et al 2022). These research outcomes are of limited value as they omit the immensely valuable unique cultural ways of knowing that Indigenous Peoples hold and express the inseparable relationship of peoples and traditions, including ancestral, spiritual and country (environment) (Benveniste & King 2018). Research has been conducted 'on' participants instead of co-designed and researched 'with' Aboriginal and Torres Strait Islander peoples (NHMRC 2018a, 2023). In Australia the National Statement (NHMRC 2023) is supplemented with guidelines for researchers to seek approval from a Human Research Ethics Committee that ensures the rights of Aboriginal and Torres Strait Islander peoples are respected and upheld (NHMRC 2018a). The guidelines are value based and six principles frame research management with '*spirit and integrity*' being at the core and interlinked with '*cultural continuity*', '*equity*', '*reciprocity*', '*respect*' and '*responsibility*' (NHMRC 2018a). In New Zealand, statutes describe appropriate consultation, collaboration and co-design with Māori peoples, authorities and/or their representatives about research involving their communities or resources (*Guidelines for Researchers on Health Research Involving Māori* Version 2 (Health Research Council of New Zealand 2010) and *Te Ara Tika Guidelines for Māori Research Ethics: a framework for researchers and ethics committee members* (Health Research Council of New Zealand 2021)).

International Regulations and Guidance

In addition to these national initiatives, the *International Good Clinical Practice* (GCP) (International Council for Harmonisation of Technical Requirements for Pharmaceuticals for Human Use 2016) standard for the conduct and reporting of clinical trials also provides guidance that has wide applicability. The international GCP standard is reflected in the Australian Therapeutic Goods Administration (TGA) *Note for Guidance on Clinical Safety Data Management* and the *Australian Clinical Trial Handbook* (Therapeutic Goods Administration 2000, 2021) and the New Zealand Medicines and Medical Devices Safety Authority (MEDSAFE). These guidelines emphasise the need for: study procedures to be carefully documented so that they are transparent and auditable, standards for recording and managing data to minimise the possibility of fraud, and a plan to disseminate the research findings in the international Committee on Publication Ethics (or COPE) standards. The COPE standards include requirements for authors to declare any conflicts of interest and standards on what constitutes authorship and the responsibilities of authors (Committee on Publication Ethics 2019). These codes are relevant for all clinical trials, and particularly trials evaluating the effectiveness of pharmaceutical products or medical devices, which must be approved for use in Australia by the TGA and in New Zealand by the MEDSAFE. In addition, all researchers and those collecting data in human clinical trials need to be trained and certified in Good Clinical Practice (GCP) every 3 years prior to and throughout the life of the research.

Evaluating and Monitoring Ethical Issues in Nursing Research

Various national and international professional nursing organisations also have a role to play in guiding nurses and midwives in the practice of research, with the International Council of Nurses (2021) **code of ethics** '*The ICN Code of Ethics for Nurses*' applying to all Australian nurses, including researchers. The Australian Nursing and Midwifery Federation (ANMF 2019) policy statement on research provides additional guidance to nurses and midwives involved in research. These documents provide the structure for ensuring accountability for nursing and midwifery research for the profession and the community, and are complementary to *National Statement on Ethical Conduct in Human Research* (NHMRC 2023) guidelines. In New Zealand, any nurse considering research involving humans is advised to first view the National Ethics Advisory Committee Guidelines (Health and Disability Ethics Committees (HDECs) 2019) before proceeding with either a local (i.e. institutional) or a national (i.e. HDECs) ethics proposal.

APPLYING THE ETHICAL CODES AND STANDARDS TO LOCAL RESEARCH

In accordance with the international standard, all Australian research that directly involves humans (or animals) must be assessed, approved and monitored by a NHMRC-registered health or university **Human Research Ethics Committee (HREC)** before the research may proceed. Human research protocols are assessed using processes and documentation as high or low risk, in accordance with the degree of risk for participants, their private and health information or bodily samples, as determined by a presubmission checklist. The research can commence only when both the HREC has approved the research proposal and the health services (referred to as research 'sites') have determined that the research meets their governance conditions and management authorise that it can proceed. Continuing the research is conditional upon the submission by the researchers and approval from HREC of an annual compliance report.

A HREC is defined as a multidisciplinary, independent body charged with reviewing research involving human participants to ensure that their dignity, rights and welfare are protected. In Australia, the HRECs review research proposals that involve human participants to ensure that they meet ethical standards and guidelines. These guidelines include the *National Statement on Ethical Conduct in Human Research*, which requires human research to undergo ethics review, in addition to setting out the requirements for the establishment, operation and membership of HRECs (Day et al 2021).

The first function of HRECs is to identify ethical issues or concerns posed by research involving human participants. This is a necessity because if all the ethical issues posed by an application are not identified then the HREC may fail to adequately protect participants in research. It needs to identify ethical issues, which has several implications for the membership and functions of HRECs. To effectively identify possible ethical issues, the committee requires several different bodies of expertise and knowledge. Firstly, the committee needs to have members who are familiar with the research areas and methodologies which are likely to come before them. This will enable them to identify methodological issues or implications that the researchers might not have identified. Likewise, if there are risks involved in the research methodology which the researchers have failed to identify, then these members are vital for being able to identify them. Ideally this means members from several different research disciplines and areas of interest (Sivasubramaniam et al 2021).

Secondly, the committee ought to have representatives from those groups who are commonly recruited as research subjects. These members are useful as they will be alert to specific concerns raised through researching these particular groups. They provide the committee with a fresh perspective, from the point of view of the participant, and they may be sensitive to concerns that the committee might otherwise neglect. So, for example, students may be more sensitive to the inappropriate usage of class time for research purposes. Lay members, in general, can be helpful in identifying issues that experts might not be sensitive to, for example complicated information being presented only in confusing scientific jargon in the information sheet. While familiarity with research methodology is very useful for ethics committees to have, it can easily blind them to the issues that lay members will identify (Brown et al 2020).

Thirdly, members from four particular backgrounds can be useful for identifying specific ethically related issues with applications. Statisticians are useful to ensure that no more people than is necessary are exposed to the risks posed by the research, and that a sufficient number of participants are being recruited to allow for a meaningful analysis. Members with experience of working with children, such as paediatricians, teachers, social workers, etc., can be useful for being able to gauge how competent a particular cohort of minors is likely to be, together with the identification of any specific issues that might be raised by researching on children. Members with a legal background can be useful for identifying any potential legal issues posed by an application. Finally, members with a formal background in ethics can be useful for picking up on more subtle ethical issues, such as issues of justice. As there are a variety of ethical theories, someone who has a formal background in ethics can also be helpful in highlighting the ethical issues from a variety of ethical perspectives, whether or not they themselves identify with those particular perspectives.

A HREC also will attempt to reduce and resolve as many, and ideally all, of the identified ethical issues as possible. This involves suggesting ways that the research can be modified, without compromising the scientific validity of the study. Again, this requires members with familiarity with a wide variety of research design and methodology, so that realistic changes can be suggested that minimally compromise the science (Brown et al 2020).

Fig. 13.1 provides a hierarchical overview of how these international, national and local ethical standards and processes are applied to an individual study.

In assessing all human research ethics applications, the HREC is particularly concerned with assessing the research within a universal **human rights** framework that considers each of the following core principles of ethical research: research merit and integrity, researcher integrity and honesty, justice, beneficence, **respect for persons** and autonomy. These six core ethical research principles to which all clinical research design, review and conduct activities should adhere are described in detail below.

Research Merit and Integrity

Human participation in research can be ethically justified only if the research has merit, is appropriately designed to answer the research question and is conducted by researchers who demonstrate integrity and maintain the integrity of the research process. Human research includes not only the direct participation of people through interviews, surveys or observations, but also the use of their information and bodily samples. All human research must be justified by its potential benefits through a process of peer review and must

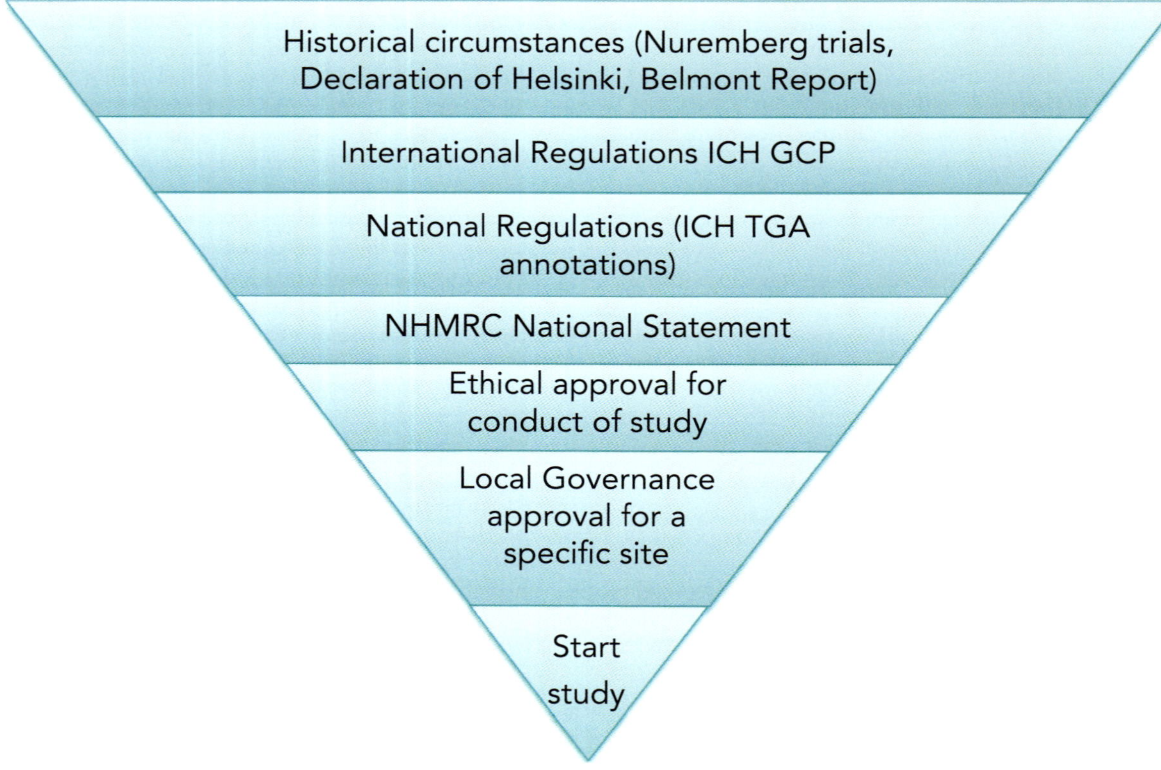

Fig. 13.1 Linkage between international, national and local ethical standards.

BOX 13.1 Criteria for Evaluating the Legal and Ethical Aspects of a Research Study

- Was the study approved by an ethics committee?
- Did participants receive full information about the purpose and nature of the study?
- What evidence is provided to indicate that informed consent was obtained from participants?
- Was the information written and discussed in a language and at the appropriate level of understanding of the participant?
- Did the researcher clearly explain any risks and their management?
- Did the researcher discuss the risk–benefit ratio?
- Did the researcher meet legal requirements?
- Is there any evidence of harassment, inducement or coercion during the consent process?
- How was the privacy of the participants maintained?
- What special protection was in place for vulnerable participants?
- Did participants have access to the results or findings of the research study?

be designed to respect and protect the individual participants. It is ethically unacceptable for people to be involved in poorly designed, badly conducted and/or dishonest research (NHMRC 2023). In the study protocol and accompanying ethics application, researchers are required to convince the HREC that their research is justifiable in that it addresses an identifiable knowledge gap, is designed to answer the research questions, has an appropriate and feasible sample size, will not expose participants to unnecessary risks or harms, and is conducted by a team with the required expertise and resources to complete the study. The detailed guidelines in Box 13.1 should assist the research consumer in evaluating the legal and ethical aspects of a research study (see also Chapter 15).

Researcher Integrity and Honesty

Researchers demonstrate integrity through the rigour of their search for new knowledge and understanding, their ability to adhere to accepted research principles and their commitment both to carry out the research honestly and to disseminate both positive and negative study results (NHMRC 2023). The integrity and honesty of a researcher is critical for the conduct, reporting and publication of reliable studies (Committee on Publication Ethics 2019). Research misconduct is evident in: *fabrication* of data or results; recording or reporting and/or *falsification* of research materials, equipment or processes; *changing or omitting* data or results such that the research is not accurately represented in the research record; and *plagiarism*, where appropriate recognition is not given to the appropriation of another person's ideas, processes, results or statements.

Research misconduct extends to include the inaccurate, false or incomplete publication and reporting of research (Wager & Kleinert 2021). In the US a definition excludes 'honest errors or differences of opinion', while another definition from the UK also includes researcher behaviours such as the misrepresentation of data, interests or involvement and failure to follow accepted procedures or to exercise due care in the handling of privileged or private information and the avoidance of unreasonable risk or harm (Holbeach et al 2023). There are many examples of the falsified claims of researchers (such as occurred in the falsification of data regarding the addictive nature of nicotine and the effects of passive smoking) within the pharmaceutical industry (as occurred in the infamous thalidomide scandal of the late 1950s and early 1960s), and unethical drug trials in Third World countries (as previously discussed). Australian and New Zealand examples of research misconduct exist, including data fabrication for a trial of the drug 'ramipril' that is used to control blood pressure and was subject to research to reduce pain in people with peripheral vascular disease amongst other studies, of which at least eight publications of research were found to be based on fabricated data and retracted (Retraction Watch 2016).

Concerns about the increasing incidence of scientific misconduct in research are reflected in the development in many countries of regulatory bodies to advise, monitor and oversee research projects involving humans, as noted above. More recently there have been a growing number of questions about pharmaceutical trials which have identified the damaging potential that conflicts of interest, whether economically or socially based, present for research involving humans (Gøtzsche 2019). Despite the considerable statutory and regulatory support and control that has been established, the continuing occurrence of scientific fraud and the failure of peer review processes continue to require careful attention and review (Holbeach et al 2023).

RESEARCH IN BRIEF 13.1

A survey of nursing research coordinators highlights the need for all nurses and midwives to be aware of the dangers of the potential for research misconduct in the clinical environment (Habermann et al 2010). Nurse research coordinators (n = 266) were invited to complete the 68-item Scientific Misconduct Questionnaire-Revised (SMQ-R), which looked at their perceptions of the workplace; the environment; the prevalence of scientific misconduct; their awareness of others about misconduct; and their reporting of misconduct, attitudes and beliefs about misconduct, and behavioural influences of misconduct (Habermann et al 2010). These participants suggested that scientific misconduct included: (a) misrepresenting data, (b) failing to explain data weaknesses, (c) selective reporting of results, (d) misuse of funds, (e) safety violations, (f) conflicts of interest, (g) agreements with sponsors not to publish data and (h) failing to obtain informed consent (Habermann et al 2010). Out of these domains, five major categories of misconduct were identified: protocol violations, consent violations, fabrication, falsification and financial conflict of interest (Habermann et al 2010). This study highlights the importance of nurses identifying and reporting scientific misconduct and why creating a safe environment where evidence of scientific misconduct is promptly reported and reviewed is critical.

The potential for ethically problematic relationships to arise between clinical researchers, including nurses and midwives, and the pharmaceutical and medical device industries is of increasing concern, in terms of both the sponsorship of research in which companies have a commercial interest and the conduct of relationships in which power imbalances are evident. It is not uncommon to find accusations of the selective reporting of research findings favourable to a corporation's products and of unspecified influence on the behaviour and attitudes of health professionals towards using and promoting such products. There are numerous examples of potential biases in nursing publications related to undeclared conflicts of interests (Lakeman 2010).

All nurses and midwives need to be aware that, despite the existence of stringent codes, unethical research practices persist; they must take all of the necessary steps to ensure that they are not implicated in charges of scientific misconduct, and they must report any evidence of scientific misconduct immediately. They need to be cognisant of what constitutes scientific misconduct and be clear about the mechanisms for reporting these transgressions (Habermann et al 2010). Organisations need to have the mechanisms in place as well as feedback loops for evidence review to ensure that research integrity is embedded in the culture of the local research environment (Habermann et al 2010).

TUTORIAL TRIGGER 13.1

- What might potentially drive a researcher or researchers to publish research that is based on corrupted data or offers misleading findings?
- Why shouldn't drug companies fund research on their own products, given that it may be beneficial not only to their target audience but also to themselves (e.g. in increased sales and profits)?
- If plagiarism is a growing problem in research reporting, do you think there should be some form of censorship or limited release on certain sensitive or nationally important research findings to stop others from stealing the ideas?
- You have been asked to investigate the experiences of Indigenous people within a large city hospital. What ethical considerations and approval processes would you need to follow to ensure that the principle of respect for cultural diversity was maintained in regard to obtaining participant consent?
- What steps should be taken to minimise any cultural harm during the data-gathering phase of the research process?

Justice

The ethical principle of **justice** requires fairness in dealing with others. It also acknowledges the broader concerns of justice in relation to research, such as recognising the responsibility of researchers to undertake research that might help explain health inequalities, or which might provide data on equitable access to healthcare. In research, it also means that participants must be provided with sufficient information to be able to give informed consent to their participation. The risks and benefits of the study must also be distributed fairly among participants and randomising participants in a controlled trial goes some way to achieving this. Research proposals, information sheets and consent forms should clearly explain the participant's involvement, the research procedures and the researcher's role and responsibilities. Research procedures should not change without the authorisation of the particular HREC and, when this is granted, further consent from the participants or participant is generally required. If the researcher promises certain benefits for participating in the study, these should be detailed and provided. Such benefits could include being sent a summary of the results or reimbursement of travel costs, but care is needed in this situation because payment of larger amounts could influence the person's decision and potentially be viewed as a possible bribe or inducement to participate.

Beneficence

The ethical principle of **beneficence** is based on the belief that the likely benefits of the research must outweigh any potential harms. People have the right to be protected from and not experience extraordinary exposure to the possibility of physical injury or discomfort, psychological injury or distress, social disadvantage, invasion of privacy or infringement of rights as a result of the research (NHMRC 2023). Researchers are required to consider and assess all of the possible risks and to devise a strategy to minimise or prevent any identified harms. While it may not be possible to remove all risks from the research process, strategies to minimise risks and explain possible benefits need to be outlined in the research protocol and ethics application. If a research topic or line of research questioning is likely to induce painful emotions or to be psychologically disturbing, such as inviting grandparents to be interviewed about their experience of losing a grandchild, the researcher must identify these harms prospectively. In addition to detailing these potentially distressing harms in the research protocol, these potential harms must also be outlined in the *Participant Information Sheet* along with the strategy for managing such harms; this may entail providing access to free counselling and to the contact details of a health professional/s that participants may wish to approach both during and after their participation in the study.

While it may not be possible to remove all risks from the research process, strategies to minimise risks and highlight possible benefits need to be outlined in the research protocol and detailed in the information provided to participants. This information may include: frequent monitoring of participants; presence of trained personnel who can respond to emergencies; coding of data to protect confidentiality; participant debriefing; continuing review and monitoring of data to ensure the study does not continue after the emergence of reliable evidence of reduced efficacy and/or safety, or actual harm to participants; exclusion of vulnerable individuals or groups from participating in research where necessary and justified; and consideration of whether alternative means for answering the research question are available, and whether participation by humans is really necessary (NHMRC 2023).

Some forms of research have the potential to produce a benefit to a person against the context of risk. For example, a person with advanced cancer might choose to be part of an experimental new treatment that offers some hope of disease control. However, in presenting the trial to the participant, neither the potential risks of the new experimental treatment nor the potential positive outcomes should be overstated. All prospective participants need to be fully informed about the study design, the experimental agent and the potential benefits and the probability of the associated risks.

The critical-thinking decision path diagram provides an example of the kind of ethical decision-making process that may be used by researchers and HREC members in evaluating the **risk/benefit** of a research study. If the risk–benefit ratio shows that the risks outweigh the benefits then it will be difficult to justify exposing participants to those risks. However, if the expected harms are minor then the study may be ethically and legally acceptable because the expected benefits outweigh these lesser harms (see Research in Brief 13.2). All risk/benefit information needs to be made clear to the participants before their consent is sought.

AN UNEXPECTED HURDLE

A school health nurse is part of a consortium of health professionals and interest groups intending to run a mental health and wellbeing campaign focusing on promoting mental health and reducing youth suicide at local high schools in a regional coastal community. Local school counsellors have provided anecdotal reports that suicidal thinking is common amongst local youth, and in the previous year there have been two suicides of young people that have rocked the local community. The nurse hopes to undertake a survey of young people to gauge the prevalence of suicidal thoughts within the local population and inform the discussion and campaign. Results will be fed back to the community of parents, teachers and students. An academic partner at the local university's School of Nursing and Midwifery is contributing to the study design. The academic expresses concern as to how members of the local ethics committee might be presented with material that might help them assess a project on a topic as sensitive as this one, with which they are likely to have had little experience.

Review the literature on talking about suicide and other sensitive topics. Beyond being equipped with the latest knowledge, which suggests that talking about suicide may be more beneficial than negative if handled sensitively, what can the researcher do to ensure that participants are safe and the ethics committee's concerns are addressed?

Respect for Persons, Their Vulnerability and Personal Integrity

Respect for each individual human being is a central tenet of human research ethics. It entails recognising the value of each individual and ensuring that all interactions are informed by that recognition (NHMRC 2023). Respect for persons requires that the individual's autonomy and capacity for self-determination and decision making is acknowledged. At the same time it requires that the interests of those with diminished or limited autonomy are protected and supported to ensure that they are not disempowered (NHMRC 2023). Potential research participants may include groups who are more susceptible to physical or psychological hurt or injury than others and hence are said to be vulnerable. Such people have diminished or no capacity to protect themselves from threats to their safety or the maintenance of their sense of personal integrity. Respect for personal integrity involves attempting to enhance the person's self-identity, paying attention to their status as subjects of experience, acknowledging who they are, and treating them with courtesy and in a way that acknowledges their worth.

Researchers in the past have recruited participants from the most vulnerable groups in society, such as the homeless, refugees, prisoners, gay men, children with intellectual disability, dying patients and ethnic minorities. Other vulnerable groups may include pregnant women, children and servicemen/women (or members of other organisations where strict hierarchy and regulatory procedures exist for 'following orders'). Overall, members of vulnerable groups have at times been treated badly by researchers; their vulnerability and sense of personal integrity have not always been respected.

Overall, involvement of vulnerable groups is not a prohibited activity as long as this is done with regard to the other core principles of conducting research, and with respect for their own personal integrity, such as appropriate consideration of consent procedures and putting into place measures to ensure they are protected if their own decision making is impaired. Concerns over the abuse of vulnerable populations in research projects have continued to emerge over the last few decades. For instance, in the 1960s Beecher (1966) published an article describing many examples of unethical or questionable behaviour in ethical studies involving various vulnerable populations. While the World Medical Association has long recommended that prisoners, being a captive population, should not be used as participants in experiments, researchers have disregarded this advice. In the 1970s it was discovered that drug companies and doctors in the United States involved prisoners in clinical experiments without informed consent, showing a 'wilful disregard' for human rights (Mitford 1973).

RESEARCH IN BRIEF 13.2

In 1996, a severe African meningitis epidemic hit Nigeria's northern states. The infectious diseases hospital in Kano State was overwhelmed because they were dealing with a measles and cholera outbreak as well. Children were being seen and treated in overcrowded halls and corridors, and the situation was described as 'chaotic'. One of the world's biggest pharmaceutical companies provided support to this struggling health service by flying in US doctors to conduct a trial of a new oral antibiotic for children with meningitis against the 'gold-standard' treatment. The team took over part of the hospital and delivered the drugs to 200 children, treating half with the new antibiotic and the other half with the recommended antibiotic. After the drug trial, the pharmaceutical company left, leaving behind some surplus drugs and equipment for the hospital. Doctors at the hospital were shocked that the company doctors were prepared to continue the research trial under such dire conditions (Boseley & Smith 2010).

TUTORIAL TRIGGER 13.2

- Should we always exclude any member of a vulnerable population from being a research subject?
- Sometimes it is argued that to do good we should accept the possibility of harm, as perhaps in the case of drug trials when there may be a degree of discomfort or unease for at least some of the subjects, but the benefits for the majority are considerable. If people are prepared to take that risk, why should we still be concerned?
- Should we ever involve participants from a 'vulnerable population' in any form of research that carries any possible risk for them?
- If children of any age are to be involved in research, shouldn't they be given the chance to accept or reject participation?
- Should those in poorer countries be used as unwilling or even willing subjects in research projects that may produce future benefits for those in richer countries?

Respect for Cultural Diversity

An individual's sense of identity and values are in part informed by membership of different groups within society, which may be distinguished by particular cultural features, ethnicity, sexual orientation, religious affiliation, employment status, disability or age. In every country (and especially in this instance in Australia and New Zealand) a wide array of culturally diverse and complex social groups exists among their respective populations. This is usually considered to be both a normal and a desirable social phenomenon since, as the UNESCO charter puts it: 'together the cultures of the world create a rich and varied tapestry'. The resulting **cultural diversity** 'expands choices, nurtures a variety of skills, human values and worldviews and provides wisdom from the past to inform the future' (United Nations Educational 2019). Yet such diversity sometimes leads to the possibility of research that reveals unintentional but problematic cultural ignorance, indifference or even bias; accordingly, anyone who wishes to perform research involving a particular group of individuals within society should be mindful of the requirement of respect for cultural diversity.

Such respect in matters relating to research begins and ends with careful and well-informed ethical consideration of all aspects of the project. Close attention needs to be given to the aforementioned ethical principles, and every aspect of the research needs to be rigorously scrutinised. Understanding and observing cultural norms, including what is culturally and linguistically salient, is vital to the successful conduction of a research study. Researchers may collaborate with members of the community being researched in order to check whether the research tools are appropriate and acceptable. Incorporating the viewpoint of the study community from the outset can improve participation and decrease research bias (Broesch et al 2020).

This is primarily because 'the effect of cultural indifference and ignorance is sometimes perceived as being disrespectful of not just the individual, but of others within that individual's cultural group, who, like Māori, may feel that their cultural identity has been "trampled upon"' (Woods 2010 p. 720). Similar sentiments have been expressed in Australia, where Aboriginal and Torres Strait Islander peoples feel that they are the most studied population in the land, but yet they remain 'generally cynical about the benefits of research and cautious towards what many perceive to be the colonial mentality or "positional superiority" ingrained in the psyche of western researchers' (Prior 2007). Members of various culturally and linguistically diverse communities in Australia and New Zealand (e.g. Pacific peoples, and Asian, Middle Eastern, Latin American, African and Continental European groups, as well as those with refugee and migrant backgrounds, international students, tourists and international visitors) may also be overlooked or poorly treated by researchers. In part, such communities may be overlooked by some researchers simply because English is not their first language and researchers conclude that they may not be able to answer questions with sufficient understanding, clarity or depth. Greater efforts need to be made to ensure that such communities are not overlooked simply on the basis of potential linguistic difficulties; researchers ought to factor into the research the costs of funding the translation of patient information material, consent forms and other study material into the appropriate languages, as well as the provision of interpreter access.

Although awareness of cultural differences that distinguish Indigenous Peoples has increased worldwide following attention from international human rights bodies, Indigenous cultural values have had little influence in shaping research agendas or methods of inquiry.

Research involving Indigenous Peoples presents additional ethical concerns because these groups may be especially vulnerable to the effects of poorly planned and inconsiderate research projects. In the past at least, such groups have often experienced the harmful effects of researcher indifference or ignorance towards their culturally sensitive ideas and practices, and this type of research has often clearly benefited the researcher more than the Indigenous Peoples who were studied. Consequently, conventional ethical procedures may not be appropriate for Indigenous Peoples because these have the potential to further disable the aspirations and integrity of those who are the focus of the research (Report of the Global Forum on Bioethics in Research 2008).

The Indigenous Peoples of both Australia and New Zealand have lobbied their respective governments and scientific communities to protect them from exploitation by researchers. As a result, guidelines for research with Indigenous Peoples now require not just respect for those cultures, but also increased mindfulness of values such as spirit and integrity, reciprocity, equality, survival, protection and responsibility (NHMRC 2023). In Australia and New Zealand, research involving Indigenous populations is governed by separate guidelines (Health Research Council of New Zealand 2010, 2021, NHMRC 2023). Consultation provides the means of establishing cooperative, collaborative and ethical working relationships between researchers and Indigenous organisations and groups.

Respect for Autonomy and Individual Responsibility (Informed Consent)

As noted above, respecting the **autonomy** of persons (their freedom to determine their own actions) acknowledges their right to make their own choices. More specifically, it acknowledges their right to hold views and to make decisions about what happens to them based on their personal values and beliefs. Individuals can exercise their autonomy only if they are free from coercion, undue influence and external restraint when making decisions. Researchers need to be respectful of the rights of participants and others, and to act to protect their autonomy (Beauchamp & Childress 2019). This means ensuring that the participant, their carers and/or persons responsible for them understand: who is leading the study and what their interests are, what the study is about and what it hopes to measure, what is involved if they agree to participate, what the risks and benefits are, how their rights and interests are protected, and any other information relevant to making an informed decision. This information is conveyed to potential participants by the lead researcher or their nominee (e.g. a study nurse). If the investigator of the study also provides direct care to the potential participant, special measures should be put in place to reduce any pressure (coercion, perceived or otherwise) for the person to agree to participate. Having another member of the research team, such as a study nurse or project officer, complete the consent process can enable the potential participant to openly consider the study. If the person is interested in the study, they are then provided with plain language information (usually in written form) and given an opportunity to ask additional questions and to think about participating in the study. They may then be asked to provide a written consent form before the study can commence, but this is not always the case and procedure can vary depending on the nature of the study. The ability to make informed decisions about participating in a study is demonstrated when an individual: (i) understands all of the issues involved in the decision including the research protocol and the risks and benefits of participation or non-participation, (ii) is capable of rationally manipulating this information, (iii) appreciates the information in the context of a patient's situation, (iv) recognises the demonstrable consistency in this process and (v) shows evidence of a voluntary and uncoerced choice (Appelbaum & Roth 1982).

This process works well for people whose first language is English, and who have good health literacy, are cognitively intact and have the capacity to provide written consent. However, seeking written consent is challenging where people may have poor literacy skills, an inadequate understanding of the research proposal owing to their age, disability or cognitive impairment, or where they find themselves in a challenging situation, such as when admitted unconscious to an intensive care unit, facing death in a palliative care unit or unable to provide consent themselves, as is the case when recruiting children into studies. Nevertheless, participants must be satisfied that all of their questions have been answered, be made aware of their right to withdraw from the study without prejudice (i.e. without adversely affecting their healthcare experience) and be allowed sufficient time for discussion with their family or significant others. In situations where written consent is not an option, other approaches can be considered, such as using an interpreter in the participant's preferred language (dialect), using a witness to confirm a verbal process was followed, using a proxy or third party consent process, and others described in further detail below.

Understanding and consent often need to be revisited, particularly if the research involves multiple study visits, procedures and/or in-depth interviews. The elements of **informed consent** listed in Boxes 13.2 and 13.3 ensure respect for autonomy and individual responsibility, and are reflected in the participant's information sheet provided to all those persons interested in the study. An example of a typical, simplified information sheet and consent form that may be used prior to any research project appears in Appendices 1 and 2, respectively. Some HRECs have a combined Participant Information Consent Form (PICF) and consent form, which can extend to several pages depending upon the nature of the research.

Australian common law and some statutes presume that an individual aged over 18 years (an 'adult') is competent, unless proven otherwise, whereas the reverse is presumed for minors aged less than 18 years (Purser & Rosenfeld 2014). A researcher must therefore be satisfied that potential study participants have capacity and are competent to consent before seeking their consent to participate. They will demonstrate these capacities by being able to maintain and communicate a choice, understand the relevant information, appreciate the situation and its consequences, and manipulate the information in a rational fashion (Agar et al 2013).

BOX 13.2 Elements of Informed Consent

- Title of agency (e.g. hospital, university, funding agency)
- Invitation to participate
- Basis for participant selection
- Study purpose or aim
- Explanation of procedures
- Description of potential risks and discomforts
- Access to treatment and compensation if injury occurs
- Explanation of potential benefits
- Voluntary participation
- Right to withdraw from the study
- Assurance of confidentiality and anonymity
- Conflicts of interest declared
- Offer to answer questions to the satisfaction of the participant
- Names and contact details for researchers, hospital or university involved and ethics liaison officer/ethics committee administrator
- Concluding consent statement or separate consent form (see Appendix 2)

BOX 13.3 Elements of Informed Consent in Research Involving Children

When inviting children to participate in any research, the investigator must ensure that the children, and where appropriate the children's parents, guardians or caregivers, have been fully informed about the research in a manner appropriate to their needs.

a. Each child must be given full information about the research in a form that he or she can readily understand.
b. Children must be advised of their right to decline participation and their right to withdraw from the research at any time without giving a reason.
c. Investigators must give the children an opportunity to ask questions and to have those questions answered to the children's satisfaction.
d. If proxy consent is required, the person giving proxy consent must also be given full information about the research and be advised of the child's right to decline participation or withdraw from the research at any time.
e. The person giving proxy consent must be given an opportunity to ask questions and have them answered to their satisfaction.

(From Peart, N., Holdaway, D., 2000. Ethical guidelines for health research with children. N. Z. Bioethics J. 1 (2), 3–9.)

A competent potential study participant will understand sufficiently what the proposed study involves, and be able to arrive at a decision about participation and clearly communicate that decision. In the case of both nursing and midwifery research, such practices should obviously be closely adhered to but, in the latter case, midwives need to be aware that any disclosure of information must include benefits and risks and details of participation for both the woman and the fetus (Ledward 2011).

While learning disabilities, stroke, dementia and mental illness may all affect a person's decision-making capacity, they do not necessarily mean that the person is not competent to consent (Etieyibo 2013, Simpson 2010). Given that capacity to consent is presumed, potential study participants would be considered 'incompetent to consent' only if they were unable to comprehend and retain the necessary information about the study procedure or treatment and were unable to weigh the information, balancing the risks and needs required to arrive at an informed choice (Keenan 2010). If a potential participant is found to be incompetent to consent, the study protocol approved by the HREC may allow researchers to seek proxy consent from someone with lawful authority to consent on the potential participant's behalf. Otherwise, the person will need to be excluded from participating (as required within a 'protection model' of consent). It is potentially possible to obtain informed consent using one of the following five differing approaches:

1. Gaining informed consent at the time of enrolment, ensuring that information on the risks and benefits of participation in the context of the person's current situation is included;
2. Gaining informed consent in advance of having the condition to be investigated, whereby the person is identified as being at risk of developing the index condition, but since that development will necessarily impact adversely on their capacity to consent, they consent in advance of developing the condition. An example of this is a study investigating the management of excessive respiratory tract secretions at the end of life. As it is difficult to predict which dying patients might experience this condition, a study could propose to assume consent by all patients with capacity admitted to a hospice for terminal care;
3. Deferring the procuring of consent, which applies in situations where the person receives the information after study participation. This type of consent is frequently used in emergency and critical care studies, but in fact there are few palliative care studies where this consent process could be justified, given that it jeopardises voluntary participation and risks over-inclusion in studies;
4. Gaining consent via proxy/person responsible in accordance with the laws of the relevant country of jurisdiction, where those laws allow for a named proxy (not necessarily the next-of-kin) to provide consent on behalf of a person who lacks capacity to provide informed consent, such as a person with dementia or delirium; or
5. Waiving consent in cases in which no information is provided to the participant, but the study has been approved by a local ethics committee. Approval to waiver consent has been largely limited to studies evaluating interventions to improve cardiac arrests and acute brain injury outcomes (Agar et al 2013).

Selecting the most appropriate method for obtaining informed consent and aligning the consent process with the source of vulnerability and level of risk requires researchers to carefully work through these consent challenges so as to ensure the broadest participation possible. To omit the possible involvement of any person from a 'vulnerable population' may be more, rather than less, detrimental to their overall wellbeing, as well as to their value within and to society (see later discussion on vulnerable populations). This also systematically excludes specific populations from participating in research and having their care based on high levels of research evidence. Also, some forms of research carry negligible risk but may confer considerable potential benefit on participants and, while rarely acknowledged, people often value the opportunity to contribute to research for altruistic reasons (Lakeman et al 2013). This is particularly the case for many palliative care participants, who often want to participate for altruistic reasons rather than any personal gain (White & Hardy 2010).

In Australia, the most comprehensive guidelines for the ethical conduct of research, and informed consent in particular, are those provided by the National Health and Medical Research Council (NHMRC) as noted above, in the form of the *National Statement on Ethical Conduct in Human Research* (NHMRC 2023) and the *Australian Code for the Responsible Conduct of Research* (NHMRC 2018b); and in specific national guidelines for Aboriginal and Torres Strait Islander communities, also covered by NHMRC (2018a). It has also been noted that similar documents are produced by the New Zealand Health Research Council (HRC 2010, 2021).

Obtaining Informed Consent for a Child's Participation in Research

Legal requirements related to a child's participation in research may vary from country to country, but there are usually strict guidelines for consent to medical procedures that act as a general guide. For instance, the legal age of adults in most Australian jurisdictions is 18 years, and so, for children under this age, consent from a parent or guardian is also required (Law Library of Congress 2007). In New Zealand, children over the age of 16 years are considered legal adults and able to give full consent for medical and/or research purposes, although under the Code of Health and Disability Services Consumers' Rights (Health and Disability Commissioner 1996), people under 16 years of age are not automatically prevented from consenting to medical, nursing or midwifery procedures, and doctors, nurses or midwives must assess each child's competency to decide whether he or she is able to give informed consent. The common law position relating to a minor's competency to consent to treatment was established by the English House of Lords decision in *Gillick v West Norfolk and Wisbech Area Health Authority [1986]* AC 112. This decision was approved by the High Court of Australia in *Secretary, Department of Health and Community Services v JWB and SMB (1992)* (Marion's case) 175 CLR 218; in Gillick, it was held that the authority of a parent decreases as their child becomes increasingly competent (Griffith 2016). Gillick prescribes that the parental right to determine their child's treatment terminates once a child under the age of 16 is capable of fully understanding the medical treatment proposed. Whether a particular child has the requisite intelligence and understanding to give a valid consent is held to be a question of fact (Griffith 2016). Although Gillick holds that a minor who has a requisite level of understanding may consent to treatment, this does not amount to a corresponding right to refuse treatment (Griffith 2016). Hence, an adolescent who is competent according to the principles established by Gillick will generally lack the capacity to refuse life-saving treatment if his/her parents are prepared to consent to it (Griffith 2016). Subsequently, child consent issues in research are considered major *ethical* issues in both Australia (the *National Statement on Ethical Conduct in Human Research* (NHMRC 2023)) and New Zealand (*Guidelines for Health Research with Children* (Ministry of Health 2007)), where considerable attention is paid to the informed consent considerations that must apply to this vulnerable group. However, all research proposals, regardless of approach, should state how consent will be obtained from potential participants.

In some cases, it may not be appropriate to gain consent in writing, such as when informal data collection methods are to be used, as sometimes happens in neighbourhood or community studies or as previously indicated, when participants in the research are illiterate or semiliterate. Other possibilities may include situations where cultural issues arise, where the research involves a sensitive issue (e.g. illegal or stigmatised activities) or where the participant's vulnerability to exposure of significant harm would increase should their identity be accidentally revealed. On the other hand, obtaining consent in research using 'naturalistic inquiry' methods, such as ethnography, might potentially lead to behavioural changes that might invalidate the study. As a result, there is debate as to whether or not researchers should inform the (prospective) observed group beforehand (Monahan & Fisher 2010). As a rule, and being mindful of what is sometimes called the 'researcher effect' or 'Hawthorne effect' (see Chapters 6 and 9), which describes the threat to the validity or accuracy of a study that can occur because of the changed behaviours of those being observed, it remains necessary to proceed with care if and when deception of any kind is being proposed within a research project. An individual's right to autonomy may be violated through coercion (force), covert (secret) data collection and/or deception (see Box 13.4). It should also be noted that there are at least some situations where it is ethically acceptable to proceed with a research project without obtaining consent from participants—for example, when the research design involves minimal risk and it is not practicable to obtain consent from each participant, such as observational surveys of the use of helmets by cyclists or seatbelts by passengers in cars. Similarly, consent is not required in the case of non-identifiable data in epidemiological research, anonymous surveys or

BOX 13.4 How an Individual's Right to Autonomy May Be Violated in a Research Project

- *Coercion* involves offering a significant reward or threatening some harm if the person does not participate. For example, students may feel pressure to participate in research conducted by academics to ensure good grades.
- *Covert data collection* occurs when participants are unaware that research data are being collected. Although covert observation and data collection may be considered acceptable if undertaken in a public place, the recording of some types of activity could have harmful consequences for the individuals being observed—especially if the activity is illegal.
- *Deception* involves misinforming participants about the nature and purpose of any intended or actual research. While it may be argued that some research designs necessarily involve some form of deception, it is still important that participants are not significantly misled or misinformed.

retrospective audits based on statistical data, rather than individual details.

In conclusion, respect for the autonomy of research participants is a complex but vitally important ethical issue.

Respect for Privacy, Anonymity and Confidentiality

Privacy

Respect for **privacy** concerns a person's right to have personal information concealed and protected from wide or public distribution by researchers. It is both a legal and an ethical requirement in Australia and New Zealand. In Australia, the *Privacy Amendment (Private Sector) Act 2000* protects personal information held by private sector organisations. Most Australian states and territories have also enacted privacy legislation that applies to state public sectors and in some cases the private sector as well. As a result, Australian researchers must access the laws on privacy relevant to their state or territory as well as the Information Privacy Principles (IPPs), which apply to the Commonwealth public sector, and the National Privacy Principles (NPPs), which apply to the private sector. In New Zealand, the *Privacy Act 1993* and its related Health Information Privacy Code 1994 apply to health and disability agencies and organisations in both the public and the private sectors (Privacy Commissioner 2020), so that any health-related research project in New Zealand is protected by privacy legislation. This legislation indicates, among other things, that personal information must be kept confidential, responses and personal details may be removed from the data if required, anonymity will be maintained (unless this is not possible) and personal information will be stored in a secure place. Ethically and legally speaking, respecting the privacy of individuals in research involves protecting their anonymity and keeping their information confidential. For example, Hilliard and O'Neill's (2010) study aimed to explore the emotions experienced by children's nurses when caring for children with burns. In accordance with privacy provisions, the nurses were advised in writing that participation was voluntary and that their anonymity and confidentiality would be preserved. Written consent was also obtained.

A source of conflict can arise when a member of the research team is also a member of the clinical team; issues related to privacy need to be clearly delineated. Researchers need to be very much aware of the need to access information as a member of the clinical team, and the separate need to access information as a member of the research team. For example, the clinical team can access the medical record of patients in order to locate pertinent clinical or personal information, but this same information cannot be accessed by the research team without the permission of the patient. If a researcher is provided with the name of a person who might be suitable for a current clinical trial and the researcher is not able to then access the medical record in order to locate a contact number, both the clinician and the researcher may have violated the privacy principles in this process. The patient will need to have been asked, and given express permission to the clinical team member, for that information to be accessed. Indeed, all patients need to have a very clear explanation as to where usual clinical care crosses to research in order to consider the boundary and the implications for their privacy.

Anonymity

Complete **anonymity** ensures that no person, not even the researcher, will be able to identify individuals participating in a study. In qualitative research, protecting anonymity can be more challenging because the researcher meets the participant face-to-face and needs to develop rapport (a relationship) with the participant in order to obtain information. This may also be the case in quantitative research. However, the participant's anonymity can be protected by using assumed names (pseudonyms) and, in any event, the research itself is written up in a fashion that protects the confidentiality and anonymity of each participant. For example, a recent phenomenological qualitative study aimed to provide insights into younger women's experiences of recovery from cancer-related breast surgery (Elmir et al 2010).

Given the small number of participants ($n = 4$), a pseudonym was used to identify each participant and to protect her identity. The researchers presented the findings in such a way as to disguise any possible connection to any personal or identifying details of any of the four individuals (Elmir et al 2010).

However, it is difficult to guarantee absolute anonymity in some research projects, especially those involving a very small group of individuals within an agency or geographical area where personal traits or identifiable responsibilities may be recognised by others within the same boundaries. This issue is a particular problem in smaller towns, localised neighbourhoods or communities where the small population and the likelihood of personal traits or activities being recognised by others may have consequences for a research participant. People who live in close proximity share so many aspects of life that research narratives may give clues to an individual's identity; in some cases, even identifying a participant's gender could compromise their privacy.

Where maintaining the privacy of organisations and participants becomes particularly challenging, the use of pseudonyms may not be sufficient. In such cases, it is recommended that the possibility of the participants' identities becoming known should be discussed with them as part of the process of gaining informed consent. While some participants will not be concerned with this, the possibility may prevent others from participating. However, the essential requirement in all such cases is the achievement of informed consent, where all of the possible advantages and disadvantages of the proposed research are made clear at the start.

Confidentiality

Maintaining **confidentiality** means that the identities of research participants will not be linked to the information they provide and, therefore, measures must be taken at all stages of a research project, including the obtaining of data, its analysis and its storage, to ensure that the identities of participants are not revealed to others. In qualitative research, maintaining confidentiality can be challenging. For example, a participant's name should not be recorded on an audiotaped interview; consequently, if someone other than the researcher will be transcribing the interview, the participant has a right to know this and to be assured that the person transcribing will sign a confidentiality declaration. If another researcher will be examining the data to confirm the credibility of the study findings, participants should be told this when their consent is being sought.

The basic requirement of protecting participants' identities by keeping the information they provide confidential applies equally to quantitative research, although the confidentiality issues are generally less problematic in research that focuses on statistics and aggregated data, rather than on material obtained through in-depth interviews, etc. However, even then, sufficient attention needs to be paid to the need for adequate confidentiality measures in such research. It is always possible that, while particular individuals may not be recognisable, certain groups of people in a particular situation or institution may be, and the researcher has to consider the role of the group within the institution, and the relationship of its members with fellow healthcare professionals. This is particularly the case when researchers are investigating their own professional group within the shared workplace (see 'Research in brief 13.3').

RESEARCH IN BRIEF 13.3

A team of midwives explored the challenges of conducting an observational study of postnatal interactions between midwives ($n = 40$) and breastfeeding ($n = 78$) women in two maternity units in New South Wales, Australia (Burns et al 2012). The duality of being both a midwife and a researcher highlighted the influence and challenges of 'identity' and 'insider' knowledge on the conduct of the research. While possessing 'insider' midwifery knowledge was advantageous in the initial 'getting in' and 'fitting in' phases of the study, unanticipated role ambiguity and moral and ethical challenges arose as a result of this 'insider' knowledge and status (Burns et al 2012). Ethical problems emerged associated with: the level of 'participating' and 'observing' that the midwife researcher could engage in, overidentification with midwifery participants, and feelings of betrayal of participant trust, regardless of the level of insider or outsider positioning (Burns et al 2012).

TUTORIAL TRIGGER 13.3

- Why is it that the principle of autonomy and an individual's right to choose are deemed to be so important in research?
- Do you think that the autonomy principle is universally desirable, or are there some people, in at least some parts of the world, who might prefer or be happy to surrender such individualised autonomy for the sake of the collective or the state?
- Consider the potentially unwanted effects of participants being made aware that they are taking part in research. Would a degree of considered deception lead to greater accuracy of the results?
- Why should the privacy concerns of a few be so important when the proposed research may benefit so many others?
- Is it always possible in all research projects to maintain someone's anonymity?

To ensure they recognise and respect privacy, anonymity and confidentiality as important legal and ethical requirements, researchers must familiarise themselves with the specific legislative and regulatory requirements appropriate to their state and nation. Researchers must then consider the ways in which some participants are susceptible to exploitation and explore the need for other protective ethical principles, such as respect for justice, beneficence, human vulnerability and personal integrity.

The roles of both the general and the specific guidelines for the ethical conduct of research and the institutional research and ethics committees cannot be overstated; both are vitally important safeguards. Sometimes, research studies published in professional journals do not provide the research consumer with detailed information regarding the ways in which the research complied with ethical procedures. This does not necessarily mean that the research was unethical. In the absence of documentation regarding ethical issues, the acknowledgment that the research study was approved by an external HREC should assure the reader that the proposal was reviewed and permission given to proceed with the study. However, *all* published research should be carefully scrutinised for reasonable evidence of ethical soundness by the nurse or midwife reader because authors, editors and publishers all have ethical obligations with regard to the publication of the results of research. These obligations include a duty to make the results of their research on human subjects publicly available, and to be accountable for the completeness and accuracy of their reports (World Medical Association 2013).

Any published research that indicates HREC or even institutional ethics approval is incomplete or vague, or does not appear to consider research limitations or contain any negative or inconclusive results, is on that account to be suspect, although it may not necessarily be unethical. However, because it is possible that someone may wish to replicate a research project or act upon the findings of the research, it is important that the published research is trustworthy.

SUMMARY

All research projects involving humans are required to be submitted to their respective institutional ethics committees before the commencement of a project. These institutional ethics committees act in the interests of research participants in order to ensure the guidelines developed by the appropriate national authority are observed. It is important for nurses and midwives to understand exactly what is meant by, and entailed in, ensuring the rights of participants and other individuals (including themselves) in the research process. Also, as research consumers, nurses and midwives need to critically evaluate research studies in order to decide whether or not ethical and legal issues have been appropriately addressed.

Adhering closely to ethical principles and procedures is an inherent part of the research process. Researchers are duty bound to clearly include details of this process in their disseminated findings. Addressing ethical issues is a vital part of research design and an integral part of the overall research process.

KEY POINTS

- Internationally agreed ethical principles in research involving human participants are: respect for autonomy, respect for privacy, respect for justice, beneficence, respect for human vulnerability and integrity, and respect for cultural diversity.
- Informed consent procedures ensure the individual's autonomy and right to self-determination are respected.
- Respecting the privacy of individuals in research involves protecting their anonymity and treating their information as confidential.
- Research misconduct involves fabrication, falsification, plagiarism or other unacceptable practices.
- Some groups of people are more vulnerable to exploitation than others and require special protection; these include children, prisoners, service people, people with mental health and learning disability issues, and pregnant women.

TIME TO REFLECT

The following exercise is based on a hypothetical study.

Aim: To enhance your research ethics skills.

Objective: To enable you to more fully appreciate desirable ethical requirements when researching a vulnerable population.

Reflect on the following: You are a clinician working in an emergency department (ED) of a regional hospital. You notice that some ED attendees appear to present frequently in varying states of intoxication with a range of alcohol-related health problems. Some attend so frequently that they know you and other members of the healthcare team by name, yet others may attend only once and not again. You are interested in why these frequent attendees seem to fail to address their problematic alcohol use and you obtain a small grant to explore the experience of people who present to the ED in a state of intoxication, their utilisation of after-care services, and their post-ED presentation drinking patterns.

Continued

TIME TO REFLECT—cont'd

Questions

1. What research designs would address the broad objectives of the study?
2. What ethical problems may be associated with obtaining informed consent for participation in the study and how might they be addressed?
3. What ethical problems might arise given that you are both a clinician in ED and a researcher, and how might these be addressed?
4. How can confidentiality and anonymity be assured for participants?

LEARNING ACTIVITIES

1. When the researcher notifies a person of any proposed participation in research, which of the following ethical requirements is most being met?
   a. Respect for justice
   b. Respect for privacy
   c. Beneficence
   d. Respect for autonomy
2. The qualitative researcher used pseudonyms when quoting the participant's narrative in the published study, and so met the main requirement for:
   a. respect for justice and equity
   b. respect for privacy
   c. beneficence
   d. respect for autonomy.
3. By selecting only unemployed men for the study and promising to pay them a substantial amount of money to be in the experimental group, the researcher did not meet the requirement for:
   a. respect for justice and equity
   b. respect for privacy
   c. beneficence
   d. respect for autonomy.
4. The researcher acknowledged in the information sheet that talking about experiences of the death of a child might be emotionally painful. By setting up access to counselling services for participants, the researcher met the requirement for:
   a. respect for autonomy
   b. respect for justice
   c. beneficence
   d. respect for privacy.
5. The main role of an institutional or regional ethics committee in Australia or New Zealand is to:
   a. protect research participants from harm
   b. protect the institutions involved from adverse publicity
   c. protect the researcher/s from criticism
   d. protect the funding body of the research.
6. Which statement is not true about vulnerable participants?
   a. Vulnerable participants are less able to understand what is involved if they take part in the study.
   b. Vulnerable participants find it difficult to understand how risky the study may be.
   c. Vulnerable participants cannot communicate their wishes about taking part in the study.
   d. Vulnerable participants are those people less likely to be harmed.
7. Research involving Indigenous Peoples has special ethical concerns because:
   a. such groups are a different culture from the rest of the population
   b. such groups have been exploited by researchers in the past
   c. such groups have leaders who may refuse access to participants
   d. such groups tend to live in remote areas.
8. Research misconduct refers mainly to:
   a. a study that has been poorly conducted
   b. a study that is unscientific
   c. errors in data analysis or interpretation
   d. fabrication or falsification of research results.
9. Informed consent in research involves:
   a. a person being informed that they are a study participant and about the nature of the study
   b. a person agreeing to participate in a study after receiving information about the nature of the study and being told the experimental drug may cure them
   c. a person signing a consent form for a research study after receiving information about the nature of the study and what it will involve for them personally
   d. a person freely agreeing to participate in a study after receiving adequate information about the nature of the study and what it will involve for them personally.
10. Therapeutic research is:
    a. research that may benefit future patients but not those acting as research participants
    b. research investigating different forms of treatment that ranks the most effective (therapeutic) to the least effective treatment
    c. the therapeutic effect experienced by participants sharing distressing experiences in qualitative studies
    d. research that benefits society.

For further content associated with this chapter visit: https://evolve.elsevier.com/cs/product/9780729596794?role=student 

APPENDIX 1 SAMPLE INFORMATION SHEET

(The information sheet is to be printed on the letterhead of the university at which you are enrolled or hospital/health service in which you are employed.)

Information Sheet

Dear ______________,

I am currently studying for my *(name of degree)* at *(name of university)*. My thesis is by research. The title of my research project is:

'Women's experiences of pregnancy in an environment of conflicting discourses about health'

Researcher: (student's name, department in which enrolled, university, suburb, state and postcode).

____

____

Telephone number: ______________________________

Email: _______________________________________

Address: ____

___________________________ Postcode: __________

I would like to invite you to consider participating in my research project. The purpose of this exploratory research project is to discover how you experience your pregnancy, and the attitudes and meanings you give to the event. Your **own** interpretation and the meaning and significance you attach to this period are important in this study.

If you agree to participate, you will be asked to attend four interviews conducted at three stages during your pregnancy (8–12 weeks, 20–28 weeks and 36–38 weeks gestation) and once following the birth of your baby. Each interview will take about 1 hour. The interviews will be conducted at a time and place convenient to both you and me.

Please understand that you are free to withdraw from participation in this research study at any time and to ask that all your records be returned to you or destroyed and not used in any way, provided that the request for destruction or return of records is made within 4 weeks of the completion of the interview.

Any complaint regarding the nature or conduct of this research may be directed to:

Ethics Liaison Officer, Human Research Ethics Committee, *(name of university, suburb, state and postcode).*

____

____

Telephone: __________________________________

Yours sincerely

(Researcher's name)

APPENDIX 2 SAMPLE CONSENT FORM

(The information sheet is to be printed on the letterhead of the university at which you are enrolled or hospital/health service in which you are employed.)

Faculty of

___

Consent Form

Title of Project: 'Women's experiences of pregnancy in an environment of conflicting discourses about health'
Name of researcher, and department address:

___

___

I *(name of participant) (please print)* have read and understood all of the information on the 'Information Sheet' and any questions that I have asked have been answered to my satisfaction.

I agree to take part in this research study on the understanding that:

I can withdraw from the study at any stage Yes/No

I agree to the four interviews being taped Yes/No

I agree to the use of any material which does not identify me in any way Yes/No

I understand that I am free to withdraw from participation in this research study at any time after *each* interview, and ask that all my records are returned to me or destroyed and not used in any way, provided that the request for destruction or return of records is made within 4 weeks of the completion of the interview.

Should I wish to discuss my participation with someone not directly involved in the project, particularly in regard to matters concerning policies, information about the conduct of the study or my rights as a participant or I wish to make a confidential complaint, I may contact:

Ethics Liaison Officer, Human Research Ethics Committee, *(name of university, suburb, state and postcode).*

___

___

Telephone: ___________ ___________

Name of participant: ___________ ___________

Date: ___________ Signature: _______ ___________

Researcher: ___________ ___________

Date: ___________ Signature: _____ ___________

ADDITIONAL RESOURCES

Australian Privacy Commissioner. https://www.privacy.gov.au/.

Curtis, E., Drennan, J. (Eds.), 2013. Quantitative Health Research: issues and methods. Open University Press/McGraw Hill Education, New York.

Fouka, G., Mantzorou, M., 2011. What are the major ethical issues in conducting research? Is there a conflict between the research ethics and the nature of nursing? Health. Sci. J. 5 (1), 3–14.

Heilferty, C.M., 2011. Ethical considerations in the study of online illness narratives: a qualitative review. J. Adv. Nurs. 67 (5), 945–953.

Houghton, C.E., Casey, D., Shaw, D., et al., 2010. Ethical challenges in qualitative research: examples from practice. Nurse Res. 18 (1), 15–25.

International Council of Nurses, 2021. The ICN Code of Ethics for Nurses. https://www.icn.ch/sites/default/files/inline-files/ICN_Code-of-Ethics_EN_Web.pdf.

National Health and Medical Research Council. https://www.nhmrc.gov.au.

New Zealand Health and Disability Commission. https://www.hdc.org.nz.

New Zealand Health Research Council. https://www.hrc.govt.nz.

New Zealand Nurses Organisation, 2019. Code of Ethics https://www.nzno.org.nz/Portals/0/publications/Guideline%20-%20Code%20of%20Ethics%202019.pdf?ver=19LQpYx8wspprjbTNt9pWw%3D%3D.

New Zealand Privacy Commission. https://www.privacy.org.nz.

Nursing and Midwifery Board of Australia, 2018. Code of Professional Conduct for Nurses in Australia. https://www.nursingmidwiferyboard.gov.au/codes-guidelines-statements/professional-standards.aspx.

Nursing Council of New Zealand. Code of Conduct for Nurses. https://www.nursingcouncil.org.nz/Public/Nursing/Code_of_Conduct/NCNZ/nursing-section/Code_of_Conduct.aspx.

Twycross, A , 2008. An interprofessional approach to the ethics of undertaking research with children. Nurse Res. 16, 3.

REFERENCES

Agar, M., Ko, D.N., Sheehan, C., et al., 2013. Informed consent in palliative care clinical trials: challenging but possible. J. Palliat. Med. 16 (5), 485–491. doi:10.1089/jpm.2012 0422

Appelbaum, P.S., Roth, L.H., 1982. Competency to consent to research: a psychiatric overview. Arch. Gen. Psychiatry, 39 (8), 951–958.

Artal, R., Rubenfeld, S. 2017. Ethical issues in research. Best Pract. Res. Clin. Obstet. Gynaecol. 43, 107–114.

Australian Nursing and Midwifery Federation (ANMF), 2019. National school nursing standards for practice: registered nurse. Retrieved from: https://www.anmf.org.au/media/x1gaxvbj/anmf_national_school_nursing_standards_for_practice_rn_2019.pdf.

Barrow, J.M., Brannan, G.D., Khandhar, P.B., 2022. Research ethics. In: StatPearls [Internet]. StatPearls Publishing, Treasure Island, FL. Retrieved from: https://www.ncbi.nlm.nih.gov/books/NBK459281/.

Batt, S., 2017. Revisiting New Zealand's 'Unfortunate Experiment:' is medical ethics ever a thing done. Ind. J. Med. Ethics 3 (2), 142–146.

Beauchamp, T.L., Childress, J.F., 2019. Principles of Biomedical Ethics, 8th ed. Oxford University Press, New York.

Beecher, H.K., 1966. Ethics and clinical research. N. Engl. J. Med. 274 (24), 1354–1360.

Benveniste, T., King, L., 2018, 'Researching together: reflections on ethical research in remote Aboriginal communities', Learn. Commun. 23, November. Retrieved from: https://www.cdu.edu.au/sites/default/files/the-northern-institute/docs/10.18793-lcj2018.23.05.pdf.

Boseley, S., Smith, D., 2010. As doctors fought to save lives, Pfizer flew in drug trial team [Press release]. The Guardian. [online] 9 Dec. Retrieved from: https://www.theguardian.com/business/2010/dec/09/doctors-fought-save-lives-pfizer-drug.

Broesch, T., Crittenden, A.N., Beheim, B.A., et al., 2020. Navigating cross-cultural research: methodological and ethical considerations. Proc. Royal Soc. B, 287 (1935), 20201245.

Brown, C., Spiro, J., Quinton, S., 2020. The role of research ethics committees: friend or foe in educational research? An exploratory study. Br. Educ. Res. J. 46 (4), 747–769.

Burns, E., Fenwick, J., Schmied, V., et al., 2012. Reflexivity in midwifery research: the insider/outsider debate. Midwifery 28 (1), 52–60.

Cartwright, S.R.; Committee of Inquiry into Allegations Concerning the Treatment of Cervical Cancer at National Women's Hospital and into Other Related Matters, 1988. The Report of the Cervical Cancer Inquiry: the report of the Committee of Inquiry into allegations concerning the treatment of cervical cancer at National Women's Hospital and into other related matters. Government Printing Office, Auckland, New Zealand. Retrieved from: https://www.nsu.govt.nz/health-professionals/national-cervical-screening-programme/legislation/cervical-screening-inquiry-0.

Committee on Publication Ethics, 2019. Promoting integrity in research and its publication. Retrieved from: https://publicationethics.org/.

Day, P.G., Satin, D., Lennon, R.P., et al., 2021. Utilizing community research committees to improve the informed consent process. Am. J. Bioethics, 21 (5), 73–75.

Elmir, R., Jackson, D., Beale, B., et al., 2010. Against all odds: Australian women's experiences of recovery from breast cancer. J. Clin. Nurs. 19 (17–18), 2531–2538.

Etieyibo, E., 2013. The case of competency and informed consent. J. Clin. Res. Bioethics 12, 2.

Gotzsche, P., 2019. Deadly medicines and organised crime: how big pharma has corrupted healthcare. CRC Press, New York.

Green, G.H., 1969. Invasive potentiality of cervical carcinoma in situ. Int. J. Gynecol. Obstet. 7 (4),157–171.

Griffith, R., 2016. What is Gillick competence? Hum. Vaccin. Immunother. 12 (1), 244–247. doi:10.1080/21645515.2015.1091548

Gustafsson, B.E., Quensel, C.E., Swenander Lanke, L., et al., 1953. The effect of different levels of carbohydrate intake on caries activity in 436 individuals observed for five years. Acta Odontol. Scand. 11, 232–264. doi:10.3109/ 00016355308993925

Habermann, B., Broome, M., Pryor, E.R., et al., 2010. Research coordinators experiences with scientific misconduct and research integrity. Nurs. Res. 59 (1), 51–57.

Health and Disability Commissioner, 1996. Code of Health and Disability Services Consumers' Rights. Retrieved from: https://www.hdc.org.nz/your-rights/about-the-code/code-of-health-and-disability-services-consumers-rights/.

Health and Disability Ethics Committees, 2019. Ethical Standards for Health and Disability Research and Quality Improvement. Retrieved from: https://neac.health.govt.nz/publications-and-resources/neac-publications/national-ethical-standards-for-health-and-disability-research-and-quality-improvement/.

Health Research Council Act 1990 (1990). Retrieved from: https://www.legislation.govt.nz/act/public/1990/0068/latest/DLM213017.html.

Health Research Council of New Zealand (HRC), 2010. Guidelines for Researchers on Health Research Involving Māori. Health Research Council of New Zealand, Auckland. Retrieved from: http://www.hrc.govt.nz/sites/default/files/2019-06/Resource%20Library%20PDF%20-%20Guidelines%20for%20Reseasrchers%20on%20Health%20Research%20involving%20Maori%20.pdf.

Health Research Council of New Zealand (HRC), 2021. Te Ara Tika Guidelines for Māori Research Ethics: a framework for researchers and ethics committee members. Health Research Council of New Zealand, Auckland. Retrieved from: https://www.hrc.govt.nz/sites/default/files/2019-06/Resource%20Library%20PDF%20-%20Te%20Ara%20Tika%20Guidelines%20for%20Maori%20Research%20Ethics_0.pdf.

Hilliard, C., O'Neill, M., 2010. Nurses' emotional experience of caring for children with burns. Journal of clinical nursing, 19(19–20), 2907–2915.

Holbeach, N., Freckelton AO QC, I., Mol, B.W., 2023. Journal editors and publishers' legal obligations with respect to medical research misconduct. Res. Ethics, 19 (2), 107–120. doi:10.1177/17470161221147440

Huria, T., Palmer, S.C., Pitama, S., et al., 2019. Consolidated criteria for strengthening reporting of health research involving indigenous peoples: the CONSIDER statement. BMC Med. Res. Methodol. 19, 1–9.

International Council for Harmonisation of Technical Requirements for Pharmaceuticals for Human Use, 2016. Integrated addendum to ICH E6(R1): Guideline for Good Clinical Practice. Retrieved from: https://www.ema.europa.eu/en/partners-networks/international-activities/multilateral-coalitions-initiatives/international-council-harmonisation-technical-requirements-registration-pharmaceuticals-human-use.

International Council of Nurses, 2021. The ICN Code of Ethics for Nurses. Retrieved from: https://www.icn.ch/sites/default/files/inline-files/ICN_Code-of-Ethics_EN_Web.pdf.

Jackson-Barrett, E., Price, A., Stomski, N., et al., 2015. Grounded in country: perspectives on working within, alongside and for Aboriginal communities. Issues Educ. Res. 25 (1), 36–49.

Jones, R.W., 2017. Doctors in Denial: the forgotten women in the 'unfortunate experiment'. Otago University Press, Dunedin.

Kampmeier, R.H., 1974. Final report on the Tuskegee syphilis study. Southern Med. J. 67 (11), 1349–1353.

Keenan, R. (Ed.), 2016. Health Care and the Law. Thomson Reuters New Zealand Limited.

Kolstoe, S.E., Pugh, J., 2023. The trinity of good research: distinguishing between research integrity, ethics, and governance. Account Res. 25, 1-20. doi:10.1080/08989621.2023.2239712. Retrieved from: https://pubmed.ncbi.nlm.nih.gov/37475134/.

Lakeman, R., 2010. Mental health nursing is not for sale: rethinking nursing's relationship with the pharmaceutical industry. J. Psychiatr. Ment. Health Nurs. 17 (2), 172–177.

Lakeman, R., McAndrew, S., MacGabhann, L., et al., 2013. 'That was helpful... no one has talked to me about that before': research participation as a therapeutic activity. Int. J. Mental Health Nurs. 22(1), 76–84.

Law Library of Congress, 2007. Children's rights: international and national laws and practice. Australia. Retrieved from: https://www.loc.gov/law/help/child-rights/australia.php.

Ledward, A., 2011. Informed consent: ethical issues for midwife research. Evid. Based Midwifery 9 (1), 23.

McIndoe, W.A., McLean, M.R., Jones, R.W., et al., 1984. The invasive potential of carcinoma in situ of the cervix. Obstet Gynecol. 64 (4), 451–458.

Milgram, S., 1963. Behavioral study of obedience. J. Abnorm. Soc. Psychol. 67 (4), 371–378.

Ministry of Health (MOH), 2007. Guidelines for Health Research with Children. MOH, Auckland. Retrieved from: https://www.hrc.govt.nz/sites/default/files/HRC%20.

Mitford, J., 1973. Kind and Unusual Punishment. Random House, New York.

Monahan, T., Fisher, J.A., 2010. Benefits of 'observer effects': lessons from the field. Qual. Res.10 (3), 357–376.

National Health and Medical Research Council Act 1992 (1992). Retrieved from: https://www.legislation.gov.au/Series/C2004A04516.

National Health and Medical Research Council (NHMRC), 2018a. Ethical Conduct in Research with Aboriginal and Torres Strait Islander Peoples and Communities: guidelines for researchers and stakeholders. NHMRC, Canberra, ACT. Retrieved from: https://nhmrc.gov.au/about-us/publications/ethical-conduct-research-aboriginal-and-torres-strait-islander-peoples-and-communities#block-views-block-file-attachments-content-block-1.

National Health and Medical Research Council (NHMRC), 2018b. Australian Code for the Responsible Conduct of Research. NHMRC, Canberra, ACT. Retrieved from: https://nhmrc.gov.au/about-us/publications/australian-code-responsible-conduct-research-2018.

National Health and Medical Research Council (NHMRC), 2023. National Statement on Ethical Conduct in Human Research. NHMRC, Canberra, ACT. Retrieved from: https://nhmrc.gov.au/about-us/publications/national-statement-ethical-conduct-human-research-2023.

Prior, D., 2007. Decolonising research: a shift toward reconciliation. Nurs. Inq. 14 (2), 162–168.

Privacy Commissioner, 2020. Health Information Privacy Code 1994. Privacy Act and Codes. Retrieved from: https://www.privacy.org.nz/privacy-act-2020/codes-of-practice/hipc2020/.

Purser, K.J., Rosenfeld, T., 2014. Evaluation of legal capacity by doctors and lawyers: the need for collaborative assessment. Med. J. Aust. 201 (8), 483–485.

Report of the Global Forum on Bioethics in Research, 2008. Ethics of Research Involving Indigenous Peoples and Vulnerable Populations. Retrieved from: https://gfbr.global/wp-content/uploads/2015/09/GFBR9.pdf.

Retraction Watch, 2019. 8th retraction appears for researcher who faked patient records. Retrieved from: https://retractionwatch.com/category/by-author/anna-ahimastos/.

Simpson, C., 2010. Decision-making capacity and informed consent to participate in research by cognitively impaired individuals. Appl. Nurs. Res. 23 (4), 221–226.

Sivasubramaniam, S., Dlabolová, D.H., Kralikova, V., et al., 2021. Assisting you to advance with ethics in research: an introduction to ethical governance and application procedures. Int. J. Educ. Integ. 17 (1), 1–18.

Therapeutic Goods Administration (TGA), 2000. Note for Guidance on Clinical Safety Data Management. TGA, Canberra, ACT. Retrieved from: https://www.tga.gov.au/resources/publication/publications/note-guidance-clinical-safety-data-management-definitions-and-standards-expedited-reporting.

Therapeutic Goods Administration (TGA), 2021. Australian Clinical Trial Handbook. TGA, Canberra, ACT. Retrieved from: https://www.tga.gov.au/sites/default/files/australian-clinical-trial-handbook.pdf.

Tuskegee Syphilis Study Legacy Committee, 1996. Final Report of the Tuskegee Syphilis Study Legacy Committee. Retrieved from: https://www.tuskegee.edu/Content/Uploads/Tuskegee/files/Bioethics/SyphilisStudyCommitteeReport.pdf.

United Nations Educational Scientific and Cultural Organisation (UNESCO), 2005. Universal Declaration on Bioethics and Human Rights. Retrieved from: https://www.unesco.org/en/legal-affairs/universal-declaration-bioethics-and-human-rights?hub=66535.

United Nations Educational Scientific and Cultural Organisation (UNESCO), 2019. Cultural Diversity. Retrieved from: https://en.unesco.org/themes/education-sustainable-development/cultural-diversity/.

Wager, E., Kleinert S., 2021. Cooperation & Liaison between Universities & Editors (CLUE): recommendations on best practice. Res. Integ. Peer Rev. 6, 6.

Waitangi Tribunal. 2020. Retrieved from: https://www.waitangi-tribunal.govt.nz/treaty-of-waitangi/.

White, C., Hardy, J., 2010. What do palliative care patients and their relatives think about research in palliative care? A systematic review. Support. Care Cancer 18 (8), 905–911. doi:10.1007/s00520-009-0724-1

Wilson, D., Mikahere-Hall, A., Sherwood, J., 2022. Using indigenous kaupapa Māori research methodology with constructivist grounded theory: generating a theoretical explanation of indigenous women's realities. Int. J. Soc. Res. Methodol. 25 (3), 375–390. doi:10.1080/13645579.2021.1897756

Woods, M., 2010. Cultural safety and the socioethical nurse. Nurs. Ethics 17 (6), 715–725.

World Medical Association, 2013. Declaration of Helsinki: ethical principles for medical research involving human subjects. JAMA 310 (20), 2191–2194.

World Medical Association, 2023. Medical Ethics Manual. Retrieved from: https://www.wma.net/what-we-do/education/medical-ethics-manual.

Zimbardo, P.G., 1972. Stanford prison experiment: a simulation study of the psychology of imprisonment. SLIDE SHOW. Retrieved from: https://web.stanford.edu/dept/spec_coll/uarch/exhibits/Narration.pdf.

14

Indigenous Peoples and Research

Lynore Geia and Nicolette Sheridan

LEARNING OUTCOMES

After reading this chapter you will be able to:

- critically reflect on the reasons that Indigenous Peoples want to reclaim their histories (and ways of being and knowing) in Aotearoa New Zealand and Australia
- explore Indigenous literature and ways of thinking about research with Indigenous Peoples
- recognise the distinctiveness of Indigenous research and where issues and methodologies intersect
- understand the implications of research for Indigenous Peoples, their lives and futures

KEY TERMS

cultural competence, p. 245
cultural safety, p. 242
Indigenous knowledge, p. 237
Indigenous research methodologies, p. 236
knowledge translation, p. 234

INTRODUCTION

Critical Indigenous inquiry is vital to social change, to economic and social justice and to practices of democracy. Indigenous and non-Indigenous researchers are central in their positioning as enquirers participating and leading in developing and conducting research that should challenge ineffective research methods and seek out more distinct research processes that will meet the need of Indigenous society, enabling mechanisms for social change.

Indigenous Peoples (Māori in Aotearoa New Zealand and Aboriginal and Torres Strait Islander Peoples in Australia) in their Indigenous contexts as cultural knowledge holders bring an *emic* view of culture that should determine how research is to be designed and implemented, amplifying the issues as they know it as 'Indigenist' researchers communing with Indigenous communities (Rigney 1999). Indigenous research must be conducted in a way that honours cultural ways of 'being and doing' through all stages, from research design and methodology through to data collection, analysis and writing up the findings (Martin 2008). It should generate knowledge and inform **knowledge translation** into action for change.

Research that embeds Indigenous concepts within research programs is judicious research. Indigenous nurse researchers bring rational and culturally relational knowledge to research in individual-centred systems of care in health, resulting in safe and effective outcomes. The imperative in taking a heuristic research approach by Indigenous nurse researchers with, and for, Indigenous people in seeking health equity for their peoples and communities cannot be overstated. Therefore, in this context, research is a moral and political road of inquiry.

In Australia, research of Indigenous context now preferences an expectation that the research is to be led by Indigenous researchers. As mandated by the Commonwealth, Indigenous research must meet the expected National Health and Medical Research Council (NHMRC 2018) criteria; all researchers must adhere to six core values of ethical research conduct: *spirit and integrity*, *cultural continuity*, *equity*, *reciprocity*, *respect* and *responsibility*, which are important to all Aboriginal and Torres Strait Islander

Peoples (pp. 2, 3). More information on these core values can be found in the link at the end of this chapter. Importantly, this is reiterated by the prestigious Australian Research Centre Indigenous (ARC) Discovery Indigenous scheme, which supports research programs for Aboriginal and/or Torres Strait Islander researchers and builds the research capacity of higher degree research students and early career researchers where all funded research must be led by an Indigenous researcher or have Indigenous researchers as Chief Investigators (CIs).

This is also the case for Māori in Aotearoa New Zealand. For decades, non-Indigenous researchers have researched Indigenous Peoples. 'When mentioned in many indigenous contexts, it (research) stirs up silence, it conjures up bad memories, it raises a smile that is knowing and distrustful' (Smith 2012 p. 1). The experience of being researched by others can cause distress to Indigenous Peoples when important issues are not understood, or ignored and not reported. Indigenous researchers taking a lead role in governance can make an essential contribution to the analysis and interpretation of research findings that impact Indigenous Peoples. One recent example of Indigenous governance in a large national study investigating equity in primary care in Aotearoa New Zealand (Sheridan et al 2023a) concluded that government funding must support underresourced Māori general practices and ensure accountability for the patient health outcomes of all Māori patients in any models of general practice.

In 2020 an independent Tribunal found the New Zealand Government had 'breached the Treaty of Waitangi by failing to design and administer the current primary healthcare system to actively address persistent Māori health inequities' (Waitangi Tribunal 2019). A cultural reform is needed to move the health and disability sector to be 'pro-equity, culturally safe, Tiriti compliant and anti-racist' (Reid 2021 pp. 7–10). Research continues to report lower life expectancy, earlier onset and higher rates of conditions such as diabetes for Māori in Aotearoa New Zealand. Indigenous research across all sectors commands moral and political agency; these are complex requisites that must be respected by all researchers. 'We as researchers cannot afford to allow the gap between Aboriginal and Torres Strait Islanders and mainstream Australia health outcomes to grow even wider' (Geia et al 2013). Aboriginal and Torres Strait Islander nursing and midwifery researchers are now leading research projects in various fields 'integrating culture and Aboriginal and Torres Strait Islander research ethics', generating knowledge of Indigenous research content and data sovereignty (Lovett 2016, Power et al 2021a, West et al 2019).

Mohamed et al (2021) maintain that the most effective way of addressing 'the persistent health disparities' is through Aboriginal and Torres Strait Islander-led research. Now Australian health research is witnessing the growth of an authoritative Indigenous research movement creating their space in what was normally held as a non-Indigenous Western research domain. However, despite these important advances, leading Indigenous researchers continue to 'stand at the door and knock' asking for recognition from a predominantly Western paternalistic research environment. This is exemplified through the distinct lack of citations of Indigenous research by non-Indigenous authors. This situation is further complicated by journals being reluctant to include cultural affiliations, adding to what Mohamed et al (2021 p. 383) assert: 'there is no systematic way of identifying Australian Aboriginal and Torres Strait Islander scholarship in the peer-reviewed literature'.

If research is to improve the lives and experiences of Indigenous Peoples, collaboration between Indigenous researchers and clinicians and Indigenous communities and institutions is pivotal. It requires intentioned conversations, deeper connections and an understanding of the liminal space where possibilities exist, where relationships are negotiated and where knowledge can be created on new terms. Research positioned in the contested space of equity and justice, despite pre-existing contexts and recriminations, creates opportunities to determine the systems that can improve our lives and environments.

Approaches grounded in the hegemony or power of 'Western ways of knowing' or 'Western ideology' provide a linear way of seeing the world that dominates and has little relevance in the lives of many Indigenous Peoples whose experience of being in the world is located in time, space and place. 'For Māori, place can involve geography, history, mythology, cosmology, personal health, spiritual healing and interdependent social connection. While each of these components or notions can be individually understood, the place of one's origin and belonging is far more than the sum they represent' (Rinehart et al 2018 p. 5). Similarly, in Aboriginal and Torres Strait Islander worldview, research involves what could be described as '*reciprocative cultural archaeology*' (Geia 2012 p. 443) where the Indigenous researcher is engaged at a deeper (heart) level with Indigenous research participants. There is a two-way flow of knowledge exchange, a reciprocity of cultural discourse that flows from the past, the present and the future. Thus, simultaneously the Indigenous researcher is also listening to their own past, present and in some sense their future in uncovering or discovering their cultural truth. The Māori term '*ako*' means to teach and to learn and recognises the reciprocal relationship of teaching and learning. Bishop (2008) uses *ako* in the context of teacher and student 'storying and restorying their realities, either as individual learners or within a group context' (p. 443). In this chapter we explain why Indigenous Peoples are seeking to reclaim their histories in Aotearoa New Zealand and Australia. By critically reflecting on literature and on contemporary research, alternative viewpoints emerge, and we believe the reader will be challenged to think in new ways about research methodologies and about Indigenous Peoples.

NEW WAYS OF THINKING ABOUT RESEARCH WITH INDIGENOUS PEOPLES

New ways of thinking about research with Indigenous Peoples raises a thought-provoking juxtaposition. Essentially in our contemporary thinking we can rightly say that Indigenous research concepts are new research paradigms being introduced to the Western research academy. However, if we take a closer examination, Indigenous research concepts rise from a deeper enduring foundation of knowledge and skills of Indigenous Peoples who practised their science for generations, enabling Indigenous Peoples to flourish by adapting to change and surviving on their lands. Hence, when we consider Indigenous research, we correctly reason this is, on the one hand, a new way of thinking in contemporary research. On the other, it is enduring old science in its emergence, an honoring of an ancient way of being and doing, where 'the new is the old and old is new', the revitilisation of knowledge that has always been in a contemporary world.

Dr Linda Tuhiwai Smith is a Distinguished Professor at Te Whare Wānanga o Awanuiārangi in Whakatane, Aotearoa New Zealand. She is Māori and from Ngāti Awa, Ngāti Porou and Tuhourangi. Smith is one of the world's most well-known Indigenous scholars and her seminal book, *Decolonizing Methodologies*, explores new ways of knowing and thinking about research with Indigenous Peoples (Smith 2012). Smith guides the reader to 'delve deeper' to gain an understanding of why **Indigenous research methodologies** matter. She identifies concerns about the context within which research problems are conceptualised and designed, and the implications of research for Indigenous participants, including communities. She raises questions about the values and practices of an academic research institution. Recently, Smith raised the significance of land acknowledgements as a commentary on Indigenous pedagogies—recognising that they can be at worst a 'tokenistic and meaningless gesture, an awkward and embarrassing display of institutional arrogance' or they can signal the beginning of a restorative process that can lead to academic institutional transformation in knowledge, teaching and research (Smith 2023).

Smith explains counter-hegemony in terms of Indigenous researchers taking power and demonstrating resistance to the dominant discourses within Western research (Smith 2007).

As is common, intellectual insights rarely occur alone. Other Indigenous scholars in Australia were journeying this same path of decolonising and privileging Indigenous voices. Likewise with other Indigenous researchers across the globe, eminent Narungga, Kaurna and Ngarrindjeri educator and researcher Professor Lester-Irabinna Rigney empowered Indigenous research in Australia through his seminal work '*Internationalization of an Indigenous Anticolonial Cultural Critique of Research Methodologies: A Guide to Indigenist Research Methodology and Its Principles*' (1999). Rigney (1999 p. 109) theorised Indigenist research and gave substance to Indigenist research methodology through three principles and rationales—that of resistance, political integrity and privileging Indigenous voices:

1. *Resistance* is the emancipatory imperative in Indigenous research whereby stories of survival, resilience and resistance to past and continuing oppression give support to the personal, community, cultural and political struggles experienced by Aboriginal and Torres Strait Island Peoples;
2. *Political integrity* in Indigenist research means that, in this time, Indigenist research should be undertaken only by Indigenous Australians who live in community and their research is done with community—thereby setting the opportunity for the political and social agenda towards the liberation of Aboriginal and Torres Strait Island Peoples. Indigenous researchers can only meaningfully connect the research with political and social pathways to change within the community;
3. *Privileging Indigenous voices* in Indigenist research is giving Aboriginal and Torres Strait Island Peoples a credible voice in national and international arenas. Indigenous researchers are able to represent the unique and distinct community voice and be accountable to their community for what they are relaying to others. Indigenous researchers are able to speak on a political level with awareness and authority about Indigenous issues.

In creating this formative research approach, Rigney brings moral and political imperative with cultural meaning to research for Indigenous researchers, giving power to their research with communities. This is made possible only through Indigenous Peoples being involved in 'defining, controlling, and owning epistemologies and ontologies that value and legitimate the Indigenous experience. Indigenous perspectives must infiltrate the structures and methods of the entire research academy ... and must look to new anticolonial epistemologies and methodologies to construct, rediscover, and/or reaffirm their knowledges and cultures' (p. 114).

In recent times, Aboriginal and Torres Strait Islander nursing and midwifery scholars have lately begun to include acknowledgement of 'Country', language and tribal affiliations in their nursing and midwifery publications as steps of taking back their power and reaffirming knowledge through a culturally restorative process in academia (Geia et al 2020, Power et al 2022). Jackson (2023) brings perspective to this new restorative move; by taking back power, Indigenous nurses and midwives are engaging in a counter-hegemonic way, disrupting the perpetuating system of the Whiteness of nursing in Australia. Jackson clarifies 'White' as so much more than a category of skin colour (Puzin 2003), and that this phrase, the Whiteness of nursing, refers to the seen and the unseen, the acknowledged and the unacknowledged discourses that shape nursing. Whiteness forms the means through which power is distributed and held in nursing, and the ways that people of all cultural backgrounds become enculturated into Western nursing (p. 819). These are still early days for Aboriginal and Torres Strait Islander nursing and midwifery academics in Australia as they take steps in taking back their power and establishing their cultural scholarly identity with nursing and midwifery integrity in developing their publishing relationships with Australian nursing and midwifery journals.

Resistance is seen in counter-strategies that are more reflective, appropriate and responsive to Indigenous research agendas. Counter-strategies or counter-hegemonies have enabled Indigenous researchers 'to tell an alternative story: the history of Western research through the eyes of the colonised' (Smith 2012 p. 2). Seminal research by distinguished Professor Graham Hingangaroa Smith (2000) found that a counter-hegemonic approach could cause a movement from a marginal position of the constructed 'other' to a more central position of inclusion. Indigenous narratives gradually find their way into the existing dominant discourse. When this happens in health research, communities take control of the agenda, design and methods, and the outcome is community owned. Counter-hegemonies are ways that decolonisation 'claims back' what has been colonised—taken or appropriated by others.

Geia et al (2013) claim space in a counter-hegemonic stance where Aboriginal storytelling or yarning, practised over thousands of years and integral to Indigenous learning, is promoted as a research methodology:

> *Aboriginal yarning is a fluid ongoing process, a moving dialogue interspersed with interjections, interpretations and additions. The stories remain in our conscious state like a thread hanging, waiting to be picked up again, to be continued, reconstructed, reinforced and once again embedded ... threads of Aboriginal and Torres Strait Island history as it moves into the present tense, its parameters within present time is filtered through the memories of the past as the two move simultaneously and at points collide and reveals fragments of the future* (p. 15).

Yarning is highly relational, and Indigenous relationality is not always dependent on face-to-face contact. Indigenous connections are inherent; thus, yarning emerges out of connections and moves into newly carved out Indigenous spaces within today's technology and is thriving in online platforms. Indigenous research methodology and methods, as with culture, are not static; Aboriginal and Torres Strait Islander Peoples are advancing and adapting their knowledge to society's changes. Riley et al (2022), citing Arnold (2016), noted that, when it comes to **Indigenous knowledge**, 'It is all too easy to ascribe such ways of knowing as being inevitably lost in the past or as being too peripheral to be of value today' but Arnold (2016) reminds us how Indigenous scholars, educators and artists have consistently harnessed new technologies to serve future generations.

For example, as a response to research during COVID, the well-known research method of storytelling or yarning was adapted to online Indigenous discourse in what is termed E-yarning (Weston 2011). Yarning online still embraces Aboriginal and Torres Strait Islander storytelling, as yarning entails 'heart' listening through connection and nuanced communication. Online technology has seen Indigenous communities of practice rise in spaces that now connect researchers and clinicians globally, from home office spaces to university spaces, maintaining the continual cyclical process of telling lived experience that is an integral part of Aboriginal and Torres Strait Islanders' oral traditions. Hence the use of yarning and 'storytelling as a research tool weaves each storyteller's truth; each individual sees the facts of their story through their own lens of experience within their family and community' (Geia 2012) giving rise to richer data.

E-yarns still carry the integrity of storytelling; this new way of doing also collaborates with research translation of Indigenous cultural connection and communication style to a different mode. The protocol of relationality is a core tenet of Aboriginal and Torres Strait Islander communication, wherever the meeting spaces; there is co-creation and a deepening of connections. However, as in anything new in research where anecdotal evidence exists, it will eventually need to give way to evaluation through empirical processes. The traditional research evidence on E-yarning is still to be generated and more research is needed on this new research methodology praxis E-yarning for research.

History is interpreted through the lens of lived experience and is influenced by power, politics, economics and social constructs. History that Indigenous Peoples experience as 'wrong' was often not perceived as wrong by colonial forces in early settler times and may not be perceived as wrong by some people today. In the Australian health context, Aboriginal and Torres Strait Islanders see colonial history as exacting harm on Indigenous Peoples, and there is a contemporary discourse with strong views on both sides—harmful and not harmful ('get over it'), hence the deep moral and political praxis. A critical aspect of decolonisation is to reclaim history—knowledge and heritage, which involves sharing stories from the past and telling stories to reclaim Indigenous realities.

Nurse researchers in Aotearoa highlighted the practice of European nurses who worked with Māori communities between 1900 and 1930 to care for those with introduced infectious diseases, among other health issues. They contended that 'in spite of the nurses' humanitarian intentions and their onerous work, their Eurocentric practice undermined the Māori way of life' (McKillop et al 2013). Two of the authors were indigenous nurse researchers (NS, DR). Data were analysed through the lens of colonial theory, critiquing the colonising effect of Native Health nurses' work in Māori communities. Previous histories of nursing practice in the colonial period of Aotearoa New Zealand have tended to describe the context within which nurses practised while the impact of the values embedded within nurses' practice has not been challenged. The assimilationist agenda of the New Zealand Health Department has been well documented. In her autobiography, Hester Maclean, New Zealand's Chief Nurse during the time of the Native Health Nursing Service, attested that European nurses rightly held superiority over all Māori people (Maclean 1932) and promulgated the 'image of nurses as "ministering angels" in colonial "backblocks"' (McKillop et al 2013 p. 2). For all Indigenous Peoples, decolonisation is about reclaiming *mana* (respect) and dignity, holding steady to Indigenous knowledge and reclaiming history as a means to embracing a more self-determined future.

We recognise the distinctiveness of Indigenous research and where issues and methodologies intersect. This is important if we are to carry new (and experienced) researchers forwards to a vision of health and social research that improves the lives of Indigenous Peoples and whole societies. Indigenous researchers, including those who are nurses and midwives, have many research methodologies available to them. Cultural knowledge and Elders can help in the stance we take towards the challenges from new technologies—for example, when we must test appropriate responses to these challenges—and those yet to be laid down.

INDIGENOUS RESEARCH: WHERE ISSUES AND METHODOLOGIES INTERSECT

Here the distinctiveness of Indigenous research methodologies, and where issues and methodologies intersect, is discussed in Australian and Aotearoa New Zealand contexts. By understanding the implications of research for Indigenous Peoples and their communities and by critically reflecting on history, traditions and ethical principles in the conduct of research, those researching in the discipline of nursing and midwifery can better understand *cultural safety* and the need for *cultural competencies*. Empowering Indigenous communities by partnering in the planning and implementation of research, especially when the research is community driven, is discussed. The contribution of Indigenous scholars (and those working closely with them) is to support Indigenous communities to engage with research on Indigenous terms and as researchers. Smith (2012) is clear:

> *Theory enables us to deal with contradictions and uncertainties ... It gives us space to plan, to strategise, to take greater control over our resistances ... It helps us to interpret what is being told to us, and to predict the consequences of what is being promised. Theory can protect us because it contains within it a way of putting reality into perspective. If it is good theory it also allows for new ideas and ways of looking at things to be incorporated constantly, without the need to search constantly for new theories* (p. 40).

Undertaking research in Indigenous contexts and with Indigenous Peoples requires the positionality of researchers to locate their own cultural and professional backgrounds within the context of the research and in relation to the communities and Indigenous Peoples engaged in the research. The chapter focuses on research-related issues for Aboriginal and Torres Strait Islander Australians and New Zealand Māori. The authors acknowledge it is important not to engage in 'pan-indigenising' cultures, except where there have been connections made by the people themselves. This chapter has been revised by two academics. Lynore Geia is a Bwgcolman, meaning many tribes one people of Palm Island and shares her cultural affiliation with her Elders who were forcibly removed in the early 1900s under the control of government from their respective Aboriginal culture and Country of the Kalkadoon, Birri Gubba, Clumpoint and the Kaurareg nation of the Torres Strait. Born on the Aboriginal community of Palm Island in Queensland, she is a Bwgcolman registered nurse and midwife who holds a PhD in Nursing and is active in community leadership. Her nursing and midwifery research, education and practice is also informed by the needs of the Indigenous community; this is translated in collaboration with community in co-designing and co-producing research that impacts on health praxis, to reduce the health inequities experienced by communities and 'Closing the Gap' in Aboriginal and Torres Strait Island health.

Nicolette Sheridan has tribal affiliations to Ngāpuhi, Te Hikutū, Te Māhurehure, Ngāti Pākau and Ngāti Rauwawe in the North of Aotearoa New Zealand. She has a PhD in Nursing and Community Health, a Master of Public Health, and is professor and Head of the School of Nursing at Massey University, Te Kunenga ki Pūrehuroa in Aotearoa. Her research interests include analysing disparities in health services between Indigenous and non-Indigenous citizens as a means of monitoring government commitment to Indigenous rights. She was the first Associate Dean Equity in the Faculty of Medical and Health Sciences at the University of Auckland, Aotearoa New Zealand.

For researchers, whether they are Indigenous or non-Indigenous, introducing who they are and their relationship to the research and the community is 'best practice' and a way of enacting cultural safety by making explicit their commitments and responsibilities. This process provides a central framing across many significant national guiding documents that have informed best practice in nursing, medicine and health-related fields and in broader Indigenous research communities. This framing occurs across the National Health and Medical Research Council *Ethical Conduct in Research With Aboriginal and Torres Strait Islander Peoples and Communities: guidelines for researchers and stakeholders* (NHMRC 2018) and the National Health and Medical Research Council, the Australian Research Council and Universities Australia *National Statement on Ethical Conduct in Human Research 2023* (2023).

Other relevant publications on Indigenous research practice include:

Commonwealth Closing the Gap Implementation Plan https://www.niaa.gov.au/2023-commonwealth-closing-gap-implementation-plan

The New National Aboriginal and Torres Strait Islander Health Plan 2013–2023 https://www.health.gov.au/topics/aboriginal-and-torres-strait-islander-health/how-we-support-health/health-plan

Australian Research Council Indigenous Discovery Grant https://www.arc.gov.au/funding-research/funding-schemes/discovery-program/discovery-indigenous

NACCHO Strategic Plan 2018–2021 https://www.naccho.org/uploads/downloadable-resources/2018-strategic-plan.pdf

The Lowitja Institute Research Ethics Hub https://www.lowitja.org.au/tools/ethics-hub/ethics-guidelines/

In 2019, *Te Mahere Whakamātāmuatanga a Rangahau Hauora Aotearoa / The New Zealand Health Research Prioritisation Framework* (NZHRS) was published as part of the implementation of the New Zealand Health Research Strategy 2017–2027. Advancing Māori health was a principle underpinning the New Zealand Health Research Prioritisation Framework (https://www.hrc.govt.nz/sites/default/files/2020-01/NZ%20Prioritisation-Framework-Te-Reo-web pdf and https://www.hrc.govt.nz/sites/default/files/2020-01/NZ%20Prioritisation-Framework-FA-web_0.pdf), which comprises two parts: the 'Health Research Domains' that frames the vision of the NZHRS with high-level health and social outcomes, and the 'Health Research Attributes' that prioritise five essential attributes of health research and roles and responsibilities for contributors.

Indigenous Qualitative, Quantitative and Mixed-Methods Research

Qualitative research methodologies (see Chapter 5) and methods are often used by Indigenous researchers to position the experience of Indigenous Peoples as of high importance. Some Indigenous researchers are challenging the notion that only qualitative research can provide an accurate picture of Indigenous Peoples' lives and experiences. Such researchers include Maggie Walter, a Trawlwoolway woman of the Pymmerrairrener Nation, and Canadian First Nations' Métis or Michif, Chris Anderson, who have long argued for a better understanding of statistics. While they have challenged the misuse of statistics in Indigenous health contexts, these researchers have advocated for more Indigenous researchers to engage in mixed-methods research that employs both qualitative and quantitative approaches (Anderson & Walter 2013) (see Chapter 12).

Sheridan (the second author) is principal investigator of a mixed-methods study funded by the New Zealand Government and Health Research Council to investigate primary care across Aotearoa to identify the model of general practice that provides the best patient health outcomes (Sheridan et al 2023a). While Te Tiriti o Waitangi (1840) guarantees equal health outcomes for Māori and non-Māori, differences are longstanding. The study included 924 (91.3%) of all general practices with 4,491,964 enrolled patients. The study found no one model of practice outperformed others across all outcomes measured, although there were statistically significant differences between models. Māori ethnicity was statistically associated with poorer outcomes (Sheridan et al 2023a). Nurses undertook more preventative care (cervical screening, cardiovascular risk assessment, PHQ9 assessment, HbA_{1c} testing) in Māori practices compared with the dominant 'traditional' model of practice that enrolled 73% of the total population. Despite those with high complex health needs receiving more clinical input, this was insufficient to achieve equity in health outcomes. Across all models, primary care need was unmet for many Māori patients. Māori patients had a higher health risk profile, despite Māori practices having similar outcomes to other models of care, except for lower immunisation rates. The study concluded that Māori practices were an expression of autonomy in the face of enduring health system failure. Funding to support under-resourced Māori practices was required, along with accountability for the health outcomes of Māori patients in all models of general practice (Sheridan et al 2023b, in press). The researchers were from five universities and research organisations; three were Māori. The Māori researchers took a lead in governance, as well as data collection, analysis and interpretation of results. They were all clinicians with knowledge in Māori health, public health, primary healthcare, statistics and Kaupapa Māori methodology. Study results are informing investment in a future model of general practice with evidence supporting improvements in patient health outcomes for Māori and other populations.

The Issue of Language—the Words We Use

> *Knowledge translation and health professional communication is often ineffective despite the many opportunities to meaningfully engage.*
>
> ***(Sheridan et al 2015)***

> *'Indigenous' is a label that has become associated with deprivation and marginalisation; however, for many of the world's Indigenous people, their [use of this identifier] ... is self-conferred by a long association with the lands [in which] they live and from which their ancestors derived their existence and identity, and a tradition of unity with the environment that is told in song, reflected in custom, evident in subsistence as well as approaches to healing and rituals associated with birth and death.*
>
> ***(Durie 2004, as cited in Pulver & Harris 2007 p. 6).***

In Australia, the term 'Indigenous' is often used by organisations that are engaged in work with Aboriginal and Torres Strait Islander Peoples. This reference is respectful and short-form for 'Indigenous Australians'.

'Aboriginal' (and variants such as 'Aboriginals' or 'Aborigines') are terms no longer used by the Australian Government and there is a range of literature that suggests such words are outdated and should not be used by researchers. These terms do not reflect the diversity of cultures and identities across Australia and should be accompanied by 'peoples' in the plural (https://www.narragunnawali.org.au/terminology-guide). 'First Peoples' or 'First Nations' are pluralised terms that show respect and are acceptable because they encompass the diversity of Aboriginal and Torres Strait Islander cultures and identities. It is considered inappropriate to use the term 'ATSI' as a short-form for Aboriginal and Torres Strait Islander Peoples, although it is appropriate if this acronym is part of an organisational name, such as 'AIATSIS'—The Australian Institute of Aboriginal and Torres Strait Islander Studies (an independent Australian Government statutory authority). Including cultural affiliation names is also appropriate and should be used respectfully in context, and most Indigenous researchers in Australia now add their cultural affiliation name to their professional biography.

Much of the collective naming of Indigenous Australians has been challenged because many people do not want the colonial name to frame their individual communities. These collective terms, while aiding national positioning, are being replaced by terms that individuals choose to reference their Country, nation, or geographic location. Dr Lynore Geia always includes her cultural affiliation or Country as a nurse and midwife, academic researcher and teacher, and leader. She proudly refers to herself as a fourth-generation Bwgcolman woman, acknowledging her birthplace and home on Bwgcolman Country (Palm Island) on the Great Barrier Reef in North Queensland near Townsville. These acknowledgements provide a context for other Aboriginal Peoples so that they know who she is and the responsibilities she holds and where she is positioned in kinship and cultural relationality with other Aboriginal and Torres Strait Islander Peoples and communities.

The use of the word 'Country' needs to be explained here; the term 'Country' has deeper cultural meanings than the word country. Country is not just a word! In Aboriginal English, Country has deep meaning—it is described as not only being a common noun, but also a 'proper noun' (Rose 1996) and a 'verb'—it carries deep meanings of Aboriginal and Torres Strait Island peoples 'living, being and doing' in right relationship and understanding of our world and its interaction with the contemporary world.

In a recent nursing publication, Wiradjuri nurse educator and researcher Tamara Power led a bold list of Indigenous nursing co-authors who scribed their Indigenous academic identity as: Ngāti Tahinga (Tainui), Bwgcolman, Kalkadoon and Djaku-nde, Aaniniiin Nation, Ngāpuhi, Cree/Métis, Beaver Lake Cree Nation, Cherokee/Creek/Lenape, Guna, Gamilaroi, and Gorreng Gorreng, Boonthamurra and Yugambeh (Power et al 2021b). The authors also prefaced the publication with an acknowledgement of Country: 'We begin by acknowledging the sovereignty of Indigenous Peoples across the Earth as the traditional custodians of Country, and their timeless and embodied relationships with cultures, communities, lands, waters, and sky. We honour children born and yet to be. We pay our respects to Elders, past and present, particularly those who led the way, allowing us to realise our own calling to be healers.' Thus, embedding cultural identity in publications is a way of decolonising the academy and making space for academic transformation.

For researchers who do not come from Indigenous backgrounds, explaining who you are, your cultural background and your work is important. As previously outlined, best-practice documents in both Aotearoa New Zealand and Australia frame this process and highlight key issues that relate to ethical engagement with communities. Researchers are also required to explain their contribution back into a community through 'knowledge transfer':

> *Understanding how people value and interpret the benefits of research is critical. While academics talk about research impact, Indigenous people talk about ethical positions and 'tangible' benefits such as responses and solutions to issues studied in research projects that are meaningful to their lives. These benefits might include the development of historical artefacts and languages that preserve culture and benefit future generations and direct benefits such as the translation of any research knowledge into more immediate relevant and consumable product.*
>
> ***(Bainbridge et al 2015 p. 6)***

Elders, Concepts and Methodologies

Elders across most Indigenous communities have responsibilities to those communities and to the land. Philosopher Aunty Mary Graham, a Kombumerri and Waka Waka Elder, has talked about belonging and the importance of a continuation of connection to country for Aboriginal Peoples (Graham 2008). Her work has positioned these responsibilities as central to what it means to be an Aboriginal person. She argues that Aboriginal communities show ethical leadership when they consider the land and the environment over their own personal needs. Elders like Aunty Mary Graham, while recognised as experts in health-related fields, have a role in guiding Indigenous communities and in engaging with the broader community. As research partners, Elders can contribute to continuous and ongoing responsibilities to culture, community and kinship, and support the interconnected relationships that link communities across states and country. While Aboriginal and Torres Strait Islander communities are not homogeneous, they share a common connection to their lands.

Well-known Nauiyu Elder Miriam Rose Ungunmerr-Baumann AM, Senior 2021 Australian of the Year, activist, writer, educator and public speaker, introduced Australia to the Aboriginal spiritual practice of *Dadirri* (pronounced da-did-ee) in 1988. Conceptualised as a way of being and doing of 'inner deep listening and quiet still awareness' on Country by the Nauiyu (Daly River) people in the Northern Territory, *Dadirri* is an enduring Indigenous practice that has been adapted and embedded in contemporary Indigenous nursing research (West, Geia). *Dadirri* is now a legitimate scholarly research methodology which supports the positioning of the researcher in 'reciprocal archaeology' where both researcher and research participant can experience an 'awareness of past, present and future belonging to Country and self in the research process'. So too, on the opposite side of the nation in Canberra, Ngunnawal and Ngambri Elder Aunty Matilda House gifted her cultural word of *Muliyan* meaning 'Eagle eye view' to the Congress of Aboriginal and Torres Strait Islander Nurses and Midwives (CATSINaM) and reminded CATSINaM to rise above in attending to the work of nursing and midwifery education and practice, to 'look across' the Country to aim at connecting with all the Schools of Nursing and Midwifery exercising Indigenous nursing and midwifery authority on matters of curricula, education and research. Elders bring vital cultural associations in research relationships that must be understood and included in research design when undertaking research on 'Country'.

Similarly in Māori society, Elders or Kaumātua have an important leadership role. Male Elders are also known as Koroua (or Koro), and female Elders are known as Kuia. Kaumātua are expected to undertake certain roles and duties within the wider family and tribal community. Traditionally, they made decisions about the whānau (family), whenua (land), the control and use of whānau property, the education of tamariki (children), and speak on behalf of whānau in tribal councils (rūnanga). Kaumātua are respected for their knowledge of tribal history and traditions and through everyday activities, and through storytelling, poetry and waiata (song), and they pass on knowledge to the younger generation. Dyall et al (2013), in the article 'Navigation: process of building relationships with Kaumātua (Māori leaders)', describes how a research project becomes more relevant when Kaumātua are effective advisers.

In Aotearoa New Zealand, Kaupapa Māori research seeks to involve Māori communities in research that privileges Māori ways of knowing, Māori language and Māori culture. Kaupapa Māori approaches to research or Kaupapa Māori research is a means by which Māori researchers can take back space from non-Māori researchers whose research is embedded within an institution of Western knowledge and power. Developed in the 1980s, Kaupapa Māori research has been described as a cultural strategy to define the perspectives, needs, practices and ethics of Māori peoples (Hoskins & Jones 2012).

Nurse academic, the late Dr Irihapeti Ramsden (Ngāi Tahu/Rangitane), is acknowledged as the architect of '**cultural safety**', a concept that defines a therapeutic relationship as safe, maintaining individual and whānau respect (mana) and empowering. Cultural safety became a requirement for nursing and midwifery courses in 1992, signalling a change in nursing education which was controversial at the time (Papps & Ramsden 1996, Ramsden 1993), but has since become increasingly recognised as essential for safe clinical practice beyond the nursing profession. Cultural safety (kawa whakaruruhau within a Māori context) is essential if health outcomes are to be improved for Māori patients and whānau. Nurses, doctors and other health workers are required to be culturally safe as well as clinically competent to improve health outcomes for Māori populations (and other populations). All health workers must be 'pro-equity, culturally safe, Tiriti compliant and anti-racist' (Reid 2021 p. 7).

RESEARCH IN BRIEF 14.1

It is well known that health disparities continue to exist between Māori and non-Māori New Zealanders. Huria et al (2014) qualitatively explored the experience and impact of racism on Māori registered nurses within the Aotearoa New Zealand healthcare system using a Kaupapa Māori research methodology. As previously outlined, Kaupapa Māori research offers an Indigenous theoretical framework that is increasingly being applied within health research to document the experiences of Māori within the health system and highlight inequity in healthcare, health outcomes and the nursing workforce. Fifteen Māori registered nurses were interviewed about their experiences of racism. A theoretical framework for understanding racism on three levels—institutionalised, personally mediated and internalised (Jones 2000)—was used as a coding frame for the analysis of data. Participants reported they experienced racism on all three levels and that this had led to marginalisation, being overworked and being undervalued. Māori nurses identified a lack of recognition of their dual nursing competencies. While their clinical skills were validated, their cultural skills—skills in Hauora Māori—were not. Experiences of racism were common. The study recommended that the nursing profession in New Zealand, and other countries, acknowledge the presence of racism within training and clinical environments and support Indigenous nurses to develop and implement dual cultural and clinical competencies.

In relation to research, the term 'by Māori, for Māori, of Māori' captures the essence of a Kaupapa Māori approach and worldview that seeks to determine a person's own destiny while maintaining wellbeing (mauri-ora). Māori language is a tāonga—a gift or treasure—because it holds knowledge and encompasses Māori culture and ways to work within cultural contexts. In terms of researcher competence from a New Zealand perspective, specific philosophies and competence are privileged by Māori through language and practices, often guided by Kaumātua (Elders) or other significant people within a community who are guardians of Māori customs and practices. These include:

- *manaaki*—show respect or kindness to
- *manaakitanga*—hospitality
- *kaitiakitanga*—helper/adviser
- *kaiāwhina*—helper, assistant, attendant
- *tikanga*—customs
- *tapu*—sacred, restricted, prohibited
- *noa*—free from tapu or any other restriction
- *tangata whenua*—people of the land
- *whakapapa*—lineage, genealogy, to layer (Ministry of Justice 2001).

There are everyday practicalities in ensuring that such protocols are observed. For example, attention to aspects of *tapu* and *noa* are critical for the acknowledgement and acceptance of *manuhiri* (visitors) to Aotearoa New Zealand communities; of engagement with communities and for ongoing trust and respectful relationships. Conditions of *tapu* could relate to formalities like: knowing who to speak to, knowing when to visit, participating in formal welcome-to-community/country, knowing where to stand, or even when to sit. Conditions of *noa* then 'lift *tapu*' through: *karakia* (a prayer), *waiata* (a song), sharing of cultural gifts and eating, and then engaging in formal and informal relationship building. Kaumātua in Māori communities ensures that processes are followed because, for them, this relates to *mana* (respect and dignity) and cultural perpetuity.

Understanding Indigenous Contexts in Australasian Research

Indigenous research processes in the Australian context have undergone a long progression of establishing its cultural authority to develop and lead Indigenous research in health industries in Australian society. The existence of organisations such as The Lowitja Institute (https://www.lowitja.org.au/), Australia's only Aboriginal and Torres Strait Islander community-controlled health research institute, is now a national formative voice for the Aboriginal and Torres Strait Islander health. Named after Yankunytjatjara Elder and Aboriginal nurse, Dr Lowitja O'Donoghue, AC CBE DSG, who is arguably Australia's most recognised Aboriginal Elder for her work in Australian nursing and

Indigenous health, the Lowitja Institute leads high-impact research, knowledge exchange and translation, and is instrumental in growing the next generation of Aboriginal and Torres Strait Islander health researchers. Its reach has extended globally, amplifying the impact of Indigenous research to improve health and wellbeing of global First Nations Peoples as well. The Institute's service to the Indigenous community rests on five key principles that reinforce their research practice with Aboriginal and Torres Strait Islander people:

1. beneficence – to act for the benefit of Aboriginal and Torres Strait Islander Peoples in the conduct of our research
2. leadership by Aboriginal and Torres Strait Islansder People
3. engagement of research end users (Aboriginal and Torres Strait Islander organisations and communities, policy makers and other potential research users)
4. development of the Aboriginal and Torres Strait Islander research workforce, and
5. measurement of impact in improving Aboriginal and Torres Strait Islander Peoples' health.

In the Australian Indigenous research context, the Lowitja Institute's research leadership is viewed as a positive gatekeeper for the wider Aboriginal and Torres Strait Islander communities advocating and reinforcing ethical practices. There is no single pan-Indigenous experience. Indigenous communities are organised nations of heterogenous groups that reflect kinship and cultural ties. There is, however, an expectation that all researchers are required to act with integrity and care and to accurately portray the uniqueness of those who consent to participate in research and share their experiences. Their responsibility is to ensure that community knowledge and information, shared in the research process, is not appropriated or reported in ways that perpetuate bias or prejudice.

RESEARCH IN BRIEF 14.2

Bwgcolman Country, often referred to as Palm Island, is home to the Bwgcolman and Manbarra people, who make up a distinct Aboriginal and Torres Strait Islander community situated 65 kilometres north-west of Townsville on the east coast of Queensland, Australia. 'Palm Island's history has been shaped by punitive government policies and practices, coercive displacement from mainland Aboriginal communities, dispossession and violence' (Geia & Lindsay 2017).

Palm Island is a resilient growing community of about 3000 people with more than half of the population (53%) under 24 years of age. However, like many Indigenous communities, social determinants of health such as employment, finance, housing and education remain inadequately addressed, leading to health and social burdens for the community. As a result, youths have sought ways of coping with these hardships through engaging in risk-taking behaviours, including substance misuse.

There was a clear need for more information, particularly about youth health risk-related behaviours. This resulted in a community-led research collaboration, a first of its kind in over 100 years with a Bwgcolman researcher (Geia, first author) and colleagues in a study titled '*The social impact of drug, alcohol and volatile substance misuse among young Aboriginal and Torres Strait Islanders and their family on Palm Island: a community survey informing a Palm Island Youth Strategy*'. The aim was to explore high-risk behaviours in youths 14–24 years of age and find solutions with the young people and community.

A mixed-methods approach was used. A survey provided quantitative data that could be numerically summed and used by the government and health services. The qualitative data collection led by Indigenous researcher (Geia) and with local research assistants was undertaken by creating a critical space for privileging the voice of Indigenous people. 'Yarning' or storytelling provided qualitative data, contextualising the numbers and meeting the need of the community to tell their stories in their way. While the two approaches are interdependent, the information collected through yarning supported a richer interpretation of data. Geia et al (2013) argue:

> *Indigenous community research must be conducted with the people and not imposed upon people. Partnership and collaboration are vital for research success. Bwgcolman youth were employed as research assistants in the fieldwork and provided an emic (insider) reality, which culturally 'grounded' study methods in terms of language and social and familial relationships. 'Murri Talk' was a method to share information between close-knit peer groups. Bwgcolman youth took part in developing the research questions, which was vital as understanding Palm Island youth culture was central to constructing a culturally sensitive data collection tool. The research assistants invited young people to participate in the survey. Data was collected after school hours and on weekends. Confidentiality and privacy were emphasised.*

Continued

RESEARCH IN BRIEF 14.2—cont'd

Maintaining cultural safety in research is paramount. The participant information sheet, for example, included: 'If sharing your story upsets you in any way, you can stop at any time and we will make sure that you get some counselling support from a person of your choice on the Island'. Relational accountability between the researcher/s, participants and wider community was demonstrated in the reciprocal research relationships that nurtured and respected culture.

Building the capacity of Indigenous youth to take ownership of meaningful and sustained change was important in this research that started at grassroots and developed as an effective intersectoral collaboration. A key finding of the research was the centrality of connection for young people with their family and cultural affiliations; these are positive findings that are now identified as cultural determinants of health, they are protective elements of Indigenous Peoples' lives that affirm identity and belonging. The findings of the research were taken back to the community and presented to the youth and services with recommendations for a way forward. Both findings and recommendations were accepted and released to the Palm Island community and those outside organisations that provide services to the community. The study findings and recommendations are now being used to inform a long-term intersectoral youth strategy led by Palm Island young people with commitment from community, service providers and governments.

RESEARCH IN BRIEF 14.3

Barclay et al (2014) present a summary of a 5-year collaborative program of maternity services for remote-dwelling Aboriginal women and their infants. The study area consisted of two large remote Aboriginal communities (Community 'A' and Community 'B', both of approximately 2000–3000 people) in the Top End of Australia and the hospital in the regional centre that provided birth and tertiary care facilities for these communities. The mixed-methods participatory approach ensured engagement of the Aboriginal communities and industry stakeholders including consumers, midwives, doctors, nurses, Aboriginal health workers, managers, policy makers and support staff. Aboriginal women, policy makers, managers and clinicians helped guide the research.

Baseline data in the two communities were obtained from 412 mothers and their 413 infants across a trajectory of care from 2004 to 2006. Substudies identified patterns of health service utilisation, discharge processes, barriers to care, adherence to guidelines and infant treatment as measures of care quality. Serious deficiencies were identified in the quality of maternal and infant health services for Aboriginal families, such as discrimination, inadequate understanding of Aboriginal culture, and deficiencies in the quality and availability of data to inform decisions. Clinical identification, management and treatment completion in infant care delivery and infant health were poor for both growth faltering and anaemia. Significant improvements were achieved—for example, by the midwifery group practice, and women's engagement with the health services through their midwives.

Māori research is rich in metaphor and analogical thinking. For example, it is suggested that the accompanying 'rhythm' of research needs to take care of the 'heartbeat' of individuals within communities. For example, a frequently referenced Māori health and wellbeing perspective, 'Te Whare Tapa Wha', is a construct that compares good health to the four sides of a whare (house) and demonstrates a 'balance between spirituality (taha wairua), intellect and emotions (taha hinengaro), the human body (taha tinana) and human relationships (taha whānau) (Ministry of Health–Aotearoa 2012a). A code for sensible living often depended on classifying activities, situations and objects as either risky (tapu) or safe (noa)' (Durie 2004 p. 12) (see Fig. 14.1). Stylistically and dynamically, Te Whare Tapa Wha demonstrates overall Māori wellbeing with a model of a whare (house) demonstrating reliance upon all four walls or dimensions of wellbeing (Durie 2004):

- *taha tinana*—physical health
- *taha wairua*—spiritual health
- *taha whānau*—family health
- *taha hinengaro*—mental health.

Indigenous health must also be part of a 'wider societal discussion that includes cultural identity, the natural environment, constitutional arrangements, socio-economic realities, and indigenous leadership' (Durie 2004 p. 16). Health promotion, if it is to be effective, must consider the quality of interaction between people and the environment and also the balance between development and environmental sustainability (p. 12). Te Pae Māhutonga, a model of Māori health promotion, represented by the constellation of stars referred to as the Southern Cross, signposts the strategic direction governments, health and education sectors, and Indigenous Peoples themselves might take. It has

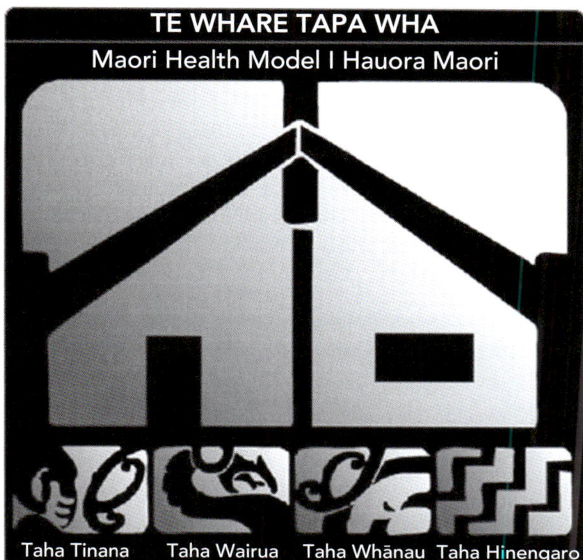

Fig. 14.1 Te Whare Tapa Whā health model (Source: Ministry of Health–Aotearoa 2012a Māori health models—Te Whare Tapa Whā. https://www.health.govt.nz/our-work/populations/maori-health/maori-health-models/maori-health-models-te-whare-tapa-wha.)

four central stars that symbolise the four key tasks of health promotion: Mauriora (cultural identity), Waiora (physical environment), Toiora (healthy lifestyles) and Te Oranga (participation in society). Te Pae Māhutonga also has two stars arranged in a straight line, which point towards the cross. These are known as the two pointers and can represent Te Mana Whakahaere (autonomy) and Ngā Manukura (community leadership). Indigenous models focus renewed and dynamic attention on the ways research can connect with people's lives and uncover health and social impacts on wellbeing (Durie 1999).

> **TUTORIAL TRIGGER 14.1**
>
> What analogy does Fig. 14.1 represent, and how can it be linked to research and ethics?

The role of 'endurance' in Indigenous Peoples' lives over generations cannot be overemphasised. Although we argue the importance of avoiding the pathologising of Indigenous Peoples, there is a need to understand the impact of colonisation on communities and the wellbeing of Indigenous Peoples (Atkinson 2002). Intergenerational trauma caused by government interventions, such as the Stolen Generations—a practice that involved the forced separation of children from their family—can leave communities suspicious of the role of government and Western organisations (Human Rights and Equal Opportunity Commission 1997).

RELATING CULTURAL COMPETENCE TO INDIGENOUS RESEARCH AND ETHICS

Cultural competence has emerged as a desired outcome in university-graduated nurses in Aotearoa New Zealand and Australia. The Nursing Council of New Zealand demands that cultural safety is a mandatory requirement for all undergraduate and registered nurses to meet. Key references include: the Code of Conduct standards and guidelines; Scope of Practice competencies and guidelines; and *Guidelines for Cultural Safety, the Treaty of Waitangi and Māori Health in Nursing, Education and Practice* (https://www.nursingcouncil.org.nz/Public/NCNZ/nursing-section/Standards_and_guidelines_for_nurses.aspx?hkey=9fc06ae7-a853-4d10-b5fe-992cd44ba3de).

Cultural competence includes notions of cultural safety, cultural respect and cultural awareness. In Australia, cultural competence has been the impetus for including Indigenous Australian perspectives and content in undergraduate curriculum since the mid 2000s (Bradley et al 2008), and the expectation to meet cultural competencies is increasingly more apparent in postgraduate education. Building cultural competence in nursing is essential to providing safe and effective care, and cultural models of health can support a deeper understanding of Indigenous Peoples' perspectives and offer a framework to guide practice. Future evaluation will be essential to determining the effects of cultural competence education on nurses' practice. Current evidence suggests there is a positive effect (see Fig. 14.3, later in this chapter).

> **RESEARCH IN BRIEF 14.4**
>
> Cultural competence—cultural respect, cultural safety and cultural awareness—is critical to reducing healthcare disparities in the healthcare system. Wepa (2003) documented the experiences of four cultural safety educators in nursing education in Aotearoa New Zealand. Participants were purposively selected on the basis of their knowledge of the research topic. An action research method offered a dynamic process for joint learning and problem solving. Two prerequisites were identified: the participants must identify a problem they wanted to investigate, and the study should be relevant and important to those involved. Six questions related to experiences and behaviours, opinions and values, feelings, knowledge, sensations. and

Continued

RESEARCH IN BRIEF 14.4—cont'd

background/demographic factors were asked about in tape-recorded semistructured interviews. Reflective diaries provided another source of data. Data were analysed using thematic analysis and three themes emerged: (1) 'feeling unprepared to teach cultural safety', (2) 'the dichotomy between enjoyment of teaching and the lack of energy to continue' and (3) 'lack of support'. Recommendations included: (1) provision of support to dialogue and network; (2) introduction of Nurse Educator Programs, (3) an increase in knowledge on cultural safety and (4) recognition of Māori cultural safety educators.

Working together with Indigenous communities requires respect, reciprocity and, above all, care. These values are integral to the nursing profession and are critical to the development of the researcher. Smith contends 'Indigenous research is a humble and a humbling activity' (Smith 2012 p. 5) and has shown that contextualising *takepu* (applied principles), and the thinking within them, guides researchers in gathering people's stories, insights and knowledge about different situations that have impacted communities over time.

Utilising *whakapapa* (connected layering) in research is about engaging with the order and processes of the purpose and construction of research, so that there is cohesion and a legitimate awareness in recognising potential disruptions for individuals and community. This awareness is required because:

> *We have a different epistemological tradition which frames the way we see the world, the way we organise ourselves in it, the questions we ask and the solutions we seek. It is larger than the individuals in it and the specific 'moment' in which we are currently living.*
>
> ***(Smith 2000 p. 230)***

It is not just about the gathering of data, but also the way that 'gathering' is utilised and how information is treated. Indigenous research draws knowledge from people and part of that process is for researchers and individuals together to facilitate a safe space to rename that knowledge in a conscious act of claiming stories from the past and naming stories from the present, in order to reclaim heritage. Reclamation of heritage by sharing stories has the capacity for healing and is decolonising (Muller 2014).

New narratives and stories must be told and recorded. There has been an overemphasis on negative stories in the media and on deficits and poor health outcomes. Stoneham et al (2014) found that reporting on Aboriginal and Torres Strait Islanders' health in Australia was overwhelmingly negative and perpetuated racist stereotypes. Future health is impacted by reporting deficits, making more important a strengths-based approach to research within the community. This can be achieved by acknowledging the good health of precolonised societies, taking opportunities to report Indigenous Peoples' stories (counter-hegemony), and supporting and encouraging the capacities that reside within people and the community. Embracing culture and recognising potential is paramount.

RESEARCH IN BRIEF 14.5

A qualitative study conducted by Chapman et al (2014) explored the perceived barriers and enablers to Aboriginal and Torres Strait Islander people accessing healthcare through one Victorian Emergency Department (ED). Ethics approval was obtained. Indigenous community members (12 women and 4 men) were invited to participate in tape-recorded semistructured focus groups/yarns. Recordings were transcribed verbatim and the analysis included coding, finding categories, clustering and identifying patterns and meaning. Three main themes emerged: Theme 1: Organisational processes (e.g. waiting, Aboriginal and Torres Strait Islander status, cultural concerns), Theme 2: Staff interactions—staff members were seen as both barriers and enablers to accessing healthcare, and Theme 3: Strategies for improvement (e.g. communication strategies, cultural awareness training, identifiable cultural features). Strategies for identifying and resolving issues when interacting with the Western healthcare system were identified as outputs from this research.

Indigenous researchers and research units continue to be instrumental in the successful implementation of processes of engagement with Indigenous Peoples. For example, Kaupapa Māori practice is manifested through attention to embracing and exercising cultural safety. Māori Nurse Educator Dianne Wepa recounts the term cultural safety being adopted following a significant *hui* (meeting)—*Hui Waimanawa*—in 1988. Wepa took the gathering to her tribal (Iwi) area—*Te Arawa*—in Aotearoa New Zealand, where she was supported by her grandparents and whānau/family who sat with her for a week. Her grandfather named the meeting *Hui Waimanawa*, 'in recognition of the tears which had been shed over the years of colonisation and to recognise the importance of the hui taking place' (Wepa 2015 p. 22). In the following year the Nursing Council of New Zealand and nursing and midwifery education providers based an understanding of cultural safety on two documents:

'*A Model for Negotiated and Equal Partnership*' (Ramsden 1989) and 'Kawa whakaruruhau: cultural safety in nursing education in Aotearoa (New Zealand)' (Ramsden 1993). Four key objectives of cultural safety were identified in Wepa (2003 p. 23) and were influenced by classroom encounters with student nurses. They are:

- not blaming the victims of historical processes for their current plights
- to examine their own realities and the attitudes they bring to each new person they encounter in their practice
- to be open-minded and flexible in their attitudes towards other people who are different from themselves, to whom they offer and deliver service
- to produce a workforce of well-educated, self-aware registered nurses and midwives who are culturally safe to practise, as defined by the people they serve.

With regard to healthcare for Indigenous Australians, Taylor and Guerin (2019) assert that it requires the non-Indigenous workforces and systems to examine themselves and consider what they can do differently, rather than always expecting Indigenous clients to change to fit the dominant culture's ways of thinking, being and doing. Indigenous health and cultural safety raise complex and challenging issues for health professionals and consumers alike. However, this should not be an excuse to fail to make the effort or to resist the very necessary notion of equitable, safe and accessible healthcare for every Australian (p. 223).

The emergence of many best-practice models in Aotearoa New Zealand and Australia suggest there is a growing strength and opportunity for Indigenous researchers to privilege their own stories for their own people, rather than having these stories told by others. In the research economy (because research attracts funding and has its own inherent economy), non-Indigenous researchers who undertake research *without* connecting with Indigenous individuals and communities are decreasing in number. Despite this, Indigenous research continues to be undertaken by individual academics in relative isolation. In 2011, all universities in Australia had a Human Research Ethics Committee to ensure the appropriateness and safety of research conducted by the staff and students of the institution congruent with the NHMRC guidelines. Twenty-one Australian universities also had additional mechanisms in place to ensure that research with Indigenous Peoples is culturally safe and employed culturally appropriate methodologies and processes. The same is true for all New Zealand tertiary educational institutions where research is undertaken.

Indigenous cultural competency activities in universities in Aotearoa New Zealand, Canada, the United States and Hawaii have more recently revealed many exemplars of culturally sound research principles, ethical guidelines, processes and protocols related to research activities and engagement with Indigenous and First Nations Peoples. Indigenous Treaty rights, as acknowledged in New Zealand, Canada and the United States, provide the platform for Indigenous self-determination over research on or about Indigenous communities and issues, with jurisdictions in Canada and the United States requiring tribal approval for all research undertaken within or about their communities. International codes of ethics such as the *Nuremberg Code* (1947), the *Helsinki Declaration* (1964), the *Belmont Report* (1979) and, more recently, the *UNESCO Universal Declaration on Bioethics and Human Rights* (2005), along with the principles of the Treaty of Waitangi, shape the changing ethical standards and professional expectations for researchers working in Māori contexts (Berglund 2012). This is explored more fully in Chapter 13.

AN UNEXPECTED HURDLE

A prospective research team has been established to overview innovative and exemplary research approaches and practice undertaken with and by Indigenous communities that are relevant to nursing and nursing practice. As part of a research team at the beginning of the research process, the team identifies that they need to establish some key guidelines and critical questions. Some of these include: 'What were the research topics and methods undertaken in Australia in recent years that deal with nursing issues and Indigenous people?', 'What constitutes good practice in nursing research and evaluation?', 'What are some of the key considerations when conducting research with Indigenous people and communities?', 'What should constitute good practice and what are examples?' and 'What are the main practical challenges associated with such practice?' Discussions are going well and some of your team working on an ethics application and Indigenous Elders have been approached to be a part of the central discussions around establishing what the community might need in the way of nursing care into the future.

At a key juncture in the discussions one of your research team becomes impatient and exhibits behaviour that could at best be described as intolerant and at worst racist. As this team member is one of the researchers that has attracted funding for this project, they are crucial to the continuation of this research work. This team member has also been told sensitive things by Indigenous community members about their individual nursing experiences.

How might you, as an ethical researcher and practitioner, approach this issue and overcome this hurdle?

What Does Culturally Competent Research Look Like?

Culturally competent research remains an evolving entity. The taken-for-granted, non-Indigenous approach to the ethical conduct of research is being challenged by the respect and inclusion recognised in, and demanded by, Indigenous rights. These rights are articulated in national and international documents. The challenge for the non-Indigenous researcher is correctly interpreting the Indigenous code of ethics and embracing the spirit of the code, and not simply paying lip-service to gain the approval of the relevant ethics committee to conduct research or gain related funding.

The health models represented in this chapter from Aotearoa New Zealand bring together the richness of language, metaphor, spirituality, connectedness and relational aspects of research and ethics that all contribute to sustainable mātauranga Māori—Māori knowledges; **Indigenous knowledge**. This knowledge is captured and utilised alongside recognition of the value of Western knowledge (Smith 2000) to highlight a specific legacy that informs relationship expectations and the guidance from past, present and future generations (Durie 1998). Aotearoa New Zealand has a further distinctive Treaty of Waitangi (Tiriti ō Waitangi) legacy out of which biculturalism is embraced, and utilising a combination of non-Indigenous concepts and those from a Kaupapa Māori stance not only provides a rich contrast for research analysis, but has been endorsed by distinguished Professor Graham Hingangaroa Smith (2000) about the legitimacy of drawing on theories to inspire, guide and support our own critical initiatives.

Indigenous ethics is intertwined with Indigenous rights. The Free, Prior and Informed Consent (FPIC) movement is a worldwide movement protecting the rights and lands of Indigenous Peoples (Barelli 2012). It broadens the concept of research by acknowledging the significance of place and land and ensures the involvement of Indigenous Peoples in decision making about research and other projects that impact them. It is not solely about consultation, acknowledging the autonomy and decision-making rights of the community. These conditions are related to research and the ethical conduct of research related to Indigenous Peoples, their land and culture.

Table 14.1 explains the implications of each component of Free, Prior and Informed Consent (FPIC) for Indigenous people and communities as articulated by Barelli (2012). Although FPIC and research are not specifically mentioned in its declaration, it is in concert with the United Nations (UN) *Declaration on the Rights of Indigenous Peoples*. For example, Article 31 of the declaration states:

> *Indigenous Peoples have the right to maintain, control, protect and develop their cultural heritage, traditional knowledge and traditional cultural expressions, as well as the manifestations of their sciences, technologies and cultures, including human and genetic resources, seeds, medicines, knowledge of the properties of fauna and flora, oral traditions, literatures, designs, sports and traditional games and visual and performing arts. They also have the right to maintain, control, protect and develop their intellectual property over such cultural heritage, traditional knowledge, and traditional cultural expressions.*
>
> ***(United Nations 2008).***

These documents recognise the rights of Indigenous Peoples to their own knowledge and to the exploration, development, recording and sharing of their ways of knowing and doing. Indigenous Peoples' right to consent to, be involved in, own and benefit from research outcomes related to and impacting on them is recognised at an international level.

TABLE 14.1 Component of FPIC for Indigenous Peoples and Communities

Term	Implications
Free	No coercion, intimidation or manipulation.
Prior	Consent must be sought sufficiently in advance of any commencement of activities and enough time should be allowed to facilitate consultation.
Informed	Indigenous people should receive information in relation to key areas and the implications of any planned activity.
Consent	Involves a process of consultation, done in good faith, with equitable participation of the Indigenous people guaranteed. Participation is through freely chosen representatives of the Indigenous people and participation is in accordance with their customs.

(Source: Barelli, M., 2012. Free, prior and informed consent in the aftermath of the UN Declaration on the Rights of Indigenous Peoples: developments and challenges ahead. Int. J. HR. 16 (1), p. 2)

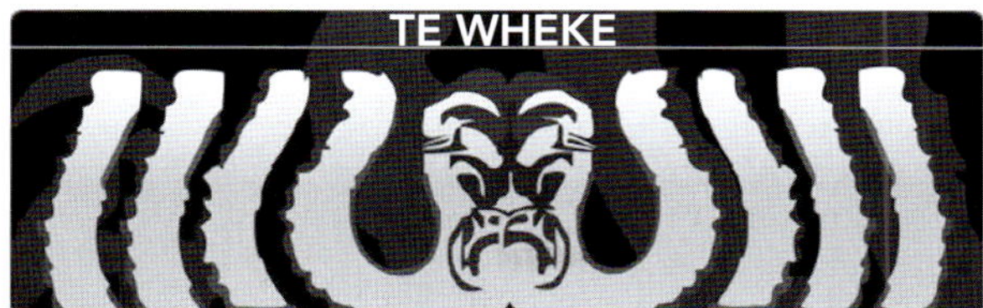

Fig. 14.2 Te Wheke health model (Source: Ministry of Health–Aotearoa 2012b Māori health models—Te Wheke. https://www.health.govt.nz/our-work/populations/maori-health/maori-health-models/maori-health-models-te-wheke)

A well-known and highly relevant model, *Te Wheke*, the octopus (Fig. 14.2), straddles the realm of research, living and health (Pere 2015). Traditional Māori health acknowledges the link between the mind, the spirit, the human connection with whānau and the physical world in a way that is seamless and uncontrived, and Pere captures this in Te Wheke. She makes strong claims between the use of the whole brain and the place of consciousness, and makes particular mention of Māori as having a high degree of intuitive intelligence. This is likely to be true of all Indigenous cultures who embrace the seamless links between the spiritual world, the physical land and people both past and present. Consideration of one without the others, or a lack of understanding of the implications of that connection, can, albeit unintentionally, lead to a breach of ethics when undertaking Indigenous research.

The concept of Te Wheke is to define family health, and doing this also defines individual health and a place in knowing. The head of the octopus represents te whānau (the family), the eyes of the octopus as waiora (total wellbeing for the individual and family) and each of the eight tentacles represents a specific dimension of health and wellbeing. The dimensions are interwoven and this phenomenon represents the close relationship of the tentacles, being:

- *te whānau*—the family
- *waiora*—total wellbeing for the individual and family
- *wairuatanga*—spirituality
- *hinengaro*—the mind
- *taha tinana*—physical wellbeing
- *whanaungatanga*—extended family
- *mauri*—life force in people and objects
- *mana ake*—unique identity of individuals and family
- *hā a koro ma, a kui ma*—breath of life from forebearers
- *whatumanawa*—the open and healthy expression of emotion (Ministry of Health—Aotearoa 2012b).

From an Indigenous worldview and a socioecological perspective, where everything is connected to everything else, the connection that Aboriginal and Torres Strait Islander Peoples have to the land, to Country and to culture through song, dance, language, stories, the Dreaming and food, for example, is deeply spiritual and akin to Māori connections through whakapapa; to whānau, hapū and iwi. Ranzijn et al (2010 pp. 36–53) offer numerous examples and explanations of the significance of the Dreaming, of creation and sacredness, of ceremonies and the telling of Story, and the impacts on Indigenous Australian lives.

What Does a Culturally Competent Researcher 'Look Like'?

Indigenous communities throughout Australia and Aotearoa New Zealand are heterogeneous and unique. For many Indigenous Peoples, knowledge about ways of doing things—protocols, rituals and heritage relationships—is tied to language acquisition and use. The displacement of individuals from community and culture, including access to language, makes acquiring cultural knowledge difficult. Language revitalisation and regeneration programs, however, have become prominent in the last decade within many Indigenous communities. In Aotearoa New Zealand, for example, connecting to whānau, hapū and iwi (family, subtribe and tribe) is being orchestrated nationally and internationally through community-held wānanga (places/sites of learning) and through the strategic plans of different iwi rūnanga (governing council/administrative group/corporation). Sometimes these initiatives have been designed to capitalise on Treaty of Waitangi settlement funds. Such initiatives are underpinned by emancipatory community action research processes (see Chapter 12) and seek to create resilience and sustainability (Ormsby-Teki et al 2011). In a contemporary world, technology has played an important part in achieving this connection—going online means that Māori anywhere in the world can exercise one of the fundamental tikanga principles—doing things right and staying connected to whānau/family. Several similar initiatives are ongoing in Australia, including the ideas around 'reawakening languages' (Hobson et al 2011).

In this chapter, links between the individual, community, hapū and iwi also have importance within Māori Indigenous research contexts and initiatives set down by Māori Research Units, such as Ngā Pae o te Māramatanga, that challenge power by questioning: 'What counts as knowledge?', 'Who has it?' and 'How will it be used?' Some Indigenous researchers have argued that quantitative and qualitative research methods do not easily allow the privileging of Kaupapa Māori theory as a resistant counter-narrative against dominant paradigms. Kaupapa Māori theory, as described by G. H. Smith (2000), with its foundations in Māori community development and the regeneration of te reo Māori has been central to the revitalisation of educational success and learning. The use of cultural knowledge strengthens cultural identity and wellbeing and is especially important for tamariki and rangatahi (Māori children and young people).

The implication is that it is incumbent upon the researcher to engage and collaborate with the relevant community to identify cultural values that are significant to a community, and then to work with that community to ensure these values are respected and upheld. This is the development of cultural competence. Cultural competence (discussed earlier in the chapter) has no universally agreed definition, but there are shared elements within the range of definitions (Ranzijn et al 2008a), which include:

- valuing diversity
- having the capacity for cultural self-assessment
- being mindful of the dynamics of cross-cultural interactions
- valuing cultural knowledge
- adapting approaches to meet cultural values and needs.

Fig. 14.3 represents the movement towards cultural competence, representing the development of cultural competence as a journey requiring an investment of humility, reflective practice and deep engagement with the Indigenous community.

TUTORIAL TRIGGER 14.2

Name three qualities that you think you would need to make you an effective and culturally competent researcher working with Indigenous Peoples/Indigenous communities.

Denzin and Lincoln (2007) integrated work by Smith (2012) and Cram (2001) to align cultural values with implications for researchers working with Māori communities (see Table 14.2). The national best-practice framework for

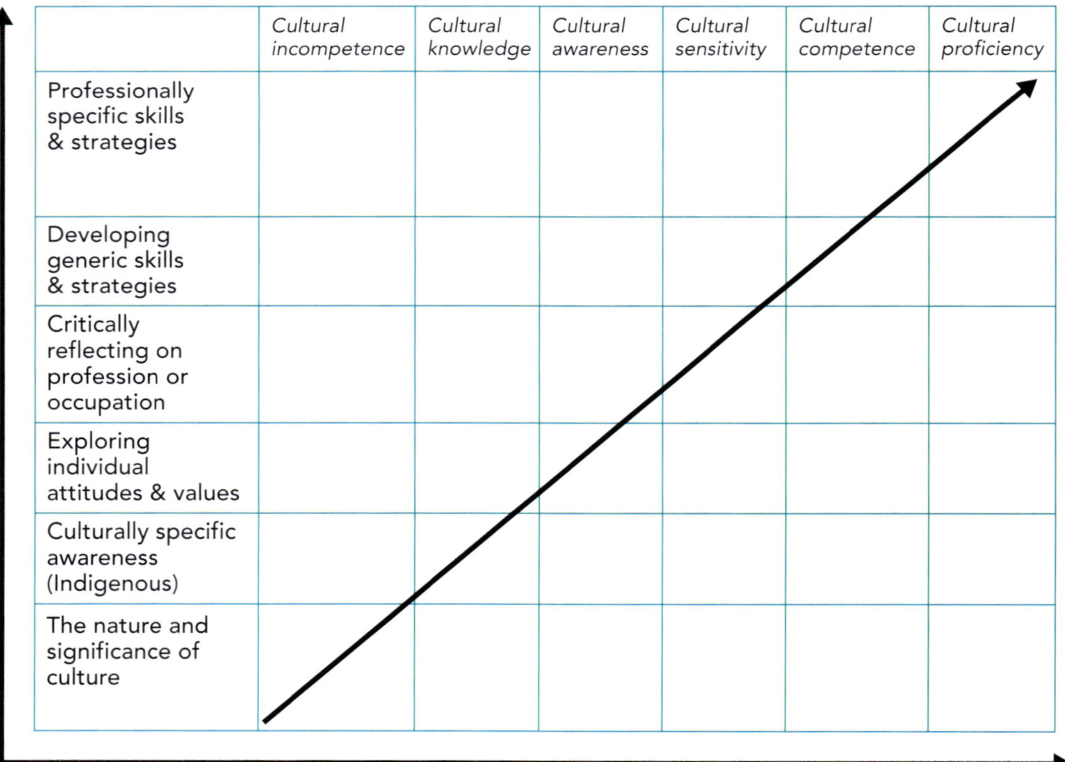

Fig. 14.3 Developing cultural proficiency (Source: Ranzijn, R., McConnochie, K., Nolan, W., 2008b. ALTC grant (2006–2008) 'Disseminating strategies for incorporating Australian Indigenous content in psychology programs throughout Australia' (CG6-50), p. 19.)

TABLE 14.2 'Community-Up' Approach to Defining Researcher Conduct

Cultural Values (Smith 2012)	Researcher Guidelines (Cram 2001)
Aroha ki te tangata	A respect for people—allow people to define their own space and meet on their own terms.
He kanohi ki te a	It is important to meet people face to face, especially when introducing the idea of research, 'fronting up' to the community before sending out long, complicated letters and materials.
Titiro, whakarongo ... korero	Look and listening (and then maybe speaking). This value emphasises the importance of looking/observing and listening in order to develop understandings and find a place from which to speak.
Manaaki ki te tangata	Sharing, hosting, being generous. This is a value that underpins a collaborative approach to research, one that enables knowledge to flow both ways and that acknowledges the researcher as the learner and not just a data gatherer or observer. It also facilitates the process of 'giving back', of sharing results and of bringing closure if that is required for a project but not a relationship.
Kia tupato	Be cautious. This suggests that researchers need to be politically astute, culturally safe and reflective about their insider/outsider status. It is also a caution to insiders and outsiders that in community research, things can come undone without the researcher being aware or being told directly.
Kaua e takahia te mana o te tangata	Do not trample on the 'mana' or dignity of a person. This is about informing people and guarding against being paternalistic or impatient because people do not know what the researcher may know. It is also about simple things like the way Westerners use wit, sarcasm and irony as discursive strategies or where one sits down. For example, Māori people are offended when someone sits on a table designed and used for food.
Kaua e mahaki	Do not flaunt your knowledge. This is about finding ways to share knowledge, to be generous with knowledge without being a 'show off' or being arrogant. Sharing knowledge is about empowering a process, but the community has to empower itself.

(Source: Smith, L.T. 2007 On tricky ground: researching the native in the age of uncertainty. In: Denzin, N.K, Lincoln, Y. (Eds), The Landscape of Qualitative Research. Sage Publications, Thousand Oaks, CA. pp. 113–144.)

Indigenous cultural competency in Australian Universities presents a detailed Māori ethical framework (Health Council of New Zealand 2010 p. 160) with a clear and informative explanation. This text, and indeed the whole document, makes for valuable reading. The framework is shown in Fig. 14.4 and one sector is elaborated in Fig. 14.5. The framework is presented in three concentric circles which represent minimal *ethical standards*, *good practice* and *best practice*. The circles are cut into four quadrants that represent four principles of Māori *tikanga* (ways of doing things): *whakapapa* (relationships), *mana* (justice and equity), *tika* (research design) and *manākitanga* (cultural and social responsibility).

TUTORIAL TRIGGER 14.3

Why do we need ethics when researching with Indigenous Peoples and in Indigenous communities?

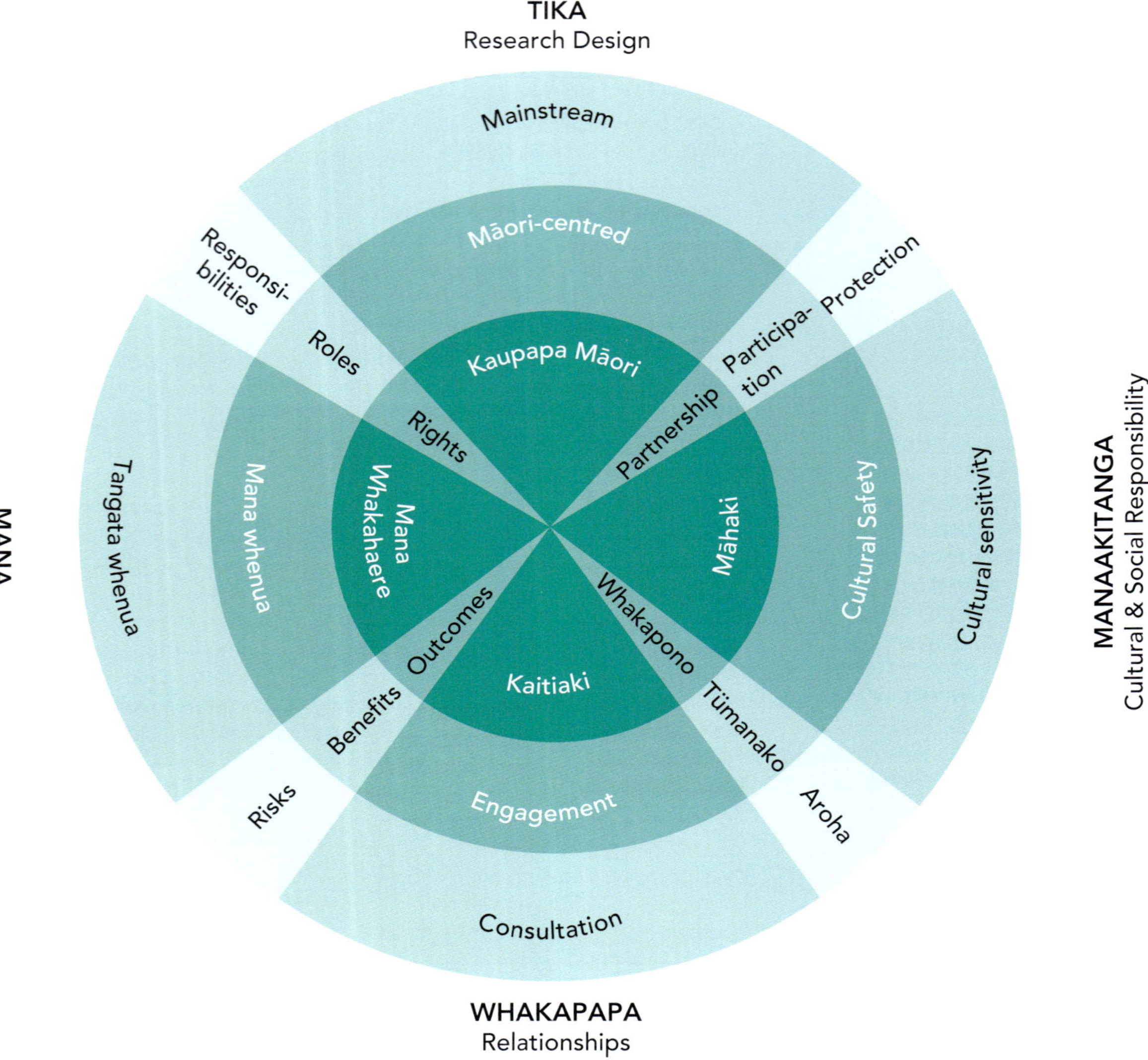

Fig. 14.4 Māori ethical framework (Source: Health Research Council of New Zealand on behalf of the Putaiora Writing Group, 2010. Guidelines for Māori Research Ethics: a framework for researchers and ethics committee members. ©Health Research Council of New Zealand.)

RESEARCH IN BRIEF 14.6

There are 'things that we know' that clearly highlight the need for health services for Indigenous populations that better serve their needs by being more culturally responsive. For instance, Ratima and Crengle (2013) state what we know of Indigenous maternal services that are mirrored 'on both sides of the Ditch'—Australia and New Zealand. Despite their high relative needs, Māori women are less likely to receive antenatal education classes and have fewer cumulative antenatal visits than non-Māori women. Māori women have reported lower levels of satisfaction with antenatal care, labour, care at birth and inequities in access to obstetric care. Key barriers to antenatal care

RESEARCH IN BRIEF 14.6—cont'd

and/or care during labour and delivery include access to information to support informed choices, insufficient numbers of independent practising Māori midwives, inadequate access to culturally responsive care including whānau-centred services, and cost barriers. Against this context, we know Māori women have expressed preferences for:

- culturally appropriate venues
- integration of customary Māori practices (e.g. mirimiri and karakia) and incorporation of:
  - a focus on spiritual needs
  - a more informal approach
  - inclusiveness of whānau
  - delivery by other Māori women
  - opportunities to share experiences, including those of older women
  - an increased emphasis on 'normal' birth.

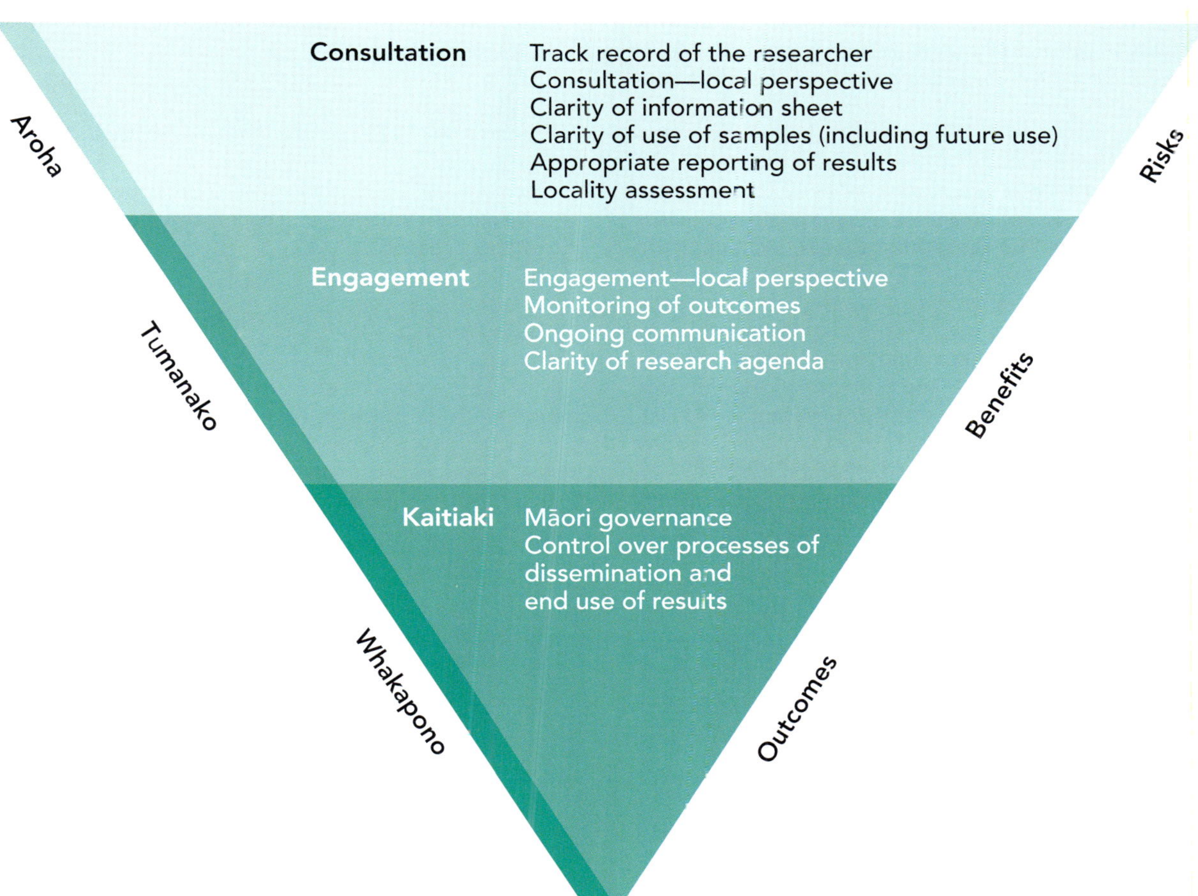

Fig. 14.5 Whakapapa (Source: Health Research Council of New Zealand on behalf of the Putaiora Writing Group, 2010. Guidelines for Māori Research Ethics: a framework for researchers and ethics committee members. ©Health Research Council of New Zealand.)

SUMMARY

This chapter asks you to begin to think about how to critically reflect on the history of Indigenous research in both Australian and Aotearoa New Zealand contexts. It is important that you understand key ideas related to what a cultural competence research model could look like. Crucial to this understanding is being able to identify **Indigenous research methodologies** and ethical processes in research. Immersing yourself in important relevant literature is necessary. Ethical research practice is a process of working together to improve the lived experience of Indigenous Peoples, and the starting point is from a position of humility (Smith 2012). Indigenous research reveals critical tools that nurses and midwives can work with; it is a matter of engaging with these tools to generate necessary changes (Geia et al 2020 p. 9). We can do this through ensuring cultural safety in graduates, addressing the lack of cultural capability in practice (Power et al 2016, Virdun et al 2013) and mobilising the cultural determinants of health in education and research.

A culturally competent researcher acknowledges hegemonic discourses and values the strengths inherent in the health and wellbeing of 'precolonial' societies. This strengths-based approach is vital to encouraging existing capabilities within Indigenous Peoples and Indigenous communities to change a narrative overwhelmed by deficits. Culture must be embraced if Indigenous Peoples and researchers are to work in partnership.

KEY POINTS

- It is important to be aware of the impact of Western research methodologies on Indigenous Peoples in Australia and New Zealand and the need for Indigenous Peoples to reclaim their history and advance Indigenous aspirations.
- Reflection on ethics is vital, as is adherence to the spirit of ethical protocols and frameworks relevant to Indigenous Peoples, including Aboriginal and Torres Strait Islander Peoples and Māori. Cultural competence is a *hikoi* (journey) and not a destination.
- Deep listening is important, as is silent engagement, when working collaboratively with Indigenous communities and Elders.
- It is important to research with (not on) Indigenous Peoples with collaborative strengths-based research models that are owned and controlled by the community.
- Decolonising methodologies—counter-hegemonies—can empower Indigenous Peoples and lead to real and sustained change.

TIME TO REFLECT

The following is based on a hypothetical study.

Aim: A nurse researcher wants to investigate the gaps in routine data collection systems, as relevant to monitoring health service to Indigenous Peoples in Aotearoa New Zealand and Australia.

Objective: To identify current indicators, and potential alternative or additional indicators, of inequalities that are social in nature and contribute to poor health outcomes.

Design: The research methods involve: (1) a literature review to identify current indicators and candidate indicators; (2) key informant interviews with Indigenous Peoples and data experts to identify additional candidate indicators and to prioritise both current and candidate indicators. Prioritising should account for do-ability, cost and estimated relative importance of the concept being measured.

Reflect on the following:

1. Why did the researcher want to establish and name inequalities that are social in nature?
2. How does the principle of non-homogeneity of Indigenous persons apply to this research?
3. What are some of the strengths and weaknesses of this study?

Questions

Reflect on the information given and answer the questions:

1. Why did the researcher want to investigate the data collection systems?
2. Who should conduct this research?

LEARNING ACTIVITIES

1. Decolonising methodologies are:
   a. owned by the colonisers
   b. counter-hegemonic
   c. simplistic and homogenising
   d. grounded in Western ideology.
2. What is the base position for undertaking research in Indigenous contexts?
   a. Ontological views of the participants should be considered, valued and acknowledged.
   b. Epistemological and axiological views should be considered, valued and acknowledged.

c. Ontological, epistemological and axiological views should be considered, valued and acknowledged.
d. Ontological, epistemological and axiological views should be considered, valued and acknowledged, including the positionality of the researcher(s).

3. Why is it important to introduce yourself as a researcher?
a. It is essential for safety.
b. It is essential for agreement.
c. It is essential for responsibility.
d. All of the above.

4. When finding out how to refer to Indigenous people it is best to:
a. call them all Indigenous no matter where they come from
b. find some current literature and read about what is considered acceptable
c. ask people themselves how they would like to be referred to
d. both b and c.

5. Elders across most Indigenous communities have responsibilities for:
a. community
b. land
c. philosophy
d. input into relation to the continuous and ongoing responsibilities to culture, community, kinship and the interconnected relationships across, and to, a community.

6. The NHMRC's best practice document is:
a. not very important
b. guidelines for ethical conduct in Aboriginal and Torres Strait Islander health research
c. only necessary when addressing specific issues that may arise when undertaking research
d. legislated by law.

7. Cultural competence includes:
a. cultural awareness
b. cultural sensitivity
c. cultural safety
d. all of the above.

8. Interpreting the Indigenous code of ethics involves:
a. initial consultation only
b. the Ethics Committee
c. a challenge for the non-Indigenous researcher in interpreting the Indigenous code of ethics, then embracing the spirit of the code
d. working with a skilled interpreter.

9. The United Nations Declaration on the Rights of Indigenous Peoples:
a. is too old to worry about even though it used to be important; it is no longer relevant
b. is only about genetic resources, seeds, medicines, knowledge of the properties of fauna and flora
c. recognises the rights of Indigenous Peoples to their own knowledge and to the exploration, development, recording and sharing of their ways of knowing and doing
d. is just about consent.

10. Cultural competence means:
a. valuing diversity and having the capacity for cultural self-assessment
b. being mindful of the dynamics of cross-cultural interactions
c. valuing cultural knowledge and adapting approaches to meet cultural values and needs
d. all of the above.

ADDITIONAL RESOURCES

Aboriginal Health and Medical Research Council (AH&MRC). https://www.ahmrc.org.au/.

Cultural safety in health care for Indigenous Australians: monitoring framework 2023. https://www.aihw.gov.au/reports/indigenous-australians/cultural-safety-health-care-framework/contents/summary.

National Aboriginal Community Controlled Health Organisation (NACCHO) Strategic Plan 2018. https://www.naccho.org/uploads/downloadable-resources/2018-strategic-plan.pdf.

National Health and Medical Research Council (NHMRC) Ethical conduct in research with Aboriginal and Torres Strait Islander Peoples and communities: Guidelines for researchers and stakeholders (2018) https://www.nhmrc.gov.au/about-us/resources/ethical-conduct-research-aboriginal-and-torres-strait-islander-peoples-and-communities#block-views-block-file-attachments-content-block-1 and The National Health and Medical Research Council, the Australian Research Council and Universities Australia, National Statement on Ethical Conduct in Human Research 2023 (2023). NHMRC, Canberra, ACT. https://www.nhmrc.gov.au/sites/default/files/documents/attachments/publications/National-Statement-Ethical-Conduct-Human-Research-2023.pdf.

New Zealand Health Research Council. Guidelines for Researchers on Health Research Involving Māori. https://www.hrc.govt.nz/resources/guidelines-researchers-health-research-involving-maori.

Taylor, K., Guerin P., 2019. Health Care and Indigenous Australians: cultural safety in practice, Bloomsbury, London.

The New National Aboriginal & Torres Strait Islander Health Plan 2013–2023. https://www.health.gov.au/topics/aboriginal-and-torres-strait-islander-health/how-we-support-health/health-plan?utm_source=health.gov.au&utm_medium=callout-auto-custom&utm_campaign=digital_transformation.

The New Zealand Health Research Prioritisation Framework. Health Research Council of New Zealand, the Ministry of Business, Innovation and Employment and the Ministry of Health. 2019. https://www.hrc.govt.nz/resources/new-zealand-health-research-prioritisation-framework.

NSW Aboriginal Health Plan 2013–2023. https://www.health.gov.au/sites/default/files/documents/2021/02/national-aboriginal-and-torres-strait-islander-health-plan-2013-2023.pdf.

REFERENCES

Anderson, C., Walter, M., 2013. Indigenous Statistics: a quantitative research methodology. Left Coast Press, Walnut Creek, CA.

Arnold, J., 2016. Walking in both worlds: rethinking Indigenous knowledge in the academy. Int. J. Inclus. Educ. 21 (5), 475-494. doi:10.1080/13603116.2016.1218946

Atkinson, J., 2002. Trauma Trails, Recreating Song Lines: the transgenerational effects of trauma in Indigenous Australia. Spinifex, North Melbourne, VIC.

Bainbridge, R., Tsey, K., McCalman, J., et al., 2015. 'No one's discussing the elephant in the room': contemplating questions of research impact in Aboriginal and Torres Strait Islander Australian health research. BMC Public Health 15, 696.

Barclay, L., Kruske, S., Bar-Zeev, S., et al., 2014. Improving Aboriginal maternal and infant health services in the 'Top End'; synthesis of the findings of a health services research program aimed at engaging stakeholders, developing research capacity and embedding change. BMC Health Serv. Res. 14, 241–249.

Barelli, M., 2012. Free, prior and informed consent in the aftermath of the UN Declaration on the rights of Indigenous Peoples: developments and challenges ahead. Int. J. Hum. Rights 16 (1), 1–24.

Berglund, C., 2012. Ethics for Healthcare, fourth ed. Oxford University Press, South Melbourne, VIC.

Bishop, R., 2008. Te kotahitanga: kaupapa Māori in mainstream classrooms. In: Denzin, N.K., Lincoln, Y.S., Smith, L.T. (Eds.), Handbook of Critical and Indigenous Methodologies. Sage Publications, Thousand Oaks, CA, pp. 439–458.

Bradley, D., Noonan, P., Nugent, H., et al., 2008. Bradley Review, Review of Higher Education Final Report. DEEWR, Commonwealth of Australia, Canberra, ACT.

Chapman, R., Smith, T., Martin, C., 2014. Qualitative exploration of the perceived barriers and enablers to Aboriginal and Torres Strait Islander people accessing healthcare through one Victorian Emergency Department. Contemp. Nurse 48 (1), 48–58.

Cram, F., 2001. Rangahau Māori: tona tika, tona pono—the validity and integrity of Māori research. In: Tolich, M. (Ed.), Research Ethics in Aotearoa New Zealand. Pearson Education, Auckland, NZ, pp. 35–52.

Denzin, N.K., Lincoln, Y. (Eds.), 2007. The Landscape of Qualitative Research. Sage Publications, Thousand Oaks, CA, pp. 113–144.

Durie, M., 1998. Whaiora-Māori Health Development, second ed. Oxford University Press, Oxford.

Durie, M., 1999. Te Pae Mahutonga: a model for Māori health promotion. Health Promotion Forum of New Zealand Newsletter 49, 2–5.

Durie, M.H., 2004. An Indigenous model of Health Promotion. Paper presented at the 18th World Conference on Health Promotion and Health Education, Melbourne, VIC. Retrieved from: https://www.massey.ac.nz/documents/483/An_Indigenous_model_of_health_promotion.pdf.

Dyall, L., Skipper, T.K., Kēpa, M., et al., 2013. Navigation: process of building relationships with kaumātua (Māori leaders). N. Z. Med. J. 126, 65–74.

Geia, L., Lindsay, D., 2017. Towards an Indigenous youth led strategy: building research capacity in vulnerable youth. 14th National Rural Health Conference, Cairns, QLD, 26–29 April.

Geia, L., Baird, K., Bail, K., et al., 2020. A unified call to action from Australian nursing and midwifery leaders: ensuring that Black lives matter. Contemp. Nurse 56 (4), 297–308. doi:10.1080/10376178.2020.1809107

Geia, L.K., 2012. First steps, making footprints: Intergenerational Palm Island families' Indigenous stories (narratives) of childrearing practice strengths. PhD thesis. James Cook University, Cairns, QLD.

Geia, L.K., Hayes B., Usher K., 2013. Yarning/Aboriginal storytelling: Towards an understanding of an Indigenous perspective and its implications for research practice. Contemp. Nurse 46 (1), 13-17.

Graham, M., 2008. Some thoughts about the philosophical underpinnings of Aboriginal worldviews. Aust. Humanit. Rev. 45, 181.

Health Research Council of New Zealand on behalf of the Putaiora Writing Group, 2010. Guidelines for Māori Research Ethics: a framework for researchers and ethics committee members. Retrieved from: https://www.hrc.govt.nz/resources/te-ara-tika-guidelines-maori-research-ethics-0.

Hobson, J., Lowe, K., Poetsch, S., et al. (Eds.), 2011. Re-Awakening Languages: theory and practice in the revitalisation of Australia's Indigenous languages. Sydney University Press, Sydney, Australia.

Hoskins, T.K., Jones, A., 2012. Kaupapa Māori: shifting the social. N. Z. J. Educ. Stud. 47 (2), 21.

Human Rights and Equal Opportunity Commission, 1997. Bringing Them Home. Report of the National Inquiry Into the Separation of Aboriginal and Torres Strait Islander Children From Their Families. Commonwealth of Australia, Sydney, NSW.

Huria, T., Cuddy, J., Lacey, C., et al., 2014. Working with racism: a qualitative study of the perspectives of Māori (Indigenous Peoples of Aotearoa New Zealand) Registered Nurses on a global phenomenon. J. Transcult. Nurs. 25, 364–372.

Jackson, D., 2023. Perpetuating the whiteness of nursing: enculturation and nurse education. In: Lipscomb, M. (Ed.), Routledge Handbook of Philosophy and Nursing. Routledge, London, pp. 392–403.

Jones, C.P., 2000. Levels of racism: a theoretic framework and a Gardener's Tale. Am. J. Public Health 90 (8), 1212–1215.

Lovett, R., 2016. Aboriginal and Torres Strait Islander community wellbeing: identified needs for statistical capacity. In: Kukutai T, Taylor J (Eds.) Indigenous Data Sovereignty. ANU Press, The Australian National University, Canberra, ACT, pp. 213–231.

Martin, K., 2008. Please knock before you enter: Aboriginal regulation of outsiders and the implications for research. Post-Pressed, Teneriffe, QLD.

McKillop, A., Sheridan, N., Rowe, D., 2013. 'New light through old windows': nurses, colonists and indigenous survival. Nurs. Inq. 20 (3), 265–276. doi:10.1111/nin.12005

Maclean, H., 1932. Nursing in New Zealand: history and reminiscences. Tolan Printing Company, Wellington, NZ.

Ministry of Health—Aotearoa, 2012a. Māori health models—Te Whare Tapa Whā. Retrieved from: https://www.health.govt.nz/our-work/populations/maori-health/maori-health-models/maori-health-models-te-whare-tapa-wha.

Ministry of Health—Aotearoa, 2012b. Māori health models—Te Wheke. Retrieved from: https://www.health.govt.nz/our-work/populations/maori-health/maori-health-models/maori-health-models-te-wheke.

Ministry of Justice, 2001. He Hīnātore ki te Ao Māori: a glimpse into the Māori world. Retrieved from: https://www.justice.govt.nz/assets/he-hinatora-ki-te-ao-maori.pdf.

Mohamed, J., Matthews, V., Bainbridge, R., et al., 2021. Who is speaking for us? Identifying Aboriginal and Torres Strait Islander scholarship in health research. Medical Journal of Australia 215 (8):383-383.e1. doi:10.5694/mja2.51281

Muller, L., 2014. A Theory for Indigenous Australian Social Work and Health. Allen & Unwin, Crows Nest, NSW.

National Health and Medical Research Council (NHMRC). 2018. Ethical conduct in research with Aboriginal and Torres Strait Islander Peoples and communities: guidelines for researchers and stakeholders. NHMRC, Canberra, ACT.

National Health and Medical Research Council, the Australian Research Council and Universities Australia, 2023. National Statement on Ethical Conduct in Human Research 2023. Commonwealth of Australia, Canberra, ACT. Retrieved from: https://www.nhmrc.gov.au/sites/default/files/documents/attachments/publications/National-Statement-Ethical-Conduct-Human-Research-2023.pdf.

Ormsby-Teki, T., Timutimu, N., Palmer, H., et al., 2011. Reo o Te Kāinga: a Ngāi te Rangi—tribal response to advancing Māori language in the home. Te Whare Wānanga o Awanuiārangi and Te Rūnanga o Ngāi te Rangi Iwi Trust, Whakatāne, NZ. Retrieved from: https://www.maramatanga.ac.nz/sites/default/files/05%20RF%2014%20Web%20ready.pdf.

Papps, E., Ramsden, I., 1996. Cultural safety in nursing: the New Zealand experience. Int. J. Qual. Health Care 8 (5), 491–497. doi:10.1093/intqhc/8.5.491

Pere, R., 2015. Te Wheke Kamaatu—The Octopus of Great Wisdom. Retrieved from: https://www.natureplaynz.co.nz/pdf/te-wheke_rosepere.pdf.

Power, T., Virdun, C., Parker, N., et al., 2016. REM: a collaborative framework for building Indigenous cultural competence. J. Transcult. Nurs. 27 (5), 439–446. doi: 10.1177/1043659615587589

Power, T., East, L., Gao, Y., et al., 2021a. A mixed-methods evaluation of an urban Aboriginal diabetes lifestyle program. Aust. N. Z. J. Public Health 45 (2), 143–149. doi:10.1111/1753-6405.13092

Power, T., Wilson, D., Geia, L., et al., 2021b. Cultural safety and Indigenous authority in nursing and midwifery education and practice. Contemp. Nurse 57 (5), 303–307. doi:10.1080/10376178.2022.2039076

Power, T., Geia, L., Wilson, D., et al., 2022.) Cultural safety: beyond the rhetoric. Contemp. Nurse 58 (1), 1–7. doi:10.1080/10376178.2022.2087704

Pulver, L.J., Harris, E., 2007. Australia and New Zealand. In: Nettleton, C., Napolitano, D.A., Stephens, C. (Eds.), An Overview of Current Knowledge of the Social Determinants of Indigenous Health. London School of Hygiene and Tropical Medicine, London, pp. 89–100.

Puzan, E., 2003. The unbearable whiteness of being (in nursing). Nurs. Inqu. 10 (3), 193–200.

Ramsden, I., 1989. A Model for Negotiated and Equal Partnership. Author, Wellington, NZ.

Ramsden, I., 1993. Kawa Whakaruruhau: cultural safety in nursing education in Aotearoa. (New Zealand). Nurs. Prax. N. Z. 8 (3), 4–10.

Ranzijn, R., McConnochie, K., Day, A., et al., 2008a. Towards cultural competence: Australian Indigenous content in undergraduate psychology. Aust. Psychol. 43 (2), 132–139.

Ranzijn, R., McConnochie, K., Nolan, W. 2008b ALTC grant 'Disseminating strategies for incorporating Australian Indigenous content in psychology programs throughout Australia' (CG6-50), p. 19. Retrieved from: https://ltr.edu.au/resources/CG650_UniSA%20_Ranzijn_Final%20report_Feb09.pdf.

Ranzijn, R., McConnochie, K., Nolan, W.. 2010. Psychology and Indigenous Australians: foundations of cultural competence. Palgrave Macmillan, South Yarra, VIC.

Ratima, M., Crengle, S., 2013. Antenatal, labour, and delivery care for Māori: experiences, location within lifecourse approach, and knowledge gaps. Pimatisiwin 10, 353–366.

Reid, P., 2021. Structural reform or a cultural reform? Moving the health and disability sector to be pro-equity, culturally safe, Tiriti compliant and anti-racist. N. Z. Med. J. 134 (1535), 7–10.

Rigney L-I (1999) Internationalization of an Indigenous anticolonial cultural critique of research methodologies: A guide to indigenist research methodology and its principles. Wicazo Sa Rev. 14 (2), 109–121. doi:10.2307/1409555

Riley, T., Meston, T., Ballangarry, J., et al., 2022. From yarning circles to zoom: navigating sensitive issues within indigenous education in an online space. Int. J. Inclus. Educ. 1–16. doi:10.1080/13603116.2022.2127501. Retrieved from: https://www.tandfonline.com/doi/abs/10.1080/13603116.2022.2127501.

Rinehart, R.E., Kidd, J., Quiroga, A.G., 2018. Southern Hemisphere Ethnographies of Space, Place and Time. Peter Lang, Oxford, UK.

Rose DB (1996) Nourishing terrains : Australian Aboriginal views of landscape and wilderness. Australian Heritage Commission, Canberra, ACT.

Sheridan, N.F., Kenealy, T.W., Kidd, J.D., 2015. Patients' engagement in primary care: powerlessness and compounding jeopardy. A qualitative study. Health Expect. 18 (1), 32–45. doi:10.1111/hex.12006

Sheridan, N., Love, T., Kenealy, T.; Care Models Study Group, 2023a. Is there equity of patient health outcomes across models of general practice in Aotearoa New Zealand? A national cross-sectional study. Int. J. Equity Health 22, 79. doi:10.1186/s12939-023-01893-8

Sheridan, N., Jansen, R., Harwood, M., et al.; Primary Care Models Study Group, 2023b. Hauora Māori – Māori health: a right to equal outcomes in primary care. Int. J. Equity Health (in press). doi:10.21203/rs.3.rs-3132255/v1. Retrieved from: file:///Users/crwyard1/Downloads/Hauora_Maori_-_Maori_health_a_right_to_equal_outco.pdf.

Smith, G.H., 2000. Protecting and respecting indigenous knowledge. In: Battiste, M. (Ed.), Reclaiming Indigenous Voice and Vision. UBC Press, Ontario, Canada, pp. 209–224.

Smith, L.T., 2000. Kaupapa Māori research. In: Battiste, M. (Ed.), Reclaiming Indigenous Voice and Vision. UBC Press, Toronto, Canada, pp. 225–247.

Smith, L.T., 2007. On tricky ground: researching the native in the age of uncertainty. In: Denzin, N.K., Lincoln, Y. (Eds.), The Landscape of Qualitative Research. Sage Publications, Thousand Oaks, CA, pp. 113–144.

Smith, L.T., 2012. Decolonizing Methodologies. Research and Indigenous Peoples, 2nd ed. Zed Books, London, UK.

Smith, L., 2023. The significance of land acknowledgements as a commentary on Indigenous Pedagogies. Occasional Paper Series 49, 6. doi:10.58295/2375-3668.1483

Stoneham, M.J., Goodman, J., Daube, M., 2014. The portrayal of Indigenous health in selected Australian media. Int. Indig. Policy J. 5, 1. doi:10.18584/iipj.2014.5.1.5

Taylor, K., Guerin, P.T., 2019. Healthcare and Indigenous Australians: cultural safety in practice, third ed. Palgrave Macmillan, South Yarra, VIC.

The New Zealand Health Research Prioritisation Framework. Health Research Council of New Zealand, the Ministry of Business, Innovation and Employment and the Ministry of Health. 2019. Retrieved from: https://www.hrc.govt.nz/resources/new-zealand-health-research-prioritisation-framework.

United Nations (UN), 2008. Declaration on the Rights of Indigenous Peoples. UN, Geneva. Retrieved from: https://www.waikato.ac.nz/__data/assets/pdf_file/0009/339885/Kaupapa-Rangahau-A-Reader_2nd-Edition.pdf.

Virdun, C., Gray, J., Sherwood, J., et al., 2013. Working together to make Indigenous health care curricula everybody's business: a graduate attribute teaching innovation report. Contemp. Nurse, 46 (1), 97–104.

Wepa, D., 2003. An exploration of the experiences of cultural safety educators in New Zealand: an action research approach. J. Transcult. Nurs. 14 (4), 339–348.

Wepa, D., 2015. Cultural Safety in Aotearoa New Zealand, second ed. Cambridge University Press, Melbourne, VIC.

West, R., Mills, K., Rowland, D., et al., 2019. Impact of a discrete First Peoples health course on students' experience and development of cultural capabilities. Higher Educ. Res. Dev. 38 (5), 1090–1104. doi:10.1080/07294360.2019.1603202

Weston, A., 2011. Development of an online Yarning place for Indigenous health workers. Aborig. Islander Health Worker J. 35 (2), 9–10. doi:10.3316/ielapa.936587281441782

15

Applying Research Knowledge: Implementing Evidence Into Practice and Policy

Alison M Hutchinson and Tracy Robinson

LEARNING OUTCOMES

After reading this chapter, the reader should be able to:

- describe the different types of evidence that inform nursing and midwifery practice
- understand the steps to implement evidence in practice
- discuss why capacity building for implementation is important to healthcare professionals and organisations
- discuss the reason for and importance of de-implementation in healthcare.

KEY TERMS

capacity building, p. 270
de-implementation, p. 267
evidence-based healthcare, p. 259
implementation, p. 262
midwifery, p. 259
nursing, p. 259

INTRODUCTION

This chapter covers two key areas: the implementation of evidence into practice and strategies for building the capacity of nurses and midwives to **implement evidence into practice**. Previous chapters in this book deal with the many ways research evidence is generated for nursing and midwifery practice. Although in this chapter we acknowledge that not all nurses or midwives need to be able to conduct research, all should be able to use the best available evidence to inform their practice. To achieve best practice in healthcare, nurses and midwives require the kinds of knowledge that a book like this brings together to enable them to engage with and learn about the implementation of evidence into practice.

RESEARCH KNOWLEDGE AND NURSING AND MIDWIFERY PRACTICE

As practice-based professions, **nursing** and **midwifery** focus on the practical processes of attending to the fundamental care needs of people who access health services. While clinical practice is focused on practical knowledge and skills, increasingly such practice is informed by a substantial research and theory base. The exponential growth in knowledge to guide clinical decision making and best practice enables nurses and midwives to draw on evidence from various sources to inform their practice. Fig. 15.1 illustrates the interconnectedness between evidence, clinical experience and patient preferences in **evidence-based healthcare**. However, this growth in research has not necessarily led to an increase in the timely adoption of research in practice and policy. Some nurses and midwives rely on their experience or knowledge gained during their initial professional training rather than current scientific findings (Ellis 2019). Indeed, one of the most consistent findings from clinical and health services research is the failure to translate research into practice and policy (Braithwaite et al 2018, Klepac et al 2022). The gap between research and practice—that is, between what nurses and midwives *do* and what the research/evidence *recommends*—has been widely discussed in the literature. Significant barriers to using up-to-date

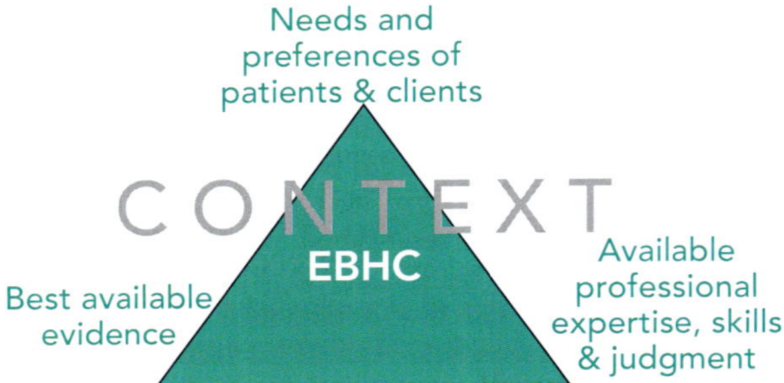

Fig. 15.1 Elements that, when combined, promote evidence-based healthcare (©JBI.)

research evidence in clinical practice persist, including lack of training, time management and research leadership (Dagne & Tebeje 2021).

TUTORIAL TRIGGER 15.1

Q) Evidence-based practice is often considered the same as 'doing or participating in research'. What does this section indicate about the role of research findings in evidence-based practice?

A) This section highlights that different types of evidence address different needs in clinical practice and acknowledges that research itself is simply one part of a larger framework requiring skills and tools for **applying** evidence in practice and **evaluating** its impact on outcomes.

Types of Evidence Used in Midwifery and Nursing Practice

Evidence-based practice is now understood as using the best-available evidence together with the clinician's expertise and the preferences and values of the person receiving care (Agency for Healthcare Research and Quality 2018). New evidence in healthcare is being generated at an ever-increasing rate and takes many forms (Duff et al 2020). Although the results of well-designed studies are an obvious source of evidence, research results are by no means the only form of evidence used in everyday practice. The experience of service users and their relevant others (e.g. designated family members or friends), the practitioner's own experiences and the nature and norms of the setting and culture in which care is being delivered are all rich sources of evidence to draw upon in making clinical decisions.

Patient-centred care consists of providing healthcare services that respect and meet the needs of service users and their caregivers, and is essential in promoting positive care outcomes and perceptions of quality of care (Kwame & Petrucka 2021). When making decisions, clinicians (often entirely subconsciously) assess the degree to which their decision will meet four criteria—that is, the extent to which the decision is:

- feasible within the context of care and the resources available
- appropriate for the person, place and time
- meaningful to the person and her/his family and community
- effective in achieving the desired outcome (Pearson 2004).

Thus, decisions about adopting evidence for practice relate to these four criteria (referred to as 'FAME') (Pearson 2004). As noted above, while research evidence indicates whether interventions are effective, this is not the only source of evidence that is important to nursing and midwifery. For example, while evidence indicates that chemotherapy may have a good outcome for some cancers, the person may choose to decline treatment because they do not wish to experience the side effects. In order to support people in making an appropriate choice, nurses and midwives need to understand the experience and feasibility of chemotherapy for people in a variety of contexts. The feasibility of chemotherapy for a person who is more concerned with quality of life and avoiding the impact of side effects differs from someone who is keen to pursue all treatment options. Hence nurses and midwives require evidence from various sources to inform their practice. It is worth noting that without appropriate, timely input from consumers as equal partners in decision making, healthcare is not evidence based.

Evidence-Based Nursing and Midwifery

Although a relatively new term, evidence-based nursing is a much older concept. Over 160 years ago, British nurse Florence Nightingale implemented regular hand washing based on evidence of the benefits for infection prevention, resulting in a substantial reduction in sepsis-related deaths during the Crimean War. More recently, the establishment of the Cochrane Library, along with the evolution of systematic review methodologies, has led to the accumulation of high-quality research evidence in the form of systematic reviews of multiple studies that address the same research question to provide a more robust answer compared with a single study alone. Systematic reviews are rapidly growing in number and provide an important source of evidence to guide practice. The rigor of evidence can be visually represented. Fig. 15.2 is typical of research 'pyramids' or 'hierarchies of evidence'. Given that the evidence quality in these representations varies, nurses and midwives also need effective skills to critically appraise and evaluate evidence (see Chapter 3).

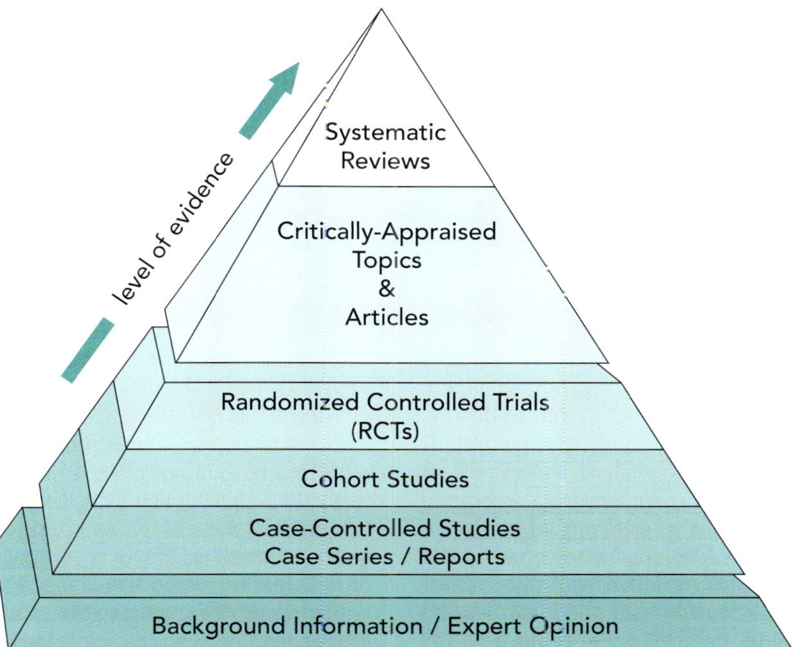

Fig. 15.2 The evidence hierarchy (©JBI.)

As more knowledge is generated through research, and as the ability to transmit information via the internet and open-access publishing increases, all clinicians have come under increasing pressure to show that they are abreast of current research evidence, and that they exhibit this by delivering care that is in line with the best available evidence. This is challenging because it is estimated that nearly one million new articles are posted on PubMed annually (Duff et al 2020).

In healthcare today, nurses and midwives have information at their fingertips via access to high-quality resources at the point of care through smartphones and other devices, and institutional libraries. Given the challenges associated with integrating clinical practice with current research evidence, as well as the unique values and circumstances of service users and caregivers (Abu-Baker et al 2021), the importance of quality assessed, synthesised information gathered through the systematic review of the international literature on a given topic cannot be underestimated (Dogherty et al 2013, MacDermid & Graham 2009, Wensing & Grol 2019).

RESEARCH IN BRIEF 15.1

While nurses and midwives are increasingly expected to engage in evidence-based practice, there is a lack of systematic review evidence about the effectiveness of evidence-informed interventions used by nurses and midwives, especially in regard to promoting decision-making knowledge and skills. Abu-Odah et al (2022) conducted a systematic review of barriers and facilitators to the translation of research evidence into clinical practice. After excluding 834 articles that did not fit the inclusion criteria, the authors included 10 papers in their review. Barriers to the use of evidence in clinical practice were identified at the micro (individual), the meso (organisational) and the macro (political) levels. Training and engaging clinicians and policy makers in research practice is needed, but limited access to resources such as research databases and the equipment required for them (such as IT infrastructure) is a significant barrier. The authors concluded that the factors driving engagement and interest in research are multifaceted, ranging from individual perceptions of the value of research to wider systemic issues such as limited clinical academic career pathways. Although research evidence is essential to improving healthcare practice (and improving patient outcomes), targeted interventions are needed to address barriers that operate at individual and organisational levels.

TUTORIAL TRIGGER 15.2

Q) Consider how you might investigate the evidence base for a clinical issue you are interested in and whether current practice is based upon that evidence.

A) Research may be the most immediate answer but is not always the most practical or responsive when taking issues of local context into consideration. Read ahead to Tutorial trigger 15.3 for additional options.

Frameworks for Implementing Evidence

Numerous frameworks are available to guide the **implementation** of new evidence into practice, including process models, determinant frameworks and evaluation frameworks (Nilsen 2015). One example of a commonly used framework is the Knowledge to Action Framework (K2A) (Graham et al 2006)—a process framework that aims to foster the translation of evidence-based interventions (i.e. programs, policies and practices) into practice. The action cycle includes a series of phases: problem identification, adaptation of knowledge to the local context, assessment of barriers to knowledge use, selection and tailoring of interventions, monitoring of knowledge use, evaluation of outcomes and sustainment of knowledge use. For this chapter, however, we use a framework developed in Australia by the Joanna Briggs Institute.

The Joanna Briggs Institute

The Joanna Briggs Institute (JBI) was established in 1996 and is the international not-for-profit research and development arm of the School of Translational Science based within the Faculty of Health Sciences at the University of Adelaide, South Australia (https://health.adelaide.edu.au/our-research/translational-health-outcomes). The Institute collaborates internationally with over 70 entities worldwide to promote and support the synthesis, transfer and utilisation of evidence by identifying feasible, appropriate, meaningful and effective healthcare practices to assist in improving healthcare outcomes. In addition, the JBI:

- develops methods to appraise and synthesise evidence through the conduct of systematic reviews and analyses of the research literature (evidence synthesis)
- disseminates information in diverse formats to inform health systems, health professionals and consumers (evidence transfer)
- facilitates the effective implementation of evidence and the evaluation of its impact on healthcare practice (evidence utilisation)
- contributes to clinically and cost-effective healthcare through the promotion of evidence-based healthcare practice (evidence utilisation).

The Institute promotes the involvement of nurses, midwives and allied health professionals in the implementation of best practice (Jordan et al 2006), and the JBI Model of Evidence-based Health Care (Jordan et al 2019, Pearson et al 2005) attempts to recognise all types of evidence (see Fig. 15.3). The model depicts the major components of the evidence-based healthcare process:

1. global health
2. evidence generation
3. evidence synthesis
4. evidence transfer
5. evidence implementation.

Evidence-based healthcare is represented as a cyclical process. It begins by deriving questions, concerns or interests from the healthcare information needs of clinicians, consumers or caregivers. It then proceeds to address these questions by generating knowledge and evidence to effectively and appropriately meet these needs in ways that are feasible and meaningful to specific populations, cultures and settings (Pearson et al 2012). Healthcare providers have access to evidence that has been appraised and synthesised, and they facilitate the transfer of evidence to service delivery settings and clinicians. The following section details the components of the model.

Evidence Generation

The evidence generation component of the model identifies discourse, experience and research as appropriate sources of evidence or knowledge (Pearson et al 2012). When nurses and midwives select evidence to inform questions in their practice, they need to select the evidence that best answers the question. When the means and purposes of evidence generation and synthesis are linked to the specific type of practice question (feasibility, appropriateness, meaning and effectiveness), that evidence has the best chance of becoming best practice. Any indication that a practice is effective, appropriate, meaningful, or feasible—whether derived from experience, expertise, inference, deduction or results of rigorous inquiry—is regarded as evidence in the model. The results of well-designed research studies grounded in any methodological approach may be more credible evidence than anecdotes or personal opinion; however, when no research evidence exists, expert opinion is seen to represent the 'best-available' evidence (Pearson et al 2012). One challenge is that current evidence generation processes focus largely on questions of safety and efficacy, and stakeholders may lack 'real-world' evidence to inform treatment decisions. For example, the requirement that people participating in traditional clinical trials do not have comorbidities means that new treatments are commonly trialled on a cohort of people who are not

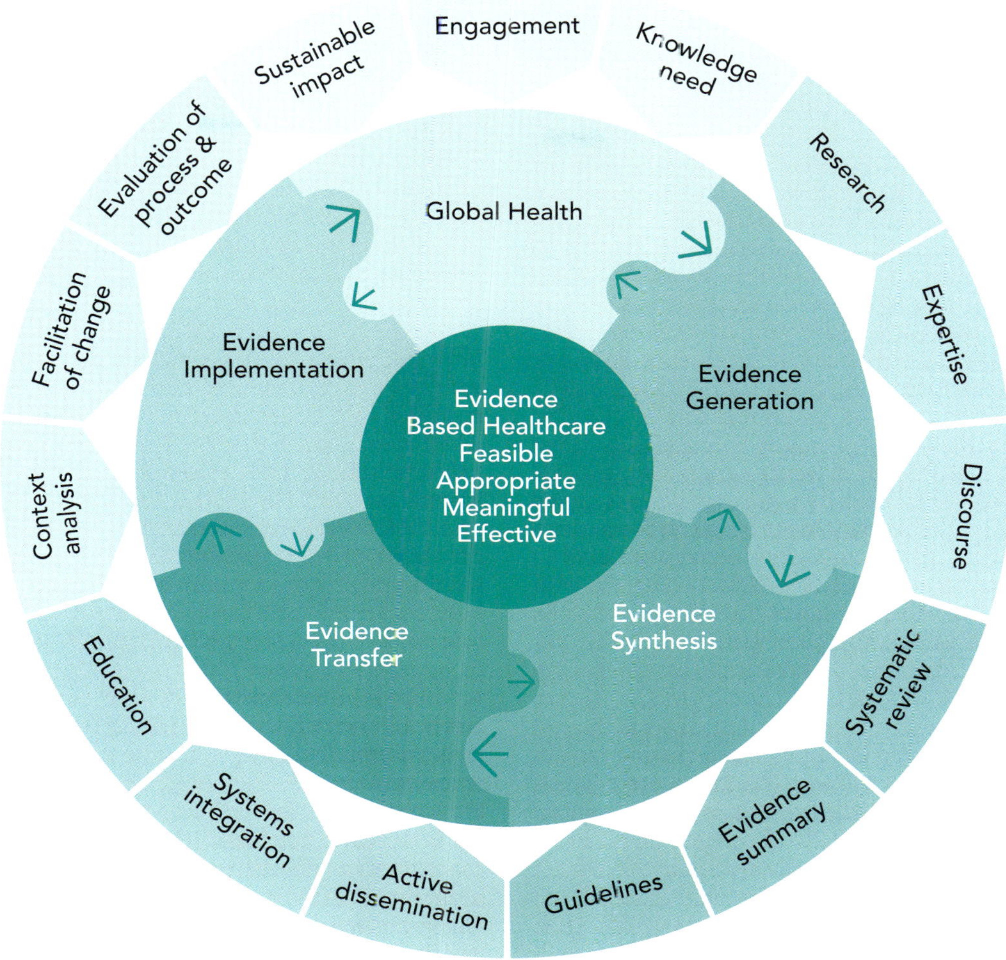

Fig. 15.3 The JBI model of evidence-based healthcare

reflective of the 'real-world' population. Service users and communities need to be active partners in the evidence generation process (National Academies of Sciences et al 2017).

Evidence Synthesis

Evidence synthesis refers to the evaluation or analysis and summary of evidence on a specific topic to aid decision making in healthcare. The model includes the concepts of the methodology, theory and conduct of systematic reviews (Jordan et al 2006, Pearson et al 2005, 2012). This element in the model is grounded in the view that evidence of feasibility, appropriateness, meaningfulness, effectiveness and economics are legitimate foci for the systematic review process, and diverse forms of evidence (from experience, opinion and research that involve numerical and/or textual data) can be appraised, extracted and pooled (Pearson 2004, The Joanna Briggs Institute 2014). Historically, methodologies for systematic review (evidence synthesis) developed rapidly in relation to the meta-analysis of numerical data to establish cause and effect measurement of outcomes (e.g. whether ice packs effectively relieve episiotomy pain). The JBI Model of Evidence-based Healthcare adopts an approach to systematic review where the findings of all good-quality research or other sources of knowledge (when the research results are unavailable) are regarded as evidence for systematic review (Pearson et al 2012).

Evidence Transfer

This component of the model is about the act of transferring knowledge to individual clinicians, health facilities and health systems globally through journals, other publications, electronic media, education and training and decision support systems (Pearson et al 2012). Evidence transfer involves more than disseminating or distributing information and includes careful development of strategies that identify target audiences—such as clinicians, managers, policymakers and consumers—and designing methods to package and transfer information that is understood and used in decision making (The Joanna Briggs Institute 2014). Central to this process is:

- developing understandable and actionable messages
- accommodating the context of a target audience's information needs
- facilitating the uptake of knowledge via pedagogic approaches suited to the knowledge needs of the specific audience (including brief educational sessions, short-course programs and more-formal education methods).

Therefore, the model depicts three major elements of evidence/knowledge transfer—education and training, information delivery and the transfer of evidence through organisational and team systems (Pearson et al 2005). For example, knowledge may move from synthesis through transfer when nurses and midwives use a systematic review of evidence for treatment options for a particular cancer, through to the development of a guideline for clinicians, followed by interactive educational sessions and, finally, a plain language summary to help inform people's treatment choices.

Evidence Implementation

This component of the model relates to the implementation of evidence in practice, as is reflected in practice and/or system change. It identifies three elements: *practice change*, *embedding evidence* through system/organisational change and *evaluating the impact* of the utilisation of evidence on the health system, the process of care and health outcomes. Based on the JBI Model of Evidence-based Healthcare (Jordan et al 2019), healthcare practitioners, policymakers and others involved in the management or delivery of care can adopt seven steps to guide the implementation of evidence into practice (Aromataris & Munn 2020), as follows:

1. Identify the practice area.
2. Engage change agents.
3. Assess context and readiness to change.
4. Review practice against evidence-based audit criteria.
5. Implement changes to practice using the Getting Research into Practice (GRiP) method that involves three stages including the evaluation of baseline audit findings, the identification of barriers and enablers to the use of evidence and the development of strategies for change (Porritt et al 2020).
6. Reassess practice using a follow-up audit.
7. Consider the sustainability of the project.

Although clear frameworks for implementing evidence exist, understanding what and where the gaps are in healthcare is challenging and scant attention has been paid to reducing low-value care and how such care might be de-implemented (Ingvarsson et al 2022).

TUTORIAL TRIGGER 15.3

Q) In the Joanna Briggs Institute Model, where does clinical audit best fit? What purpose does clinical audit fulfil that informed your decision?

A) Clinical audit fits within the 'evidence utilisation' element of the model as it focuses on the implementation and impact of best practice on healthcare practice and patient outcomes.

EVIDENCE IMPLEMENTATION BY NURSES AND MIDWIVES IN ORGANISATIONAL CONTEXTS

This chapter has explained the components of a model for evidence-based practice; however, research shows that context has an important influence on the implementation of research into practice and policy. The context in which implementation occurs can affect the success of implementation by perpetuating outdated practices, influencing how clinicians respond to any planned change and modifying how the strategy works. Although numerous theories and frameworks include context as an element, their definitions of context vary.

Given the lack of clarity about context, Squires et al (2023) used a meta-synthesis of three interrelated studies to produce the Implementation in CONtext (ICON) framework. This framework reflects context across three levels: micro (individual), meso (organisational) and macro (external to the organisation). Across the three levels are six domains of context that collectively include 22 core attributes of context (Table 15.1). This highlights the complexity and breadth of context as an enabler or barrier to implementation efforts and provides guidance on contextual attributes that could be considered when planning, monitoring and evaluating the implementation of evidence into practice and policy.

TABLE 15.1 Implementation in Context Framework

Levels	Domains	Attributes
Micro	Actors	Patient/client consumer population Service provider population
Meso	Organisational climate and structures	Economic arrangements Elements of organisations Organisational climate
	Organisational social behaviour	Physical and technological resources Internal relationships
	Organisational response to change	Organisational culture Organisational change processes
	Organisational processes	Receptivity to change Communication processes Evaluation activity Governance Leadership Management Organisation of work System processes
Macro	External influences	Community influences Intercommunity/interorganisational/intersectoral relationships

EVIDENCE IMPLEMENTATION

Analysis of the implementation process from published studies suggests it follows a particular sequence (see Box 15.1). Evidence implementation models, such as the JBI Model illustrated earlier in this chapter, can be read and understood as a cyclical process; however, evidence implementation in clinical practice is more dynamic and iterative than can be conveyed in a model. Identifying a gap between practice and the existence of relevant, high-quality evidence should trigger efforts to adopt a reliable process to implement the evidence into practice.

This section presents a case example of an implementation initiative to illustrate how healthcare professionals can move from choosing a topic, preparing for practice change, developing an implementation plan and working through data collection, implementation and evaluation. The case study illustrates the steps and processes that help achieve success in implementation. While the focus of this section is on implementation, the principles are also relevant to de-implementation—for circumstances when a policy or practice is no longer consistent with the best-available evidence and needs to be ceased because it is not beneficial, or it is harmful.

Implementation models and frameworks, such as the JBI Model, specify including external, high-quality synthesised evidence to inform both the clinical issue and the implementation strategy. Numerous high-quality resources are available online (see the end of the chapter for resources) where evidence can be accessed to inform implementation. Additionally, clinical practice guidelines and standards for practice guide best practice. To support the translation of evidence into practice, clinicians may draw on local context-specific, organisational and social/professional resources including personal experience, colleagues, organisational knowledge, policy and organisational leaders. Our case study illustrates the steps of the JBI evidence implementation approach.

Identifying the Practice Area

All Australian hospitals are accredited by the National Safety and Quality in Health Service Standards; this case study illustrates the process of implementing one element of the Delirium Clinical Care Standard (Australian Commission on Safety and Quality in Health Care 2021). For the purposes of this case study, the specific guideline element we focus on is 'early identification of risk of delirium'. This element requires that people with known risk factors for delirium are identified on admission to hospital using a validated tool.

Engaging Change Agents

In recognition of the need to implement the standards organisation-wide, efforts to implement elements of the Delirium Clinical Care Standard into practice were co-designed by a working group with representatives from all health service sites and clinical departments, key professional groups and the quality unit. A governance structure was established with clear reporting lines, vertically and horizontally, and responsibility and accountability for implementation was allocated.

Assess Context and Readiness for Change

In this scenario, there was a clear imperative for implementing the Standard. To understand existing practices across the organisation, audits were conducted to determine which tools were used and by which professionals for delirium risk assessment. Audits were also undertaken to assess the frequency of tool usage.

Review Practice Against Evidence-based Criteria

After collating these data, an evidence review was conducted of all tools in use and other tools reported in the literature. The review aimed to understand the properties of existing tools. Consideration was given to the feasibility, appropriateness, meaningfulness and effectiveness of the available tools using the FAME Framework (Jordan et al 2019). In considering *feasibility*, the working group reviewed factors such as cost associated with use of the tool or whether it was freely available, ease of use, number of items, time required to administer the tool and availability in different languages. In assessing the *appropriateness* of the tools, consideration was given to their fit in different contexts across the organisation and how they could be incorporated into the workflow and routines in a wide range of areas, such as the emergency department, general medical wards and subacute care settings. When considering the *meaningfulness* of the tools, the evaluation centred on how different health professional groups and those working in different areas would use the tools in their work routine to inform their practice. Finally, regarding *effectiveness*, the working group considered existing evidence concerning the psychometric properties of the tools, including their reliability, sensitivity and specificity.

With this knowledge, extensive discussions took place to determine the most appropriate tool for use across the organisation; the 4AT tool (Bellelli et al 2014) was selected. This tool was chosen because it is free, brief (four items), takes less than 2 minutes to complete, is easy to use, requires no special training, is validated and is available in a wide range of languages. Once the working group decided to recommend the 4AT, the recommendation was advanced through the governance structure to the executive for final approval. With the final approval in place, the implementation plan was developed.

Implement Change to Practice

To ensure the 4AT was implemented across the organisation, the working group, which, as noted above, purposefully included representatives of all professional groups, health service sites, clinical departments and the quality unit, collaborated on designing the implementation plan. Representation from all areas and professional groups was critically important to ensure the plan was comprehensive, and it took account of the nuances of different groups and their functions and processes and the contextual distinctions across the different settings. The plan included required actions, who was responsible, expected outcomes and timeframes.

The first component of the plan was a communication strategy, which was designed to ensure that all clinicians were informed of the plan to adopt the 4AT across the organisation and the expectations regarding its use. An education module about delirium and using the 4AT was developed and loaded onto the learning management platform. A promotional campaign was undertaken to make personnel aware of the module and the expectation for its completion. Completion rates were monitored, and reminders were sent to those who had not completed the module within a specific timeframe. Managers were also sent reports on their area's education module completion rates. In conjunction with the launch of the education module, existing policies were revised to include the 4AT and specify when the tool was to be applied and the required actions, depending on the patient's score. The electronic medical record was also revised to include fields for recording the 4AT assessment results and prompts to use the tool for patients that met the eligibility criteria.

Reassess Practice

The Quality Unit implemented an audit and feedback program to monitor the use of the 4AT. An audit plan was developed, incorporating guidance on the frequency of audits, the number of records to audit across the health service, who should conduct the audit, the audit tool and the mechanism for reporting and feedback of the results. Champions were identified for each ward and department, and their role in supporting implementation was documented and communicated. They received from the Quality Unit the local area audit feedback reports on the 4AT completion rates. Depending on the feedback report results, the champions worked with the local area manager to promote use of the 4AT, monitor education module completion rates and support health professionals to use the 4AT and/or complete the education module.

Consider Sustainability

To promote sustained change, ongoing monitoring (audits) and feedback on use of the 4AT continues and remedial actions are taken in areas in which rates are not optimal. All newly recruited clinicians must complete the education module in their orientation program. Existing staff members are required to complete the education module annually, which is monitored via audits and through individuals' annual performance management.

Section Summary

For illustration purposes, in this case study we focused on implementing one element of the Delirium Clinical Care Standard (Australian Commission on Safety and Quality in Health Care 2021): the 'early identification of risk of delirium'. A multifaceted implementation strategy comprised organisation-wide communication, education, change to policy, feedback and reminder systems. This implementation effort was part of a much larger initiative to implement all elements of the Standard. The complexity of implementing a range of elements within a single standard across an

BOX 15.1 Choosing Wisely Recommendation of the Australian College of Nursing

- Don't replace peripheral intravenous catheter unless clinically indicated.
- Don't restrict the ability of people with diabetes to self-manage blood glucose monitoring unless there is a clinical indication to do so.
- Don't routinely administer antipyretics with the sole aim of reducing body temperature in undistressed children.
- Don't use urinary catheters to manage urinary incontinence unless all other appropriate options have proved to be ineffective or to prevent wound infection or skin breakdown.
- Don't initiate plain X-ray for foot or ankle trauma unless criteria of the Ottawa Ankle Rules are met.

(From: Choosing Wisely Australia, 2016b. Australian College of Nursing. Recommendations. https://www.choosingwisely.org.au/recommendations/acn1)

entire organisation cannot be underestimated. The imperative to implement the Standard to comply with accreditation requirements was a key driver for implementation in this case study, and much implementation work does have the advantage of such imperatives to underpin the effort. In such cases, creating tension for change is necessary and assessing the readiness for change is critically important to the timing of implementation efforts. Tension for change can be created by appealing to hearts and minds by drawing on local evidence and comparing the results with best-practice expectations, providing real-life examples of individual patient outcomes when best practice is not followed and providing a clear and compelling account of existing evidence that informs best practice. Tools such as the Organisational Readiness to Change Assessment (Helfrich et al 2009) and the Checklist to Assess Organisational Readiness for Evidence Informed Practice Implementation (Barwick 2011) are available to assess the readiness for change so that the timing of implementation is optimised.

LOW-VALUE CARE AND DE-IMPLEMENTATION

It is as important to reduce or eliminate low-value care as it is to implement high-quality evidence into policy and practice. Low-value care provides little to no benefit to the patient, is potentially harmful or the costs outweigh the potential benefits. **De-implementation** refers to the discontinuation or cessation of practices determined to be of low value (Harris et al 2017, Upvall & Bourgault 2018, Verkerk et al 2018). The Organisation for Economic Co-operation and Development (OECD) estimated that 20% of public health expenditure is for low-value care (Organisation for Economic Co-operation and Development (OECD), 2017). Other research has indicated that approximately 30% of medical expenditure in the United States of America (USA) is for unnecessary care (Committee on the Learning Health Care System in America & Institute of Medicine 2013). Thus de-implementation of low-value care is necessary to improve care quality, reduce waste and promote the sustainability of limited resources (Harris et al 2017).

As a key initiative to reduce low-value care, the Choosing Wisely campaign was launched in 2012 in the USA (Choosing Wisely Australia 2016a). The Choosing Wisely movement has since spread internationally and has been adopted in over a third of OECD countries, including Australia and New Zealand (OECD 2017). As part of the campaign, specialty groups are invited to identify 'Top 5' lists of practices that meet the definition of low-value care and to promote their de-implementation. The campaign's initial focus was on the medical profession; however, the movement has now expanded to include other professional groups, such as nurses and midwives (Choosing Wisely Australia 2016b, Texas Board of Nursing 2016).

The Australian arm of Choosing Wisely (https://www.choosingwisely.org.au/) now comes under the auspices of the Australian Commission on Safety and Quality in Health Care. In the professions of nursing and midwifery, several low-value practices have been identified. For Australian nurses, the Australian College of Nursing has identified the Top 5 recommendations (Choosing Wisely Australia 2016b) (Box 15.1), including their rationale and supporting evidence. The New Zealand College of Midwives has similarly identified its Top 4 recommendations for midwives (New Zealand College of Midwives 2013) (Box 15.2).

One of the initiatives of the Choosing Wisely campaign was the development of five questions (Box 15.3) for patients to help them decide whether to undergo a test, treatment or procedure. The questions are intended to help promote a conversation with health professionals about key considerations when making such decisions.

De-Implementation Process and Strategies

Research has shown that developing and disseminating recommendations about low-value care are insufficient to change practice (Rosenberg et al 2015). Thus planned

BOX 15.2 Choosing Wisely Recommendation of the New Zealand College of Midwives

- Don't automatically initiate continuous electronic fetal heart rate monitoring during labour for women without risk factors: undertake intermittent auscultation (IA) first.
- Don't offer women with uncomplicated pregnancies a routine early first trimester ultrasound for dating purposes.
- Unless the mother has diabetes, in the absence of other clinical concerns, ultrasound scans should not be routinely offered to check whether a baby is bigger than normal for its gestational age.
- In term and preterm infants who do not require resuscitation at birth, delay umbilical cord clamping for at least 3 minutes or until the cord has stopped pulsating (whichever is longer).

(From: Choosing Wisely Australia, 2016b. Australian College of Nursing. Recommendations. https://www.choosingwisely.org.au/recommendations/acn1)

BOX 15.3 Choosing Wisely Questions

- Do I really need this test, treatment or procedure?
- What are the risks?
- Are there simpler, safer options?
- What happens if I don't do anything?
- What are the costs?

efforts to implement the recommendations for cessation of low-value care are required; van Bodegom-Vos et al (2018) describe two types of de-implementation. The first occurs when a practice is substituted or replaced with another practice. An example of this may be refraining from administering an antipyretic to an undistressed febrile child and, instead, removing extra layers of clothing. The second occurs when a practice is ceased or removed and an alternative practice is not substituted. An example of this may be refraining from routinely offering an ultrasound for dating purposes for women with uncomplicated pregnancies early in trimester one.

Norton and Chambers (2020) propose two other types of de-implementation: reducing and restricting practices. Reducing a practice may involve reducing the frequency of an intervention. An example of this may be the replacement of a peripheral intravenous cannula only when clinically indicated rather than after a certain number of days. Restricting a practice includes restricting based on certain conditions such as a population, professional group or setting. An example of this may include caesarean sections being restricted according to specific criteria. Van Bodegom-Vos et al (2017) note that abandoning low-value practices is more complicated than adopting new practices, even when evidence confirms the former practice's lack of benefit or potential harm. They, therefore, argue that strategies to de-implement practices may not be the same as those used to implement new practices. The barriers and enablers to each process may be different, necessitating different strategies and processes.

While de-implementation strategies may not take the same form as implementation strategies to translate evidence into practice or policy, some general principles are consistent between the two goals. First, a planned approach should be adopted. Second, the strategies should be tailored to identified barriers and enablers and the context in which the practice change is occurring. Third, the strategy should be feasible, acceptable, meaningful and effective ('FAME') (Pearson 2004). Norton and Chambers (2020) note that some strategies may be unique to de-implementation, particularly if the barriers are unique. Examples include reassuring patients that changes in their condition will not be missed, system changes to eliminate flags or prompts to take action, and financial disincentives. Authors of a recent systematic review of the evidence for de-implementation strategies to reduce low-value nursing practices found that education (including educational meetings, educational outreach visits and educational material) was the most frequently used strategy (Rietbergen et al 2020). Other strategies used in de-implementation efforts included audit and feedback, clinical guidelines and local consensus processes. These are all strategies that are also used in implementation efforts. The practices being de-implemented included restraint use, inappropriate antibiotic prescribing, unnecessary urinary catheter use, unnecessary liver function test ordering and unnecessary antipsychotic prescribing.

Summary

Clinical practices that have limited evidence for their efficacy continue to be performed. De-implementation is one of many terms used in the literature to describe the removal or reduction of costly or potentially hazardous approaches to care (Burton et al 2019). Although there is some transferability of the theory and frameworks between implementation and de-implementation, the factors that shape both processes are likely to be different and work in different ways.

BUILDING CAPACITY FOR EVIDENCE-BASED PRACTICE

Capacity is key to the success of implementation efforts. Organisational capacity refers to whether the organisation has the requisite resources, including information systems, skilled personnel, equipment, space, systems, processes and time to implement evidence and sustain the change. As noted previously, the organisation's readiness for change should be assessed prior to an implementation effort.

Individual capacity refers to having the knowledge, skills, time and resources to enable the adoption of the evidence. Many studies have demonstrated that nurses have positive attitudes towards evidence-based practice and recognise its usefulness (Pitsillidou et al 2021, Saunders & Vehviläinen-Julkunen 2016, Stokke et al 2014); however, the gap between evidence and its routine application in practice persists. A survey of 61 nurses revealed that 72.1% had not attempted to apply evidence in practice (Duncombe 2018). This suggests that nurses' capacity to use evidence may not always align with their favourable attitudes towards evidence-based approaches to practice. The contexts in which clinicians work, including various factors such as the systems, culture and leadership support, will also influence their practice. A review of the evidence of nurses' readiness for evidence-based practice showed that, although nurses had positive attitudes towards evidence-based practice, they reported that their skills and knowledge were inadequate, and they consequently did not use the best available evidence in practice (Saunders & Vehviläinen-Julkunen 2016).

Competence in evidence-based practice has been defined as 'the ability to ask clinically relevant questions for the purpose of acquiring, appraising, applying and assessing multiple sources of knowledge' (Labrague et al 2019). Researchers also refer to 'dynamic capabilities' to describe clinicians' capabilities to adjust to change when providing evidence-based care in a complex, diverse and dynamic environment (Huo et al 2022). Huo et al (2022) argued that such behavioural capabilities are necessary to implement evidence into practice and undertook a concept analysis of 'dynamic capabilities' for evidence-based practice. They found that personal (e.g. evidence-based practice competence and motivation) and infrastructure-related factors (e.g. resources including evidence, equipment, personnel and funding) were requirements for dynamic capability. The identified attributes of dynamic capability were sensing (capability to detect changes in the environment, including patient preferences, relevant evidence, policies and relevant technologies), learning (capability to acquire new knowledge and understand the evidence), integration (capability to change the environment and reorganise resources to enable integration of evidence into practice) and coordination (capability to coordinate resources and allocate tasks, e.g. provide clear guidance, secure leadership support and provide feedback). In terms of consequences of dynamic capability for evidence-based practice, improved patient outcomes, reduced expenditure and improved job satisfaction were identified.

Capacity-Building Approaches

Capacity building for evidence-based practice begins during undergraduate education. Strategies to build capacity for evidence-based practice among clinicians are varied, including education in various forms (e.g. educational outreach, educational meetings, problem-based learning), training, assessment or audit and feedback, reminders, peer networking and incentives. While numerous strategies are used to promote evidence-based practice capacity, nurses and midwives report various challenges in implementing evidence in practice. Such challenges include a lack of knowledge, training, skills and resources (Dagne & Beshah 2021). Educational strategies have been the most commonly used approach to build capacity for evidence-based practice amongst nurses and midwives. Authors of a recent systematic review identified three key forms of educational interventions: multifaceted educational strategies, including mentoring and tutoring; single component strategies, including online delivery; and multifaceted educational strategies based on five steps of evidence-based practice. The authors concluded that computer-based approaches were the most cost effective and efficient (Portela Dos Santos et al 2022).

A Cochrane review of the evidence for teaching health professionals critical appraisal skills indicates there is potential for low-intensity critical appraisal teaching to improve health professionals' knowledge to a modest extent (Horsley et al 2011). More-recent research has shown that strategies based on actions (e.g. audit and feedback, and reminders) and educational interventions are more likely to be successful in promoting the implementation of evidence into routine practice, compared with persuasion-based strategies such as consensus processes and opinion leaders. The authors concluded that combining interventions is more likely to be influential in promoting evidence use (Johnson & May 2015).

In the field of public health, systematic review evidence for capacity-building interventions identified the need for organisations to consider not just the interventions offered to personnel, but also the mechanisms for delivery, the audience and the purpose (DeCorby-Watson et al 2018). Six types of capacity-building interventions were identified: (1) internet-based instruction, (2) training and workshops, (3) technical assistance, (4) self-directed learning, (5) communities of

TABLE 15.2 Programs for Capacity Building in Implementation of Evidence Into Policy and Practice

Program	Mode and Country	Link
Joanna Briggs Institute Evidence Implementation Training	In-person, Australia	https://jbi.global/education/evidence-implementation-training
Training in Dissemination and Implementation Research in Health (TIDIRH)	In-person, Australia	https://ncois.org.au/training/
Training Institute for Dissemination and Implementation Research in Cancer (TIDRC)	Open access, international	https://cancercontrol.cancer.gov/is/training-education/training-in-cancer/TIDIRC-open-access
Monash Centre for Health Research and Implementation: Masterclass in Implementation Science and Effective Healthcare Improvement in Practice	In person and online	https://www.monash.edu/medicine/mchri/training/courses

practice and (6) multi-strategy interventions. Authors of a scoping review found the most common features of interventions for implementation of **capacity building** were in-person or online didactic teaching, mentorship and consultation with experts and practical activities such as field placements. Of the 14 studies included in the review, all showed improved knowledge, implementation ability, productivity and satisfaction (Juckett et al 2022).

Nurses and midwives are uniquely positioned to lead implementation efforts because they have an intimate understanding of the healthcare setting, systems and processes, and the barriers to and enablers of change, and they play a prominent role within the broader multidisciplinary team. Thus investment in training nurses and midwives to participate in and lead implementation efforts is essential. Several programs are on offer to build the capacity of nurses and midwives for implementation (Table 15.2).

TUTORIAL TRIGGER 15.4

Q) The gap between attitude to best practice and routine use of best practice can be addressed through capacity-building strategies. Identify four strategies that relate to capacity building.

A) Four strategies highlighted in this chapter include: (1) the education of individuals in fundamentals of understanding research methods, (2) skills teaching in specific tools and resources for best practice, (3) active participation in service improvement projects that are guided by evidence-based methods, and (4) organisational commitment to facilitation, mentorship and capacity building among staff.

SUMMARY

Strategies to improve the effectiveness and quality of healthcare have emphasised the need to implement new research and evidence into clinical practice and service delivery. This chapter has outlined the concepts and activities of implementing evidence into practice and policy and, through a case study, highlighted how a conceptual framework facilitates applying research knowledge to practice. There is a need to build the capacity of all clinicians and policy makers to appraise and implement new evidence and to demonstrate that their practice is based upon the best available evidence. Many practice questions are not addressed in the literature and, therefore, nurses and midwives draw on other sources of evidence to inform their practice, including their own professional experience and the desires and preferences of their patients. The use of frameworks such as the JBI model provides a roadmap for translating evidence into practice.

Implementation of evidence into practice requires midwives and nurses to have specific knowledge and skills. However, without organisational capacity in the form of support, resources for education and training, as well as a research culture, nurses and midwives will struggle to implement evidence into practice. Thus clinician capacity coupled with organisational capacity for implementation is a necessary prerequisite for successful implementation.

KEY POINTS

- Evidence is information and knowledge that, when applied in the right context for decision making about the care of individual patients, promotes evidence-based practice.

- Evidence for practice needs to be valid and reliable. Well-conducted systematic reviews are currently the preferred type of evidence for policy and practice.
- Having evidence available without training and equipping ourselves with the knowledge and skills in how to reliably implement is one of the barriers to better healthcare.
- Building organisational capacity for best practice includes culture change as well as education and training of individual staff.

TIME TO REFLECT

Aim: To identify implementation strategies for the following best-practice recommendations:

- Introduction of a multidisciplinary multifactorial intervention program including a falls risk alert card, an exercise program, an education program and the use of hip protectors
- Use of one-to-one patient education packages including information on risk factors and preventive strategies for falls as well as goal setting
- Introduction of a targeted falls risk factor reduction intervention that includes fall risk factor screening
- A fall prevention exercise program as a stand-alone intervention which comprises tai chi, functional movements and activity visualisation.

Objective: To audit current practice of falls prevention within the acute clinical setting, to improve practice in the prevention of falls in accordance to the best-available evidence, to implement interventions according to the findings; to improve compliance, accuracy and sustainability and to re-audit to identify further change.

Design: Clinical audit using evidence-based audit criteria:

1. Fall risk assessment is completed upon admission.
2. Fall risk assessment is completed upon transfer.
3. Reassessment occurs when there is a change in condition or following a fall.
4. Patients who have experienced a fall are considered at high risk for future falls.
5. Healthcare professionals have received education regarding falls assessment and prevention strategies.
6. Targeted interventions are implemented according to risk factors.

Reflect:

a. Was clinical audit the right approach for the stated objectives?
b. Do the documented criteria measure the stated objectives?
c. Would the indicators for assessment described above be useful in your experiences in clinical practice? If not, why not? Consider what aspects of the ward practices; culture or routines might act as barriers.
d. What is the strength/weakness of this design?

Time to Reflect: Answers

a. While clinical audit is sometimes confused with research, the basic premise is that research establishes new knowledge while audit examines current practice for compliance against known best-practice standards. Some audits require ethical approval, some research is not on patients; there is therefore often some 'grey' in the distinction between audit and research.
b. The criteria are based upon whether the assessments were completed, and the timing of completion. While this does meet the standard required for best practice, it also raises the issue of *how* the standard would be measured. Confirming whether it was completed may require observation of the assessment as it occurs, since the standard does not include comment on the documentation of completion of assessment. This may add to the complexity of audit data collection in order to establish compliance with the criteria on assessment.
c. Only you can answer this question—don't skip this; take a few minutes to write down your response to the following:
   i. Could it be useful—yes or no?
   ii. Why did you answer that way?
   iii. What aspects of the structure, hierarchy or organisational culture were you thinking might act to either make it possible or act as a barrier?
d. Clinical audits based on best practice provide an objective benchmark to establish whether current clinical practice is evidence based or not. This is more reliable and rigorous than basing audit criteria on opinion, or on standards that have not been developed from the best-available evidence. However, audits tell us only the degree to which we comply with a standard. They do not have explanatory power in the same way that research does.

LEARNING ACTIVITIES

1. Evidence to inform policy or practice comes from:
   a. the publications of learned experts in a clinical specialty
   b. empirics, including experimental and qualitative research as well as discourse and opinion
   c. experimental research that produces statistics and quantifies clinical outcomes.
2. The FAME scale addressed:
   a. feasibility, by which is meant whether something is easy or hard to do
   b. feasibility, by which is meant practice change is considered in light of the cultural context
   c. feasibility, by which is meant both the context of care and the available resources.
3. Evidence-based practice is a combination of:
   a. research evidence combined with clinical expertise and recognition of patient preferences within a given context
   b. expert advice from top research professors or researchers, plus organisational policy and guidelines
   c. easily accessible instructions for practice, plus recommendations from patients on their preferences.
4. The hierarchy of evidence is:
   a. a theoretical hierarchy of the quality of evidence
   b. a hierarchy of study designs that when properly conducted are associated with different levels of reliability for clinical decision making
   c. a useful indicator that less evidence exists the higher up the pyramid one follows.
5. The JBI Model positions:
   a. evidence generation as the central process in evidence-based healthcare
   b. evidence synthesis as the central process in evidence-based healthcare
   c. evidence transfer as the central process in evidence-based healthcare
   d. evidence utilisation as the central process in evidence-based healthcare
   e. evidence-based healthcare as central to all of the above.
6. Evidence synthesis is:
   a. using a rigorous and transparent method to craft clinical questions, identify evidence, establish its validity and present summaries of findings
   b. scanning the literature or using citation alerts to pick up on the most recent topical publications
   c. updating our knowledge by reading Wikipedia
   d. writing summaries of literature on specific clinical questions.
7. Evidence transfer in the JBI Model of EBHC:
   a. follows on from evidence generation
   b. is the use of specific strategies to ensure evidence is communicated to the right group using strategies appropriate to that group
   c. is the interpretation of research findings into other languages.
8. Implementation of best practice:
   a. is based on the conduct of locally relevant and rigorous research
   b. is based on reading recent journal articles and implementing their recommendations
   c. is based on knowledge transfer strategies combined with method for utilisation as depicted in the JBI Model of EBHC.
9. Capacity building for evidence-based healthcare:
   a. is not particularly important; simply telling people about best practice is enough
   b. is an organisational strategy that includes a focus on culture as well as individual staff education and training
   c. is a process of educating staff and providing examples of published research.
10. Research evidence cited in this chapter indicates that nurses and midwives have positive attitudes to evidence-based healthcare, but:
    a. report that they lack skills in conducting research
    b. report that the steps of problem identification and question development are the biggest barriers
    c. report that specific skills for EBHC are the area where ongoing training and development is required.
11. Implementation of best practice is achieved by:
    a. identifying priority issues, conducting systematic reviews and implementing the findings
    b. identifying research that fits a clinical need and evaluating the impact on patient outcomes
    c. undertaking important topics of research led and conducted by nurses or midwives
    d. identifying issues in practice, accessing relevant evidence, using targeted implementation strategies combined with specific facilitation of staff engagement in the process
    e. undertaking quality improvement projects that facilitate organisational accreditation.

ADDITIONAL RESOURCES

BMJ—evidence-based nursing. https://ebn.bmj.com/.

Nursing World. OJIN—The impact of evidence-based practice. https://www.nursingworld.org/MainMenuCategories/

ANAMarketplace/ANAPeriodicals/OJIN/TableofContents/Vol-18-2013/No2-May-2013/Impact-of-Evidence-Based-Practice.html.

The Agency for Health Care Quality and Research National Guideline Clearing House. https://www.guideline.gov/.

The Canadian Institute of Health Research Knowledge Translation Clearinghouse. https://ktclearinghouse.ca/.

The Joanna Briggs Institute. https://joannabriggs.org/.

REFERENCES

Abu-Baker, N.N., AbuAlrub, S., Obeidat, R.F., et al., 2021. Evidence-based practice beliefs and implementations: A cross-sectional study among undergraduate nursing students. BMC Nurs. 20 (1), 13. doi:10.1186/s12912-020-00522-x

Abu-Odah, H., Said, N.B., Nair, S.C., et al., 2022. Identifying barriers and facilitators of translating research evidence into clinical practice: a systematic review of reviews. Health Soc. Care Commun. 30, e3265–e3276. doi:10.1111/hsc.13898

Agency for Healthcare Research and Quality. 2018. Evidence-Based Decision Making. doi:10.46658/JBIMES-20-01. Retrieved from: https://www.ahrq.gov/prevention/chronic-care/decision/index.html.

Aromataris, E., Munn, Z. (Eds.), 2020. JBI Manual for Evidence Synthesis. JBI, North Adelaide, SA. Retrieved from: https://synthesismanual.jbi.global.

Australian Commission on Safety and Quality in Health Care, 2021. Delirium Clinical Care Standard (revised 2021). Retrieved from: https://www.safetyandquality.gov.au/sites/default/files/2021-11/delirium_clinical_care_standard_2021.pdf.

Barwick, M, 2011. Checklist to Assess Organizational Readiness (CARI) for Evidence Informed Practice Implementation. Hospital for Sick Children, Toronto. Retrieved from: https://melaniebarwick.com/wp-content/uploads/2019/01/CARI-Checklist_for_Assessing_Readiness_for_Implementation-BARWICK.pdf.

Bellelli, G., Morandi, A., Davis, D.H.J., et al., 2014. Validation of the 4AT, a new instrument for rapid delirium screening: A study in 234 hospitalised older people. Age Ageing 43 (4), 496–502. doi:10.1093/ageing/afu021

Braithwaite, J., Hibbert, P.D., Jaffe, A., et al., 2018. Quality of health care for children in Australia, 2012–2013. JAMA. 319 (11), 1113–1124. doi:10.1001/jama.2018.0162

Burton, C., Williams, L., Bucknall, T., et al., 2019. Understanding how and why de-implementation works in health and care: research protocol for a realist synthesis of evidence. Syst. Rev. 8 (1), 194. doi:10.1186/s13643-019-1111-8

Centers for Disease Control and Prevention (CDC), 2014. Applying the Knowledge to Action (K2A) Framework. CDC, US Dept of Health and Human Services, Atlanta, GA.

Choosing Wisely Australia, 2016a. Eliminating Unnecessary Tests, Treatments & Procedures. Retrieved from: https://www.choosingwisely.org.au/.

Choosing Wisely Australia, 2016b. Australian College of Nursing. Recommendations. Retrieved from: https://www.choosingwisely.org.au/recommendations/acn1.

Committee on the Learning Health Care System in America & Institute of Medicine, 2013. In: Smith, M., Saunders, R., Stuckhardt, L., (Eds.). Best Care at Lower Cost: the path to continuously learning health care in America. National Academies Press, Washington DC. Retrieved from: https://www.ncbi.nlm.nih.gov/books/NBK207225/.

Dagne, A.H., Beshah, M.H., 2021. Implementation of evidence-based practice: the experience of nurses and midwives. PloS One, 16 (8), e0256600. doi:10.1371/journal.pone.0256600

Dagne, A.H., Tebeje, H., Mariam D. 2021. Research utilisation in clinical practice: the experience of nurses and midwives working in public hospitals. Reprod. Health, 18, 62. doi:10.1186/s12978-021-01095-x

DeCorby-Watson, K., Mensah, G., Bergeron, K., et al., 2018. Effectiveness of capacity building interventions relevant to public health practice: a systematic review. BMC Public Health 18 (1), 684. doi:10.1186/s12889-018-5591-6

Dogherty, E.J., Harrison, M.B., Graham, I.D., et al., 2013. Turning knowledge into action at the point-of-care: the collective experience of nurses facilitating the implementation of evidence-based practice. Worldviews Evid. Based Nurs. 10 (3), 129–139. doi:10.1111/wvn.12009

Duff, J., Cullen, L., Hanrahan, K., et al., 2020. Determinants of an evidence-based practice environment: An interpretive description. Implement. Sci. Commun. 1 (1), 85. doi:10.1186/s43058-020-00070-0

Duncombe, D.C., 2018. A multi-institutional study of the perceived barriers and facilitators to implementing evidence-based practice. J. Clin. Nurs. 27 (5–6), 1216–1226. doi:10.1111/jocn.14168

Ellis, P., 2019. Evidence-Based Practice in Nursing—Transforming Nursing Practice, fourth ed. Sage Publications, London.

Graham, I.D., Logan, J., Harrison, M.B., et al., 2006. Lost in knowledge translation: time for a map? J. Contin. Educ. Health Prof. 26 (1), 13–24.

Harris, C., Allen, K., King, R., et al., 2017. Sustainability in Health care by Allocating Resources Effectively (SHARE) 2: identifying opportunities for disinvestment in a local healthcare setting. BMC Health Serv. Res. 17 (1), 328. doi:10.1186/s12913-017-2211-6

Helfrich, C.D., Li, Y.-F., Sharp, N.D., et al., 2009. Organizational readiness to change assessment (ORCA): Development of an instrument based on the Promoting Action on Research in Health Services (PARIHS) framework. Implement. Sci. 4 (1), 38. doi:10.1186/1748-5908-4-38

Horsley, T., Hyde, C., Santesso, N., et al., 2011. Teaching critical appraisal skills in healthcare settings. Cochrane Database Syst. Revi. 11, CD001270. doi:10.1002/14651858.CD001270.pub2

Huo, M., Zhao, B., Li, Y., et al., 2022. Evidence-based practice dynamic capabilities: a concept derivation and analysis. Ann. Transl. Med. 10 (1), 22. doi:10.21037/atm-21-6506

Ingvarsson, S., Hasson, H., von Thiele Schwarz, U., et al., 2022. Strategies for de-implementation of low-value care—a scoping review Implement. Sci. 17 (1), 73. doi:10.1186/s13012-022-01247-y

Johnson, M.J., May, C.R., 2015. Promoting professional behaviour change in healthcare: what interventions work, and why?

A theory-led overview of systematic reviews. BMJ Open 5 (9), e008592. doi:10.1136/bmjopen-2015-008592

Jordan, Z., Donnelly, P., Pittman, E., 2006. A Short History of a Big Idea. The Joanna Briggs Institute, North Adelaide, SA.

Jordan, Z., Lockwood, C., Munn, Z., et al., 2019. The updated Joanna Briggs Institute Model of Evidence-based Healthcare. Int. J. Evid. Based Healthcare 17 (1), 58–71. doi:10.1097/XEB.0000000000000155

Juckett, L.A., Bunger, A.C., McNett, M.M., et al., 2022. Leveraging academic initiatives to advance implementation practice: a scoping review of capacity building interventions. Implement. Sci. 17 (1), 49. doi:10.1186/s13012-022-01216-5

Kwame, A., Petrucka, P.M., 2021. A literature-based study of patient-centered care and communication in nurse-patient interactions: barriers, facilitators, and the way forward. BMC Nurs. 20 (1), 158. doi:10.1186/s12912-021-00684-2

Labrague, L.J., McEnroe-Petitte, D., D'Souza, M.S., et al., 2019. A multicountry study on nursing students' self-perceived competence and barriers to evidence-based practice. Worldviews Evid. Based Nurs. 16 (3), 236–246. doi:10.1111/wvn.12364

MacDermid, J.C., Graham, I.D., 2009. Knowledge translation: putting the 'practice' in evidence-based practice. Hand Clin. 25 (1), 125–143, viii. doi:10.1016/j.hcl.2008.10.003

National Academies of Sciences, Engineering, and Medicine; Health and Medicine Division; Board on Health Sciences Policy; Forum on Drug Discovery, Development, and Translation, 2017. Improving Evidence Generation for Decision Making on Approval and Use of New Treatments: Some Stakeholder Priorities. In: Real-World Evidence Generation and Evaluation of Therapeutics: Proceedings of a Workshop. National Academies Press, Washington DC. (US). Retrieved from: https://www.ncbi.nlm.nih.gov/books/NBK441693/.

New Zealand College of Midwives, 2018. Practice updates. Retrieved from: https://www.midwife.org.nz/midwives/professional-practice/practice-updates/.

Nilsen, P., 2015. Making sense of implementation theories, models and frameworks. Implement. Sci. 10, 53. doi:10.1186/s13012-015-0242-

Norton, W.E., Chambers, D.A., 2020. Unpacking the complexities of de-implementing inappropriate health interventions. Implement. Sci. 15 (1), 2. doi:10.1186/s13012-019-0960-9

Organisation for Economic Co-operation and Development (OECD), 2017. Tackling Wasteful Spending on Health. Retrieved from: https://read.oecd-ilibrary.org/social-issues-migration-health/tackling-wasteful-spending-on-health_9789264266414-en#page1.

Pearson, A., 2004. Balancing the evidence: incorporating the synthesis of qualitative data into systematic reviews. JBI Rep. 2 (2), 45–64. doi:10.1111/j.1479-6988.2004.00008.x

Pearson, A., Wiechula, R., Court, A., et al., 2005. The JBI model of evidence-based healthcare. Int. J. Evid. Based Healthcare 3 (8), 207–215. doi:10.1111/j.1479-6988.2005.00026.x

Pearson, A., Jordan, Z., Munn, Z., 2012. Translational science and evidence-based healthcare: a clarification and reconceptualization of how knowledge is generated and used in healthcare. Nurs. Res. Pract. 2012, 792519. doi:10.1155/2012/792519

Pitsillidou, M., Roupa, Z., Farmakas, A., et al., 2021. Factors affecting the application and implementation of evidence-based practice in nursing. Acta Inform. Med. 29 (4), 281–287. doi:10.5455/aim.2021.29.281-287

Klepac, B., Krahe, M., Spaaij, R., et al., 2022. Increasing research evidence translation and utilisation to improve health outcomes: policy evidence brief 2022-02. Mitchell Institute, Victoria University, Melbourne, VIC. doi:10.26196/0bck-q209

Porritt, K., McArthur, A., Lockwood, C., et al. (Eds.), 2020. JBI Handbook for Evidence Implementation. The Joanna Briggs Institute, North Adelaide, SA. Retrieved from: https://jbi-global-wiki.refined.site/space/JHEI.

Portela Dos Santos, O., Melly, P., Hilfiker, R., et al., 2022. Effectiveness of educational interventions to increase skills in evidence-based practice among nurses: the EDITcare Systematic Review. Healthcare 10 (11), 2204. doi:10.3390/healthcare10112204

Rietbergen, T., Spoon, D., Brunsveld-Reinders, A.H., et al., 2020. Effects of de-implementation strategies aimed at reducing low-value nursing procedures: a systematic review and meta-analysis. Implement. Sci. 15 (1), 38. doi:10.1186/s13012-020-00995-z

Rosenberg, A., Agiro, A., Gottlieb, M., et al., 2015. Early trends among seven recommendations from the Choosing Wisely campaign. JAMA Internal Med.175 (12), 1913–1920. doi:10.1001/jamainternmed.2015.5441

Saunders, H., Vehviläinen-Julkunen, K., 2016. The state of readiness for evidence-based practice among nurses: an integrative review. Int. J. Nurs. Stud. 56, 128–140. doi:10.1016/j.ijnurstu.2015.10.018

Squires, J.E., Graham, I.D., Santos, W.J. et al. The Implementation in Context (ICON) framework: a meta-framework of context domains, attributes and features in healthcare. Health Res. Policy Sys. 21, 81 (2023). doi:10.1186/s12961-023-01028-z

Stokke, K., Olsen, N. R., Espehaug, B., et al., 2014. Evidence based practice beliefs and implementation among nurses: a cross-sectional study. BMC Nurs. 13 (1), 8. doi:10.1186/1472-6955-13-8

Texas Board of Nursing, 2016. Texas nurses selected to pilot Choosing Wisely® Campaign. Texas Board of Nursing Bulletin. Austin, TX. Retrieved from: https://www.bon.texas.gov/pdfs/newsletter_pdfs/2016/January2016.pdf.

Upvall, M.J., Bourgault, A.M., 2018. De-implementation: a concept analysis. Nurs. Forum 53 (3), 376–382. doi:10.1111/nuf.12256

van Bodegom-Vos, L., Davidoff, F., Marang-van de Mheen, P.J., 2017. Implementation and de-implementation: two sides of the same coin? BMJ Qual. Saf. 26, 495–501.

Verkerk, E.W., Tanke, M.A.C., Kool, R.B., et al., 2018. Limit, lean or listen? A typology of low-value care that gives direction in de-implementation. Int. J. Qual. Health Care 30 (9), 736–739. doi:10.1093/intqhc/mzy100

Wensing, M., Grol, R., 2019. Knowledge translation in health: How implementation science could contribute more. BMC Med. 17 (1), 88. doi:10.1186/s12916-019-1322-9

SECTION 3

What You Need to Know About Research if You Want to Conduct Research

16

Writing Research Proposals and Grant Applications

Nicolas H Hart, Darren Haywood and Raymond J Chan

LEARNING OUTCOMES

After reading this chapter, you should be able to:

- describe key considerations for writing research proposals and grants
- outline the process for preparing and submitting a research proposal or grant
- identify the significance of the topic and potential outcomes
- identify funding agencies appropriate for nursing or midwifery research studies
- prepare a draft research proposal according to a specified format.

KEY TERMS

budget, p. 287
consumer engagement, p. 289
funding agencies, p. 276
grants, p. 290
human research ethics committee (HREC), p. 276
informed consent, p. 285
intellectual property, p. 278
preliminary work, p. 279
theoretical or conceptual framework, p. 284
timeframe, p. 283
track record, p. 277

INTRODUCTION

As a grant writer you are required to argue the significance of your presented topic and outcomes in an interesting and engaging way—this is an art. The *art* implied refers to writing style, coherence, knowledge of the research problem/question, clarity and readability. Although you need a great story, it also needs to be fundamentally underpinned by rigorous science to support your argument. The *science* refers to the techniques and methodological rigor involved in writing a proposal, while providing evidence as to why the presented research team is best placed to conduct the study. A research proposal or grant can be used for a number of purposes, for example: (1) to gain competitive research funding, (2) to complete a higher degree course or (3) to inform a study protocol or **human research ethics committee (HREC)** application. This chapter describes the major components involved in developing a research proposal or grant. The stages for preparing and submitting a research proposal or grant are presented in a way that will facilitate familiarity with the information required by institutional ethics committees and **funding agencies**. Information regarding appropriate funding agencies for nursing and midwifery is also provided, though many funding opportunities are now interdisciplinary.

WHAT IS A RESEARCH PROPOSAL?

A research proposal and/or research protocol is a succinctly written document justifying the need for a project and how the aims of the project will be achieved and sustained. There are international resources and guidelines that many institutional and research publications require researchers to use. You must review these and find the most appropriate reporting guidelines prior to formally planning your research proposal. They will guide the structure of your proposal; please see https://www.equator-network.org/. The format of the proposal is influenced by the specific purpose of the research and by the audience for whom it is intended.

The proposal must demonstrate that:

- the investigator, or research team, is competent to undertake the research, which is often demonstrated through track record
- the topic is important and that the findings will have impact, for example, to benefit patients or a particular group, to advance or generate new knowledge
- the design, method and timeframe are feasible and appropriate
- the risk–benefit for participants is acceptable
- participant anonymity, confidentiality, safety and right to withdraw are protected
- if the proposal is submitted as part of a higher degree, there is assurance from the head of department that the student will have appropriate supervision and access to the required facilities
- funding requested is reasonable.

PLANNING A PROPOSAL, PROJECT OR GRANT APPLICATION

Writing a proposal, project or grant application requires considerable preparation, time, skill and teamwork. Writing a successful proposal is not something that should be done by one person. Novice researchers benefit by attending research seminars and conferences, participating in research interest groups and being members of professional associations. It is imperative to keep up to date about health and healthcare priorities through reading the research literature, talking to researchers with similar interests, and through participating in professional groups and social media. As with any project, planning is an important preliminary stage.

This stage can involve:

- reading the relevant evidence-based literature in your area of interest (see Chapter 3)
- identifying and clarifying a researchable topic (see Chapter 4)
- applying a research approach to address the research question or objectives (see Chapter 13)
- describing the impact, significance, translation and outcomes of the project
- identifying the requirements for submission to a particular HREC (see Chapter 13)
- consulting resource personnel available to advise on the development and submission of the proposal (e.g. academic colleagues, clinicians, ethics office staff).

Teaming up with the Right Mentor

Teaming up with the right mentor for your planned project or application is vital for success in all stages. Once you have a research area that you are interested in pursuing, finding the right mentor in that area will support your thought processes and execution of the range of tasks that are required to see a project go from an idea through to completion and dissemination. But what makes a mentor 'right' for you? Chan and Hart (2023) suggest that the right mentor should ideally be someone who has not only a **track record** of success in the research area (e.g. demonstrated expertise, successful grants in a similar stream), but also someone who has the capability (i.e. capacity, ability and motivation) to provide you with high-level mentorship and contribute to your application or proposal. Sometimes it is beneficial to have multiple mentors who may have different expertise and who may work together in a mentorship team. This can be helpful as having a mentorship team can not only mean that you are provided with well-rounded mentorship but also help alleviate some of the time commitment (capacity) for each mentor. If you do have a mentorship team, it is recommended to define the specific roles and expectations for each mentor and to define a lead mentor from the outset (Chan & Hart 2023). Now that you know your research area, and have the right mentor/mentorship team, you can select a specific research topic.

Selecting a Topic

From the beginning, it is critical when formulating your research topic that you take a step back and look at the bigger picture. Where does your research problem sit within the context of local, national and global research environments? It is fundamental to do your homework and examine your research problem within existing evidence-based literature and similar research currently being undertaken. Conceptualising a quality research topic is an important yet sometimes challenging task. It is important to select a topic that has the potential for you to demonstrate novelty, significance and urgency for the proposed research (Chan & Hart 2023).

- ***Novelty*** refers to the extent to which the proposed research is original, unique and innovative.
- ***Significance*** refers to the importance, relevance and potential impact of the proposed research.
- ***Urgency*** refers to the immediate need or time sensitivity of achieving the proposed research outcomes

It is important to remember, however, that, while having a research topic that provides the potential to display novelty, significance and urgency is critical, it is just as important that the proposed project is shown to be feasible and of high scientific quality (Chan & Hart 2023). Even the most innovative and seemingly impactful proposed research will not be looked upon fondly by funding reviewers, or HRECs, if it is not clearly feasible within your particular context (resources, environment and capability) and of high scientific quality.

Keeping these points in mind, there are a number of critical factors involved when thoughtfully selecting a research topic. These include the following:

- Adopt a teamwork approach to brainstorming and incubating real-world, clinical problems and pragmatic solutions.
- Anchor your research topic within the context of the highest-level, good-quality evidence available.
- Adopt a mindset that is flexible and pragmatic.
- Remember that you cannot fix the world—select a specific piece of the puzzle that is achievable and manageable within the scope of the resources available.
- Formulate your research question and hypothesis, which may not be easy. Seek advice early and leave plenty of time. Clear research questions and hypotheses are critical when you develop your research methodologies.
- For a novice researcher, it is strategic to be part of a collaborative and high-performing research team. You will likely need to express a passion and enthusiasm for engagement and hard work.
- Collaboration is key to success—you may need to seek interdisciplinary and cross-institutional collaboration, outside of your discipline or institution, for these collaborative opportunities.
- As a nurse or midwife you will need to articulate what your expertise is and how your contributions can value-add to a research team. See also Chapter 4.

Developing Your Research Team

To successfully obtain funding for your project, and to conduct the planned research, it is important to develop the right research team. Chan and Hart (2023) suggest that a planned research team should be developed *prior* to a suitable grant scheme for your project opening and suggest that an early career researcher (ECR) use their mentor/mentorship team's networks to develop their research team while they build their own networks. The best research teams (a) have completed previous research together, (b) have members that complement each other's skill sets and (c) have members at various stages in their careers. However, you should not recruit your entire research team too early in the process or at a too-rapid pace. Choosing the wrong team members for your project may greatly impact your likelihood of successfully obtaining funding owing to the often-limited number of chief or co-investigators you may include on an application. When choosing your research team members, Chan and Hart (2023) suggest reflecting on five questions:

1. Will the collaborator make a meaningful contribution to the grant scheme?
2. Will the collaborator be seen as a weak link in the team?
3. Does the collaborator have a good reputation as a collegiate team member?
4. Is there any discipline-specific perspectives that are key to the proposed research?
5. Is the collaborator recognised as a national or international leader in the field for their area of contribution?

Further, there has been increased recognition of the utility of partnering with consumers and patient advocates in investigator roles on grant applications (Forsythe et al 2019, Price et al 2022), and in the process of preparing research proposals (in the absence of available investigator roles), as well as throughout the entire research trajectory (planning, preparation, proposal, acquisition, delivery, completion, analysis and dissemination). This partnering should show how the proposed project has been genuinely informed by and thoughtfully involved consumers and other end-users, and that they are, and will be, involved in all phases of the research. Ultimately, building your research project team requires a strong time investment and careful consideration. Consumers or other types of end-users are an essential part of the modern research landscape in health and medical research and must have meaningful involvement.

Format Requirements for the Proposal

Most grant applications, academic institutions or industries will have a standard format, which you will need to investigate prior to starting your proposal. A separate standard form requiring different information may be required by a hospital HREC (see Chapter 13). These forms may differ from those used by funding agencies, who usually provide their own application forms.

Some tips:

1. Seek advice from the HREC administrative officer.
2. Follow grant guidelines and university research office advice.
3. Review guidelines, particularly in relation to funding priorities and scheme scope.
4. Find an academic mentor to support writing an initial application or proposal.
5. Consult the National Health and Medical Research Council (NHMRC) or a funding body if there is a standardised proposal/protocol template.

Intellectual Property

Intellectual property is defined as the property of your mind or proprietary knowledge, and has implications for research planning, conduct, completion and utilisation post-completion that may differ according to whether you are a student or staff member of a university, or a clinician researcher within your hospital and health service. Information about intellectual property may be obtained from the intellectual property office or legal department of your institution. It is important the students and staff members as early-career or clinician researchers understand exactly what these conditions mean. Issues surrounding intellectual property are important when applying for external funding, and it is your responsibility to seek clarification before embarking on writing a proposal. The *National Principles of Intellectual Property Management for Publicly Funded Research* document can be found at https://www.nhmrc.gov.au/about-us/resources/national-principles-ip-management-publicly-funded-research. It is a condition of funding from the NHMRC and Australian Research Council (ARC), among other research funding agencies, that universities and hospitals or health services observe the national principles. A major responsibility of Universities Australia is the monitoring of government legislation and policies regarding ownership and copyright materials by its staff and students. These principles are mirrored in Committee on Publication Ethics (COPE) publications (https://publicationethics.org/intellectualproperty).

As a researcher, it is important to understand your rights and obligations should your research have the potential for patentable inventions or any other discoveries that have commercial value. Such innovations or discoveries may arise out of research conducted by higher degree students, early-career researchers and clinician researchers. Any researcher who is engaged in work that may result in discoveries is usually included as one of a team with senior academic researchers undertaking funded research of a commercial nature (although this is not always the case), thus formal discussions with pre-established agreements among the lead researcher, senior researcher, research team and any lead or partner organisations are vitally important to establish from the outset. All researchers will come up against copyright provisions and publication related to their work. In the age of digital media and digital theses, your research may be considered to have been published if it is freely available electronically through open-access publication and electronic repositories required by funders such as the NHMRC and ARC. Journal publishers will often set a requirement that manuscript submissions have not been published previously elsewhere. This does not preclude publishing different aspects of the same study. As a wise student you should check first with your supervisor or institutional librarian how your thesis will be archived and made available.

Preliminary Work

Often, preliminary data from earlier work, developed through **systematic reviews** or **pilot studies,** are required to establish the need for subsequent work. A research proposal may be required for this initial small-scale study, or these systematic reviews or pilot studies may form a component of a larger proposal (i.e. a program of work). A pilot study evaluates the feasibility of the procedure or proposed instruments. For example, if new protocols or procedures were being introduced into a clinical area, it is important that the nurses or midwives become familiar with the new procedures and understand what is required of them. A pilot study would highlight any ambiguities or misunderstandings the staff may have and systematically capture any potential barriers or facilitators that may be implemented to improve feasibility and quality of the next phase of research. When new procedures are understood, implementation in the clinical area is likely to result in less stress for the nursing and other staff and enhance the acceptance, conduct and performance of the project.

Funding agencies often expect applicants to have undertaken previous work in the topic area, whether a systematic review or pilot study, to ensure they have the relevant expertise, domain knowledge and feasible capacity to deliver the proposed research. An example is the development and completion of a pilot randomised controlled trial to evaluate the feasibility of delivering a telehealth cancer-related fatigue model for cancer survivors in one geographical location (Ladwa et al 2022) as a precursor to the expansion of this model of care to multiple locations nationwide in a future larger-scale study with feasibility suitably demonstrated. The advantage of running a pilot study is that feedback learning can be applied to existing protocols before commencing larger-powered research.

Increasingly, the academic publishing landscape is changing in relation to the publication of either systematic reviews or pilot studies in nursing and midwifery peer-reviewed journals. Systematic reviews must be registered with the PROSPERO. Pilot studies must be registered with the Australian New Zealand Clinical Trial Registry (ANZCTR). The ANZCTR is an online registry of clinical trials being undertaken in Australia, New Zealand and elsewhere. See https://www.anzctr.org.au/ for further information. It is worthwhile considering registering your pilot study with the ANZCTR at the time of your proposal writing and ethics application if you intend to publish your pilot study data in a credible academic journal.

WRITING A PROPOSAL

A proposal involves adept writing skills—that is: clarity, logic, order, coherence and a clear understanding of the purpose for which the proposal is written. Developing drafts and discussing the proposed study with mentors, supervisors and peers is essential and will highlight any limitations or weaknesses in the proposed research. However, before you start writing your proposal, it is critical to have a strong understanding of the target grant scheme objectives and selection criteria (Chan & Hart 2023).

Understanding the Objectives and Selection Criteria

Having a detailed understanding of the objectives of the scheme and the associated assessment criteria is required prior to writing a proposal. Prior to writing your proposal, you will need to develop an understanding of how your proposed project 'fits' the scheme's objectives and selection criteria, in addition to the potential funding amounts and duration. Regularly, the objectives, selection criteria and funding parameters of a scheme may not perfectly fit your proposed project. However, you may be able to adaptively develop your proposal to better fit the fixed objectives, selection criteria and funding parameters prescribed by the scheme. If you and/or your research team feel as though there are too many compromises to your planned project to have it fit the scheme's objectives, criteria and funding parameters, it is likely that the scheme is not the right fit. In these cases, it may be better to search out/wait for alternative funding opportunities that may better fit the proposed project. Once you have found a grant scheme that is applicable to your project and have a clear understanding of the grant scheme objectives, selection criteria and funding parameters, you can start writing proposal drafts.

Writing Drafts

Writing drafts can involve first sketching out the research idea (Attard 2018), which can then be developed in a stepwise manner such as the following:

1. Write your working research question.
2. Talk with colleagues.
3. Read the literature.
4. Ask yourself: What is known? What could I feasibly research? Would this be new? And who would care?
5. Go back to the beginning and refine your working research question.

Keep doing this until you have a good research question and overall design before writing the detailed proposal that will include breaking the research question down into smaller researchable parts. An organised researcher will make sure there is time to have a proposal reviewed by others during development and prior to submission. You should assume that the committee (e.g. faculty, hospital, grant review panels and university boards) reviewing your proposal will have a limited knowledge of your specialised research area. This will help you focus on writing comprehensively and clearly, with minimal jargon. Importantly, the time and effort spent thinking about the topic is never wasted. Even a proposal that is rejected should become the basis for a reworked proposal. Many proposal reviews include a rejoinder process where the researchers see the assessment made by the reviewers with the opportunity to respond before the decision is made whether or not to approve. It is a fact that more grant proposals in competitive schemes get rejected than accepted. Data from the NHMRC reveals that only between 11% and 25% of applications are funded. All experienced researchers are familiar with their proposals being rejected and it is unusual for a proposal to be funded at the first submission. It is important to use the assessment information gained through the grant evaluation process to improve the application in those areas that assessors had identified as a weakness, which could be in the study rationale, design, team or outcomes.

A research proposal is evidence of the investigator's writing skills. However, good writing alone will not necessarily equate to a stellar research proposal. Success in writing a research proposal may be seen as an indication of how thoroughly the researcher has understood, conceptualised and communicated the information relating to the research topic in a well-thought-out plan. It is a good idea to write a draft about the purpose, significance and potential usefulness of the study. Begin by asking yourself: 'What is the purpose of the study?' and 'What is it that I want to know about the topic?' Identifying the aims assists in clarifying your thoughts and provides a basis for discussion with colleagues and/or lecturers. The appropriateness of the study in terms of feasibility, practicality, budget, availability of resources and facilities and supervision can then be considered with the benefit of enhanced clarity.

Generally, the following structure and content are required:

- The title of the research project.
- The investigators (names, qualifications, position or employment).
- An abstract or summary (about 250 words).
- A statement of the problem being investigated.
- The significance or importance of the project.
- A literature review or background of the topic.
- The aims and objectives of the project.
- Assumptions and definitions.
- The research plan or design showing evidence of rigour, which will ensure a logical, systematic, sound and accurate study (e.g. methodology, samples and sampling (selection of participants, inclusion/exclusion criteria), setting, procedure, instrumentation, data collection and data analysis).
- Ethical issues (including the participant information sheet and informed consent form).

- Dissemination of the findings.
- The budget (including justifications for line items).
- The investigator's details such as an abbreviated 'two-page CV' or statement of track record (usually previous grants, publications and awards). A table of contents may be required for a lengthy proposal.

The structure and content of a research proposal for both qualitative and quantitative proposals are basically the same, although differences are likely in the 'research plan/method' section when writing about:

- Recruitment of participants (e.g. random sample, purposive sample and snowballing) (see Chapter 6 for qualitative approaches and Chapter 9 for quantitative approaches).
- The kinds of relationship with participants and major tasks of the researcher (e.g. avoiding coercion in participant recruitment if a lecturer surveys students, dealing with possible bias).
- The purpose of the research (e.g. testing hypotheses, instrument development and theory building).
- The research design (e.g. intervention study, observation study).
- Data collection strategies (e.g. interventions, tests, audiotapes, field notes from memory, transcripts of conversations and audit trails).
- Data analysis procedures (e.g. descriptive or inferential statistics, data reduction and development of thematic coding tree).
- Dissemination of findings (conference presentations and journal articles, proactive research translation activities with clinicians, managers and policy makers).

In the next section, we discuss each component of the research proposal in more detail.

Research Proposal Components

Project Title

Give your project a working title that is clear, descriptive and succinct. The title should be informative but not too long as this may result in confusion about the specific question or issue. Similar to a journal article title, the proposal title should include the study participants, concept/s or variable/s being studied, the research approach and the intervention used (if any). Having an attractive study acronym can be useful to gain media attention for the study and potentially useful in attracting research participants. Study acronyms can be helpful, as these are both memorable for end-users and can be easily shared easily across social media. A few examples include INFORM-AF (a study evaluating an educational intervention for atrial fibrillation), FRAME-HF (a study examining frailty in the heart failure setting) and TEXT-ME (a study examining SMS text messages for patients living with cardiovascular disease). An online acronym generator may be helpful to help create your study title. Specific terms used in the title will need to be defined in the proposal. Initially, the use of a working subtitle may be useful—for example, 'An investigation of the factors and their impact on the quality of parenting for at-risk first-time parents'. During the course of writing a proposal, your thinking may change and it may be necessary to modify the working subtitle as well. The final title of your project could well be: 'Factors that impact on the role of first-time parents'. Compared with the subtitle, the final title is not as explicit and specific. A broad title can be acceptable to capture the topic and the reader's interest.

'*Keywords*' are also commonly required in proposals and grant applications. Keywords are specific terms or phrases that represent the main topics, themes, concepts or subjects within the research. Keywords are used to categorise research and make the research discoverable via search engines. Appropriate keywords are important to ensure your proposal or grant application is correctly categorised (which may impact the review process) and accessible to the right readership. An example is that in Crocker et al's (2023) proposal to explore the attraction and retention of staff within the public mental health services. Crocker et al (2023) used the keywords 'mental health personnel', 'career choice', 'recruitment', 'retention' and 'turnover intention'.

The Investigators

Proposal reviewers need to assess the ability of the investigators in the research team to undertake the research. Information about the research team should include name, qualifications, employment position and area of expertise as a minimum. In some instances (e.g. NHMRC and MRFF grants), a two-page track record that includes a short biography and a publication and grant record (research track record) are necessary for each chief investigator. All authors on the research team should provide intellectual capital to the research project—that is, they must actively participate in the project and contribute to the generation of knowledge. The research team is comprised of principal or chief investigators and associate investigators. Chief investigators carry the main responsibility for the research while associate investigators are engaged because of specific skills or resources that they bring to the project (e.g. recruiting patients, data analysis, formulation of clinical or policy recommendations or critical to research translation). On some proposals, all investigators are required to sign that they have contributed to and approved the application. Also, the head of the department from where the research will be conducted may have to sign off on the proposal indicating that the research will be supported. For information about some unfortunate episodes of 'honorary', 'guest' or 'ghost' authorship to persons in authority who provided no academic input to the research and related publications see: https://publicationethics.org/intellectualproperty.

Abstract

An abstract or summary is typically about 250–300 words long and describes the aims and methods of the proposed study. Abstracts can be either unstructured (or narrative) or structured. Many funders or publishers will require a structured abstract that usually follows these subheadings: (1) Background and significance, (2) Aims and objective, (3) Design and method, (4) Results and discussion and (5) Conclusion and implications.

It is often useful to begin the introductory paragraph with a succinct problem statement and the research question. A problem statement should address the question of significance and innovation—to put this simply, 'So what?' and 'Who cares?' This should address why the problem is an issue and why funders should want to fund this research. In this way, the topic or key sentence provides the focus and alerts the reader from the outset to the point of the proposal. Having explained what the proposal is about, the next point is to describe how to address the issue or answer the research question. In some cases, keywords or disciplinary field codes may be required. For example, the key words given in the systematic review by Hickman et al (2019) titled 'Key elements of interventions for heart failure patients with mild cognitive impairment or dementia' were 'mild cognitive impairment', 'dementia', 'heart failure' and 'nurse-led interventions'. It may be helpful to align your keywords with MESH (medical subject) headings. (See https://meshb.nlm.nih.gov/ for more information.) Review panels sometimes use the abstract to make a basic determination about the value of the proposal. It is good advice to write your abstract last, after the proposal has been completed when all the relevant information is at hand.

Statement of the Problem and Justification for the Project

This section of the proposal informs the reviewer about the need for the study. A statement, sometimes called 'the plain English language statement' or 'lay person description', should provide the rationale and justification for undertaking the project. This is often referred to as the 'So what?' or 'Why does it matter?' The clarity required for the plain language statement will be the same for proposals that use a quantitative or qualitative research approach. The research question should be stated and an indication given of the pragmatic value—that is, how you think the findings of the study will be useful (e.g. will it benefit patients, advance knowledge and/or influence protocols and policies?) and what the implications are of the knowledge gained for the field (e.g. theory building and expanding the knowledge base). The justification should also explain how your project will be different from other studies. The paucity of published research is often included as a justification for undertaking research, although you should avoid the cursory use of this claim, as reviewers will want you to be specific about how your research will add to what is already known. In this section it is critical to clearly and concisely demonstrate the *novelty*, *significance* and *urgency* of your proposed research (Chan & Hart 2023). Further, it is important in this section to detail the return on investment for the proposed project. Return on investment refers to the benefits or value to be obtained from the resources to be invested in your project. It is important that you understand the perspectives of the funders with regard to return on investment. While some funders may prioritise the return on investment at an individual patient level, others might emphasise the return on investment at the organisational or societal level. However, regardless of their perspective, you will need to demonstrate the value of your proposed research. In your proposal, 'value' may defined in various ways, encompassing both monetary and non-monetary aspects. Chan and Hart (2023) suggest the use of the 'quintuple aim for healthcare improvement' (Nundy et al 2022) when describing your project's value and return on investment. The quintuple aim describes that you should detail how your proposed research will:

1. improve population health and outcomes
2. enhance care experiences
3. enhance care team wellbeing
4. reduce costs
5. advance health equity.

Additionally, a financial return on investment calculation may be useful to argue for the cost value of your proposed research. A return of investment calculation can estimate the projected financial impact of successfully achieving your research outcomes versus the amount of funding and resources you are asking for. These calculations are often undertaken by health economists, who may take into account factors such as potential cost savings associated with your proposed research outcomes including healthcare costs, absenteeism from work and productivity gains (e.g. see Snowden et al (2020)).

Literature Review

A critical literature review is documented to identify the current knowledge about the topic and place the research problem in context. Reviewing the literature helps to conceptualise the research problem (see Chapter 3). The literature review demonstrates your ability to critically evaluate the information and should convince the relevant committee that the proposed research addressing the knowledge and methodological gaps is important and necessary. Reasons for undertaking the research should be based on an analysis of the gaps in the reviewed literature (e.g. the current state of research about your topic, the inappropriateness of design and/or tests administered, gaps in knowledge, conflicting or inconclusive findings and problems with the samples, such as the numbers, selection or profile). It is usual to focus on recent studies but also include older works if these are seminal or if little research has been conducted in the area. The literature review should also describe the designs used in previous studies, as these can be the basis for justifying your study design. Imposed word limits mean that the literature review needs to be a focused and concise critique of the state of knowledge in the particular field and the methods used in previous research. In general, the broader evidence from national data and policy will be put into the problem statement and justification section (which could also be called the introduction or background), whereas the previous research studies will be placed in the literature review.

TUTORIAL TRIGGER 16.1

Explain the intent of a literature review in the development of a research proposal.

Aims and Objectives of the Project

Aims are usually broad and are a statement of purpose. Research objectives should be specific and explicit, and describe the activities employed to achieve the aim(s). Both aims and objectives should be feasible, achievable and unambiguous. The purpose of the project should be very clear—that is, why the intended project is important in itself and what the benefits might be. In writing the proposal, the investigator must be ever mindful of the congruency between the aims and objectives and the plan of the project within the given **timeframe** (see Chapter 4).

When considering the aims and objectives of the project, it is important to remember that these aims constitute the boundaries of the research. The aims guide the ways in which data are collected and analysed. For example, if the aim is to find out whether nurses or midwives coming from a night's work think as clearly as they do after a night's sleep, an objective might be to administer some kind of cognitive test, which will measure thinking ability. These issues are important because other nurses or midwives may want to replicate or repeat the design and test(s) to see whether they obtain the same results. If, on the other hand, your aim is to find out how women experience and cope with breast cancer, the design will probably include a face-to-face interview at different times (e.g. at diagnosis, following surgery and 3 months after surgery).

Assumptions and Definitions

Assumptions and definitions should be clearly stated to avoid ambiguity or confusion, and variables should be operationally defined where appropriate. To ensure appropriate objectives (researchable outcomes), it is important that the assumptions and definitions are clearly stated. For example, if the plan is to administer a *self-care* intervention to a group of patients, a verified assumption that should have been covered in the literature review may be that many people want to learn how to care for themselves. People may then be defined in terms of health status, ethnicity, education, age and cultural background. A researcher may define the concept of *self-care* as the acceptance of responsibility by individuals for their care in those activities of daily living considered appropriate for their particular health status. There may well be other definitions of self-care. However, an important point is that having chosen a particular definition considered appropriate for the project, the researcher can then decide how best to operationalise the concept. That is, the conceptual definition is translated into a form that can be measured (see Chapter 4).

AN UNEXPECTED HURDLE

As a clinician researcher you have a groundbreaking research idea that you hope will help address a real-world clinical problem. You attend the library, where the librarian assists you in undertaking a comprehensive literature search. It reveals that there are quite a few published studies addressing your idea; however, some are nearly 20 years old. The librarian introduces you to the professor of nursing at your hospital. They advise you that your research question is too broad, your idea may have little impact and your proposed study may not be feasible.

Outline three key strategies that you would employ as a novice researcher to ensure best use of your time, feasibility and success of your research. Your response should consider factors such as research team, frameworks to inform your research and resources.

Research Plan

The research plan is the most important section of the proposal, providing the principal description of the study—detailing the research design, method and involvement of the study participants. The method includes the design, sampling (how participants will be recruited) and sample

RESEARCH IN BRIEF 16.1

An example illustrates how two different definitions of frailty would lead to different operational concepts and hence measures. Yang et al (2018) conducted a cross-sectional study to look at frailty status among older people living in urban communities in Wuhu, China. As part of this study the authors used the Edmonton Frail Scale (EFS) to measure frailty. However, as there is no globally agreed-to frailty measure, the authors had to justify why they chose this specific definition of frailty to operationalise. In this instance, compared with other clinically feasible frailty tools, as the EFS does not require any specialised training to administer it was considered the most appropriate within a community setting. This study found that, among 306 older Chinese residents, 14% of people displayed some level of frailty. If a different measure of frailty was used, it is likely that the outcome prevalence would be different. Any researcher using a concept with multiple definitions must decide how best to operationalise these concepts. When the empirical definitions have been clearly stated by the researcher, someone reading about the research is able to evaluate the findings (i.e. comparing 'like with like' outcomes across different studies and time).

profile (inclusion and exclusion criteria), intervention (if appropriate), ethical issues, measuring instruments (including reliability and validity), procedure, data gathering (describe what data will be collected and method of data collection), data analysis techniques (these should correspond with the objectives of the project) and the projected timeframe for the stages of the project. Be prepared to write several drafts of the research plan prior to submission. As with other sections of the proposal, it is important to present the plan in detail; this section can be refined and shortened later if necessary. The design and timeframe must be carefully explained in order to convince reviewers that the research approach and methods entailed in the proposal are the most logical and appropriate for this particular research question.

Each research approach has its own philosophy and theoretical or conceptual framework and strategies for data collection and analysis. The main consideration is always to find the research design and approach that will best answer the research question(s). Articles included in these previous chapters illustrate how the investigators have matched their research designs to their research question/s. These chapters should be carefully read and understood prior to writing a proposal. Whether a qualitative or quantitative design is chosen, bear in mind the feasibility of the project in terms of access to the sample(s), ethical issues, financial restraints and timelines.

Inclusion of a Theoretical or Conceptual Framework

The importance of a **theoretical or conceptual framework** is in linking the proposed study to the previous knowledge about the concept of interest. As applied disciplines, nursing and midwifery can legitimately use appropriate frameworks from the social or physical sciences s well as from within the discipline.

Finding an appropriate theoretical or conceptual framework for a study can be challenging. Many research studies benefit from specific theoretical or conceptual frameworks that can importantly underpin the design of an intervention, or evaluation of a program (i.e. effectiveness-implementation trials). For example, a large body of research that has aimed to improve health professional practice has been informed by the COM-B framework (Michie et al 2011). This framework consists of three specific components: capability (C), opportunity (O) and motivation (M), which are claimed to determine the performance of a target behaviour (B). Designing your study informed by a theoretical or conceptual framework such as the COM-B framework can facilitate your choice of methodology, intervention design and analysis. For example, the use of the COM-B framework specifies the theoretical mechanisms of change and informs interventional targets (i.e. capability, opportunity and motivation), measures used to assess the interventional targets and analysis techniques used to examine change in the interventional targets, as well as their specified theoretical relationships (Mullan et al 2023). Similarly, most studies incorporating implementation science will incorporate the RE-AIM framework (Glasgow et al 2019). RE-AIM is a planning and evaluation framework that seeks to quantify the reach (R), effectiveness (E), adoption (A), implementation (I) and maintenance (M) of a particular intervention. In the nursing context, this may be a new nurse-led or nurse-enabled model of care (Chan et al 2023) as an example.

Utilising a theoretical or conceptual framework can facilitate your demonstration that your proposed research builds upon prior literature and can inform both theory and practice. The use of a theoretical or conceptual framework will also allow the direct comparison of outcomes to related research that has used the same framework. While there are many benefits of including a theoretical or conceptual framework in proposed research, some research projects do not benefit from being grounded within any particular theoretical or conceptual framework and do not include a framework within their development or completion. These types of studies are often referred to as *atheoretical research*. These studies are typically pragmatic in nature and not informed by any framework (although they may be informed by theoretically grounded research). The choice of whether to include a theoretical or conceptual framework in your proposed research depends upon many factors, including the availability of applicable evidence-based frameworks and whether the available frameworks would facilitate the achievement of the study aims and objectives. You should discuss the possible inclusion and choice of a theoretical or conceptual framework with your mentor/supervisor and research team and be guided by their advice.

TUTORIAL TRIGGER 16.2

You are discussing with your nursing colleagues whether to include a theoretical/conceptual framework within your proposed study. List some of the 'pros' of including a framework and the key considerations when choosing whether to include a framework within your proposed study.

Timeline

Timelines should be included. Submitting a timetable identifying the various stages of the research project's key activities (e.g. literature review, ethics and governance application, database design and development, advertising and participant recruitment, data collection, data analysis, report writing, results dissemination) will do much to satisfy the funding body that you have carefully and realistically thought through your plan of action and that you have a good understanding of the project requirements and duration. A useful technique for incorporating a timeline is a Gantt chart, which also provides a quick overview of the progress of key activities. A Gantt chart is a visual project planning and management chart that displays the schedule of tasks and activities in a project over time. Gantt charts can be more or less complex and detailed, depending on your needs and their purpose. While a Gantt chart for a high-level funding application might include most tasks and be large and detailed, a Gantt chart for an HREC application for a small-scale project might be more basic and only include the main tasks to be completed.

Ethical Considerations

For further reading, refer to Chapter 13: Ethical and legal issues in research.

Informed Consent

Informed consent is the process by which participants who are recruited for a research study are informed, at their particular level of comprehension, about the nature

RESEARCH IN BRIEF 16.2

The objective of a study by Kularatna et al (2023) was to understand the attributes of breast cancer follow-up care preferences. The researchers used a discrete choice experiment survey where 14 breast cancer survivors and 6 clinicians were asked to read a list of 16 key attributes of breast cancer follow-up care and rank these from most to least important. For each participant, the attributes were scored from 16 (least important attribute) to 1 (most important attribute). Kularatna et al (2023) then calculated the average scores for each of the 16 attributes across all of the participants. The attribute with the highest average score was seen as the most important attribute, while the attribute with the lowest average score was seen as the least important attribute. They found that the top two prioritised attributes were (no. 1) the patient receiving clear and simple information and (no. 2) information sharing between clinicians/providers. The two least prioritised of the 16 key attributes included (no. 15) including cultural components and (no. 16) connection to networks and community organisations. This study provided important information that may improve the prioritisation of the key follow-up care attributes for breast cancer survivors.

of the study, the purpose, the demands, the interventions (if required) and the risks and benefits to them. It is based on being provided with adequate information so that participants understand what is expected of them alongside the risk and benefits of participation. Participants should be provided with an information sheet (a plain English language summary about the project) and a consent form (see Chapter 3). Any questions raised by the participants or their proxy must be answered clearly and unambiguously in order for them to make a decision about whether or not to participate. It is desirable that consent should be obtained in writing. Information about informed consent and other ethical and legal issues can be found in Chapter 13 and *The National Statement on Ethical Conduct in Human Research* (NHMRC, ARC & AVCC 2007). In addition to the ethical issues relating to all research participants, specific issues arise in research involving certain categories of people—for example, Indigenous Peoples, women who are pregnant and the human fetus, people with cognitive impairment or mental illness, people highly dependent on medical care and unable to give consent, prisoners, military personnel, and children and young people (see NHMRC, ARC & AVCC 2007). No investigator may involve a person as a research participant before obtaining legally effective informed consent from them or from their legally authorised representative. The language of the consent form must be clear and understandable for the individual or group concerned. People *must not* be coerced into participating, nor may researchers collect data on people who have explicitly refused to be involved in a study. An ethical violation of this principle occurred when an audit conducted in 1994 indicated that medical data on at least three dozen women were collected and analysed without authorisation, against the women's expressed wishes (Snowdon 1994).

As more research is being conducted in large healthcare institutions (e.g. a state or regional Department of Health), there is a requirement for ethical approval as well as a requirement to have a site-specific assessment conducted as a part of the ethics review process. There are also state-specific bodies such as The Research Ethics and Governance Information System (REGIS), which supports ethics and governance management of human research projects within all NSW public health organisations. REGIS is a joint initiative between eHealth and the Office for Health and Medical Research (https://www.medicalresearch.nsw.gov.au/regis/).

The following points must be considered when planning a research project and care taken that they are addressed in the proposal:

- Recruitment should include detailed information about the participants' particular role in the study and a clear indication of timelines.
- Individuals should not be involved in research without asking them whether or not they wish to participate.
- Information should not be withheld from participants.
- Information provided should not be misleading.
- Participants should not be made to do or say things that violate their moral standards or expose them to mental or physical stress.
- Anonymity and confidentiality of participants, organisations and institutions should be maintained, and if this is not possible then people should be informed of this before being asked to participate.
- Privacy should not be invaded.
- Benefits should not be withheld from the control groups, which means that the intervention might be given to these participants after the study.
- Results should be made known to participants.
- Known and anticipated long-term effects of the study on the participants should be declared.
- The informed consent of the participant should be gained.
- The welfare of laboratory animals or other animals participating in the project should be covered.
- Storage and safety of data should be addressed.

TUTORIAL TRIGGER 16.3

You are proposing a research project to your department. You have been asked by the department committee to justify the research design and ethical and governance matters in your proposal.

What factors would you consider?

Dissemination of Findings

All research and quality improvement regardless of significant results or findings should be disseminated. What is working and what is not working is important to inform future projects. Publishing these results and presenting them at relevant conferences is an obligation to improve not only the science of nursing and midwifery but also healthcare. Without dissemination of results and lessons learned, the work is invisible and can result in others doing the same work, which is not an efficient use of limited resources. The proposal application form will often require information about how the findings will be disseminated. This could include dissemination through scientific conferences, public lectures and peer-reviewed academic refereed journal articles. Nowadays, it is quite common for researchers to develop a dissemination plan: new and innovative dissemination methods may include a radio interview, a podcast, a blog on social media or creating a YouTube animation about your findings. The Conversation (https://theconversation.com/uk) is a media and news outlet that works with academics and researchers to create stories around their work. This style of dissemination is becoming more popular to better engage the general public with findings of publicly funded research. (See Chapter 19 for information on presenting, publishing and disseminating research.)

Research translation and implementation science is core to nursing practice—as a profession, all nurses and midwives have an obligation at their different levels to contribute and articulate their role in improving patient care. This involves a proactive and targeted dissemination of research findings to healthcare policy makers, managers, clinicians and, if appropriate, patients for implementing these findings into practice. The process requires more than simply making a conference presentation or writing a paper, which are passive strategies. Proactive and targeted dissemination requires knowing who is important to make practice changes and then developing communication with them. Ideally, this communication would be throughout all stages of the research from conceptualisation to completion so that people feel some connection and commitment to the research. Contemporary thinking is that research translation involves a partnership between the researchers and those who have an interest in the research. For some types of research, this is described as research exchange, meaning a two-way communication between the researchers and those with the research interest about the research question, design, what the findings mean and then the recommendations. Participatory co-design methods are quickly becoming more popular to design and better plan research. These can involve authentic partnerships and engagement with the research participants and end-users.

Budget

A detailed itemised account of all expenditures (e.g. personnel, equipment, travel, accommodation, printing, telephone charges, photocopying and stationery) is required by funding agencies when applying for a grant. The university may also charge a fee for managing a research account. Some funding agencies stipulate that a university must manage the account. In this event, it is important to add the appropriate on-costs (15%–45%) for this purpose. This figure should be discussed with the university research office. In their application for funding, the NHMRC *Guidelines for Funding* stipulate six categories/levels of Personnel Support Packages (PSP): non-graduate personnel, junior graduate research assistant, experienced graduate research assistant, experienced postdoctoral researcher, senior experienced postdoctoral researcher and senior researcher. Formats and salary scales do vary from one funding source to another and relevant information will be provided on each form. Fig. 16.1 shows an example of a simplified, abbreviated **budget** justification form. A useful guide to preparing a budget can be found in Chapter 12 of Aldridge and Derrington's (2012) The Research Funding Toolkit, where they state that all items in the budget should have been mentioned in the proposal. This provides the real justification that all budget items are needed.

The financial remuneration is designed to cover all salary and salary on-costs (e.g. workers' compensation, payroll tax and leave loading) and some additional support for minor maintenance, such as phone/fax, stationery, computer hardware and software. On-costs can also vary between research assistants, clinical trial nurses, administrative and technical staff, and casual or fixed term employees from one institution to another and should be added on to the basic salary. These range in cost but can be up to an additional 25%–30% of base salary costs. It is important to factor these into wage and salary estimations, as this can impact project delivery and feasibility.

References and Appendices

References should be contemporary and arranged in a standard format. This is most frequently the Harvard system (author–date system, e.g. Smith & Barton 2011) or Vancouver system (numbered system, e.g. Smith & Barton[1]).

> **TUTORIAL TRIGGER 16.4**
>
> Imagine this scenario:
>
> Congratulations! You have completed your research study and your clinical trial of a new nurse-led, self-management intervention for patients living with chronic obstructive pulmonary disease was shown to decrease symptom burden, improve quality of life and reduce hospitalisation and mortality. This is great news. Your academic paper has also been accepted for publication in a high-ranking, credible peer-reviewed journal. This research has taken 4 years to complete. You want your research to make an impact in clinical practice and research a broad audience of patients, clinicians, policy makers and the wider general public.
>
> ***As part of your proposal, what dissemination strategies and activities would you plan to promote your research findings to reach a broad audience?***

Whichever format is used, consistency is the key element. Increasingly, online resources will be used as references and the reference format may also include the date the information was accessed, as well as the other bibliographical details. Using electronic bibliographic referencing tools such as Endnote, Mendeley or Refworks is strongly recommended. Your library should be able to provide guidance on how to access and use these systems.

Appendices will include a participant information sheet and consent form, as well as other documents such as recruitment materials (e.g. posters, flyers, planned emails and social media posts), case report forms, questionnaires, instruments or an interview and focus group guides that will be used in the research. Some ethics and governance offices may charge a submission fee for processing investigator-initiated research—it is important to check this with the office prior to submitting an application.

Letters of Support or References

Letters of support and references will be required from department heads or higher degree research supervisors and external funding agencies to verify that the research is achievable and appropriate resources are available from the department/university and/or hospital. Letters of support may also be required by external organisations or universities should the nature of the research project warrant support from particular groups. For example, in clinical research studies based within hospitals' studies, there are levels of entry and access to participants that have to be negotiated with the governance office within the organisation in order to be on site and access medical records and visit patients if you are not a hospital employee.

PERSONNEL $	
Principal Researcher	
Research Assistant Level 3 to assist with data collection for 6 months	
Salary $3,000/mth × 6 months = $18,000 + benefits	
Salary total	18,000
Consultant for statistical analyses (20 hours @ $150 ph)	3,000
Personnel TOTAL	$21,000
SUPPLIES	
Photocopy (printing of questionnaires)	300
Telephone	50
Postage (400 questionnaires @ $1.50)	600
Equipment rental (computer) supplied by Faculty	
Supplies TOTAL	$950
TRAVEL	
Conference air travel interstate (Sydney)	320
Hotel accommodation ($195 × 3 nights)	585
Meals × 3 days ($45 per day)	135
Local travel (400 kms @ 65c p km)	260
Travel TOTAL	$1,300
TOTAL	**$23,250**
POTENTIAL ON-COSTS FOR MANAGING THE BUDGET	
(varies between agencies — at 20%) On-costs at 20% = $4,650	$4,650
TOTAL BUDGET	**$27,900**

Fig. 16.1 A sample of a budget justification form

COMMON PITFALLS IN PROPOSALS

You should realise by now that writing a successful proposal takes time and attention to detail. A rushed proposal is a waste of time, can lead to a misreading of guidelines and criteria, may see a weak justification for doing the study, may result in an unconvincing literature review and may be poorly expressed. Proposals will be rejected when there is a poor logical fit between the problems, research questions and study design, when there are budget problems (e.g. lack of detail and inaccurate costings) and when there is a failure to demonstrate the feasibility, practicality and applicability of the proposed study. The National Institute of Nursing Research has identified the following common mistakes in research proposals (Tully 2014), with some of our own included:

- Aims:
  - Too ambitious.
  - Unfocused research question.
  - Unclear direction.
- Significance:
  - No advance on knowledge.
  - Lacks compelling rationale.
  - Inadequate value proposition.
  - No or little perceived impact.

- Design:
  - Too much or too little detail relative to the maximum word count.
  - Feasibility not shown or not adequately justified.
  - Lacks quality indicators or innovation in design.
  - Lack of discipline, specialty or methodological expertise in team (content or method).
  - Lack of demonstrable, thoughtful and consistent **consumer engagement**.
  - Does not clearly or completely answer the research questions.
  - Unclear or unjustified use of measurement tools or outcome measures.
- Environment:
  - Little institutional support or poorly articulated institutional support.
  - Weak research environment and mentorship.
  - Insufficient resources to conduct the research.
  - Inadequate formalised partnerships with other organisations or institutions.
- Other:
  - Missing or inadequate knowledge translation.
  - Unclear evaluation or mitigation of project risks versus value.
  - Does not clearly adhere to the guidelines or requirements of the proposed scheme.

Fig. 16.2 gives 10 tips for successful grant writing (Chan & Hart 2023).

SUBMITTING A PROPOSAL FOR REVIEW

With effective planning, with a suitable timeframe for proposal development and with informal review and refinement, a completed rigorous proposal can be submitted on time. Check the submission requirements, particularly the frequency of meetings, due dates for submission to the ethics

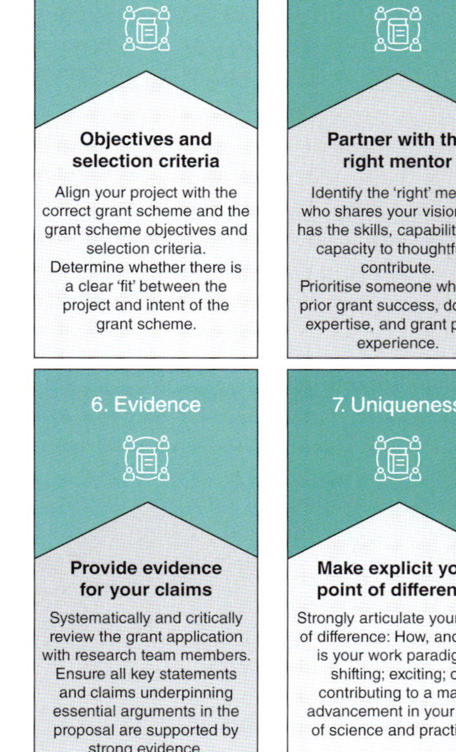
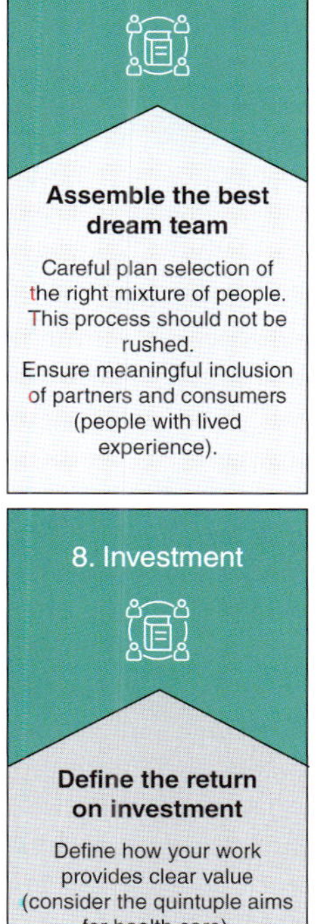
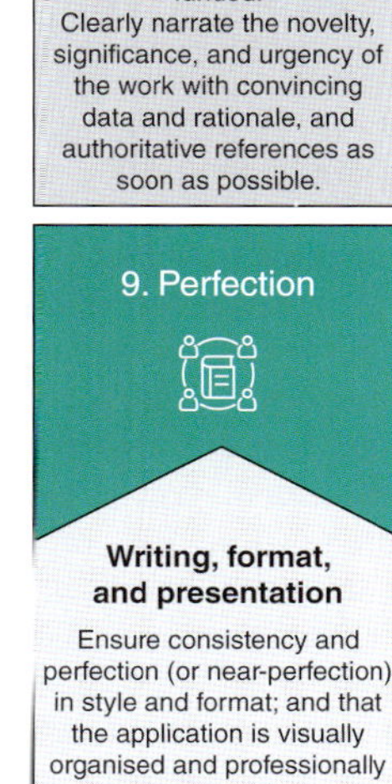
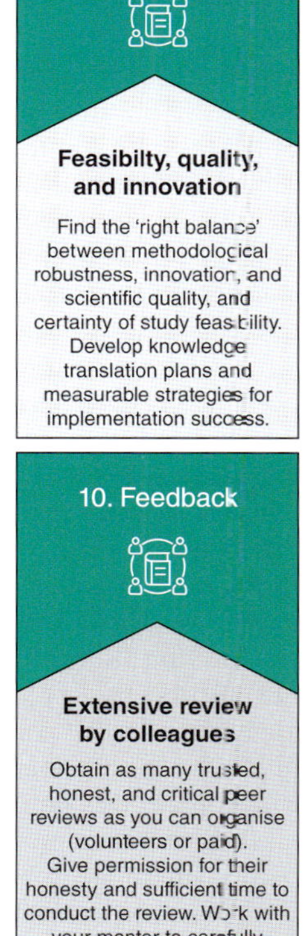

Fig. 16.2 Successful grant writing

office and whether online, email attachment or paper copies of the proposals are requested.

It is smart planning to get someone who is not connected to your proposal to read and provide feedback. It is also a good idea to put the proposal away for a few days and then re-read with fresh eyes. When you are doing this you could ask the following questions:

- Have we answered the 'So what?' and 'Who cares?' questions to demonstrate the significance of the research?
- Are the research design and methods appropriate?
- Have we explained that we have the skills and resources required to conduct the research?
- Have we described the likely outcomes?

Online Submissions

Most funding agencies and universities have their application forms and guidelines for submitting research proposals online. The guidelines provide step-by-step information to ensure that you address all the requirements. It is useful to read all guidance carefully well before preparing your grant application and gain familiarity with the platform to avoid last minute mishaps and potential delays in submission.

Research Committee Review and HREC Review

In some institutions, there are two different committees that review research proposals—namely, a research committee and an HREC. In the first instance, the proposal is reviewed by the research committee. If approved, the proposal is then submitted to the HREC. In some institutions, both committee functions are incorporated into one.

The membership of university and hospital research committees is generally composed of staff from the respective institutions. However, membership of HRECs and AEECs is specified by government bodies. Submitted proposals are reviewed by the relevant committee (e.g. hospital, scholarship board, university or funding organisation) and discussed at a committee meeting. In general, research and ethics committee meetings are planned in advance and the dates on which the committees meet are often provided by the institution online. Although not common, a researcher may be invited to speak about their proposal at the committee meeting. Regardless, a written reply is sent advising the outcome of the committee review. The proposal may be approved, clarification or additional information may be requested, modification or amendments may be required or the proposal may be rejected.

Following rejection of a proposal, some funding agencies permit a resubmission to give the researcher an opportunity to answer their questions. A resubmitted proposal should be written as comprehensively and clearly as the original, with all questions and requirements answered. A comprehensive resubmission is important as committee members change and the resubmitted proposal may be considered by new reviewers.

Funding Sources

Nurses and midwives in Australia and New Zealand seeking financial assistance to pursue academic interests and funding for research projects have a number of options.

Small Grants

For a novice researcher, small internal seed **grants** are often made available for staff of universities or healthcare institutions and for nurses, generally through professional nursing organisations and interest groups. If you have never applied for a grant before, securing funds for $5000 can be a learning experience in what it takes to both win a grant and then manage a grant. Healthcare services (such as hospitals) and universities often offer internal funding schemes to their employees/students. These internal funding schemes can vary widely across organisations and departments in terms of objectives, selection criteria and funding parameters. It is a good idea to ensure that you are on the 'mailing list' of your organisation and department's research and grants office. That way you will receive information on any upcoming internal (and external) funding opportunities. For those who wish to undertake research through a Master's Degree or a PhD, seeking a scholarship is a good place to start.

While not research grants specifically, many community grants include a research component and this can also be a way for a new researcher to get a start. The Parliamentary Library of the Parliament of Australia provides a guide to community grants in every state, and can be accessed at: https://www.aph.gov.au/About_Parliament/Parliamentary_departments/Parliamentary_Library/pubs/rp/rp2223/Quick_Guides/CommunityGrants .

Public Sector Competitive Grants

Most public sector research funding in Australia is through the NHMRC and the ARC, and in New Zealand through the Health Research Council of New Zealand and the Ministry of Business, Innovation and Employment. These sources provide funding for individuals in their research training through postgraduate scholarships, early-career fellowships and career development awards. For research projects specifically, funds are available through project, program and research centre schemes. Applications for all of these research grants are usually highly competitive.

Non-Government Organisation Grants

There are hundreds of non-government organisation grant schemes in Australia and New Zealand; for example, the Australian Cancer Research Foundation, the Australian

College of Nursing, the Stroke Foundation, the Australian Rotary Health Research Fund, Kidney Health Australia, the National Breast Council Foundation and the National Heart Foundation of Australia offer grants for research (biomedical and education/health promotion). Numerous charitable organisations in New Zealand offer funding—for example, the WellcomeTrust, the Cancer Society and Family Planning. Many non-government organisation schemes have specific research priorities.

SUMMARY

Research proposals may be written to undertake a higher degree, apply for financial assistance to undertake a research project, comply with nursing/midwifery degree course requirements or apply to an ethics committee for approval to conduct a research project. Research ideas can come from the clinical or administrative areas, reading literature and networking at conferences. Grants may be available from universities, government agencies and non-government agencies. Funding agencies' research priorities must be considered when applying for funding. Faculty research priorities, appropriate supervision and facilities are important when planning a project. Each ethics committee or funding body may have specific requirements regarding application forms and format. Proposals must adhere to the standards for research for the nursing and midwifery professions, the codes of ethics and the codes of professional conduct for nurses and midwives. Crafting effective research proposals and applying for related research grant funding are time-consuming tasks but, done well, offer many benefits to emerging and established researchers.

KEY POINTS

- A research proposal provides a detailed and reasoned explanation of the research problem and question, the design, recruitment, participant profile, exclusion and inclusion criteria, data analysis and data collection methods.
- A proposal may be written for a higher degree committee, a department or faculty research committee, an HREC, a hospital research committee or a funding agency.
- Researchers (academic staff and students or clinician researchers) must be aware of their rights and obligations in relation to intellectual property.
- Legally effective informed consent must be obtained from each participant in the research project.

TIME TO REFLECT

George, A., Dahlen, H.G., Blinkhorn, A., et al., 2018. Evaluation of a midwifery initiated oral health-dental service program to improve oral health and birth outcomes for pregnant women: a multi-centre randomized controlled trial. Int. J. Nurs. Stud. 82, 49–57.

A midwifery-initiated oral health dental service program was developed to address gaps in oral health promotional interventions during pregnancy. The study aimed to assess the effectiveness of a midwifery-initiated oral health dental service program to improve dental services, oral health knowledge, quality of oral health, oral health status and birth outcomes of pregnant women. A multicentre randomised controlled trial design was used. Pregnant women attending their first antenatal appointment, ≥18 years old and who had a single low-risk pregnancy between 12 and 20 weeks' gestation were recruited from three metropolitan public hospitals in Sydney, Australia. A total of 638 pregnant women were allocated to three groups using block randomisation (n = 211)—control group, intervention group 1 (n = 215), intervention group 2 (n = 212)—and followed up until birth. Study investigators and data collectors were blinded to allocation. Intervention group 1 received a midwifery intervention from trained midwives involving oral health education, screening and referrals to existing dental pathways. Intervention group 2 received the midwifery intervention and a dental intervention including assessment and treatment from cost-free local dental services. The control group received oral health information. Primary outcome was uptake of dental services. Secondary outcomes included oral health knowledge, quality of oral health, oral health status and birth outcomes. Substantial improvements in the use of dental services, women's oral health knowledge, quality of oral health and oral health outcomes were identified. The midwifery-initiated oral health dental service program improved the uptake of dental services and oral health of pregnant women.

Questions

Reflect on the information given and answer these questions:

1. What is the research design?
2. Is the design appropriate for this study?
3. What are the independent (intervention) and the dependent variables? Are these sufficiently defined?
4. Does the recruitment strategy satisfy the usual ethical standards?
5. Are the strengths of the study sufficient to address the problems that were given to justify it being conducted?

LEARNING ACTIVITIES

1. A literature review of your topic should be conducted:
   a. only if you don't know enough about your topic
   b. once you have identified your research problem/topic
   c. after you have written your proposal
   d. after you have sought permission from faculty to proceed.
2. A research proposal is written principally for the purpose of:
   a. satisfying the requirements of a committee
   b. laying out a logical plan of the various parts of the project
   c. passing the research topic in university
   d. all of the above.
3. What does 'operationalising objectives' mean?
   a. Providing definitions for the concepts.
   b. Translating objectives into measurable and observable phenomena.
   c. Identifying the feasibility and potential value of a study.
   d. Supporting your research plan.
4. What key aspects do you need to demonstrate about your planned research?
   a. Novelty
   b. Significance
   c. Urgency
   d. All of the above
5. Most successful researchers work in teams because:
   a. it shares the work around
   b. it makes the project more enjoyable
   c. it builds the research track record to be competitive
   d. funders prefer this.
6. Theoretical or conceptual frameworks are particularly useful to:
   a. inform the cost of a project
   b. inform the interventional targets of a project
   c. inform your study timeline
   d. include in all studies.
7. Some procedures for protecting the rights of your participants are:
   a. assuring them that you will not publish their data
   b. a letter of explanation, informed consent and ethics approval for the study
   c. being friendly and honest with them
   d. telling them that information about them will be kept in a locked room somewhere.
8. The funding agency needs to be persuaded that you:
   a. enjoy reading and writing proposals
   b. think research is an important academic activity
   c. are qualified to carry out your research design
   d. can get time off work to do the research.
9. Two key preliminary steps in writing a research proposal are:
   a. spending a lot of time reading
   b. attending conferences and talking to colleagues
   c. finding aims and operationalising objectives to fit your research design
   d. identifying a feasible research question and finding a design that will answer the research question.
10. Committees usually make decisions about proposals on the basis of:
    a. how long they take to read them
    b. their purpose, clarity, logic, standard and appropriateness
    c. how important they think your topic is
    d. how relevant the research problem is to the faculty's strategic research plan.

For further content associated with this chapter visit: https://evolve.elsevier.com/cs/product/9780729596794?role=student. 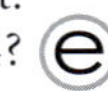

ACKNOWLEDGEMENT

The 7th edition authors (Nicolas Hart, Darren Haywood and Raymond Chan) would like to thank and acknowledge Louise Hickman, Caleb Ferguson, Jeffrey Fuller and Zevia Schneider for contributions to this chapter in previous editions of the text.

ADDITIONAL RESOURCES

Australian Directory of Philanthropy Australia 2006 (lists over 370 foundations and trusts with their contact details and funding preferences). https://www.philanthropy.org.au.

Funding agencies (lists can be accessed through Google). https://www.google.com.au/search?hl=en&q=Australian+Funding+Foundation&btnG.

Gledhill, S., Mannix, J., MacDonald, R., et al., 2011. Nursing and midwifery research grants: profiling the outcomes. Aust. J. Adv. Nurs. 28 (3), 14–21.

Health Research Council of New Zealand. http://www.hrc.govt.nz/.

Higdon, J., Topp, R., 2004. How to develop a budget for a research proposal. West. J. Nurs. Res. 26 (8), 922–929.

International Committee of Medical Journal Editors (ICMJE). https://www.icmje.org/.

Jensen, A., Lidell, E., 2009. The influence of conscience in nursing. Nurs. Ethics 16 (1), 31–42.

Mauthner, M., Birch, M., Jessop, J., et al., 2002. Ethics in Qualitative Research. Sage Publications, Thousand Oaks, CA.

Ministry of Business, Innovation and Employment, New Zealand. https://www.mbie.govt.nz/.

National Health and Medical Research Council (NHMRC), 2023. Human Research Ethics Application (HREA) https://hrea.gov.au/.

National Institute of Nursing Research. Research Funding Tips. https://www.ninr.nih.gov/researchandfunding/sbir-sttr/sb-tips
NHMRC (2023) National Statement on Ethical Conduct in Human Research (2023). https://www.nhmrc.gov.au/about-us/publications/national-statement-ethical-conduct-human-research-2023.
Penrod, J., 2003. Getting funded: writing a successful qualitative small-project proposal. Qual. Health Res. 13 (6), 821–832.
Universities Australia. https://universitiesaustralia.edu.au/.

REFERENCES

Aldridge, J., Derrington, A., 2012. The Research Funding Toolkit. Sage Publications, Los Angeles, CA.
Attard, N., 2018. WASP (Write a Scientific Paper): writing an academic research proposal. Early Hum. Dev. 123, 39–41.
Chan, R.J., Hart, N.H., 2023. Top 10 tips for research grant writing: a guide for nurses and allied health professionals. Sem. Oncol. Nursing 39 (2). 151394. doi:10.1016/j.soncn.2023.151394
Chan, R.J., Crawford-Williams, F., Crichton, M., et al. 2023. Effectiveness and implementation of models of cancer survivorship care: an overview of systematic reviews. J. Cancer Surv. 17 (1), 197–221. doi:10.1007/s11764-021-01128-1
Crocker, K.M., Gnatt, I., Haywood, D., et al. 2023. The impact of COVID-19 on the mental health workforce: a rapid review. Int. J. Mental Health Nurs. 32 (2), 420–445. doi:10.1111/inm.13097
Forsythe, L.P., Carman, K.L., Szydlowski, V. , et al. 2019. Patient engagement in research: early findings from the Patient-Centered Outcomes Research Institute. Health Aff. 38 (3), 359–367. doi:10.1377/hlthaff.2018.05067
George, A., Dahlen, H.G., Blinkhorn, A., et al., 2018. Evaluation of a midwifery initiated oral health-dental service program to improve oral health and birth outcomes for pregnant women: a multi-centre randomized controlled trial. Int. J. Nurs. Stud. 82, 49–57.
Glasgow, R.E., Harden, S.M., Gaglio, B., et al. 2019. RE-AIM planning and evaluation framework: adapting to new science and practice with a 20-year review. Front. Public Health 7, 64. doi: 10.3389/fpubh.2019.00064
Kularatna, S., Allen, M., Hettiarachchi, R.M., et al. 2023. Cancer survivor preferences for models of breast cancer follow-up care: selecting attributes for inclusion in a discrete choice experiment. Patient 16 (4), 371–383. doi:10.1007/s40271-023-00631-0
Ladwa, R., Pinkham, E.P., Teleni, L. , et al. 2022. Telehealth cancer-related fatigue clinic model for cancer survivors: a pilot randomised controlled trial protocol (the T-CRF trial). BMJ Open 12 (5), e059952.
Michie, S., Van Stralen, M.M., West, R., 2011. The behaviour change wheel: a new method for characterising and designing behaviour change interventions. Imp. Sci. 6 (1), 1–12. doi:10.1186/1748-5908-6-42
Mullan, B., Liddelow, C., Haywood, D. , et al. 2022. Behavior change training for health professionals: evaluation of a 2-hour workshop. JMIR Form. Res. 6 (11), e42010. doi:10.2196/42010
National Health and Medical Research Council (NHMRC), Australian Research Council (ARC), Australian Vice-Chancellors' Committee (AVCC), 2007. National Statement on Ethical Conduct in Human Research. Canberra, ACT: Australian Government. Retrieved from: https://archive.epa.gov/osa/hsrb/web/pdf/2-supplement1-excerpt-australian-national-statement-ethical-conduct2007.pdf.
Nundy, S., Cooper, L.A., Mate, K.S., 2022. The quintuple aim for health care improvement: a new imperative to advance health equity. JAMA 327 (6), 521–522. doi:10.1001/jama.2021.25181
Price, A., Clarke, M., Staniszewska, S. , et al. 2022. Patient and public involvement in research: a journey to co-production. Patient Educ. Couns. 105 (4), 1041–1047. doi:10.1016/j.pec.2021.07.021
Snowdon, J., 1994. Breast cancer study monitored patients against their wishes. Houston Chron. 22, 1994.
The Research Ethics and Governance Information System (REGIS). Retrieved from: https://www.medicalresearch.nsw.gov.au/regis/.
Tully, L. 2014. National Institute of Nursing Research: Writing a successful grant application. Retrieved from: http://www.ninr.nih.gov/sites/www.ninr.nih.gov/files/Module3WritingaSuccessfulGrantApplication.pdf (accessed September 2019).
Yang, L., Jiang, Y., Xu, S., et al., 2018. Evaluation of frailty status among older people living in urban communities by Edmonton Frail Scale in Wuhu, China: a cross-sectional study. Contemp. Nurse 54 (6), 630–639.

17

Managing a Research Project: Roles and Processes

Nathan J Wilson, Christopher Patterson and Rebecca O'Reilly

LEARNING OUTCOMES

After reading this chapter, you should be able to:

- understand the multiple processes and different strategies required to manage a research project
- identify how to set a research project up for long-term success, in its operation, dissemination and closing
- outline how to manage human, financial and other resources over the life of a research project
- describe the vital importance and responsibility that comes with leading research projects
- summarise research career strategies that can lead to research success.

KEY TERMS

budget, p. 296
ethics, p. 295
human research, p. 295
knowledge translation, p. 303
marketing, p. 299
recruitment, p. 296
research funding, p. 295
research report, p. 309

INTRODUCTION

Being a research leader confers both great opportunities and responsibilities and, whether one is an undergraduate student with an interest in getting some work as a research assistant or is working in a postdoctoral role, understanding the key issues related to managing research projects is important. After applying for research funding—a time-consuming and large endeavour that often results in not being funded—if the news from the funder is positive there is a flurry of activity to get the project started. Being funded for a research project after many years of applying can be career changing as it offers the researcher an opportunity to generate new and exciting evidence that would otherwise not be possible. Most crucially, however, getting funded is not an end point, and managing a research project is a major responsibility. The onus is on the lead researcher not only to conduct the study in a rigorous manner as outlined in the research proposal, but also to ensure that the research project team operates to the highest ethical standards. Achieving this outcome requires the lead researcher to be more than a content and research design expert. That is, there is a need to be across the detail of signed legal agreements, setting up and monitoring employment contracts and understanding a myriad of employment regulations. Lead researchers manage often large budgets while operating within sometimes complex financial guidelines and ensuring that project milestones are met at specific time-points over the life of the project. This chapter unpacks some of this detail, not to overwhelm the novice or budding researcher, but rather to offer a glimpse into how being a researcher is an exciting and important career goal that requires many diverse leadership skills. First, the chapter focuses on setting the project up to succeed, then it gives some necessary detail about conducting a research project, and finally it provides an overview of the final stages of a research project. This detail is intersected with some opportunities for critical reflection and some activities for a tutorial-like session.

SETTING THE PROJECT UP FOR SUCCESS

Funders

Securing **research funding** is not only about generating great ideas with national significance, but also about seeking funding from the right funder—one that is likely to fund your ideas as opposed to one that is unlikely to do so—of which there are many. In Australia, research funds are divided into four broad categories: (1) nationally competitive grants (e.g. the National Health and Medical Research Council (NHMRC), the Australian Research Council (ARC)), (2) public sector research and development funding (e.g. the Department of Health), (3) industry funding (e.g. a national disability service) and (4) Cooperative Research Centres (CRCs) (e.g. the Autism CRC). Each scheme and every funder will have some differing contractual requirements, likely to be directly linked with timeframes and/or deliverables, which are vital to know about and understand. Thankfully, most universities and research institutes have teams of lawyers and accountants who are there to assist with the reviewing and signing of any research contracts, as well as to set up accounting systems, meaning researchers can get on with what they are good at!

Most commonly, the research contract is referred to as a funding agreement, where there is usually a range of conditions attached. The funding agreement covers a number of important areas, but typically funders want to be sure that the awarded funds are spent as agreed, that the stated milestones are met and that the research project is completed on time. Milestones are usually linked with a concrete deliverable, or event, and are crucial to the ongoing conduct of a study where more funds are not released until the milestone is satisfactorily met. Funding agreements will also usually have a clause or agreement on intellectual property, including publishing rights. Intellectual property refers to rights resulting from intellectual activity not only in scientific endeavours, but also in the arts, literary and industrial fields (National Health and Medical Research Council (NHMRC) 2021). Although many might think that intellectual property relates to inventions, designs, trademarks and novel discoveries, it also includes scientific works that are produced, such as peer-reviewed journal articles where authors retain ownership but copyright is assigned to the publisher. In nursing and health research, an example of where intellectual property rights become very important includes the development of a standardised scale, where a commercial benefit might be desired by the authors. For instance, many standardised scales are free to use, as the authors want their scale to be used, but some authors earn considerable income from the sale of their scale.

Human Research Ethical Approval

An essential consideration prior to commencing a research project that involves human participants is that all **human research** conforms to *The Australian Code for the Responsible Conduct of Research* (NHMRC 2018a) and the *National Statement on Ethical Conduct in Human Research* (NHMRC 2023). If your research participants are Australian Indigenous Peoples and/or communities, you must also conform with the *Ethical Conduct in Research with Aboriginal and Torres Strait Islander Peoples and Communities: guidelines for researchers and stakeholders* (NHMRC 2018b). Chapter 13 covers ethical principles, but this chapter delves into the *Human Research Ethics Application* (HREA), without which you cannot proceed with your research.

There are many *Human Research Ethics Committees* (HRECs) in Australia, often located within universities, local health districts and hospitals. Choosing the right HREC depends on a number of criteria, some of which are listed below:

- type of research you are conducting—some research must be registered with the NHMRC (e.g. clinical trials and human embryo research)
- state and/or territory research legislations and/or policies
- research team members' professional affiliations
- research funding bodies' requirements for funded research, and
- participant recruitment site/s.

Some research projects will require more than one HREC approval. For example, if you are a researcher undertaking research within a hospital setting by a team where the chief investigator is affiliated with a university and another is affiliated with the hospital, then both institutions may require separate HREAs. The HREC affiliated with the chief investigator will advise of specific requirements in these cases.

Completing and submitting a HREA can be an arduous process. It requires a lengthy application with detailed information about your proposed research methodology and methods, and ethical conduct that you will uphold throughout your research journey, including dissemination of research findings. Achieving **ethics** approval can take many months and so these timeframes should be considered when planning a project. Several supporting documents will be needed, including participant information sheets, participation consent forms, interview questions guide and/or survey questions. A risk strategy to support research staff members who will be working in the field and/or collecting sensitive data should also be developed. In Australia, the NHMRC have developed an electronic HREA form that is required by many HRECs. The HREA form is a concise application developed to facilitate timely and efficient ethics review for research involving humans, and to assist researchers to consider the ethical principles of the project, including those pertaining to the level of risk (Commonwealth of Australia 2021). A risk is a potential for harm, discomfort or inconvenience to the participants, and risk levels are described in Table 17.1.

Clinical Trial Research Ethical Approval

Nurses and midwives may be involved in clinical trial research (O'Brien et al 2022). A participant in a clinical trial is being asked to take a new or existing treatment, or a medical intervention targeted at preventing, treating or managing various diseases or medical conditions (Department of Health and Aged Care 2021). In addition to the usual HREA, clinical trials involving unapproved therapeutic goods (drugs, medical devices and biologicals), are also subject to *The Therapeutic Goods Act 1989* and *The Therapeutic Goods Regulations 1990*, as well as requiring approval via *The Clinical Trials Notification* scheme, and *The Clinical Trials Approval* scheme (Department of Health and Aged Care 2020, 2021). As part of the HREA, a clinical trial will require the submission of the trial protocol. This allows the HREC to determine that the clinical trial is as safe as possible, is using correct and most appropriate means of measurement and that the results are likely to be meaningful (Department of Health and Aged Care 2020). Once you have received HREC approval for your research, be it a clinical trial or other human research, you can commence with your **recruitment**, data collection and analysis. However, ethical requirements do not stop here; there will be ongoing ethical requirements throughout the conduct of your project.

Ethics Committee Reports

For the duration of an approved research project, you will be required to submit progress reports, usually annually, and a final report to the HREC. This is for monitoring the ethical conduct and safety of the research, and show that your research has conformed to the approved research protocol. Most HRECs will have a standard template to complete for the annual and final reports. See the end-of-chapter Additional resources for examples of annual and final report templates. Reports include a number of key pieces of information, but as a minimum they require the researcher to report whether there were any adverse outcomes, participant withdrawals or complaints. Participant recruitment is another important piece of information, where there are usually questions about whether recruitment was as expected, higher or lower, and whether the methods are still the best to conduct the study. In addition, the report may ask what outputs have been published or reported.

TABLE 17.1 Research Risk Levels

Risk Level	Description
Minimal	'No risk of harm or discomfort; potential for minor burden or inconvenience*' (NHMRC 2023 p. 14).
Low	'No risk of harm; risk of discomfort (+/− foreseeable burden)' (NHMRC 2023 p. 14).
Higher risk	More than low-risk research that can result in physical, psychological, cultural, social, economic or legal harm, and must be reviewed by a HREC (NHMRC 2023).

Managing a Research Budget

Managing a research **budget** starts well before any research project begins. It is important to carefully plan and manage a research budget to ensure a project can be accomplished and completed on time. The best time to start planning a budget is as soon as you know you are going to be conducting a research project. Planning is important to consider the scope of the project. Funds provided are usually specified by the funder, and do not always cover every aspect of the proposed project. For example, some funders will not cover the cost to travel to conferences; others will cover this cost but not the cost associated with the chief investigator's time (rather this is covered without charge by the investigator's employer). Before a project begins it is important to estimate potential costs of the project. Budget items usually include research staff salaries, PhD stipends, advisory group costs, fieldwork travel reimbursement costs and open-access journal fees. There may also be fees to purchase standardised questionnaires, and funds to reimburse participants for their time and the costs for specialist advice such as from a biostatistician or a health economist.

When providing budget details to stakeholders, especially when seeking funding, it is important to be specific and justify all costs. This could mean breaking down project costs into specific tasks (such as those for participant recruitment, data collection, data analysis and dissemination), and providing detailed and realistic costings. Budget items such as staff salary on-costs (which covers things such as workers' compensation and maternity leave, accounting for approximately 25% of salary costs) and institutional research overheads (possibly 20%–30% to research costs) need to be factored in for some grants. Not all funders allow institutional overheads to be added to a budget, and so it is vital to check these matters before you apply. Avoiding over- or underspending is important and so time must be taken to get the budget right at the outset.

Starting the budget-planning process as soon as possible provides time to gather the necessary information and offers the researchers time to consult with stakeholders and identify the best possible prices. Allowing time in the planning phase to have a budget reviewed is also an important consideration, particularly for novice and early-career researchers, as some organisations have research office staff who can help create a budget and prepare the project for budget management. Managing a budget requires a thorough understanding of any funding conditions and reporting requirements. Effective strategies for budget management include, but are not limited to:

- monthly monitoring of income and expenditure, and comparing this with the planned budget
- highlighting possible budget variations early on and discussing this with study team members and the funder
- being flexible and making adjustments as needed, but in keeping with the project plan.

Concurrent and detailed tracking of spending is recommended, as this can promote the research team's ability to identify and address any spending issues and facilitate timely budget reporting as required. A project timeline should make provisions for reporting requirements as regular and/or detailed reporting requirements. This includes the frequency of budget reports for the funder as well as the timing and necessities within the final budget reconciliation.

THE RESEARCH TEAM

A diverse and strong research team with complementary research, communication and leadership skills is an important factor directly related to the team's performance and impact (Cheruvelil et al 2014). The research team is made up of investigators who write and submit the grant proposal, through to the wider team that is needed to conduct the research project once funded. Although the investigators are decided upon before a grant application is submitted, it is vital to first reflect on the typical make-up of the investigator team and how it is formed (Ghamgosar et al 2023). More often than not, it is difficult to get research funding unless the chief investigator (see Table 17.2 for a description of roles and responsibilities) is an expert in the topic area with a strong track record of grants, publications and impact in the area. In fact, the investigator team is ranked when grant applications are reviewed and, although there are arguments about how this process can be problematic (Vavrycuk 2018),

TABLE 17.2 Roles and Responsibilities of Research Team Members

Role	Responsibilities
Principal Chief Investigator	Otherwise referred to as the project leader, oversees the overall conduct of the research project and is accountable for project outcomes. Will most often be a senior and experienced researcher, often with a professorial title.
Other Chief Investigators	Provide specific support to the project, whether this is through content or methodological expertise, and have a defined role/task within the research project.
Partner Investigators	Often a lived-experience expert or an industry partner with content expertise and access to experts and/or participants. Can also be a partner from an overseas university, where Chief Investigator status is precluded.
End-users	The people who are going to benefit from the research project, often via direct participation in an advisory/governance group and/or as participants.
Research Associate, Project Manager	To lead the conduct of the research project under the direct supervision of the principal Chief Investigator, usually a junior researcher who has recently completed a research degree (e.g. Honours, Master or PhD).
Research Assistant	Paid employee to carry out specific research tasks, such as recruitment, data collection and data entry.
Research students (PhD, Masters, Honours)	Some projects have embedded Masters/PhD scholarships where the candidate conducts a specific part of the overall project, but can also be Honours students who are affiliated with the investigators.
Associate Investigator	Although usually associated with national competitive health grants, associate investigators are often an early-career researcher without adequate expertise or track record to be a chief investigator, but who is added to the team by the Chief Investigator to offer specialised input into one part of the study and to be mentored by the investigators.

forming a strong team is important. The chief investigator will form a team with complementary expertise that conveys to the funding body that the team is the best-possible team for that project. For example, if a study was a national survey of people with diagnosed mental illness and type 2 diabetes, then a complementary team of investigators might be led by an expert in mental health and chronic illness. Other investigator/s would require expertise in type 2 diabetes—perhaps an early-career researcher with emerging expertise in mental health research being mentored by the chief investigator, and a methodological expert such as a statistician. Taking this one step further, if the study also wanted to explore the economic impact of having a diagnosed mental illness and type 2 diabetes, then a health economist would be a good addition to the team.

Once the project has been funded, then the investigators will recruit research personnel to fill the various roles as listed in Table 17.2. Emerging researchers who want to pursue a research-based career should consider a pathway that takes them from finishing a research degree through to getting contract work as a research assistant, and then as a research associate working on larger research teams. This not only offers the benefit of learning how to work in various teams, but also allows development of a range of research skills that will broaden the early-career researcher's worldview. What is becoming increasingly important is the inclusion of end-users in research teams, usually referred to as patient and public involvement in research, which dates back to the Alma-Ata Declaration in the late 1970s (WHO 1978). In fact, the inclusion of members of the public in research is becoming increasingly mandated, or at least noted as best practice, in health research (Department of Health 2005). This approach gives a 'voice' to the end-users, and their involvement can be during the design of the project and writing the grant application through to participation in lived-experience advisory groups across the life of a project (see, for example Tapsell et al 2020 and Cashin et al 2023). Crucially, it envisages a working relationship that is developed across the course of a project and can include the employment of an end-user within the research team through to the dissemination of research outputs towards the end of the project (Jackson et al 2020).

Research Staff

The recruitment and preparation of research staff is a part of project management. The decision of what and when research staff are brought on board is one that requires consideration, for it has an impact on the project budget, project accomplishment and team culture (Ghamgosar et al 2023). It is also necessary to ensure early discussion of workload and deliverable expectations, and the authorship of any outcomes such as journal articles. The overall goal of recruitment should be to build as strong a research team as possible within budget and project constraints that best promote the accomplishment of the project.

The safety of research staff is a paramount concern, and all studies need to consider how researcher safety can be maintained, in particular for fieldwork in remote and complex settings (Barr & Welch 2012). A researcher safety protocol identifies hazards or risks and offers a framework to support the researcher who is collecting data. Guidance for the development of safety protocols has been produced by the Auckland University of Technology (2023). Questions that researchers should consider when planning a safety protocol include:

- Where is the research being undertaken?
- Who will be collecting the data and interacting with participants?
- How familiar is the researcher with the social or cultural context of the research?
- How safe are the activities in which the researcher is taking part?
- What level of access to support is available?
- What emergency plans are in place? Who can help?

Unforeseen adverse events in research are a potential for the participants and for researchers (see, for example, Vallury et al 2021). Consideration needs to be given to ensuring that the researchers collecting data are experienced, or at a minimum practised, at conducting research as professionally and safely as possible. Research leads and supervisors, particularly where qualitative interviews or observation are part of the study, should provide novice researchers with the opportunity to practise or pilot data collection approaches to prepare them for possible participant scenarios, including challenging and distressed participant responses. Some forms of research require conducting assessments of participants, whether these are psychological (depression screening) or physical (vital signs). Consideration about having a second person in attendance, to witness the assessment, can help to maintain researcher safety.

Researchers are ethically responsible for protecting participants in their studies. An essential part of any research project is considering the ethical implications of the research being undertaken and the planning of steps to prevent and mitigate against any negative impact on participants (see Chapter 13). This is of particular importance in the context of participant trauma and inequality, and the ongoing management of a research project requires the researcher to be reflexive and to continuously review the ethical implications of their work. Protecting participant vulnerability requires continuous focus. It also requires the promotion of participant self-determination.

Protecting and promoting self-determination and Indigenous knowledge and authority, and acknowledging vulnerability and trauma, is a core feature of the *AIATSIS Code of Ethics for Aboriginal and Torres Strait Islander Research* (Australian Institute of Aboriginal and Torres Strait Islander Studies (AIATSIS) 2020). Principle 1 of the Code details that the 'recognition of, and respect for, Aboriginal and Torres Strait Islander peoples' right to self-determination is fundamental to all research conducted in Australia'. It details that it is the responsibility of researchers to understand the meaning of self-determination, the rights articulated in the United Nations Declaration on the Indigenous Peoples and how these rights can be recognised in research.

Recognising the potential negative impact of health research on participants in the context of trauma, socio-economic, cultural and structural issues, Edelman (2023) adapts trauma-informed and resilience-informed approaches to care and research to develop the *Trauma and Resilience Informed Research Principles and Practice* (TRIRPP). According to Edelman (2023 p. 70), 'TRIRPP offers a framework from which to approach research with the explicit intention of addressing intervention-generated inequalities'. The principles are:

- Take active steps to seek participation from disenfranchised groups and individuals.
- Unite with social justice, tackling deprivation and health inequalities.
- Frame the researcher–participant relationship as relational.
- Empower individuals and communities through choice and agency.
- Emphasise strengths and resilience.
- Minimise retraumatisation.
- Recognise the potential impact of trauma and adversity in all participants.
- Strive to be culturally competent and promote safety.

Researcher wellbeing also needs consideration and requires ongoing and reflexive focus, often with supervisory or peer support (Six 2020). Moran and Asquith (2020) and Williamson et al (2020) discussed the impact of vicarious or secondary trauma in research—traumatic stress responses that can develop in people when exposed to the traumatic experiences of others. For researchers, vicarious trauma can be caused by a variety of factors, including sustained, repeated exposure to traumatic research material, a strong emotional connection to the participant as a victim and a sense of responsibility to help (Moran & Asquith 2020). Williamson et al (2020) discuss several strategies that can be used to prevent and mitigate vicarious trauma in researchers including:

- providing training on secondary trauma including the signs and symptoms
- creating a supportive research environment
- providing opportunities for debriefing and stress management, and
- ensuring that researchers have access to professional support.

CONDUCTING THE PROJECT

Project Launch

Similar to **marketing** a product, your launch is where you are marketing your proposed research. The research project launch will mark the beginning of the implementation of your research protocol, commencing with recruitment of participants. The key stakeholder audience for your launch includes end-users, other researchers, practitioners, journalists and the general community (Klar et al 2020). Durham et al (2014) defines a research stakeholder as '... any person or group who influences or is influenced by the research' (p. 12), but also includes those who can influence the outcome and impact of your research. Stakeholder engagement should also ensure balanced participation by all relevant stakeholders, and recognition that not all stakeholders will have the same interests or motivations to be involved with your research project. In addition to engaging key stakeholders, a well-planned research project launch increases the potential to:

- target recruitment of appropriate participants
- attract potential added funding
- build the research team by enticing interested experts (researchers or practitioners)
- showcase your area of research and develop a following (further promoting your research), and
- set the stage for greater success in dissemination of your research findings.

How do you Launch Your Research Project?

Your research project can be launched in a number of different ways. Some researchers will promote their research project at a formal event, such as a conference or a webinar. Others may engage traditional means through your university (or other workplace) media services or journal press releases (Klar et al 2020). In today's technological world, an opportune method to launch your research project, and one that is fast growing, is the use of social media platforms (PLOS 2020). Social media provides you, as a researcher, with one of the most direct routes for sharing and tracking your research with a wider audience. For instance, in 2019, there were 7.7 billion people worldwide and at least 3.5 billion online, equating to one-in-three people worldwide using social media platforms. While such platforms are changing how people access information (Ortiz-Ospina 2019), you should approach use of social media thoughtfully and check the journal guidelines for social media use, as well as the organisation that provided your HREA and the terms and conditions of the selected social media sites. Considerations for which social media platform to use includes selecting the platform that will best suit your research needs and your area of expertise; where your best connections will be and how to build these. It is also important to create your own social media profile and to stay active and engage frequently on the social media platforms you use to promote your research.

There are many social media platforms available for researchers to use, and various benefits to the use of such platforms for launching your research and disseminating your findings/results (see Table 17.3). Commonly used social media sites by researchers include, but are not limited to, the following:

- *ResearchGate* (https://www.researchgate.net): this is used by 20 million researchers from diverse sectors in over 190 countries to connect, collaborate and share research (Research Gate 2008-2023); it allows researchers to upload presentations, working papers and research proposals, to ask questions or answer questions posted by other researchers, to make direct contact with other researchers and authors, and to request their published papers not available via Open Access or not subscribed to by your university library (Adhikari et al 2020).
- *Academia.edu* (https://www.academia.edu/about): this online database allows researchers to share research papers, monitor analytics around the impact of your research and follow other researchers and academics; it is a good database to search for potential grants (Adhikari et al 2019).
- *Mendeley* (https://www.elsevier.com/products/mendeley): this offers a free referencing management program as well as an academic social network to collaborate online with other researchers and discover the latest research; it is another good database for access to potential grants (Adhikari et al 2019).
- *LinkedIn* (https://www.linkedin.com): this is a popular website for professional networking and creating links with others who have similar interests and expertise; it supports posting of photos, videos and presentations, and creating links—for example, to your research project participant information sheets or surveys (Adhikari et al 2019).
- *X* (https://twitter.com): this supports locating new research and sharing your own research; it offers networking with other researchers and facilitates promoting your research to a wider non-academic audience, and engagement in academic discussion, conferences, talks and events using hashtags (Royal Melbourne Institute of Technology (RMIT) 2023).
- *Facebook* (https://www.facebook.com/): this is the largest social media platform worldwide—2.4 billion followers in 2019 (Ortiz-Ospina 2019); its benefits include access to a large and diverse range of potential research participants; it is an inexpensive and effective way to utilise snowball sampling for participant recruitment, with easy integration of links for surveys or other research documents (Kosinski et al 2016).

TABLE 17.3 Benefits to Using Social Media Platforms in Research

Benefit	Rationale
Visibility	Builds, improves and promotes your public profile and increases citation metrics.
Reach and impact	Extends your potential participation pool; direct and quick way to communicate your research to a wider audience.
Network	Assists in developing relationships with other researchers and potential collaborative partnerships.
Being informed	Facilitates keeping up to date with new research in your discipline.

(Adapted from RMIT 2023)

While there are many benefits to the use of social media, there are also some negatives. For example, setting up and maintaining your profile is time consuming and requires some effort (Adhikari et al 2020), and some potential research participant profiles may introduce bias through social desirability and intentional misrepresentation. Additional pitfalls of using social media platforms are the demographic heterogeneity of the site's users, a lack of face-to-face contact that can decrease participants' accountability and, where cultural differences exist, there may be misunderstanding of instructions for participating in the research (Kosinski et al 2016, Ortiz-Ospina 2019).

Participant Recruitment

The recruitment phase of your research project is a crucial element to the success of your research. Your recruitment strategy is largely determined by the research methodology, the topic/subject matter, objectives and theoretical underpinnings, potential participants and the context. The majority of research designs that involve participation by people (such as surveys, interviews, focus groups, observation and health or behavioural interventions) will require the research to consider a number of questions, as listed below:

- *'Who will be recruited?*
- *How will participants be identified and recruited?*
- *Will the potential participants be screened?*
- *What is the impact of any relationship between researchers and potential participants on recruitment?*
- *How will the recruitment strategy facilitate obtaining the consent of participants?*
- *How will the recruitment strategy ensure that participants can make an informed decision about participation?*
- *Are there any risks associated with the recruitment strategy for potential participants or for the viability of the project?'*

(NHMRC 2023 p. 28)

Once the recruitment strategy has been determined, contact between the research team and potential participants for expression of interest in participating in the research, screening for inclusion or exclusion of participants, and preparing to seek informed consent from selected participants are required. There may be more than one recruitment strategy for a single project—for example a mixed-method research design, or where discrete or vulnerable participants are required.

There are a number of strategies you can use to communicate your research project to potential participants. As discussed previously, social media platforms are a commonly used method for recruitment. Other strategies include flyers or notices placed in locations where potential participants that meet the inclusion criteria would frequent; advertisements in other media sources, such as newspapers or radio broadcasts (NHMRC 2018a). Regardless of how recruitment occurs, it is essential that all steps within the recruitment strategy adhere to the ethical principles of justice and respect. This involves ensuring that the inclusion and exclusion criteria are justifiable and fair so as not to exclude individuals or groups; the assurance of a fair distribution of benefits and burdens; fair treatment of all participants; respect towards cultural beliefs and values, privacy and confidentiality; and obtaining informed consent with consideration of the participants' capacity to provide such consent (NHMRC 2023). The ethical principle of respect within research also includes considering the needs of minority groups or vulnerable people (NHMRC 2018a).

Vulnerable People

While ethical considerations for your research project during the recruitment, conduct and dissemination of findings/results pertain to all participants in your research, there may be additional considerations required for participants who are from vulnerable groups. The World Medical Association (2018) has defined vulnerable groups based on the Declaration of Helsinki definition, stating that 'Some groups and individuals are particularly vulnerable and may have an increased likelihood of being wronged or of incurring additional harm.' Similarly, in the context of conducting research in Australia, vulnerable people are considered those at a greater risk of exploitation or are unable to protect themselves from harm (Commonwealth of Australia 2018). It is important that researchers and HREC consider the degree to which potential participant populations might be overresearched or may require special consideration or protection, and balance this with the participants' option to exercise self-determination to consent to participate (NHMRC 2023). The NHMRC (2023) has specified ethical considerations for research participants who are considered to be at a greater risk of harm, discomfort or inconvenience and therefore considered to be at greater than a low risk (see Table 17.4).

Managing Complaints

There is an expectation, both nationally and internationally, that all research will be conducted in a manner that is responsible, ethical and with integrity. The NHMRC *Code for the Responsible Conduct of Research* (2018a) provides a framework for responsible research conduct by Australian researchers. By following this framework, assurance is provided that your research is of high quality, meets ethical standards and gains community trust (NHMRC 2018a). Despite your best intentions, however, there may be complaints raised about

TABLE 17.4 Specific Participants Classified as Above Low Risk for Research

Section 4 Chapter	Vulnerable Group
4.1	Women who are pregnant and the human fetus
4.2	Children and young people
4.3	People in dependent or unequal relationships
4.4	People highly dependent on medical care who may be unable to give consent
4.5	People with a cognitive impairment, an intellectual disability or a mental illness
4.6	People who may be involved in illegal activity
4.7	Aboriginal and Torres Strait Islander Peoples
4.8	People in other countries

(Adapted from NHMRC 2023)

your research. These can be made by a participant, another researcher or a staff member of an institution. The principal researcher on the approved HREA will usually be the initial contact person to receive responses, questions and complaints about the research. In addition, there should be a process independent from the researcher/s for managing complaints (NHMRC 2018a). It is usual practice to include contact details of the approving research ethics committee for concerns or complaints about a research project to be raised during the recruitment phase of your project.

Managing the Study Data

Data management is a critical component of a research project (Kanza & Knight 2022). According to the Australian *Code for the Responsible Conduct of Research* (NHMRC 2018a) it is the responsibility of researchers to 'retain clear, accurate, secure and complete records of all research including research data and primary materials' (p. 4). It is the responsibility of research institutions, such as universities, to 'provide access to facilities for the safe and secure storage and management of research data, records and primary materials and, where possible and appropriate, allow access and reference' (NHMRC 2018a p. 3).

Planning for data management—which includes data collection, monitoring, storage, archiving and eventual destruction—should occur as early as possible, and before data are generated. All research projects require a formal data management plan (DMP), which should be submitted with the ethics application. A DMP is a document that outlines how data will be handled during and after a research project. By taking the time to create a DMP, researchers can help to ensure that their data is well managed, accessible and secure. According to the NHMRC's guide *Management of Data and Information in Research* (NHMRC 2019a) it is the researchers' responsibility to manage data, and thus a DMP is strongly encouraged. Researchers should also consider developing a DMP based on the FAIR Guiding Principles for scientific data management and stewardship (Wilkinson et al 2016). This approach aims to support knowledge discovery and innovation by promoting the sharing and reuse of data, including across multiple disciplines. Applying to the FAIR principles means researchers ensure their data is **F**indable, **A**ccessible, **I**nteroperable and **R**eusable.

A DMP should be developed as early as possible in the research process and should include, but not be limited to, details regarding:

- physical, network, system security and any other technological security measures
- policies and procedures
- contractual and licensing arrangements and confidentiality agreements
- training for members of the project team and others, as appropriate
- the form in which the data or information will be stored (e.g. cloud-based, hard drive or paper-based)
- the purposes for which the data or information will be used and/or disclosed
- the length of time that data is stored (the minimum is 5 years, but it can be 15 years for some clinical trials)
- the conditions under which access to the data or information may be granted to others, and
- what information from the data management plan, if any, needs to be communicated to potential participants (NHMRC Australia 2019a p. 5)

Consideration also needs to be given to the retention and publication of data, managing confidential and other sensitive information, and ensuring researchers engage in relevant data management training (NHMRC 2019a).

Research Dissemination via Reports and Written Publications

Considerable responsibility is placed on appropriate and timely dissemination of research (NHMRC 2018a). Funded research projects are usually not considered complete until the results are made available to the public. In addition to the formal report that is usually required by your funder, often to ensure you get the final instalment, there are three broad choices when it comes to written dissemination of your research results: (1) accessible report with a DOI, (2) published peer-reviewed journal articles and (3) a 'how to' workbook for intervention-based studies. The primary consideration is that not everyone can get access to academic journals unless they are open access, but regardless of open or other access the written style of a peer-reviewed journal article can be a barrier for many who do not have expertise in reading and understanding research data. Therefore, it is usually good practice to ensure that your research is published both in peer-reviewed scientific journals as well as in accessible reports. By way of an example, a study about nurses who work with people with intellectual disability to promote better health and wellbeing outcomes used both approaches; as the audience was likely to be nurses, families, service providers and people with intellectual disability, an accessible report was published (see Wilson et al 2019) as well as a peer-reviewed journal article (see Wilson et al 2020) for academic audiences.

When thinking about written dissemination, authorship is a crucial area that can, sometimes, be difficult to navigate if some team members over- or underclaim their writing role. The NHMRC (2019b) provides excellent guidance on this issue, of which every researcher should make theirself aware. Fundamentally, any author listed on a publication needs to have had a significant intellectual or scholarly contribution to the research and agree to be an author. Typically, the author who has led the writing of the particular publication and conducted most of the work to generate the publication will be first author. Oftentimes, the last author will be the overall research leader for the project, and in health and medical research last authorship is considered just as important as first authorship.

Other Forms of Dissemination and Knowledge Translation

Just as there are multiple choices when it comes to publishing written outputs from your research, there are many choices to be made when it comes to other forms of dissemination and **knowledge translation** activities. Crucially, the researcher's goal should be to get the findings to the people who can use them and, as noted previously, not everyone can access academic journals and so other forms of knowledge translation are very important. This is where conferences, seminars and workshops come into play, yet each of these has its differences, strengths and weaknesses! Oftentimes, researchers can get too fixed on large research-focused conferences that are affiliated with a national, or international, scientific association—in part as they usually offer published conference abstracts that can be good to help flesh out your CV, but also as they are often held in glamorous overseas cities. Of course, travelling to Rome or Rio for a 10-minute presentation is more than appealing; however, such events are not usually attended by end-users and practitioners who are likely to want to know about, and use, your results. By way of providing a short summary, Table 17.5 offers a descriptive summary of some of these different forms of dissemination, many of which research teams will need to organise themselves. The range of approaches to translating the results of your research are all-important, and all research teams should endeavour to disseminate their research through as many approaches as possible.

Each of the approaches listed above can also be supported by different social media outlets, whether this is from posting updates from a conference to your own networks, advertising a workshop you are organising via social media, or offering short snippets of what people can expect to learn from a CPD webinar. In addition, creating co-presentation opportunities for end-users can be a powerful way to help to convey your results and messages about impact at the individual and community level—for instance, supporting an end-user to present a short personal vignette and impact statement at a conference co-presentation.

Research Project Amendments

There may be times throughout the conduct of your research project where changes arise that require an amendment. A research ethics amendment will usually take the format of a formal written submission for approval that details the amendment type and rationale submitted to

TABLE 17.5 Different Knowledge Translation Approaches

Sector	Strategy	Knowledge Translation Approach
Academic	Conferences	• Oral and/or poster presentations at national and international scientific conferences Strategic approach to different academic audiences, such as nursing-specific (e.g. Australian College of Nursing) and topic-specific (e.g. diabetes-specific) conferences
Professional	Seminars, webinars and workshops	• Professional seminars (e.g. health department-led) and topic-based round-tables • Continuing professional development webinars (e.g. nurses, occupational therapists, GPs) 'How to' workshops for specific audiences (e.g. how to embed an intervention into practice for disability support workers)
Community	Community forums	Small community-based forums for different audiences (e.g. carers or families, teachers or community leaders)
All sectors	Social media	Promoting outputs via a range of social media platforms to engage with a wider international audience who may not access other forms of knowledge translation

the HREC/s that approved your HREA. Most ethics offices have managers who can advise you on what changes to your research require an amendment and how these can be best communicated. Amendment approvals are needed for a number of reasons and can include, but are not limited to, changes that *(i) are proposed or undertaken in order to eliminate immediate risks to participants; and (ii) may increase the risks to participants; or significantly affect the conduct of the research, or (iii) change the scope of the project.* (NHMRC 2023 p. 100). Some specific examples of what would require a research ethics amendment include:

- adding or removing investigators/researchers from the team
- any changes to the research design that will necessitate edited participant information sheets and consent forms
- new methods to recruit participants, and
- changing the location of research.

Amendments for Clinical Trials

Some research designs, such as a clinical trial that involves therapeutic goods (medicinal products or medical devices), will carry a higher risk for participant safety. While such research will have participants' safety monitoring procedures in place (a requirement for HREA), they may still carry a risk for the safety to the participants. Where a significant safety issue presents in clinical trial research, such as adverse reactions to a new drug, urgent measures would need to be put in place that may involve a temporary halt or termination of the trial.

WRAPPING THE PROJECT UP

Closing the Research Project

Managing a research project requires consideration of how the project should come to an end. Planning a project's close should always be a part of its design and delivery and should begin at the project's inception. Closing a project is different from exiting the field or completing data collection. It is the end of the total project. What that means, or how that may be measured, is a discussion necessary for all stakeholders—particularly the researchers involved. A project end may be defined by the dissolution of funding or other resourcing, changes in researcher circumstances, the fulfillment of obligations and contracts, or the shifting of priorities, be they internal or external to the project. A project may end unexpectedly. This was experienced globally with the disruption caused by isolation requirements with COVID-19. It could also be experienced because of the sudden end of a specific project's funding (Tay 2023). However, a project may reach a natural end, one where closure was expected. No matter the circumstances regarding expectations, consideration is needed as to when and how the project is called to an end, including who informs of the project's end and who is informed.

Once the decision has been made to end the project, the exit strategy should be initiated. A proactively planned closure allows for a considered approach—one that is not rushed and provides time to adequately address all significant features of a project.

When planning for the end of a project, consideration should be given to:

- the providing of final reporting to stakeholders and funders
- the closing of financial accounts and finalising of any outstanding transactions
- the opportunity to reflect on the management and delivery of the project
- the stock-take of data and its storage, including making it accessible to others
- any complementary means of dissemination and translation of findings and knowledge ensuring access by a wider community, and
- any planning for follow-on projects.

Proper consideration should be given to 'closing the loop' with research participants. Closing the loop means providing closure to participants at or near the end of a project, and this can be achieved by informing participants about the project's outcomes, its dissemination and translation, and their contribution to the research, and providing the opportunity for them to raise any concerns and ask any questions. Researchers could also seek participants' feedback on the research project. Such engagement may also enhance their trust in research and encourage future participation. Research participants play an integral role in any study and, by effectively closing the loop with participants, researchers honour the ethical responsibilities of treating participants with dignity and respect throughout the research journey.

Post-Ethics Approval Reporting

Throughout your project, you will also be required to submit reports to the HREC that approved your research project. Your HREA will have an expiration date. When submitting your HREA, you will be required to identify a project completion date. The period of time for which a project will be granted ethics approval differs for each HREC. However, many HRECs understand that a longer duration for the research to be undertaken may be required. In this case the Chief Investigator must submit a request for an extension that will be submitted and considered by the HREC.

RESEARCH IN BRIEF 17.1

Many people with an intellectual disability are prescribed psychotropic medication to help manage challenging behaviours, despite the limited evidence for their effectiveness. Disability support staff members play an important role in this area of practice as they have some influence over the types of support strategies offered. An education program for disability support staff was developed—called the *Short-Term Psycho-Education for Caregivers to Reduce Overmedication of People with Intellectual Disabilities* (SPECTROM)—and was piloted for feasibility with Australian disability support staff in 2022. The results showed that disability support staff knowledge about psychotropic medications increased significantly after the training (Wilson et al 2023). Nevertheless, these staff members felt that this was a very complex area of practice and that they may need mentoring and support from health professionals, such as skilled registered nurses, to implement a program to help individuals who might want to reduce their psychotropic medications (Barrett et al 2023). These small studies offer a starting point, but funding needs to be obtained to see whether such an educational intervention leads to fewer psychotropic medications being used by people with intellectual disability and challenging behaviours. That is, although more knowledgeable staff is a good outcome, it is not the core outcome for this wider program of research. To collect outcomes from people with intellectual disability, once funded, will require a very detailed ethics application as issues of consent, capacity and risk are vital to get right.

RESEARCH IN BRIEF 17.2

Domestic violence (DV) is a concern for pregnant and postnatal (perinatal) women and their babies. Assessing perinatal women for DV by their healthcare providers (HCPs) is important in both identifying DV and providing supportive care and services appropriate for the woman and her circumstances. Despite this, HCPs can be reluctant to enquire about DV. Usanov et al (2023) reported on the qualitative findings of a sequential mixed-methods study that aimed to explore HCPs' perspectives on factors that influence women to disclose DV and screening practices for DV of HCPs. Participating HCPs worked in a region where there was a high population of vulnerable groups—notably high rates of unemployment, Aboriginal people, people with disability and people with culturally and linguistically diverse backgrounds—all risk factors for DV. Findings suggested that better policies and systems are needed that can support HCPs to ask about DV during their clinical practice. One suggestion was for mandatory training for all HCPs about DV to enhance their capacity to know about the complex issue and how to respond. A noted gap was knowledge about working with women from culturally and linguistically diverse communities and understanding cultural barriers to discussing DV.

RESEARCH IN BRIEF 17.3

Many research projects are planned for the short to medium term owing to various factors such as funding limitations and the availability of personnel. However, it is important to consider the potential for a project to continue and collect longitudinal data, particularly when studying phenomena that allow for investigation over time and that may evolve or change over a long-term period. The continuance of a research project can allow for the collection and investigation of longitudinal data, providing valuable insights into trends, patterns and changes that may not be captured in short-term studies.

One such example is that of the Australian research project from the University of Wollongong: Recovery Camp (see, for example, Tapsell et al 2021). Starting in 2013, the Recovery Camp project was a small-scale, short-term project where preregistration nursing students attended a 5-day, 4-night therapeutic recreation-based mental health clinical placement, alongside people with lived experience of mental illness. The research had a singular focus: understanding how an innovative and immersive clinical placement experience influenced the professional learning and mental health work intentions of preregistration nursing students (see Moxham et al 2015). Continuance of the project, however, has allowed for the expansion of the scope of research to investigate the broader experience of students (including stigma, confidence, competence and help-seeking) and the experience of people with lived experience of mental illness (e.g. hope, leisure boredom, recovery, goal attainment). Longitudinal data are now also available enabling researchers to observe and analyse changes that have occurred over an extended period, allowing a more comprehensive understanding of outcomes (such as self-reported measures of hope).

AN UNEXPECTED HURDLE

A small and funded study comparing individual chronic health histories and the economic costs of different models of care was effectively stopped because of multiple changes in managerial staffing over a 12-month period—the 'gatekeepers' who enable access to some research participants. The participants trying to be reached via the gatekeepers were adults with severe to profound intellectual disability and associated chronic and complex health problems living in different models of supported accommodation. Many hours, and budgeted staff time, had been dedicated to getting a complex ethics application approved and visiting multiple managers and staff teams to talk about the study, with no participants recruited. After 1 year, the study evolved into a single case study as the grant funds ran out. Nevertheless, the resulting publication (Wilson et al 2021) offered the first-ever economic evaluation of a registered nurse-led model of care and, despite the outcome being different to the planned project, the team was able to pivot and still produce a meaningful output.

TUTORIAL TRIGGER 17.1

Getting research funding often takes many years and many small projects to gradually build evidence in support of research ideas and to develop a track record of working with other researchers. What are some ways that an early career academic—such as a lecturer in nursing—can start to build evidence in an area of interest? Choose a research topic (e.g. reducing stress in undergraduate university students) and, when discussing possible solutions with your peers, think about the different levels of research evidence.

Answers: Conducting literature reviews, as they do not require any research participants and can be undertaken with support from research students and other academic staff. Academics can team up with other colleagues and do small qualitative studies together. Descriptive surveys are a good way to generate research data quickly and cheaply. Develop honours projects that future honours students might be interested in undertaking.

TUTORIAL TRIGGER 17.2

You have been asked to lead a small research team to provide some evaluation data to an organisation that supports women and their children escaping family and domestic violence (FDV). They have recently been allocated funding to build a safe house for short-term, transient accommodation with on-site FDV speciality services in an inner regional area. The new accommodation will provide safe housing to a number of vulnerable groups, one of these groups being Aboriginal women and their children. Your HREA has been approved by the HRECs of the university you work for and the organisation responsible for the safe house. You will be collecting data from both the DFV service providers and the women who access the safe housing. Data will be collected from approximately 10 women clients via focus group interviews between 3 and 5 months after they first moved into the safe house accommodation. The group consists of a mix of women who identify as Aboriginal, women with young children and also pregnant women. What are some of the ethical risks involved in this project and how you would manage these?

Answers: The participants are all considered to be within vulnerable groups and so this will require added care and attention when conducting the research. The issue of beneficence will be important owing to the sensitive nature of the research, in particular the potential for triggering retraumatisation where immediate professional support should be available to respond to any distress. The privacy and safety for the women clients of the safe house is paramount and making sure that their identity and location is protected will be essential.

SUMMARY

This chapter has explored the range of often-complex issues that need to be considered when managing a research project. Crucial to the success of a research project is detailed planning before, during and at the end of the project. Research has the power to transform lives, but a lot can go wrong during a research project and vigilance at all stages is a must. Importantly, the management processes summarised here are key research skills that, similar to all skills, must be learnt and refined over time, and that complement the other skills outlined in this textbook.

KEY POINTS

- Setting a project up for success involves the formation of a team with complementary expertise.
- Most researchers will seek expertise from other departments and personnel—such as finance, legal and ethics experts—to ensure project success.
- Ethics approval and managing a project ethically are vital parts of the research process.
- Data management starts before the project and ends well after the project.
- Research budgets can be complex, can change during the course of a project and all funds must be reconciled ethically and appropriately.
- Dissemination of research outputs is a large responsibility and should be conducted in a manner that conforms to accepted publishing standards.

TIME TO REFLECT: INCIDENTAL RESEARCH PARTICIPANTS

In this activity, we reflect on the ethical implications of conducting health research and what this means for researchers, participants and what we have termed 'incidental participants'. To date, little has been written about the ethical dilemmas that arise in carrying out field research, especially in settings where vulnerable people, such as those diagnosed with mental health illnesses or issues, may unwittingly come into contact with researchers and research participants. Fig. 17.1 offers a diagrammatic representation of the unnatural setting that can emerge in health research with vulnerable groups.

Background

This ethnographic study of Patterson (2020) focused on the point of time in which a specially qualified registered nurse engages with a person who is very likely experiencing psychological distress and/or mental illness. Due to its absolute relevance to the study, the researcher endeavours to observe such a situation. Thus, through the process of applying for ethical approval, it is likely that the researcher would, at times, be in proximity with and interact with people experiencing psychological distress and/or mental illness.

To give ethics approval, the ethics committee required detail about the potential risks associated with a population group who were not the intended study participants. Specifically, the ethics committee asked: how would the researchers ensure that 'patient welfare [would] be maintained' even though 'patients [were] not intended to be participants'? Given the likelihood of research existing where the design brings a researcher and participants into direct or indirect interaction with vulnerable population groups, it could be assumed that 'incidental participants' were a significant area of inquiry. Nevertheless, there is a dearth of literature on the matter. Further, there is no guidance on the issue from either the *National Statement on Ethical Conduct in Human Research* (NHMRC 2023) or the *Australian Code for the Responsible Conduct of Research* (NHMRC 2018a).

Drawing from Reeves et al's (2008) notion of researcher detachment, it was presented to the satisfaction of ethics committees that, through the data collection process, the

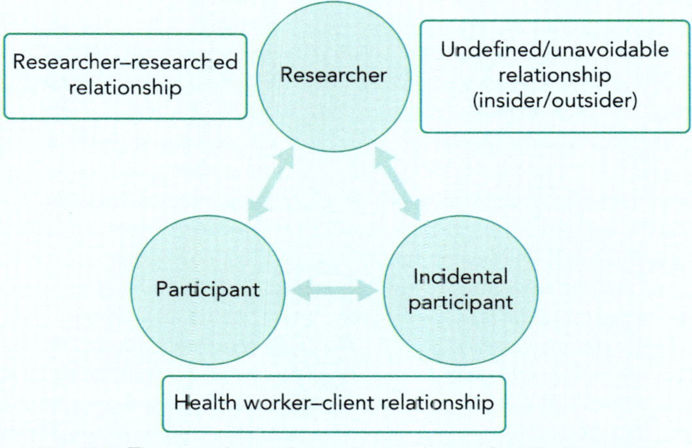

Fig. 17.1 The complex and unnatural context of applied research

TIME TO REFLECT: INCIDENTAL RESEARCH PARTICIPANTS—cont'd

researchers would demonstrate detachment by explicitly identifying themselves to all, including 'vulnerable' persons who were experiencing psychological distress and/or mental illness and were receiving intervention or assessment. Further, to safeguard the autonomy of the vulnerable persons, verbal permission was always sought to be present, where the role as an observer of the registered nurse was made clear to all.

Ethical Dilemma

In one situation, given the particulars of how the nurse and participant engaged one another, the researcher was unable to explicitly identify theirself. The situation that then unfolded generated concern that the researcher had absolutely and negatively intruded not only on the natural setting of the nurse–client interaction, but also on the space and wellness of a person. The following is a personal account of this situation, recorded in a field diary:

> *The situation I found myself in today, I did not expect. I was with John for the assessment of a man. For one and a half hours I sat at the man's kitchen table, next to John, present while John conducted a comprehensive mental health assessment with a man who had never before come into contact with mental health services. For one and a half hours I tried to ensure that my presence was negligible; receding to the background to watch the natural setting from what I call a 'present distance'. At the closure of John's assessment, the man commented on how he found the general process of discussing his situation and mental health difficult. He then turned to me and stated 'especially with you sitting there silent'.*
>
> ***Personal Account***

Reflective Activity

- What ethical concerns do you have about the researcher's decision not to identify theirself to the participant?
- How might the researcher's presence have impacted the nurse–client interaction?
- Is a researcher responsible for the protection of 'incidental participants'? If so, why?

LEARNING ACTIVITIES

1. *Human research ethical approval:* the main role of an institutional or regional ethics committee in Australia or New Zealand is to protect the:
   a. research participants from harm
   b. institutions involved from adverse publicity
   c. researcher/s from criticism
   d. funding body of the research.
2. In Australia which of the following situations would require a Human Research Ethics Application?
   a. Any research that involves human participation.
   b. Running a poll to determine food preference for an event you are organising.
   c. Recording the scores of a sports team to submit to the competition organisers.
   d. Research that uses information found freely in public domain such as published biographies.
3. You are a Clinical Nurse Specialist and will be conducting a clinical trial on a new, unapproved compression bandage. Which of the following must be included in the human ethics research approval process?
   a. The Clinical Trials Approval (CTA) scheme
   b. The Clinical Trials Notification (CTN) scheme
   c. The Therapeutic Goods Act 1989
   d. All of the above
4. *Project launch:* you have organised a project launch event for a research project you are leading. The research project is to showcase a series of short, online modules for busy, primary-based healthcare providers on opportunistic enquiry and intervention for family and domestic violence. Key reasons for launching your project include:
   a. increasing your personal social media followers
   b. keeping the project within your own professional circle
   c. engaging key stakeholders and assisting with participant recruitment
   d. hosting a social event for your work friends.
5. *Participant recruitment:* recruiting participants is an exciting stage of your research. It signifies the beginning of your data collection. Many strategies can be used to recruit participants but, whichever strategy used, the researcher/s must adhere to the ethical principles of:
   a. justice and respect
   b. accountability
   c. fidelity and veracity
   d. research rigour.
6. *Vulnerable people:* research involving Indigenous Peoples has special ethical concerns because such groups:
   a. are a different culture from the rest of the population
   b. have been exploited by researchers in the past

   c. have leaders who may refuse access to participants
   d. tend to live in remote areas.
7. Which of the following groups would not be classified as a vulnerable group for the purposes of inclusion in research?
   a. People who may be involved in illegal activities
   b. Aboriginal and Torres Strait Islander People
   c. Men and women aged 18 years or older who are deemed competent
   d. Women who are pregnant and the human fetus
8. *Managing complaints:* which of the following documents provides a framework for assuring the conduct of research is of high quality and meets ethical standards?
   a. NHMRC *National Statement on Ethical Conduct in Human Research* (2023)
   b. The NHMRC *Safety Monitoring and Reporting in Clinical Trials Involving Therapeutic Goods* (2016)
   c. World Medical Association *Declaration of Helsinki—ethical principles for medical research involving human subjects* (1964)
   d. NHMRC *Guide to Managing and Investigating Potential Breaches of the Australian Code for the Responsible Conduct of Research* (2018c)
9. The *first* stage of managing a complaint raised about the conduct of a research project is to:
   a. interview the complainant
   b. undertake a preliminary assessment
   c. make recommendations for corrective actions
   d. refer the complaint for an investigation.
10. *Research project amendments:* which of the following changes to a research project *would not* require a research ethics amendment to be submitted?
   a. Adding publicly available literature details into your **research report**
   b. Changes to the research team
   c. Funding agreement changes
   d. Adding a data collection site

ADDITIONAL RESOURCES

Australian Institute of Aboriginal and Torres Strait Islander Studies. https://aiatsis.gov.au/.

Examples of ethics forms and report templates. https://www.health.act.gov.au/research/research-ethics-and-governance/hrec-reporting.

Human Research Ethics Applications: Welcome—NHMRC Portal. https://hrea.gov.au/.

Social Media: use in research. https://www.rch.org.au/uploadedFiles/Main/Content/ethics/Social%20Media%20(use%20in%20research)%20Guideline.pdf.

REFERENCES

Adhikari, S.D., van Teijlingen, E.R., Regmi, P.R. et al., 2020. The presentation of academic self in the digital age: the role of electronic databases. Int. J. Soc. Sci. Manage. 7 (1), 38–41 doi:10.3126/ijssm.v7i1.27405

Auckland University of Technology. 2023. Researcher Safety Protocol. Retrieved from: https://www.aut.ac.nz/__data/assets/word_doc/0004/181597/Researcher-safety-protocol-guide-032019.docx#:,:text=The%20main%20purpose%20of%20a,minimise%20and%20manage%20those%20risks.

Australian Institute for Aboriginal and Torres Strait Islander Studies (AIATSIS), 2020. Code of Ethics for Aboriginal and Torres Strait Islander Research. AIATSIS, Canberra, ACT. Retrieved from: https://aiatsis.gov.au/sites/default/files/2020-10/aiatsis-code-ethics.pdf.

Barr, J., Welch, A., 2012. Keeping nurse researchers safe: workplace health and safety issues. J. Adv. Nurs. 68 (7), 1538–1545. doi:10.1111/j.1365-2648.2012.05942.x

Barrett, M., Jorgensen, M., Deb, S., et al., 2023. Staff perceptions following a training programme about reducing psychotropic medication use in adults with intellectual disability: The need for a realistic professional practice framework. J. Appl. Res. Intellect. Disabil. (36) 3, 486–496. doi:10.1111/jar.13070

Cashin, A., Kersten, M., Howie, V., et al. 2023. The experience of facilitating inclusive research advisory groups with parents and people with intellectual disability and/or autism spectrum disorder. Adv. Nurs. Sci. Apr. 20. 1–20. doi:10.1097/ANS.0000000000000497. Online ahead of print.

Cheruvelil, K.A., Soranno, P.A., Weathers, K.C., et al., 2014. Creating and maintaining high-performing collaborative research teams: the importance of diversity and interpersonal skills. Front. Ecol. Environ. 12 (1), 31–38. doi:10.1890/130001

Commonwealth of Australia (2018). Vulnerable People. Commonwealth of Australia, Canberra, ACT. Retrieved from: https://www.acnc.gov.au/tools/topic-guides/vulnerable-people.

Commonwealth of Australia (2021). The Human Research Ethics Application. Commonwealth of Australia, Canberra, ACT. Retrieved from: https://www.nhmrc.gov.au/research-policy/ethics/human-research-ethics-application-form.

Department of Health, 2005. Stakeholder Engagement Framework. Department of Health, Canberra, ACT.

Department of Health and Aged Care, 2020. How clinical trials work. Commonwealth of Australia, Canberra, ACT. Retrieved from: https://www.australianclinicaltrials.gov.au/about/how-they-work.

Department of Health and Aged Care, 2021. Clinical Trials Handbook. Commonwealth of Australia, Canberra, ACT. Retrieved from: https://www.tga.gov.au/resources/resource/guidance/australian-clinical-trial-handbook.

Durham E., Baker H., Smith M. et al., 2014. The BiodivERsA Stakeholder Engagement Handbook. BiodivERsA, Paris, France. Retrieved from: https://www.biodiversa.org/1223/download.

Edelman, N.L. 2023. Trauma and resilience informed research principles and practice: a framework to improve the inclusion and experience of disadvantaged populations in health and social care research. Health Serv. Res. Policy 28 (1), 66–75. doi:10.1177/13558196221124740

Ghamgosar, A., Nemati-Anaraki, L., Panahi, S., 2023. Barriers and facilitators of conducting research with team science approach: a systematic review. BMC Med. Educ. 23 (1), 638. doi:10.1186/s12909-023-04619-0

Jackson, T., Pinnock, H., Liew, S.M., et al., 2020. Patient and public involvement in research: from tokenistic box ticking to valued team members. BMC Med. 18, 79. doi:10.1186/s12916-020-01544-7

Kanza, S., Knight, N.J. 2022. Behind every great research project is great data management. BMC Res. Notes 15 (1), 20. doi:10.1186/s13104-022-05908-5

Klar, S. Krupnikov, Y. Ryan, J.B., et al., 2020. Using social media to promote academic research: identifying the benefits of twitter for sharing academic work. pLoS One 15 (4), e0229446. doi:10.1371/journal.pone.0229446

Kosinski, M., Matz, S., Gosling, S.D., et al., 2016. Facebook as a research tool. Retrieved from: https://www.apa.org/monitor/2016/03/ce-corner#.

Moran, R.J., Asquith, N.L., 2020. Understanding the vicarious trauma and emotional labour of criminological research. Methodol. Innov. 13 (2), 205979912092608. doi:10.1177/2059799120926085

Moxham, L., Liersch-Sumskis, S., Taylor, E., et al., 2015. Preliminary outcomes of a pilot therapeutic recreation camp for people with a mental illness. Ther. Recr. J. 49 (1), 61–75.

National Health and Medical Research Council (NHMRC), 2016. Safety Monitoring and Reporting in Clinical Trials Involving Therapeutic Goods. Commonwealth of Australia, Canberra, ACT. Retrieved from: https://www.nhmrc.gov.au/about-us/publications/safety-monitoring-and-reporting-clinical-trials-involving-therapeutic-goods#block-views-block-file-attachments-content-block-1.

National Health and Medical Research Council (NHMRC), 2018a. Australian Code for the Responsible Conduct of Research. Commonwealth of Australia, Canberra, ACT. Retrieved from: https://www.nhmrc.gov.au/sites/default/files/documents/attachments/grant%20documents/The-australian-code-for-the-responsible-conduct-of-research-2018.pdf.

National Health and Medical Research Council (NHMRC), 2018b. Ethical Conduct in Research with Aboriginal and Torres Strait Islander Peoples and Communities: guidelines for researchers and stakeholders. Commonwealth of Australia, Canberra, ACT. Retrieved from: https://www.nhmrc.gov.au/about-us/resources/ethical-conduct-research-aboriginal-and-torres-strait-islander-peoples-and-communities.

National Health and Medical Research Council (NHMRC), 2018c. Guide to Managing and Investigating Potential Breaches of the Australian Code for the Responsible Conduct of Research. Commonwealth of Australia, Canberra, ACT. Retrieved from: https://www.nhmrc.gov.au/sites/default/files/documents/reports/guide-managing-investigating-potential-breaches.pdf.

National Health and Medical Research Council (NHMRC), 2019a, Management of Data and Information in Research: a guide supporting the Australian Code for the Responsible Conduct of Research. Australian Research Council and Universities Australia. Commonwealth of Australia, Canberra, ACT.

National Health and Medical Research Council (NHMRC), 2019b. Authorship: a guide supporting the Australian Code for the Responsible Conduct of Research. National Health and Medical Research Council, Australian Research Council and Universities Australia. Commonwealth of Australia, Canberra, ACT. Retrieved from: https://www.nhmrc.gov.au/sites/default/files/documents/attachments/Authorship-Guide.pdf.

National Health and Medical Research Council (NHMRC), 2021. National Principles of IP Management for Publicly Funded Research. Commonwealth of Australia, Canberra, ACT. Retrieved from: https://www.nhmrc.gov.au/about-us/resources/national-principles-ip-management-publicly-funded-research.

National Health and Medical Research Council (NHMRC), 2023. National Statement on Ethical Conduct in Human Research. Commonwealth of Australia, Canberra, ACT. Retrieved from: https://www.nhmrc.gov.au/about-us/publications/national-statement-ethical-conduct-human-research-2023.

O'Brien, C., Furlong, E., Coughlan, B., et al., 2022. Building research capacity and culture: exploring nurses' experience of implementing a nurse-led clinical trial. J. Nurs. Manage. 30 (4), 1002–1010.

Ortiz-Ospina, E. 2019. The rise of social media. Retrieved from: https://ourworldindata.org/rise-of-social-media.

Patterson, C., 2020. Situated knowledge of the client's experience: the ethnography of the involuntary admission decision. Thesis (PhD (Nursing)), University of South Australia, Adelaide, SA.

PLOS. 2020. Media Toolkit for PLOS Authors. Retrieved from: https://plos.org/wp-content/uploads/2020/12/Media-Toolkit-for-PLOS-Authors_REV.pdf.

Reeves S., Kuper, A., Hodge, B.D., 2008. Qualitative research methodologies: ethnography. BMJ, 337, a1020. doi:10.1136/bmj.a1020

Royal Melbourne Institute of Technology (RMIT), 2023. Social media for researchers. Retrieved from: https://rmit.libguides.com/socialmedia.

Six, S., 2020. Anticipating doing a study with dying patients: an autoethnography on researcher well-being. Int. J. Qual. Method. 19 (4). doi:10.1177/1609406920967863

Tapsell, A., Patterson, C., Moxham, L., et al., 2021. Informing work-integrated learning through Recovery Camp. Int. J. Work Integr. Learn. 22 (1), 73–81.

Tapsell, A., Martin, K.M., Moxham, L., et al., 2020. Expert by experience involvement in mental health research: developing a wellbeing brochure for people with lived experiences of mental illness. Issues Ment. Health Nurs. 41 (3), 194–200.

Tay, A., 2023. How to wrap up research projects gracefully. Nature 615, 549–550. doi:10.1038/d41586-023-00377-7

Usanov, C., Keedle, H., Peters, K., et al., 2023. Exploration of barriers to screening for domestic violence in the perinatal period using an ecological framework. J. Adv. Nurs. 79, 1437–1450. doi:10.1111/jan.15560

Vallury, K.D., Baird, B., Miller, E., et al., 2021. Going viral: researching safely on social media. J. Med. Internet Res. 23 (12), e29737. doi:10.2196/29737

Vavrycuk, V. 2018. Fair ranking of researchers and research teams. PLoS One 13 (4), e0195509. doi:10.1371/journal.pone.0195509

Wilkinson, M., Dumontier, M., Aalbersberg, I., et al., 2016. The FAIR Guiding Principles for scientific data management and stewardship. Sci Data 3, 160018. doi:10.1038/sdata.2016.18

Williamson, E., Gregory, A., Abrahams, H., et al., 2020. Secondary trauma: emotional safety in sensitive research. J. Acad. Ethics 18, 55–70. doi:10.1007/s10805-019-09348-y

Wilson, N.J., Lewis, P., Whitehead, L., et al., 2019. A national survey of Australian nurses who work with people with intellectual and developmental disability: report to the Professional Association of Nurses in Developmental Disability, Australia (PANDDA) Inc. School of Nursing and Midwifery, Western Sydney University, NSW. doi:10.26183/5d76e6d07efab

Wilson, N.J., Collison, J., Feighan, S., et al., 2020. A national survey of nurses who care for people with intellectual and developmental disability. Aust. J. Adv. Nurs. 37 (3), 4–12. doi:10.37464/2020.373.120

Wilson, N.J., Reeve, R., Lin, Z., et al., 2021. The financial costs of registered nurse led relationship centred care: a single-case Australian feasibility study. Disabilities 1, 331–346. doi:10.3390/disabilities1040023

Wilson, N.J., Barratt, M. Jorgensen, M. et al., 2023. Training support workers about the overmedication of people with intellectual disabilities: an Australian pre–post pilot study. J. Intellect. Disabil. Res. 67 (6), 519–530. doi:10.1111/jir.13023

World Health Organization (WHO). 1978. Declaration of Alma-Ata: International Conference on Primary Health Care; September 6–12, Alma-Ata, USSR. WHO, Geneva.

World Medical Association. 2018. Declaration of Helsinki—ethical principles for medical research involving human subjects. Retrieved from: https://www.wma.net/policies-post/wma-declaration-of-helsinki-ethical-principles-for-medical-research-involving-human-subjects/.

18

Writing and Presenting Research Findings

Dean Whitehead and Rebecca Feo

LEARNING OUTCOMES

By the end of this chapter, you should be able to:

- identify the importance of research dissemination (sharing the findings of research) as part of the overall research process and for improving clinical practice
- explore the nature of the tasks associated with publishing research findings
- understand how to avoid many of the traditional barriers associated with publishing research findings and, therefore, increase the possibility of successful dissemination/publication
- identify different formats, other than journal publication, by which research findings can be disseminated/presented to a wider audience.

KEY TERMS

conference presentations, p. 321
dissemination of research/conceptual findings, p. 313
dissemination plan, p. 318
peer workshops, p. 312
poster presentations, p. 324
research dissemination, p. 313
writing for publication, p. 312

INTRODUCTION

> *If people cannot write well, they cannot think well, and if they cannot think well, others will do their thinking for them.*
>
> ***(George Orwell)***

Writing about nursing and midwifery practice for publication is a skill that can be learned over time. As one of the most famous writers of the 20th century, George Orwell, described in his dystopian science fiction novel *1984*, people who do not write for themselves lose the ability to think for themselves. However, for many, **writing for publication** is not a natural process. Rarely are high-distinctions students, for instance, born with the capacity to write well to a targeted scholarly (and lay public) audience. It is, more often, a skill that is learnt. So it is a further skill set that is required and therefore there is a need for a chapter such as this.

This chapter outlines the benefits of writing for nurses and midwives as well as for the wider public at large. It discusses the various modes of dissemination (means of sharing research) for research findings (including **peer workshops**, professional conferences and journal publications) and provides helpful 'tips' for developing a writing style as an engaging author. It presents these tips not just to share personal/shared ideas and arguments but also as a means to assist career progression.

THE BENEFITS OF WRITING FOR NURSES AND MIDWIVES

As Williams (2015) states: 'Writing for publication ... allows nurses [and midwives] to share their excellent practice and ideas with others; to benefit those who use our services.' That sums up the main reasons to write and share our writing with others—namely, to express and promote good practice and creative ideas with a wider professional and public (health consumer) audience. Doing so:

- provides a means to express values, desires and ideas for change, to educate others so that they benefit from other views and insights. It can stimulate transformation and change so that things/self do not get 'stuck' in time (i.e. traditional practice, tacit knowledge and hierarchy)
- encourages communication, connection and participation in a scholarly community
- facilitates professional and personal growth
- becomes a means to 'do good for others' and promote ourselves as practitioners who engage with and promote new knowledge.

The Importance of Research Dissemination

The main reason to disseminate research findings is to influence and change practice. If research findings are not widely shared, then only the researchers themselves and a few 'insiders' (i.e. supervisors and local colleagues) benefit from the knowledge gained. Since nursing and midwifery research aims to improve client care and enhance practice and culture, it is essential that research outcomes are communicated widely. Patient care will not improve without the widest **dissemination of research/conceptual (theory-based) findings**. Effective nursing and midwifery **research dissemination** becomes a vital and key vehicle for empowerment to best serve the public (Eckert et al 2022).

Research in the 'Academic' Setting

Universities remain the main social institutions to generate research. However, clinical and 'industry' settings are also important (i.e. hospital and public health settings). In this respect, the traditional saying of 'publish or perish' is well known in settings outside of Higher Education (Holland & Watson 2021a). 'Publish or perish' refers to the fact that established, mid- and early-career researchers (ECRs) are expected to publish their research findings, with publication (in terms of both quality and quantity) forming part of their Key Performance Indicators (KPIs). For many researchers, publishing is also a moral and ethical obligation. The critical question is asked, 'Why would researchers conduct research and then not attempt to share their important findings?'

Within academic settings, the need to share research findings is further reinforced by individual and institution-wide research 'rankings' and 'metrics' (see later in this chapter). These metrics demonstrate the overall performance, visibility and collective impact of research produced by individuals, teams and healthcare institutions, with research publications and other forms of dissemination forming a key part of the assessment. At the organisational or institutional levels, the research performance and impact of universities are monitored in a variety of ways. In Australia, this is assessed through the Australian Research Council's Excellence in Research Australia (ERA) program (https://www.arc.gov.au/excellence-research-australia), though it should be noted that the ERA exercise was being officially phased out in 2023. However, at the time of writing, its replacement has not fully come about, which means ERA remains the 'default' for now. In New Zealand, the Tertiary Education Commission does the same through its Performance Based Research Fund (PBRF) program (https://www.tec.govt.nz/funding/funding-and-performance/funding/fund-finder/pbrf/). There are also important international rankings for universities, with a major focus on research and publication impact. These include the Times Higher Education World University Rankings (https://www.timeshighereducation.com), QS World University Rankings (https://www.topuniversities.com) and CWUR World University Rankings (https://cwur.org). Most of these ranking systems also break down rankings into disciplines. Hence, readers can view how a university ranks overall, in terms of research, and how nursing and midwifery ranks between universities.

At the individual researcher level, research performance and impact are measured through a variety of means, again relying heavily on assessments of the quality and quantity of research dissemination. Researcher metrics (rankings) include the *H*-index, available through both Scopus and Google Scholar, which focuses on how many times a researcher's publications have been cited by others. An *H*-index of 20, for instance, means an author has at least 20 publications that each have been cited by other published studies at least 20 times. Other metrics include ratings on academic social media sites and research repository databases, such as ResearchGate, Education.Edu and ORCID (see later in this chapter). A common metric is the quality of journals to which researchers submit their research findings. These metrics include impact factors, which focus on the number of citations received for publications within a given journal, and quartile (or Q) rankings, which rank journals within a specific field based on their impact factors and other citation metrics (also see later in this chapter). *SCImago* is a leading example of this latter type (https://www.scimagojr.com/).

Publishing research findings is also a key component of securing research funding. A large proportion of research activity requires some sort of funding—both internal and external to the organisation in which the researcher(s) works. Where the researcher has already actively researched and disseminated widely, then it establishes a reputation for individual researchers and their collaborators. This raises the confidence of funding providers that the researcher(s) will undertake future research faithfully and complete what they set out to do with recognised outcomes that can directly impact practice (see Chapter 15).

Given the importance of research dissemination to the performance and reputation of research organisations and institutions, as well as for individual researchers, nursing and midwifery researchers must find ways to publish their research findings to a wide range of audiences (Oermann & Hays 2018). Failing to publish regularly in appropriate forums can mean nursing and midwifery researchers will lose on two main counts: (1) their CV/resume begins to stall and (2) their position within their institution begins to lose relevance if their work is neither raising the research profile of their institution nor contributing to practice change/impact.

Research, Publishing and the Higher Degree Research Student

Many nurses and midwives will continue their undergraduate studies with postgraduate studies. A good proportion of these studies will be research higher degree (RHD) programs. Research dissemination is significant because it allows RHD students to fulfil the requirements of their studies. Nurses and midwives who undertake higher degree studies are often motivated to publish to advance their careers. Holland and Watson (2021) and Gimenez (2024) point out that writing for publication is often important for the career development of nurses and midwives via the higher education route. More so now, RHD students are encouraged to publish as they progress throughout their degrees (i.e. publication of systematic reviews—see Chapter 3) rather than, as not so long ago, tending to publish towards the end of the degree/research project.

Undergraduate students can also benefit from publishing. Hayter's (2021) book chapter is devoted to demonstrating how students can turn assessments/assignments into publications. While such students are beginning researchers, they bring the benefit of 'fresh eyes' to problems that might be entrenched or taken for granted and no longer critiqued by more-experienced nurses or midwives. Undergraduate students are also often keen consumers of research (as the discipline has just recently been presented to them during their training program) and are likely to have something worthwhile to communicate via nursing and midwifery journals, peer workshops, or conferences (Mitchell 2018). Box 18.1 outlines some of the available journals and conferences that welcome student involvement. They often welcome personal and anecdotal accounts of a clinical incident or activity, case studies, reflections on practice, letters and general literature reviews or theoretical/conceptual papers—using the best-available research literature to support these. Keeping a diary or journal during clinical placements might provide rich material on clinical issues to share more widely.

BOX 18.1 Journals and Conferences That Welcome Student Involvement

Journals	Conferences
Contemporary Nurse	Australian College of Nursing
Nursing Review	Australian College of Mental Health Nurses
Neonatal, Paediatric and Child Health Nursing	
Kai Tiaki Nursing New Zealand	

RESEARCH IN BRIEF 18.1

Hawkes et al (2016) explored 'writing across the curriculum' (WAC) as a strategy in which writing instruction occurs in classes outside of composition, literature and other English courses—to better disseminate assignment- and research-related information. Their literature review was conducted to identify and synthesise the peer-reviewed literature about WAC in nursing education. They identified and included 48 articles that discussed WAC. Most of the articles described writing courses in nursing programs, strategies to teach writing to nursing students and writing activities (research/theses) or assignments within nursing courses. They found that high-level evidence examining the impact of writing strategies and exercises in courses and occurring across the curriculum was lacking. Only 18 (37.5%) of the articles were evaluative, and most of the databased articles were either author observations or perceptions of changes in students' writing ability or low-level research studies. They concluded that strategies and courses intended to promote writing skills of nursing undergraduate and research students were documented, but further evaluation is needed to determine which are the most effective.

TUTORIAL TRIGGER 18.1

Recall a clinical incident that you think others might benefit hearing about. Perhaps it is a story of success, failure or redemption. It could be a cautionary tale that future students or clinicians could benefit from learning about, so that elements within the story can be avoided or resolved in the future. Taking care to keep confidential matters private, write about the incident and share it in a student discussion forum such as an online blog. Readers of the forum might wish to appraise the story for the following factors relevant to dissemination: 'Does the story resonate with you?', 'Does the story show you something you did not previously know?', 'Could the story be useful to share with others?', 'Where you identify what could be improved upon, could this be the beginning idea for future research?', and 'If so—what might that research look like?'

Disseminating Research Findings Through a Range of Formats/Forums

Research findings can be shared in several different ways using a variety of formats. Publishing findings in research journals is a vital and main resource, but is only one of the available options. Other formats are, for instance: local meetings, forums, workshops or symposia, and at state, national or international conferences in oral (spoken) and/or poster formats. Increasingly, open discussions, 'round-tables' and expert panels are becoming more common at conference events. There is also the option to promote topical findings through various media (i.e. university media, radio, television and online forums). We can look to authors such as Archibald et al (2023) who advocate arts-based approaches that can provide an understanding of priorities by providing an engaging and expressive means of stimulating meaningful dialogue reflective of participants' lived experiences. Their study sought to determine the priorities and preferences of youth, parents or caregivers, newcomers and immigrants, and Indigenous community members regarding the use of eHealth in supporting their mental health using an innovative arts-based priority-setting method.

In the immediate locality, forums such as peer-sharing workshops are useful and more 'intimate' approaches. The benefits include raising awareness among peers of the changes at the local and wider level, role modelling and contributing to ongoing local conversation about improved practices to create a dynamic, scholarly, open and change-focused work culture (Gimenez 2024).

TUTORIAL TRIGGER 18.2

Prepare a 15-minute talk for your work colleagues on your actual/hypothetical completed project as a proposal for a peer workshop. If you are using PowerPoint, limit your slides to 10 and the lines on each slide to no more than four to six bullet points—alongside accompanying images/graphics. For each slide, explain what the problem was that your study aimed to explore or resolve, the approach you took, your main findings and future implications—and consider how best to get this across to the targeted audience.

TUTORIAL TRIGGER 18.3

A university lecturer suggests to a student that one of their assignments is of such a high standard that they should consider submitting it for publication as a literature review. What steps would the student need to take to ensure that it would be suitable for submission to an academic journal, rather than it being just an excellent assignment?

Translating and Disseminating Research Findings for Clinical Practice

Just because research findings are available in the public media does not necessarily mean that they are always useful for clinical practice. A problem for many potential writers is that they find it difficult to translate the findings and outputs of their research into an understandable and publishable format that directly applies to practice (Williams 2015). If researchers find it difficult to effectively promote their findings, then it is most likely that those who read them will have difficulty in translating reported findings into practice.

There are seminal texts that identify the common barriers that prevent nurses and midwives from using research findings in their practice environments (e.g. Leeman et al 2006, Walsh & Downe 2006). They might be a little dated now, but they remain relevant in helping nurses and midwives to translate research findings into the practice environment. The barriers to research utilisation that these texts identify are:

- an absence of information on how to implement the intervention(s) outlined in the study
- too much emphasis on persuading the reader of the internal validity of findings
- an absence of information on cost and cost effectiveness of interventions
- a lack of exploration of underlying theory
- minimal guidance on the process applied to 'deciding' the population or setting
- a lack of fidelity of the whole process.

Oermann and Hays' (2018) text also assists by suggesting ways that these common barriers can be overcome by nursing and midwifery researchers. These suggestions include:

- collaborating with other practitioners (sound-boarding and proofreading)
- selecting a title that attracts clinical attention
- writing 'catchy' abstracts that convince nurses and midwives to read the research in its entirety
- writing introductions that are aimed at clinicians
- presenting the clinical purpose of papers early on
- writing methods sections with clinicians in mind
- presenting the results clearly and concisely—avoiding technical language
- focusing the discussion and recommendations on clinical implications and outcomes
- including relevant information on cost and cost effectiveness (if available), as well as implementation strategies.

This type of information enables students, academics and clinicians to interpret **dissemination of research findings** in a more understandable, targeted and meaningful way.

TUTORIAL TRIGGER 18.4

Before reading on, what perceived barriers would prevent you from publishing in a peer-reviewed health professional journal? Do they fit with the points under the following discussion 'Barriers to publishing'? To what extent are these barriers real or imagined?

Barriers to Publishing

While we are mainly addressing the issue of publishing in academic/professional journals here, similar principles apply to any related writing process that involves peer review (e.g. conference abstract submissions).

It might appear negative to begin a section on publishing findings with the potential barriers to publication. However, by identifying and avoiding the main barriers of the publication process early on, half of the issues are already addressed. Lessons and skills learned at this stage will help the writer to avoid potential frustrating problems and enhance the eventual written outcome (Gimenez 2024, Holland & Watson 2021). This, in turn, is more likely to result in a successful publication. Hanrahan et al (2010) list what they view as the most common barriers to research publication as:

- *personal characteristics*—dislike of writing, inexperience, lack of confidence, anxiety, lack of motivation and perseverance, inefficient work habits, other priorities and poor writing skills
- *writer's block*—thinking about doing things, but never actually getting around to doing them, and not knowing exactly what to write about
- *perceived/actual lack of time and/or resources*
- *role conflict*—such as conflicting expectations, 'perfectionist' expectations and difficulties working with constructive criticism and feedback.

Next, we explain these potential barriers in more detail.

Lack of Confidence and Experience

For many authors, their first publication might be their most demanding. It is often a 'catch-22' situation. When authors are at their most vulnerable or least confident and would most benefit from possessing skills that are likely to produce a successful publication, they tend to lack such skills or the confidence to apply them. Many novice researchers and authors, therefore, do not put forward their findings for publication because of a lack of confidence and experience (Holland & Watson 2021). This can be referred to as the 'glass ceiling' effect whereby the researcher feels they can climb a developmental ladder only so far before they encounter an impenetrable barrier. For some, this barrier might exist at the first rung of this imaginary ladder. This 'barrier' is mostly not an actual physical barrier, but more an internally constructed emotional/psychological one. For the hesitant first-time author this perception might mean that the individual never really gets started, despite their best intentions to progress. Most potential authors should appreciate, however, that if they do not at least try to publish then they will never gain the required experience.

Fear of Failure or Rejection

Many beginning authors are also novice researchers. In this situation, potential authors might feel that their findings are either not relevant or significant enough to 'deserve' publication—or that if they submit an article for publication then their attempts will potentially be subjected to 'automatic' rejection and/or demoralising scrutiny (Watson 2021a). This very rarely happens—unless the 'attempt' is poor quality and the process has not been well thought through (Gimenez 2024). Authors might have their work rejected but, usually, there is feedback and indication as to why and how to change things to improve the original manuscript submission. It is often obvious to reviewers and editors who are the beginning researchers and, in most cases, they will extend deliberate assistance rather than undermine confidence.

Fear of Scrutiny—Peer Reviewers and Editors

Often there is a perception that journal peer reviewers and editors are an elite gathering of 'gatekeepers' who are in place to maintain an impeccable standard for research. This is simply not the case. Reviewers are often volunteers who juggle their normal working commitments with a desire to share their experiences and support others. Busy people are fallible too. This means that some editors and reviewers will be seen as 'poor' compared with others, but this should be measured against the fact that they also normally hold full-time busy positions for which they get no compensatory time for reviewing or editing (Browne 2014). This said, it is also equally true that reviewers often offer highly comprehensive, supportive and constructive feedback that very much assist the process of publication.

The notion that all published research must be good-quality research because it has passed through the peer review and editorial process is highly flawed. Reviewers and editors cannot know everything. Even in the pages of the most highly regarded nursing and midwifery journals, there is as much poor-to-moderate quality research as there is good-to-excellent quality research. For this reason, the research consumer should always be critical when reviewing the research literature (see Chapter 3).

TUTORIAL TRIGGER 18.5

To assist, we include a brief summary (Box 18.2) of what the broad literature says people should do to help them write and disseminate. For each recommendation, provide practical ways that they can be achieved.

Overcoming the Barriers Towards Publication

Now that the potential barriers to publication have been identified, they can hopefully be avoided. It is equally useful to identify what factors assist the process of successful publication of research findings. They include those that follow and complement Hanrahan et al's (2010) helpful list of strategies to help the novice author get started. These are as follows:

- Start with a small manageable publication: book reviews, opinion letters, clinical procedures and case studies are considered entry opportunities for publishing.
- Start with a poster presentation; build towards oral presentations and manuscripts.
- Write about something you are interested in/passionate about.
- Write with a group.
- Write with an experienced writer or mentor.
- Participate in student–faculty collaborations.
- Start with a title and work from there.
- Then progress to your research methods process and work from there.
- Schedule time for writing.
- Remember to regularly back up, save and clearly file your draft article manuscripts as you work on them. 'Losing' work (or rewriting old files) can be very demotivating.

See Box 18.3 for more pointers on preparing your manuscript.

Publishing Research as Part of the Research Process

Research is not complete until it is appropriately shared in the public domain (Watson 2021a). Disseminating study results is part of the research design and process and not

BOX 18.2 Recommendations and Strategies to Help Students Write Research Findings

What the Literature Says	Practical Solutions and Strategies
Find time to write	Hold 'Shut up and write' sessions at work—and outside of work. Managers provide incentives to nurses and midwives to attend writing sessions. Arrange 'writing retreats' away from the usual distractions that allow feedback.
Convert writing flaws into writing flair	Bring in a writing expert to provide a drop-in session to diagnose and prescribe solutions. They are often available in your own institution—especially library staff. Share sessions where authors talk about their successes and failures. Are there common reasons for both?

BOX 18.3 Developing a Manuscript for Publication

- Ensure the title is a concise and descriptive statement reflective of the manuscript.
- Draft an outline of the manuscript for direction, including the structure of sections.
- When writing as a team, assign sections, tasks or roles for members—but maintain a 'single' and overall voice during editing.
- Ensure that 'authorship' priority is predetermined—that is, who is lead author, subsequent authors and 'final' author (which may be consultant author), depending on contribution.
- Develop a timeline for completion of stages, drafts and the target date for submission.
- Attract and maintain a reader's interest by stating the purpose and aims early on.
- Provide a comprehensive but concise background to the topic, including a justification for the study.
- Use simple sentence structure to maintain reading clarity.
- Provide content linkages between sentences and between paragraphs to maintain flow.
- Maintain the original intent throughout the paper, with logical linkage between the title, purpose, approach, findings and discussion.
- An abstract or summary is a self-contained précis of the manuscript, using appropriate keywords, and is often written (or at least completed) last. Sometimes journals ask for a bulleted list of 'key points' to summarise.
- Find a target journal that has a history of supporting novice authors.
- Carefully check the 'house style' of the journal and adapt the manuscript accordingly (i.e. citation style, headings used, word count, abstract and title page format, etc.).

separate from it. Therefore, with the planning of all research, it is useful to have in mind the type of dissemination format and potential audience. Often this is known early on within a study. Yet Brownson et al (2013) report that researchers spend less than 10% of their time on these activities. A way to ensure you devote time to this process is by developing a **dissemination plan**. The key questions to consider are: the goal (what is the purpose or objective of disseminating the research findings?), the target audience (apart from the participants who may have been provided with 'lay summaries' of the findings, who else would benefit from knowing about the findings?), the medium (what are the most effective ways available to you of communicating and reaching intended/best targeted people/groups?) and the best execution of putting the plan in action (Gimenez 2024).

In addition, a useful exercise is to write up research as it progresses in such a way that it already 'copies' targeted academic journal house styles (these styles provide guidance relating to the presentation of a journal article, including referencing, figures and tables, etc.). For those undertaking research for higher degrees and who present their work in the form of a report or thesis, writing two versions (one for publication and one for the university submission requirement) is a labour-saving technique. Heinrich (2011) refers to the related process of 'chunking it' to summarise and create articles from large written projects. In the case of completing a higher degree (especially at the PhD level), it is a good idea to prepare and submit one or more article(s) for publication while still engaged in the study and then include it in the final thesis reference list. Some PhDs are based on the researcher's existing publication profile—what are usually called 'PhD by publication' or 'PhD by portfolio' awards. It has also become more common to include a combination of traditional theses content complemented 'with' publications (i.e. the literature review chapter also containing a published systematic review).

RESEARCH IN BRIEF 18.2

Tornwall and McDaniel's (2022) Q methodology (see Chapter 12) explored Doctor of Nursing Practice (DNP) students' self-perceptions of scholarly writing skills before and after a scholarly writing course. Twenty-six DNP students with either a Bachelor's or a Master's degree in nursing were the participants. The study concluded that effective instruction in scholarly writing for DNPs should include explicitly directed prewriting activities, frequent opportunities to give and receive feedback, and training on management of emotional aspects of writing.

Be Confident of Your Ability to Publish and in the Quality of Your Research

If one has invested the time, personal resources and effort into conducting successful research, the chances of successful publication-related outcomes are high. Getting published is just part of the overall 'research game'. Being confident in the knowledge that, if the correct forum for publication has been chosen and that the conducted research is sound and of good quality, the chances of eventual success are in the researcher's favour. Well-structured, well-designed and well-conducted research has a much higher chance of being published (Clark & Thompson 2012). Another tip is acknowledging the context and motivation to write. As Grympna (2007 p. 1) wisely states '... the best writing comes from an internal need to write rather than simply from an external need to publish'.

Many researchers view the peer review process as intimidating and something to be wary of. However, reviewers are mostly researchers who enjoy offering the benefit of their experience to help others and, in doing so, to help generate higher quality nursing and midwifery research publications for professional consumption. The peer-reviewing platform should not be a place to undermine research but rather to assist and support would-be authors in developing and improving the quality of their submitted research, and to assist in making it more likely to impact practice.

Start Small and Work Your Way Up

An author's first publication could be seen in the pages of high-ranking nursing and midwifery journals, such as the *International Journal of Nursing Studies*, *Journal of Clinical Nursing*, *Journal of Advanced Nursing*, *Journal of Nursing Scholarship*, *Midwifery* or *Women and Birth*. In fact, Clark and Thompson (2012) suggest the mantra 'aim high, aim wide'—but caution is also advised. Rejection from journals such as those just mentioned might not simply reflect the fact that a submission lacks quality, but rather that much higher levels of competition dictate the quality thresholds for acceptance. Choosing 'high-end' journals to 'learn the trade' can be a risky route. However, if rejection from a highly ranked journal poses no problem for the author, submission to these journals can be attempted. The expertise of reviewers and the quality of review are often high with these types of journals and so, even with rejection, useful commentary can be acquired to improve the manuscript for submission elsewhere. That said, be aware that, in a highly competitive editorial environment, many journals now perform a 'desk-top' review, so if a manuscript submission is not seen to be 'of standard' or scope then it will be rejected before it goes out to wider review.

For some, chances might be higher of getting article acceptance within more specialised discipline-focused journals. This fact should be considered against usually smaller readerships and, sometimes, lower quality rankings (see later in this chapter). An important point to remember with all peer-reviewed journals is that it is rare for original manuscript submissions to be accepted on first submission draft. Reviewers, even if supporting 'broad' acceptance of a first-draft submission, will nearly always recommend amendments to be made before final editorial acceptance is suggested.

'Starting small' also refers to the fact that writing a full research article is not the only publication option available. Many journals (e.g. the *Journal of Clinical Nursing* and *Journal of Advanced Nursing*) offer the scope to submit a summary of research or a 'brief report'. In this case, a summary of research findings (usually a page or two) is presented. It is, however, suggested that this option best serves ongoing research, and is used to promote the fact that the results will later be published as a fuller version.

Work With Others

Much as it is recommended earlier in this book that beginning researchers work with more experienced researchers, the same is so for beginning authors. In any professional endeavour, it is better to learn from those with experience than to start alone in the unknown. Experienced authors and researchers are often looking to engage with others in good-quality research and often do not have the time and resources to come up with all the ideas themselves. Approaching experts with a sound proposal can often result in a positive response and possible collaboration. Another consideration here is that, in securing research funding (see Chapter 16), funding agencies will usually look to the publication record of the lead researcher/s for credibility and dissemination experience before releasing funds. Often, experienced authors are approachable and value the opportunity to share their skills and experiences. A well-planned communication approach and a positive outlook can provide valuable opportunities for the novice researcher and writer. It is also more realistic as a beginning author, and yet still very useful to be named the third, fourth or even fifth author in a good-quality publication.

What if English Is Your Second Language?

While not always fair and equitable, the reality is that most journals that target an international audience are often presented as English language only. For those whose first language is not English but are highly proficient in English, this might not be an issue. Helpfully, Bomar (2014) has developed a 'writing toolbox', which includes useful advice such as:

- Select, read and be familiar with an article written in English that models the type of scientific writing, the

AN UNEXPECTED HURDLE

The Director of Research in a local university's School of Nursing and Midwifery looked at ways of raising the school's research profile and increasing publication 'outputs'. The Director decided to set up regular monthly meetings for staff to come together and share their experiences, support each other and report any potential research/writing projects that could be shared. Initially, the sessions were well attended and created much discussion. However, over time, they reduced in both frequency and attendance—and resulted in no 'formal' dissemination outputs.

- Could anything have been done prior to starting the publication meetings, other than just having the meetings, to have made them more focused and productive?
- Once started, could the meetings have been approached differently to ensure that they were less likely to 'come to a halt' and that there was clearer evidence of dissemination outputs?

RESEARCH IN BRIEF 18.3

Shellenbarger et al (2018) sought to understand undergraduate baccalaureate nursing students' knowledge, skills and attitudes towards scholarly writing. The study was based on their observation that nursing students often demonstrate basic oral and written communication skills and have varying levels of skill with scholarly writing. However, they suggested that current approaches within preregistration nursing (and midwifery) might not fully prepare students for scholarly writing expectations. They used a quantitative correlational descriptive approach (see Chapter 8) with a national US sample of 125 undergraduate nursing students who self-assessed their knowledge, skills and attitudes with respect to scholarly writing over a 2-month period. The project also sought to determine the association between writing knowledge, skills and attitudes and participants' demographic variables. They found that participants believed they knew the basic components of scholarly writing. However, they had difficulty managing the emotional aspects of writing, such as feeling vulnerable or exposed to critique. Select personal and demographic variables were not associated with scholarly writing self-assessment, indicating that other factors might influence scholarly writing development. The authors suggested that nursing faculties and schools should provide students with opportunities to practise writing and to incorporate ungraded practice activities, to help students develop scholarly writing confidence and skills.

research design and concept that you are planning to write about.

- Assemble a contact list of native English colleagues who might read your papers before submitting to a journal. On social media and professional websites, connect with L2 scholars who have similar writing, research and specialty interests. (L1 is used to refer to the student's first language, while L2 is used in the same way to refer to their second language or the language they are currently learning.)
- Attend or create a writing network group in your workplace, professional organisation or with scholars from a variety of nations.

Know Your Medium

For the readers of this book, the most common places for publication will be academic nursing and midwifery or broader health-related journals. General guidelines for authors on manuscript style and submission will be found online on journal homepages. Some journals occasionally run special editorials or commentary on how to ensure the best possible outcome for publication in their journals. Quite commonly, journals will also put out a timely call for 'special theme' editions—for instance, the *Journal of Advanced Nursing* (2024) 'Nursing for a Healthy Planet and People'—https://onlinelibrary.wiley.com/page/journal/13652648/homepage/call-for-papers/healthy-planet and *Journal of Clinical Nursing* (2024) 'Generative AI in Nursing and Healthcare—https://onlinelibrary.wiley.com/page/journal/13652702/homepage/call-for-papers/si-2023-000702

Most journal editors, while often very busy, welcome the opportunity to discuss manuscript proposals before submission. However, few authors take advantage of this opportunity. Editors are usually best placed to know what they want in their journals and when they want it. Initial consultation with journal editors can save a lot of time and frustration in the publication process.

Keep It Simple, Keep It Brief

Most journals will specify a certain word limit for submitted research articles—often up to around 8000 words, but more usually 3000–5000 words. A great deal of work goes into conducting research and this means there is usually much to report and write about. Five thousand words or so is not a lot of words to achieve this task. Stages of the research process, therefore, can only be summarised in terms of the main activities. Journal word limits are particularly challenging when writing for a nursing and midwifery audience. Nursing and midwifery research is often published with high levels of description of the whole process from beginning to end, especially in the methodology sections. This is because many target readers of nursing and midwifery journals might not yet be active research consumers or overly familiar with research terminology (e.g. undergraduate students reading research for assignments). In many medical journals these levels of description are not included in the expectation that the readers are more familiar with research language and processes.

An essential skill for effective presentation of research findings for publication and for conforming to journal word limits is that of summarising—the same skill needed for critical evaluation. Writing briefly is important. Many new authors are under the impression that, to get an article accepted in a top-rated nursing journal, they must write either very *eloquently* or technically, or both, which can often take up a lot of words. This is a misconception. Most journal editors will insist that submissions are written in a concise, clear, coherent, uncomplicated and approachable manner (Gimenez 2024), making it easier for readers with differing levels of expertise and familiarity with research to read through and understand the journal article.

Be Patient and Persevere

For those who do submit manuscripts for publication, the experience of getting published is often one of patience and perseverance. Getting published is rarely a quick process. One or two rejections and subsequent modifications later can see a publication in print several years after the research was started. This is another good reason to write up research for publication as research progresses rather than after completion. The initial peer review process can be time consuming (between 6 and 12 weeks, and often much longer), while recommended amendments might take further months to complete, and might not be confirmed as final until several months after that. With *major amendment* recommendations, the revised manuscript might go back to the original peer reviewers for further review. All manuscripts, therefore, are best viewed as 'works in progress'. Being aware of 'wait times' with publishing and being patient rather than giving up will help you to navigate through the publication process and increase your likelihood of publication success (Davidhizar et al 2006).

The Process and Structure of Writing for Peer-Reviewed Publication

Now that the potential barriers and the means to overcome these have been explored, it is useful to begin thinking how an author can set out to plan and complete the writing process—through to the submission phase and beyond. The following information acts both as a summary of points made earlier in this chapter and as further elaboration on process and structure (Box 18.4).

BOX 18.4 Submission to Acceptance

- *Find a suitable journal*—consider scope of journal, house style, impact factor, etc.
- *Submit online*—following author guidelines and submission guidelines.
- *Depending on journal protocol, editorial 'desk-top review' (filtering)*—before deciding if manuscript goes out to 'full review' or not, *or* manuscript is assigned a review number and goes out to full review. Usually, two to three reviewers are assigned and it goes out to 'blind' review (i.e. the reviewers do not know each other or communicate with each other).
- *Depending on various factors, full manuscript review*—on average, this takes 6–12 weeks. It can be shorter or longer with many journals.
- *When all reviewers have completed, the results are sent to the author*—there are generally several outcomes: (1) Accept with no revisions (very rare), (2) Accept with minor revisions, (3) Accept with moderate revisions, (4) Accept with major revisions, (5) Reject (with the option to re-submit), or (6) Reject (outright). Note: the word 'accept' may not be there (i.e. a journal may ask for revisions—but that still may not mean that it will be accepted). A common outcome is 'accept with major revisions'. With several reviewers, they may offer different review outcomes. One may say minor revisions, and another may say major revisions. This is 'normal'.
- *If invited to, the author is expected to address all reviewers' comments*—making changes and/or offering 'rebuttal' (a defence/reason as to why a suggestion is not appropriate/possible) so that they are clearly identified 'in-text' of the revised manuscript. Journals also often request for a separate 'summary table', which sequentially lists each reviewer comment and identifies what changes have occurred and where. The manuscript is then returned via the same online submission process, and the manuscript is designated the same review number, but usually denoting 'R' (meaning 'revision') to identify that it is not the original submission. This process can occur more than once, depending on whether the editor/reviewer deems the revisions are adequate, or not.
- *If the final outcome is rejection*—this is not a 'disaster'. Go to the next 'appropriate' journal, adjust for their scope and house style, etc., and repeat the process, knowing that the manuscript should be improved from addressing the previous reviewers' comments.

Academic writing spans a range of purposes; from abstract writing for **conference presentations**, dissemination at conferences by poster or verbal presentations (see later in this chapter), through to full-text papers in peer-reviewed journals or books. Writing for publication in a refereed journal can also take several forms—a review paper, a clinical paper describing a practice or a series of clinical cases, a scholarly or theoretical paper discussing a concept or phenomenon of disciplinary interest, or a report of a research study. The focus of discussion here will be on the last form—a journal-based research paper.

Selecting a Journal

One is advised to select a list of journals to target for submission early in the writing process. Clark and Thompson (2012 p. 2373) highlight the importance of this step in stating '... the world of academic publishing has changed profoundly. Risks and opportunities abound like never before. Most crucially: publications no longer all count Making good choices about where to publish has never mattered so much.' This is especially the case more recently with most journals moving to *open access* (see later) models (Watson 2021b). While you must submit your manuscript to only one journal at a time (following copyright laws), it is important to consider other options if the first journal rejects your paper. This will generally mean targeting other journals of similar scope and house style so that a resubmission will not require a major rewrite. When determining a list of suitable journals, a range of issues needs to be considered, including:

- matching the manuscript topic, approach and target audience to the journal's scope, intent and readership
- identifying the submission process, including the journal's timelines for peer review and publishing accepted manuscripts
- determining whether the impact factor and quartile ranking of the journal are important in this instance (see later under 'Journal impact factors').

Identifying an appropriate journal to target can be assisted by asking experienced colleagues and reviewing previous issues of the journals for the style and scope of articles already published. Journal readership is important for authors to consider in terms of focus (national versus international application), scope (general discipline versus specialty knowledge) and orientation (clinical and/or academic). Most journals provide information for potential authors that note the types of manuscripts considered, the requirements for the manuscript (e.g. word count, heading structure, in-text citation and reference list format) and submission processes (Gimenez 2024). This information is usually readily available on the website of the journal or publisher (see Chapter 3 for examples of journal websites).

If undecided, it is advisable for you to contact the journal's editor to gauge their interest in your manuscript.

Manuscript submission processes vary considerably between journals and publishers. They range from emailing the manuscript directly (as an attachment) to the editorial office or, more commonly, completing online submission through the journal's website (Browne 2014). The type of process used by different publishers will also influence the time for peer review and feedback to the authors. This varies widely and many journals state their 'average' processing times within the author instructions. Many journals now also post 'in press' articles online as 'early view'. These articles are complete versions of the final article that has been accepted by the journal for publication except that they are still in a 'queue' waiting to be assigned to a specific future volume of the journal. These in press versions are often posted 6 months or more before they are assigned to a particular journal volume. They can be cited and tracked using their given Digital Object Identifier (DOI) number.

Scheme of publication pipeline. Increasingly, given the delays often associated with publishing, it is important for nursing and midwifery researchers to develop and maintain an ongoing publication plan. The aim is to have several writing projects in various stages of development and submission in targeted journals, rather than writing one manuscript after the other (see Fig. 18.1). Some nursing and midwifery texts are specifically devoted to managing this process—for example, Gimenez (2024) and Holland and Watson (2021a).

Journal quality rankings. The Excellence in Research for Australia (ERA) and the Performance-Based Research Funding (PBRF) exercise in New Zealand monitor impact in relation to research outcomes in universities. University funding from government is reliant on how well an institution's overall research scores in this regular monitoring. It should be noted, however, that the ERA exercise was being officially phased out in 2023. However, at the time of writing this chapter, its replacement has not fully come to fruition, which means ERA remains the default monitoring approach for now.

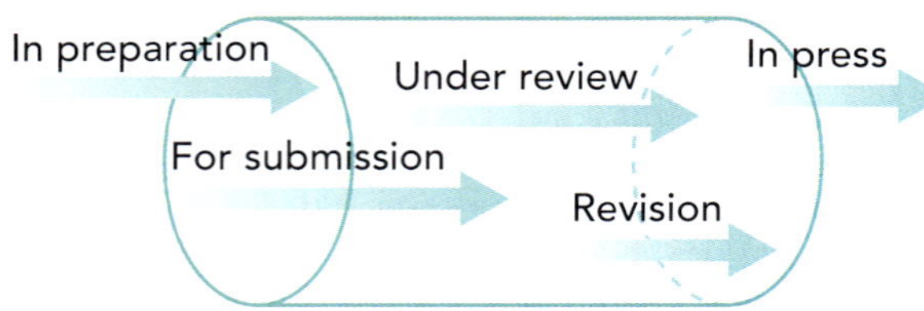

Fig. 18.1 Schema of publication pipeline

One important, but disputed, measure of 'impact' and 'quality' of research publications and of journals themselves is the journal citation rate. Citation indexes were first developed in the 1950s to measure the average citations of articles in journals. Currently, the Journal Citation Reports (JCR) (Clarivate Analytics—https://jcr.clarivate.com/jcr/home) and the SCImago Journal Rank (SJR) (a subdivision of Scopus—https://www.scimagojr.com) are two of the most popular sources for citation indexes and have similar functions and formats.

JCR provides a journal impact factor, which reflects the mean number of citations for articles published within a given journal over the last 2 years. JCR has both 'science' and 'social science' editions, which provide discipline-specific lists of journals, detailing the impact factors and other information such as an 'immediacy index' (how quickly an average article in a journal is cited) and 'cited half-life' (the rate of continuing citations to a journal's articles). SJR produces the SJR Indicator as well as quartile rankings. The SJR indicator is the number of weighted citations received within a given year per article within a journal, averaged over the previous 3 years. Quartile rankings provide a measure of the top journals within given subject fields. For those wanting to make a career out of publishing, it is worthwhile targeting those journals that have high citation indices (i.e. impact factors and quartile rankings) to give published work the most visibility.

Open-access journals. In more recent times, the health sciences have witnessed a dizzying 'explosion' of journals that have either become or emerged as online-only or 'open access' (i.e. viewing a journal article without paying for it), or both. This caters well for the market of personal electronic devices and the rapid growth of social media. This is inevitably paving the way for increasingly diverse platforms and forums for researchers to share, debate and disseminate their findings. There are different models of open access—mainly related to levels of access, copyright issues and fees charged (Clark & Thompson 2012, Watson 2021b). While the move to open access publishing is generally welcomed, in a crowded and competitive market, there are of course sceptics. As Griffiths (2014 p. 689) argued, when it comes to open access, 'all that glitters is not gold'. Predatory and unscrupulous publishers who will publish just about anything for the right fee try to promote themselves as legitimate journals—often having very similar names to established and reputable journals.

Many open-access journals (including many of the legitimate ones) also do not have impact factors or JCR/SJR rankings. That said, there are established, highly ranked and respectable mainstream open-access publishing companies—for example, PLoS Medicine, titles that cluster under the BioMed Central (BMC) company and SAGE Open journals. The authors of this chapter are respectively Associate Editors for *BMC Public Health* and for *BMC Health Services Research*—both well-respected, well-ranked and competitive journals. Over 2023–2024, the Council of Australian University Librarians (CAUL) has worked with major publishing houses (e.g. Elsevier, Wiley, Hindawi) to develop the *CAUL Consortium*. This Consortium works to negotiate Read & Publish (R&P) agreements, enabling libraries to support students, academics and researchers with useful scholarly content, and providing authors the opportunity to publish open access immediately on acceptance, and free of any transactional article processing charges (APCs)—https://caul.libguides.com/read-and-publish. These publishing organisations offer similar R&P agreements across the New Zealand universities.

Developing and Refining a Manuscript

Box 18.3 outlines a range of issues to address when developing a manuscript (article/paper) for publication. It is important to consider both aspects of content and those of format when developing the work. Writing the content can be relatively straightforward, with some of the early material (background, literature review, methods used) already developed for other purposes (such as an ethics proposal). The format includes the overall structure and sections of material flow, which might be guided by the journal's requirements (e.g. in-text reference format and reference list style).

The two common types of reference style (each with numerous variants) are:

- author–date style ('Harvard', also 'APA', favoured by humanities and social science journals, including many nursing and midwifery journals)
- numbered style ('Vancouver', favoured by biomedical and some nursing journals).

These styles dictate the in-text referencing style (author and date cited in parentheses, or a superscript number, respectively) as well as the format of the reference lists (references are listed in alphabetical order, or in numerical order as cited in text, respectively). There are benefits and limitations of each style. It is best to note how these are presented in the house style or author guidelines of a targeted journal (especially in reference lists), as subtle variations exist between journals.

Another aspect to consider during development of the background and discussion material is 'author orientation' in sentence structure. The types of author orientation are 'strong', 'weak' and 'no' orientation (see Table 18.1). Another factor to consider here is the preference for writing from the first-person (personalised), third-person (distant) or passive-voice (assumed) perspective (Wiley 2016). Choosing one stance, justifying it and being consistent throughout is the overall recommendation.

Progressive refinement occurs through multiple drafts of the manuscript. This might include using functions in the word-processing software, such as 'track changes' and 'insert comments' to facilitate editing and communicating in a writing team. Self-editing is an important experiential skill to develop and refine as a writer. Allowing time between the completion of a draft and the next edit enables you to review with a 'fresh critical lens' and see where improvements could be made. Wiley Publications (2016) offer a useful guide titled *Writing for Publication: an easy-to-follow guide for nurses* (https://onlinelibrary.wiley.com/pb-assets/assets/14667657/Writing_for_Publication-1509467251000.pdf).

Once you (an individual writer or a team) are satisfied with the development of the manuscript to almost-completion, it is useful to then engage a 'critical friend' to review the quality of the manuscript. This aspect of informal review can be achieved through a 'publication syndicate'

TABLE 18.1 Comparison of Author Orientation in Sentence Structure

Type	Description	Example[a]
Strong	Primary focus is on what the authors said or did; the author therefore takes a prominent position in the sentence.	'Elsevier (2016) concluded that a comparison of previous studies was problematic because of varying study methodologies.'
Weak	Information is again presented as the author doing it or writing about it, although the author details are placed outside the grammatical structure of the sentence.	'A conducted comparison of previous studies was shown to be problematic because of varying study methodologies' (Elsevier 2016)
None	Information is presented as fact, and author details located outside the grammatical structure of the sentence.	'Previous studies were problematic because of varying study methodologies' (Elsevier 2016).

[a] Using an author–date reference style.

(Gee 2011, Williams 2015)—a small group of colleagues who review each other's work in progress on a regular basis in a safe and collegial manner. The aim of these refinement and editing processes is to produce a manuscript that reflects clarity and correctness and enhances the likelihood of publication.

Submitting the Manuscript

An important consideration is to follow journal guidelines closely. Guidelines might be supplied by the editor or offered as 'author instructions' in the pages of a journal (hard copy or online). Guidelines are usually clear and unambiguous. As Silver (2009 p. 11) states, 'It is important to understand publishing protocols and how editors expect prospective authors to present their work for consideration'. While this might seem an obvious requirement, it is worth stressing here. Murray (2009) has stated that often authors do not follow the guidelines offered and, therefore, this calls into question whether authors really do look at them or seek them out in the first place. Writing and formatting as requested might mean the difference between seeing your submission in print (or online) in a timely manner and a much slower process with content returned for reworking or checking. In competitive journals it could mean the difference between your manuscript being sent for review and simply being rejected.

When you are satisfied that the manuscript is complete and satisfies the journal's submission requirements, then follow the submission processes outlined by the journal, including the submission format, need for a cover letter, assignment of copyright of the material to the journal's publisher and so on. The journal's editorial office usually sends an acknowledgment of receipt. Waiting for feedback can be a lengthy process, so check the stated timeframe for peer review and follow up with the editor after that time has lapsed. They might do the same with you if they require feedback—that is, between several reviews. This 'transition time' is a good time to commence another writing project and/or complete others already in process. It is a good idea to keep the publication process going.

Receiving and Responding to Peer-Review Feedback

The common decisions for a manuscript from a journal editor/s are: acceptance (plus or minus minor revisions), major revisions (requiring response to substantive comments by the reviewers) and rejection, with similar variations across journals and publishers. Acceptance of the manuscript for peer review (or rejection) can also occur at the initial submission stage to the editor. If an editor decides that the submitted manuscript is not suitable for the journal, they might not send it out for review and notify the researcher that this is the case. If the manuscript does go out to review, depending on the editor and the journal, a compilation of the reviewers' comments or the original review from each of the peer reviewers will be sent to the first author only or to the entire author team (Hanrahan et al 2010). Remember that reviewer comments (should) relate to the manuscript, not to you as a person—so try to be objective when you receive the feedback and when you address their comments. Most manuscripts require some form of revision prior to acceptance by the journal, so consider this aspect as part of the usual process for article writing. Respond to each issue raised by the peer reviewer(s) in a systematic way—either defend your position in an objective, justifiable way or comply with the suggestion by modifying the text. Follow the editor's instructions and resubmit in a timely manner.

After your first round of revisions there might be a further review, again by the peer reviewers, requiring some response from the author/s. At some point, a final decision will be made by the editor to accept or reject the manuscript. If the former, the editor will detail the publication process including the possible timeframe for publication and when the author will be involved in various processes—such as copyediting of the page proofs. This process usually has a tight timeframe, sometimes requiring the author to respond within 48 hours by emailing the annotated corrected page proofs to the editorial office. You might be dealing with several different individuals throughout this process—for example, the editor (or subeditors), copyeditors, typesetters and administrators.

Other Forums for Research Dissemination

It can potentially take a year or more for an academic research-based article to find its way into journal print—even with the advent of open access. This is from conception, through submission, then peer review, possible rejection, then resubmission to another journal, more peer review revisions, final acceptance, journal panel editing, proofing and then placement in the volume 'queue' (in press) of a journal for eventual publication. This is not always the case but, in such an eventuality, the use of other dissemination forums, either in place of or in association with journal publication, is desirable.

Publishing in academic journals, while generally regarded as the most effective way to reach a broad audience and ensure the rigour of the final product, is not the only means/media through which researchers can disseminate their study findings. Other means include posters and oral presentations at local clinical forums and local, national and international conferences. Some might apply for this type of presentation as first choice. Either way, **poster presentations** can be a very useful means of disseminating findings—with the added benefit that the posters can be displayed elsewhere later—for example, on university and hospital corridor noticeboards (Gimenez 2024). Well-designed posters can provide a creative, eye-catching and detailed means of communicating research findings.

Although potentially reaching much smaller audiences, the above-stated presentation options are still important for disseminating research findings, especially if used in conjunction with presenting findings in academic journals. They generally allow the extra advantages of personal interaction, networking and problem solving. For some, acceptance of an abstract submission for a conference and subsequent publication in conference proceedings marks the beginning of their publication career (Gimenez 2024). However, it is important to point out that the effort, patience and diligence required for publishing in academic journals are also required for oral and poster presentation formats.

There is little nursing- or midwifery-related literature that relates to the writing of abstracts and presenting for oral forums and conferences. Draper (2021), however, offers sound advice in relation to oral and poster presentation in terms of avoiding barriers and presenting effectively by:

- reviewing the proposed presentation with experienced colleagues
- ensuring that the content does not marginalise or discriminate and avoids offensive humour
- reviewing for potential legal or ethical issues (i.e. sensitive or confidential information)
- ensuring that content complies with professional and organisational codes and standards
- ensuring that due acknowledgment is given to all contributors to research projects—not just presenters
- ensuring that both benefits and limitations to research findings are presented
- ensuring that departmental heads are informed of the forum and have a copy of the presentation.

For effective presentation, it is advisable to:

- use a wide range of presentation material (i.e. graphics, photos, videos, links, etc.)
- ensure the use of visuals, colour and sound does not 'swamp' or take the place of the intended information
- ask departmental audiovisual/technical/marketing services to offer their expertise
- use concise and relevant information alongside 'catchy' titles and headings.

While some avenues for disseminating research findings have been discussed in detail, there are other ways of reaching not only nursing and midwifery audiences but also wider community audiences—for example, press releases, community radio, magazines, newspapers and so on. One therefore should be mindful of all possible avenues for disseminating research findings. The mantra 'all publicity is good publicity' applies in this case—within the context that it is appropriate and professional dissemination.

As hinted at earlier, the increasing expansion and popularity of social media and related forum-sharing options—web publishing, podcasting, blogging, wikis, etc.—provide fertile ground for increasing innovation and scope to share findings (Murphy & Cowman 2012, Watson 2021a). Ferguson and Jackson (2014 p. 79), however, highlight caution in relation to issues of intellectual property and the use of social media. They ask the question, 'If it's posted, is it published?' O'Connor et al (2022) investigated the opinions of undergraduate nursing students in relation to 'digital professionalism' on social media as a means of highlighting good practice when disseminating information on social media such as Facebook, Instagram, Snapchat, etc.

Academic social media is now recognised as an important 'mainstay' of disseminating research information and increasing a researcher's portfolio and profile. Perhaps the most 'popular' academic media site is Research Gate (RG)—https://www.researchgate.net/. It is a social platform that invites researchers (from novice through to very experienced) from around the world to share their experiences and findings, report on current projects, ask forum questions for feedback, etc. Feel free to check out the RG site of one of the authors (https://www.researchgate.net/profile/Dean-Whitehead) as an example. Other related sites are also competing in this space, such as academic.edu (https://federation-au.academia.edu/DeanWhitehead), LinkedIn, etc. Other academic media forums directly report publications and their impact collectively (i.e. ORCID, Google Scholar, Mendeley, etc.). X (formerly Twitter) is also used by researchers, journals and publishers to inform the research community and wider public about the dissemination of new research findings. Some journals ask authors for 'tweetable' abstracts and enable authors to include their 'X (Twitter)' handles as part of the manuscript submission process. There are also X (Twitter) and other social media-related metrics that researchers can use to demonstrate the reach of their research and its findings outside of academic circles. Topically, O'Connor et al (2023) present their systematic review on the use of artificial intelligence (AI) in nursing and midwifery (see following Time to Reflect). At the time of the publication of this text, the use of AI across healthcare disciplines in practice and education is 'hotly' contested and debated, for both its advantages and its disadvantages.

SUMMARY

Disseminating research findings, whatever media are used, is an integral part of the research process. It is understandable why some researchers do not promote their findings to a wider audience, for reasons such as time constraints and lack of confidence in findings and the competitiveness of the publication process. These, however, are often 'perceived' barriers and can be overcome with careful planning. Effective researchers will have in mind, from the beginning stages of their research, a well-planned strategy for how, when and where they will disseminate and promote their research findings. Research dissemination is usually seen as the final stage of the research process. That said, the process is often viewed as cyclical. Dissemination of research findings does not always represent closure of research projects, but 'rebirth' of the next project.

KEY POINTS

- The sharing of research findings is an integral part of the research process and needs to be planned and structured early on in any research study. Dissemination of findings is often viewed as a moral and ethical obligation of the nurse or midwife researcher to present their research for critical scrutiny so as to benefit the public, peers and colleagues.
- Disseminating research findings is necessarily a rigorous process. Expectation of authors might be high but success does not always follow (at least not immediately). Careful planning and perseverance, however, are essential to eventual success.
- Authors do not have to restrict themselves to a narrow range of media (i.e. academic journals) to promote their research. There exist many different formats at discipline/setting-specific or generic levels.
- Presenting research findings adds to the overall database for supporting nursing, midwifery- and healthcare services-based knowledge.

LEARNING ACTIVITIES

1. The common expression that relates to what researchers should do with their study findings is:
   a. always publish
   b. make them known
   c. publish or perish
   d. get the knowledge 'out there'.
2. Many potential nurse and midwife researchers appear reluctant to write up their research for publication, often because:
   a. they do not write well
   b. they have already presented their findings at a clinical forum
   c. they can contribute to the clinical area in other ways
   d. they fear scrutiny and rejection of their article.
3. On average, how much time do researchers spend on dissemination activities?
   a. More than 10%
   b. Less than 10%
   c. More than 20%
   d. Less than 20%

TIME TO REFLECT

O'Connor, S., Yan, Y., Thilo, F.J.S., et al., 2023. Artificial intelligence in nursing and midwifery: a systematic review. J. Clin. Nurs. 32, 2951–2968. doi:10.1111/jocn.16478

Aim: Topically, the aim of the systematic review (see Chapter 3) study by O'Connor et al (2023) was to synthesise the current literature related to the use of artificial intelligence (AI) in nursing and midwifery.

Objectives: To identify potential benefits where AI techniques were applied in real-world nursing and midwifery settings.

Design: One hundred and forty articles were included in the systematic review. Nurses' and midwives' involvement in AI varied, with some taking an active role in testing, using or evaluating AI-based technologies; however, many studies did not include either profession. AI was mainly applied in clinical practice to direct patient care (n = 115, 82.14%), with fewer studies focusing on administration and management (n = 21, 15.00%) or education (n = 4, 2.85%). Benefits reported were primarily potential, as most studies trained and tested AI algorithms. Only a handful (n = 8, 7.14%) reported actual benefits when AI techniques were applied in real-world settings.

Reflect on the following:

- Do you know of the use of AI in clinical settings? What is it being used for? What are the ethical, legal and social implications for the use of AI in healthcare?
- The review states 'Curricula need to be developed to educate the professions about AI, so they can lead and participate in these digital initiatives in healthcare.' What is the current national situation, across Australasian higher education institutions, on the use of AI across undergraduate and postgraduate programs—both for teaching and for assessments?

Questions

Reflect on the information given and answer the questions:

- What was the review design?
- Does the review offer useful insight as to where current and future primary research related to AI in nursing and midwifery could be conducted? If so, is this happening already? What does it look like?

4. All published nursing and midwifery research findings are important because:
   a. it is important to implement them in the practice area
   b. they encourage all nurses to conduct research
   c. they add to the sum of nursing and midwifery knowledge
   d. they provide an outlet for good writing skills.
5. The Excellence in Research for Australia (ERA) and the Performance-Based Research Funding (PBRF) exercise in New Zealand have:
   a. made it easier to publish research
   b. highlighted the importance of nursing and midwifery research
   c. made research findings more credible
   d. asserted the prominence of measures of impact in relation to research outcomes.
6. The most common styles of referencing are:
   a. Harvard, APA and Vancouver
   b. Yale, APA and Ottawa
   c. West Point, APA and Toronto
   d. UCLA, APA and Ontario.
7. Undergraduate nursing and midwifery students should welcome the opportunity to participate in a research study because:
   a. they can then write their own research proposal
   b. they can meet other nurses and midwives doing research
   c. they can learn, at first-hand, aspects of the research process
   d. they can tell their colleagues about it.
8. It is helpful to consult colleagues who have research publication experience when you have started writing an article because:
   a. you can tell them all about your research
   b. they will probably enjoy the opportunity to share their knowledge and experience with you
   c. they can point out the weaknesses in your article
   d. the journal editor wants to know that you have had help with your article.
9. One of the main barriers to dissemination is where researchers 'put off' or delay the writing up of their study findings. This is called:
   a. withdrawal
   b. pre-emption
   c. procrastination
   d. effect heuristic.

For further content associated with this chapter visit: https://evolve.elsevier.com/cs/product/9780729596794?role=student

ADDITIONAL RESOURCES

International Academy of Nursing Editors. Writing for publication. https://nursingeditors.com/resources/writing-for-publication/.

International Committee of Medical Journal Editors (ICMJE). ICMJE meets to refine its *Recommendations for the Conduct, Reporting, Editing and Publication of Scholarly Work in Medical Journals*. https://www.icmje.org/.

Royal College of Nursing (UK). Getting your research published. https://www.rcn.org.uk/Professional-Development/research-and-innovation/Get-a-research-paper-published.

REFERENCES

Archibald, M., Makinde, S., Tongol, N., et al., 2023. Experiences and priorities in youth and family mental health: protocol for an arts-based priority-setting focus group study. JMIR Res. Protoc. 12 (1), e50208. doi:10.2196/50208

Bomar, P.J., 2014. How to create a 'writing tool box' for scholars writing in English as a second language. Int. J. Nurs. Pract. 20, 1–8.

Browne, N.T., 2014. Writing for nursing publication. J. Pediatr. Surg. Nurs. 3 (2), 51–57.

Brownson, R.C., Jacobs, J.A., Tabak, R.G., et al., 2013. Designing for dissemination among public health researchers: findings from a national survey in the United States. Am. J. Public Health 103, 1693–1699.

Clark, A.M., Thompson, D.R., 2012. Making good choices about publishing in the journal jungle. J. Adv. Nurs. 70, 2373–2375.

Davidhizar, R., Dowd, S.D., Harris, A., 2006. Evaluating and choosing journals and editors – a guide for authors. Nurse Author Ed. 16 (1), 1–3.

Draper, J., 2021. Writing a conference abstract and paper. In: Holland, K., Watson, R. (Eds.), Writing for Publication in Nursing and Healthcare: getting it right, second ed. Wiley-Blackwell, Oxford, UK, pp. 24–43.

Eckert, M., Rickard, C.M., Forsythe, D., et al., 2022. Harnessing the nursing and midwifery workforce to boost Australia's clinical research impact. Med. J. Aus. 217 (10), 514.

Ferguson, C., Jackson, D., 2014. If it's posted, is it published? Intellectual property, conference and social media. Collegian 21, 79–80.

Gee, R.M., 2011. Writing for publication: a scholars' group approach. Nurse Author Ed. 21 (3), 1–4.

Gimenez, J., 2024. Writing for Nursing and Midwifery Students, fourth ed. Bloomsbury Publishing, London, UK.

Griffiths, P., 2014. Open access publication & the International Journal of Nursing Studies: all that glitters is not gold. Int. J Nurs. Stud. 51, 689–690.

Grympna, S., 2007. Publish or perish: confessions of a new academic. Nurse Author Ed. 17, 1–3.

Hanrahan, K., Marlow, K.L., Aldich, C., et al., 2010. Dissemination of Nursing Knowledge: tips and resources. University of Iowa College of Nursing, Iowa City.

Hawkes, S.J., Turner, K.M., Derouin, A.L., et al., 2016. Writing across the curriculum: strategies to improve the writing skills of nursing students. Nurs. Forum 5 (4), 261–267.

Hayter, M., 2021. Writing for publication: turning assignments into publishable works. In: Holland, K., Watson, R. (Eds.), Writing for Publication in Nursing and Healthcare: getting it right, second ed, Wiley-Blackwell, Oxford, UK, pp. 122–143.

Heinrich, K.T., 2011. Chunk it: how to turn large written projects into articles. Nurse Author Ed. 21 (3), 4–7.

Holland, K., Watson, R. (Eds.), 2021. Writing for Publication in Nursing and Healthcare: getting it right, second ed. Wiley-Blackwell, Oxford, UK.

Leeman, J., Jackson, B., Sandelowski, M., 2006. An evaluation of how well research reports facilitate the use of findings in practice. J. Nurs. Scholarsh. 38, 171–177.

Mitchell, K.M., 2018. Constructing writing practices in nursing. J. Nurs. Educ. 57 (7), 399-407. doi:10.3928/01484834-20180618-04

Murphy, P., Cowman, S., 2012. The World Wide Web and its potential for publication. In: Holland, K., Watson, R. (Eds.), Writing for Publication in Nursing and Healthcare: getting it right. Wiley-Blackwell, Oxford, UK, pp. 209–223.

Murray, R., 2009. Writing for Academic Journals, second ed. Open University Press, Milton Keynes, Berks.

O'Connor, S., Odewusi, T., Mason-Smith, P., et al., 2022. Digital professionalism on social media: the opinions of undergraduate nursing students, Nurse Educ. Today 111, 105322. doi:10.1016/j.nedt.2022.105322

O'Connor, S., Yan, Y., Thilo, F.J.S., et al., 2023. Artificial intelligence in nursing and midwifery: a systematic review. J. Clin. Nurs. 32, 2951–2968. doi:10.1111/jocn.16478

Oermann, M.H., Hayes, J.C. 2018. Writing for Publication in Nursing, fourth ed. Springer, New York.

Shellenbarger, T., Gazza, E.A., Hunker, D.F., 2018. Advancing scholarly writing of Baccalaureate nursing students using the knowledge, skills, and attitude self-assessment for writing development. Nurse Educ. Today 69, 109–112.

Silver, J., 2009. Secrets of successful writers. Nurse Author Ed. 19 (4), 9–12.

Tornwall, J., McDaniel, J., 2022. Key strategies in scholarly writing instruction for Doctor of Nursing practice students: a Q-methodology study. Nurse Educ. Today 108, 105192. doi:10.1016/j.nedt.2021.105192

Walsh, D., Downe, S., 2006. Appraising the quality of qualitative research. Midwifery 22, 108–119.

Watson, R., 2021a. The basics of writing for publication and the steps to success: getting started. In: Holland, K., Watson, R. (Eds.), Writing for Publication in Nursing and Healthcare: getting it right, second ed. Wiley-Blackwell, Oxford, UK, pp. 7–22.

Watson, R., 2021b. Open access and open science. In: Holland, K., Watson, R. (Eds.), Writing for Publication in Nursing and Healthcare: getting it right, second ed. Wiley-Blackwell, Oxford, UK, pp. 202–215.

Wiley, 2016. Writing for Publication: an easy-to-follow guide for nurses. Wiley-Blackwell, Hoboken, NJ. Retrieved from: https://onlinelibrary.wiley.com/pb-assets/assets/14667657/Writing_for_Publication-1509467251000.pdf.

Williams, B., 2015. Support for nurses in writing for publication. Nurs. Times 11 (9), 15–17.

19

A Research Project Journey: From Conception to Completion

Elizabeth Brogan and Jane Maguire

LEARNING OUTCOMES

By the end of this chapter, you should be able to:

- understand the application of mixed-methods approach (see Chapter 12) used in research projects
- identify how to plan a research project in a logically structured and sequenced manner—from start to the end
- understand how teams work together to define and achieve common project research goals
- appreciate how findings and results are used, and influence and impact health professionals in different health-related settings
- understand an entire research project from design to dissemination and be able to articulate the details of the project to appreciate the constituent parts that make up the whole process.

KEY TERMS

Behaviour Change Wheel, p. 330
COM-B model, p. 332
experienced nurse, p. 331
healthcare research, p. 330
mixed-methods research (MMR), p. 329
new graduate nurses, p. 329
qualitative research, p. 333
quantitative research, p. 333
research project, p. 329
transition to practice program (TPP), p. 330

INTRODUCTION

The purpose of this final chapter is to enhance what other authors have written about in the 18 previous chapters by detailing a recent mixed-methods **research project** from the beginning research idea through to eventual dissemination of findings. When the first draft of this chapter was written in early 2023, the project had been completed for 24 months and several publications produced. The chronological sequence of events and the details of this project are presented here. The project used both quantitative and qualitative methodologies within the mixed-methods (MM) design approach (see Chapter 12) and therefore aligns closely with most of the chapter topics in this textbook. Specifically, this chapter reports the application of a study that used a sequential exploratory **mixed-methods research (MMR)** implemented over two phases. Fig 19.1 describes the sequential exploratory design used in the Start Healthy and Stay Healthy Intervention. Fig 19.2 describes the sequence of the study as related to the chapters in this book.

The Start Healthy and Stay Healthy Workplace Health Promotion Intervention project emerged from engagement with new graduates that included formative research that explored their *diet and physical activity* behaviours and attitudes towards *health promotion interventions.*

New graduate nurses (i.e. registered nurses with less than 12 months clinical experience) are the next generation of the nursing workforce; however, they face numerous challenges in Australia, including a population with an increased demand for high-quality healthcare, an ageing nursing workforce and a global nurse shortage (Nursing and Midwifery Board of Australia 2023,World Health Organization 2019). They also face several barriers

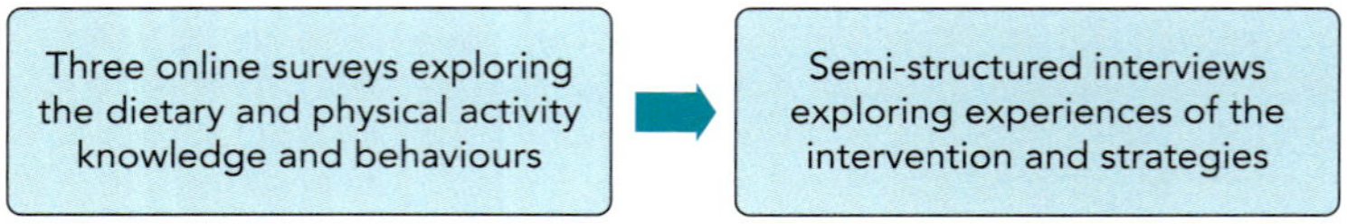

Three online surveys exploring the dietary and physical activity knowledge and behaviours	→	Semi-structured interviews exploring experiences of the intervention and strategies

Fig. 19.1 Sequential exploratory design used in Start Healthy and Stay Healthy

Methodology		Methods	Further information
Quantitative	⇨	Data collection	Chapters 8 and 9
Qualitative	⇨	Data collection	Chapters 5 and 6
Integration	⇨	Of quantitative and qualitative findings	Chapter 12

Fig. 19.2 Sequential exploratory design (Adapted from Creswell et al 2017.)

to participation in healthy dietary and physical activity behaviours during their transitional year of practice, including shift work, the regular availability of discretionary foods at the workplace and fatigue (Brogan et al 2021, Gifkins et al 2018).

A preliminary review of the relevant literature identified that most research focused on diet and physical activity behaviour of nurses, along with workplace health promotion interventions designed to improve nurses' health behaviours (Lavoie-Tremblay et al 2014, Torquati et al 2017, Tucker et al 2011). None of the review studies focused specifically on the diet and physical activity behaviours of new graduate nurses or delivered targeted diet and physical activity workplace health promotion interventions for this cohort. Therefore, this study sought to examine the diet and physical activity behaviours of new graduate nurses and implement a workplace health promotion intervention embedded into a **transition to practice program (TPP)** to assist new graduate nurses to adopt and maintain healthy lifestyle behaviours from career commencement.

The Start Healthy and Stay Healthy intervention is informed by the **Behaviour Change Wheel**, and aimed to assist new graduate nurses working in one Australian Local Health District to establish healthy dietary and physical activity behaviours. Briefly, it included face-to-face education sessions, the use of a fitness tracker and twice-weekly messages. Participants completed three online surveys: at orientation, 6 weeks and 6 months. A subsample participated in semistructured interviews to explore their experience of the intervention.

THE STUDY PROJECT—CHAPTER-BY-CHAPTER

Chapter 1—The Significance of Nursing and Midwifery Research and Evidence-based Practice

The growth of knowledge within the nursing and midwifery discipline occurs through engagement in research projects, which then leads to translation, implementation and dissemination of findings and results.

Knowledge growth occurs via the exploration, investigation and discovery of new insights and understanding, which enables the advancement of nursing practice, promotes evidence-based practice and improves outcomes for healthcare consumers. Knowledge growth also bridges the gap between researchers and consumers of **healthcare research**, including healthcare professionals, policy makers and patients. Knowledge can be translated in many ways; for example, in this project the Start Healthy and Stay Healthy intervention was incorporated as a core element of the TPP offered by the Local Health District.

Implementation of new knowledge in nursing research is a crucial step in improving patient outcomes and changing clinical practice. Implementation involves practical application of new knowledge; this may be through pilot testing, education sessions and integration of revised clinical policies, procedures and protocols. Furthermore, the implementation of new knowledge involves a multidimensional approach, which may include education, policy changes, technological advancements and collaboration among stakeholders to ensure an effective and sustainable integration of research findings into clinical practice.

Dissemination of research findings is a critical and final stage in the research process. The significance of disseminating research findings is in sharing outcomes and research results with the broader healthcare community and beyond healthcare to policy makers and governments. It also contributes to the overall body of knowledge and facilitates healthcare professionals to remain up to date with current evidence and best-practice guidelines. In this project the findings were disseminated via conferences and manuscripts (see Chapter 18 for details).

Another key aspect of the research process is the formation of the research team, which may include researchers from across disciplines in the healthcare workforce and outside the multidisciplinary team. Other important groups to participate in research are patients, family members and caregivers both as participants and as lived-experience researchers engaged in co-design research projects. Collectively, research, professional expertise and lived-experience experts constitute 'evidence-based practice' (see Chapter 12).

This project was conducted by a team of four researchers who brought a diverse range of clinical research experience and expertise to the project. Two expert researchers and a novice or early-career researcher (ECR) were trained in the discipline of nursing and worked in the academic setting. The remaining team member was a biostatistician. The diverse clinical and research experience of this team brought together an expert nursing workforce researcher, an expert obesity and nursing researcher and an **experienced nurse** (i.e. a registered nurse with greater than 12 months clinical experience) educator who has worked closely with new graduate nurses during their transitional year of practice. The combined experience and expertise of this research team created a collaborative environment for exploring the implementation of targeted workplace health promotion interventions for new graduate nurses, while also leveraging their diverse expertise to gain a more comprehensive understanding of the topic and generate innovative solutions and recommendations for promoting healthier behaviours among new graduate nurses.

The ECR was also the project lead under the supervision of the two expert nursing researchers. One strategy to ensure the ongoing contribution of new knowledge to the disciplines of nursing and midwifery is the supervision and support of ECRs. This may occur through two pathways. The first is a formalised PhD program, as was the case in this project, or more informal mentoring of ECRs through engagement on small research projects or grant applications conducted within the academic or clinical setting. Alternatively, research teams may consist of members from the multidisciplinary healthcare team, or patients and caregivers as individuals with lived experience, as this draws on their diverse knowledge, experiences and clinical expertise.

The experience levels and professional diversity of the research team was an appropriate combination to implement a workplace health promotion intervention that supported new graduate nurses to adopt and maintain healthy diet and physical activity behaviours from career commencement. Therefore, a sound understanding of the dynamic challenges faced by new graduate nurses was a pertinent element of this process and was addressed by this research team.

RESEARCH IN BRIEF 19.1

To investigate the barriers and enablers to healthy eating and participation in regular physical activity, along with participation in workplace health programs, Brogan et al (2021) conducted a qualitative study with new graduate nurses working across a variety of clinical settings during their first year of clinical practice. Semistructured interviews informed by the socioecological model were conducted with 24 new graduate nurses. Four key themes emerged as barriers to healthy eating and physical activity; these included meal times, shift work, the work environment and work culture. High interest in engaging with workplace health promotion programs was also found. A lack of time and shift work often led to increased snacking behaviours to maintain energy; fatigue also reduced motivation to be physically active before or after work. The workplace and culture influenced the consumption of foods that were quick to consume but often nutritionally poor. Positive attitudes towards engagement with health promotion programs were also reported by participants. Overall, individual, interpersonal and organisational factors may negatively influence the diet and physical activity behaviours of new graduate nurses and the development of a targeted intervention may assist new graduate nurses to navigate these barriers to healthy behaviours.

Chapter 2—An Overview of Research Theory, Process and Design

In this project, the research theory was identified and chosen prior to commencing the study proper. The researcher chose the Behaviour Change Wheel because it provides a systematic and evidence-based approach to understanding and influencing behaviour change. In the context of workplace health promotion interventions, the Behaviour Change Wheel offers a structured framework to identify the determinants of behaviour, design appropriate interventions and evaluate their effectiveness. By using the Behaviour Change Wheel, interventions can be tailored to address the specific needs and challenges of the workplace environment, considering factors such as organisational culture, social influences and individual motivation.

At the centre of the Behaviour Change Wheel (Fig. 19.3) is the **COM-B** model, the central premise of which is that, for an individual to engage in behaviour change, they need to have the **c**apability to engage in the behaviours, the **o**pportunity to perform the behaviour and sufficient **m**otivation (Michie et al 2014 p. 59). The use of a theoretical framework is advocated by leading researchers in implementation science (Atkins et al 2017, French et al 2012, Michie & West 2013) as well as the UK's Research Council for the development and implementation of complex interventions (Campbell et al 2000, Craig et al 2008, Moore et al 2015).

In this study, the Behaviour Change Wheel was used to systematically select appropriate behaviours and strategies for implementation into Start Healthy and Stay Healthy intervention. The Behaviour Change Wheel was used to inform the selection of the target behaviours, namely diet and physical activity, along with the intervention strategies, specifically three face-to-face education sessions, twice-weekly text messages and the provision of an activity tracker (Fitbit Flex2™). The Behaviour Change Wheel also guided the selection of policy options to ensure stakeholder engagement within the Local Health District.

This theory was coupled with the process of MMR design (see Chapter 12) because it allows for a comprehensive understanding of the research topic. By incorporating the chosen theory within an MMR design, researchers can gather quantitative data to examine patterns, trends and statistical relationships, while also exploring qualitative data to capture rich, contextual information, individual experiences and in-depth perspectives (Creswell et al 2018, Halcomb & Andrews 2009).

During the planning stages of this project an MMR approach was selected, specifically a sequential exploratory design. This design was chosen as it enabled the research team to explore in depth the feasibility of embedding a workplace health promotion intervention into an existing TPP, while also examining the acceptability of the intervention and its strategies to support the participants to adopt and maintain healthy dietary and physical activity behaviours during their transition year of practice.

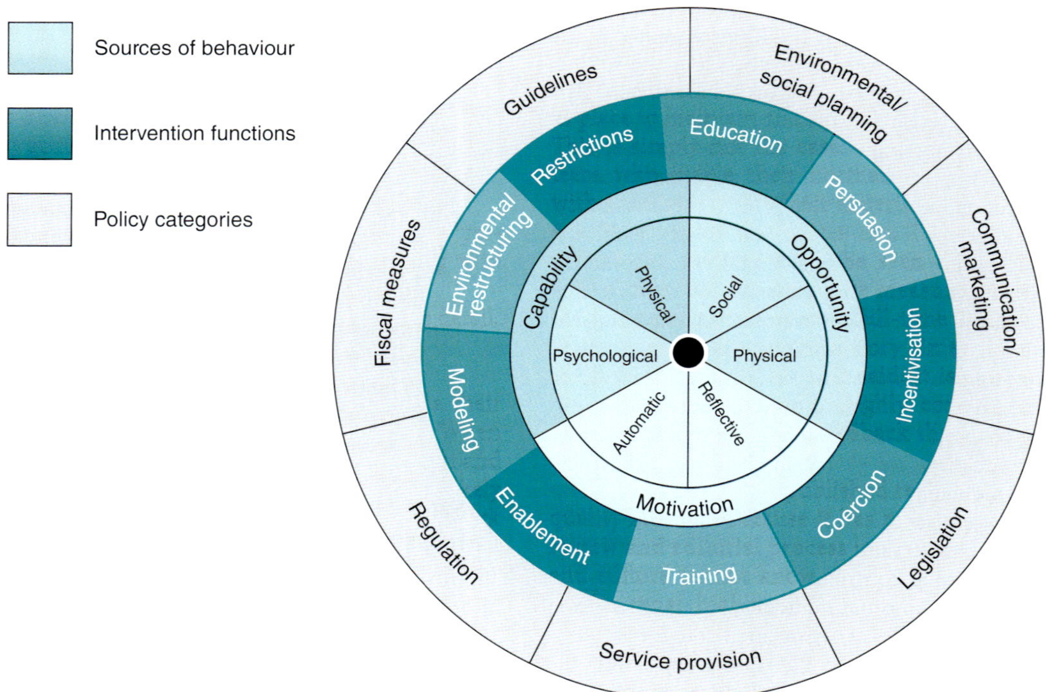

Fig. 19.3 The Behaviour Change Wheel: a system for selecting interventions and policies from an analysis of behaviour (From Michie & West 2012, with permission.)

Sequential exploratory designs are increasingly being used in healthcare research as they enable the researchers to answer complex questions, which may not be answered using quantitative or qualitative methods alone (Creswell et al 2018, Halcomb & Andrews 2009). Another important aspect of MMR is the priority assigned to the **quantitative research** and **qualitative research** components (Andrew & Halcomb 2009, Creswell & Plano Clark 2017) (see Chapter 12).

In this project, equal priority was given to the quantitative and qualitative data, as the project explored the feasibility and acceptability of the Start Healthy and Stay Healthy intervention (see Fig. 19.1). Data integration is central to MMR, as part of sequential exploratory design data integration occurs after analysis of the quantitative and qualitative data sets (Andrew & Halcomb 2009). For this study, data integration was the final stage of analysis of the findings and occurred after the completion of separate quantitative and qualitative data analysis; data integration also guided the discussion of the research findings.

TUTORIAL TRIGGER 19.1

Imagine that you wanted to conduct a similar project using a mixed-methods approach and a nursing lead team. What workplace issue would interest you the most? What type of methodologies and methods would you be most likely to adopt? Who would you be likely to include in your research team?

Chapter 3—Searching and Reviewing the Research Literature

All projects require a critical review of the literature to be conducted at various time-points along the research project process. For example, the problem being investigated requires a preliminary literature review to gain a comprehensive understanding of the existing knowledge and research related to the topic. Conducting a literature review helps researchers identify the gaps, trends and key findings in previous studies while avoiding duplicating previous research. This is typically followed by a more comprehensive, systematic approach review and may be a scoping review, narrative review or a systematic review. This is needed to clearly define the existing evidence base for the problem or phenomenon being explored or investigated. In addition, this supports the rationale for the project and its aims and choice of methodology.

In this exemplar project, an initial search of the literature was conducted to summarise what was already known regarding workplace health promotion programs that targeted nurses. Two systematic reviews were found: the first, conducted by Chan and Perry (2012), found only three interventions that targeted nurse's health behaviours and only one aimed to increase physical fitness (Yuan et al 2009); a second review, conducted by Torquati et al (2017), identified nine studies that targeted the diet and physical activity behaviours of registered nurses, assistants in nursing and student nurses. However, neither of these reviews identified any studies that specifically targeted the diet and physical activity behaviours of new graduate nurses, nor did they implement a workplace health promotion intervention to support them to develop healthy behaviours during their transition year of practice.

Despite the provision of targeted health promotion interventions for registered nurses, the literature did highlight the lack of a targeted workplace health promotion intervention for new graduate nurses during their transitional year of practice. This information helped to inform and prepare a comprehensive review of the literature, examining workplace health promotion interventions among non-nursing and nursing populations.

Three databases (CINAHL, Medline and Scopus) were searched using MeSH terms keywords and free text to identify eligible studies. Keyword searches covered common terms used in the workplace and health promotion literature (e.g. workplace health promotion program, workplace health promotion intervention, lifestyle intervention, diet, physical activity, and diet and physical activity). A second search was conducted using the list of identified key terms across all three databases, and finally a manual search of the relevant reference list and reviews was conducted. The inclusion criteria were focused on interventions conducted at workplaces, adults aged over 18, involving registered nurses and targeting diet, physical activity singularly or in combination, and published in English between 2008 and 2020. All study types were eligible for inclusion (quantitative, qualitative and mixed-methods research).

The Mixed-Methods Appraisal Tool (MMAT) (Hong et al 2018) was used to assess the various study designs including randomised, non-randomised and qualitative studies. The quality of included studies varied, with high scores associated with implementing the intervention as planned, participants being representative of the target population and appropriate data collection tools used to measure whether a change in behaviour occurred. Overall, the critical appraisal found some evidence that interventions which targeted the diet and physical activity behaviours of non-nursing and nursing populations were associated with positive behavioural change (Gilson et al 2013, Lavoie-Tremblay et al 2014, Tucker et al 2011).

Chapter 4—Identifying Research Ideas, Questions, Statements and Hypotheses

In addition to the extant literature in the case of nursing and midwifery disciplines, there may be other clinical concerns that are driving the need for research inquiry. In this project, the preliminary idea for this research study evolved from the researcher's perspective and experience. This was a clinical career working with new graduate nurses and delivering TPPs. During this time a deterioration in the health behaviours of some new graduates was noted. The researcher was driven to find a solution to support new graduate nurses during their transitional year. It was considered possible to implement a workplace health promotion program that would assist new graduate nurses to start their careers in a healthy state and remain healthy.

However, before a workplace health promotion intervention could be considered, the researcher understood that it was important to conduct exploratory research with new graduate nurses to identify what, if any, barriers and enablers to participation in healthy dietary and physical activity behaviours were being experienced. This was considered the best starting point as well as exploring what graduate nurses' attitudes were towards workplace health promotion programs. Therefore, in 2016, an exploratory qualitative research was conducted (Brogan et al 2020) to answer the following research question: *'What are the barriers and enablers that influence the diet and physical activity behaviours of new graduate nurses and what are their attitudes towards engagement in workplace health promotion programs?'*

The key findings from this 2016 study indicated that shift work, a lack of time, the work environment and culture impacted on their diet and physical activity behaviours. Generally, the participants indicated they would be interested in participating in a targeted workplace health promotion program.

Informed by this research, a pilot intervention was developed and delivered during the 2017 TPP offered by a teaching hospital in Sydney NSW (Brogan et al, under review). The pilot aimed to answer the following research question: *'Would a workplace health promotion intervention that targets their diet and physical activity behaviours be acceptable to new graduate nurses?'*

Eighteen new graduate nurses agreed to participate in the study; they received a face-to-face education session delivered during their transition to practice orientation day, twice-weekly text messages, access to a private Facebook group and an activity tracker (Brogan et al, under review). The findings suggested that it was feasible to deliver the intervention, with participants reporting they found the program to be acceptable with improvements to diet and physical activity engagement reported by some participants (Brogan et al, under review).

Informed by the findings from the 2016 and 2023 studies, the larger Start Healthy and Stay Healthy Intervention was designed with the aim of answering the following question: *'What are the diet and physical activity behaviours of new graduate nurses?'* and to explore the acceptability of embedding the Start Healthy and Stay Healthy intervention into a TPP.

Frequently, within MMR designs, the overarching question is broken down into manageable components specific to the different methodologies and/or stages. In the case of this example project, the research questions for now included:

1. What is the health knowledge of new graduate nurses?
2. What are the diet and physical activity behaviours of new graduate nurses?
3. Is the delivery of a targeted workplace health promotion intervention embedded into a TPP feasible?
4. Are the intervention strategies acceptable to new graduate nurses?

Chapter 5—Common Qualitative Methods

There are numerous qualitative methods available to collect qualitative data, including observation, field notes, interviews, focus groups and descriptive non-analytical surveys. In this study, semistructured interviews and descriptive surveys were employed.

Analysis of this data is predominantly *descriptive exploratory*, with the qualitative findings used to answer the study's questions related to the acceptability of the Start Healthy and Stay Healthy intervention, and its strategies, along with any barriers experienced by participants to engagement in healthy dietary and physical activity behaviours. Descriptive exploratory methodology seeks to adopt general qualitative principles and does not require a specialised or an in-depth knowledge or the addition of further theories, frameworks or philosophies (Whitehead et al 2016). This methodology enables researchers to gather rich data that are narrative, driven from the sample population, and analysis of that data using thematic or content analysis to explore the meaning within the findings (Whitehead 2016). It can be used to assess needs, for questionnaire development, in MMR and to understand first-hand experiences, the outcomes of which might lead to further exploration (Vaismoradi et al 2013, 2016, Whitehead et al 2016).

Chapter 6— Data Collection and Sampling in Qualitative Research

The data collection phase for this research project was typical for a qualitative study, as it involved semistructured interviews with nurse participants. The text derived from these interviews forms the primary source of data for this study.

Data Collection

In the qualitative stage of the project, telephone interviews were conducted with the new graduate nurses at a prearranged time using the mobile phone numbers provided by participants and audio recorded with the consent of the participants. Data collection was guided by a set of in-depth, semistructured, open-ended questions informed by previous research conducted with new graduate nurses (Brogan et al 2021) and the review of the literature. The participants were encouraged to share their experiences of the intervention and any barriers to participation.

The audio-recorded interviews lasted between 20 and 35 minutes. Each transcript was transcribed verbatim. Verbatim transcription aims to preserve participants' experiences by using their own words without interpretation (Braun et al 2015, DePoy & Gitlin 2015). Checking, using the following questions, was undertaken by the first author to verify accuracy and to enable familiarisation with the data.

1. Was it a good approach to interview participants using their mobile phone?
2. What may have occurred to make the outcomes of the interviews different if the authors had conducted focus groups instead of semistructured interviews?

Sample

Participants from the intervention group (those who received the start healthy and stay healthy program) were purposely recruited to participate in the semistructured interviews. Congruent with a qualitative design, purposive sampling was identified as the most appropriate strategy to recruit participants who possessed the required knowledge and experience of the phenomenon under investigation (Doyle et al 2020). The recruitment strategy involved a free text invitation at the end of the 6-month survey. This method was chosen because it was a convenient and accessible way for participants to express their interest in participating in the semistructured interviews, ensuring a smooth recruitment process. Interested participants provided their mobile number, and a text message with a link to the participant information sheet and consent form was then distributed to participants. Twelve new graduates agreed to be interviewed, the majority of whom were female, and their ages ranged from 21 to 36 years, which is a representative sample of new graduate nurses.

Chapter 7—Analysing Data in Qualitative Research

There are several steps required before analysis of qualitative data should proceed. The researchers' perspective needs to be articulated and raised as a source of bias in the analysis and interpretation phase. It is impossible to completely take the researcher's own set of values and perspective away from the qualitative research process, so it is vital that the researcher's perspective is clarified and considered in terms of how it may influence that interpretation of the data.

Prior to the commencement of data analysis, the researchers in this study had to acknowledge and examine their preconceived ideas and biases towards the data, as each researcher was an experienced registered nurse and the first author had extensive experience working with and educating new graduate nurses in a previous role. To increase the researcher's objectivity, three strategies were utilised: research reflexivity, recording of field notes prior to, during and post interview, and cross-checking interpretation of results with other researchers. Reflectivity views the researchers as both an insider and an outsider occurring on a continuum and requires the researcher to monitor for the impact their personal views, bias and experiences may have on the research so as to minimise its impact on the findings (Berger 2015, Fienfter-Rosenbluh 2017).

Traditionally, recording of the notes has been recognised as an integral part of qualitative data collection, with nurse researchers using the notes as a supplementary source of data and to enhance the context for analysis (Creswell 2007, Phillippi & Lauderdale 2018). Field notes often include research impression and prompt the researcher to closely observe responses and the environment, and they facilitate the preliminary ideas for the identification of codes and themes (Phillippi & Lauderdale 2018). However, field notes and researcher reflexivity do not replace the formal transcribing, and checking of transcripts increases the depth and breadth of the researcher's understanding of the participant's experiences (Braun et al 2015). Interview recordings were transcribed by a professional company, with the first author checking each transcript against the audio recording for completeness.

The six-step model described by Braun and Clarke (2013) was used to understand the transcripts. Based on thematic analysis, this model helps to preserve the meaning of participants' words and is particularly beneficial when using the pragmatic approach of MMR. After rereading transcripts and sorting data, eight open codes were identified within the transcripts, which were further refined to three themes. The codes fell under the themes of *Influence from colleagues and peers, The work environment* and *Engagement in Start Healthy and Stay Healthy* (the intervention), and these themes represented the experiences and challenges faced by participants.

Chapter 8—Common Quantitative Methods

Common quantitative methods used in research include surveys, experiments, observational studies and secondary data analysis. For example, surveys involve collection of data through questionnaires to gather information from a sample of participants. The use of quantitative methods offers a systematic and objective approach to research, allowing for generalisability and statistical inference.

For Start Healthy and Stay Healthy, the first stage of this project comprised three online surveys distributed at baseline (orientation), 6 weeks and 6 months. The aim of the surveys was twofold: first, to assess the level of health knowledge and physical behaviours among new graduate nurses and, second, to examine whether participation in the intervention supported participants in adopting and maintaining healthy behaviours during their transitional year of practice.

The online surveys comprised five sections:

1. introduction and demographics
2. health knowledge
3. dietary intake
4. physical activity and sedentary behaviour
5. the impact of shift work on diet and physical activity.

An additional section was included in the 6-month survey: Activities during Start Health and Stay Healthy. To determine whether shift work affected the participants' diet and physical activity behaviours, they were asked at 6 weeks and 6 months, firstly, whether shift work influenced their diet or physical activity, using a yes or no response. If yes was selected, the participants were asked to select from a drop-down list of 13 options (e.g. Lack of time, No meal break, Overtime, No tearoom, Cost). Two open-ended questions were also included in the 6-week and 6-month questionnaires. These questions were informed by the formative research with new graduates described in Brogan et al (2021).

Open-ended questions, particularly those located at the end of specific sections and before further closed questions, can motivate respondents to share their thoughts freely and in their own words (Züll 2016 p. 2). Participants were asked 'Do you feel shift work has impacted on your diet or physical activity behaviours?' If they responded yes, they were then asked, 'Could you briefly describe in what ways?' using a free text box. If the participants selected 'no', they proceeded to the next section of the survey.

Chapter 9—Data Collection and Sampling in Quantitative Research

The goal of sampling is to obtain a representative sample that accurately reflects the characteristics of the population, allowing for generalisation of findings. It is important to ensure that the selected sample is representative of the population so as to enhance the external validity and generalisability of the research findings. As part of Start Healthy and Stay Healthy, convenience sampling was used to recruit participants for the quantitative phase of the study. The study was originally designed to include an intervention and a comparison group; however, when this strategy failed (see 'An unexpected hurdle' for an explanation of what went wrong during sampling and how it was overcome), it was decided to analyse the findings from the intervention group only.

As the aim of this study was to determine the feasibility of embedding the Start Healthy and Stay Healthy intervention into a TTP program in an attempt to support new graduates to participate in healthy diet and physical activity behaviours during their transitional year, a total of 99 new graduates participated in the study and 68 participants completed all three surveys. The mean age of the participants was 25.6 years; the sample was predominantly female (82%) and was born in Australia (77%).

AN UNEXPECTED HURDLE

New graduates are commencing a role that involves assimilation into a new work environment, with new responsibilities, and is often associated with changes to previous established routines and behaviours. Moreover, it is often the first time many of these nurses will work a 24/7 rotating roster including night duty. This research project intended to use an intervention/comparison group research design to measure the efficacy of the intervention. However, an unexpected hurdle with the control group presented itself, as participation with the intervention and completion of the online surveys was not a compulsory component of the TTP program.

Participants from the comparison group received the same 20-minute face-to-face education session and were then invited to complete the baseline survey. However, the response rate for the comparison group was particularly low at baseline, and remained consistently low at 6 weeks and 6 months. The investigators agreed that conducting a between-group statistical analysis was not feasible given the low numbers. Instead, group comparisons were made only among intervention group participants who had completed all three surveys. The intention was to determine the feasibility of embedding the intervention into an existing program and its effectiveness to support participants in healthy behaviours.

Quantitative data collection and study validity are crucial in nursing research, ensuring accurate and reliable findings. Careful planning of data collection methods and maintaining study validity are essential to accurately measure and represent the phenomenon under investigation. Data collection for Start Healthy and Stay Healthy occurred during the orientation session; participants were provided with a study flyer, and on the back of the flyer and the last slide of the presentation was a QR code that the participants could scan, and it would take them to the online survey. The first page of the survey included a copy of the participant information sheet, and participants were required to click 'I CONSENT' prior to commencing the survey at each of the three time-points. To encourage participants to provide honest responses regarding their dietary and physical activity behaviours, the surveys were anonymous, with participants identified by a unique ID number developed in RedCap.

The 6-week and 6-month surveys included additional sections of questions regarding shift work and the intervention strategies. The questionnaires have some limitations, including untested criterion validity, and the measures were self-reported, so were subject to recall and social desirability bias. However, the survey was pilot tested on a purposive sample of new graduates to address these limitations. Additionally, self-reported measures have been used in previous interventions targeting nurses' diet and physical activity behaviours (Happell et al 2014, Torquati et al 2018). (© 2014 Commonwealth of Australia as represented by the Department of Health and Aged Care).

Chapter 10—Assessing Measuring Instruments

The selection of instruments for the quantitative phase was informed by previous work conducted with new graduate nurses (Brogan et al 2022) and the workplace health promotion literature. The online survey consisted of questions from two tools: the *NSW Population Health Survey* (NSW Government 2018) and *Short Form of the International Physical Activity Questionnaire (IPAQ-SF)* (Craig et al 2003).

The surveys were distributed using the REDCap, an online electronic software program (Version 8.11). This software enables researchers to easily develop and disseminate data collection survey tools and directly import results into statistical packages for analyses. It is user friendly, as it requires no additional software for participants to access the survey (Harris et al 2009, Obeid et al 2013, Wright 2016).

The survey consisted of five sections: introduction and demographics, health knowledge, dietary intake, physical activity and sedentary behaviour, and the impact of shift work on diet and physical activity. An additional section was included in the 6-month survey: activities during Start Health and Stay Healthy. Each section contained a variety of questions from a 5-point Likert scale to free text options, to enable participants to record food consumption and levels of physical activity, with specific instructions provided at each question and the start of each section.

The baseline questionnaire consisted of 40 questions, and the 6-week questionnaire had 42, as it included additional questions regarding the impact of shift work on diet and physical activity. The 6-month questionnaire had 51 questions: the basic 40 questions, plus the 2 additional questions about shift work and 9 more about the activities delivered during the intervention. Questions from the 2018 NSW Health Population Survey were used to collect data on health status ($n = 2$), nutritional knowledge ($n = 5$) and dietary consumption ($n = 10$) (NSW Government 2018).

The instructions, question wording, number order and response options remain unaltered to maintain reliability. They target changes in participants' knowledge about the components of a healthy diet, any change in the participant's consumption of fruit, vegetables and breakfast, and any change to the consumption of takeaway and discretionary foods including sugar-sweetened beverages. The IPAQ-SF has been used extensively in research on physical activity (Deng et al 2008, Kurtze et al 2008, Moghaddam et al 2012). The IPAQ is freely available at https://plos.figshare.com/articles/journal_contribution/International_physical_activity_questionnaire_short_form_/21566338 and researchers do not require permission before use. For these reasons, the IPAQ-SF was used to measure the participants' engagement in physical and sedentary behaviours.

The IPAQ was used to measure the participants' engagement in walking continuously for at least 10 minutes per day and their levels of moderate and vigorous physical activity (MVPA), along with time spent sitting at each of the three time-points. Participation in MVPA was reclassified as per Australia's Physical Activity and Sedentary Behaviour Guidelines for Adults (18–65 years). Low-level physical activity is defined as 'activities that do not require any effort and [during which] conversation is possible and classified as less than 150 minutes of physical activity per week'.

Moderate intensity activities require some effort, but conversation is possible. Examples include brisk walking, swimming, social tennis, dancing etc. Vigorous activities make you breathe harder or puff and pant (depending on fitness). Examples include aerobics, jogging and many competitive sports. Accumulate 150 to 300 minutes (2½ to 5 hours) of moderate intensity physical activity or 75 to 150 minutes (1¼ to 2½ hours) of vigorous intensity physical activity, or an equivalent combination of both moderate and vigorous activities, each week. (© 2014 Commonwealth of Australia as represented by the Department of Health and Aged Care).

Chapter 11—Analysing Data in Quantitative Research

The analysis of data in quantitative research is a critical phase that enables nurses to derive meaningful insights and draw valid conclusions from their research studies. IBM SPSS Statistics 27.0, a data analysis software package, was utilised to perform quantitative data analysis for the Start Healthy and Stay Healthy project. This software provided the necessary tools and functionalities to effectively analyse the collected data, allowing for appropriate statistical analysis. Initially, for each survey, files were created to make data handling easier, and three individual data files were then merged into one database, which was used for the analysis of quantitative data, and a master codebook was developed.

Descriptive statistics were used to present demographic and outcome data for the study population. All dietary and physical activity variables were presented as categorical data, as frequency and percentages, and were analysed using Cochran's *Q*-test to determine whether there was a change over time. In the event of a statistically significant Cochran's *Q*-test, a McNemar's test was carried out between each pair of time-points: baseline versus 6 weeks, baseline versus 6 months and 6 weeks versus 6 months. McNemar's tests can be considered similar to paired *t*-tests, but are for dichotomous rather than continuous dependent variables (Pallant 2020); *p*-values of <0.05 were considered statistically significant. There was no adjustment for multiple testing, because this was an exploratory study.

Chapter 12—Mixed-Methods Research

As highlighted in Chapter 12, MMR can involve a variety of techniques and has many strengths, such as the multiple methods of triangulation and data integration that can be utilised. This project led with a quantitative phase to capture and measure the health knowledge, health behaviours and the effectiveness of the Start Healthy and Stay Healthy intervention strategies (see Fig. 19.2). A qualitative phase followed to explore in depth the participants' experience of the intervention along with barriers experienced. In accordance with a sequential mixed-methods study, quantitative data collection and analysis was completed prior to commencement of the qualitative phase and integration of the findings. Equal priority and independence were given to each data collection method and the findings from the quantitative data did not inform the collection of qualitative data.

Chapter 13—Ethical and Legal Issues in Research

Researchers have a responsibility to consider the risks and benefits for potential participants in a research project, and these must be clearly articulated as part of an ethics application prior to conducting the research project (see Chapter 13). For this study, ethical approval was sought from the Clinical Research Ethics Committee at Sydney Local Health District. The ethics application included the provision of a participant information sheet, which outlined the study's requirements, risks and benefits, a signed consent form, the data collection tools for the quantitative and qualitative phases, and participant inclusion and exclusion criteria (Box 19.1).

Participation in the study was voluntary and was not a condition of their employment as a new graduate nurse. Participants were informed they could withdraw from the study at any time without fear of consequences or negative impact on their employment. Participants were also informed that all data collected as part of the study would remain confidential and would be de-identified for the purpose of reporting the results, with quotes from the open-ended questions and interviews represented by participant ID and age only. An additional site-specific application (SSA) was submitted as part of the ethics application to seek permission for the research team to visit the four sites within the local health district.

The aim was to deliver the orientation and recruitments session, distribute the activity trackers and run the three face-to-face education sessions. It was also to contact participants via their personal mobile phones via text message twice weekly for a period of 6 months, along with contacting them to organise and conduct the semistructured interviews. Prior to the completion of each online survey (baseline, 6 weeks and 6 months), participants were provided with a brief reminder synopsis of the risks and benefits associated with survey completion; consent was then sought by asking participants to click 'I AGREE' prior to completing each survey.

For the semistructured interviews, participants were provided with a written participant information sheet and consent form prior to the interview being conducted. At the time of the interview, participants received a brief verbal synopsis of the risks and benefits, and verbal consent was obtained to perform the interview and audio record the interview. Participants were identifiable only by their participant number (the order in which the interviews were conducted) and their age. The risk of harm was

BOX 19.1 Inclusion and Exclusion Criteria

Inclusion Criteria

New graduate nurses who are employed by the Local Health District and are on the 2019 transition to practice program

Exclusion Criteria

New graduate nurses who were not employed by the Local Health District or not participating on the 2019 transition to practice program considered minimal for both the online surveys and the interviews, with the greatest risk/inconvenience being the time spent completing the survey (6–10 minutes) and the interviews (15–30 minutes).

Chapter 14—Indigenous Peoples and Research

This study did not actively aim to recruit Indigenous participants in either phase. However, it is acknowledged that within the target population of new graduate nurses there could have been Indigenous new graduate nurses, and this was also highlighted in the ethics applications. To our knowledge, no one who volunteered to participate in this study identified as being Indigenous.

Chapter 15—Applying Research Knowledge: Implementing Evidence into Practice and Policy

Over the past 10–15 years there has been an increased interest in developing workplace health promotion programs that target health behaviours. There are several reasons for increased popularity and delivery of health promotion intervention at the workplace, including its convenience as the target population is easily accessible and minimal changes to infrastructure are required, including established methods of communication for participant recruitment and follow-up (Hubley & Copeman 2018). Furthermore, the evidence suggests that a workplace health promotion program is an effective strategy to improve employees' health behaviours, including diet and physical activity (Dodson et al 2018, Hubley & Copeman 2018, Paskett et al 2016).

Interventions have also reported positive changes to experienced nurses' health behaviours (Lavoie-Tremblay et al 2014, Torquati et al 2017, Tucker et al 2011) and more recently those of new graduate nurses (Brogan et al 2022), thus highlighting the importance of not only exploring the current health behaviours of experienced and new graduate nurses but also continuing to develop and deliver workplace health promotion programs for nurses into the future to ensure they start healthy and stay healthy for the entirety of their careers.

This study implemented the Start Healthy and Stay Healthy intervention to assist new graduate nurses to establish healthy dietary and physical activity behaviours from career commencement. The findings presented here are an integration of the quantitative and the qualitative findings in line with a sequential mixed-methods study. The findings were integrated using a socioecological model and published literature. Briefly, the socioecological model developed by McLeroy et al (1998) consists of four levels: individual, interpersonal, organisational and policy, and is frequently used to develop and evaluate health promotion interventions across diverse settings and population groups, including interventions focused on diet and physical activity behaviours (Glanz & Bishop 2010, Golden & Earp 2012, Richard et al 2011).

The findings of this study revealed that, in general, new graduate nurses possessed a satisfactory level of knowledge regarding the recommended servings of fruits, vegetables and daily kilojoule intake. However, there was a notable increase in knowledge regarding physical activity guidelines observed between the baseline and 6-month assessments (Brogan et al 2022). Similarly, mixed results were found for engagement in healthy diet and physical activity behaviours, with some of the new graduates adopting and maintaining healthy behaviours, including regular consumption of fruits and low consumption of discretionary foods (Brogan et al 2022).

However, similar findings were not found for vegetable intake, with low consumption reported from baseline to 6 months; this is consistent with previous research among experienced nurses, who also did not consume the recommended serves of vegetables (Brogan et al 2022, Happell et al 2014, Malik et al 2011). Similar findings were reported for physical activity among participants with low levels of engagement in low-to-moderate physical activity; however, encouragingly some participants increased time spent walking (in leisure time) (Brogan et al 2022). This finding is consistent with previous research that found nurses generally do not engage in the regular physical activity (Chin et al 2016, Perry et al 2016, Schneider et al 2019).

Another important finding was that, within the first 6 months of employment, shift work led to fatigue that reduced the participants' ability to establish healthy dietary and physical activity behaviours. Participants reported consuming discretionary foods to boost energy levels and offset fatigue, despite an awareness of the importance of limiting consumption of these foods. This result is consistent with other studies' findings that both experienced and new nursing graduates consume discretionary foods to combat fatigue, particularly during night shift (Gifkins et al 2018, Phiri et al 2014, Power et al 2017).

Participation in healthy behaviours is not only influenced by personal factors. The findings of this study suggest that interpersonal relationships both positively and negatively influenced the participants' ability to participate in healthy dietary and physical activity behaviours and maintain engagement with the intervention. Supportive interpersonal relationships were associated with an increased sense of accountability, and this increased their desire to engage in healthy behaviours. There are similarities between the attitudes expressed by participants and those described by Power et al (2017) and Gifkins et al (2018), who found that the support of colleagues can improve engagement in healthy lifestyle behaviours among nurses. However, not all peer interactions improved the participants' dietary behaviours. The findings of this study confirm those of previous research (Phiri et al 2014, Power et al 2017) that nurses regularly consume discretionary foods within the workplace. The current study found that consumption of discretionary food increased between 6 weeks and 6 months, attributed to its frequent availability at nurses' stations and regular consumption by colleagues who were experienced nurses.

The exemplar project Start Healthy and Stay Healthy intervention and the strategies used to support new graduates to adopt and maintain healthy behaviours from career commencement reports several encouraging findings. Participants did not find the intervention to be burdensome, demonstrating its acceptability (Brogan et al 2022). A plausible explanation for this result is the intervention being embedded into the existing TPP as a standard component of the new graduate year. The feasibility and acceptability of the approach by participants has important implications for the delivery of future interventions (Boamah & Laschinger 2015, West et al 2007).

Another strength of the intervention was that it did not require participants to change too many behaviours at once or make substantial changes to their existing behaviours. Other research that used targeted interventions to produce improvements in diet and physical activity behaviours support this finding (Brunet et al 2020, Torquati et al 2018, Tucker et al 2011). Most participants indicated that the intervention helped them adopt and maintain healthy dietary behaviours and increase and/or maintain participation in regular physical activity (Brogan et al 2022).

The quantitative results reported that 75% of participants at 6 months had improvements in dietary and physical activity behaviours possibly attributed to engagement with the intervention, and this was reinforced in the qualitative findings (Brogan et al 2022). For example, the helpfulness of the intervention was related to acting as a prompt or reminder to monitor their behaviours. Finally, the intervention assisted participants to view their health as a priority during their transitional year, instead of focusing only on developing their clinical and time management skills (Brogan et al 2022).

RESEARCH IN BRIEF 19.2

In 2018, Torquati et al aimed to support nurses to promote improvements to the participants' diet and physical activity behaviours. Nurses working across two metropolitan hospitals in Australia were invited to participate in the 3-month pilot program. A total of 500 nurses were contacted and 65 nurses expressed an interest, with 47 participating in the intervention. The average age of participants was 41.4 years and they had on average 18.3 years of experience, which is representative of nursing cohorts. Most participants were registered nurses ($n = 22$), with the remaining participants including clinical nurses/nurse managers ($n = 14$), nurse educators ($n = 5$) and assistants in nursing or assistant midwives ($n = 6$). The intervention targeted diet via a study Facebook group where participants were encouraged to swap recipes, find a colleague with whom to participate in physical activity and share motivational content.

Changes to physical activity were targeted via access to an app and the provision of a pedometer. The intervention was guided by social cognitive theory, goal setting and control theory. Changes to physical activity measured using an accelerometer, and changes to diet were measured using the Food Frequency Questionnaire and the Australian Recommended Food Score. The results indicate that there was a significant increase in moderate-to-vigorous physical activity ($p = 0.1$) and an increase in daily step count ($p = 0.04$); however, no significant decrease in sedentary time was reported ($p = 0.7$) and a significant improvement to fruit and vegetable consumption was also reported ($p = 0.04$).

Feedback from participants at 3-month follow-up included that pedometers and the Facebook group were appropriate intervention strategies; however, the app was considered less useful, or participants stopped engaging with it, a short time after the intervention commenced. Post-intervention semistructured interviews were conducted with 14 participants; the findings suggested that the intervention improved their awareness of healthy dietary behaviours, but some felt that changing more than one behaviour at a time was too difficult. Overall, these findings provided further evidence that nurses need targeted health promotion interventions to assist them to engage in healthy diet and physical activity behaviours.

Chapter 16—Writing Research Proposals and Grant Applications

Writing proposals and grant applications in nursing research is an essential step to not only secure funding for research projects, but also enable nurses to conduct rigorous studies, advance knowledge in the field and ultimately improve patient care and outcomes. When developing the proposal for Start Healthy and Stay Healthy, a crucial factor to consider was that it not only constituted a workplace health promotion intervention but also formed a significant part of a PhD project. Therefore, it was imperative to create a well-defined research plan that effectively conveyed the necessity for the intervention and demonstrated the feasibility of conducting the study. In this project a research protocol was published (Brogan et al 2020).

The study protocol included an overview of the theoretical framework that informed the intervention, the study's methods including design, participants, data collection and analysis, along with the intervention design and strategies (Brogan et al 2020). The study proposal also informed the ethics application that was required to conduct the study and attend the varied sites across the Local Health District. The development of the study proposal was informed by a comprehensive search of the literature. A $5000 grant was awarded by the Local Health District to fund the intervention strategies embedded into Start Healthy and Stay Healthy.

Chapter 17—Managing a Research Project: Roles and Processes

The planning and management of a research project will begin before the first search of the literature or seeking out colleagues or external new experts to join the research team. It begins when you have that initial 'idea' and then you continue to think about that 'idea' and you develop and refine it into a topic, then a question, and finally it becomes something that is actionable and achievable. Once the preliminary thinking is completed, it is important to note that this critical 'thinking' does not end here. It will be an ongoing and vital part of conducting and managing any research project.

Scheduling and planning time to conduct the research phases includes writing up the research findings. These two stages are distinct, yet interconnected, as you will be writing during all the research phases of the project. For the Start Healthy and Stay Healthy study, there were three key components that required specific project management. First was the design and construction of the research study: defining the research question, searching the literature, selecting an appropriate methodology and well-aligned theoretical framework; also identification of the target population, sampling options, a feasible study setting, inclusion and exclusion criteria, identifying data collection tools and appropriate methods for data analysis, and finally, before commencing the study, obtaining ethical approval.

The development of a clearly articulated study protocol is an essential part of any research project to support and guide researchers to stay on track during the management of a research project. The study protocol is sometimes compared to a baker's recipe, as it outlines key elements that are required to successfully conduct the research and subsequently complete the project. It also assists researchers to avoid unnecessary or additional ingredients that will not progress the project towards completion. Another advantage of presenting a well-written study protocol is that the researcher may have the opportunity to publish the study protocol prior to publishing the findings from the research project, as was the case with the Start Healthy and Stay Healthy project (see Brogan et al 2020).

Another aspect that required project management during this study included the requirement of the first author to complete a higher degree by research. This Doctor of Philosophy had inherent requirements associated with a program of study at this level, including but not limited to hurdle requirements, milestones and submission deadlines. Each of these elements also needed to be considered when planning and reviewing the projects timeline. Lastly, the Start Healthy and Stay Healthy intervention included three distinct subphases: design and development, implementation and delivery of the intervention, which occurred for a period of 6 months, and the evaluation phase.

Start Healthy and Stay Healthy consisted of three intervention strategies and two planned intervention groups (intervention and comparison) (Brogan et al 2022). During development, regular consultation and meetings were held with the nursing executive of the Local Health District, the Workforce Education Management team and the nurse educators who have direct contact with the new graduate nurses during the delivery of the program. Obtaining stakeholder support for this project was essential because without the new graduate nurses we would have been unable to deliver the intervention or conduct the study. The intervention and comparison groups received the same 20-minute face-to-face education session during the TTP orientation day; the intervention group also were provided with three additional 20-minute face-to-face education sessions delivered during the compulsory TTP study days, twice-weekly text messages for a period of 6 months and an activity tracker (Fitbit Flex2). The text messages were delivered in an AM/PM then PM/AM schedule to ensure new graduates working night duty were not consistently awoken in the morning and they targeted their diet, physical activity, motivation and self-monitoring behaviours. The activity tracker aimed to increase their motivation to be physically active and to enable self-monitoring of behaviours. The comparison group received a one-off 1-hour mindfulness session to assist them with managing the challenges of transitioning from student to registered nurse.

Another important aspect when managing a research project is coordination and management of the research team members. For Start Healthy and Stay Healthy the team consisted of a (former) doctoral candidate and nurse academic and two nursing professors, each of whom had academic responsibilities, service responsibilities and supervision of several other PhD and Master of Research students. A key strategy when working in research teams is clear communication and allocation, and accountability for completion of tasks; this role generally resides with the research lead or chief investigator. In summary, management of the research project requires researchers to be across several different tasks and activities at any one time to ensure the project is delivered on time and within the budgetary requirements of any grant or funding received.

TUTORIAL TRIGGER 19.2

If you were putting together a research team for a project like this, who do you think should manage the project? What kind of skills or experience does that person need?

Chapter 18—Writing and Presenting Research Findings

The research project we have discussed in this chapter has been disseminated in manuscripts to peer-reviewed journals in nursing, as well as at nursing conferences. Peer-reviewed journals are considered to be higher-quality research than non-peer-reviewed journals because each manuscript is reviewed and critiqued before it is accepted for publication.

- *Qualitative findings:* One manuscript concerns the qualitative methodology, methods and findings of formative work that assisted in the development of the Start Healthy and Stay Healthy Intervention. Exploring the barriers and enablers to participation in healthy diet and physical activity behaviours formed an important part of this research project. Workplace health promotion interventions are complex to design and often difficult to implement, requiring organisational and participant buy-in to lead to the desired behaviour change. Therefore, designing an intervention without seeking the thought and opinions of the target audience can result in an intervention that does not meet the needs of the target audience; presenting the voices of those interviewed is also an essential and key consideration (Brogan et al 2020).
- *Study protocol:* Another manuscript details the study protocol phase of the project. The study design along with the theoretical framework and study intervention were provided in greater depth than can be presented in the intervention results (Brogan et al 2021).
- *Primary results:* The findings from the intervention were then published, including the diet and physical activity behaviours of new graduate nurses along with the feasibility and acceptability of the Start Healthy and Stay Healthy intervention (Brogan et al 2021).
- *Primary results of quantitative study:*
- A poster presentation (Brogan et al 2021) highlighting the intervention findings was presented at the 5th Annual Australian Nursing and Midwifery Conference on 6–7 May 2021 in Newcastle.
- Oral presentation of the qualitative formative work (Brogan et al 2020) was presented at the International ACORN & ASIORNA Conference, on 23–26 May 2018 in Adelaide.
- An oral presentation of the intervention findings (Brogan et al 2021) was also presented at Council of Deans Nursing and Midwifery (Australia and New Zealand), Sunshine Coast on 29–30 March 2022, Australian College of Operating Room Nursing Online Conference November 2022, NSW Operating Theatre Association Conference March 2023 and 19th National Nurse Education Conference Gold Coast on 7–9 June 2023.

RESEARCH IN BRIEF 19.3

The recent pandemic has had a significant impact on not only the delivery of workplace health promotion programs but also the health of the nursing workforce. Rangel et al (2023) conducted an observational study to explore diet, physical activity and sleep behaviours of nurses working rotating shifts and caring for patients during the COVID-19 pandemic. A total of 57 nurses were observed across 10 hospitals in the USA; participants wore wrist actigraphs and pedometers to measure sleep and step counts, with their diet measured via a 7-day electronic food diary. The findings indicate that participants, on average, did not meet the recommended amount of sleep with night-duty nurses ($n = 23$), sleeping significantly less compared with day nurses ($n = 34$). Both the day and night nurses reported poor dietary behaviours and just under half of day ($n = 13$) and night ($n = 8$) nurses reported not engaging in the recommended amount of physical activity. Rangel et al (2023) suggests the promotion of healthy behaviours among nurses is required—especially when the workforce faces heightened challenges such as the COVID-19 pandemic, which further limits the nurse's ability to engage in healthy behaviours.

SUMMARY

This chapter has highlighted the importance of supporting the next generation of the nursing workforce to adopt and maintain healthy behaviours from career commencement. Conducting formative work to explore the barriers and enablers, along with new graduate nurses' attitudes towards health promotion programs, enabled the research team to design and develop an intervention that was appropriate. Exploring the current diet and physical activity behaviours of new graduate nurses provided valuable insight into the changes that occur during the first 6 months of employment as a nurse. Alongside was testing the feasibility and acceptability of the Start Healthy and Stay Healthy Intervention for new graduate nurses. Workplace health promotion interventions play an important role in supporting not only new graduate nurses but all nurses to engage in healthy behaviours to ensure their longevity in the nursing profession. The Start Healthy and Stay Healthy Intervention was adopted by the Local Health District and now forms part of their TPP delivered to new graduate nurses during their first year of clinical practice.

KEY POINTS

- Research comprising both qualitative and quantitative methods is valuable, and its findings are used to further our knowledge of the role of health promotion in nursing.
- The use of an MMR approach can result in more-robust outcomes to guide the development and evaluation of workplace health promotion programs for new graduate and experienced nurses.
- This study has demonstrated the importance of supporting new graduate nurses to adopt and maintain healthy behaviours from career commencement, as healthy dietary and physical activity behaviours can be established within the first 6 months of employment.
- This study demonstrates that research which is translated into practice can be conducted by PhD students/early-career researchers with the right support and research supervision.
- We have captured the difficulties experienced during recruitment and delivery of the intervention. Specifically, the challenges of transitioning from a student to a registered nurse and the demand and negative impact of shift on new graduate nurses are important considerations for any future research projects involving this cohort. However, they are one of the most important groups in nursing because they are our future nurses, leaders and clinicians.

TIME TO REFLECT

To write the 'Research in brief' sections in this chapter, the literature was searched for relevant evidence-based resources from Australia or New Zealand. The criteria were that the articles should be written by workplace health promotion interventions and studies exploring nurses' diet and physical activity behaviours in peer-reviewed journals published within the last 7 years. More specifically, the articles should target nurses and focus on non-nursing populations when delivering workplace health promotion interventions. While a couple of articles have been mentioned in this chapter, they were primarily written by non-nurses, and this highlights the importance of nurses designing, developing and implementing targeted workplace health promotion interventions as nurses have an unique understanding of the workplace challenges and cultures that may contribute to the establishment of healthy or unhealthy behaviours by nurses. The best research questions, as with the overarching question for the project in this chapter, come from a burning desire to understand more about how to support the next generation of the nursing workforce to look after their own health from career commencement because we need our new graduate nurses to ensure we have long-term workforce sustainability and can meet the rising demand for healthcare by our ageing population and individuals with chronic disease and comorbidities.

Reflect on the following: A study from Queensland explored whether registered nurses' health behaviours were in line with the Australian Recommendations and what were the barriers to healthy lifestyle behaviours among experienced nurses (Heidke et al 2020). A cross-sectional survey of nurses working in public and private hospitals in regional Queensland was invited to complete an anonymous survey. A total of 123 nurses responded to the survey; the results indicated that 42% of participants self-rated their health as good. Only 18% of participants reported they consume five vegetables per day; however, 61.7% reported consuming two portions of fruit per day. Ninety-nine participants responded to the physical activity questions and the findings suggest that only 24% of participants engaged in the recommended 150 minutes of moderate physical activity per week. These behaviours are known risk factors for the development of chronic diseases such as obesity. The participants also reported that a lack of time and shift work negatively impacted on their ability to engage in healthy behaviours. A proportion of participants felt their personal behaviours did not have a direct influence on their ability to provide health education to patients.

Questions

1. Why is it important for nurses to engage in and role model healthy behaviours?
2. Reflect on the information given and answer these questions:
   a. What was the research design?
   b. In terms of results, why is it important to understand the current health behaviours of nurses?
   c. What is one strategy that could be implemented to increase vegetable consumption among this nursing population?

 For further content associated with this chapter visit: https://evolve.elsevier.com/cs/product/9780729596794?role=student

REFERENCES

Andrew, S., Halcomb, E., 2009. Mixed methods research for nursing and the health sciences. Wiley Online Library. Retrieved from: https://onlinelibrary.wiley.com/doi/book/10.1002/9781444316490.

Atkins, L., Francis, J., Islam, R., et al., 2017. A guide to using the Theoretical Domains Framework of behaviour change to investigate implementation problems. Implement. Sci. 12 (1), 77.

Berger, R., 2015. Now I see it, now I don't: researcher's position and reflexivity in qualitative research. Qual. Res. 15 (2), 219–234.

Boamah, S. A., Laschinger, H., 2015. The influence of areas of worklife fit and work-life interference on burnout and turnover intentions among new graduate nurses. J. Nurs. Manag. 24 (2), E164–E174. doi:10.1111/jonm.12318

Braun, V., Clarke, V., 2013. Successful Qualitative Research: a practical guide for beginners. Sage Publications, Thousand Oaks, CA.

Braun, V., Clarke, V., Terry, G., 2015. Thematic analysis. In: Rohleder, P., Lyons, A.C. (Eds.), Qualitative Research in Clinical and Health Psychology. Palgrave Macmillan, Hampshire, pp. 95–114.

Brogan, E., Duffield, C., Denney-Wilson, E., 2020. Start Healthy & Stay Healthy a workplace health promotion intervention for new graduate nurses: study protocol. Collegian 27 (5), 573–580. doi:10.1016/j.colegn.2019.12.005

Brogan, E., Rossiter, C., Duffield, C. , et al., 2021. Healthy eating and physical activity among new graduate nurses: a qualitative study of barriers and enablers during their first year of clinical practice. Collegian 28 (5), 489–497. doi:10.1016/j.colegn.2020.12.008

Brogan, E., Rossiter, C., Fethney, J., et al., 2022. Start Healthy and Stay Healthy: a workplace health promotion intervention for new graduate nurses: a mixed-methods study. J. Adv. Nurs. 78 (2), 541–556.

Brunet, J., Tulloch, H.E., Phillips, E.W., et al., 2020. Motivation predicts change in nurses' physical activity levels during a web-based worksite intervention: results from a randomized trial. J. Med. Internet Res. 22 (9), e11543.

Campbell, M., Fitzpatrick, R., Haines, A., et al., 2000. Framework for design and evaluation of complex interventions to improve health. BMJ. 321 (7262), 694–696.

Chan, C. W., Perry, L., 2012. Lifestyle health promotion interventions for the nursing workforce: a systematic review. J. Clin. Nurs. 21 (15/16), 2247–2261. doi:10.1111/j.1365-2702.2012.04213.x

Chin, D.L., Nam, S., Lee, S.-J., 2016. Occupational factors associated with obesity and leisure-time physical activity among nurses: a cross sectional study. Int. J. Nurs. Stud. 57, 60–69. doi:10.1016/j.ijnurstu.2016.01.009

Craig, C.L., Marshall, A.L., Sjostrom, M., et al., 2003. International Physical Activity Questionnaire: 12-country reliability and validity. Med. Sci. Sports Exerc. 35, 1381–1395.

Craig, P., Dieppe, P., Macintyre, S., et al., 2008. Developing and evaluating complex interventions: the new Medical Research Council guidance. BMJ. 337, a1655.

Creswell, J.W., 2007. Qualitative Inquiry and Research Design. Sage Publications, Thousand Oaks, CA.

Creswell, J.W., Plano Clark, V.L., 2017. Designing and conducting mixed methods research, third ed. Sage Publications, Thousand Oaks, CA.

Deng, H., Macfarlane, D., Thomas, G., et al., 2008. Reliability and validity of the IPAQ-Chinese: the Guangzhou Biobank Cohort study. Med. Sci. Sports Exerc. 40 (2), 303.

Department of Health, 2014. Australia's Physical Activity & Sedentary Behaviour Guidelines for Adults (18–64 years). Retrieved from: https://www.health.gov.au/resources/publications/physical-activity-and-sedentary-behaviour-guidelines-adults-18-to-64-years-fact-sheet?language=en.

DePoy, E., Gitlin, L.N., 2019. Introduction to Research-EBook: understanding and applying multiple strategies, sixth ed. Elsevier Health Sciences, Maryland Heights, MO.

Dodson, E.A., Hipp, J.A., Lee, J.A., et al., 2018. Does availability of worksite supports for physical activity differ by industry and occupation? Am. J. Health Promot. 32 (3), 517–526. doi:10.1177/0890117116668795

Doyle, L., McCabe, C., Keogh, B., et al., 2020. An overview of the qualitative descriptive design within nursing research. J. Res. Nurs. 25 (5), 443–455.

Finefter-Rosenbluh, I., 2017. Incorporating perspective taking in reflexivity: a method to enhance insider qualitative research processes. Int. J. Qual. Methods 16 (1), 1609406917703539

French, D.P., Stevenson, A., Michie, S., 2012. An intervention to increase walking requires both motivational and volitional components: a replication and extension. Psychol. Health Med. 17 (2), 127–135. doi:10.1080/13548506.2011.592843

Gifkins, J., Johnston, A., Loudoun, R., 2018. The impact of shift work on eating patterns and self-care strategies utilised by experienced and inexperienced nurses. Chronobiol. Int. 35 (6), 811–820. doi:10.1080/07420528.2018.1466790

Gilson, N.D., Faulkner, G., Murphy, M.H., et al., 2013. Walk@Work: an automated intervention to increase walking in university employees not achieving 10,000 daily steps. Prevent. Med. 56 (5), 283–287. doi:10.1016/j.ypmed.2013.01.022

Glanz, K., Bishop, D.B., 2010. The role of behavioral science theory in development and implementation of public health interventions. Ann. Rev. Public Health, 31, 399–418.

Golden, S.D., Earp, J.A.L., 2012. Social ecological approaches to individuals and their contexts: twenty years of health education & behavior health promotion interventions. Health Educ. Behav. 39 (3), 364–372.

Halcomb, E.J., Andrew, S., 2009. Practical considerations for higher degree research students undertaking mixed methods projects. Int. J. Mult. Res. Approaches 3 (2), 153–162.

Happell, B., Platania-Phung, C., Scott, D., 2011. Placing physical activity in mental health care: a leadership role for mental health nurses. Int. J. Ment. Health Nurs. 20 (5), 310–318. doi:10.1111/j.1447-0349.2010.00732.x

Happell, B., Stanton, R., Hoey, W., et al., 2014. Cardiometabolic health nursing to improve health and primary care access in community mental health consumers: baseline physical health outcomes from a randomised controlled trial. Iss. Ment. Health Nurs. 35 (2), 114–121.

Harris, P. A., Taylor, R., Thielke, R., et al. 2009. Research electronic data capture (REDCap)—a metadata-driven methodology and workflow process for providing translational research informatics support. J. Biomed. Inform. 42 (2), 377–381. doi:10.1016/j.jbi.2008.08.010

Heidke, P., Madsen, W.L., Langham, E.M., 2020. Registered nurses as role models for healthy lifestyles. Aust. J. Adv. Nurs. 37 (2), 11–18. doi:10.37464/2020.372.65

Hong, M., De Gagne, J.C., Shin, H., 2018. Social networks, health promoting behavior, and health-related quality of life in older Korean adults. Nurs. Health Sci. 20 (1), 79–88. doi:10.1111/nhs.12390.

Hubley, J., Copeman, J. 2018. Practical Health Promotion. John Wiley & Sons, New York.

Kurtze, N., Rangul, V., Hustvedt, B.-E., et al., 2008. Reliability and validity of self-reported physical activity in the Nord-Trøndelag Health Study—HUNT 1. Scand. J. Public Health 36 (1), 52–61.

Lavoie-Tremblay, M., Sounan, C., Trudel, J.G., et al., 2014. Impact of a pedometer program on nurses working in a health-promoting hospital. Health Care Manag. 33 (2), 172–180. doi:10.1097/HCM.0000000000000010

Malik, S., Blake, H., Batt, M., 2011. How healthy are our nurses? New and registered nurses compared. Br. J. Nurs. 20 (8), 489–496. doi:10.12968/bjon.2011.20.8.489

McLeroy, K.R., Bibeau, D., Steckler, A., et al., 1988. An ecological perspective on health promotion programs. Health Educ. Behav. 15 (4), 351–377. doi:10.1177/109019818801500401

Michie, S., Atkins, L., West, R., 2014. The Behaviour Change Wheel: a guide to designing interventions. Silverback, London.

Michie, S., West, R,. 2012. Behaviour change theory and evidence: a presentation to Government. Health Psychol. Rev. 7 (1), 1–22. doi:10.1080/17437199.2011.649445

Moghaddam, M.B., Aghdam, F.B., Jafarabadi, M.A., et al., 2012. The Iranian version of International Physical Activity Questionnaire (IPAQ) in Iran: content and construct validity, factor structure, internal consistency and stability. World Appl. Sci. J. 18 (8), 1073–1080. doi:10.5829/idosi.wasj.2012.18.08.754

Moore, G.F., Audrey, S., Barker, M., et al., 2015. Process evaluation of complex interventions: Medical Research Council guidance. BMJ. 350, h1258.

NSW Government, 2018. NSW Population Health Survey Questionnaire 2017. NSW Government, Sydney, NSW. Retrieved from: https://www.health.nsw.gov.au/surveys/adult/Documents/questionnaire-2017.pdf.

Nursing and Midwifery Board of Australia (NMBA), 2023. Annual Report. Retrieved from: https://www.nursingmidwiferyboard.gov.au/News/Annual-report.aspx.

Obeid, J.S., McGraw, C.A., Minor, B.L., et al., 2013. Procurement of shared data instruments for Research Electronic Data Capture (REDCap). J. Biomed. Inform. 46 (2), 259–265. doi:10.1016/j.jbi.2012.10.006

Pallant, J., 2020. SPSS survival manual: a step by step guide to data analysis using IBM SPSS, seventh ed. Routledge, London.

Paskett, E., Thompson, B., Ammerman, A. S., et al., 2016. Multi-level interventions to address health disparities show promise in improving population health. Health Aff. (Millwood) 35 (8), 1429–1434. doi:10.1377/hlthaff.2015.1360

Perry, L., Gallagher, R., Duffield, C., et al., 2016. Does nurses' health affect their intention to remain in their current position? J. Nurs. Manag. 24 (8), 1088–1097. doi:10.1111/jonm.12412

Phillippi, J., Lauderdale, J., 2018. A guide to field notes for qualitative research: context and conversation. Qual. Health Res. 28 (3), 381–388. doi:10.1177/1049732317697102

Phiri, L.P., Draper, C.E., Lambert, E.V., et al., 2014. Nurses' lifestyle behaviours, health priorities and barriers to living a healthy lifestyle: a qualitative descriptive study. BMC Nurs. 13 (1), 38. doi:10.1186/s12912-014-0038-6

Power, B.T., Kiezebrink, K., Allan, J.L., et al., 2017. Understanding perceived determinants of nurses' eating and physical activity behaviour: a theory-informed qualitative interview study. BMC Obes. 4 (1), 18.

Rangel, T., Saul, T., Bindler, R., et al., 2023. Exercise, diet, and sleep habits of nurses working full-time during the COVID-19 pandemic: an observational study. Appl. Nurs. Res. 69, 151665.

Richard, L., Gauvin, L., Raine, K., 2011. Ecological models revisited: their uses and evolution in health promotion over two decades. Ann. Rev. Public Health, 32, 307–326.

Schneider, A., Bak, M., Mahoney, C., et al., 2019. Health-related behaviours of nurses and other healthcare professionals: a cross-sectional study using the Scottish Health Survey. J. Adv. Nurs. 75 (6), 1239–1251. doi:10.1111/jan.13926

Torquati, L., Pavey, T., Kolbe-Alexander, T., et al., 2017. Promoting diet and physical activity in nurses: a systematic review. Am. J. Health Promot. 31 (1), 19–27.

Torquati, L., Kolbe-Alexander, T., Pavey, T., et al., 2018. Changing diet and physical activity in nurses: a pilot study and process evaluation highlighting challenges in workplace health promotion. J. Nutr. Educ. Behav. 50 (10), 1015–1025. doi:10.1016/j.jneb.2017.12.001

Tucker, S.J., Lanningham-Foster, L.M., Murphy, J.N., et al., 2011. Effects of a worksite physical activity intervention for hospital nurses who are working mothers. AAOHN J. 59 (9), 377–386. doi:10.3928/08910162-20110825-01

Vaismoradi, M., Turunen, H., Bondas, T., 2013. Content analysis and thematic analysis: implications for conducting a qualitative descriptive study. Nurs. Health Sci.15, 398–405.

Vaismoradi, M., Jones, J., Turunen, H., et al., 2016. Theme development in qualitative content analysis and thematic analysis. J. Nurs. Educ Pract. 6 (5), 100–110.

West, S. H., Ahern, M., Byrnes, M., et al., 2007. New graduate nurses adaptation to shift work: can we help? Collegian 14 (1), 23–30.

Whitehead, D., Dilworth, S., Higgins, I., 2016. Common qualitative methods. In: Schneider, Z., Whitehead, D., LoBiondo-Wood, G., et al. (Eds.), Nursing and Midwifery Research, Methods and Appraisal for Evidence-Based Practice, fifth ed. Elsevier, Chatswood, NSW, pp. 93–110.

World Health Organization (WHO), 1998. Health Promotion Glossary. WHO, Geneva. Retrieved from: https://www.who.int/health-topics/health-promotion#tab=tab_1.

World Health Organization (WHO), 2019. Health Workforce; Nursing and Midwifery. WHO, Geneva. Retrieved from: https://www.who.int/news-room/fact-sheets/detail/nursing-and-midwifery.

Wright, A., 2016. REDCap: a tool for the electronic capture of research data. J. Electron. Resour. Med. Libr. 13 (4), 197–201. doi:10.1080/15424065.2016.1259026

Yuan, S.-C., Chou, M.-C., Hwu, L.-J., et al., 2009. An intervention program to promote health-related physical fitness in nurses. J. Clin. Nurs.18 (10), 1404–1411. doi:10.1111/j.1365-2702.2008.02699.x

Züll, C., 2016. Open-ended questions. GESIS Survey Guidelines. GESIS – Leibniz Institute for the Social Sciences, Mannheim, Germany. doi:10.15465/gesis-sg_en_002. Retrieved from: https://www.gesis.org/fileadmin/upload/SDMwiki/Zuell_Open-Ended_Questions.pdf.

INDEX

D

E

F

J

K

L

M

Q

S

W

X

Y

Z

Fleye DESIGN

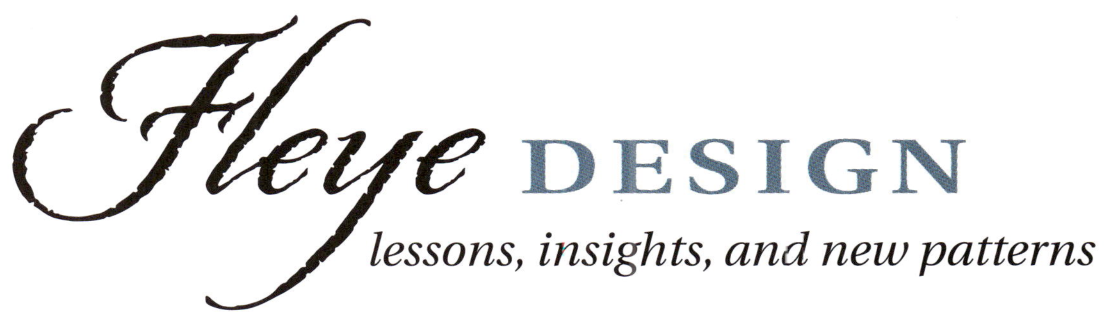

Fleye DESIGN

lessons, insights, and new patterns

BOB POPOVICS
JAY NICHOLS

Introduction by Ed Jaworowski
Foreword by Nick Curcione

STACKPOLE
BOOKS

To my wife, Alexis, for your understanding and your undying support

---

Published by
STACKPOLE BOOKS
An imprint of The Globe Pequot Publishing Group, Inc.
64 South Main Street
Essex, CT 06426
www.stackpolebooks.com

First edition

Photos by Jay Nichols and Bob Popovics unless otherwise noted
Images in "Common Baits of the Atlantic" by Richard King unless otherwise noted

Library of Congress Cataloging-in-Publication Data

Names: Popovics, Bob, author. | Nichols, Jay, author.
Title: Fleye design : lessons, insights, and new patterns / Bob Popovics, Jay Nichols ; introduction by Ed Jaworowski ; foreword by Nick Curcione.
Description: First edition. | Mechanicsburg, PA : Stackpole Books, 2016. | Includes index.
Identifiers: LCCN 2015035683 | ISBN 9780811713238
Subjects: LCSH: Fly tying. | Flies, Artificial.
Classification: LCC SH451 .P67 2016 | DDC 799.12/4—dc23 LC record available at http://lccn.loc.gov/2015035683

Printed in India

Contents

Acknowledgments

Thank you to everyone who made this book a treasured experience for me.

Jay Nichols, how did you ever stay so calm and relaxed for so long? This one's for you.

Nick Curcione, you've stood by me since the day I met you. I knew you were something special, and you never disappointed me. That says it all.

Ed Jaworowski, you're not just a friend or fishing partner, but also a brother. Your constant guidance throughout the years has been immeasurably helpful.

Lefty Kreh, you're always helping me, always caring about me, and always pointing me in the right direction. Most of all, you are always Lefty!

Richie King, you were there from my first day with a fly rod. I have learned and still learn from you. We have lots of great old memories, and it is special to see your life's work here, in "our" book.

Dave Skok, you're my favorite fly tier. I've had the privilege to watch you flourish through the years. Don't lose that Squid Fleye!

Capt. Paul Dixon, you always come through. You have been instrumental in my exposure to so much in this saltwater fly-fishing world. A true friend.

Jonny King, what a talented man you are—Princeton lawyer, jazz man, and extremely talented fly tier. In a few short years, we have shared tons of fly-tying discourse. It's been my great pleasure.

David Nelson, you're Mr. Magic at the vise, with fantastic tying creativity. You're also the best restaurateur I know.

Blane Chocklett, from the Gummy Minnow to the Game Changer, your creative energies continue to grow. You're a great person through and through.

Steve Farrar, you're one of my closest friends and tying companions. We've sat through a lot of great tying-table discussions over the years. The pleasure was all mine.

Tom Lynch and Colin Archer, your photos entertain, illustrate, and save the memories. Thank you so much.

My sincerest thanks to my friends Lance Erwin, Dick Dennis, Joe Carey, Tom Lynch, Shell E. Caris, Andy and Lily Renzetti, Rich Belanger, Jerry Siem, Ned Lunt, Rick Pope, Lou Tabory, John Abplanalp, Tom Earnhardt, Donnie Jones, Gary Graham, Bob Clouser, Dan Blanton, John Zajano, Mike Martinek, Capt. Geno Quigley, Al Quattrocchi, Capt. Jaime Boyle, Capt. Amanda Switzer, Capt. Brian Horsley and Capt. Sarah Gardner, Dr. Richard Fort, and John Kravchak. We have fished, laughed, and shared our lives together. I've been blessed with all you've done for me. Over the years, you have opened your homes to me, lent me your boats and gear, afforded me trips of a lifetime, and always welcomed my friends. I am eternally grateful.

To all the fishing clubs everywhere, thank you for sacrificing your time to promote friendship through fishing.

Finally, I want to especially thank all of you who shared in the experience of the Tuesday nights at my home in Seaside Park, New Jersey, from 1986 to 1992. You made those nights the best of my life.

Foreword

The fly-fishing world makes for some strange bedfellows. Though I've been at it for over forty years, I'm a fly tier with only mediocre talent, writing the foreword for a fly-tying book authored by one of the sport's masters, Bob Popovics. Obviously, my credentials as a fly tier were not the impetus for Bob asking me to write this foreword. Instead, it was a product of the kinds of bonds that are forged among devotees of this sport. In all the years I've spent in the fly-fishing community, I've found that participating in an activity we all love is the initial spark that draws people together. Talent is not the primary consideration within this community. What matters most is that you enjoy what you're doing.

One of the enduring attractions of fly fishing is that it is multidimensional. You can derive enormous satisfaction honing skills in any area that happens to strike your fancy: presentation strategies and casting; fish-fighting, knots, rigging, and leader construction; the ability to read the water and adapt to changing conditions; and of course, fly tying. Though his fame stems from his incredible skill and creativity at the fly-tying bench, Bob has mastered all aspects of fly fishing.

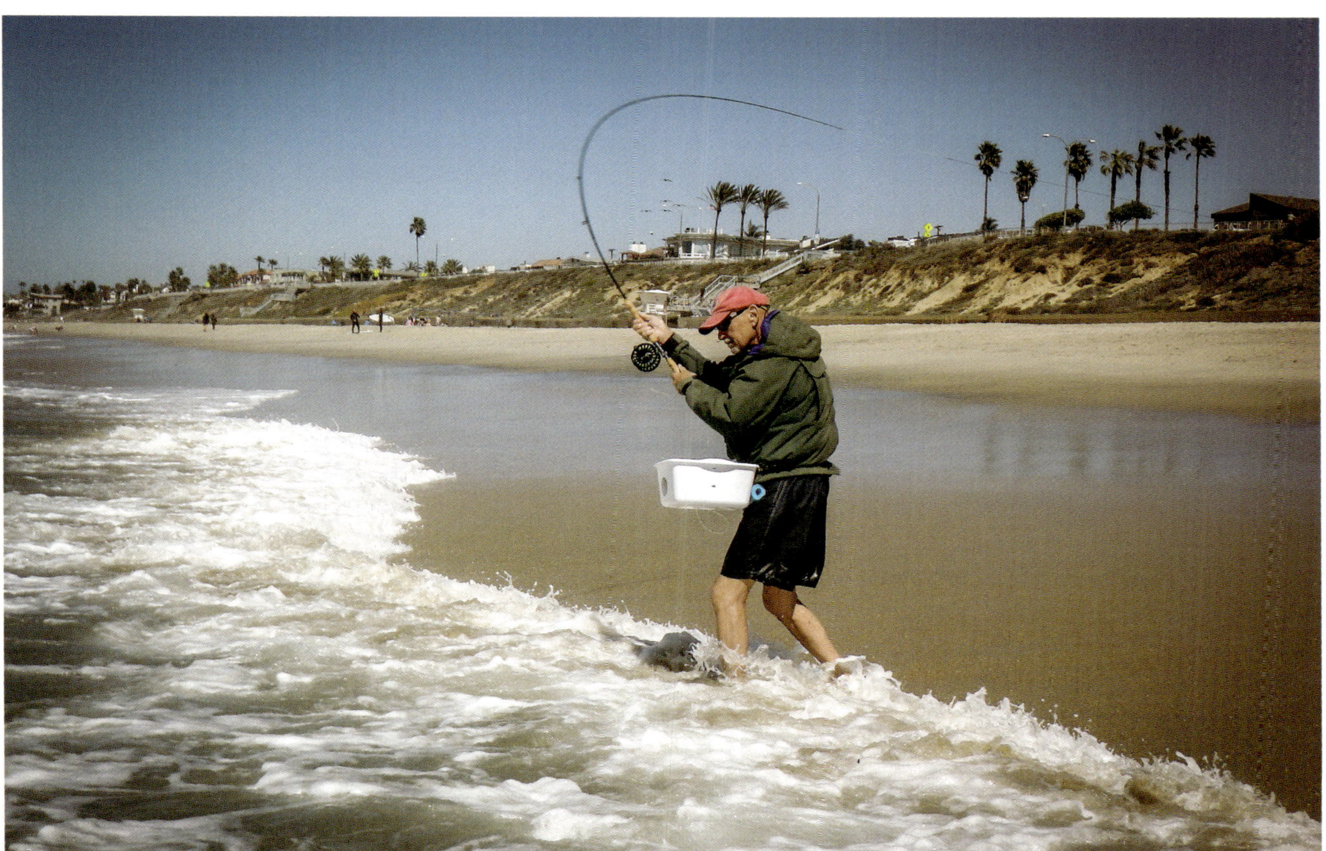

Fishing the surf where the open sea rolls in to meet the shore is a magical environment that has been a favorite of Bob's and mine from the very beginning of our fly-fishing careers. Often one of the major challenges is getting the fly the required distance, and two-handed fly rods can be a great asset. TRAVIS VAN DER LINDEN

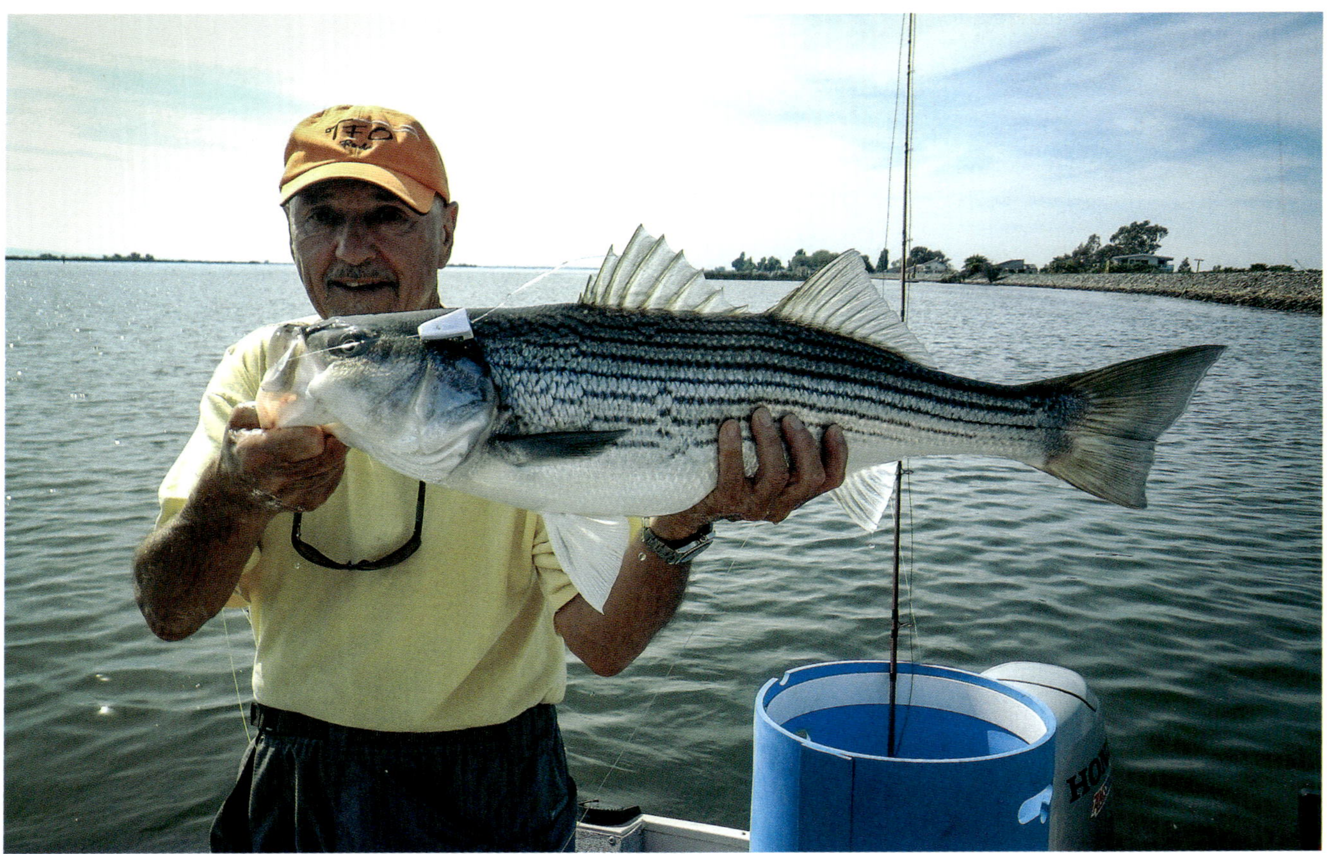

Because it has so many qualities going for it, the striped bass is one of the most sought-after species on a fly fisher's wish list. Typically it's readily accessible in both fresh and salt water practically all across the country, it can be enticed with an endless variety of offerings from your fly-tying bench, and when one engulfs your fly it can exhibit aerial displays and a pulling power that make for a very exciting contest. NICK STRELCHEK

I've stood with him on his beloved New Jersey Shore and watched him launch seemingly effortless long-range casts into howling wind. However, even though these tend to be normal conditions on his home waters, it's not all heave-and-haul with Bob. He can also execute casts with speed, accuracy, and finesse. We've logged many fun-filled trips stalking stripers in the skinny water off Martha's Vineyard and the east end of Long Island, where Bob, a hulking ex-Marine, manifests the stealth and deftness of a seasoned flats angler. Bob can also subdue fish with the best of them. On his first trip to Baja, he fought bull dorado boatside with the efficiency of someone who's fished blue water all his life.

Before I knew the man, I was aware of his flies (which he calls fleyes). I saw early versions of Bob's Surf Candy, which soon became my go-to pattern for bonito in the harbors and kelp beds of Southern California. I nailed one of my largest yellowtail ever (30-pound class) off San Benito Island on a copy of his Shady Lady Squid. Soon after, our mutual friend and mentor, Lefty Kreh, started telling me about Bob. I was anxious to meet him. The opportunity finally came at a fly show almost two decades ago. Much like Lefty, Bob is a genuine people person, and his warm, affable personality instantly drew me to him. Soon, we established a close friendship and have been fortunate to share many great times together on and off the water.

When you get to know him you will soon realize that Bob is a man of many talents, and two themes that pervade all his work are attention to detail and a relentless devotion to what he's trying to accomplish. Sit down to a meal at the Shady Rest—the restaurant that Bob owns and operates—and you'll find his philosophy reflected in everything that's served. His Fra Diavolo sauce is the best I've had anywhere, and the spare ribs will humble many maestros of the backyard barbeque. When the climate is right, linger outside and admire his rose garden. It's a work of art that he plants, prunes, and nourishes with care and commitment rivaling that of a professional botanist. Not many realize that Bob derives as much satisfaction from tending his roses as he does from working at his fly-tying desk.

However, all these credentials aside, it is Bob's imaginative, insightful, and innovative fly patterns that have earned him accolades from saltwater fly fishers all over the world. In the fly section of my book *Tug-O-War: A Fly-Fisher's Game*, I said that the one fly tier who has influenced me the most is Bob Popovics. I'm sure you could fill a phonebook with the names of people who echo the same sentiment. Not only was Bob one of the first to make innovative use of materials like epoxy (which he has now replaced with a much better product, Tuffleye) and silicone, but his patterns are designed from the beginning to be the ultimate deception, enticing fish into striking. Each fly's construction, its proportions, its movement in the water, its color, and its sink rate are designed to arouse the fish's attention.

After nearly twenty-five years of fishing these patterns, most of them the product of my own humble fly-tying efforts, I can testify that they do indeed produce results. Of all his creations, Bob's silicone series is my favorite, and I've taken species on them that run the spectrum from northern pike to sailfish. I first started fishing them in Baja, where I caught wary roosterfish. When roosters are actively feeding or being enticed with a bait-and-switch technique, they'll take many patterns. However, Siliclones are the only flies I've used that consistently draw roosters when they're simply cruising the shoreline. To me, that's the kind of test that truly reveals the effectiveness of a pattern.

Back in the days when smoking was more prevalent, I can recall instances when a cigarette butt tossed casually overboard drew an immediate response from bonito that were crashing bait on the surface. Of course, no one would jump to the conclusion that cigarette butts were a hot choice for those fish. Unfortunately, many judge flies solely on the basis of their performance during favorable conditions like these, when the fish will eat anything. But the true measure of a fly's attractive potential is if it elicits a consistent response when there is no blitz—when your quarry is being selective. It is in this latter, more common scenario that Bob's patterns have repeatedly proven themselves. This book is an invaluable guide whether you're an experienced or novice angler because it will enable to you to tie Bob's patterns for yourself. Those of you who have experienced it know full well the satisfaction derived from catching a fish on a fly that you tied. For me, the supreme compliment in this respect is when Bob picks up one of my flies and asks, "Did you tie this, Nick?"

Nick Curcione
Coronado, California, 2015

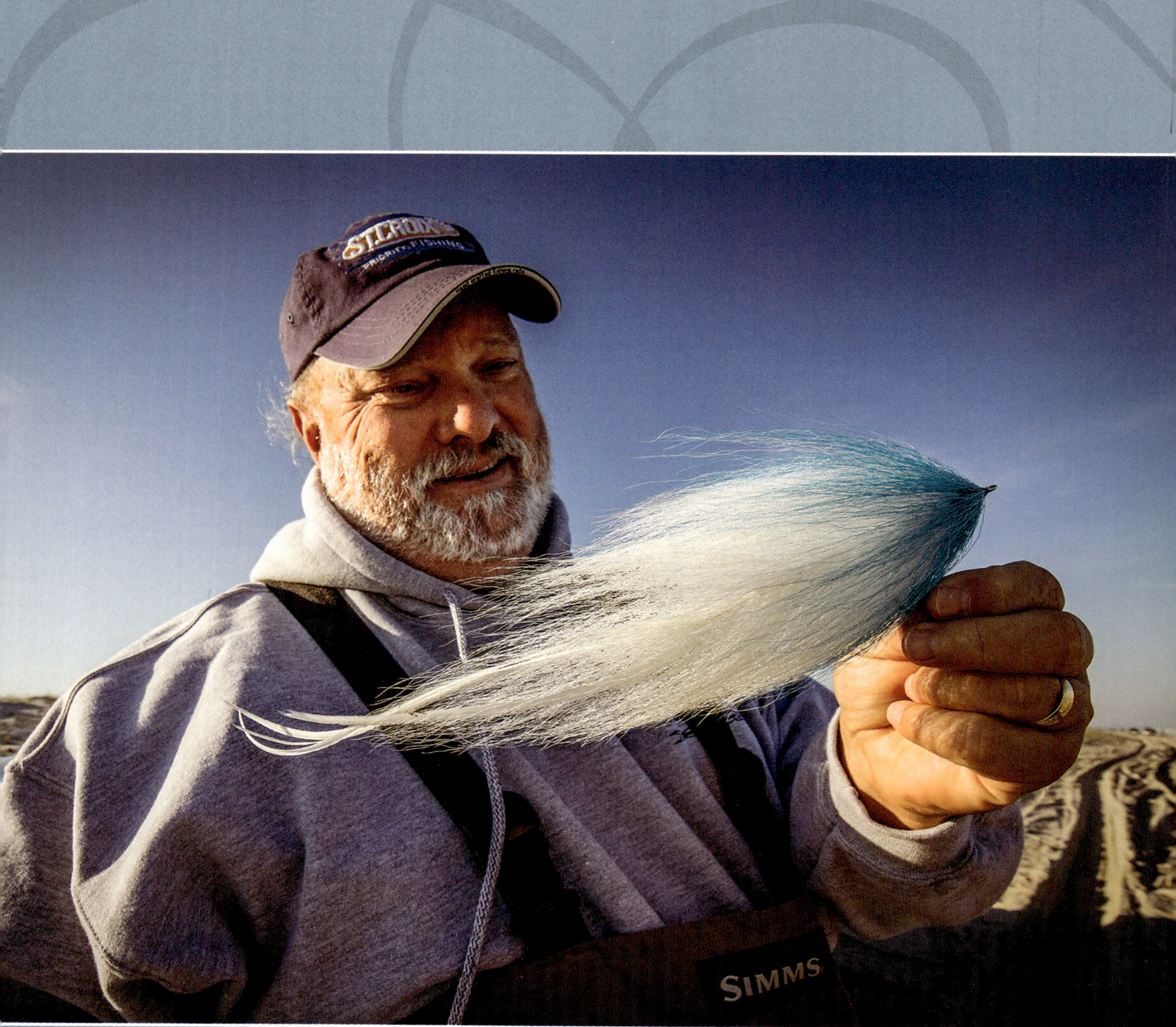

Bob checks out his Beast Fleye, Island Beach State Park, New Jersey, November 2011. "It's a beautiful fly. Has a very natural taper from shoulders to belly. It really came together well, and though the one that I am holding in the picture was still heavy, it was a start." TOM LYNCH

The Popovics School

Three of us—Bob Popovics, Bill Dickson, and I—stood on the north jetty of New Jersey's Barnegat Inlet. We had been testing and swimming flies, discussing their designs, and taking note of their behavior in the water. Bob's version of a Lefty's Deceiver showed an obvious difference from Bill's and mine. Out of the water, all of the flies showed slight variations in appearance and form, which was to be expected. However, Popovics's flies all swam with a subtle and distinctive movement. Then, as now, I'm at a loss for words to capture that look in the water. They possessed life. It wasn't just a side-to-side wiggle or shimmy; lots of flies have that. I recall asking Bill, "What is it about Bob's flies?" His answer, I came to realize, is the key to all the Pop Fleyes: "He's just seen too many baitfish."

For years, Bob had tossed a huge cast-net for mullet in the surf and developed a reputation for his skill. I recall his trying to coach me about netting—I was an abject failure at that game! While I strained to see the fish right at my feet, Bob could pick out a small pod, even one or two individual fish, working down the surf line at an incredible distance. He had a sense of form and presence, a natural and visceral awareness of baitfish structure and movement. He was simply more in touch with the nature of baitfish, and he's spent his fly-tying career sharing that gift with the rest of us. That's an important dimension of this book. He has given birth to what I can legitimately call the "Popovics school" of fly tying, for he has clearly influenced notable tiers like Jonny King, Dave Skok, Steve Farrar, David Nelson, Blane Chocklett, and others—all great in their own right.

The Popovics School of Tying

So, what defines the Popovics school? Saying that it is a way of seeing—a way of thinking—is too vague, for although it involves a mind-set, it has to be experienced. That's not a cop-out; I'm struggling to put into words that indefinable something at the heart of Pop Fleyes.

We originally applied the moniker Pop Fleyes to the earliest Surf Candies, but the term came to encompass the full range of Bob's creations, and it was the title for the first book we penned together, *Pop Fleyes*, which documented those fleyes' development. The stylized spelling emphasized the fact that eyes were a key component in most of the Pop(ovics) designs. This book, *Fleye Design*, deals not so much with the eye of the fly, but rather the eye of what Bob humorously calls the "teyer." Taper is an essential element in the concept. Bob senses and appreciates taper, whether in an individual saddle hackle, a single hair from a deer tail, a bunch of hairs, or the overall taper of the finished fly. From the start, he has been almost obsessed with what he calls the "flow" of a fly—the relationship of the various parts to one another. The whole is more than the sum of its parts, for it possesses a completeness, a unity, and a harmony that none of the parts has in itself.

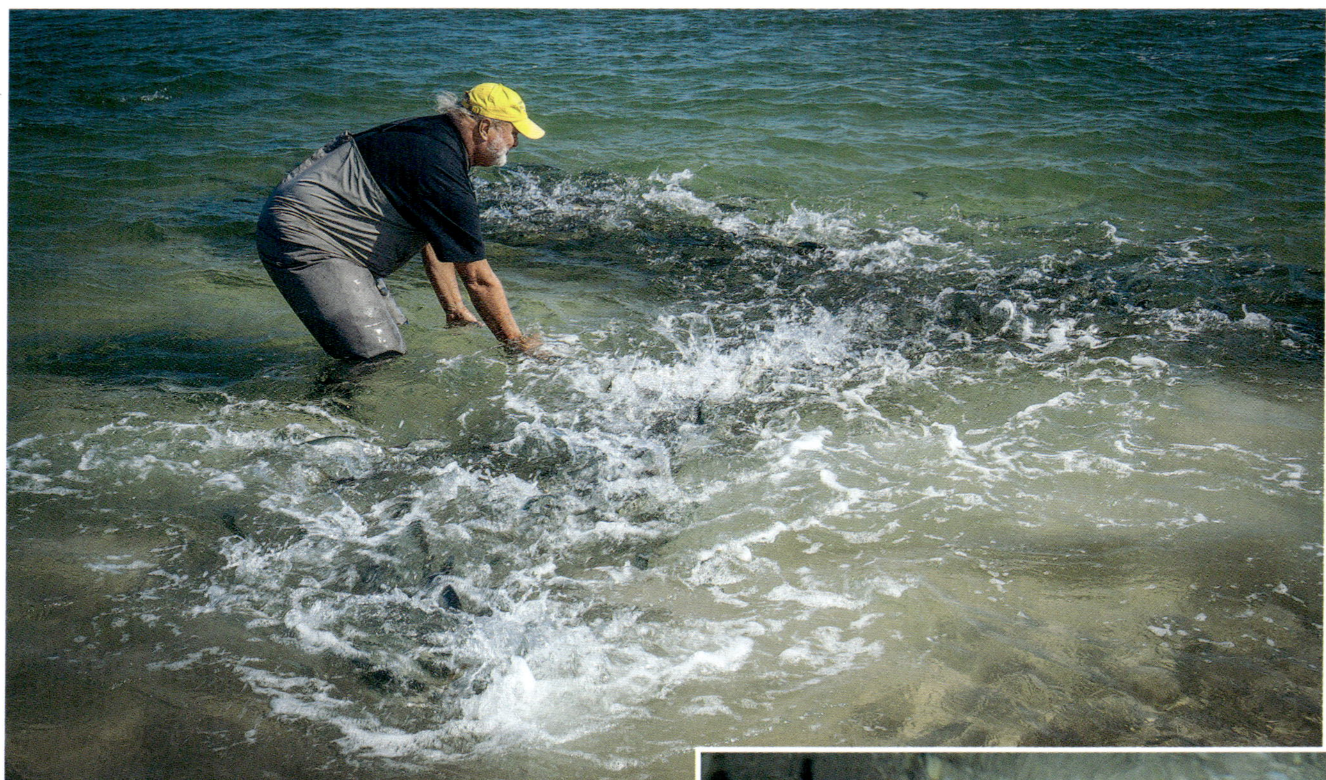

Bob loves to film fish, baitfish, and his fleyes. He began filming bluefish blitzing on bay anchovies and other baits in the 1980s. In this photo, taken in 2009, he was recording the behavior of a school of menhaden (or bunker), when a pod of jumbo bluefish suddenly rushed onto "the set" and interrupted his movie making. ED JAWOROWSKI

Right: Each Pop Fleye design is tested under fishing conditions to make sure it has the desired action in the water. I took this picture in the New Jersey surf while Bob was actually filming this large Bucktail Deceiver's movements. ED JAWOROWSKI

Historic Perspective

The Popovics school evolved through trial and error, but it has its genesis in design, and Bob's design has its roots in that natural sense of form—and life—that he gained from all those years of studying baitfish. Coupled with this talent is an uncanny sense of the potential of various tying materials. Few people, for example, appreciate the variations in the texture of bucktail fibers in terms of thickness and steepness of taper, as well as variations from different parts of the tail. Two words embody Bob's approach to tying: "What if?" *What if I tie it in at this angle, or bend it like this, perhaps splay it, or fold it back? No, that's no good; what if I do it like this?* I recall the narrator of a documentary about Leonardo da Vinci saying that if we looked at a portrait of a man and noticed that he had six fingers on his hand, most people would react to it on aesthetic grounds, saying, "It doesn't look right." But Leonardo would immediately and instinctively observe, "It won't work right." Bob has some of that.

His mind wants to go somewhere; he has a vision. But he lets the material teach his fingers how to get there. Bob toys, pokes, and prods the materials until they tell him something. It is almost maddening to watch him stroke the hair or feathers of a fly on which he is working. Stroke, stroke, stroke. Studying and stroking. "Bob, you only stroked that one twenty times. It needs a few more," I would tease. He'd smile, turn the fly this way and that, and then give it a few more strokes. Each session at the vise was a learning process, discarding this, rejecting that, but leading ultimately to *eureka*, like Thomas Edison, who said he never had a failed experiment; he simply found 10,000 ways that didn't work.

The Big Bunker

In his earliest tying experiences, Bob relied on natural materials, as few synthetics had yet been incorporated into the fly tier's arsenal. To tie a large menhaden or "bunker" fly, his first original concept, he employed two vises with a strand of stiff mono stretched between them. By flipping the bobbin around the mono, he attached numerous tufts of bucktail in succession above and below. After adding tinsel and tail feathers, he attached the mono to the hook shank. Traditional thinking dictated that the materials should be tied directly on the hook. Yet Bob saw the fly as something apart, almost as if he were fashioning a baitfish that was then impaled on a hook through its nose, akin to live-lining a herring or menhaden to entice striped bass—another type of fishing at which he excelled. He finished off the front of his fish with chenille and with more hair on the shank. Even back then, he sensed that eyes were an important component, for the Big Bunker sported heavy glass eyes.

The construction process was tedious and time-consuming, the result a bit heavy—air-resistant and unwieldy to cast—but it broke new ground. It had a wide profile, which was novel, and was a full 11 inches in length, at a time when a sleek 6-inch fly was considered large. Bob even entertained the idea of using three strands of mono: one to form the arch of the back, one the midline of the body, and one tracing the curve of the belly, all decorated with short bunches of bucktail.

Surf Candies

Years later, Bob would take one of those numerous tapered bunches of deer tail and fasten it directly onto the hook shank, with every fiber adjusted in length to create a near-perfect baitfish silhouette. This time however, his quest was for a durable facsimile of a small baitfish. Bluefish savaged bucktail and feather streamers in short order. Until then, a tier would occasionally use epoxy to protect thread wraps on conventional fly patterns, but no one had fashioned entire fly bodies of epoxy. Some had made feeble attempts, but none gained wide acceptance, because no one had persevered with the material until they learned all the subtle nuances of using it. I still marvel at Bob's early versions, most of them now yellow with age. Some had bucktail wings. A few also had long, tapered saddle hackles used in combination with the hair.

As for durability, I still remember the day Lance Erwin, one of the most talented surf anglers I know, excitedly handed Bob a fly that had accounted for more than twenty bluefish and was still producing. The bucktail was quite chewed, but the body, scarred and scraped, was intact. A light coating of Sally Hansen Hard As Nails restored the body to near-new condition. The first prototypes had emerged from the crucible of combat steeped in glory. So, the age of epoxy flies was born. Ironically, those earliest experiments didn't have eyes.

Almost immediately, however, Bob became obsessed with finding more durable wing material and seeking more realism. First, he replaced bucktail with new, translucent, synthetic hairs like Ultra Hair and Super Hair. He arrived at perfection by ignoring it until the end; he never trimmed materials to their final length until the fly was finished. Then he meticulously nipped the points of virtually every hair with the tips of his fine-pointed scissors until the fly assumed its final form. Self-sticking decal eyes, covered with a thin film of epoxy, soon replaced the painted eyes that he originally added. Anglers appreciated how the new flies realistically mimicked the translucence of certain baits like bay anchovies ("rainfish") and Atlantic silversides or spearing. Colored dyes and glitter for sparkle were mixed into the epoxy to further suggest features of the natural baits. Along the way Bob experimented with silver transfer tape and metallic silver marking pens to create reflectance reminiscent of the naturals. He eventually developed Fleye Foils to achieve these features more easily. Realism, durability, flash, translucence, subtle color blending, and tying consistency could now be readily achieved.

Subsequently, Bob perfected other innovative techniques. The Spread Fleye was simply genius. He allowed the epoxy to partially cure and set, then squeezed it between his moist finger and thumb to force it into a flat disc shape. The hairs spread out into a wide, but thin profile. This produced a great butterfish imitation instantly, obviating the need to tie in multiple pieces of hair along

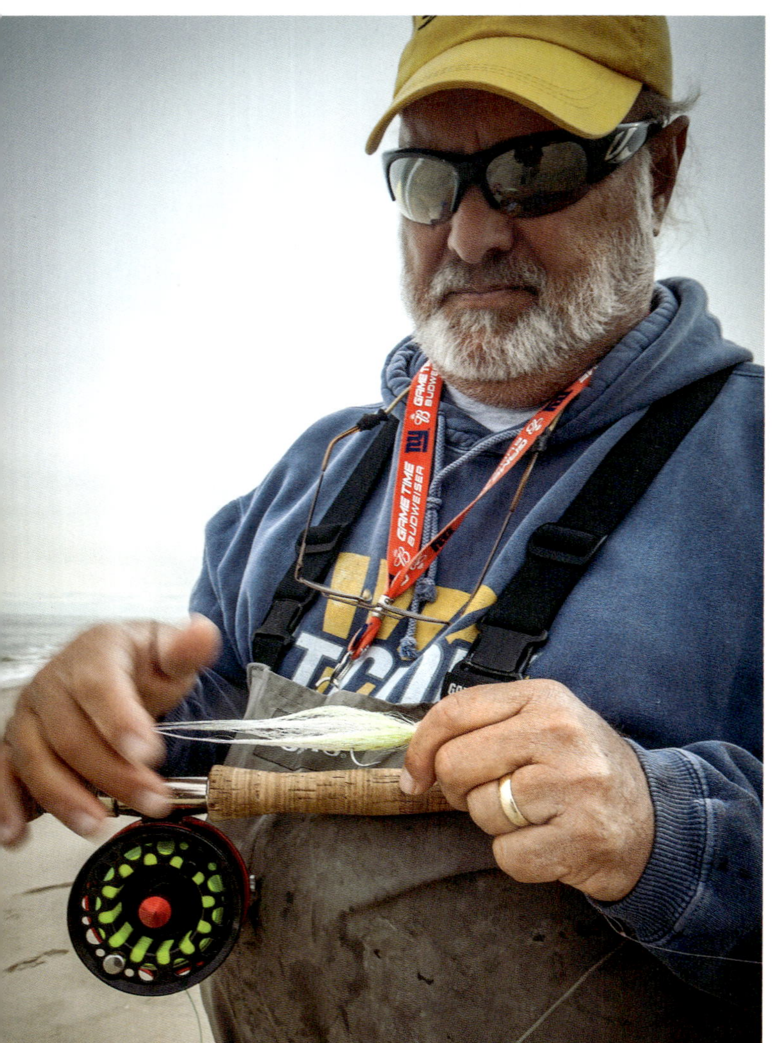

Never satisfied with his creations, Bob continually refines and modifies his designs. Although he had been tying Bucktail Deceivers since the 1990s, here in 2009, he examines how well one of his variations has stood up to the rigors of fish and the surf at Sandy Hook, New Jersey. ED JAWOROWSKI

the top and bottom of the hook shank. A more involved, but more versatile, technique was the actual sculpting of epoxy fly bodies with a dubbing needle. Although he often used a rotary drying wheel to turn flies while the epoxy cured, he understood that the cross section of flies produced in this way would always be round. He therefore resorted to holding each fly in his hand while applying or removing small amounts of epoxy here and there to thicken or thin out parts of the artificial baitfish. By turning and rotating the flies in his fingers to control the distribution of the epoxy until it set, he learned how to make flat-sided imitations to replicate wider-profile baitfish. This meticulous hand sculpting taught him the value of using five-minute epoxy, rejecting the thirty-minute variety, which, although it delayed eventual yellowing, cured far too slowly, as well as the one-minute variety, which didn't afford enough time to complete the shaping he wanted.

More than twenty-five years ago, Bob and I attended the Fly Tackle Dealers Show, held in Boston that year. I told him to bring along an assortment of his epoxy fleyes. Bob looked on, while I showed them to select exhibitors. They drew an enthusiastic response from tier after tier. With a backhand sweep, I scattered the flies across the table in front of Dick Stewart's booth. Dick, himself a great tier, was at that time editor of *American Angler* and *Fly Tyer*. He went up and down the line, fingered and studied several, and said to me tersely, "Write it up." The piece entitled "Pop Fleyes" appeared in a 1990 issue of *Fly Tyer*. The rest, as they say, is history. Plastic bodies caught on, and epoxy flies of every ilk began to appear across the country. The newly redubbed "Surf Candy," named after a colorful hard candy Bob kept in a bowl on his fly-tying table, earned its place in tying history, along with other groundbreaking innovations like Lefty's Deceiver, Clouser's Deep Minnow, the Dahlberg Diver, and the Muddler Minnow. Countless tiers since have produced their own versions, but nearly all trace their lineage back to those original Surf Candies.

I've given this somewhat detailed account of the development of epoxy flies to show that design doesn't normally evolve along a straight road; it comes in fits and starts. But Bob's well of creativity was far from dry.

Three Dimensions

One of the most significant steps in the development of Pop Fleye designs came with the concept of what we called "3D fleyes." Synthetic hairs were long, but they were uniform in thickness, lacking the taper that materials such as bucktail hair provided. Yet Bob wanted to benefit from the synthetics' translucence, variety of colors, and durability. So he tied in numerous bunches, varying in bulk and length, of the same synthetic hairs he had used in the Surf Candies, strategically placed on the top, bottom, and sides of the hook shank. He built in a head, shoulders, a broad back, rounded belly, and a thin back end.

Much as a wood-carver will draw an outline on a block of wood, then whittle away the excess material until the desired figure appears, Bob sculpted a fish from the shaggy mass of hair he had built up, deftly using the very points of his scissors. I remember thinking, as I watched him develop a realistic baitfish imitation from the raw material: *He stroked and stroked the bucktail to life; now he snips and snips the nylon hair into shape.* It was like watching a gardener shape a bonsai tree. The results were amazing. From the front, the fly tapered top to bottom. Viewed from the top, it tapered nose to tail, and from the side it revealed the natural, subtle tapers of the genuine article.

I vividly recall handling one of Bob's 3D mullet. For years, I had spent endless nights fishing for large bluefish in the New Jersey surf with whole and cut bait. Four- to six-inch white or "finger" mullet were my favorite bait. With my eyes closed, I gently squeezed and turned the fly around in my fingers, feeling the shoulders, head, and belly. I remember thinking that it felt just like a real fish. Eventually, Bob realized that the 3D fleyes were too labor-intensive and time-consuming, but they certainly gave the tier a sense of shape, taper, proportion, volume, and mass, as well as facility with the use of scissors. These valuable lessons would be put to good use as Bob continued evolving newer designs such as Bob's Banger, Schoolies, Jiggies, and Siliclones.

Siliclones

A significant example of marrying natural and synthetic components was the Siliclone, constructed of bucktail and a body of trimmed sheep fleece covered in a layer of silicone caulking. Bucktail, tied out the back and then along the sides of the hook, achieved the tapers integral to all Popovics Fleyes. The body consisted of densely packed bunches of sheep fleece trimmed to a velour-smooth texture. Over this were two layers of smooth silicone. In the way that Bob attached the bucktail and trimmed the fleece, you can recognize techniques developed and lessons learned in the Kinky Fibre and 3D fleyes: the material tied around the shank, the inner flash, the incredible scissor work.

The Siliclone was originally tied to imitate the small white mullet. The bodies and heads could be round, triangular, or any shape the tier wanted. The buoyancy of the silicone produced flies that wake semisubmerged, like the time-honored Atom plugs fished by surf casters. I had a number of successes on pitch-black nights retrieving Siliclones extremely slowly for striped bass in waters

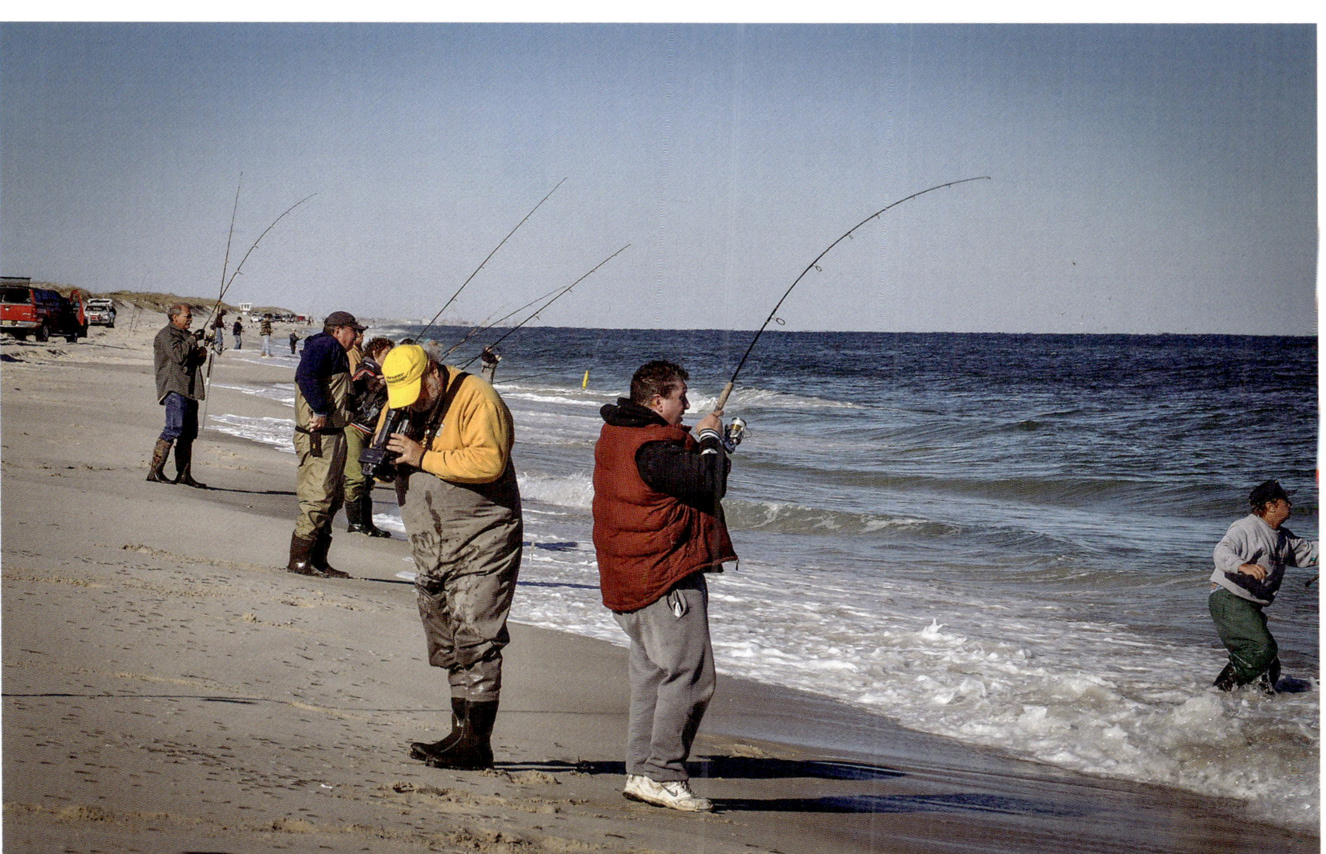

While surf fishermen are busy fighting striped bass, Bob is absorbed in filming baitfish washed onto the shore. November 2010, Island Beach State Park, New Jersey. ED JAWOROWSKI

around Sandy Hook, New Jersey. In addition to novel construction, shape, and performance, these flies offered other options. If the hollow air pockets in the fleece under the silicone gradually absorbed water, became heavy, and ran slightly deeper, you could simply squeeze out the water and restore it to a higher-floating swimming lure. If you wanted it to run a bit deeper, you could squeeze it first, then push it underwater and release the pressure. This would cause the fly to suck in water. The distinctive *splat* these flies make when they smack the surface makes them particularly attractive to striped bass in foamy whitewater around jetties. You could also repair cuts caused by toothy fish with a dab of silicone smeared over the tear. But Bob hadn't yet exhausted the potential of the Siliclone.

I vividly recall the time Bob called me and said somewhat forlornly, "Ed, I've run out of ideas."

"No you haven't, Bob, you've just temporarily run out of problems to solve."

"Well, what do we really need?"

"A fly that actually swims. Not one that simply undulates or waves in the water, but something that resembles a Rapala, Bomber, or one of those other lipped swimming plugs."

I knew tiers who had experimented with the idea, using artificial fingernails appended to the front of flies, even curved sections cut from plastic drinking cups. None were practical. I thought it would take Bob weeks or months to come up with a solution. He called me a day later and floored me when he said he had licked the problem. He immediately realized that he had been one tiny step from the solution. He fashioned a Siliclone, but instead of finishing it with a smooth, round front, he tied in an extra bunch of sheep fleece, pulled it down into a beard, coated it with more silicone, and trimmed it to shape. The lip was an integrated part of the whole fly, not a separate appendage, and the new Pop Lips worked like magic. It cut a 6-inch-wide swath as it moved enticingly side to side. It required no manipulation of rod or line, simply a constant hand-over-hand retrieve. I recall his adding rubber legs to one version and swimming it in the pool at a fly-fishing show. Observers were astounded. I have never seen any lure of any type with so much action. Everything on that fly moved.

Back to the Future

All the synthetics worked well for their purposes, yet none behaved quite the same way as natural materials, or possessed their individuality. In a sense, Bob has come full circle, moving from simplicity to complexity, and now back to a simpler form. More and more, he returns to the materials with which he began his fly-tying journey, employing the best of what past experience has taught him.

History has a way of repeating itself, but always in an altered state. Even though "Mr. Epoxy" still ties his Surf Candies, he now frequently uses Tuffleye acrylic rather than epoxy. The two materials have a number of differences. Bob had to exploit those differences to learn the potential of each. All the Pop Fleye designs of the past forty years or more have contributed something to the concepts and techniques you'll see demonstrated in the subsequent chapters of this book. This is the start of a new period of evolution.

If you have a serious interest in tying and want to benefit from the lessons that Bob has learned over the years, you are fortunate to have Bob himself as teacher. Other tying instructors will invariably say something like, "Put a hook in the vise, and tie along with me, step by step." Bob doesn't simply give "do this" instructions. He assures that everyone in the class has a clear perception of where they are headed before they take the first step. He tells a class, "Watch me tie the entire fly first, step by step." He clearly explains the how and why of each step, fielding questions on the way. Students are focused on the construction, freed from the anxiety of their own projects. By the time he completes the fly, they have a clear understanding of each component. When it comes to tying their own versions, students understand why they are to attach a material or thread precisely one-third of the way back from the eye, not halfway. They know where they are headed and how each step contributes to the whole. The lesson: have an image—a design in sight—and making whatever adjustments you must, systematically bring it to realization. I saw beginners in Bob's classes who had never tied a fly turn out results as good as anything that experienced tiers, including myself, could produce.

Obviously, that approach isn't possible in the pages of a book. However, flies are modular creations, so Bob has placed lessons in the early chapters, encouraging drills in each of the critical techniques that will be incorporated into a number of finished flies. Despite being something of a free spirit when it comes to imagination, he's disciplined in applying the principles and practicing until he gets it right. Mastering musical scales and chords, or mastering the compulsory school figures in competitive skating, are not far-fetched parallels, for they teach the components of the finished product. This kind of thoroughness and discipline owes something to Bob's

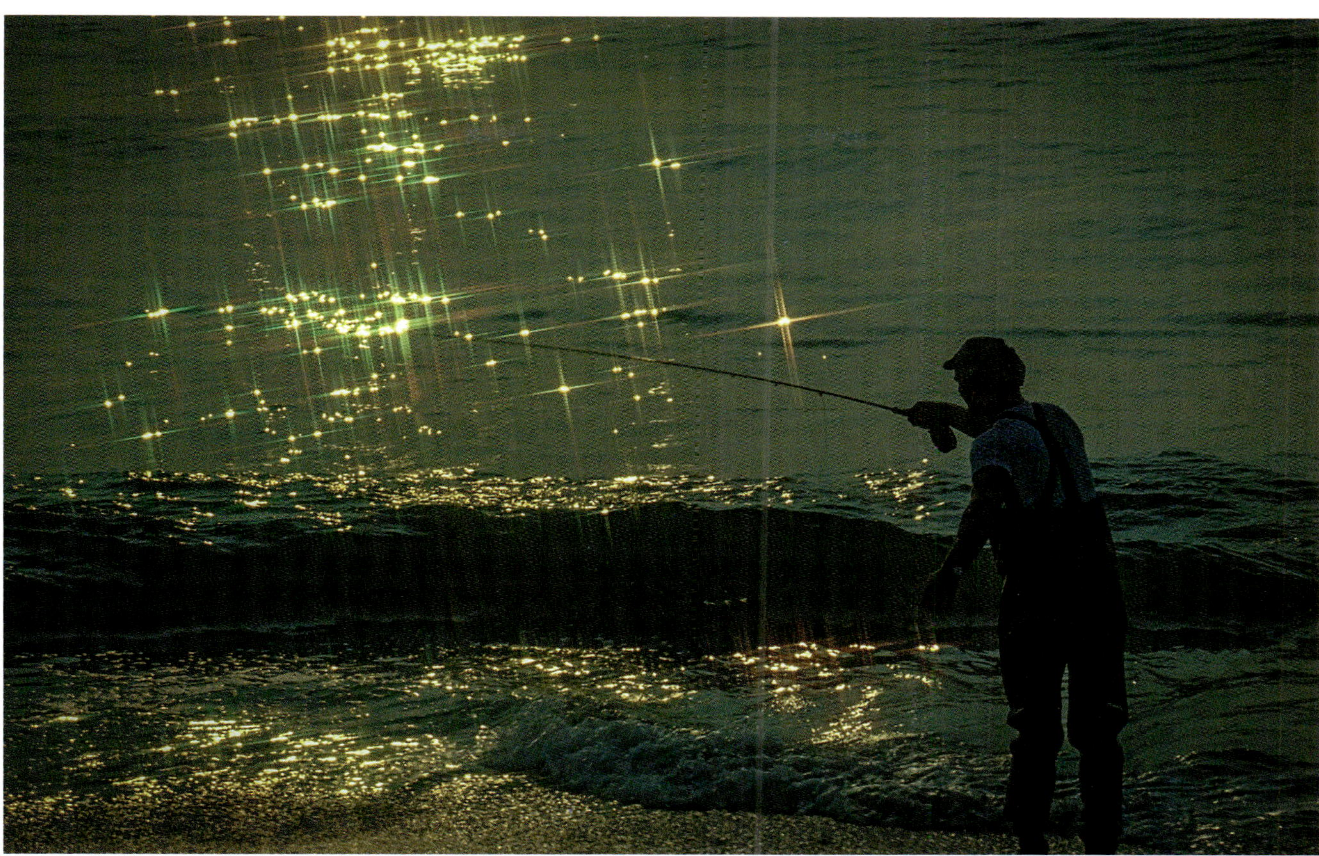

At the time I took this photo of Bob fishing at Island Beach, New Jersey, nearly forty-five years ago, he was already using a modified design of the venerable Ka-Boom-Boom Popper. ED JAWOROWSKI

participation in competitive skating as a youngster, and later to his Marine training.

The Popovics *Fleye Design* approach is true art—a living, organic process, not merely a mechanical one. Bob doesn't tie so much as create. He's an ad-lib tier, and his products, like jazz music, are never there, but always in the process of becoming something else. His tying is fluid, endlessly adapting, as he seeks to match the materials to his vision. For this reason, he would make a terrible commercial tier. He could never clone fifty dozen exact duplicates. The individuality of each fly obsesses him. Just as cane rod makers appreciate the individual nature of each culm of bamboo, Bob recognizes that natural fibers and feathers are not all the same; they must be handled as individuals.

Fly tying may be a largely mechanical process, but the art behind the process is what *Fleye Design* is all about. If anyone considers my analysis of Bob Popovics's approach too philosophical to be applied to something as seemingly mundane as making fishing lures, he may be right, but only if he treats this sport as a whim, a frivolous entertainment. However, those who undertake it with passion, who appreciate its subtleties, and who want to master this skill, would hardly agree. I don't profess to fully understand this creativity, any more than I can understand the talent a great composer or painter, but I have observed it for decades, and I admire and appreciate it. Hopefully you will too, after reading Bob's explanations and instructions and studying Jay Nichols's magnificent photos.

Ed Jaworowski
Chester Springs, Pennsylvania
June 2015

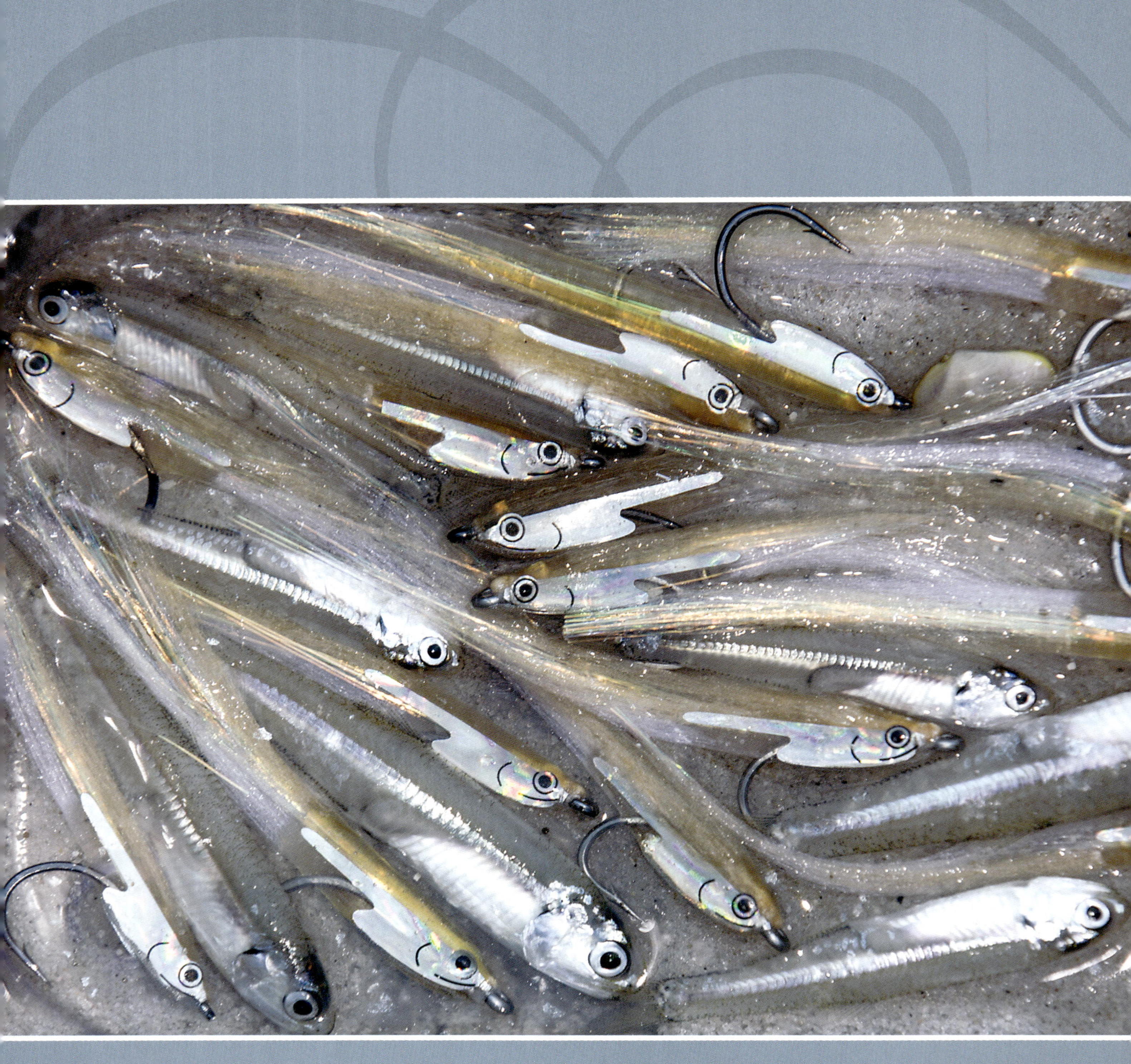

Bay anchovies and Fleye Foils. While the shape of the natural is fairly easy to imitate, its translucence requires that the tier pay attention to certain details that stand out: eyes, belly sac, stripe, and color. TOM LYNCH

Common Baits of the Atlantic

by Richard King

Baitfish

Baitfish are the indispensable food source for every gamefish we strive to catch, and the models for the lures and fly patterns we use to catch them. With short lifespans and immense populations, baitfish thrive on the food and protection afforded by intertidal estuaries. Some, like mullet and mossbunker, will enter as larvae, while others, such as the silverside and killie families, are born there. But all will spend their first season of life in estuaries, growing to no more than 6 to 8 inches in a single season.

Though the species discussed here are from a single Northeastern estuary—the Barnegat Bay estuary—they can be found up and down the coasts and estuaries of the United States. Through the years, species like spearing, grass shrimp, and bunker have inspired numerous fly patterns. And while not every species exists in every location, other members of the same genus, family, or form do. But what's just as important are their life cycles and habits, such as when and where their concentrations are greatest—from day to night and season to season—because that's where these patterns will be most effective.

The species discussed on the following pages are the most common forage of the Barnegat Bay estuary, but they're definitely not limited to that area. In fact these species, or other members of their genus or family, thrive in immense populations throughout the world. Ninety percent of the organisms of the ocean are said to live within 200 miles of the shoreline. The reason is simple: an immense nutrient flow pours from estuarine tributaries into bays and inlets, and it explodes into a food chain so immense that it attracts juveniles of all species of fish through their first year of life. Yes, there are all manner of forage throughout the surf and oceans, but it's here in estuaries that their biosynthesis begins.

Silversides (Family Atherinidae)

Of all the forage fish, it seems that the silversides (commonly called "spearing") dominate, with massive populations and year-round presence. Of the many species of this family that exist around the world, the Atlantic silverside and the inland silverside live in the Barnegat Bay estuary.

Atlantic Silverside (*Menidia menidia*)

Appearance: Greenish back with a pearl to white belly and a bright silver stripe running from the pectoral fin to tail. To 6 inches.

Range: Surf, ocean, and estuary from Nova Scotia to southern Florida.

Description: The silverside is our most important inshore forage fish throughout its range and by far our most imitated saltwater baitfish. From as far back as I

The Tier's Eye

SILVERSIDE (AKA SPEARING)

Fleye Choice: Silverside Surf Candy, olive over white.

Shape: Silversides are generally 2 to 4 inches, streamlined—almost like a comet.

Main Features: These baits are translucent, with prominent eyes (silver with black pupil), a silver stripe, and a belly sac that is half the length of the body with a square shape at the end. They have an oval to round cross-section, especially in the forward portion of the body. Overall, an imitation's taper should never get larger (fatter or higher) than the point at which it leaves the hook; it gets thinner on its way back.

Materials: Use sparse bucktail or translucent synthetic fibers such as Super Hair and Fluoro Fibre, with silver flash in between the colors. A hook with a short to moderate-length shank is fine; due to the sparse amount of material, keeling is not a factor.

Colors: Natural color combinations of light olive or gray over white work well. Attractor colors include chartreuse over white, pink over white, and pink and chartreuse.

Fishing Notes: Movement is not a priority when designing a fly to imitate silversides, but capturing the translucency is. Translucency allows prominent body features to stand out such as a belly sac, eyes, and a stripe. They swim in all areas of the water column, including hugging the bottom in the shallows or riding high in deeper water. The fly line that you use dictates your position in the water column, though variations can include a Jiggy for deeper water. To imitate silversides on the surface, you can use a slider, such as a very skinny Banger. When you're fishing and you see flashes of silver as the bait sprays out of the water, double the size of the flash that you see for the overall length of the fly that you choose.

can remember, January to December, if you saw baitfish, there was a 90 percent probability that you were seeing Atlantic silversides (*Menidia menidia*). And whereas populations of other forage are often inconsistent, there's never been a time I can remember when populations of silversides have been anything but immense. Reaching a maximum length of 6 inches in a short two-year lifespan, and with massive replenishing populations through all seasons—sometimes in locations that have no other forage fish of comparable type or size—the silverside is a premiere food source for important gamefish, like striped bass, bluefish, and weakfish.

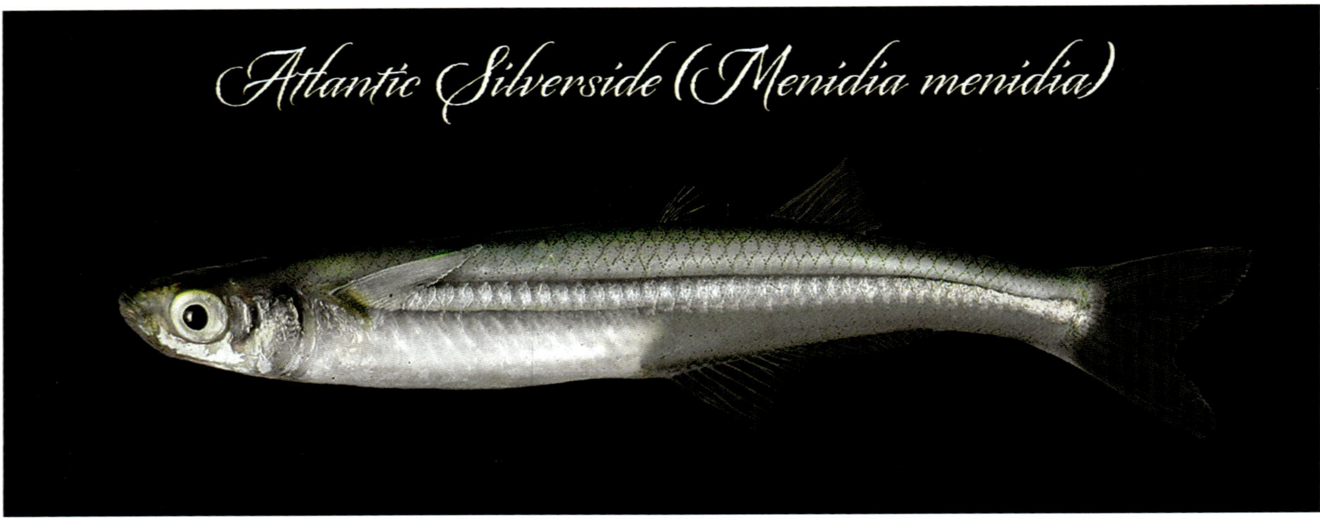

Adults reenter the estuary in early spring, having spent the winter in the adjacent surf, growing from juveniles to adults of 4 to 5 inches. As the waters warm in April, they begin their passage through the bay up into the tributaries, breeding as they go. Then they go back again, exiting in early July and bringing with them the larger striped bass that gorged on them throughout the spring. Encountering this cycle each spring was the way saltwater fly rodding began for many of us. In spring, water temperature matters. Early spring finds the silversides moving up through deeper waters, along with the striped bass that follow them. As the waters warm to 55 degrees, around mid-April, they begin moving through the shallows.

Juveniles swim throughout Barnegat Bay and in brackish tributaries from spring to December, depending on water temperature. The fish are larval in the spring, $^{3}/_{4}$ to $1^{1}/_{2}$ inches by early July, and 3 to $3^{1}/_{2}$ inches by the flood tides of August and September. Then, they create massive backlogs near inlets before moving into the adjacent surf, and ocean, though they'll remain numerous but in decreasing numbers until the end of the year. Even at their smaller size in early July, silversides' immense numbers feed the same species of gamefish that followed the breeding silversides earlier.

Unlike adults, the juveniles are nocturnal, favoring deep water and channels during daylight hours, but moving into shallow coves, creeks, and sand bars at night. Then, each morning, just before gray light, they'll pour out of these creeks into their deep-water daytime habitat. This is their daily time of greatest vulnerability to predators. Watching these immense schools make their final exodus into the adjacent surf in the predawn hours of the flood tides of late August and September is a fantastic sight.

It's been my experience that the difference between success and failure in fly rodding these nighttime shallows and creeks in early summer has been the size of the fly. Any spearing pattern under 2 inches produced fish, while anything larger didn't. And though I usually targeted striped bass, this has also held true for bluefish in the daytime. But as summer moves on and the juveniles grow larger, the size of the fly becomes less of a factor.

Inland Silverside (*Menidia beryllina*)

Appearance: To 4 inches, with a deeper anal fin with only 16 rays, compared to 24 to 26 rays in Atlantic silversides. Much smaller in the spring than the 4- to 5-inch Atlantic silversides.

Range: Bay and estuary only from Maine to Florida and the Gulf Coast (also introduced to West Coast).

Description: Similar in appearance and lifespan to the Atlantic silverside, the inland silverside is slightly smaller, at 4 inches max. Though salinity tolerant, favoring the lower salinities of tributaries, they can be found mixed in with breeding Atlantic silversides each spring as they move throughout the estuary.

Whereas the Atlantic silversides migrate to the surf and ocean in fall and winter, the inland species never leaves the estuary. But while the inland silverside's populations are comparatively smaller, in the Northeast, their range throughout the United States is greater, extending beyond Florida to the Gulf Coast and Texas.

White Mullet (*Mugil curema*)

Appearance: A thick, elongate, laterally compressed fish. Olive back and silvery sides. Large, tough scales. Juveniles to 6 inches. Adults to 18 inches.

Range: Throughout the East Coast of the Western Atlantic, from Nova Scotia south to Bermuda, and the Gulf Coast to Brazil; also the West Coast from California to Chile.

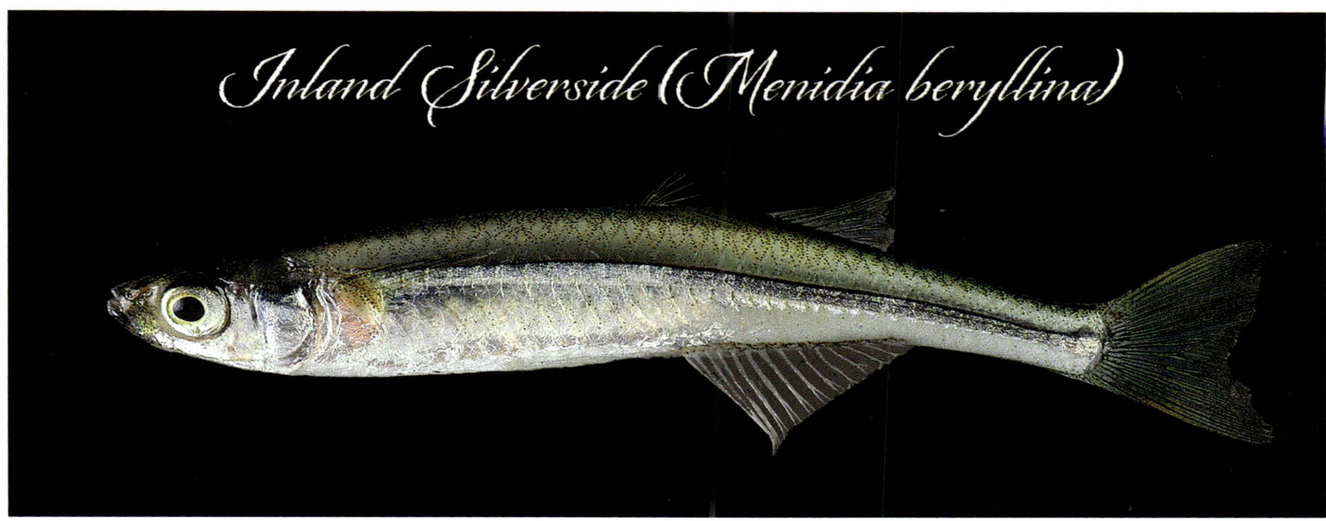

The Tier's Eye

MULLET

Fleye Choice: Bucktail Deceiver, BULKhead Deceiver, Bob's Banger, Siliclone.

Shape: Mullet are 3 to 8 inches long with a complex shape. They are bulkiest in the front. The rear portion is flatter, and it becomes more round and robust toward the shoulders and head.

Main Features: In addition to the distinct shape, the fish has prominent eyes, silver with black pupil. It also has a blue dot or blue color near the pectoral and a large, powerful tail.

Materials: I like to use bucktail, with or without feathers, for a strong silhouette with volume and a subtle amount of flash.

Colors: Natural colors include olive, gray, or tan and white, with subtle greens and blues and lots of silver. Attractor colors include a red head with a white body.

Fishing Notes: Because mullet go to the surface to escape, a fly that rides high works best. The prominent, powerful tail is a key to the speed at which the fish can swim, and fast retrieves are often best. A BULKhead, Siliclone, or Banger covers the presentations closer to the surface. At night, mullet tend to slow down and mill at the surface, so slower presentations near the surface are best, but keep the wake (retrieve) even—no stripping and no pauses. A flat profile Bucktail Deceiver stays on top and sinks slower.

Description: Whereas silversides of the right size for gamefish like striped bass, bluefish, and weakfish are available through all seasons and habitats, the white mullet, being bred offshore, enters the estuary in winter, at little more than a few millimeters. Though it has a lifespan of nineteen years, it only spends its first year in an estuary, growing to little more than 6 inches. The white mullet grows up in the secluded depths of bays and lagoons, where it's rarely seen until late August. Once they reach 4 to 6 inches, white mullet gather in massive schools in shallow coves and tidal creeks, preparing for their September exit into the surf. From September through October, as they hug the beach on their long migration south, white mullet become a prime target for schools of resident striped bass and bluefish. But even with their immense populations in this migration period, they are no easy meal for any gamefish. With their toughly scaled bodies and acrobatic agility, they truly are the tarpon of all forage fish. An extremely agile jumper, the white mullet is able to jump 2 feet from a standing start.

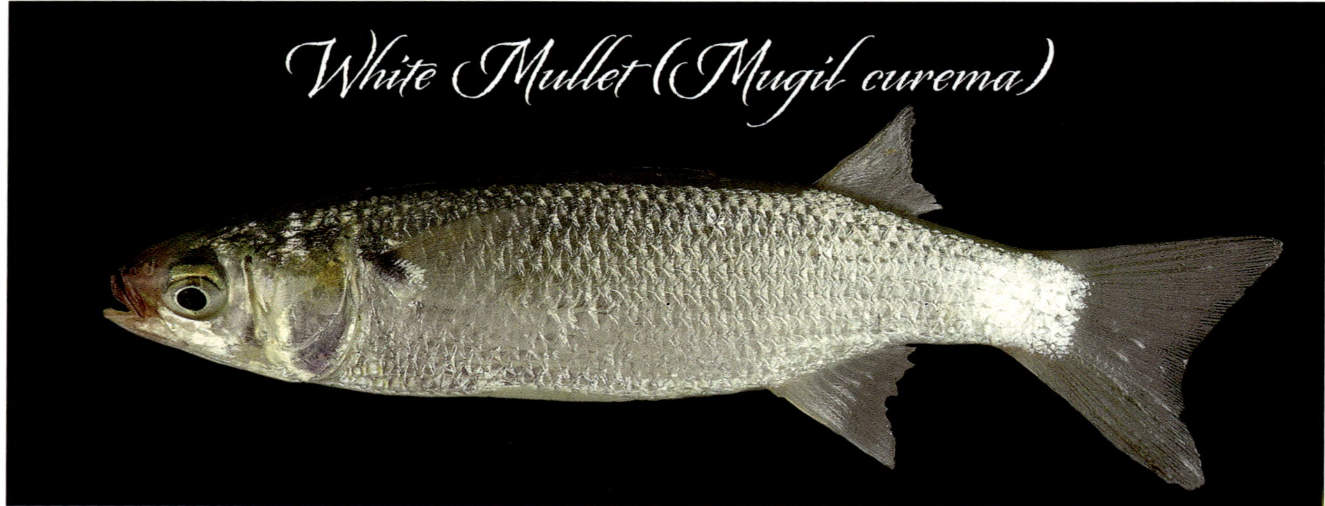

White Mullet (Mugil curema)

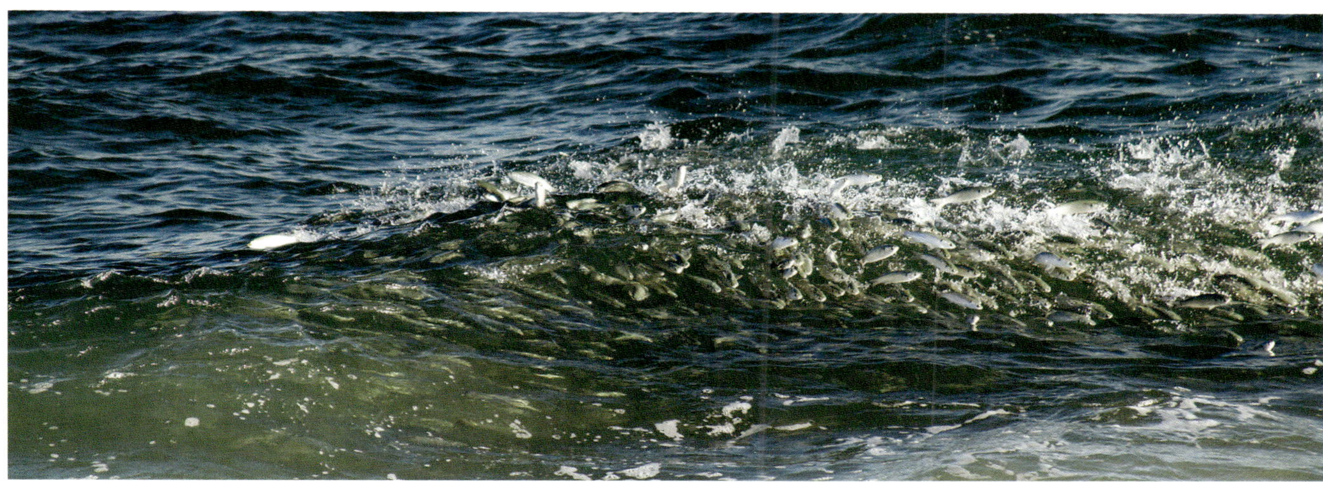

Migrating mullet burst from a wave in full panic mode at Island Beach State Park, New Jersey. The mullet were likely being attacked by bluefish or striped bass. This image was shot during the mullet run in September. This mullet school was only about 10 feet from the the shoreline when the predatory fish hit them. TOM LYNCH

Herrings and Menhadens (Family Clupeidae)

This is the family of some of our largest and deepest patterned forage species. Long used as the "silver bullet" bait for trophy-size striped bass, species like mossbunker and herring are also the patterns for our deepest body flies.

Alewife Herring (*Alosa pseudoharengus*)

Appearance: An extremely laterally compressed fish that is approximately three times as long as deep with a sharp saw-edged belly. They have a dark gray to green back with silver sides and a dark spot just above the middle of the gill plate. Juveniles are translucent; adults become more opaque. Adults to 12 inches. Juveniles to 5 inches.

Range: Newfoundland to North Carolina.

Description: Though the frantically splashing schools of alewife herring of a few years ago are rarely seen anymore, they still represent an important presence in the Barnegat Bay estuary. Alewife are anadromous, and each spring they swim up rivers and creeks from their ocean habitat to breed in tidal fresh waters. They leave behind the juveniles to spend their first season in the estuary and return to the ocean in May, where they often become the tragic bycatch of the Atlantic herring fishery, accounting for their diminished numbers. The juveniles grow up in the habitat where they were born, reaching 3 to 5 inches by September, when they, like many other juveniles, will exit into the ocean. Though little is known about their oceanic movements, like any forage concentration moving through narrow inlets, they become targets for major gamefish like stripers, blues, and weakfish.

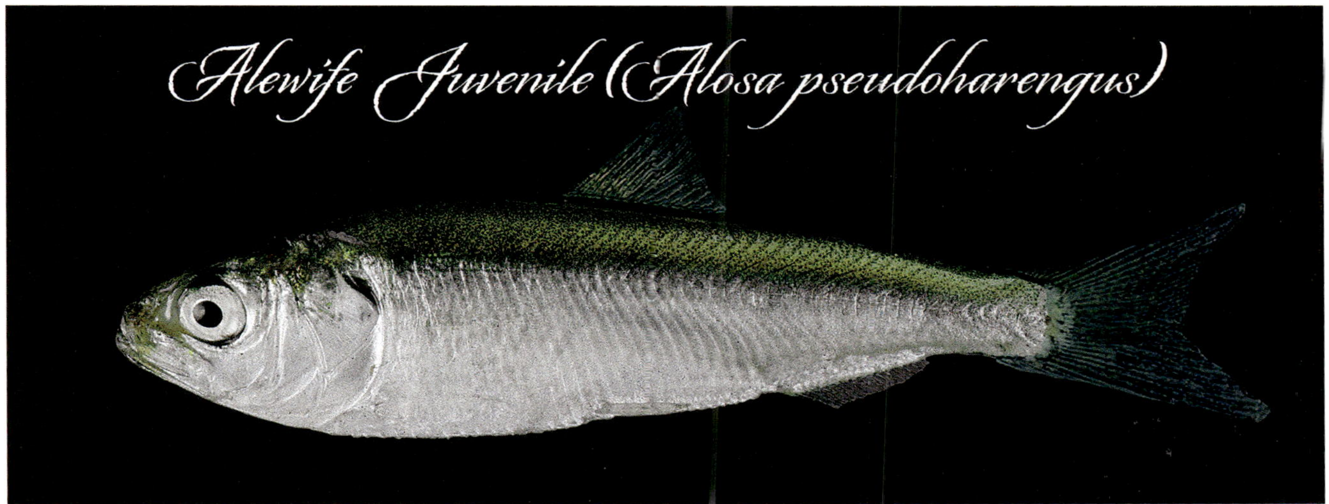

The Tier's Eye

MENHADEN (AKA BUNKER, POGY)

Fleye Choice: Hollow Fleye.

Shape: Bunker can range from 3 to 14 inches. When they're small, they're relatively thin, but as they get larger, they get heavier and thicker, though they are still symmetrical with their top half more or less the same as their bottom half.

Main Features: Menhaden have a symmetrical taper from head to tail. They have a large eye that is high and above their middle, a pronounced spot behind the gill, and other spots that are irregular from fish to fish that are above the median line. The gill area almost looks armor-plated and reflects lots of blues, pinks, and yellows.

Materials: The naturals are so flashy that if I'm going to put a lot of flash in a fly, it's usually a bunker imitation, although I'm not sure this makes a big difference. Use a bigger and heavier hook for proper keeling because of the amount of material on the hook shank and because you retrieve this fly quickly. Use more fibers on top of the hook shank to help it keel better, but maintain a proper silhouette.

Colors: All white with varying amounts of yellow (lots of yellow in the tail), tan, or golden bronze tops with buff-colored sides and white bottoms.

Fishing Notes: Bunker swim in schools throughout the water column. When they get separated from the school, they will then swim quickly and erratically—you want to match that movement with your retrieve.

Atlantic Menhaden, aka Peanut Bunker (*Brevoortia tyrannus*)

Appearance: Laterally compressed oval shape. Depth about 25 percent of its length. Back greenish, with brassy to silver sides. A large black spot directly behind the gill plate with a series of smaller black spots to base of tail. Juveniles 3 to 4 inches. Adults to 14 inches.

Range: Nova Scotia to Southern Florida where its range overlaps with the Yellow Fin Menhaden (*Brevoortia smithi*) that inhabits the Gulf waters.

Description: Like the white mullet, menhaden (also known as "peanut bunker") are born offshore in fall and winter and swim into the estuary when they're no more than 1/3 inch long. They spend the summer growing to about 3 or 4 inches in the lower salinities of tributaries and creeks, where they become prey for salinity-tolerant

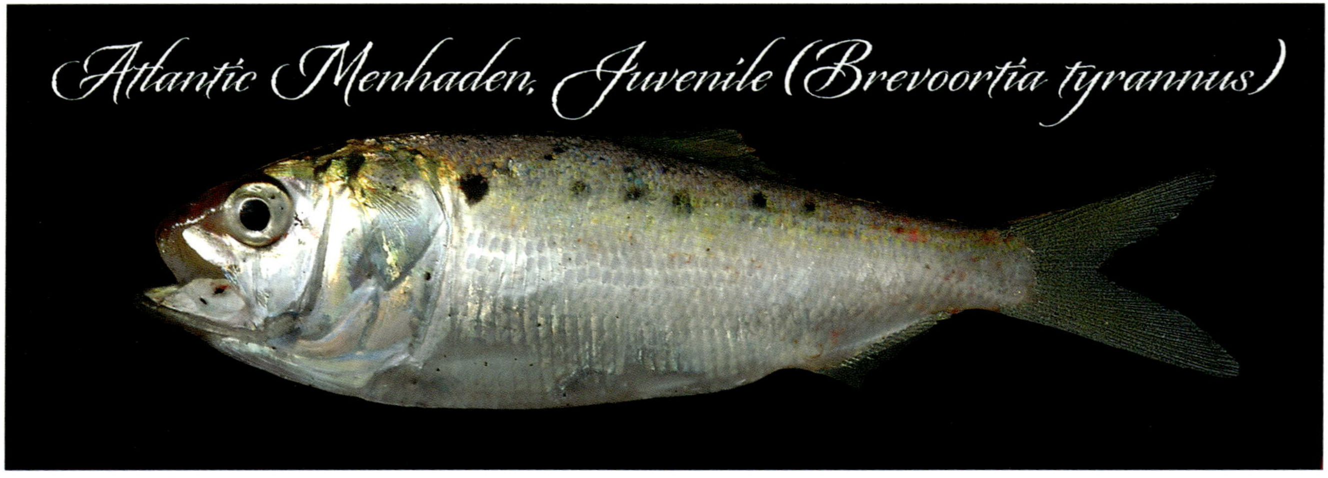
Atlantic Menhaden, Juvenile (Brevoortia tyrannus)

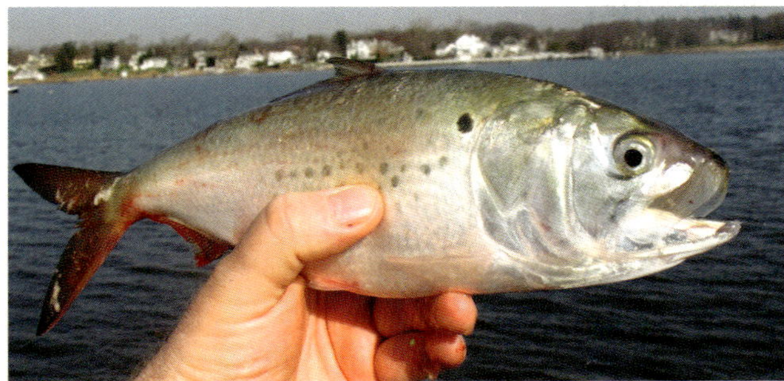

Adult menhaden COLIN ARCHER

juvenile gamefish. Then, like silversides and mullet, menhaden begin moving through the lower tidal creeks and channels around mid-October, and out into the ocean, joining populations from estuaries up and down the coast as they make their southern passage. They join the adults for the winter. Now, with peanut bunker joining the fall's mix of forage species already mentioned, the surf is primed for gamefish, giving this season some of the finest fly rodding of the year.

Adults migrate north in the spring and south in the fall. All menhaden, being inshore fish, return to their bays of origin each season, but they only spend a couple of weeks in Barnegat Bay in spring, favoring larger, deeper bays. But their migrations in deeper water are nothing short of amazing, as they're followed by 20- to 50-pound-class striped bass and large bluefish. If it wasn't for the food chains of shallow-water estuaries and the juvenile peanut bunker they produce, these spectacular deeper-water migrations wouldn't exist.

Bay Anchovy (*Anchoa mitchilli*)

Appearance: Laterally compressed elongate body with blunt nose. A greenish back, translucent sides with a reddish cast. Schools appear as a large reddish patch in the surf before wintering. Adults to 4 inches. Juveniles to 2 inches.

Range: From Maine south through the Florida Keys into the Gulf of Mexico and to the Yucatán Peninsula.

Description: Also called "rainfish," the bay anchovy has a similar life cycle to the Atlantic silverside. They

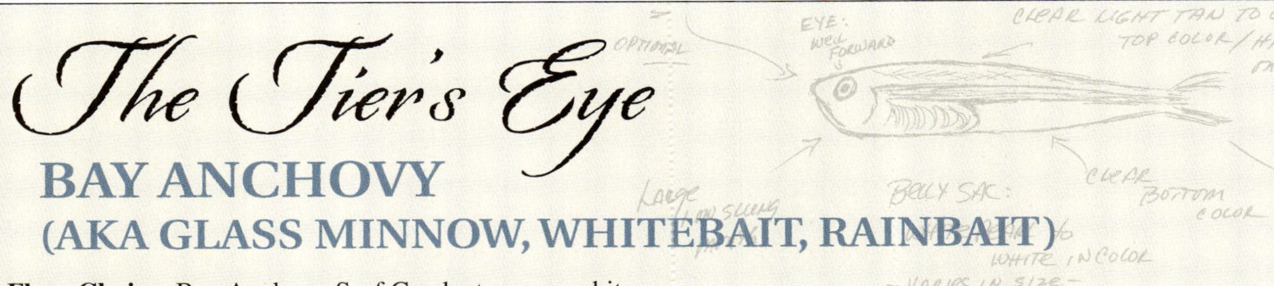

The Tier's Eye

BAY ANCHOVY (AKA GLASS MINNOW, WHITEBAIT, RAINBAIT)

Fleye Choice: Bay Anchovy Surf Candy, tan over white.

Shape: Bay anchovies are 2 to 5 inches, with an even, streamlined shape almost like a comet.

Main Features: This fish has a prominent eye (silver with a black pupil), stripes, and a belly sac that looks like it is only one-third to one-half of the body. The stripe is not as prominent as the stripe on the silverside, and the body has a flat cross section. The overall taper of the fly should never get larger (fatter or higher) than the point at which it leaves the hook, and it gets thinner on its way back.

Materials: Use the same materials you did for the silverside: sparse bucktail or translucent synthetics such as Super Hair, Fluoro Fibre, and saltwater Angel Hair, mixed with gold pearl flash. The hook should have a moderate-length to short shank. There will be a sparse amount of material, so keeling is not a factor.

Colors: Normally, you want to use a tan color, though the optimal color can change depending on light. On bright, sunny days try a fly the color of an amber beer; for hazy days or low-light conditions, use a lavender hue. Attractor colors include chartreuse, pink, or pink and chartreuse (tutti frutti). As the frenzy becomes more intense and the bait gets pushed to the surface, it seems the naturals turn darker brown to almost a rusty orange-brown as they rush to the surface, and you see a rich golden tint to the flash as they break the surface, not silver. They are absolutely gorgeous baits to watch.

Fishing Notes: The bay anchovy is one of the most common baitfish that I see. If you can understand and imitate this bait, you can take your patterns almost anywhere in the world and be successful. As with the silverside, fly line, not fly design, will dictate your position in the water column, not fly design, though you can tie variations, such as Jiggies. As with silversides, double the size of the flash that you see for the overall length of the fly that you fish.

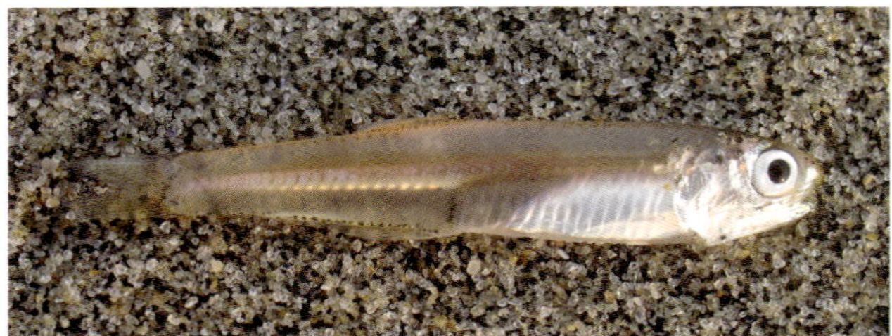

Bay anchovy COLIN ARCHER

winter in the ocean and return around April as 3- to 4-inch adults, and then breed throughout spring and summer. Juveniles then grow to about 2 inches before beginning their winter migration into the surf and ocean around October. Whereas silversides can be found throughout the Barnegat Bay estuary and adjacent surf, bay anchovies seem to favor lower salinities and tidal fresh water, except when migrating in or out. Many studies call bay anchovies the most numerous forage fish of East Coast estuaries, though in the Barnegat Bay estuary they are outnumbered by populations of Atlantic silversides, which can be found in all salinities.

Though the bay anchovy provides an important food source for juvenile gamefish in the lower salinities of the estuary, they are most important to the fly rodder in October when they migrate into the surf. Though their populations are not dependable each year and are reported to be declining, some of Barnegat's most memorable fall surf seasons have come as the result of the bay anchovy's massive fall surf concentrations.

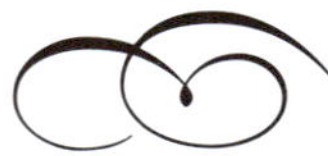

Now, are these the only forage fish in the Barnegat Bay estuary? Of course not! The estuary is both a nursery and a sanctuary for many small species. The only determining factors as to what percent they make up of the diet of local gamefish are the size of their populations and their availability by season, habitat, and habits. In this I believe the species and families we've discussed here to be the most important, either as targeted prey of the water column or as common prey of opportunity for foraging. But, by far, these baitfish are not the only forage species in the bay.

Crustaceans (Subphylum Crustacea)

Most saltwater fly rodding is based on the life cycles of "forage fish," yet how often do saltwater anglers think about "forage crustaceans"? Though different in appearance and life cycle, they live in immense populations, and like forage fish, they're a link in the food chain that feeds every important gamefish species we target. Whether crabs or shrimp or smaller crustaceans like amphipods and isopods, crustaceans are a food source that gamefish—from striped bass to kingfish—will rarely pass up.

Most crustaceans, with a few exceptions, are marine animals, meaning they live in saline waters throughout the world, and all crustaceans have an exoskeleton, which means that to grow they have to shed their shell. Shedding usually takes place near the flood tides of the new and full moons through spring and summer. The process of shedding (especially in crabs) gives off a smell that few fish can resist.

Shrimps (Infraorder Caridea)

The infraorder Caridea includes our most important shrimp species, such as the shore shrimp aka the grass shrimp (*Palaemonetes vulgaris*), the sand shrimp (*Crangon septemspinosa*), and the true grass shrimp (*Hippolyte* sp.).

Shore Shrimp, aka Grass Shrimp (*Palaemonetes vulgaris*)

Appearance: An elongate laterally compressed shape and a long dagger-like rostrum with eight to eleven dorsal teeth coming out from the head. First two pairs of walking legs are clawed, with the second pair the longest, and with a movable tooth on the claw. Five pairs of pleopods

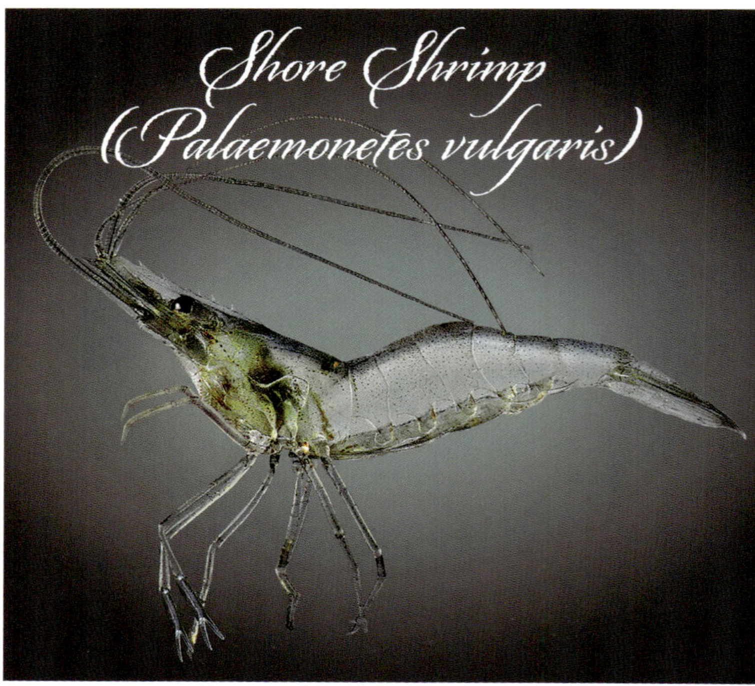

The Tier's Eye

GRASS SHRIMP

Fleye Choice: Ultra Shrimp.
Shape: 3/4 to 1 1/2 inches—smooth, no bumps.
Main Features: The natural has small eyes, very fine antennae, and a translucent appearance. It's more important to imitate the look from behind than from the side.
Materials: I like rubber legs or strands of Super Hair for legs; Tuffleye; and a size 2 to 1/0 hook.
Colors: Effective colors include clear, olive, tan, and chartreuse (with legs to match).
Fishing Notes: You need both floating and sinking shrimp patterns. Grass shrimp float with the tide and often cling to seaweed or grass-covered structure, such as pilings. When imitating sand shrimp, fish your flies along the bottom using a jig hook and lead eyes.

(swimmerets) under the tail that are also used to hold their fertilized eggs. Almost transparent right after shedding, but later take on a light translucent brownish color, and orange eye stalks. Size to 1 1/2 inches.

Range: Massachusetts south to the Gulf of Mexico.

Description: Pull a seine net anywhere on the shores of Barnegat Bay, or take a scoop off any sod bank, and you'll most likely catch a grass shrimp. It's the most numerous and important forage species of its type in the Barnegat Bay estuary. Being salinity tolerant, they inhabit the lowest salinities of brackish water, although their greatest populations seem to favor the higher salinity concentrations of the lower bay and salt marsh.

Their habit of clinging to submerged grasses (primarily eel grass) is where grass shrimp get their nickname, but they'll cling to any kind of submerged structure, which makes the submerged roots of sod banks and the macro algae that lines them an ideal habitat for immense populations. On almost any given summer night, wherever you look, you'll find grass shrimp clinging to grass beds and sod banks as their eyes glow in the beam of your spotlight, like a deer's eyes in the headlights of a car.

Shore shrimp use their legs to cling to structure and walk on the bottom and their swimmerets to swim in the water column. But when threatened, their most important defense is to shoot backward with a powerful downward thrust of their telson (tail), often skipping right out of the water. This, along with their sharp-pointed rostrum, may aid in the grass shrimp's escape from smaller fish, but they really have no defense against major predators like weakfish and striped bass in an open-water current.

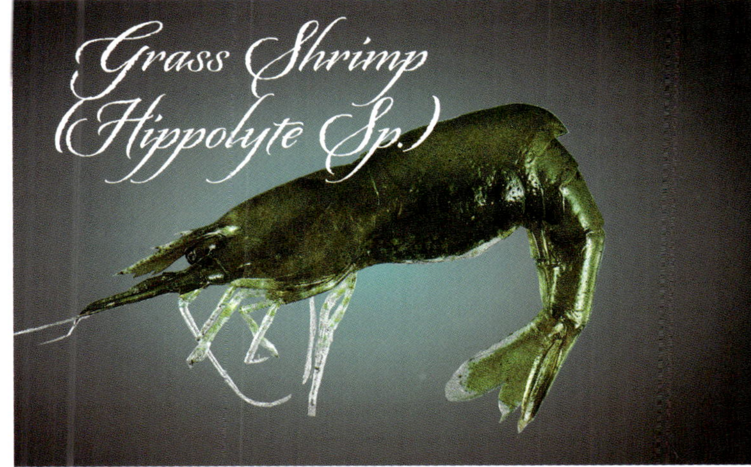

We may not think about it much, but currents are the arteries of estuaries, without which little life could exist. Currents come from tributaries, wind, and tides. They carry oxygen, nutrients, food, and—especially relevant here—grass shrimp. Whether it's the rips that occur in tidal creeks where the water goes from slow and shallow to fast and deep, around bends and sandbars during waxing tides (increasing toward new and full moons), or the loose wrack lines of grass carried by the powerful, wind-driven currents so prevalent in Barnegat Bay, they're the conveyer belts of small prey, and a dinner bell for predatory gamefish. This is the way grass shrimp move, whether they intend to or not, and it's when they're most vulnerable—but it's not the only time they're vulnerable.

With such large populations wherever they're found—in currents, grass beds, sod banks, or anywhere else—

grass shrimp are a primary food source for everything, including weakfish, striped bass, fluke, flounder, and blackfish, just to mention a few. I've even found them to be the primary prey of the lined seahorse.

The true grass shrimp looks similar to the shore shrimp, laterally compressed with a short dagger-like rostrum. It has a seemingly deformed hump where the thorax meets the tail. Though commonly "eel grass" green, they also come in dark brown, or a mottled combination. They grow to approximately 3/4 inch.

Less prevalent than shore and sand shrimp, the true grass shrimp often goes unnoticed due to its green coloration. It's found in eel grass beds and algae throughout the lower Barnegat Bay and has roughly the same habits as the shore shrimp, along with the same predators.

Sand Shrimp (*Crangon septemspinosa*)

Appearance: Sharply tapered and oval from above, and a shallow rectangular shape from the side. Unlike the shore shrimp, the sand shrimp is compressed dorsal/ventrally and lacks the dagger-like rostrum. Its body is slightly translucent with a mottled sandy brown color. Size to over 2 inches.

Range: Nova Scotia to Florida.

Description: Often, when the stomach contents of striped bass seem to be filled with shore shrimp, closer inspection might show them actually to be sand shrimp, a viable food source that is often confused with shore shrimp. Being less salinity tolerant than shore shrimp and needing a relatively sandy bottom, sand shrimp make the lower Barnegat Bay estuary their primary habitat. They move into the shallows in early spring and leave in late fall. Being nocturnally active (as you may begin to see that most forage are), sand shrimp bury themselves in the sand during the day and come out at night to feed. They're said to be omnivorous, but they're primarily predators using their two large, hooked claws to catch prey. They're often found with grass shrimp, but never far from the bottom—that is, until the water temps begin to fall into the low sixties, when, like many other creatures of the bay, sand shrimp begin moving through the tidal currents and into the deeper waters outside the inlet. As they do, they become the prime target for every predator in the bay, including striped bass and especially weakfish. I doubt that any fish could be more adapted to feeding on small crustaceans with its two fangs on the upper jaw and slower, more focused nature for hunting sod banks and grass beds.

Mantis Shrimp (Order Stomatopoda)

Stomatopoda is a unique order that includes *only* mantis shrimp species. Though there are many species worldwide, most live in tropical waters. Only one is common

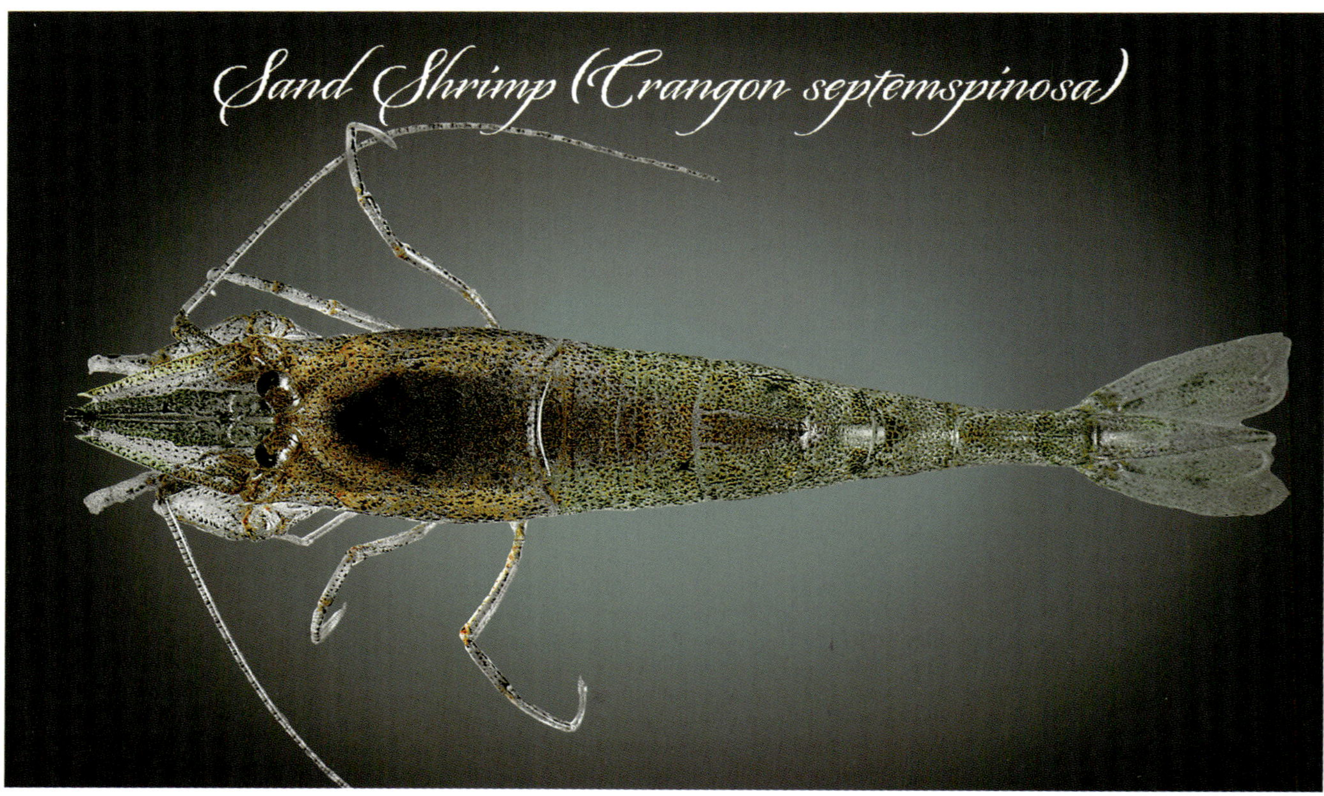

to our East Coast estuaries: *Squilla empusa*. Like other members of this order, its most distinguishable (and fascinating) attributes are its ultra powerful praying mantis–like claws, hence the name mantis shrimp.

Mantis Shrimp (*Squilla empusa*)

Appearance: Compressed dorsal/ventrally and shaped like a lobster with the telson (tail) being the widest part of the body. Five pairs of thoracic legs with one pair a long toothed claw used as a gripping spear with five teeth, which is said to have the power to break thick glass or a poorly placed finger. Size to 10 inches or more.

Range: Maine to South America.

Description: The mantis shrimp, though a true crustacean, is not, as the name implies, a true shrimp. It's something you might not consider as a forage species—in fact, you might not consider it at all. So secretive is the mantis shrimp that it's rarely ever been seen by the most seasoned of bay men, and it's mentioned here mainly because the one way it is often found is in the stomach contents of the striped bass. Though mantis shrimp populations may not be enormous, they're a lot larger than their occurrence would indicate.

Mantis shrimp are nocturnally active and live in holes dug in the mud and sod. They hunt by ambushing everything from grass shrimp to small fish, using spearlike claws said to have the power to break aquarium glass or pierce a clammer's finger, yet, despite this, the mantis shrimp seem to have little defense against foraging striped bass.

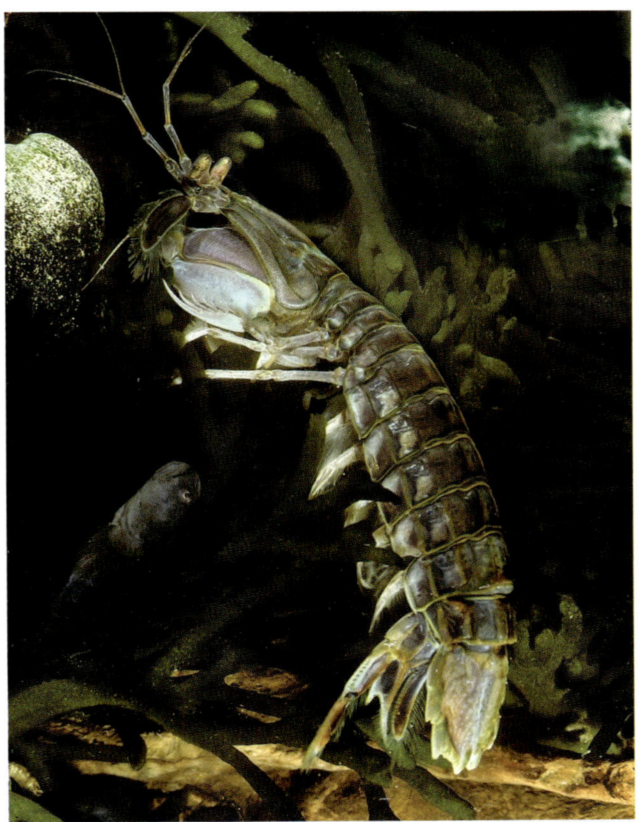

Mantis shrimp

True Crabs (Infraorder Brachyura)

True crabs are compressed dorsal/ventrally with an almost cylindrical carapace over five pairs of legs, including one pair of claws, with movable jaws. Thousands of species exist throughout the world with dozens or more in the Barnegat Bay estuary and East Coast.

They are our largest decapod crustaceans, known as one of the most advanced crustaceans for their successful size and for elimination of segments into a carapace that protects not only their head parts but also their short tails. (Their tails are actually tucked under their shells. Brachyura means "short tail.")

With their huge populations, and vulnerability during "shedding," their value to the food chain comes as no surprise.

Blue Claw Crab (*Callinectes sapidus*)

Appearance: Shell is wider point-to-point than it is long. Legs and claws are blue with red tips. Back is brownish, and belly is white. Paddle-like rear legs. Size to 10 inches.

Range: From Nova Scotia to Florida, Texas, the West Indies, and Uruguay.

Lady Crab (*Ovalipes ocellatus*)

Appearance: Shell is about as wide as it is long. Legs and claws yellow to orange. Shell is yellowish with small dark spots. Paddle-like rear legs. Size to 4 inches.

Range: From Cape Cod to South Carolina. (Note: at the southern edge of its small range a similar crab, the calico crab, *Hepatus epheliticus*, begins its range in the same habitat, which extends to Florida and the Gulf States.)

Description: Though we generally think of crabs as a food source for humans, they're also eaten by gamefish. Though hard crabs are preyed on heavily throughout their life cycle, they are most vulnerable after shedding. Because of their hard exoskeleton, crabs have to shed their shell to grow larger, which leaves them soft and defenseless until the new shell hardens. Crabs shed primarily on the flood tides of the new and full moon in the warm months of spring and summer, with the sheds of April and May being the largest. The frequency of shedding depends on age, so younger crabs, with a greater need for growth, may shed every couple of weeks, while adults shed only a couple times a year. When the new shell-like skin has been growing under the old shell for about a week, the crab sheds, becoming soft, vulnerable, and about 25 percent larger. To make things worse for the crabs (and better for their predators), shedders give off an aroma that no fish can resist, and once it sheds, all a crab can do is hide and wait until it hardens, which could take as long as three days.

All crabs have this vulnerability, as proven by the stomach contents of fish like striped bass and weakfish. But out of all crabs, the ones best known as prey for gamefish are the blue claw and the lady crab (commonly called the calico crab). Each has a special attribute not found in other crabs: a pair of paddle-like rear legs that allow them to swim. The blue claw, being salinity tolerant, uses the entire lower and middle Barnegat Bay estuary but is not found in the surf, whereas the lady crab thrives there and is the only true crab that does. Being nocturnally active, it buries itself in the sand in the daytime and comes out at night to hunt. But, though burying may protect it from the sun, it does little to protect it from burrowing striped bass that make lady crabs their preferred prey on the brightest days of summer.

The blue claw is, without a doubt, the largest and most numerous crab in the estuary. In fact, it has to be at least $4^{1}/_{2}$ inches or more point-to-point just to be legal for human consumption. But fortunately for forage consumption, three-quarters of these crabs are 1- to 3-inch juveniles, which, unlike adults, may shed as often as twice a month, making each flood tide throughout spring and summer a prime time for predation.

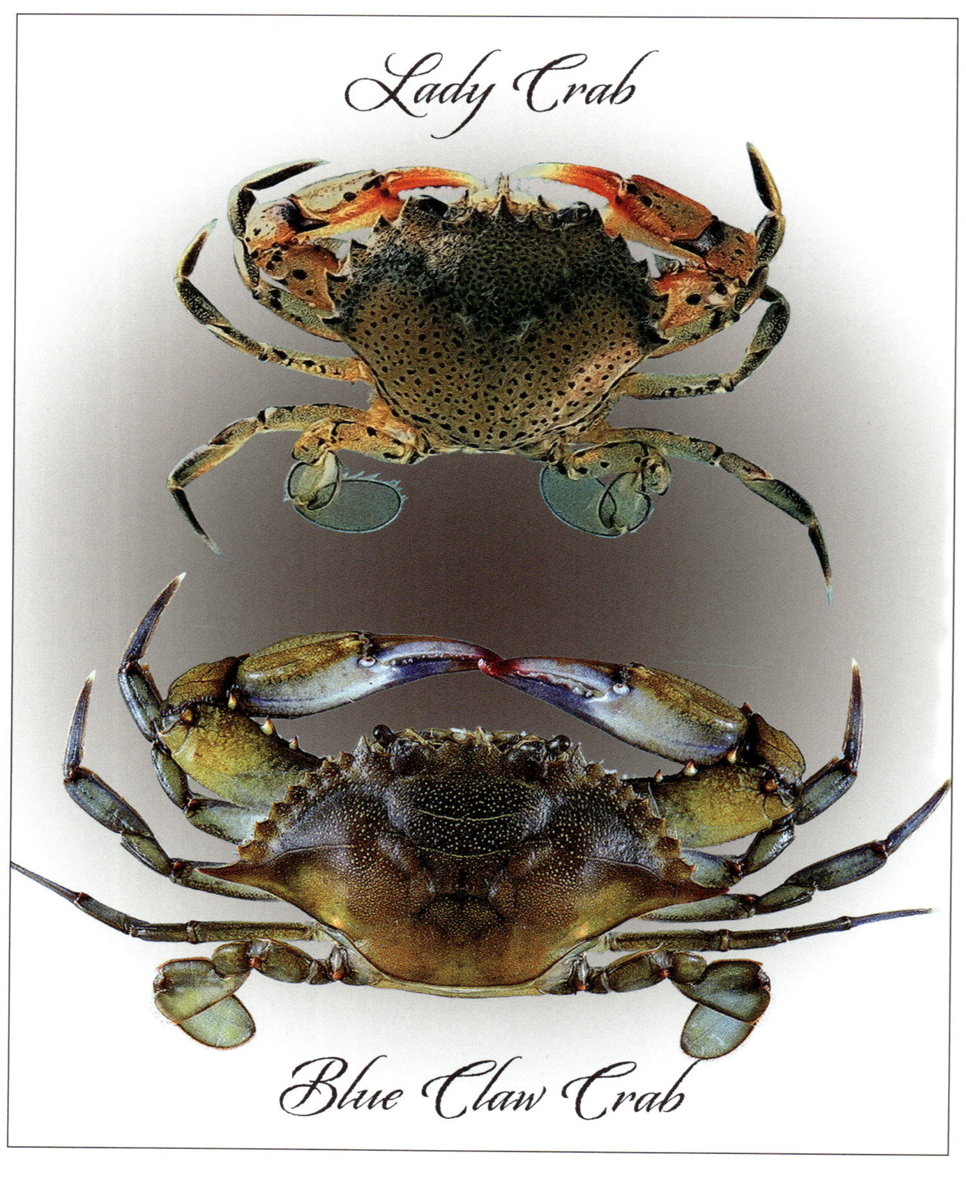

Marine Worms (Class Polychaeta)

Polychaetes are a different kind of invertebrate forage species, from the phylum Annelida. They can be distinguished by the pairs of parapodia (leglike extensions) on each segment, sensory organs, and sharp pincers on the head. Though not as easily seen as other forage, they're just as indispensable to the food chain. But of the hundreds of estuary worm species, two are so important, not only to the food chain but to fishermen, that an industry was created just to supply sport shops up and down the coast: blood worms and sand worms.

Blood Worm (*Glycera dibranchiata*) and Clam Worm (*Nereis* sp.)

Appearance: Wormlike body lined with "parapodia" (false feet) on each side from head to tail, used either for swimming or as gills. Being predators, these worms have pincher-like appendages and short antennae on the head. Color is similar to earthworms, reddish to bubblegum. Size 2 to 8 inches or more.

Range: Gulf of St. Lawrence to the Gulf of Mexico.

Description: Of the many types of worms in Barnegat Bay, the most common are of the class Polychaeta, and of those, the most common are the blood worm and the clam worm, which include many species. It's fascinating to encounter these worms when they're swarming. Often mislabeled a "worm hatch," what's really going on during a swarm is that the worms are decomposing and breeding at the same time. As their body breaks down, sperm and eggs are released, and the worm finally dies. Swarming generally takes place in currents, whether they're generated by wind or tide. Barnegat Bay runs north and south, so the strong southerly winds of spring and summer create equally strong parallel currents; these are the times when blood worms swarm, breed, and die. Swarming can readily be identified by the large flocks of laughing gulls seen picking the worms from the surface. These swarms may sometimes last all afternoon, and the worms become an easy food source for springtime stripers.

Clam worms, on the other hand, choose the nocturnal tidal currents around the time of the "dark moon" (new moon) to swarm, as they drift through tidal creeks until the tide ebbs. But the result is the same: decomposition, fertilization, and death, often a result of the predatory gamefish picking worms off the surface with a distinct popping sound. It's hard to know when swarming will happen, aside from that it happens close to a summertime new moon. But, for both blood worms and clam worms, even if they're not swarming, they remain an important prey item, as they're foraged off their bottom habitat around grass beds and mud flats. A simple fly pattern of a 2- to 3-inch piece of chenille-like material with a small black head can make the difference between success and failure.

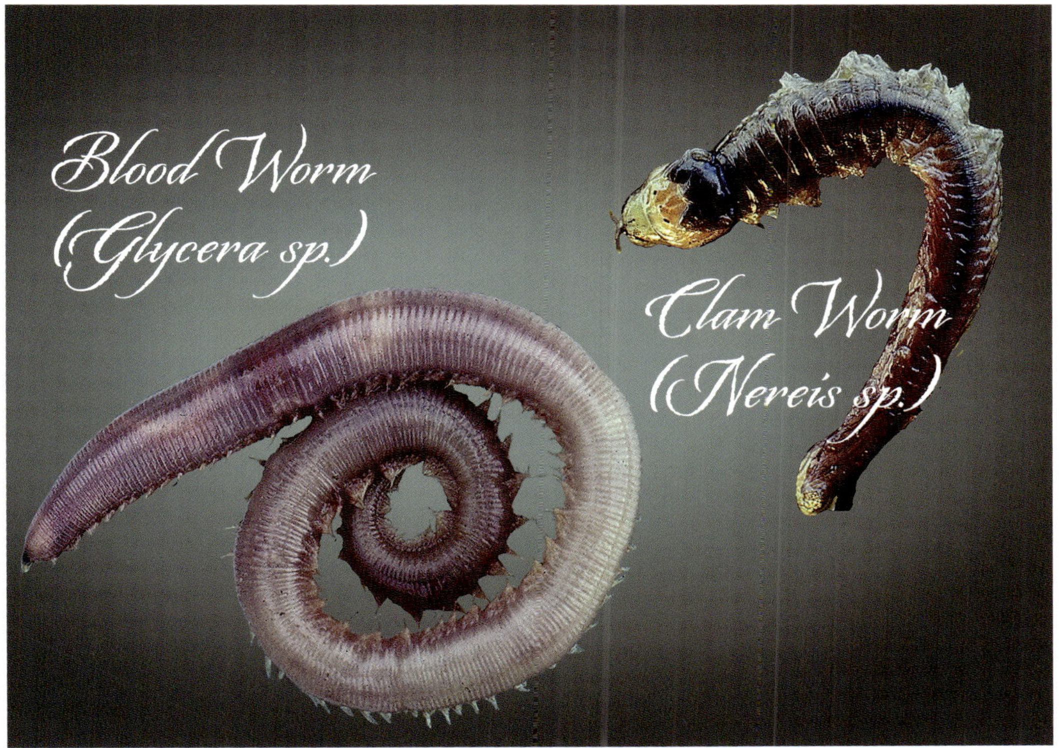

PART I

Essential Tying Techniques

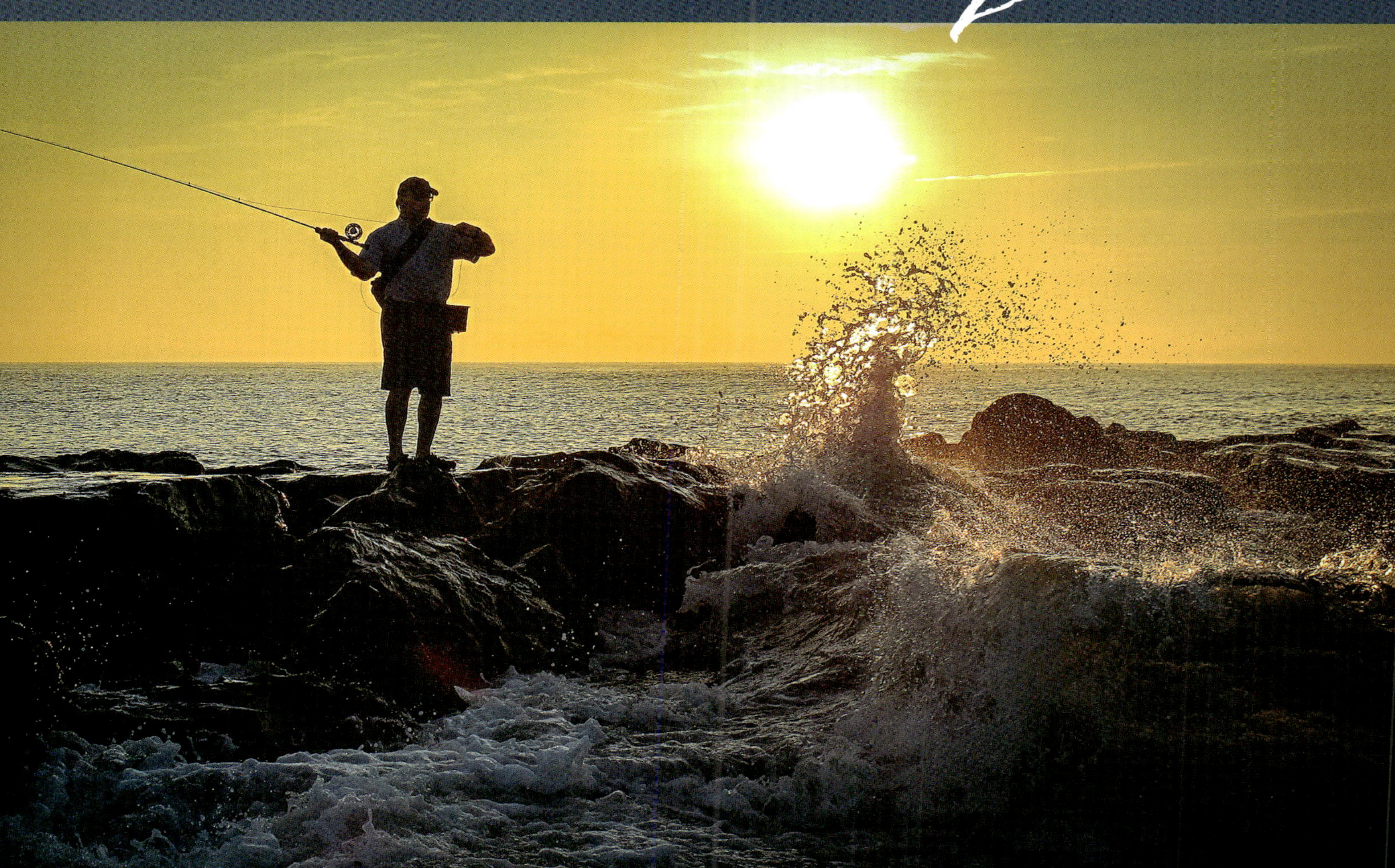

Good fly tiers must understand not just the bait that they intend to imitate, but also the behavior and habits of the fish that prey on them. Predator fish prefer chaotic water as they come in searching for bait. Both baitfish and crustaceans get confused, exhausted, or dislodged when fighting currents and wave action along the beach and rocks. COLIN ARCHER

Chapter 1

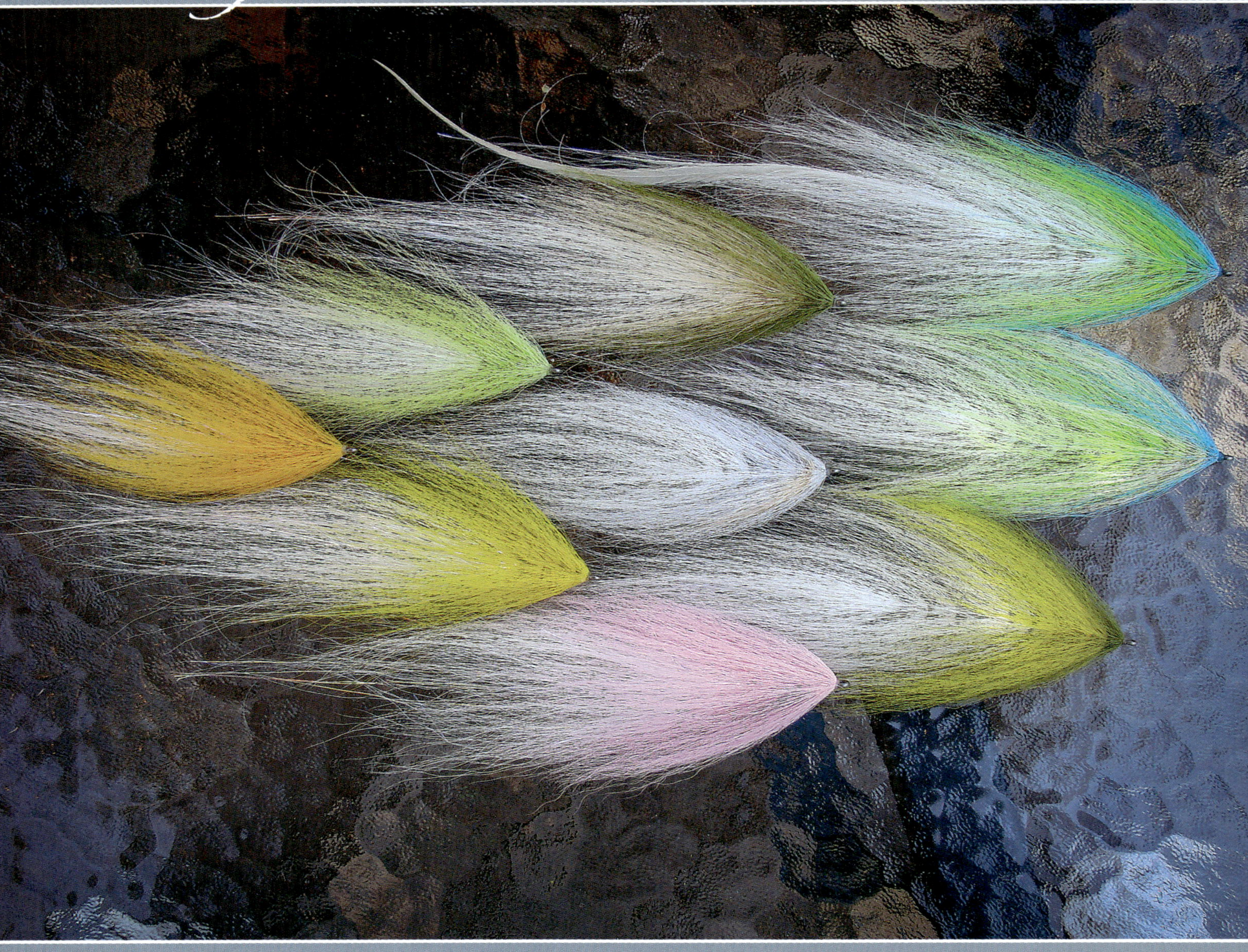

These are all Beasts—extremely large Hollow Fleyes. Hollow Fleyes constantly challenge the tier, but the more you tie them, the better you get. Take your time, observe how the bucktail reacts, and try to understand what causes what—are you using too much bucktail, did you remove all the short hairs, are you wrapping evenly around the shank, and are your tapers good? Stay aware of how the material responds to your technique, keep practicing, and you will achieve good results.

Working with Bucktail

In this section of the book, I won't cover all the techniques necessary to tie flies—other books do that well. Instead, I'd like to emphasize certain techniques that are important to master to tie the fleyes that I show in this book through a series of exercises and tutorials intended as practice drills. Once you master the techniques, you'll be well on your way to adapt and react to the different characteristics of the materials that you are using. You can stop worrying about the technique itself and free your mind for more creative endeavors—when tying with bucktail, for instance, you can focus on creating a fly with shape and taper, one that represents your particular vision. My best advice for any new tier, after being a better observer and getting to know the baits that you are trying to imitate, is to practice your techniques. The more techniques you know, the more tools you have at your disposal to solve fly-tying and fly-fishing problems. Tying techniques are nothing more than solutions to a problem.

Mother Nature still produces state-of-the-art tying materials, and many of the techniques and flies in this book will focus on using bucktail. Bucktail is inexpensive and versatile, and when dyed, it comes in a wide range of colors. Walk into any fly shop, and you'll generally find one wall reserved for a variety of them. To the new tier, these colorful displays look about the same from tail to tail, but a seasoned tier will spend a long time searching through the packs to find the perfect tail for the fly in mind. This is a primary reason for buying your bucktails in person and not online, where colors could be different than described and you don't have the chance to inspect the tail for the characteristics that you desire.

No one bucktail is perfect for every fly. When I choose my bucktails, I already have in mind the flies that I am going to tie with them. For instance, if I want to make some sand eel patterns, I want straight and thin hairs, so I will look for an olive bucktail and a white bucktail with those types of fibers. If I am looking for bucktail for Bangers, I don't want straight and thin fibers; instead, I look for wavier fibers with a little more volume to better coordinate with the thickness of the Banger head.

One magical thing about bucktail fibers is that they have an inherent taper—individual hairs are thicker at the base and finer at the tip. This natural taper allows the bucktail to pulsate or move enticingly through the water. Man has not yet been able to successfully replicate this trait with synthetic materials, and bucktail flies have an action in the water that is still hard to outdo or imitate. The action of the tips in a properly designed fly is unparalleled, and the more tips that you can add to the fly (in a Bucktail Deceiver or Hollow Fleye for instance), the better the action. Even sparse flies obtain greater action as the water swims through the hairs. The action of bucktail is subtle, natural, and never overstated, and you can easily accent it, if you wish, with a subtle amount of fine feathers, flash, or synthetics to create different effects.

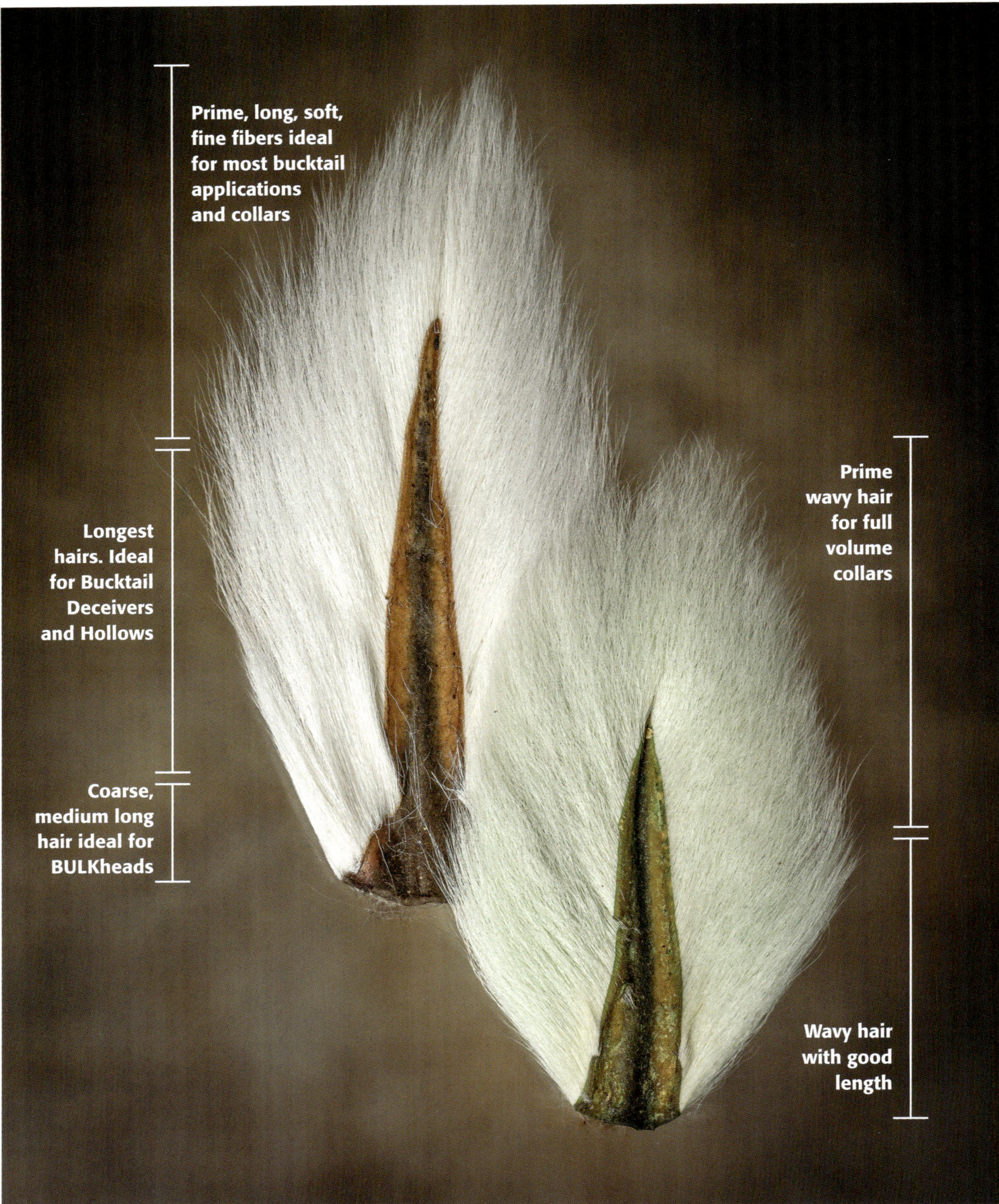

The white tail on the left is perfect for Hollows, Bucktail Deceivers, and BULKheads. It has fine, mostly straight fibers at the top of the tail and the coarse, long fibers at the base are ideal for BULKheads. Use the longest hairs in the middle of the tail wisely. The tail on the right has wavy, fine fibers. The top half of the tail has superb fibers for easily achieving a full collar on a fly.

Hair Characteristics

Fiber length is probably the easiest attribute to assess at a glance. Fibers on most bucktails are commonly 2 to 5 inches, but occasionally you can find tails with 6- or 7-inch hairs, and they are coveted. Most tails will have longer hairs at the base and shorter ones toward the tip; however, within any given section of the tail there will not be a wide range of fiber lengths, so you must have an inventory of multiple tails to cover more tying situations. This may seem trivial, but I often see tiers try to tie short flies with the tips from long fibers. The fly always lacks something in the end because it does not have the proper taper and bulk that short fibers from short hair would provide. So, remember: a short fiber is not the same as a fiber cut short. If you want shorter flies, you must use shorter hairs, or the fly will suffer.

On a fly such as the Bucktail Deceiver, where the first few ties establish the length of the fly, long fibers are very important. However, sometimes the longest fibers come from the base of the tail and are hollow. When using these fibers, I manage their tendency to flare by using a sparser amount. Another alternative is to use synthetic fibers for the first few ties.

The next aspect of bucktail to consider is the conformation of the hairs. Ramrod-straight hairs are ideal for slender bait imitations such as sand eels. Fuller flies, such as pilchard- or bunker-style patterns, benefit from wavy hairs because the kinks create more space and volume for a broader profile without extra material. I generally choose wavier fibers for collars on fleyes such as the Bucktail Deceiver when I want to provide the dimension and bulk that contribute to the fly's action and overall taper.

Texture is also important. The finest and softest hairs are often at the top of the tail while the longest, coarsest fibers are at the bottom. Coarse fibers will readily flare when tied tightly or spun, and though this characteristic is not desirable in many instances, sometimes you can use this to your advantage, such as when tying BULKhead Deceivers, building density in the collars of Hollow Fleyes, or tying flies with "soft" spun heads.

I prefer to work with softer fibers because they are usually finer with nicely tapered tips, and this type of hair usually "behaves" when tied on to the hook shank. Coarse hairs generally flare a lot and are harder to control. The trade-off is that the longest fibers are also often coarse, so it is worth learning to work with them.

Selecting and Cutting Hair from a Tail

When cutting fibers from a bucktail, many tiers grab a chunk of fibers at the base, cut them, and then preen out the shorter fibers. Not only does this require the extra step of removing the shorter fibers that came up with the clump, but those shorter fibers could be saved for other flies down the road.

After observing thousands of bucktails, I noticed one common trait from tail to tail. The short hairs that we often remove from a chosen clump of bucktail do not just grow randomly among the long hairs. The shortest hairs grow closest to the brown fibers, and they gradually increase in length as they move away from the brown hairs. Close inspection reveals that there are maybe as many as four different lengths of fibers that make up the tail. By pulling the long fibers away from the tail by their tips, and then preening away the shorter fibers, you can isolate the longer fibers for the fly that you are tying and leave the shorter fibers on the tail for another day.

SAVING THE SHORT STUFF

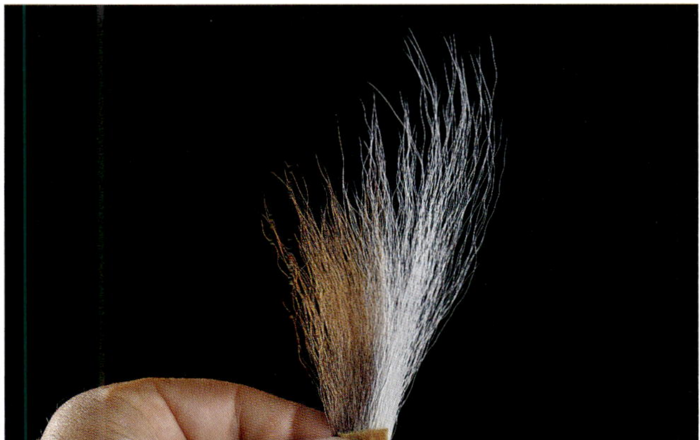

1. This crosscut section of bucktail illustrates the progressing lengths of fibers from the brown to the white. On a white-tailed deer, the top of the tail is brown, and the underside is white. The shortest white fibers are closest to the brown fibers, while the longer white fibers are farthest away from the brown fibers (before the tail is boned). So if I open that bucktail up, I can find some nice short fibers adjacent to the brown fibers.

(continued)

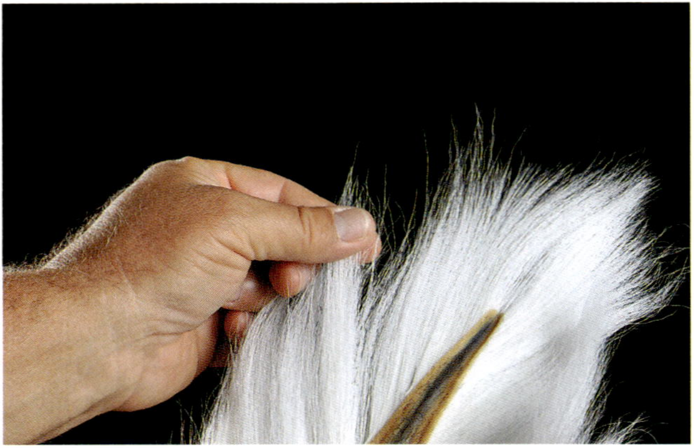

2. Instead of grabbing the fibers at the base of the clump, grab the tips with your left hand (if you are a right-handed tier).

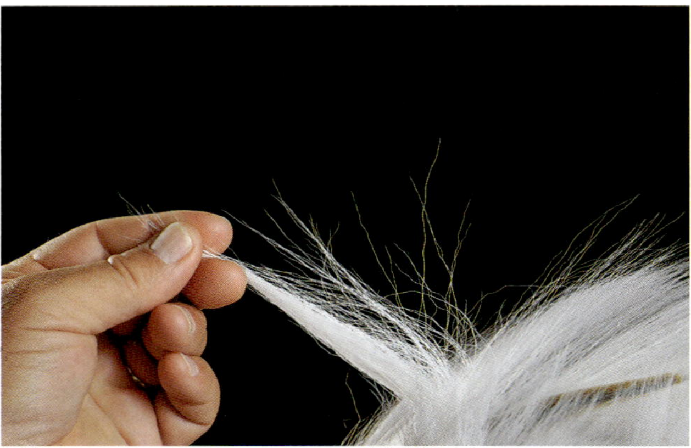

3. As you pull the longer fibers, all the shorter fibers will fall away.

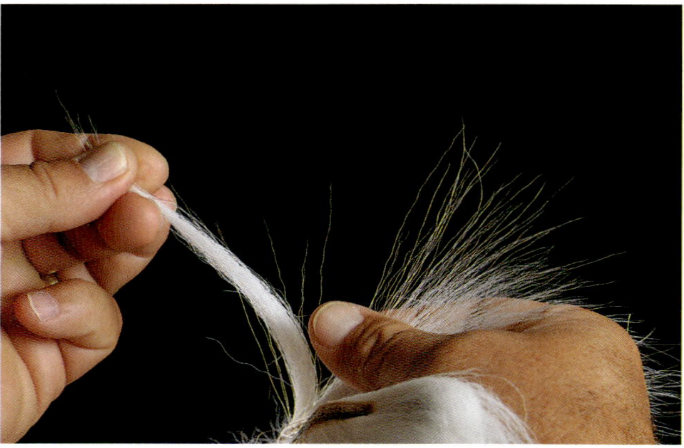

4. As you continue to pull the bunch with your left hand, help separate the shorter fibers by peeling them away with your right hand.

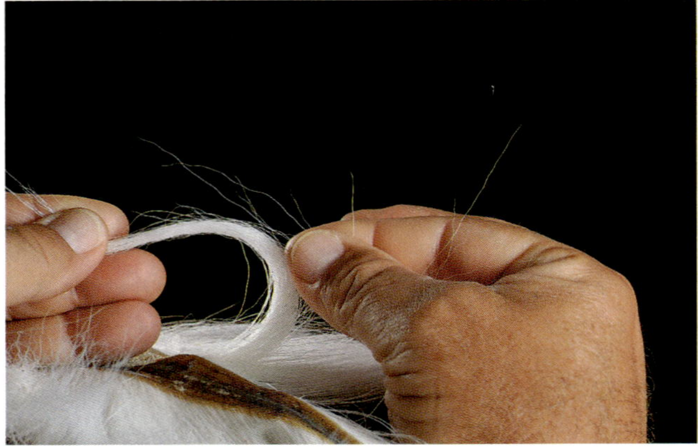

5. Keep preening the shorter fibers away by getting a little closer to the hair tips so that you can access more short fibers.

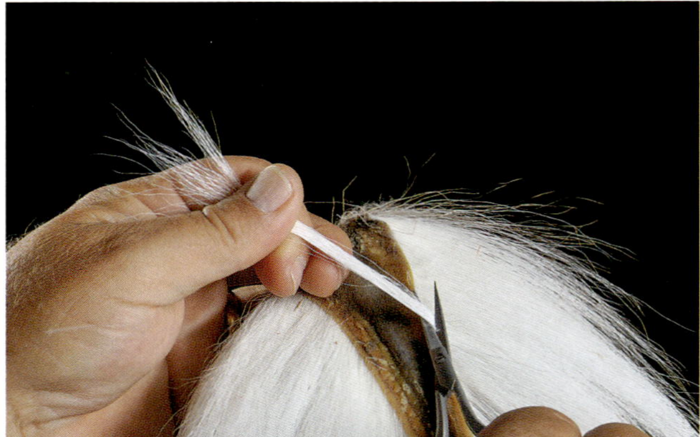

6. When only long fibers remain in your left hand, cut them from the tail and leave the short fibers on the tail for a future fly. Remember, a short fiber is not the same as a long fiber cut short.

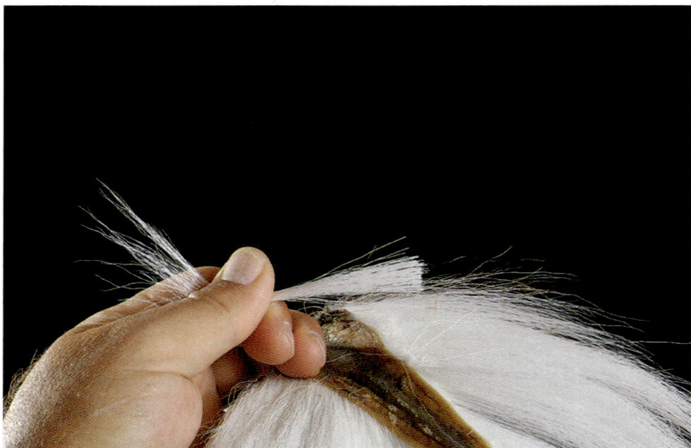

7. Now you are ready the cut the fibers at their bases. They will all be close to equal length.

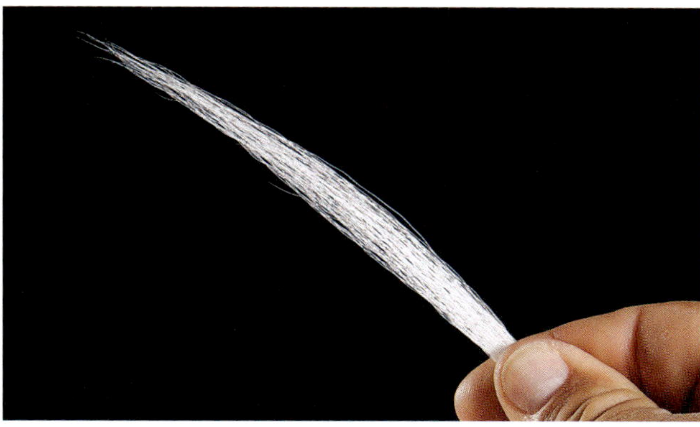

8. Your bundle should have fibers generally the same length, but with enough variance to provide natural taper. For the flies that we are going to tie in this book, you do not ever want to even the tips with a hair stacker.

Working with Bucktail Tips

Most tiers commonly cut an entire clump of fibers from the tail by grasping them at the base, rather than preening the shorter fibers out in the method previously shown. If you do this, and you need to find a way to get a good bunch of fibers or achieve better hair count in smaller bunches, then try this technique.

This sequence shows a typical method of selecting, cutting, preening, and aligning hairs. But it more closely relates to achieving a denser, shorter length. Notice the final length versus the original cut. You're not just removing the short hairs but also using the short hairs to increase hair volume by grouping tips of a similar size range together. You do not want to align all the tips; just take out the "outliers"—the shortest and the longest fibers.

EVENING BUCKTAIL TIPS

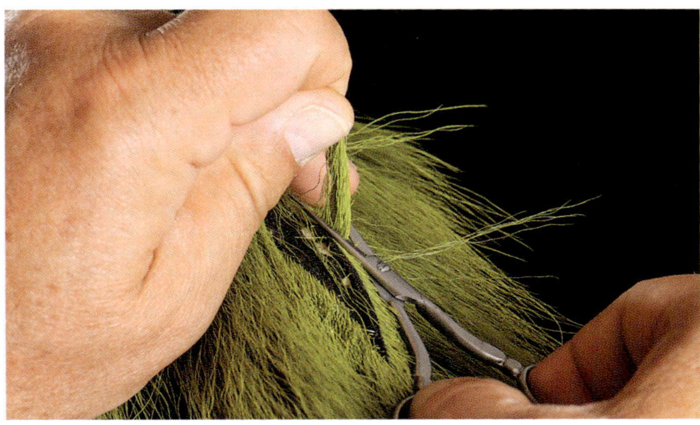

1. Select your bunch and cut as close to the tail as possible.

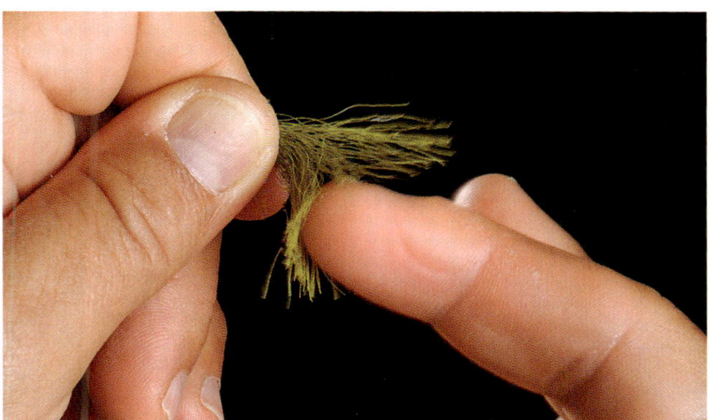

2. Swipe your fingertip through the base of the fibers to remove some of the fluff and to disengage the shortest fibers. Your left hand should be holding the clump firmly. It is critical to always remove the fluff from the base of the bucktail fibers. I will often use a small dog brush for this purpose. This fuzz is especially prominent near the base of the bucktail, where you would be selecting the fibers for a BULKhead Deceiver.

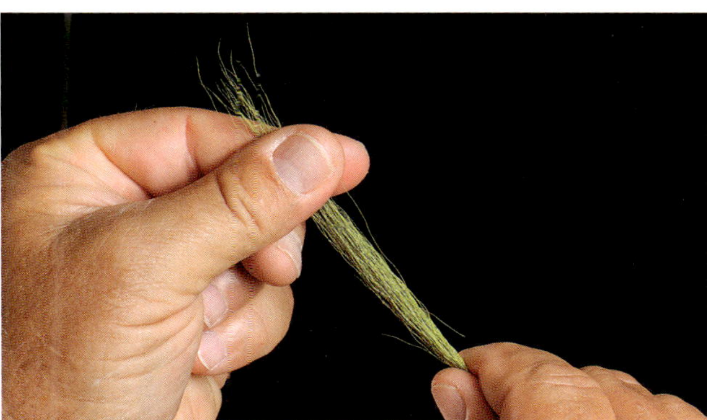

3. Hold the clump firmly near the tips, and pull at the bottom with your other hand to remove the short fibers.

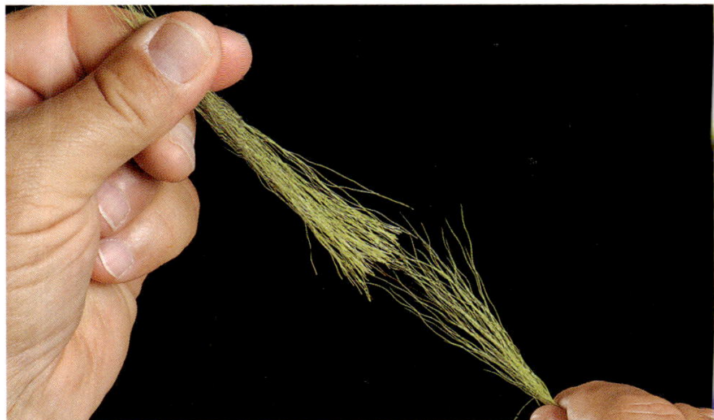

4. At this time, you can choose to keep the sparse longer hairs and discard the shorter hairs or to blend the two different lengths to make a shorter, fuller bucktail wing.

(continued)

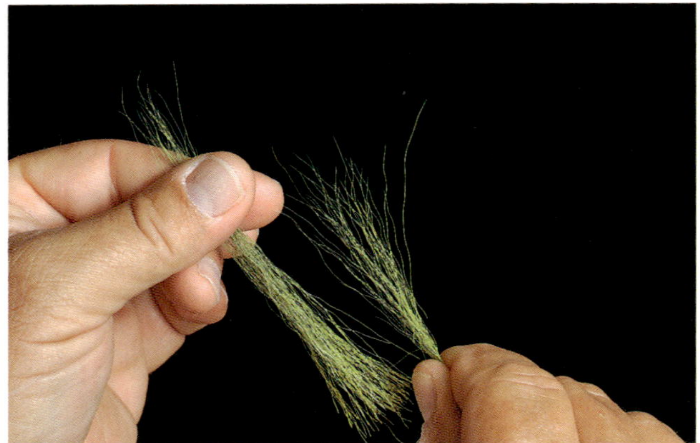

5. With the short hairs removed and now in your right hand, you are ready to match the tips. My alternative method keeps the fibers on the skin for later use.

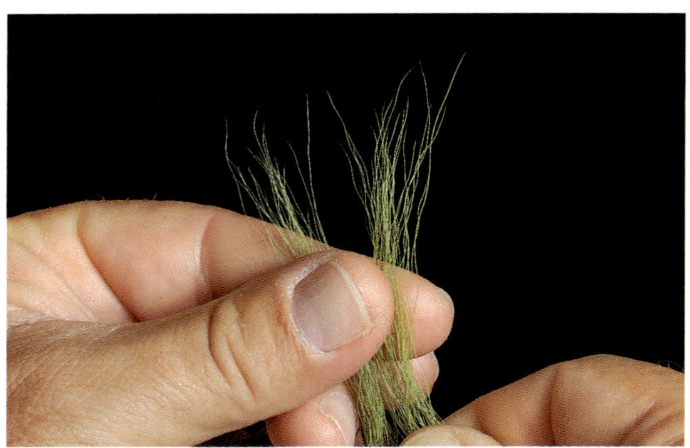

6. Align the two lengths at the tips to use the shorter fibers rather than throwing them away, and get a larger bunch of fibers if needed. Reposition your fingertips, and grab the fibers at the bottom of the shortest fibers before cutting them.

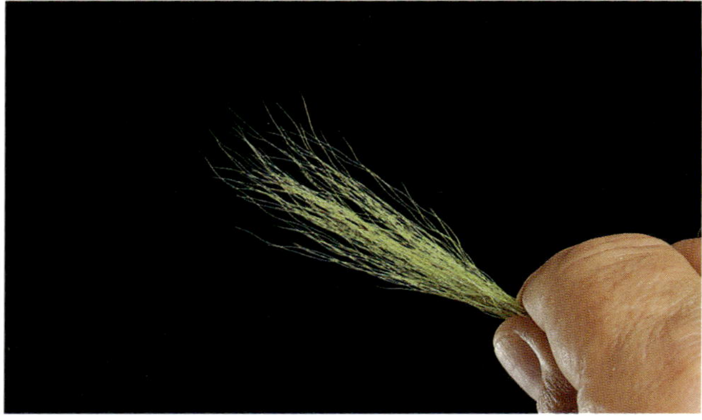

7. The new clump should look like this. Your goal is not to have all the tips perfectly even, as if you had put them in a stacker. You still want to maintain slightly different lengths that look more natural.

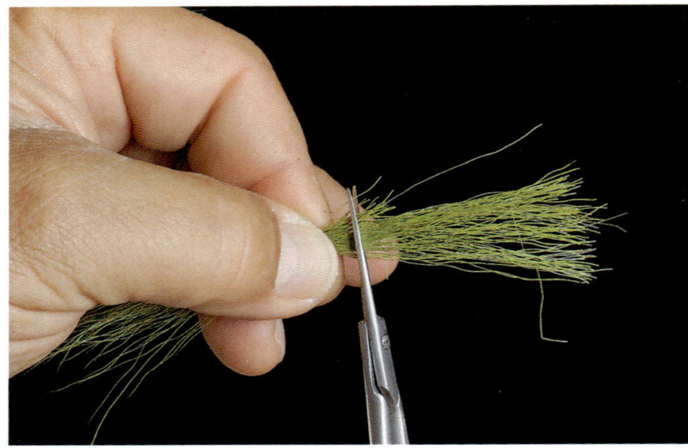

8. Trim the uneven butts at the end of the shortest fibers.

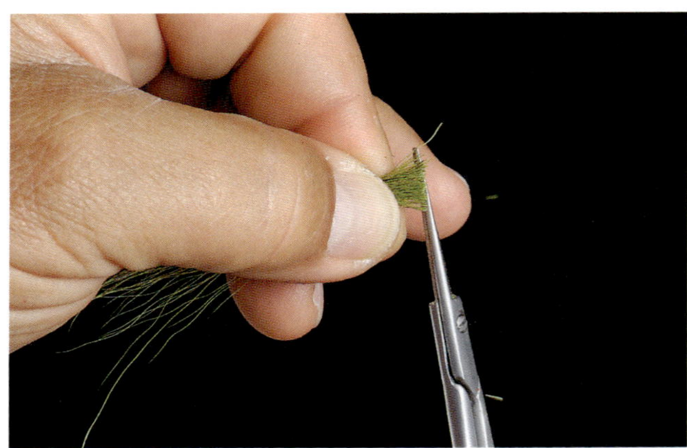

9. Make sure that you cut straight across the fibers. Every time I prepare a bundle of bucktail to be tied to the shank, I trim the butts straight. Serrated scissors are best because the serrations grip the material and prevent it from sliding during the cut.

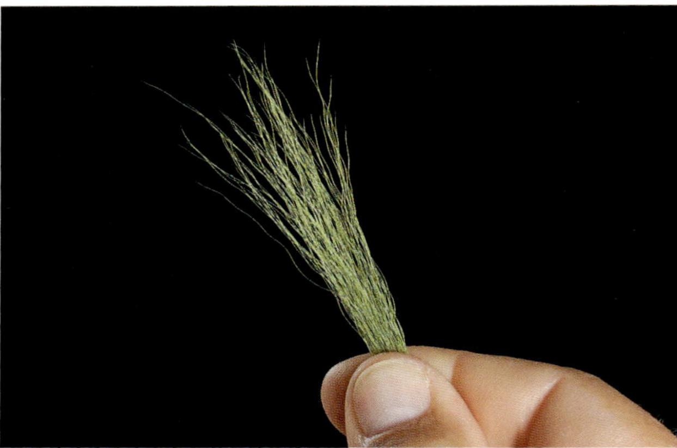

10. The remaining bundle of fibers should have tips relatively aligned, and the bundle should be nice and full.

Introducing Taper

Taper starts with the individual fiber and continues through to the finished fly. One of the keys to creating beautiful flies, in my opinion, is to follow a few simple design rules: use natural fibers with built-in taper, tie in progressively shorter lengths of fibers, and consider that most baitfish do not get thicker past the shoulders.

Another trick to getting your flies in shape is to tie in bundles of fibers that have a natural variance in length, while still being in the same overall size range. When you gather a clump of fibers, you want to avoid stacking them, and instead retain the natural variance of length in any given clump. Most of the time, as long as you don't actually stack the fibers, you will be okay, but if you have straight tips or want to introduce even more taper into a bundle, you can shift the fibers with your thumb and forefinger to create tapered ends.

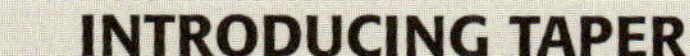

INTRODUCING TAPER

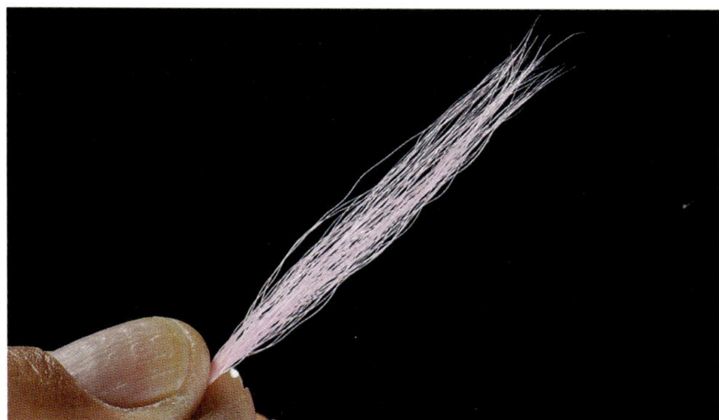

1. In this bundle, the tips are aligned too much, and they look like a paintbrush. When tied on to the shank, they will not look natural.

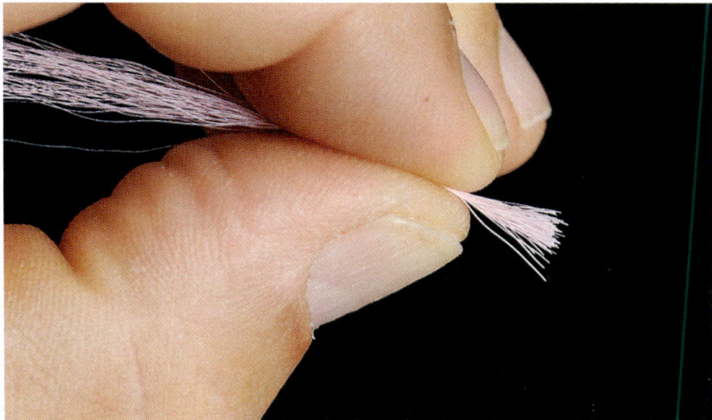

2. Note here how the butts of the bucktail fibers are even.

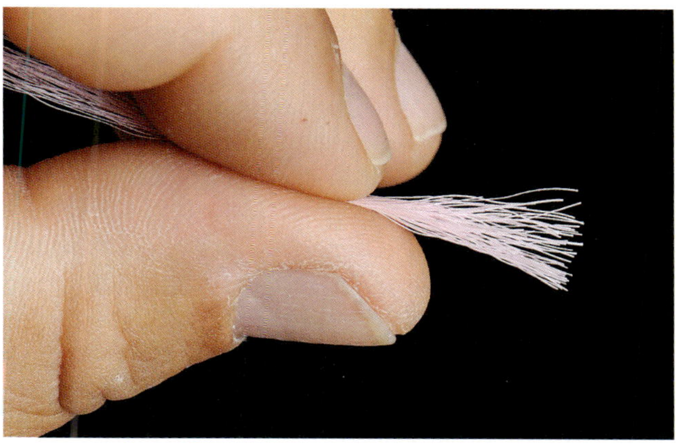

3. To add taper to the tips, hold the butts firmly between your fingertips and slide them in opposite directions to reposition the butt ends in progressive lengths.

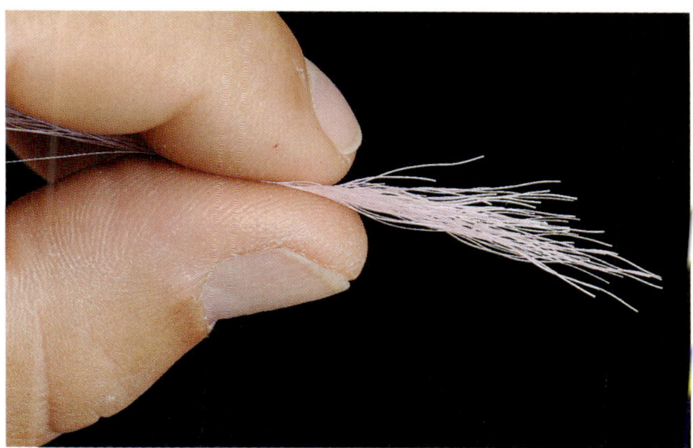

4. Keep pushing for more taper. It takes only about 1/4 to 1/2 inch of movement.

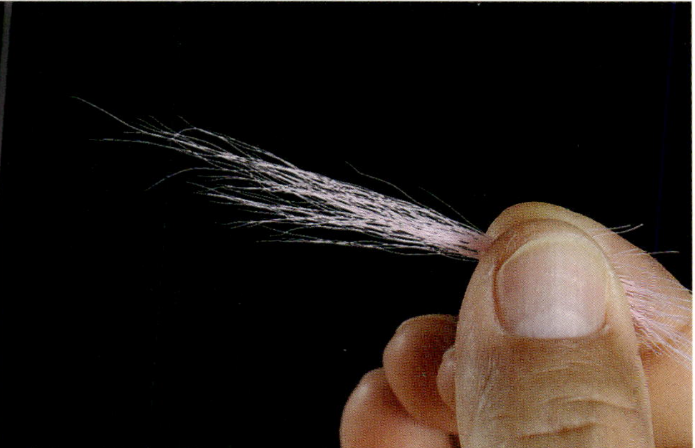

5. The fiber tips are now all different lengths. Before tying these fibers in, I will cut the butts even where my fingertips are in this photo.

Blending Bucktail Fibers

Blending fibers is not only aesthetically pleasing to the eyes of the tier, but since nothing in nature is one color, especially the sides of fish, it can also help to better approximate multihued bait. When I use this technique, I generally just blend the top colors and leave the belly white. I mostly blend fibers in larger flies, and not in smaller patterns. I feel that larger baits show more color shifts on their backs.

Blending fibers has more of an effect on the tier than the fish, I think, but even though it is a low priority in my design, I do like the way that it looks on certain flies. I do not have any favorite color combinations per se, or recipes. I just do what satisfies me at the time, which is often influenced by the bucktail that I have on hand. Blending bucktail and other materials is a good technique to have at your fingertips and may help you achieve the results that you desire in your flies.

BLENDING BUCKTAIL

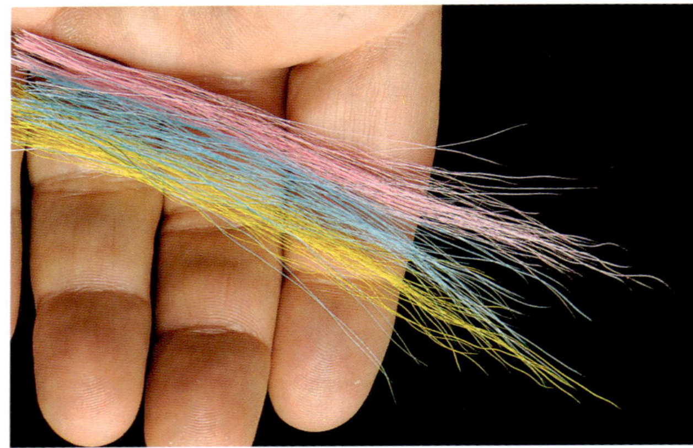

1. Choose three different bucktail colors of equal length, and place all three clumps in your palm. I picked colors that would show up well for this exercise; these are probably not colors that I would blend together in a fly pattern. Pick fibers that have approximately the same length and characteristics. For instance, you do not want to mix straight with wavy fibers.

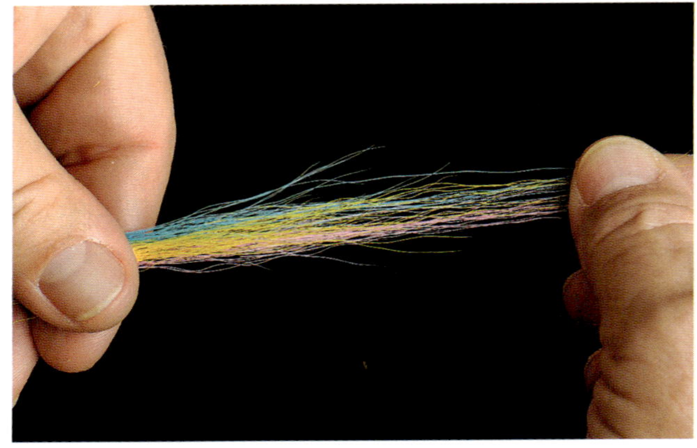

2. Holding the bases firmly, pull the fibers out by their tips with your right hand, and place them on the table.

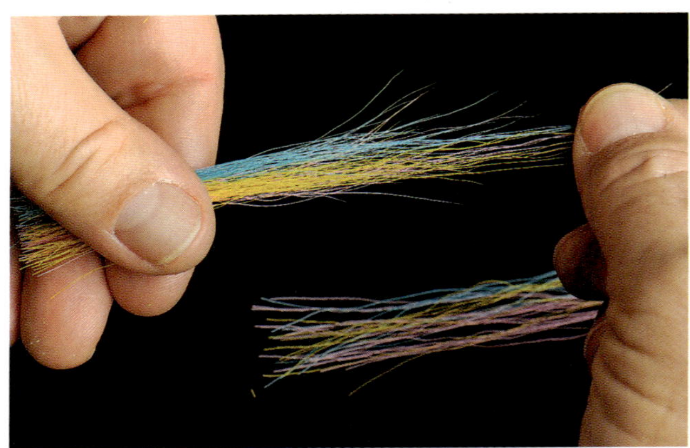

3. Repeat this until all the fibers are on the table, as if you are dealing out a deck of cards.

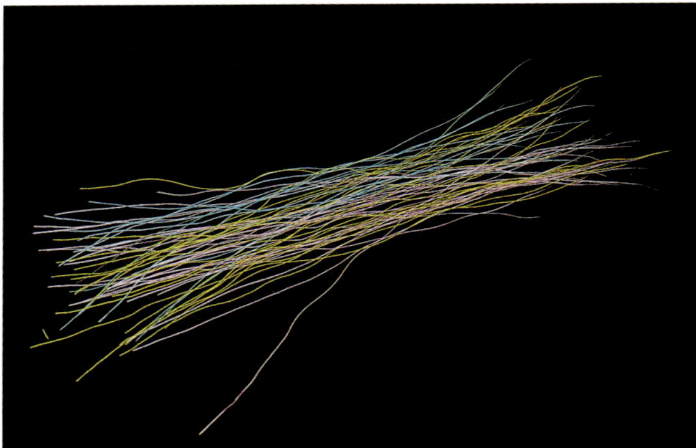

4. The fibers should be mixed fairly well by now, but keep repeating this process until you are satisfied.

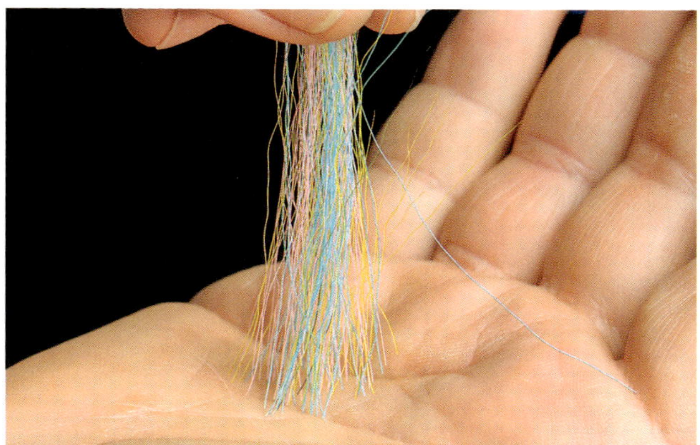

5. After repeating the process a few more times, the fibers are mixed really well. Even the butt ends by dropping (not patting) the fibers butts first onto your palm numerous times. Because you are stacking the butts and not the tips, you retain the slightly different lengths that lend to the overall taper.

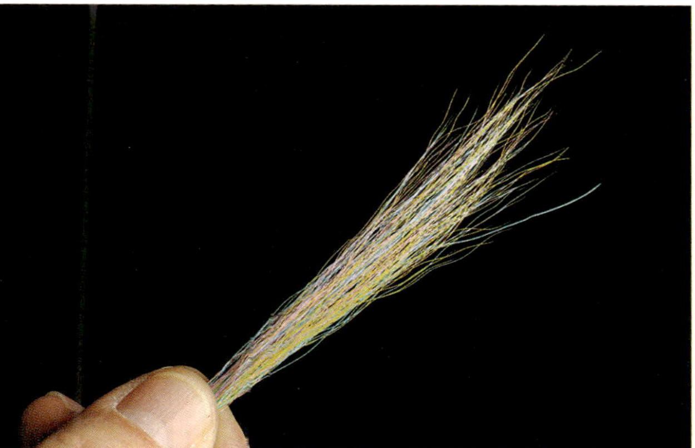

6. Preen any loose fibers from the bundle by holding the ends and gently grabbing and pulling the tips of the longest fibers with your material hand. Once you have the fibers blended the way that you like, you can measure and trim them as you would with any other bucktail bundle. Even though you are blending fibers and combining them, keep the clump sparse. Make sure to cut the ends square.

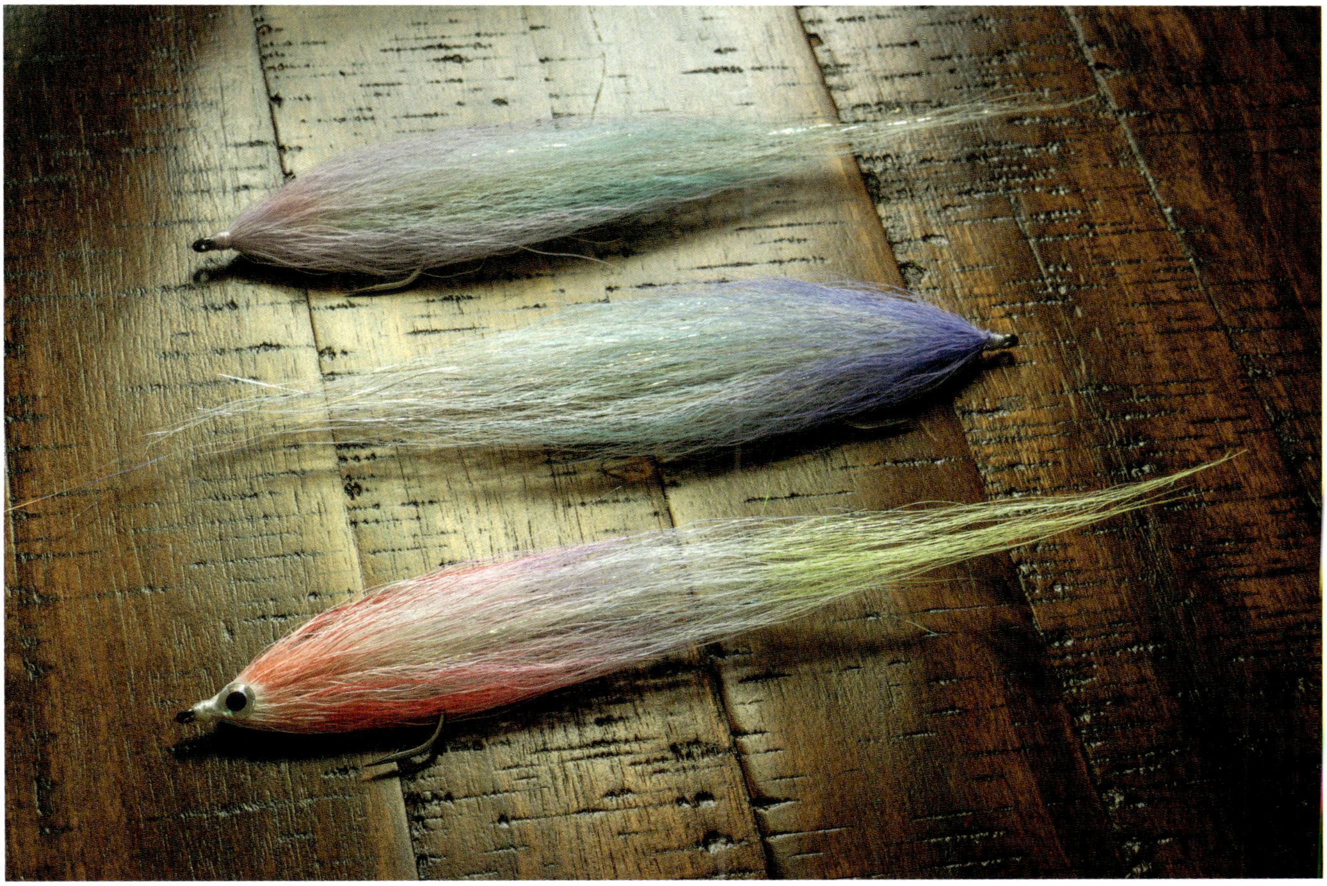

For me, taper is always a primary concern, but that doesn't mean you can't experiment and have fun with color. The top two fleyes demonstrate different approaches to blending fibers, while the bottom rainbow Bucktail Deceiver uses white bucktail with color-dyed tips.

Chapter 2

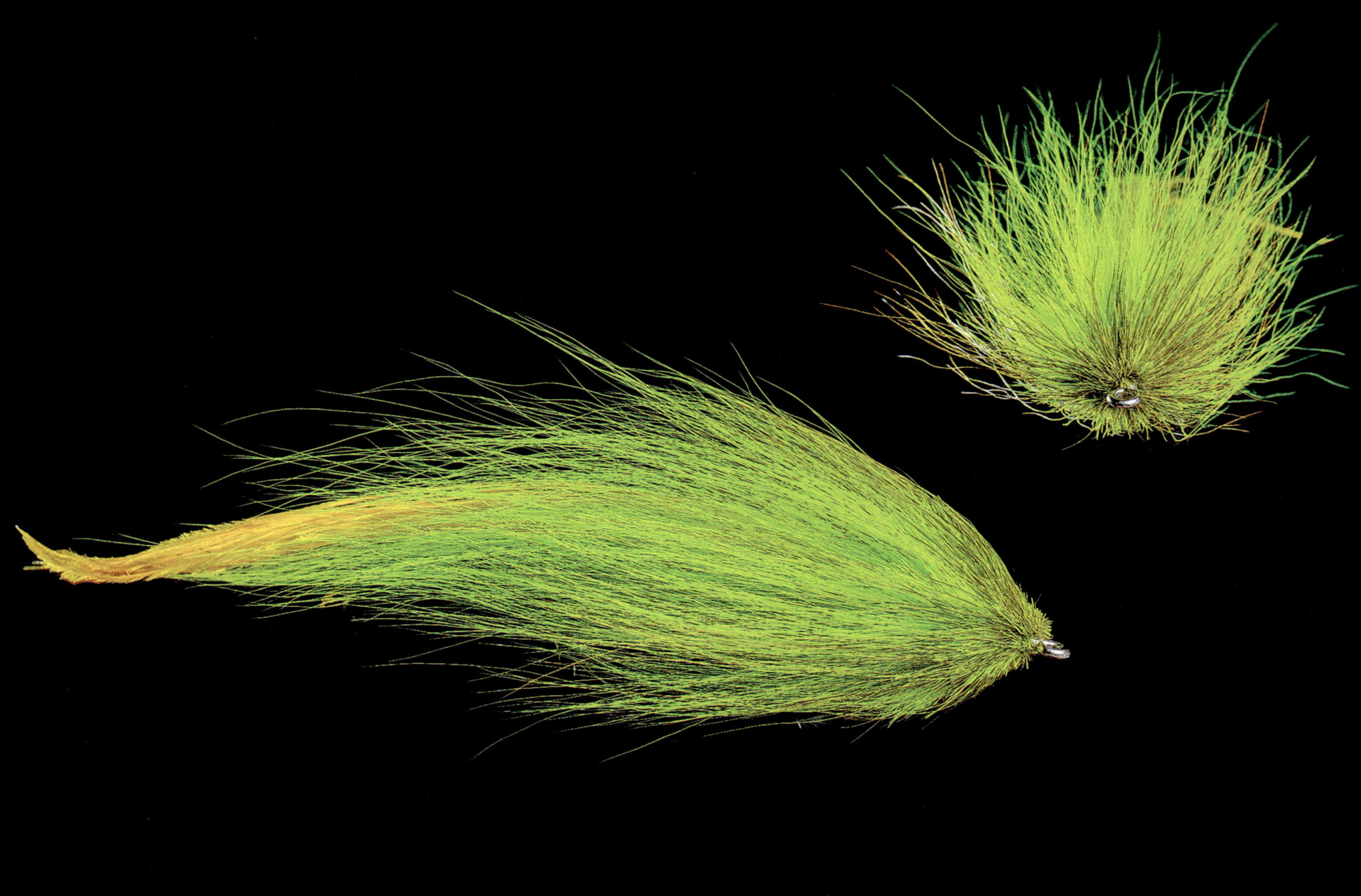

BULKhead with yellow ostrich feathers tied around bucktail. Note the triangular-shaped head on the front of the fly, which is formed by squeezing the bucktail as you tie it in.

Controlling Bucktail and Other Materials

As a fisherman, I don't want to spend excessive amounts of time at the vise. If possible, I much prefer to streamline my tying. One of the ways that I have learned to do this is to vastly simplify the process by which bucktail is tied in on a fly like the Bucktail Deceiver, which requires a complete distribution of fibers around the shank. The drills in this chapter focus on how to quickly and efficiently distribute bucktail around the hook shank as well as how to control the profile of the fibers by manipulating the fibers with your material hand while you relax and tighten the tension on the monofilament thread. I most often demonstrate these techniques when showing other tiers the different shapes of, and the possibilities with, the Bucktail Deceiver, but you can apply these techniques to any fly tied with bucktail.

I will cover four shapes here, described by how the fly looks when viewed from the front—round, narrow, flat, and triangular. Once you master these techniques you can introduce shape into your own patterns in an almost infinite number of ways, all of which not only affect the overall profile of the fly but also the way that it fishes.

In these sequences we are also going to cover some fundamentals of working with bucktail that will be repeated throughout the book.

1. When preparing the bucktail fibers to be tied in, always remove the shorter fibers from the clump and then trim the butts square.
2. When securing bucktail to the hook, always wrap at right angles to the hook shank. Even the slightest angle can botch the even distribution of hair.
3. After the clump is tied in, add head cement to the butts before wrapping over them. This step ensures maximum durability.

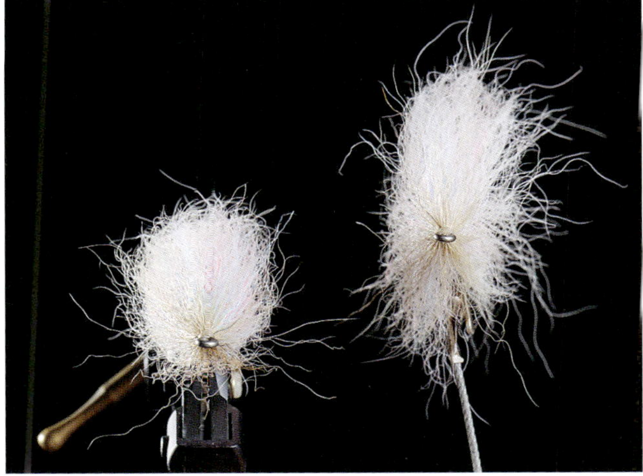

Some possible ways of achieving shape with bucktail, viewed from the front. Even the basic round shape on the left can have subtle variations, which you can create by the way you pull snuggly to apply side-to-side pressure to the bucktail when you tie it in.

ROUND

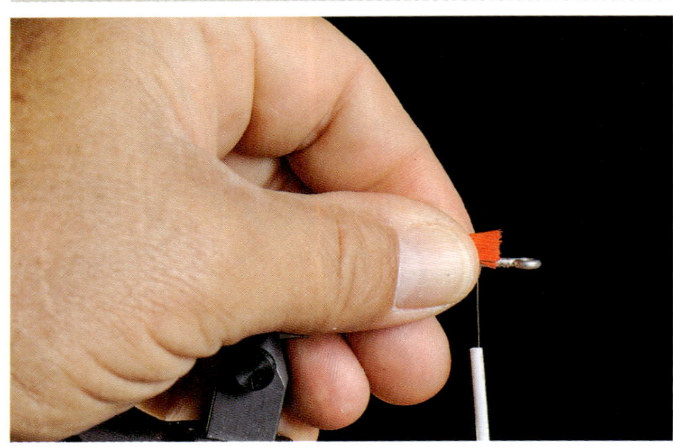

1. First, we will tie the bucktail in and then distribute it 360 degrees around the shank, which is the basic technique for the Bucktail Deceiver. Use a hook with a moderately long shank and start the thread at the forward portion of the hook so that you can avoid the barb and focus on the technique. When you tie the actual fly, you will have to work in and around the hook point. Remove all the short hairs from the bucktail clump and cut the butt ends even. Hold the clump at the tie-in position with your material hand, exposing 1/4 inch of butts to be tied down.

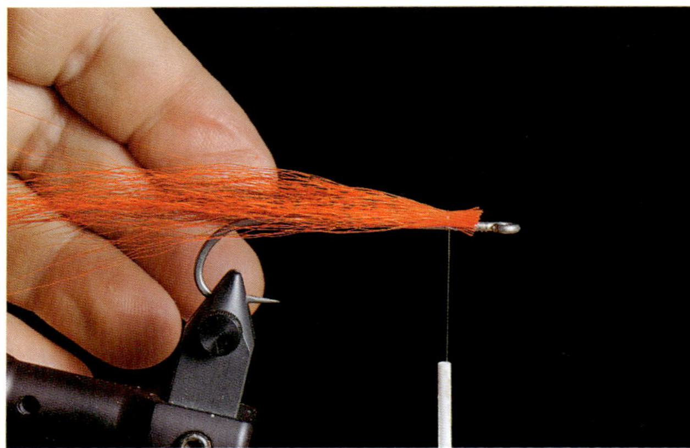

2. Take two or three thread wraps over the butts with light tension and allow the weight of the bobbin and thread spool to keep the material in place, on top of the hook shank. The thread must go straight up and over the fibers, not at an angle, or you will not get evenly distributed fibers. A lot of tiers overlook this important tip.

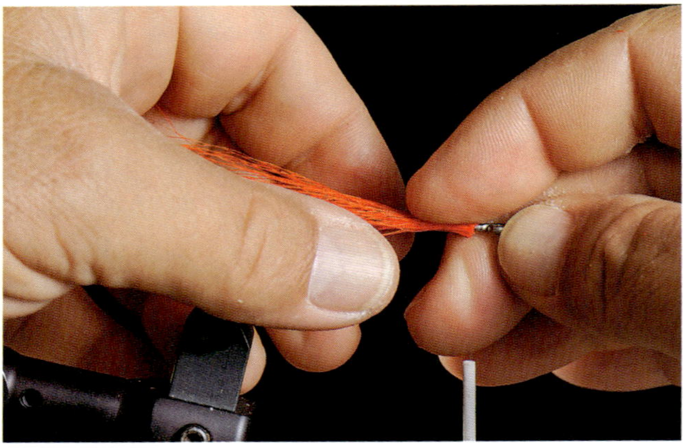

3. While the fibers are still under light thread tension, lightly press the fibers down with your fingertip to ease them around the shank in one movement. Squeeze the fibers from the top and bottom at the same time to get them to start surrounding the shank. Then, press from side to side to move the fibers around more. If the fibers aren't 360 degrees around the shank, relax the tension on the thread, adjust the fibers, and then tighten it. This sequence of relax, reposition, and retighten is the key to controlling the distribution of fibers. While this technique can be done with regular thread, monofilament thread has a spring to it that makes it much more efficient in my experience.

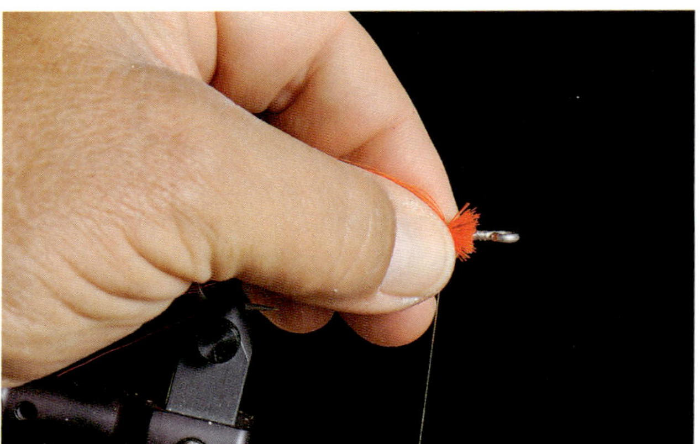

4. Once the fibers are completely and evenly distributed around the shank, hold them firmly and tighten the thread by pulling straight down. Take about four to five wraps around the fibers to help secure them.

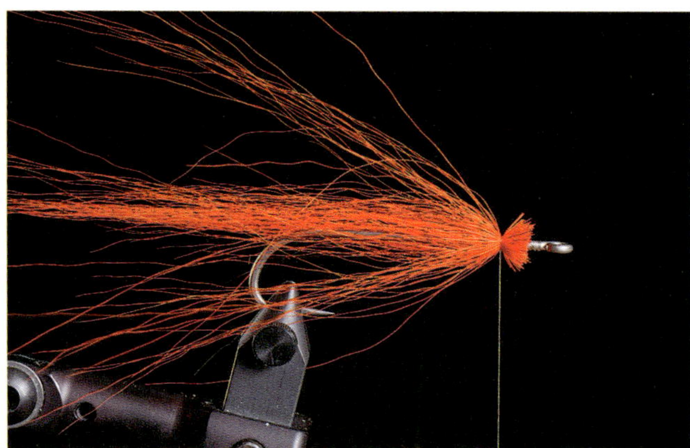

5. This is the basic, general tubular shape for the Bucktail Deceiver.

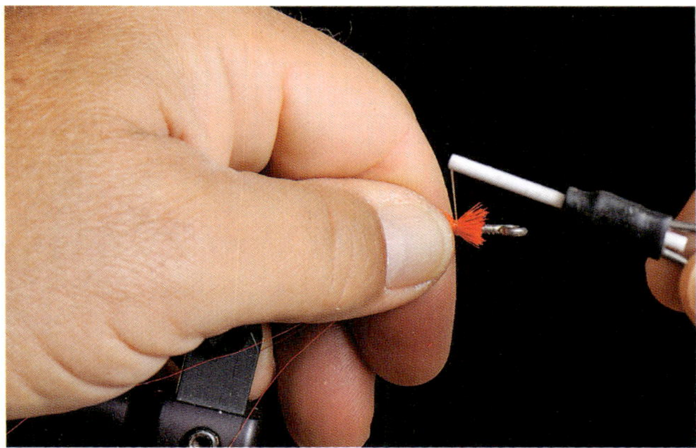

6. Apply head cement to the butts and wrap over them. When you are tying in the clump of bucktail right at the bend, you might find it helpful to use a bodkin to better distribute the fibers around the hook bend.

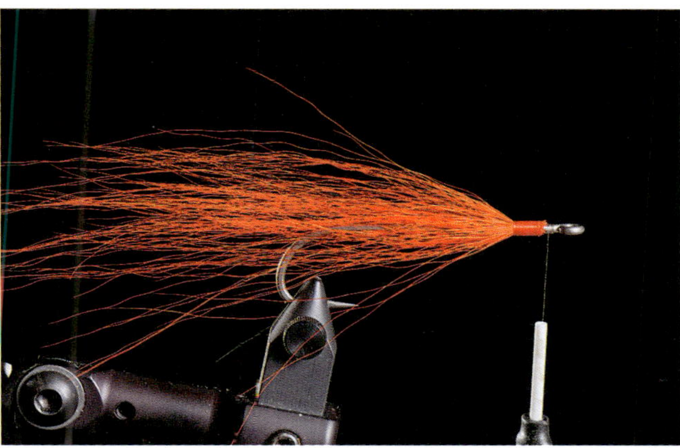

7. Wrap evenly to create a level surface onto which you can tie the next step. When you cut the bucktail straight and tie it down with even wraps, you create a flat, level surface.

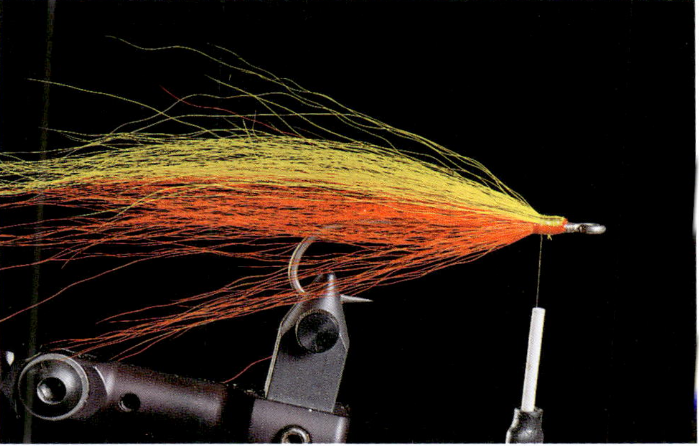

8. Notice how the platform from the previous tie of bucktail provides an even base for the next bunch of fibers. When tying on multiple materials, you must make sure that the base on which you tie them is parallel to the shank, as if it was part of the shank itself.

NARROW

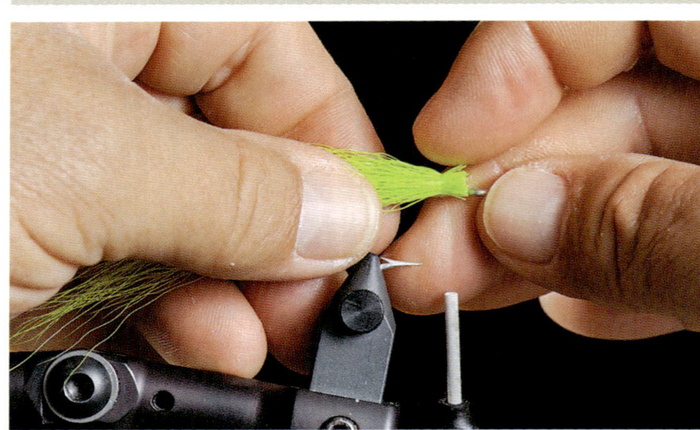

1. In the next few steps, I am going to show you how to manipulate the bucktail to create a narrow (when viewed from the front) and broad shape (from the side) typical of a herring. We are starting with the bucktail prepared and attached to the shank in the same way as before.

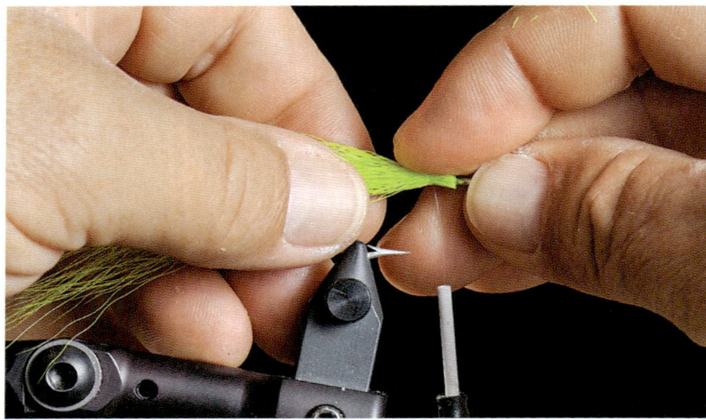

2. Both hands should work in concert as you distribute the fibers 360 degrees around the shank. Apply pressure with your right hand while controlling fibers with your left hand.

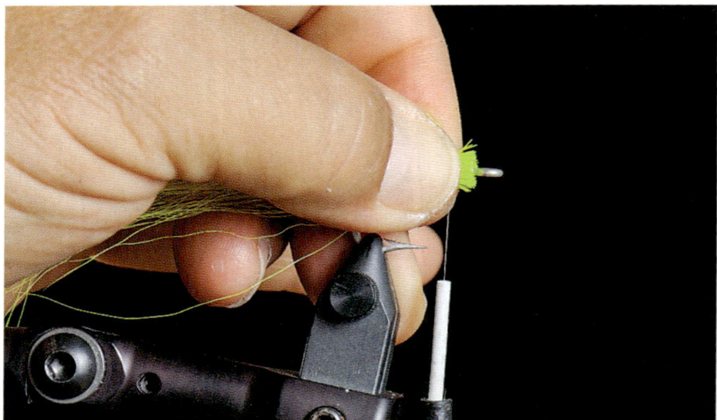

3. Once the fibers are evenly distributed around the hook shank, loosen the thread pressure and squeeze the hairs with your material hand tightly from each side to push more fibers on top and underneath the shank.

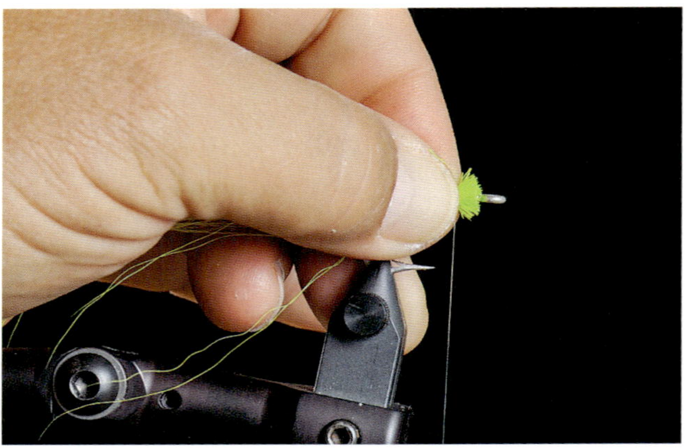

4. Tighten the thread while still squeezing the fibers.

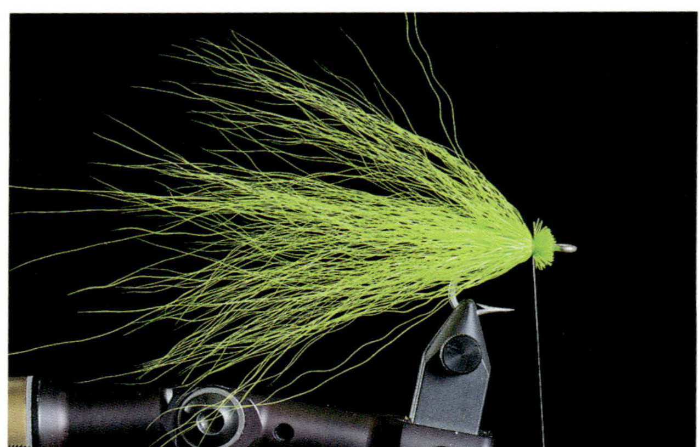

5. The fibers should be flared wide, when viewed from the side. You can build an entire fly with fibers tied in this way.

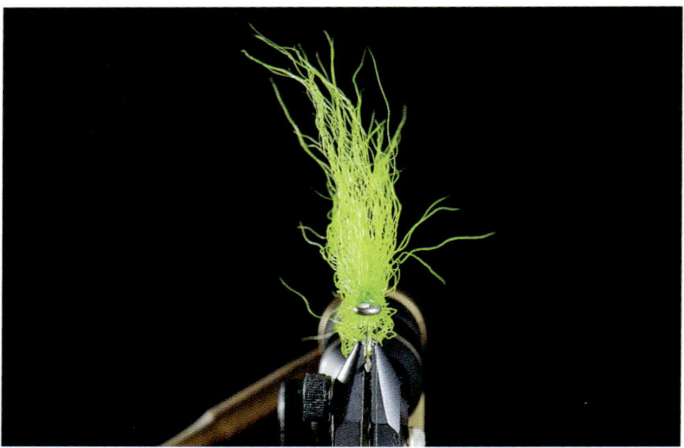

6. When viewed head on, the fibers will be at the 12 to 6 o'clock position and the fly will have a high, narrow profile.

FLAT

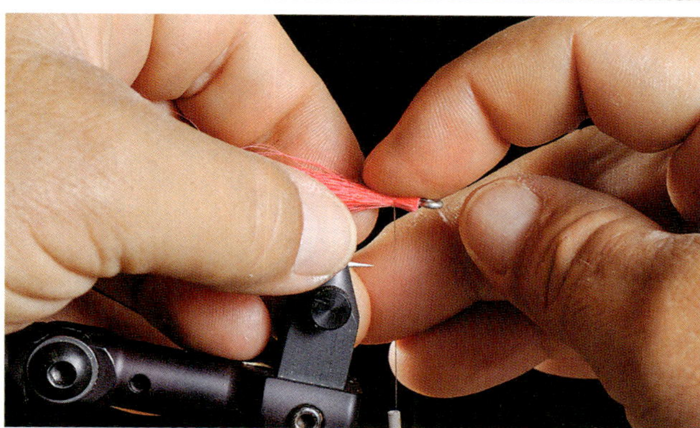

1. Instead of squeezing the fibers from the side, you can squeeze the top and bottom of them to create a flatter profile, which is important when you want to design a fly that sinks slowly and fishes higher in the water column. The steps are the same as before until the point that you squeeze the fibers into position and tighten them down. Take a few loose thread wraps around the butts. Press down to distribute the fibers around the hook shank.

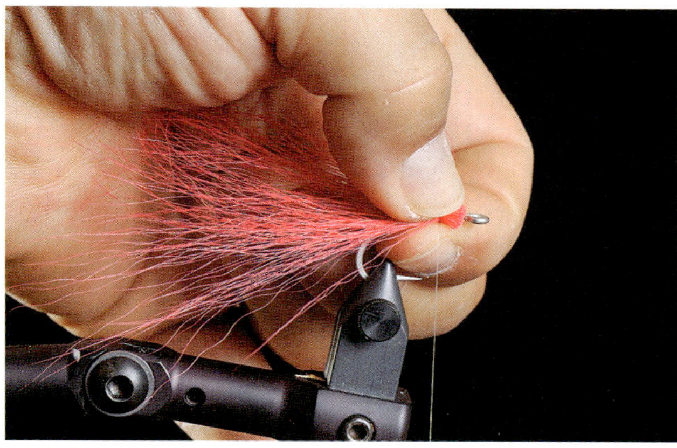

2. Squeeze the fibers from the top and bottom so that they flare.

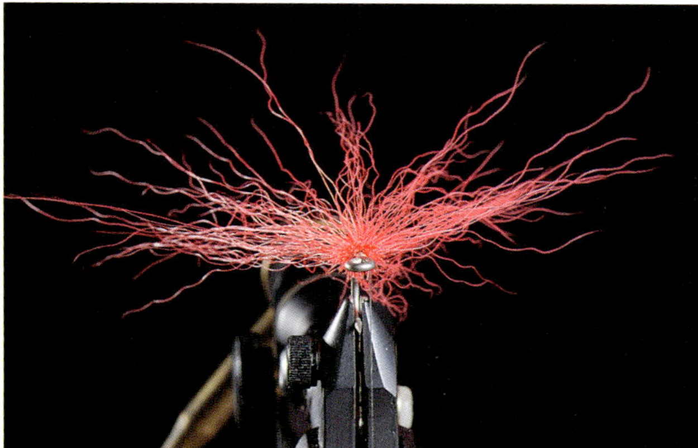

3. When viewed head on, the fly has a wide, flat profile with the fibers mostly at 3 and 9 o'clock.

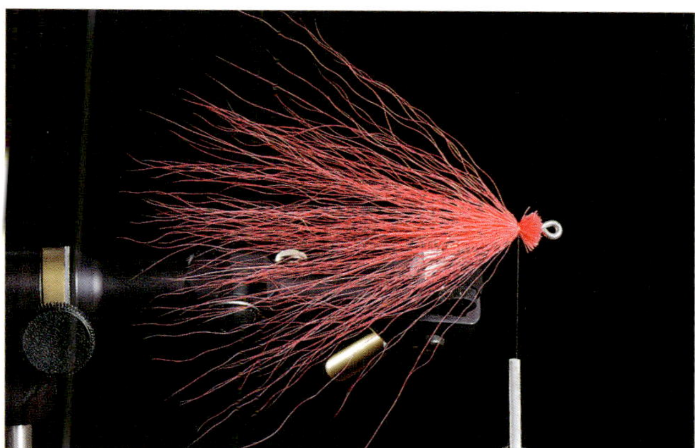

4. View from above. This technique is helpful when creating shoulders on the sides of the Bucktail Deceiver, 3Ds, Bangers, and Siliclones.

TRIANGULAR

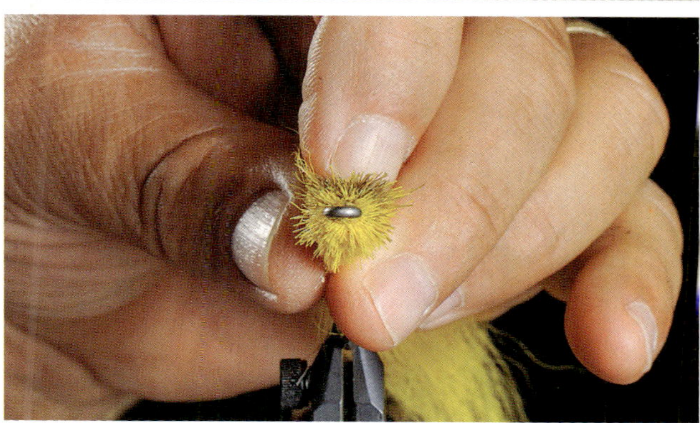

To get a more triangular shape, such as when tying the BULKhead Deceiver, you can pinch the fibers as shown as you lash them down. This achieves a flatter top and a deeper, V-shaped belly. I do not have any thread in this picture so that you can better see what my fingers are doing.

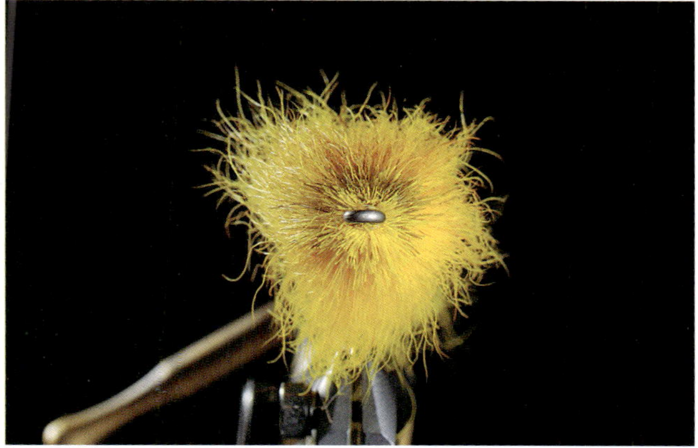

Note how the fly is more flat on top with a V-shaped belly. See also page 35 for a discussion of fly shapes.

Tying in Flash

I include flash here because I use it often, and I reference the following tips a number of times in the fly-tying tutorials in Part 2. I find that it is much easier and efficient to tie in the entire length of flash well ahead of where you want it to be positioned in the fly and then to wrap back over the folded portions. This allows you to tie in long lengths of flash without trimming them and also allows you to control the distribution of the flash around the shank.

TYING IN FLASH

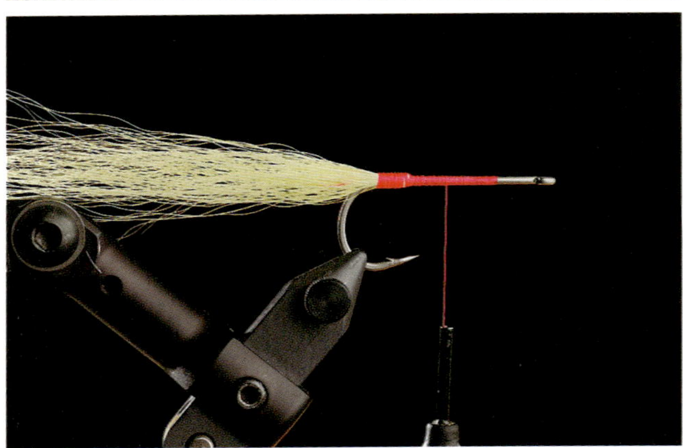

1. Insert the hook into the vise. Cover the entire shank with thread. Tie in the bucktail wing, and wrap the thread forward to about 1/4 inch ahead of the tie-down area. After you tie in the flash, you will be wrapping back over it, so this distance is necessary for working room.

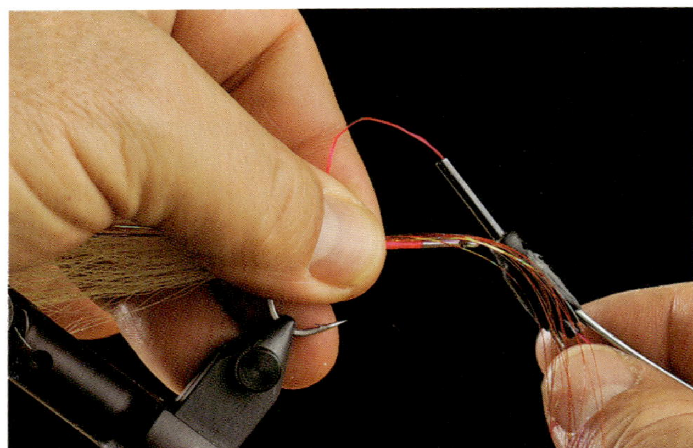

2. Trim the flash from the bundle, keeping in mind that you will be doubling it. Tie in the flash in the middle of the bunch, leaving equal lengths on each side of the tie-in point.

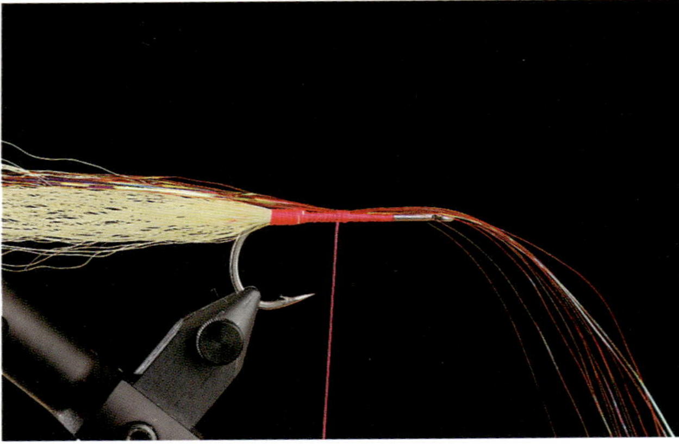

3. By tying the flash in this way, you don't need to waste time trimming the exact length you need from the bundle. Also by taking whole lengths of flash from the bundle, you can keep the bundle orderly and without random lengths of flash, which would be harder to work with.

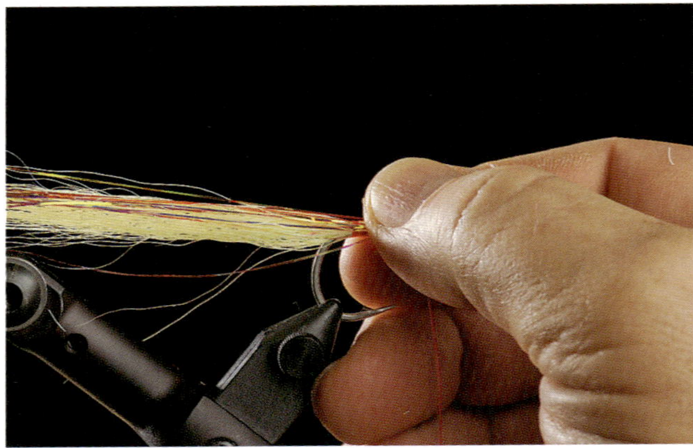

4. Once you tie the flash down, spread it with your thumb to distribute it around the shank.

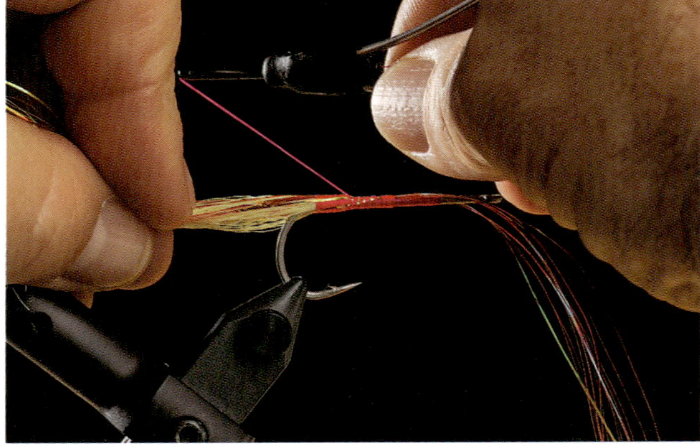

5. As you hold the flash with your material hand, keep it spread around the bucktail. This will help you get a nice flow of flash and bucktail on the finished fly. While still holding the flash in the desired position, start wrapping the thread back over the flash.

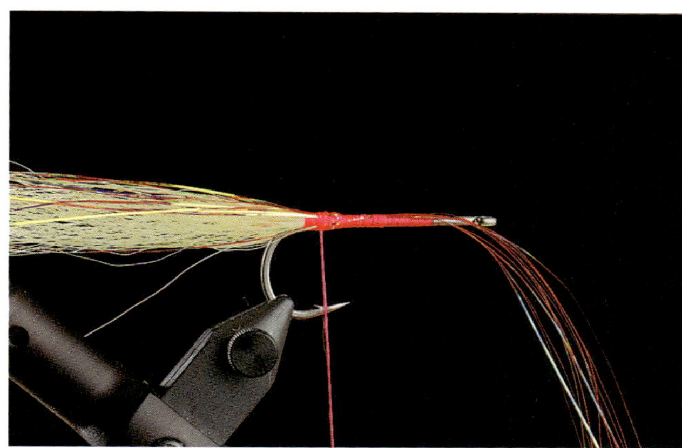

6. When you tie down the flash, leave the thread in that position.

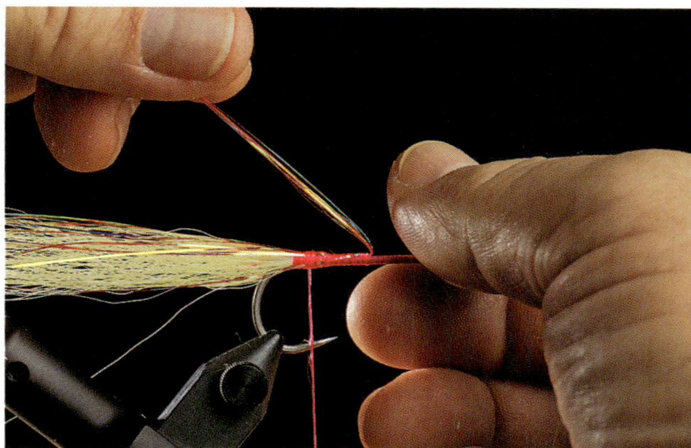

7. Fold back the other half of the flash.

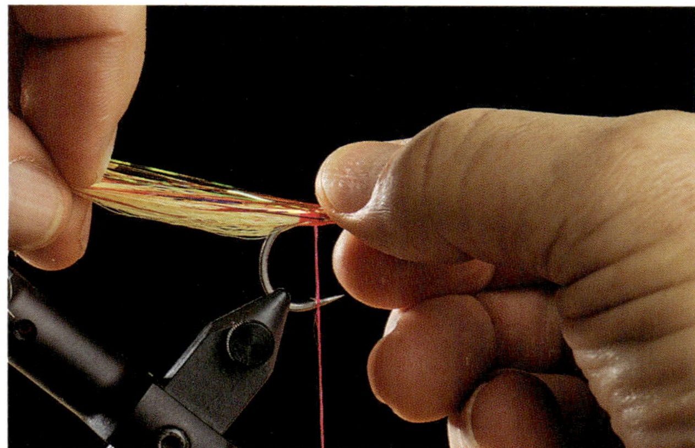

8. Spread it with your thread hand.

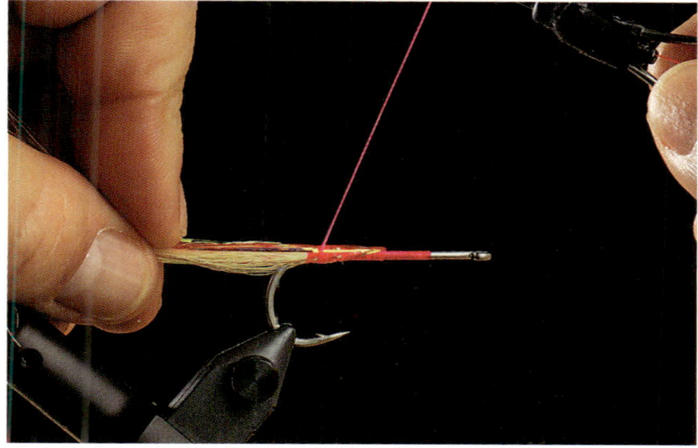

9. Wrap over the spread flash to secure it. Doing this allows you to lash the flash in the best position for the fly. Wrap the thread forward to your next tie-in point.

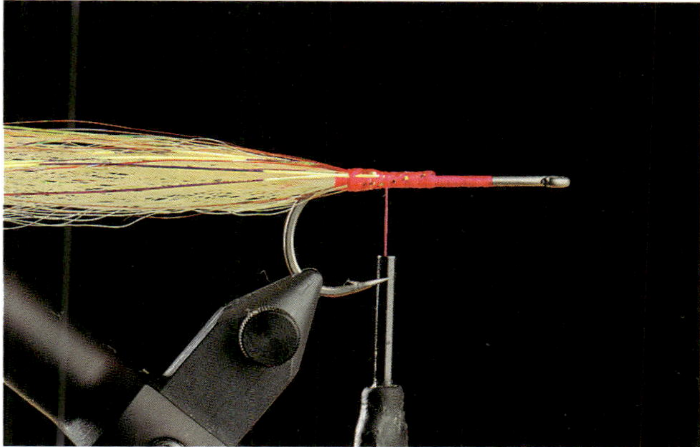

10. Tying in the flash this way gives you a more balanced distribution of flash and bucktail. The key is to tie the flash well ahead of where you ultimately want it to be, which gives you room to control the material on the shank.

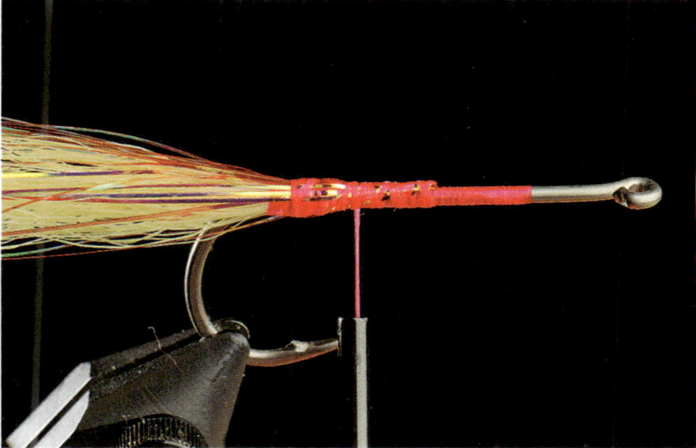

11. By using this technique you can quickly and easily position the flash exactly where you want it.

Chapter 3

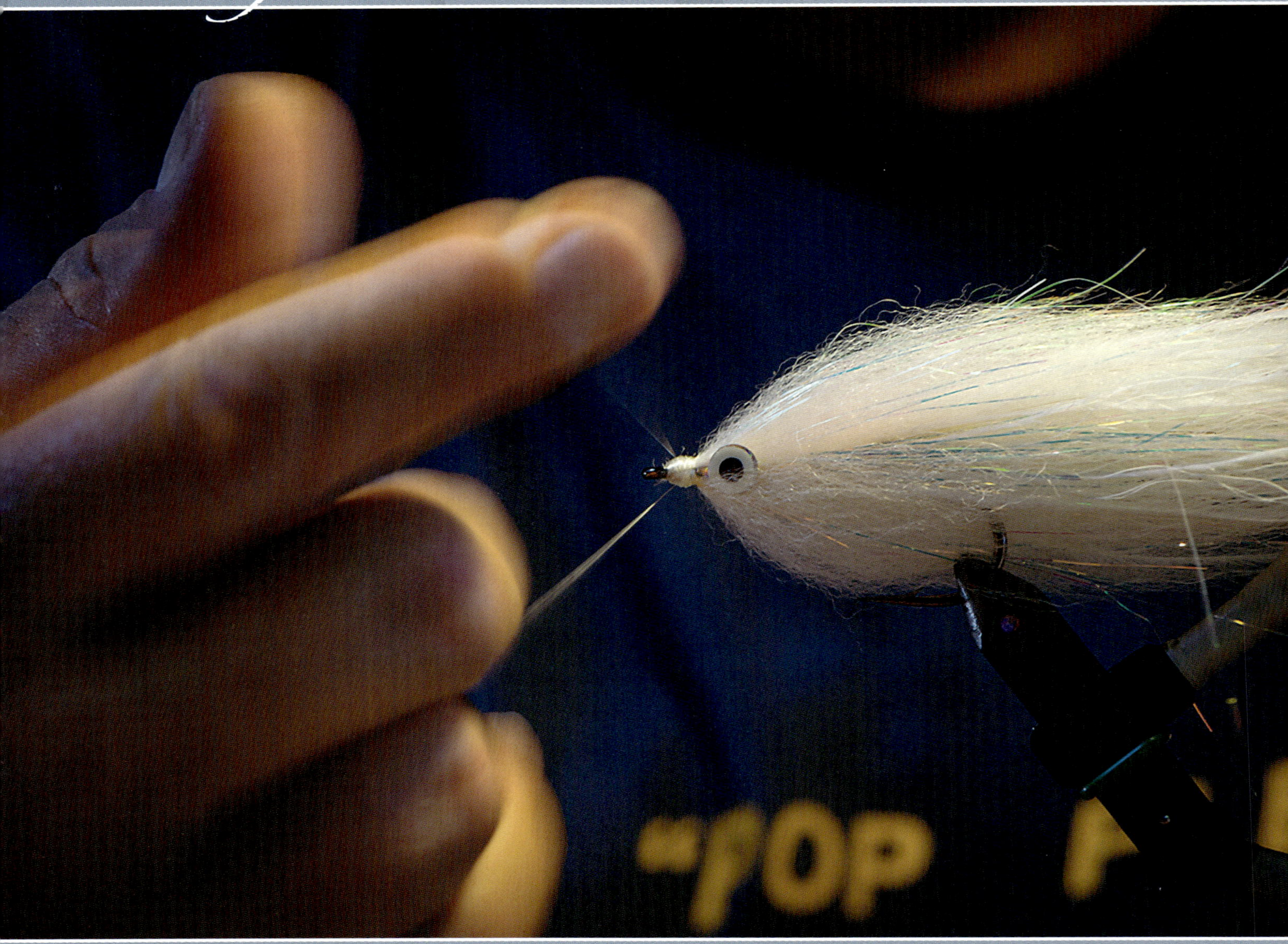

Finishing touches on a Bucktail Deceiver tied with thin layers of fleece between bucktail to softly expand the collar's volume.

Putting It All Together

In this chapter I am going to take an in-depth look at three key fleyes—the Bucktail Deceiver, Hollow Fleye, and BULKhead—to focus on certain techniques and important concepts in their construction. One of the reasons that I am isolating techniques for some of the fleyes is not only to emphasize their importance, but to provide a lot of detail for readers new to these patterns.

We already covered the specific technique of distributing bucktail fibers around the shank quickly, which is central to fleyes such as the Bucktail Deceiver and Hollow Fleye. Here I want to emphasize the importance of taper by tying a complete Bucktail Deceiver so that you can focus on the end result, the goal, of the overall fly and better understand how each tie works together. The key to this fly—and the key to many of the patterns in this book—is to use gradually shorter lengths of hair as you progress up the shank to create a smooth taper. In this tutorial I am using different colors to highlight the different lengths.

BUCKTAIL DECEIVER

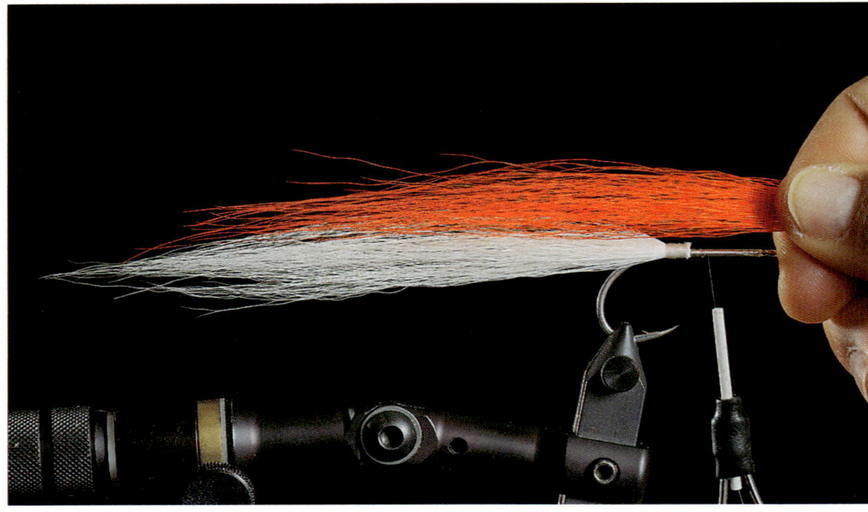

1. Insert the hook into the vise, attach the thread, and prepare your first clump of bucktail by removing the shorter fibers and trimming the butts even. Starting just ahead of the hook bend, tie in the bucktail clump on top of the shank and then distribute the fibers completely around the shank. Before wrapping over the butts, apply head cement to them.

Select another clump of bucktail fibers and measure them so that they are just shorter than the first bunch that you tied in. Transfer the bunch to your material hand and cut them to length, making sure that the butts are even.

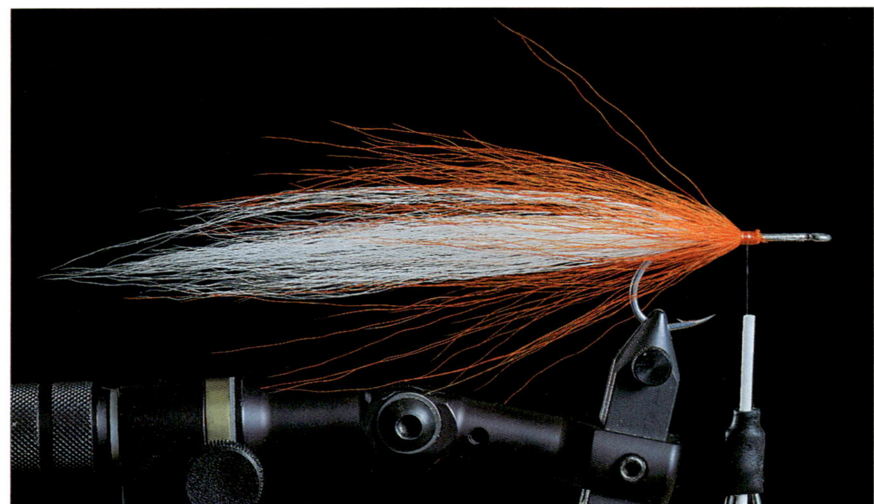

2. Tie in the second bunch of bucktail and then distribute the fibers completely and evenly around the shank. As with the first bunch, apply head cement to the butts before wrapping over them with thread.

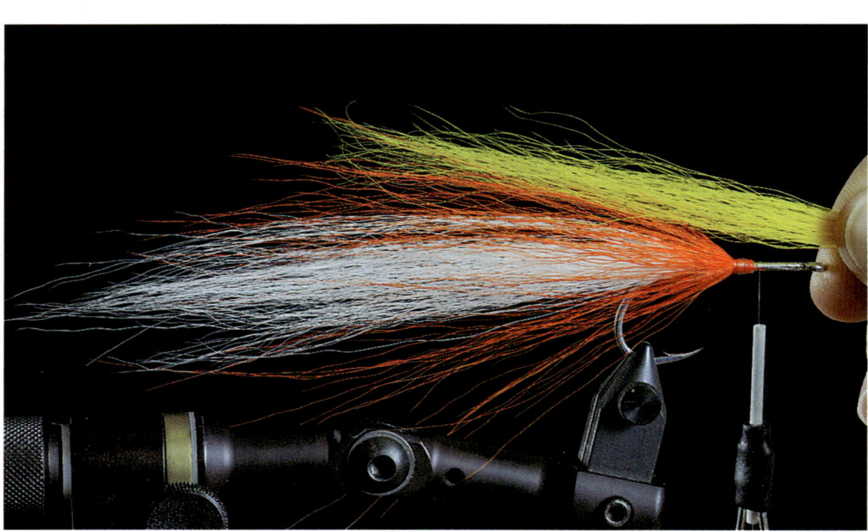

3. Move the thread ahead about 1/4 inch. Select another bunch of fibers and measure them so that they are just a little shorter than the previous bunch. Closer spacing contributes to a fuller profile; open spacing helps to attain a thinner profile. In both cases, the amount of fibers you choose to include in each bunch contributes to the overall shape, so choose the right amount of material for the profile that you have in mind.

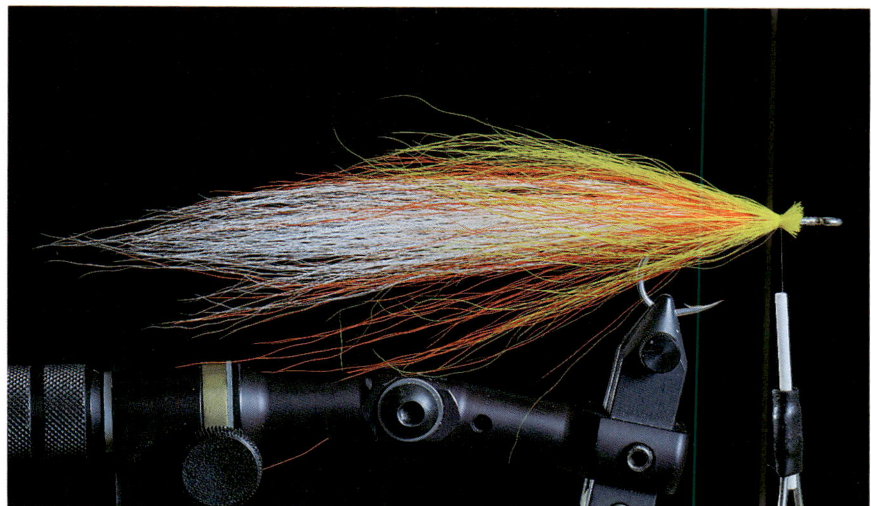

4. Distribute the fibers around the hook shank and secure them. Add cement to the butts and then wrap a smooth flat base over them to prepare for the next tie.

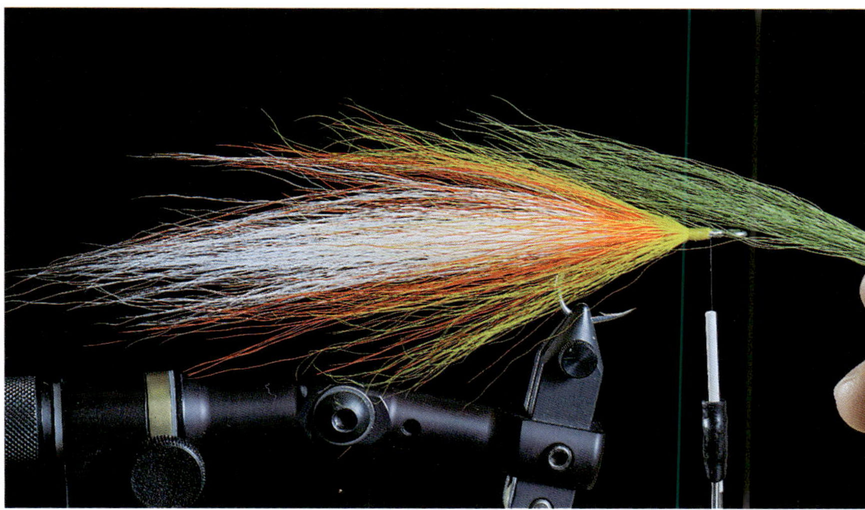

5. The taper should be smooth and subtle. If each bucktail is tied too far apart, then the fly will look like a staircase.

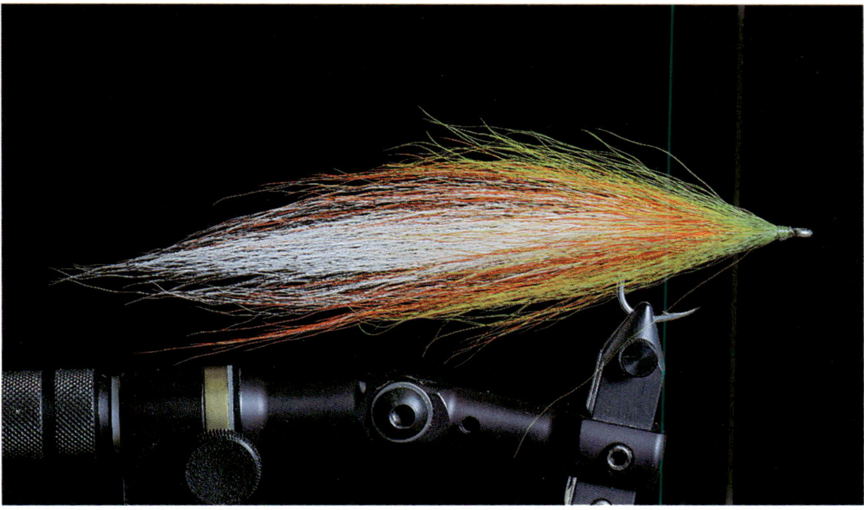

6. A well-tied Bucktail Deceiver has a natural progression of bucktail tips throughout its length and has smooth lines—no unsightly bulges.

(continued)

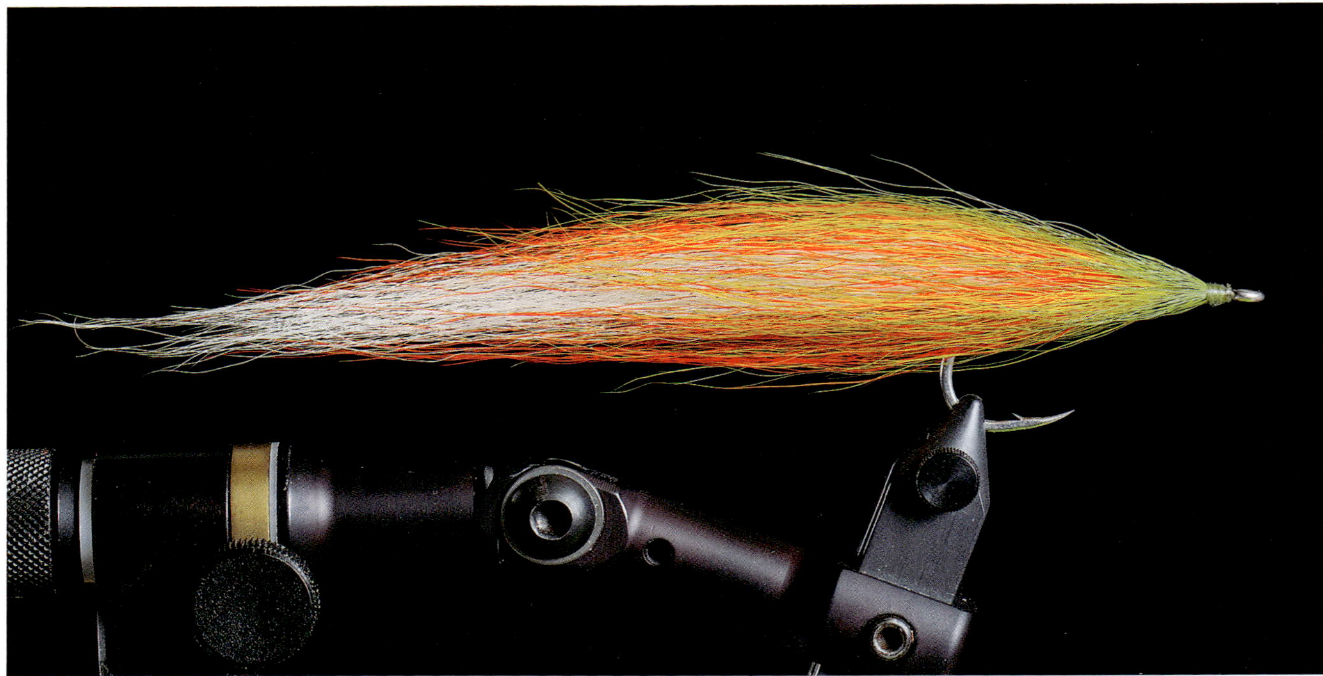

I keep a glass of water at the tying bench and wet every fly that I tie to tame the fibers. Once the fly dries completely, the once-straight tips curve inward slightly and the shape comes together nicely.

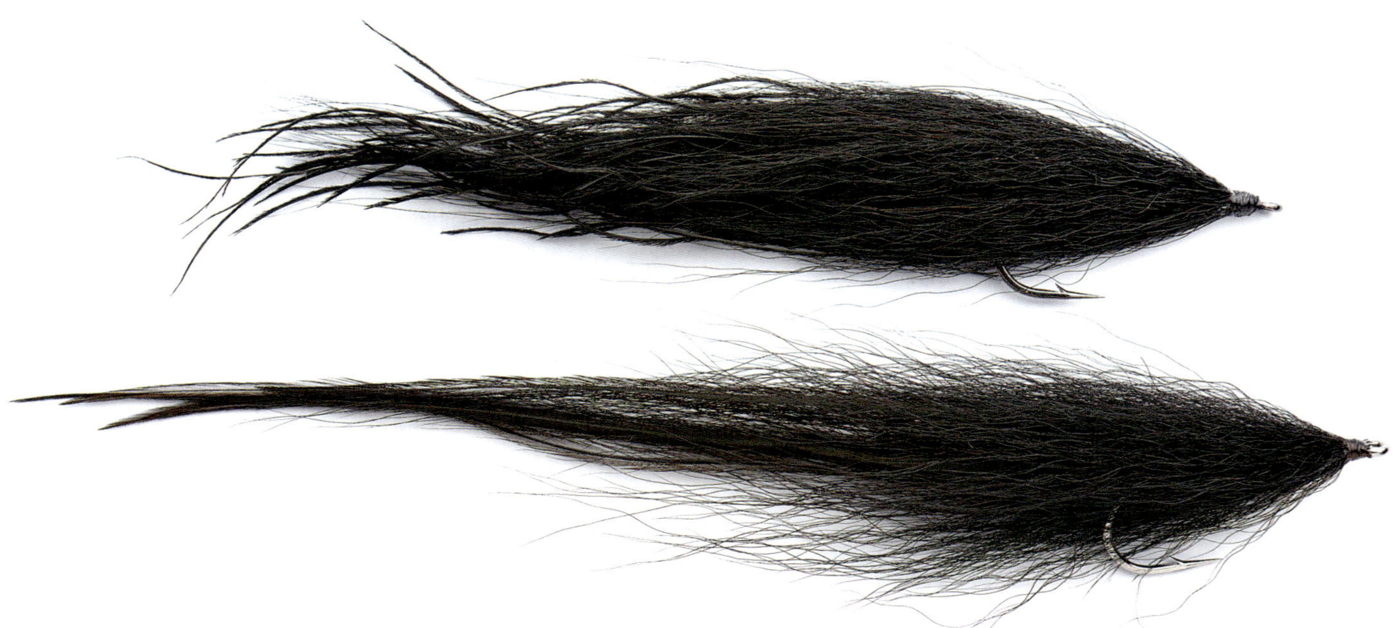

Predators such as striped bass are often looking up at night. I tied these BTDs specifically for night fishing. The thin saddles and long ostrich provide extra movement, the black bucktail provides contrast against the sky, and the very short hairs on the collar help prevent fouling. The collar is also flared to each side to help the fleye stay at or near the surface during the retrieve.

Hollow Fleye Technique

Before I discovered the Hollow Fleye technique, I built height and volume into the fly with multiple, adjacent bunches of hair or synthetic material along the shank. I also used epoxy in the case of the Spread Fleye to achieve height. While those techniques still serve a purpose, the Hollow Fleye technique allows you to achieve a full and complete baitfish shape with a minimal amount of material. Instead of tying in the fibers the conventional way, with the tips extending to the rear of the fly, in the Hollow Fleye you tie in the fibers so that the tips extend toward the hook eye. After tying them down, you bring the thread in front of the fibers and wrap back over them to control their angle. So while with a traditional fly you flare or build up the fibers to create the profile, with the Hollow technique, you begin with the fibers at 90 degrees to the shank and you wrap back over them to achieve the angle you desire. Throughout, you are in complete control of the material and can easily adjust the angle by adding or taking away thread wraps. We will tie a complete Hollow Fleye on page 117. In this exercise I want to focus on the basic hand movements and manipulation of materials because the technique is so fundamental.

Though you can use a wide range of bucktail fibers for this technique, the best fibers are fine and soft, with a moderate amount of wave to them. After you select and cut the bunch from the tail, make sure that you remove most of the shortest hairs, which only get in the way and throw off the overall flow and taper of the fly. You do want to retain some of the shorter (but not the shortest) hairs, for reasons that I explain in the Hollow Fleye chapter.

When you tie in the fibers, it is essential that you get an equal 360-degree distribution around the hook shank. I continually use my fingers to preen the fibers and better distribute them. Once you make your wraps, double-check to make sure that the fibers are evenly spaced so that you will have a better end result. Another key thing for getting the best results is that once you start to get the thread up in front and control the dam, make sure that all your wraps are straight around and not at an angle. If your wraps are angled, when you fold the fibers back, one side will fold in, and the other side will stay open. One other important tip is to tie with a sparse amount of material, which makes the hair easier to control.

HOLLOW FLEYE

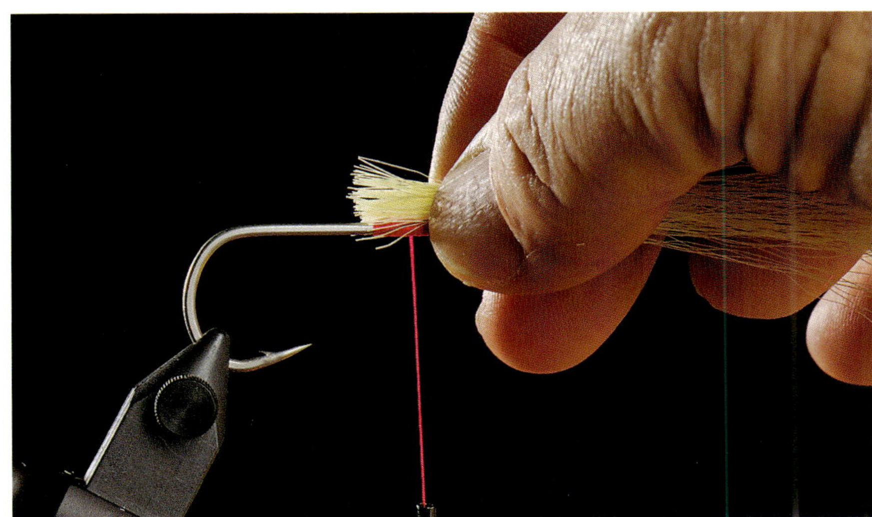

1. Insert the hook into the vise. Wrap a solid thread base on the hook shank. (The thread used here is for illustration purposes only. I always use monofilament thread.) Select fibers from the bucktail that are hollow at the bases. I find that retaining some of the hollow portion of the fibers makes them lay back easier, so be sure you don't cut that portion out. Remove most of the shortest hairs, and cut the butts square so that about 1/4 inch of butts are exposed. Hold the bucktail with your tying hand (right hand) with the butts toward the bend.

(continued)

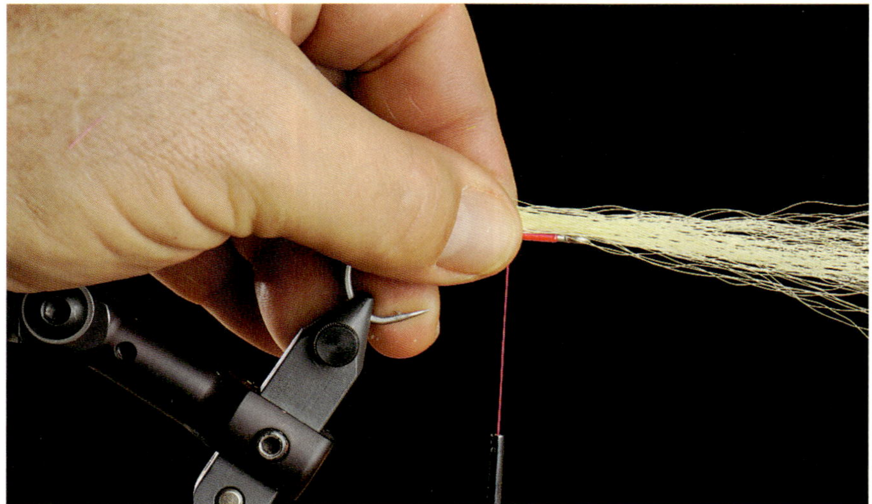

2. While still holding the bucktail with your right hand, reach in with your left hand and trap the fibers with your fingertip. During this handoff of materials, do not shuffle the fibers. Hold the material firmly in place with your material hand, so the fibers don't roll or slide around before you secure them.

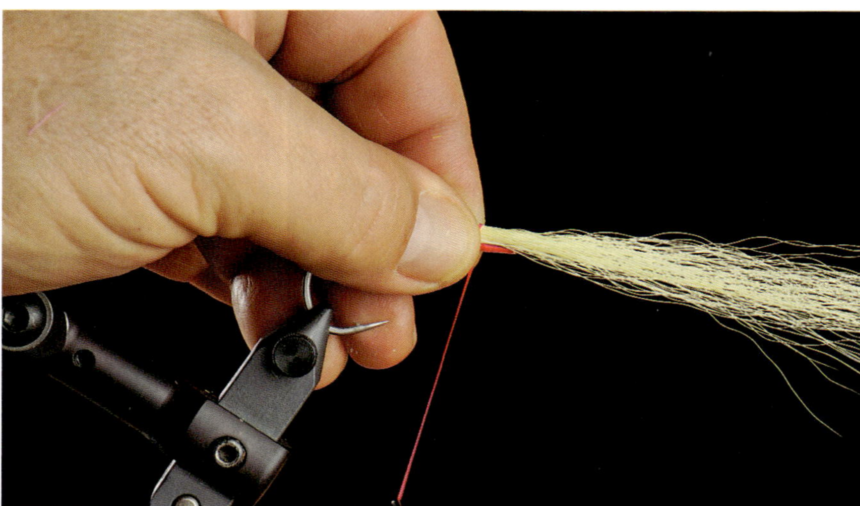

3. While still holding the butts firmly, begin wrapping the thread around the fibers. The thread should be close enough to the fingertips of your material hand that you can feel the thread as you wrap it. Don't let go until the three gathering wraps are completed. Once you make three wraps, do not pull tight. Soft tension is necessary at this time.

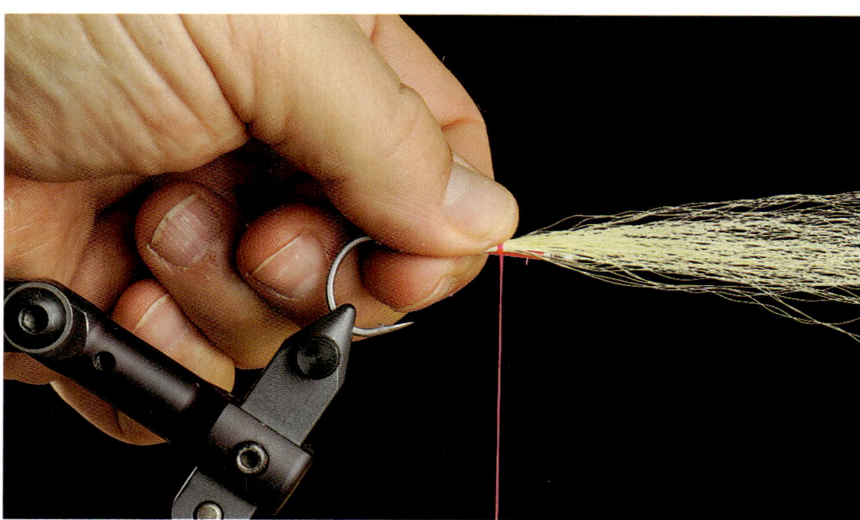

4. Note how straight the thread wraps are. Wrapping at an angle messes up the distribution of fibers. As the weight of the bobbin holds the fibers in place, push down on the fibers to begin distributing them around the shank so that the fibers completely and evenly encircle the shank. Nice, soft fibers make this easier, but with practice you can even get stiff fibers to cooperate. Sparse bunches of bucktail are easier to control and generally better than heavier ones, though bulkier flies may require bunches with more fibers in them, which take a bit more practice to distribute evenly.

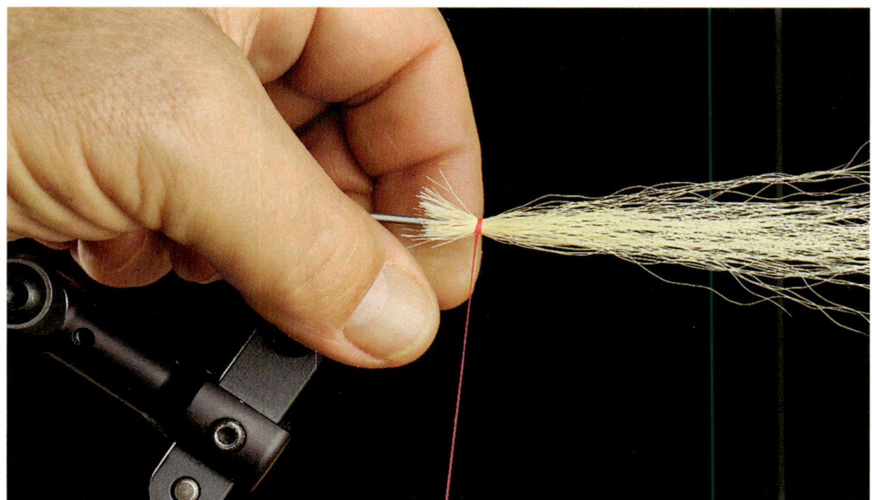

5. You not only want the fibers to completely encircle the hook, but you also want them to be evenly distributed and balanced.

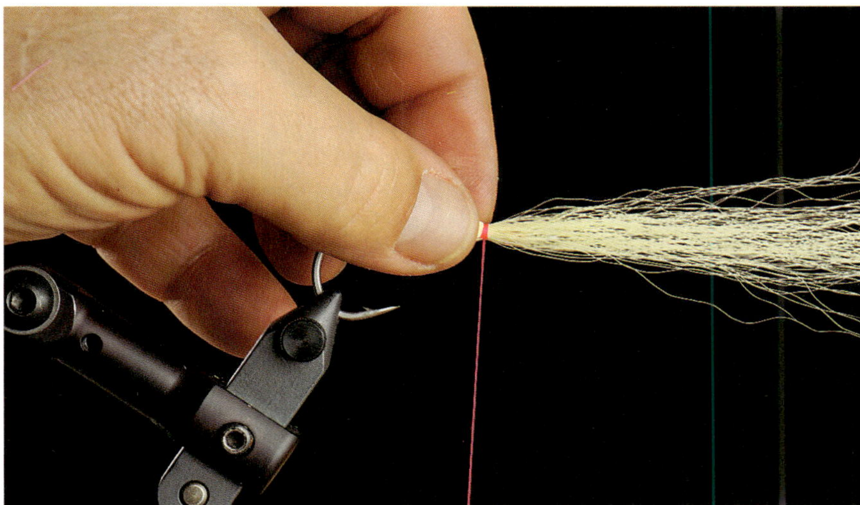

6. Hold the butts firmly with your left hand while wrapping the thread to secure the fibers. It is critical that you wrap at right angles to the shank (straight up and around) to keep the fibers straight and symmetrical.

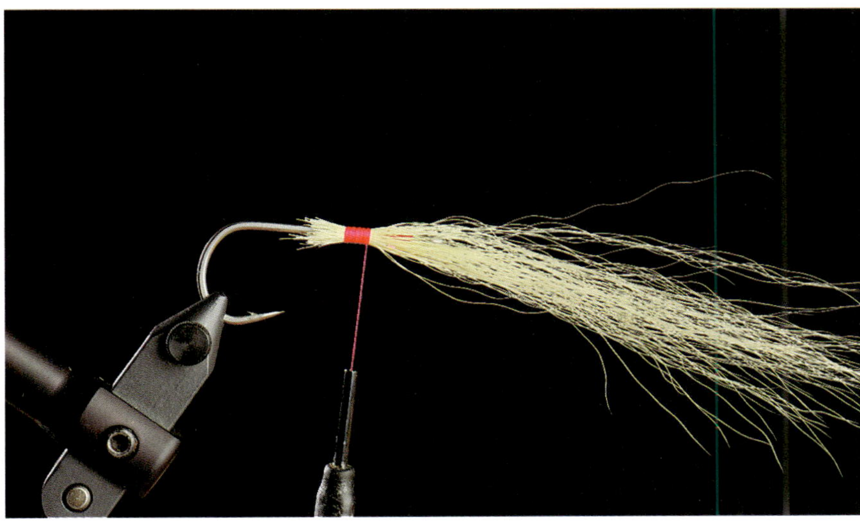

7. Wrap the thread about 1/4 inch toward the hook bend, and then wrap forward to the beginning tie-in point. Having the thread here makes it easy to bring the thread in front of the fibers in the next steps. From here on out, I will call this point the transition point. If the thread slips back during the next few steps, bring it back to this point before drawing it forward through the fibers.

(continued)

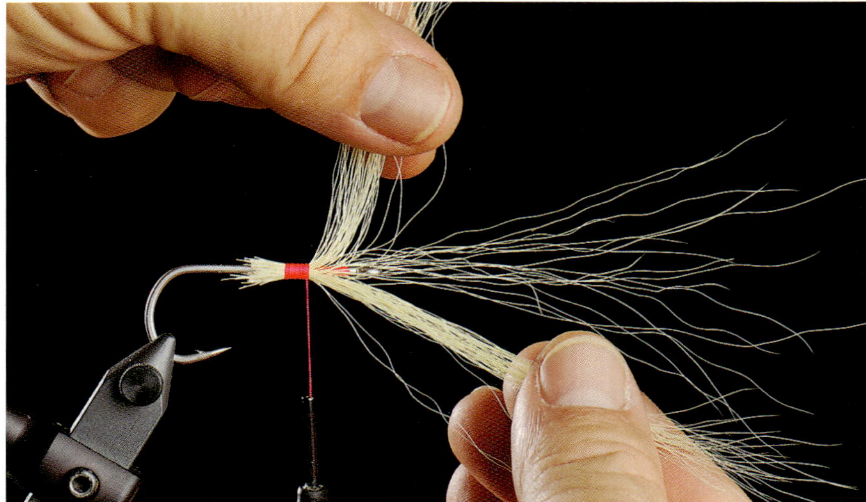

8. Spread the fibers evenly by pulling them outward and separating them. I already know that the fibers are evenly distributed around the shank, but here I am helping them open up so that it is easy for me to get in there with the pushing tool.

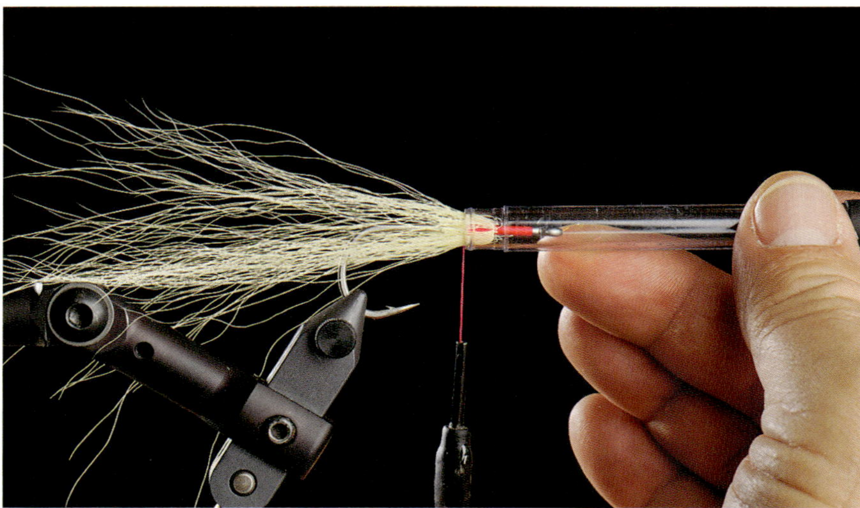

9. Slide a pushing tool—here, simply an empty pen case, clear so that I can see the 360-degree distribution—over the shank and against the base of the fibers to push them to the rear. Tip: If tying on a pedestal vise, use your left hand to hold the shank and steady the vise as you push back with your right. You only need to push the fibers back far enough so that it is easy to grab them with your left (material) hand.

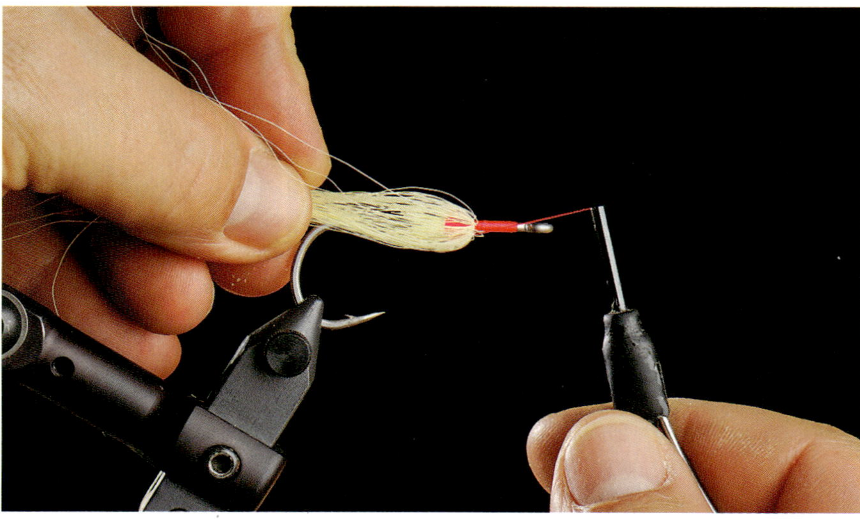

10. Grab the fiber tips with your material hand and pull them back so they are almost parallel to the shank. Make sure the thread is at the transition point, raise it parallel to the shank, and bring it through the fibers.

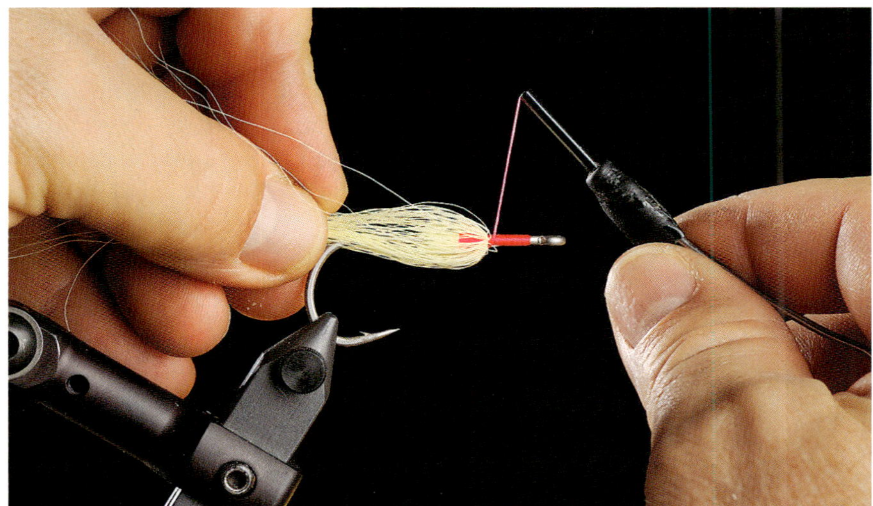

11. Once the thread passes through the bucktail, bring the bobbin back and up, and take two or three wraps at the base. Then, let the bobbin hang. Keep the fibers taut with your left hand throughout this process. You have made the transition from the rear to the front.

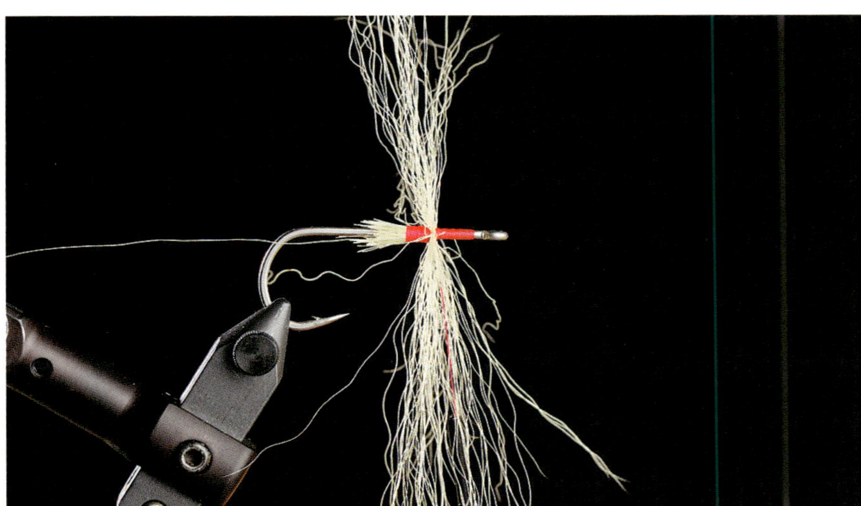

12. Once you release the fibers with your left hand, the fibers will go perpendicular to the hook shank. Up until this point, you are just getting the material in position. Stage one is complete, and you can now begin creating the right angle for the taper of your fly.

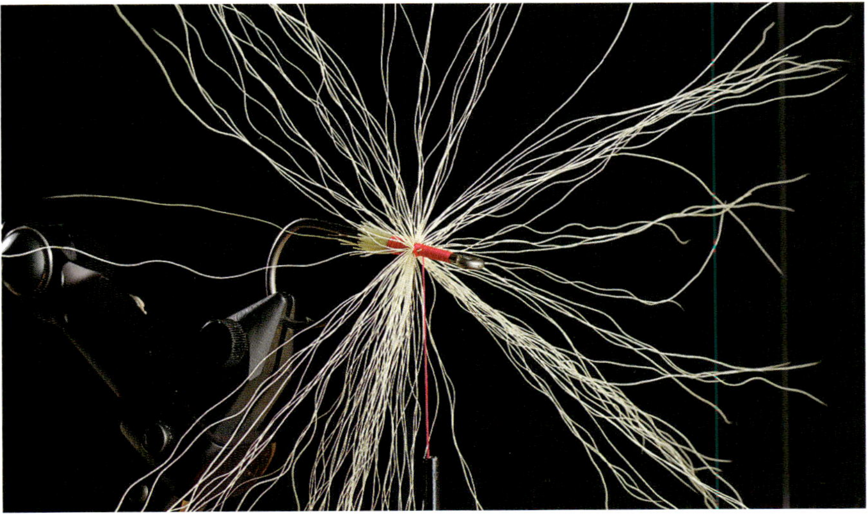

13. This is how stage one should look for each tie, before you adjust the angle with the thread. At this stage, I am constantly separating and preening the fibers to make sure they are distributed to my liking.

(continued)

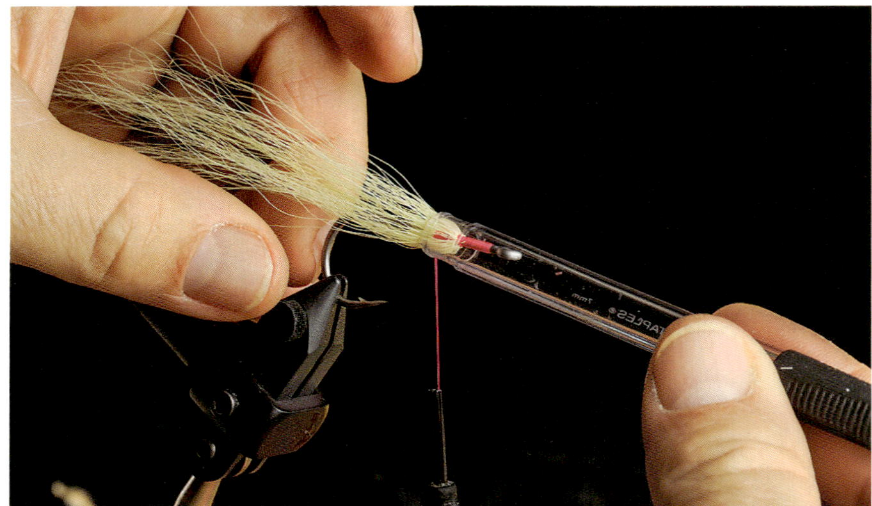

14. Now you will begin stage two of the Hollow technique—controlling the angle of the bucktail fibers with thread wraps. Push the fibers back with your tool, making sure that the fibers remain evenly distributed. The clear pen case helps here to check alignment of the fibers.

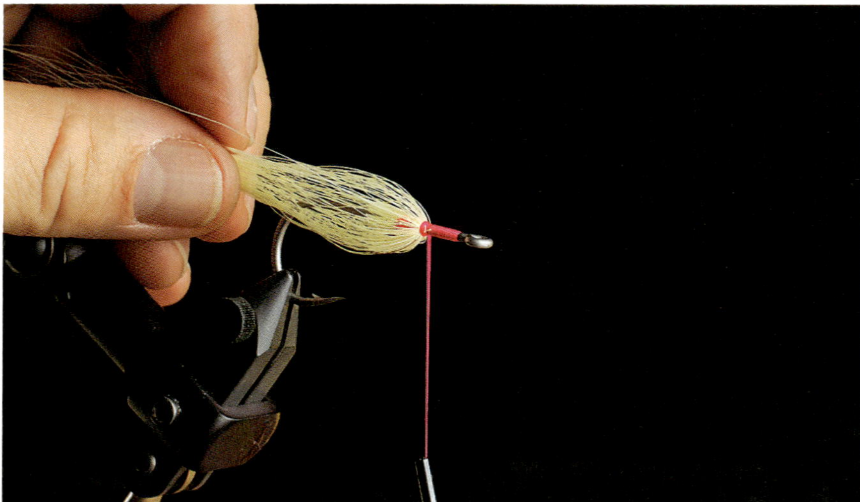

15. Grasp the fibers with your left hand and remove the pushing tool. Notice that the fibers are parallel to the hook shank and the thread is in position to begin building the dam of thread at the base of the fibers to control the angle. Holding the fibers back with your left hand, start wrapping back only one thread thickness at a time, which is enough to affect the angle.

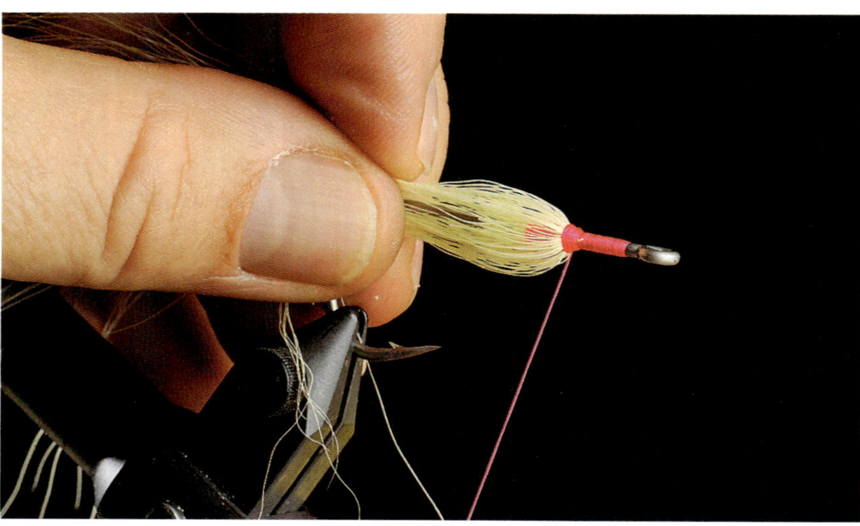

16. Wrap more thread up and down the dam to decrease the angle of the fibers. You can only go up the dam so much before you have to go down to ensure there is a thread base to prevent the ramp from collapsing. The ramp must be structurally sound. You have to constantly evaluate this on your own, but as a general guideline, after six or seven wraps, you need to go back down and come back up. But, more often than not, you will be able to get the angle you desire with that many wraps. Some bucktail might be harder to work with and resist your efforts; in that case, you need to get more aggressive with it and come back down and back up more. While you make the ramp, be sure that your wraps are straight and not at an angle.

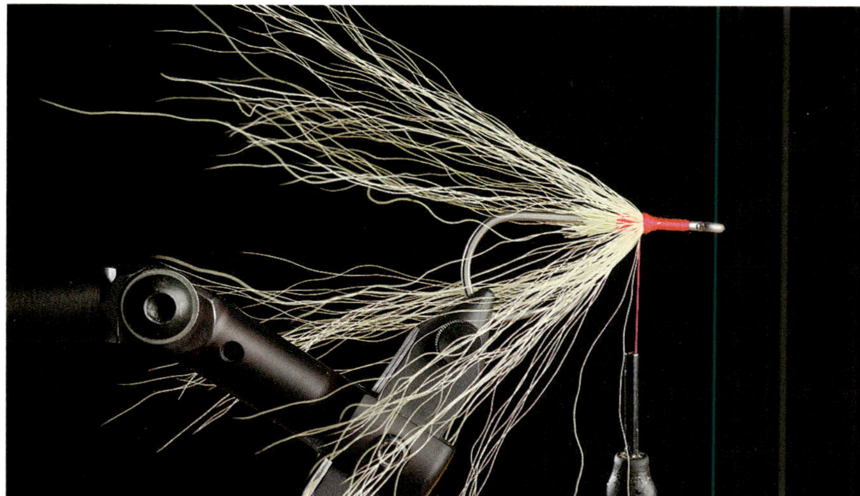

17. To achieve a progression of tapers that will imitate a baitfish profile, the rear of the fly has the smallest angle and each successive angle will be a little bit higher, with progressively shorter fibers used.

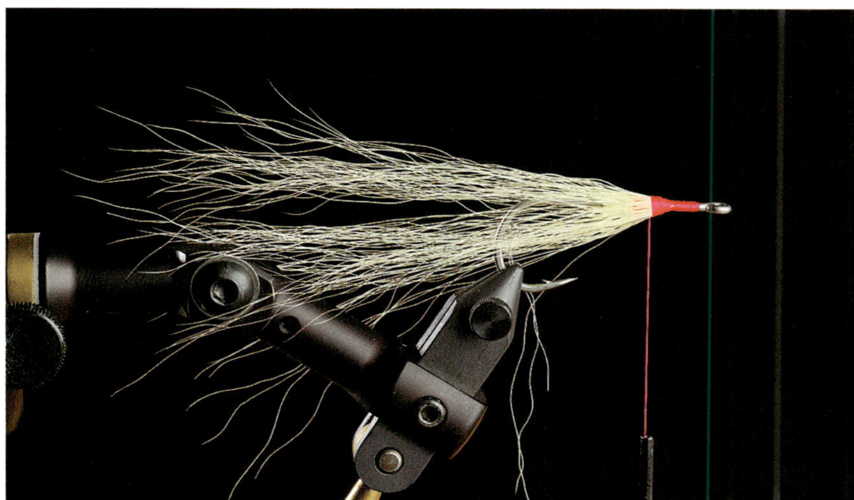

18. This photo shows fibers down all the way under the thread. These lower angles are best for the rear portions of the fly.

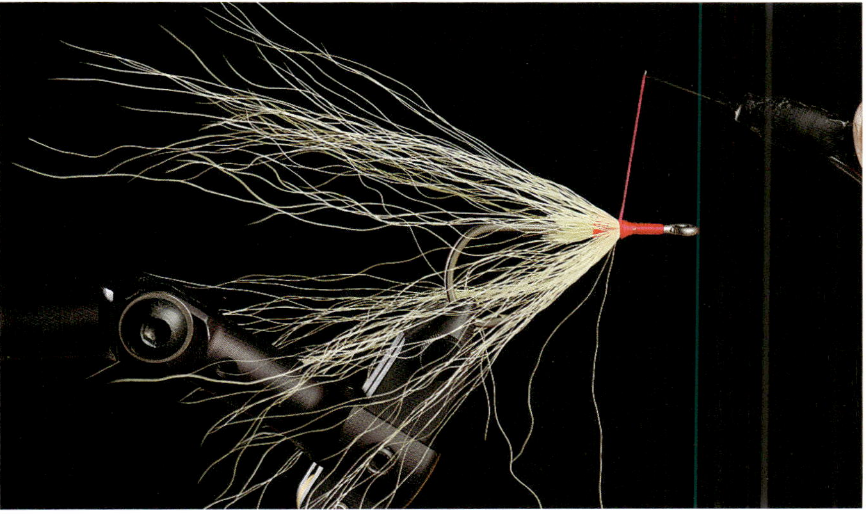

19. Now unwrap one revolution at a time. You can watch the angle of the hairs increase. This precise control of angles is key to the Hollow Fleye technique and shows how you are in complete control throughout the process.

BULKhead Technique

The BULKhead is a tying technique where you retain the hollow butts of the bucktail fibers and use them to create bulk in the front of a fly. This bulk not only provides a full profile, but it also pushes water, which can be a trigger for many predatory species. Additionally, by combining a smoothly tapered, sparse rear wing with the forward bulk, you can enhance a fly's movement. Water courses over the head, creating additional turbulence that sets the tail moving. This basic design concept—bulk in front and sparse, continuous taper in the rear—will enhance the action of almost every fly that you tie, if that is the effect that you desire.

The most common variation of this fly is the BULKhead Deceiver, but I often employ the BULKhead technique in Beasts, Hollow Fleyes, and other patterns. When tying the BULKhead Deceiver, the rear of the fly is tied exactly the same as you would the regular Bucktail Deceiver. The only difference is in how the forward portion is formed. I will elaborate on this further in chapter 9, but BULKheads are fairly spontaneous, seat-of-the-pants types of flies that I will tie only if I have bucktail that works well. When I do set out to tie one, I try not to overthink them. When I take my time with them or follow a strict pattern, it usually ends up in the garbage. So keep that in mind.

The best hairs for this style of tying come from the base of a tail. The ideal fibers are coarse enough to flare easily, but are also relatively thin so that you can easily control their angle with thread wraps (often you will need to wrap back over the butts to get a 45- to 60-degree angle). It is common in spun-hair patterns to cut off the tapered tips, but in this technique I use them to contribute to the bulk and shape of the head. Therefore, the fibers that you choose must still be long enough from butt to tapered tip to contribute to the overall taper of the fly.

Trimming technique is an important part of finishing a good-looking BULKhead, but paradoxically, part of the technique is not being overly concerned with it—you do not want to trim too much. I trim each step going forward, just a little, trimming the ends irregular to help give a more natural look to the inside. Be very careful not to trim the tips and destroy the length necessary to fill out the head shape. Once you arrive at the desired bulk and the overall fullness of the head, the fly should have the correct shape, only with the hidden bulk underneath. I will also do a little more trimming by first wetting the head and then trimming any short fibers that stick out through the longer ones. Just a few snips will do the job.

BULKhead

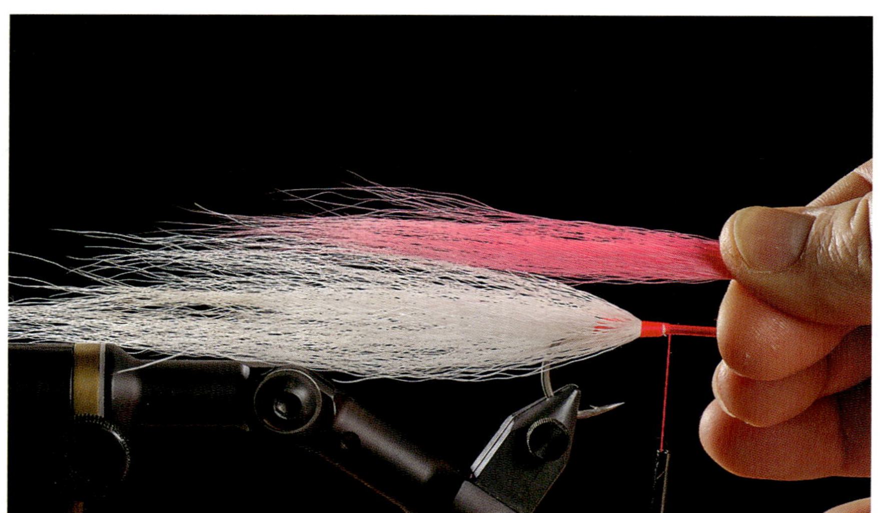

1. The rear portion of the BULKhead is the same as the Bucktail Deceiver. When you select the fibers for the forward portion of the fly, measure them so that they are shorter than the fibers preceding it and continue the taper that you have established.

The best fibers are long and have fairly hollow bases that will flare when tied on the hook shank. These come from the bottom portion of the tail. Be sure to clean out any fuzz from the base of the fibers, and snip the ends square.

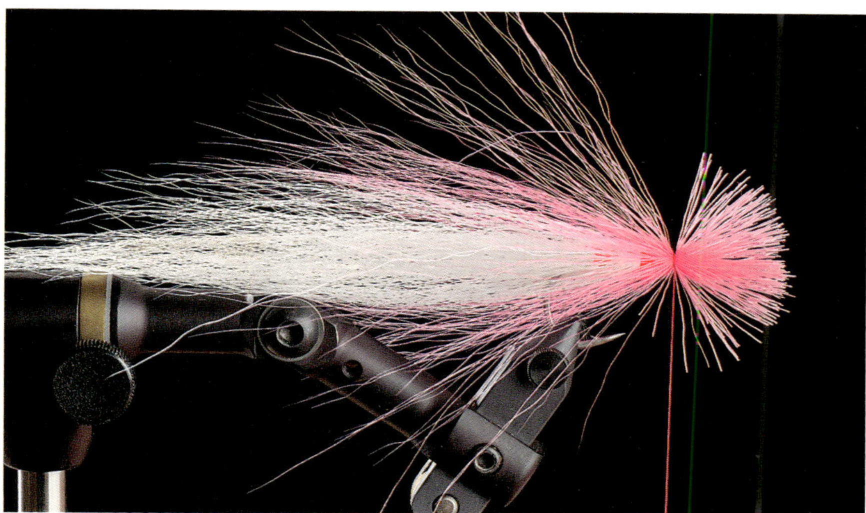

2. When you tie in the clump of fibers, leave ample butt ends (about an inch here) to create the inner bulk of the head.

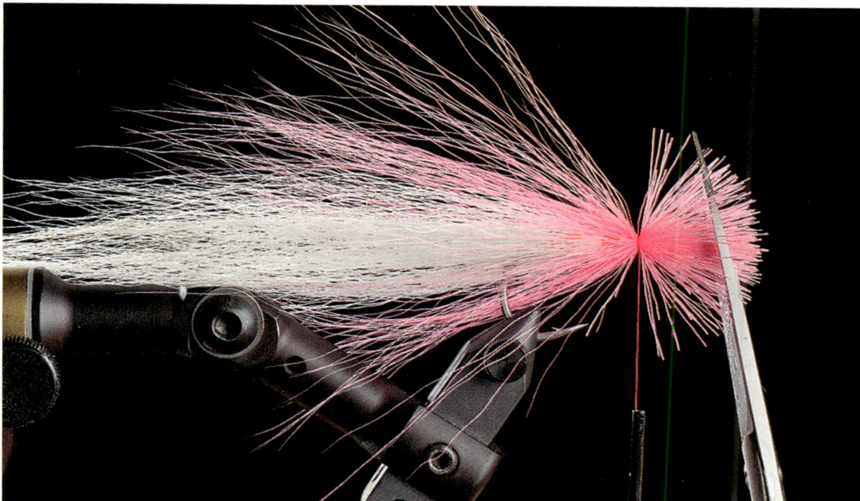

3. Snip some of the inner fibers from the butts so that when you push them back in the next step, you have a conical, rather than a circular, head.

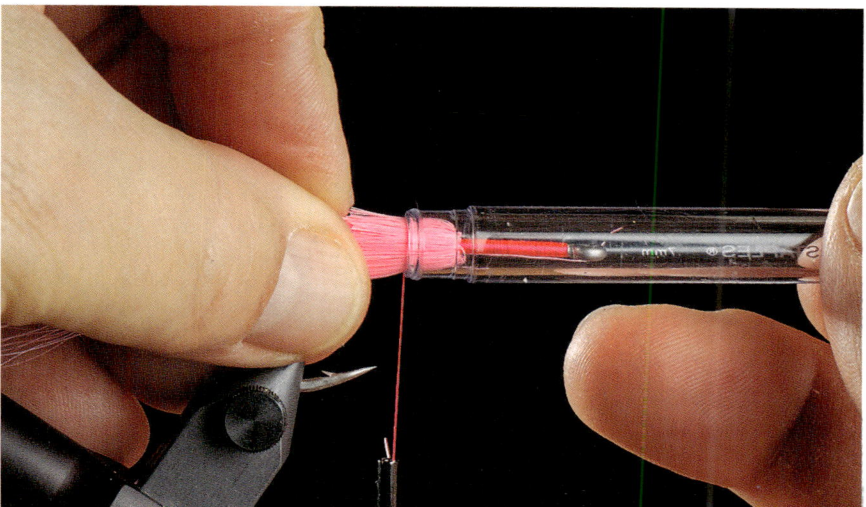

4. Push the fiber butts back with your tool and grasp them with your material hand.

(continued)

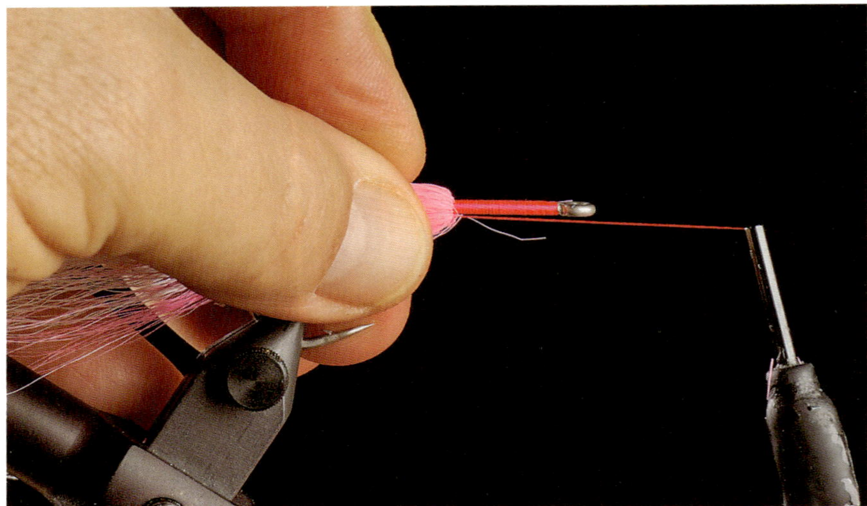

5. Bring the thread forward with the thread parallel to the shank, just as you would for the Hollow Fleye. Hold back the fibers with your material hand during the crossover move.

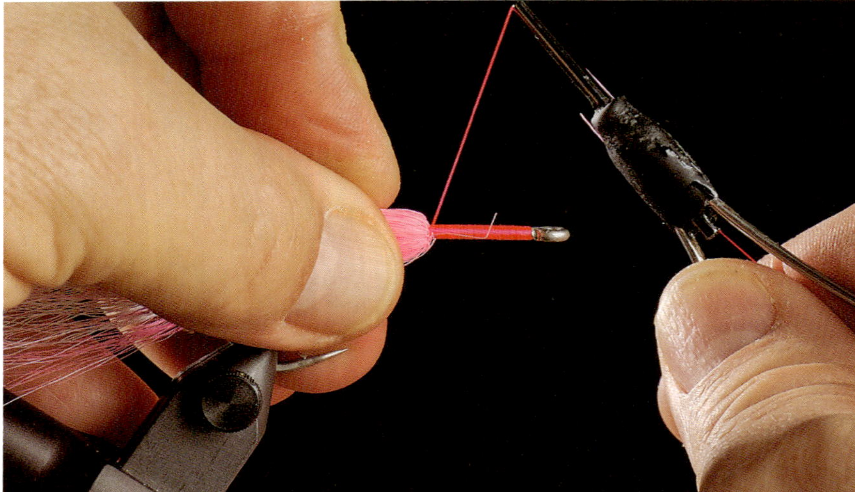

6. While continuing to hold the butts back with your material hand, build a thread dam at the base of the fibers.

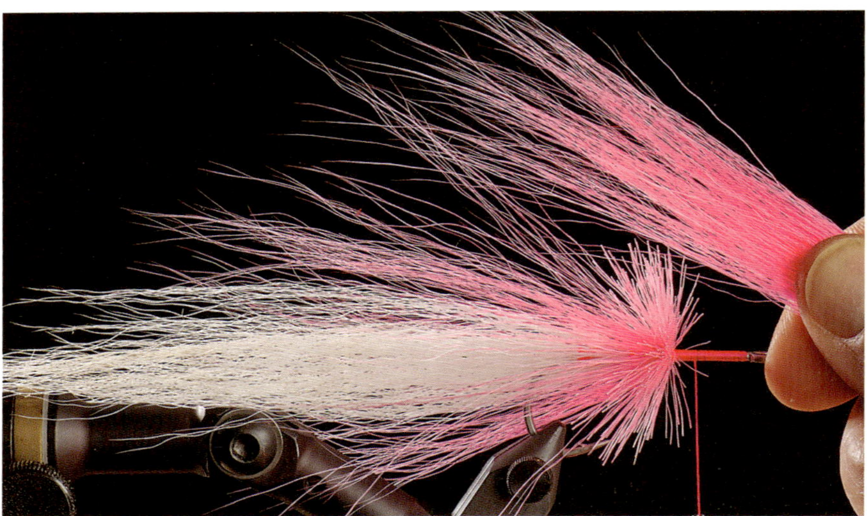

7. Notice the orientation of the fiber butts, and also note the uneven lengths. This will help create an inner taper. Select another clump of bucktail from the base of the tail, and measure it so that it is shorter than the previous one.

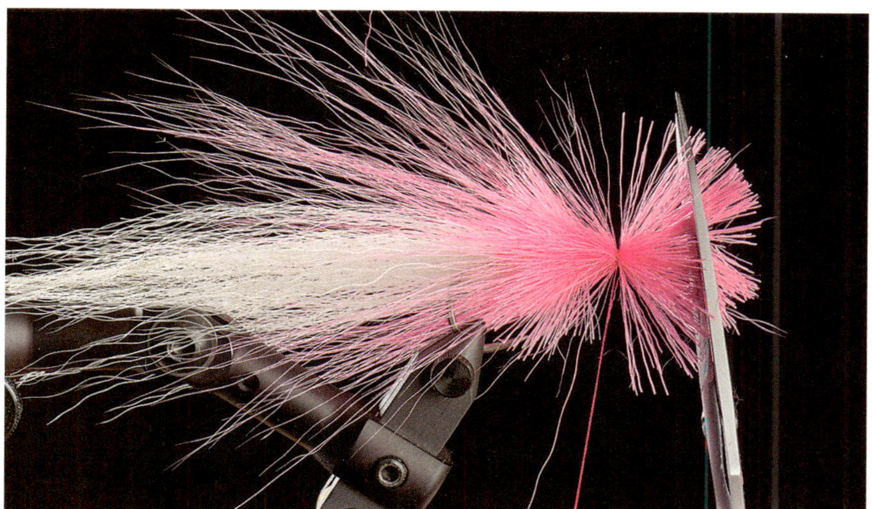

8. Tie in the clump the same way that you did the first bunch and then trim the butts.

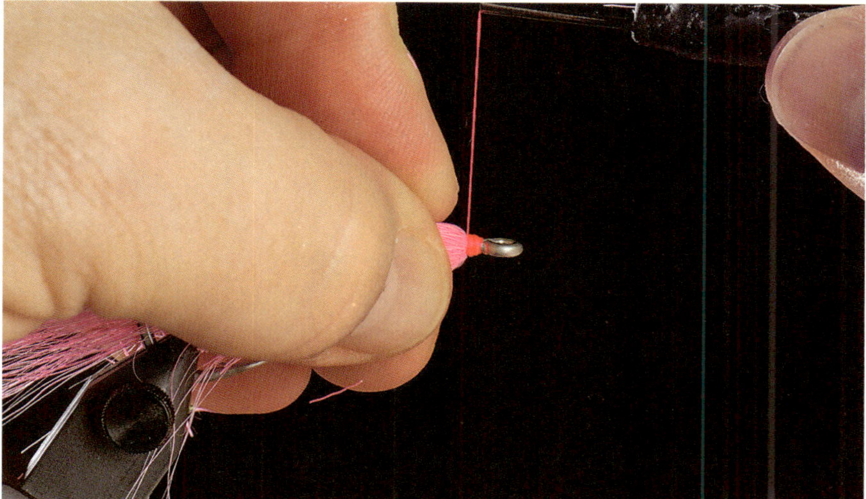

9. Bring the thread forward, dam up the fibers, and tie off the thread.

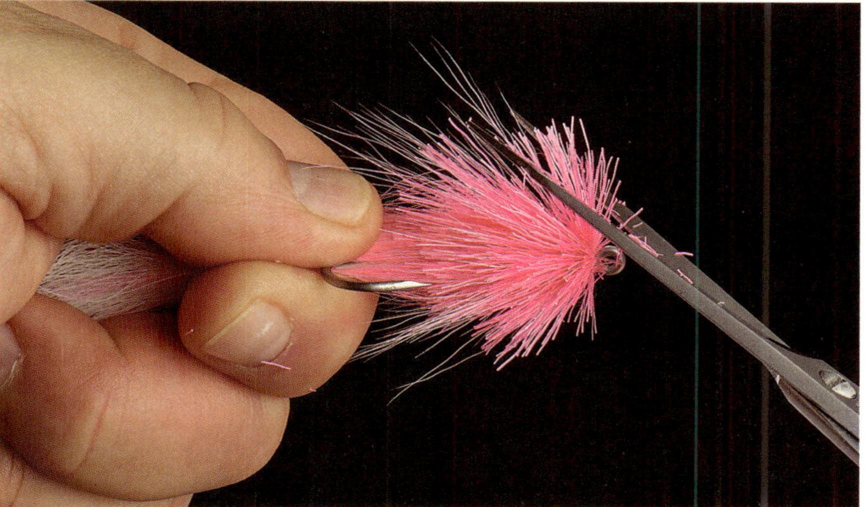

10. When trimming the flared butts in the head, protect all the tapered tips.

(continued)

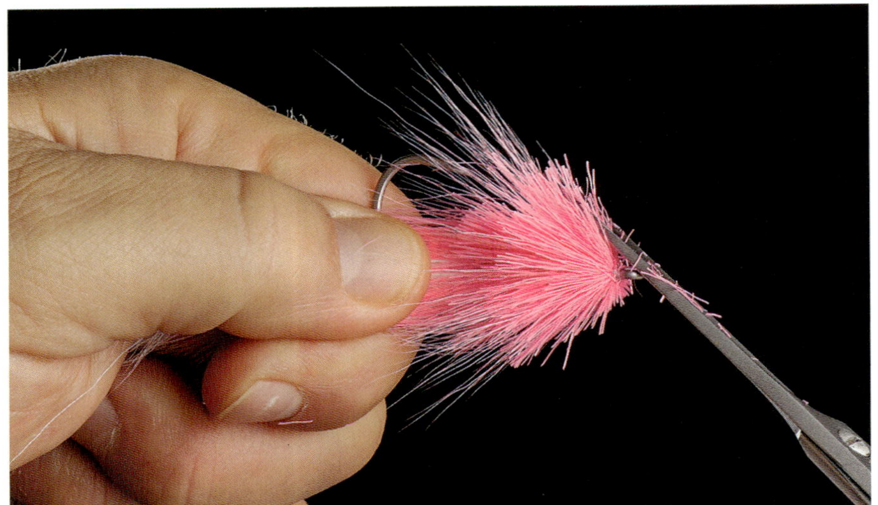

11. Trim the hairs at a fairly wide angle. You do not want to cut into them at too shallow of an angle and ruin the profile of the head. Snip very carefully. Use the hook eye to steady your cuts.

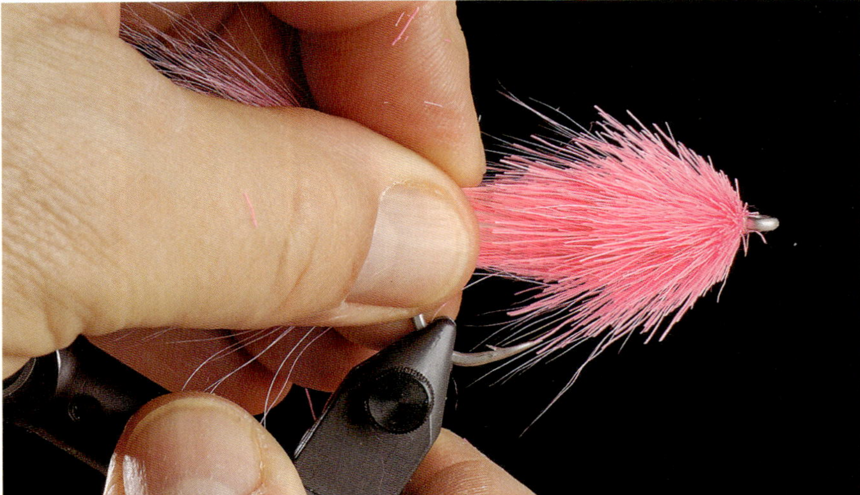

12. As the head takes shape, continue to hold the tips while you trim.

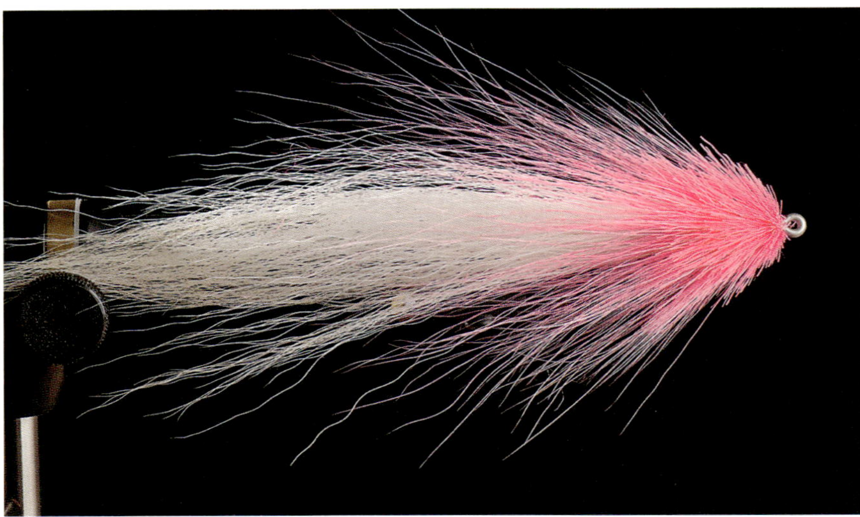

13. The finished fly will most likely have an unkempt appearance. Do not try to make it look perfect, just try to obtain an overall sense of taper.

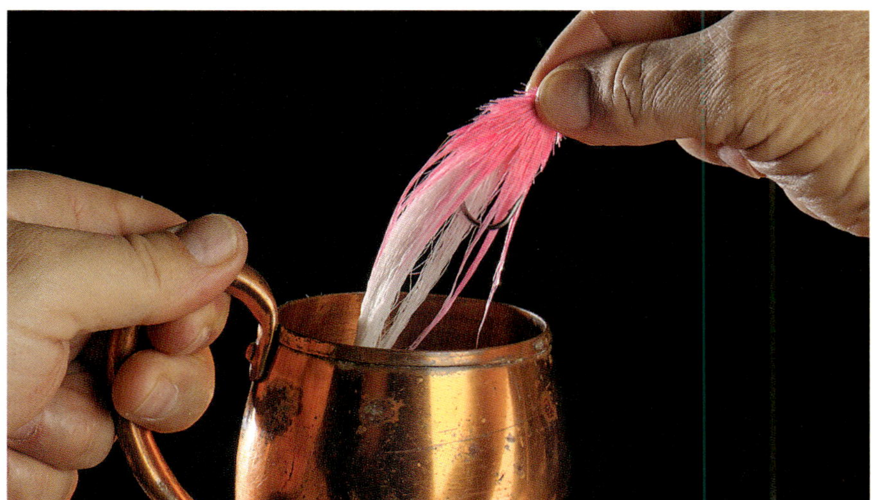

14. Wet the fly to make it easier to spot any wayward fibers.

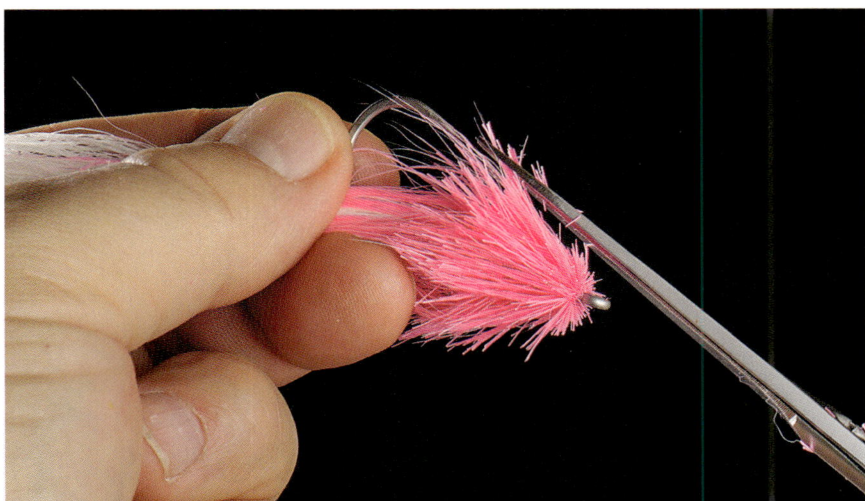

15. Give the fly a final trim, if necessary. It does not have to look rough, but rough is acceptable. Final trimming is just a little snip here or there to eliminate any obvious stray hairs.

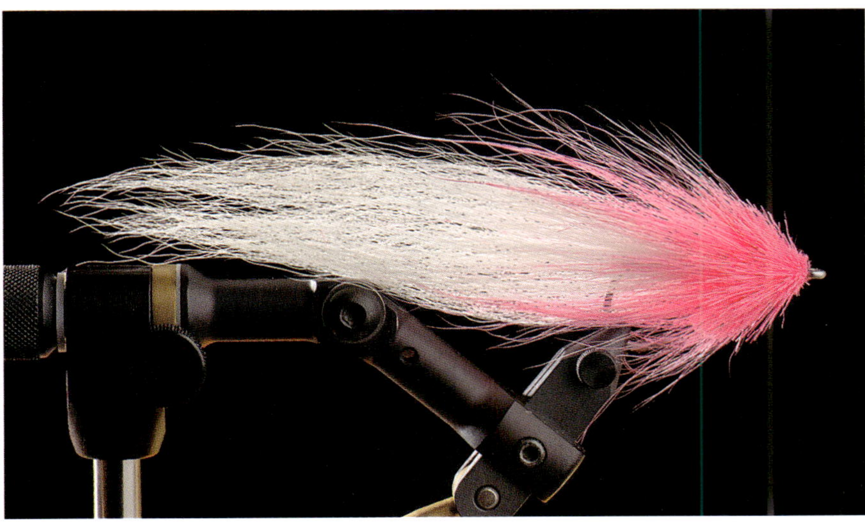

16. The finished BULKhead. You can see how it comes into shape after it has been wet and then dried. The BULKhead is a little awkward to tie in the beginning, but once mastered it will reward you—fish love them.

Chapter 4

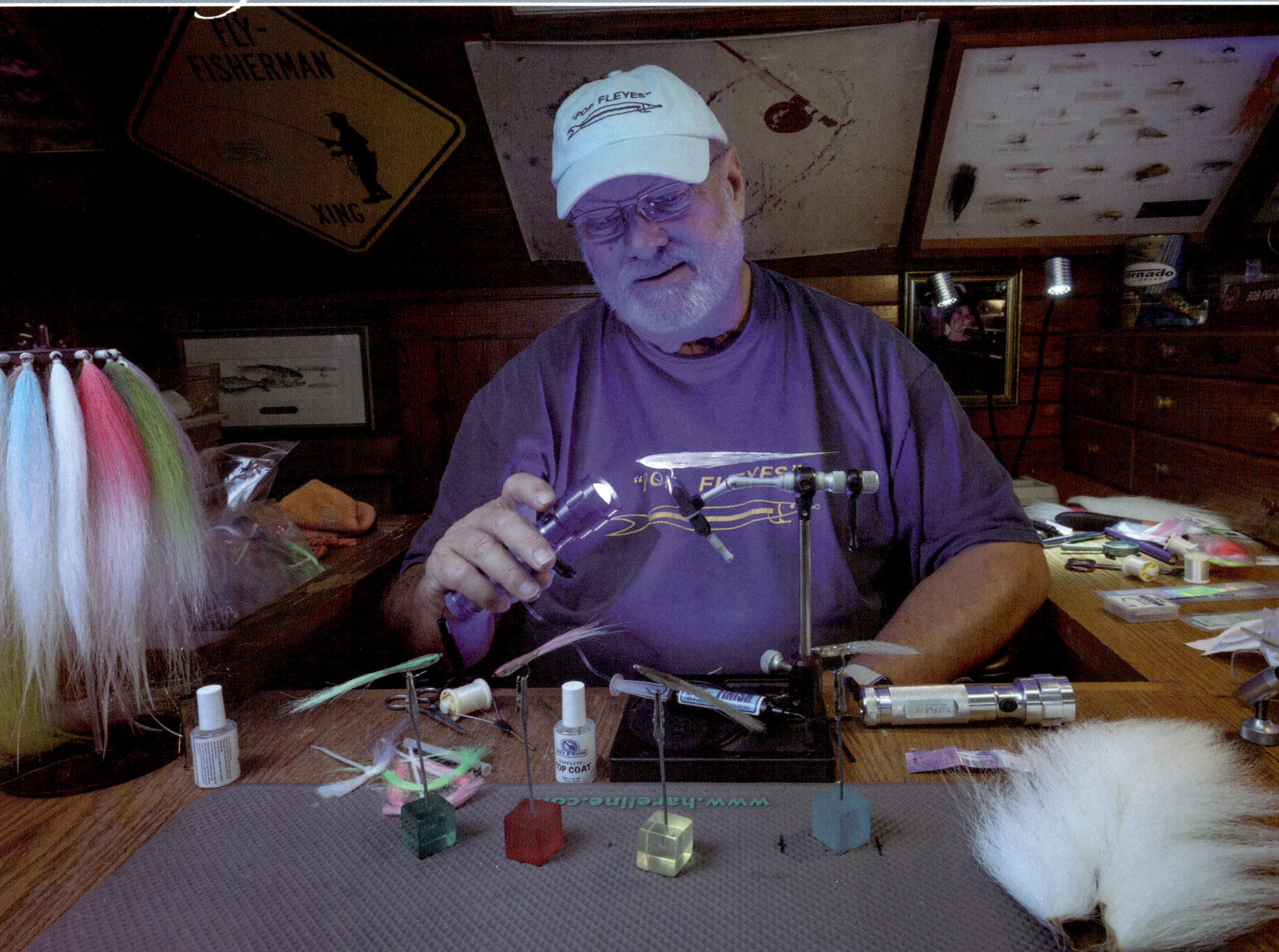

Blue light special. Light-cured acrylics such as Tuffleye have made it easier for fly tiers to shape and strengthen their flies without the hassles of epoxy.

Working with Light-Cured Acrylics

Light-cured acrylics are a superb substitute for epoxy in fly-tying applications because they remain fluid until you harden them with a special light. Depending on the manufacturer, the light required is a blue light or UV light. I like to use Tuffleye, which is cured with a blue light. Light-cured acrylics come in different viscosities for different applications; Tuffleye is available in Core (thick) and Finish (thin), as well as Flex, which remains flexible when it hardens. In the Surf Candy below, I am using Core, which most closely resembles the consistency of epoxy. I use the Flex for the Shrimp and Crab patterns shown later.

Tuffleye comes in syringes with curved tips, which you can use like a bodkin to apply the gel to the fly. Whereas with epoxy, I used to have to put the epoxy on the pad and then apply it to the fly with a bodkin, I can put the Tuffleye directly on the material and manipulate it with the syringe. While you do not need to mix Tuffleye like epoxy, you must make sure that it is fully cured with the blue light. However, you don't have the limited working time of epoxy. I have applied the Core to a fly, went downstairs for a cup of coffee, went back to the vise and made some adjustments to the fly, and then cured it with the light. Try that with epoxy!

One interesting virtue of Tuffleye is that it gets clearer as the sunlight hits it. I recently checked out a half-dozen Candies that I placed in a clear plastic bag on my dashboard in the sun for over six months, and I found no signs of yellowing. This is the direct opposite of epoxy. Sunlight causes epoxy to turn prematurely yellow, and for some, this ruins their flies. Patterns tied with light-cured acrylic remain clear and vibrant from year to year, season to season.

We will discuss Tuffleye in more detail in chapter 12, but I want to look closely at some key techniques when working with it.

Tuffleye Tips

- Cover the entire shank with thread, or some other material, so that the acrylic has something to adhere to and the fly won't spin on the hook shank.

- Use multiple coats to start. Don't try to build the fly all at once. One of the beautiful things about light-cured acrylics is that they allow you to work at your own pace.

- To properly cure the resin to yield a hard, clear fly, hold the light close to the resin, cover small parts of the fly slowly and methodically, and light the resin for at least twenty seconds. Be patient with the light and hold it very close, within 1/4 inch of the gel. Give it time to work. As an example, if I am tying a small Surf Candy, that body might be 1/2 inch to 3/4 inch long, so it would take me probably 12 seconds to do one side. Don't just wave the light back and forth and expect it to cure properly. Be deliberate and take your time.

- Weak power is one of the causes of acrylic that doesn't cure properly. Use fully charged batteries or purchase a light that runs on AC power.

- Only wipe off the tacky layer on the last coat (if doing two or more coats). According to Tuffleye, their resins cure from the inside out, and the oily layer that remains on the surface is a bonding layer that allows subsequent layers to be added, which fully bond to those underneath. If the material isn't properly cured or this layer isn't removed when the fly is finished, the surface can be contaminated by a number of chemical reactions.

- Pre-tie your blanks, and then apply the acrylic to all the flies for faster, more efficient tying. To batch-tie Surf Candies, I'll place them in clip stands, maybe six at a time, and apply the gel to all of them at once. I make minor adjustments for the final shape, then light them up as I go down the line, resulting in a bunch of hardened Surf Candies very quickly. A dozen Surf Candies would take me two solid hours at the vise using epoxy, but now I can complete that amount in thirty minutes or less.

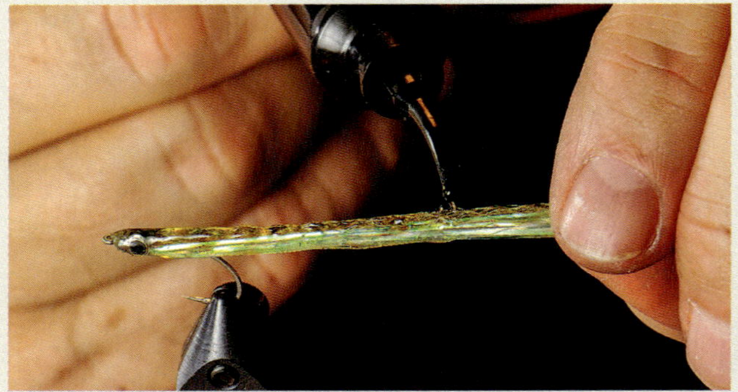

Here I am extending the gel well past the hook using Tuffleye Flex. It may go on uneven at first, but you have plenty of time to smooth it out before you hit it with the light.

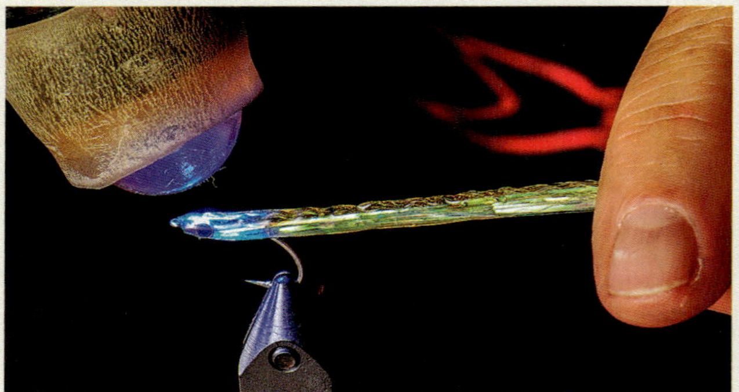

When applying the Tuffleye, you always have to use two hands. Hold the material taut until the acrylic is set. The advantage of the acrylic is that you get a lot more control than with epoxy, since you can set it when you are ready rather than working at the mercy of the material. This is a huge leap forward.

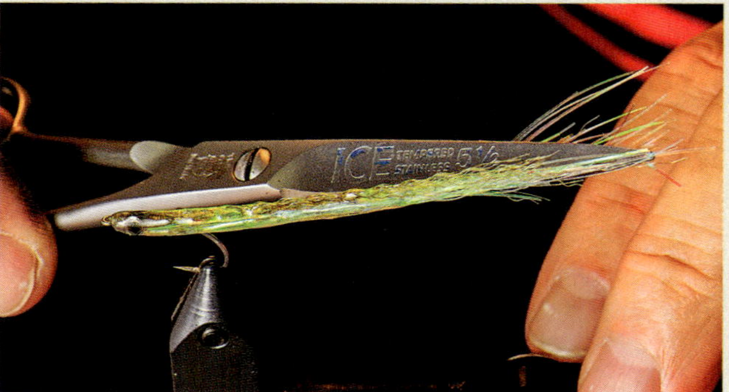

One of synthetics' biggest advantages is the fact that the tier can trim the fly to shape. Using serrated scissors, cut *with* the fiber direction to step-cut the ends. Cutting against the grain might be quicker, but you run the risk of cutting too deep. Be sure to hold the fibers close to the ends to cut cleanly.

ACRYLIC SURF CANDY

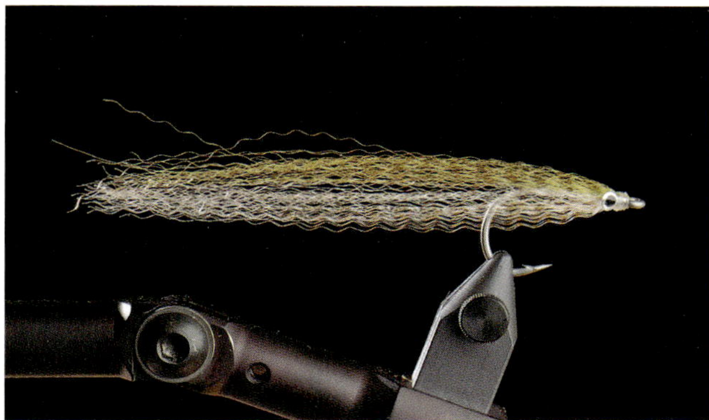

1. This fly is complete and ready for the light-cured acrylic. In general, I prefer translucent synthetic fibers for the body, as Surf Candies most often imitate smaller, more translucent baits. FisHair, Super Hair, Steve Farrar's Flash Blend, Iceabou, and Craft Fur are all great for this. Even though the materials are only tied down at the front of the hook, I covered the entire shank with thread so that the acrylic has something to adhere to.

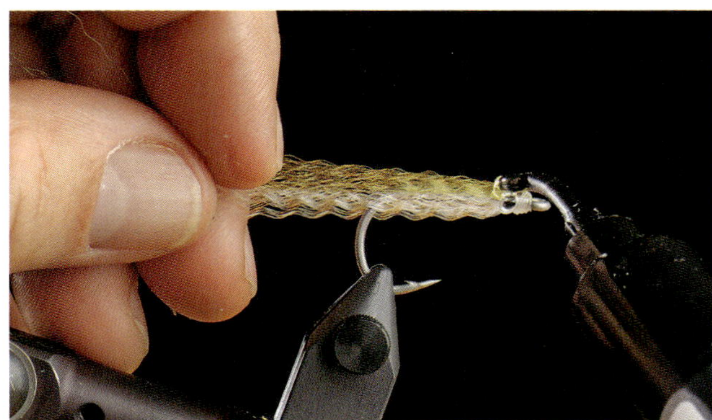

2. Hold the wing firmly to the rear with your material hand, and apply gel from the front of the fly (at the eye of the hook) to the back. Your left hand must maintain control of the wing throughout the entire process. As I push the gel out, I also press into the fibers until I can feel the hook shank with the tip to ensure I am getting complete penetration, quickly.

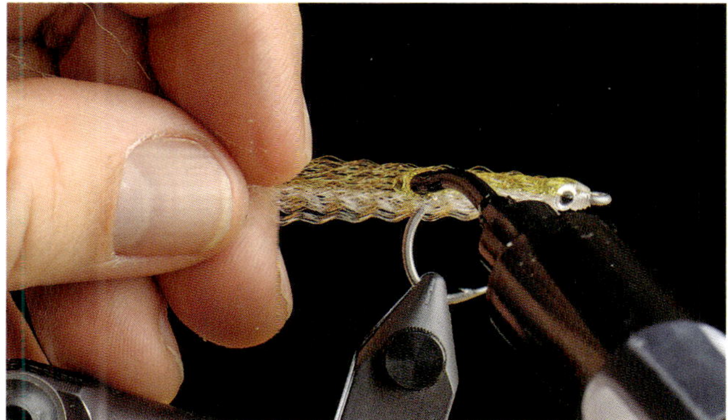

3. Press gel into all the fibers, and distribute the gel from the hook eye to about 1/4 inch past the hook bend. To keep the gel flowing, be sure to maintain pressure on the syringe as you move the tip across the fly.

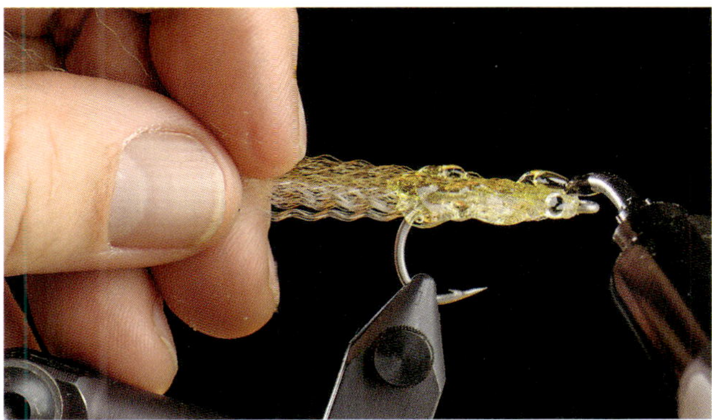

4. Apply the gel on all sides and keep it as balanced as you can. Use a liberal amount of gel to make it easier to distribute it along the shank with the bodkin in the next step. Tiers get into trouble when they use "just enough." I like to have enough gel on there so that I can move it around the shank to get the shape that I want.

When applying the gel to the fly in the first coat, I like to push the material into the fibers enough so that I hit the hook shank with the tip of the syringe. To help the gel penetrate, I will often pulsate the fibers, expanding and contracting them by pushing and pulling gently from the rear with my left hand.

(continued)

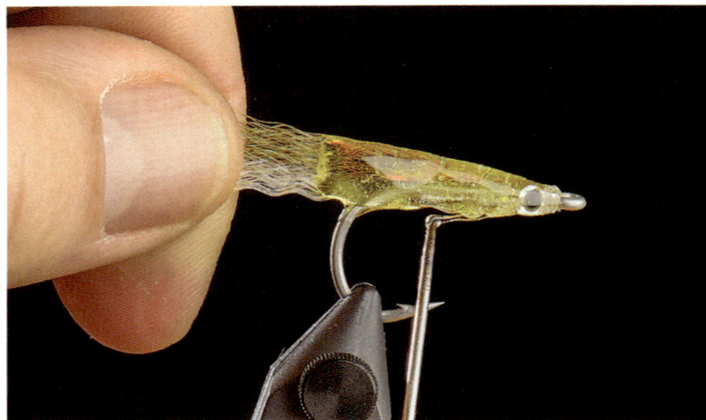

5. Using a bodkin, distribute the gel to even any bulges. Keep the tip perpendicular to the shank and draw the gel smoothly forward or back. If you don't use enough gel, you just end up pushing it from one spot to the other. Use enough so that you can control it easily but not so much that it drips off the fly.

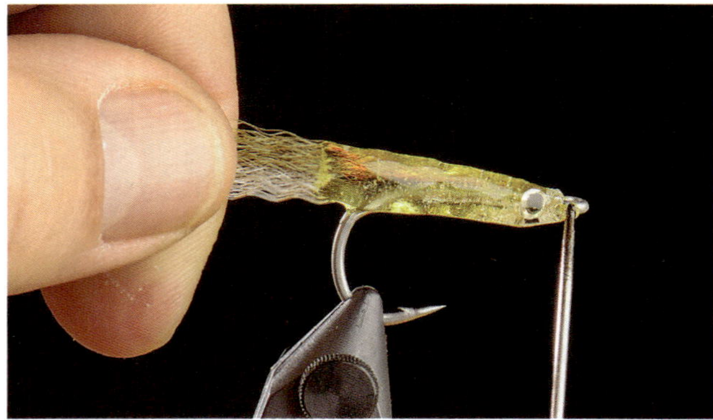

6. Keep distributing the gel until you are satisfied that all gaps are filled. If this is the first time you are tying these flies, you might be better off using multiple coats to build up the proper body. Set the basic shape with a thin coat, and then add other coats to achieve the results you desire. I often just build the fly with one coat but here will demonstrate how to build up several coats.

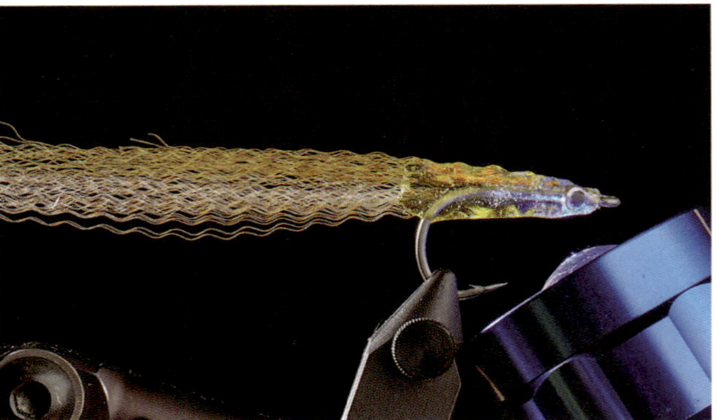

7. The Core, as long as you don't use too much, stays in place until you cure it with the light. Hold the light within 1/4 inch of the gel, and move slowly from the eye of the hook to the rear—in one direction. Do all four sides in the same deliberate manner: left, right, top, and bottom. Going slowly and staying close ensures that the gel cures properly. This first coat sets the shape; subsequent coats smooth out the body.

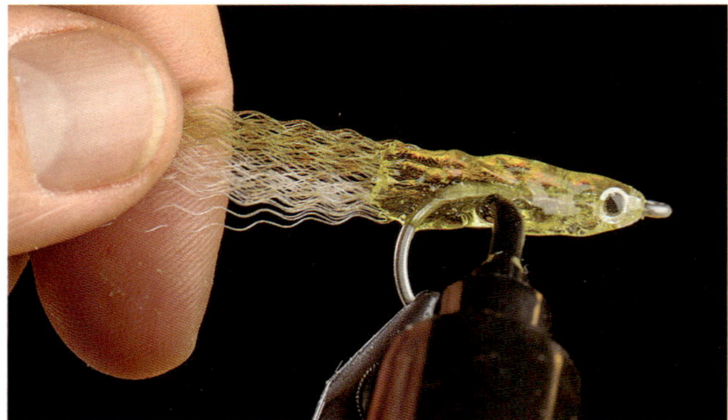

8. Apply a second coat in the same manner as the first, but this time instead of worrying about penetrating fibers, just fill in any gaps. You should have already set the basic shape of the fly in the first application.

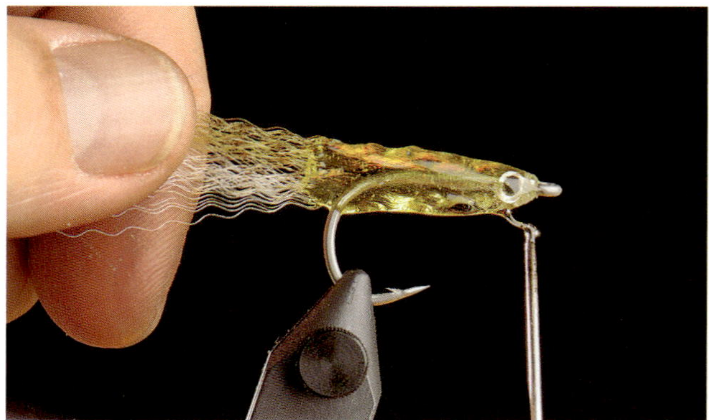

9. I like to use a bodkin to draw and distribute the second coat of acrylic around the fly and fill any gaps.

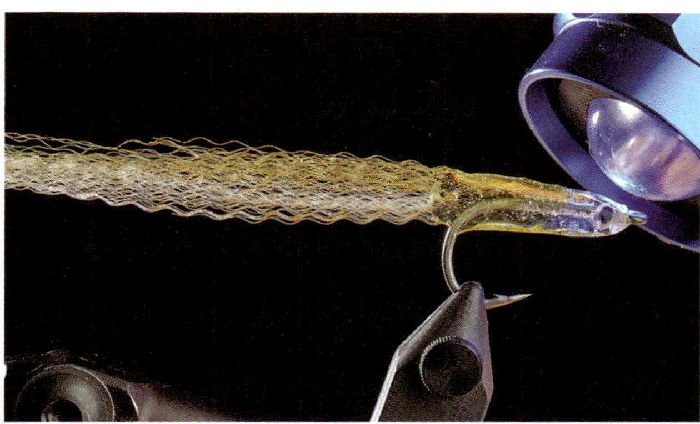

10. Set the acrylic with the light in the same deliberate manner as you did the first time through.

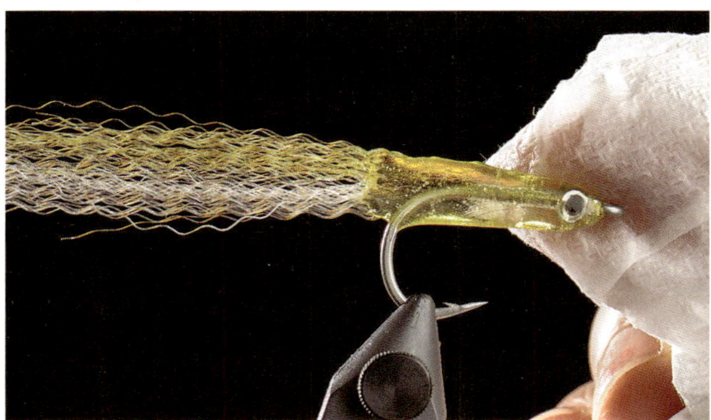

11. Apply rubbing alcohol to a paper towel and wipe off the tacky residue from left to right so that you are wiping away from the untreated fibers. Apply Top Coat or Sally Hansen Hard As Nails.

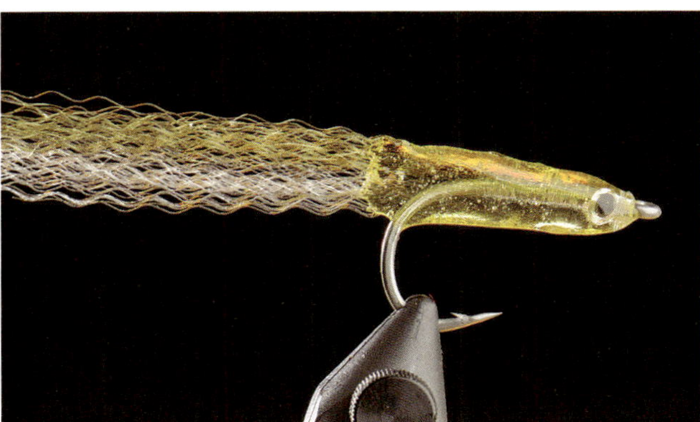

12. After I apply Top Coat or Hard As Nails, I will sometimes color the belly with silver nail polish, but that is a completely optional step.

ACRYLIC ULTRA SHRIMP

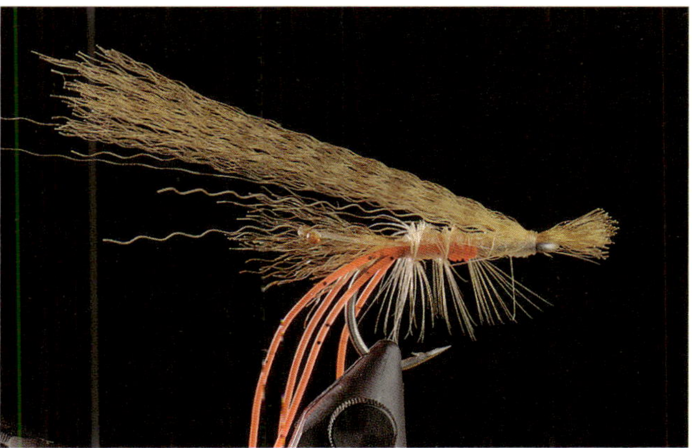

1. Just as with the Surf Candy, we have already tied the basic form of the Ultra Shrimp and are here going to go over the basics of applying the light-cured acrylic—this time the Flex. The extra length of the carapace provides a handle to grasp and control the fibers and keep your fingers away from the gel as you work.

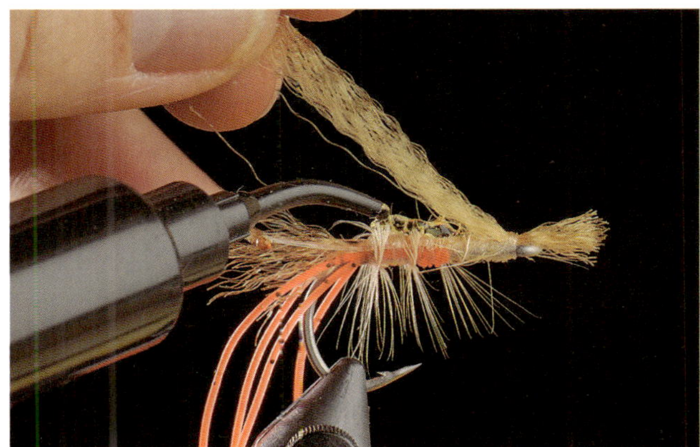

2. Lift the carapace and place a liberal amount of acrylic along the shank. You are not making a skim coat here. You want the entire carapace to be solid and stuck to the shank. Then, pull the carapace into the gel to be sure that you have covered it thoroughly.

(continued)

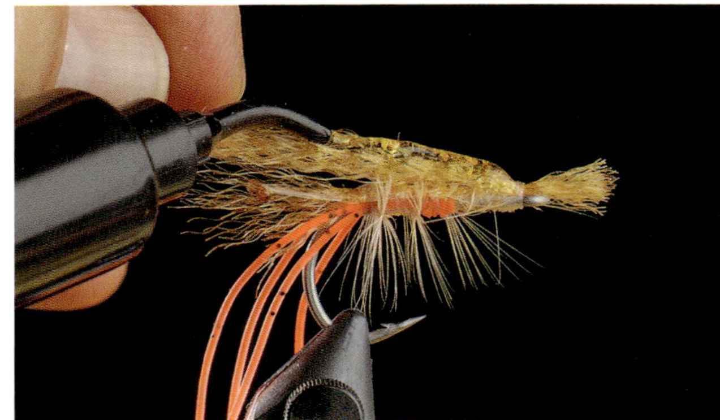

3. Add more gel to the top of the carapace. Move the gel along the length of the fly, poking it into the fibers with the tip of the applicator. In the photo, I am still holding the carapace taut with my material hand. You must maintain control over the fibers at all times. Note the gap just under the carapace, which you will close in the next steps.

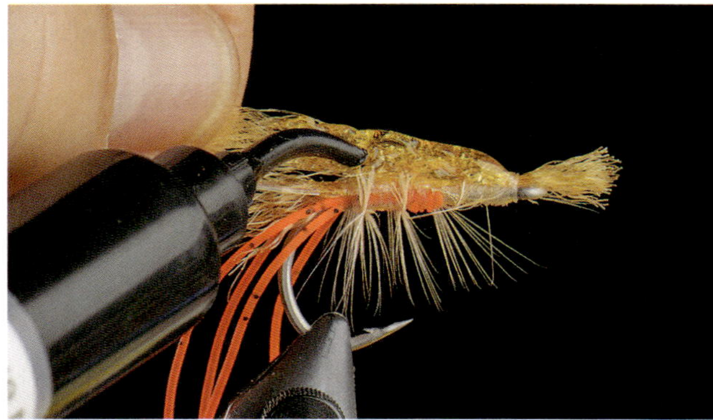

4. The gel should not go much past the hook bend at this stage. Be sure to apply gel to any indentations. I'm not necessarily adding more gel—though I might—but I am using the tip to evenly distribute the gel. Look to keep a balanced amount on each side.

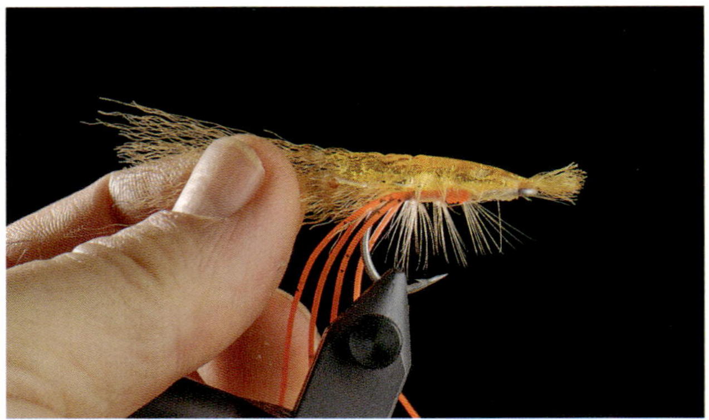

5. Manipulate the fibers to better distribute the gel and get the shape that you want. This also helps you visualize the proper angle of the carapace to best achieve the natural appearance of a shrimp. Manipulate the lower fibers to close the gap without destroying the natural, upward angle of the carapace. Note that while I am pulling the fibers down to close the gap, the top fibers are still straight and in line with the slightly upward angle of the carapace above.

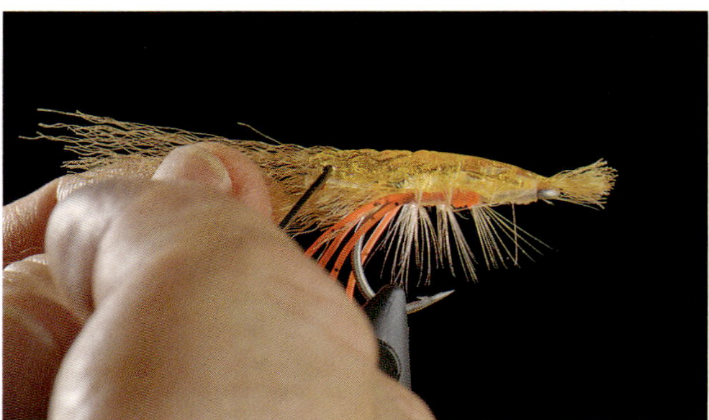

6. Using a bodkin, fine-tune the distribution of gel into the fibers around the eye.

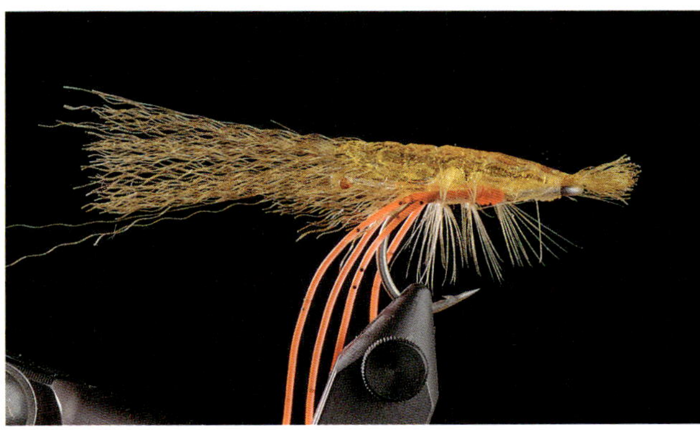

7. The light-cured acrylic on the fly is ready to be set. Verify there is no gap between the carapace and the hook shank, and that gel coats all the thread wraps in the front of the hook where you tied down the carapace. Also, note that the carapace has an angle of about 35 to 40 degrees from the hook shank. This angle is easier to see in the next step.

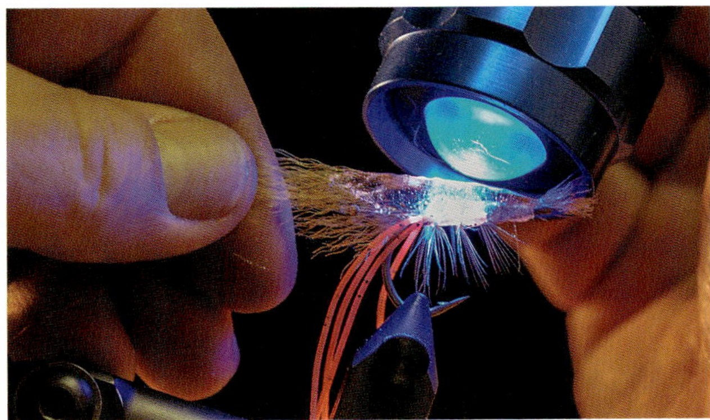

8. Holding the fibers at the desired angle, start to set the gel with the light. Hold the light close and move it slowly over the entire body—top, bottom, and both sides. Wipe alcohol on the body just as you did with the Surf Candy to remove any tackiness, and apply Top Coat or Sally Hansen Hard As Nails. Trim the carapace at an angle, removing your handle.

ACRYLICS FOR SHAPE: CRAB

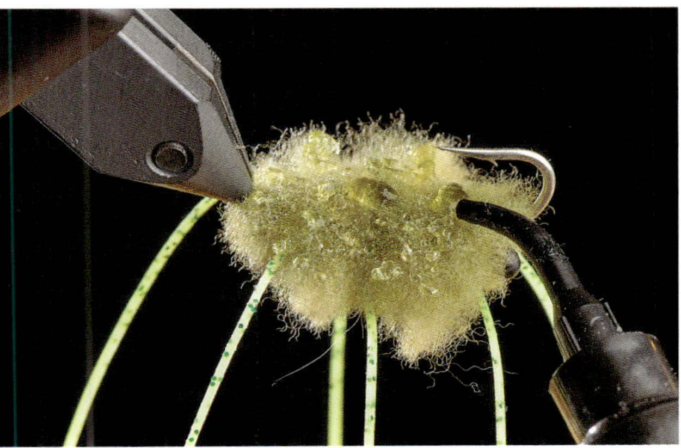

1. You can also use light-cured acrylics to give shape to softer materials. In this application, Tuffleye Flex helps firm up the shape of the crab. Apply small dollops of gel randomly across the top. Once you have dotted the entire back of the fly, distribute the gel with a bodkin.

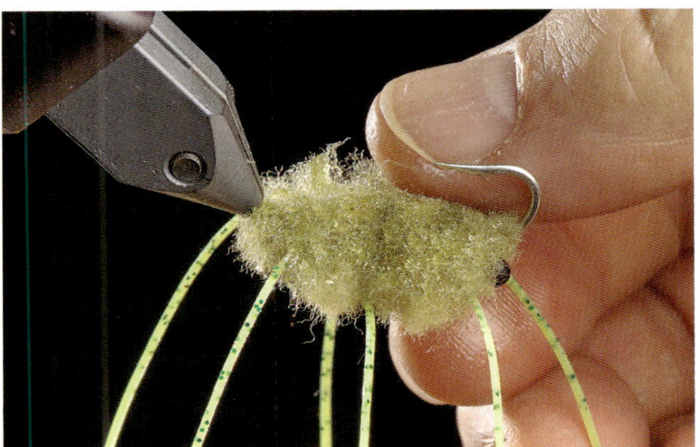

2. Wet your thumbs and then pat down the fibers and gel to distribute the gel around the crab top.

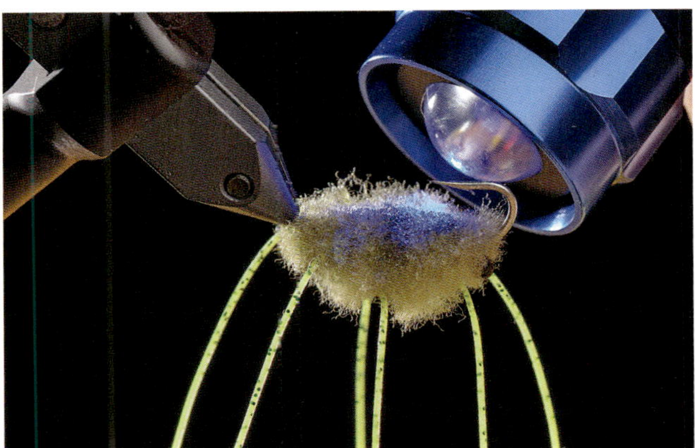

3. Set the acrylic with the light. A version of this technique also works well with the Worm Fleye.

Spread Technique

The technique used to create Spread Fleyes is terrific for creating broad, extremely thin imitations that are both realistic and easy to cast. With light-cured acrylics, this technique has become a lot easier and a lot less anxiety-ridden than when we did it with epoxy. You are no longer at the mercy of epoxy's curing time to spread and hold the fibers; you can spread them when you are ready to. The main point behind this technique is that you spread the fly in two stages: first spread the top, then the bottom. As with Surf Candies, and other fleyes, the acrylic must completely penetrate the fibers. As we show later on in the book, you can use this technique inside the fly as well as at the head.

SPREAD TECHNIQUE

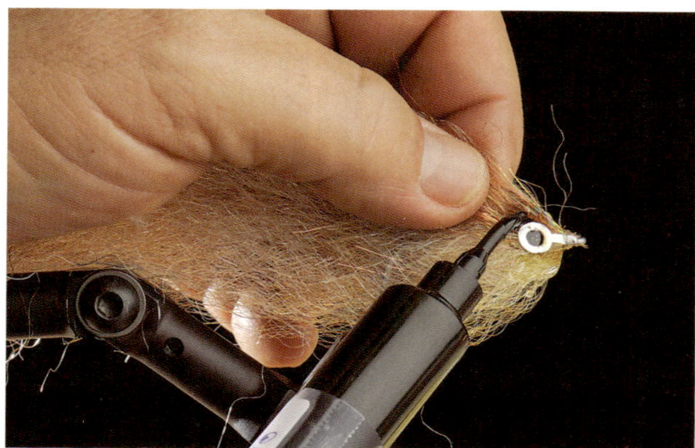

1. While spreading out the fibers, start to apply the light-cured acrylic to the nose area, barely past the eye. Work the gel into the fibers as well as the area underneath the eye.

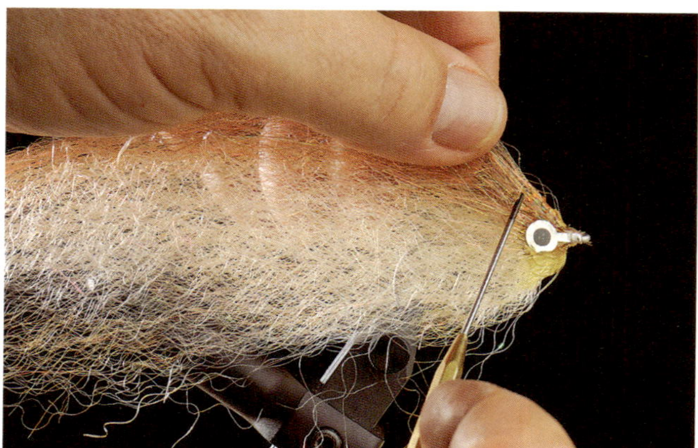

2. Once you have applied a base coat, apply more light-cured acrylic as needed to get a nice coating, making sure that it penetrates the fibers thoroughly. Open up the fibers with a bodkin to increase the width of the fly and to help distribute the acrylic. The bodkin is also helpful for controlling drips or final shaping.

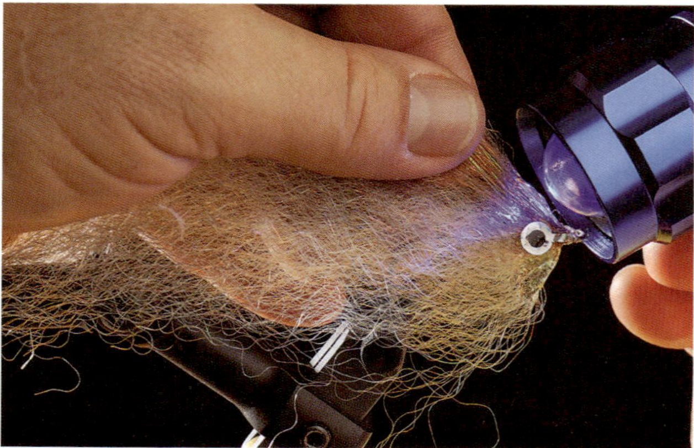

3. While holding the fibers firmly upward in the desired shape, set the area above the shank with the blue light just enough to maintain the shape. It will take a bit of practice to learn how long to hit it with the light to only partially cure it.

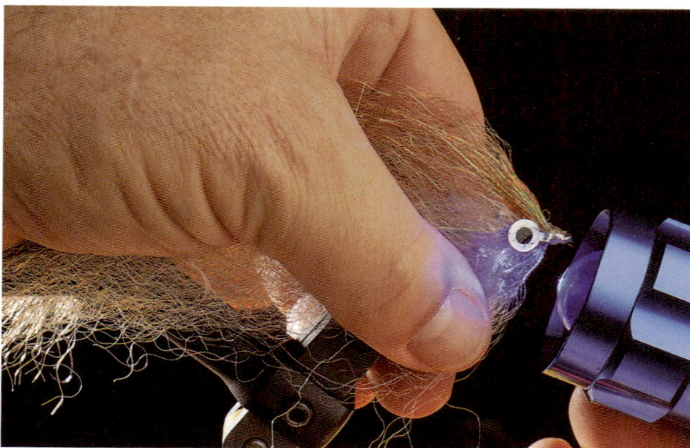

4. Next, do the same underneath. When you are happy with the shape of both the top and bottom, set them completely with more light. These first two applications set the initial shape. You can go back and reapply more gel as needed. For the complete tying steps of a Double Spread, see page 200.

PART II

The Patterns

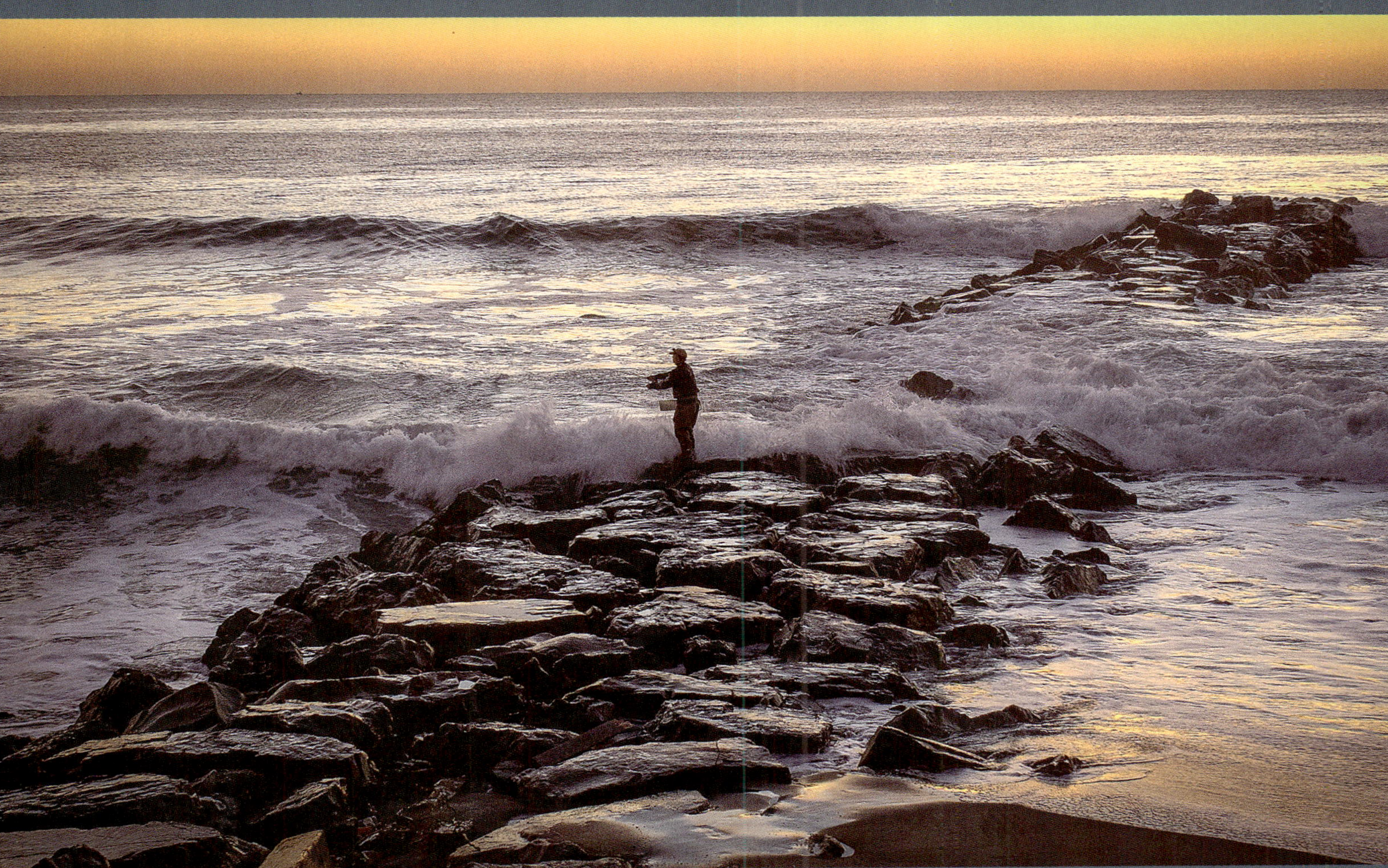

Good design means much more than a good-looking fly in the vise. For instance, effective saltwater patterns must not only catch fish, but they must withstand the rigors of the saltwater environment. COLIN ARCHER

Chapter 5

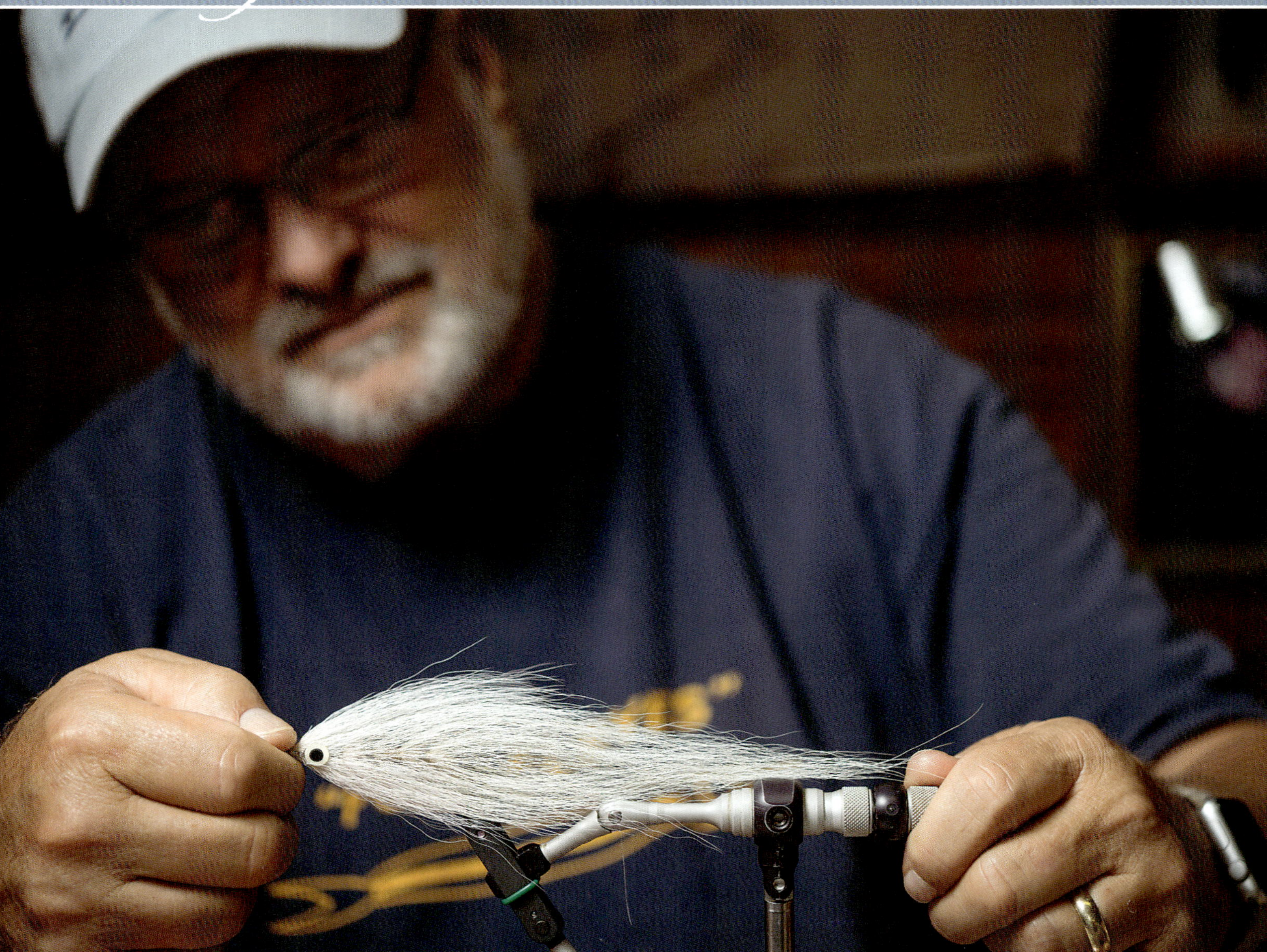

One of my original Hollow Fleyes. This version shows a bit more open angle of the bucktail, creating a nice bunker/herring shape.

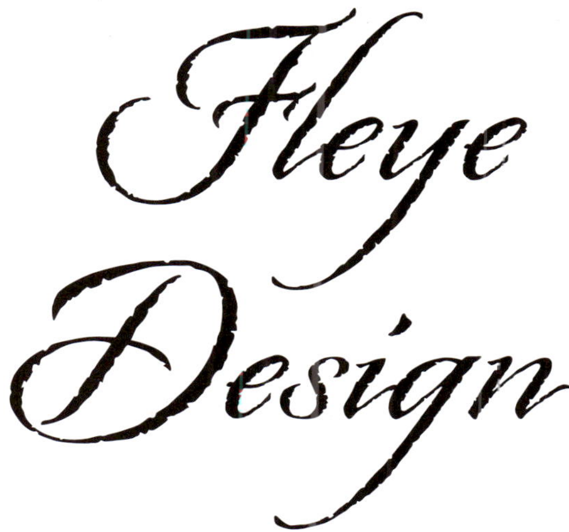

Fleye Design

Catching a fish on a fly that you tied yourself can be exciting and very satisfying. Tying flies often leads to tying flies of your own design instead of merely replicating others' patterns, and for me, the main motivation to design my own patterns is to solve fishing and tying problems, such as how to make my fleyes more durable, or how to make them swim better or cast easier. In my opinion, trying a new way just for the sake of doing something different will get you nowhere, and merely changing colors doesn't qualify as a new design.

Be a Better Observer

Fly design begins with keen observation, and the tier must be intimately familiar with the bait he is trying to mimic. Everything, including size, shape, distinctive physical features (such as spots, lines, eye position or size, translucent or opaque colors), and habits (swimming characteristics, survival tactics, and habitat), becomes important not only in the design of the fly but also in how it is fished. The Surf Candy, for example, arose out of a series of simple observations. Small baits are translucent, with prominent eyes, bellies, and flash. Until epoxy, it was difficult to re-create that combination of translucency and extreme durability. Now light-cured acrylics push the envelope further.

By observing the baits in their natural settings, you can get an idea not only of how they look in the water, but also of the types of water that they frequent, which in turn will influence your fishing strategy. Look closer, and you will probably notice that they look different depending on the overall light and even the time of day or season of the year. Watch them when they are scared and being attacked by a predator. How they react then will determine how you design the fly for action or to swim in a certain part of the water column, as well as how you ultimately present and retrieve the fly.

What are the bait's most noticeable characteristics besides size and silhouette? Large or small eyes, stripes or barred markings, translucent flesh or solid opaque bodies are some considerations to build into the design. Does the fly need action in the water, or is it intended to be retrieved quickly where action is not so important? Is flash necessary, and if so, how much? Is realism advantageous, or will a simple design be enough for success? These considerations are like optional equipment. Some elements become necessary, and some remain ornamental. Either way, I feel that it is important to keep the design simple while you try to capture as much of the bait's essence as possible.

Learn on your own, and also listen to the experiences of others, but with reservation. It is important to question conventional thinking. For instance, a generally accepted

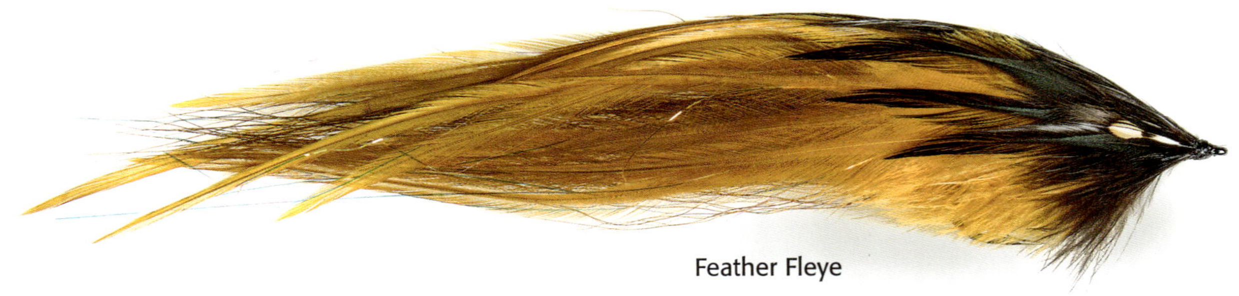

Feather Fleye

The Feather Fleye

A Study in Practical Design

The Feather Fleye is sculpted from many lengths of feathers to create a beautiful, naturally tapered fly. As with the BULKhead, the Feather Fleye was a way for me to use up a lot of material that I had lying around. In the case of the BULKhead, it was the hollow hair toward the base of the tail; on the Feather Fleye, it was the shorter feathers that I previously had no use for. When I tied them in progressively shorter lengths, shingling them around a palmered feather, it created a fly that felt almost like a little bird in the hand, and in the water the many feather tips pulsed with life.

But, in my opinion, frugality doesn't override the fly's major flaws. The Feather Fleye looks good in the vise and in the water, and it does catch fish; however, it not only takes too long to tie but it is heavy to cast. The Bucktail Deceiver, or the Semper Fleye Deceiver, which has feathers in it, is simpler to tie, and is just as effective and beautiful with a lot less time involved. So in the final analysis, I deemed the Feather Fleye impractical and stopped tying and fishing it. However, it taught me the shingling techniques that I use for the Feather Fleye Squid.

A successful, well-thought-out design constantly undergoes critical scrutiny by its creator, and the process is often ongoing. One simple rule of thumb: change a design only to improve it. Not all designs go right, and not all flies pass muster just because they look good.

rule when picking out a color scheme for a fly is to use a darker material over a lighter one. Backs are dark; bellies are light. But, in shallow, clear water or for bait just under the surface on sunny days, the tops of bait will appear brighter than the undersides. Also, many baits are broader at the tops of their bodies, which means their undersides are in shadow and look dark. Time of day and angle of the sun can be critical, and when you take these things into consideration, you then begin to make changes as you observe more from trip to trip.

Another misconception that is easily corrected through observation is that a finished fly must be wet to look like it does in the water. I have watched countless people dip a fly in the water and then point to the fish-like taper, but that is misleading. How you see your fly in the vise is exactly what it looks like in the water. All you have to do is drop it in a pan of water after you tie it. There you'll see the answer. When you move the fly, it doesn't collapse as much as you think either. It only pulsates slightly.

What does this mean to you as a tier? If you want a taper in your fly, you must tie it in so that you can see it in the vise. The Bucktail Deceiver began first as an idea, or realization, that the fly in the water will look like the fly in the vise. This might not seem like a big deal, but for me it was an important step in creating form and taper in my finished fleyes.

It's important not only to observe the baits and the fish that are your quarry, but also to observe your flies in the water after you tie them. Performance in the water is the final test. For me, fishing comes first; I do not think that flies are simply pieces of art to be looked at. On and in the water, you will find out whether you succeeded, and

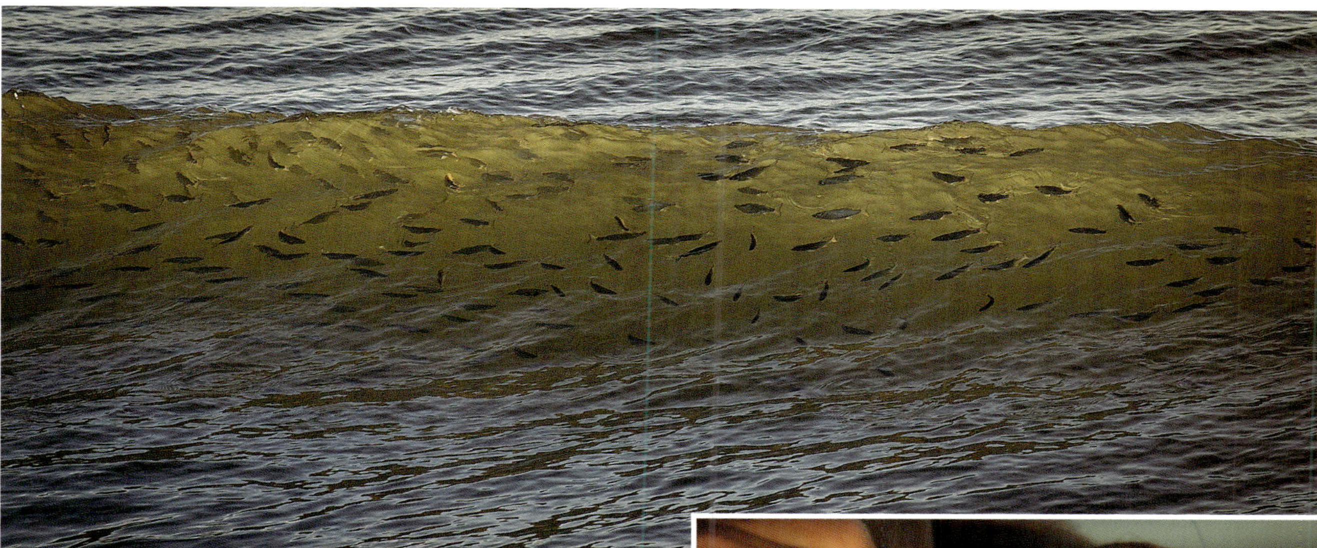

Mullet in the waves. Mullet are a great food for predator fish because they are usually found in good numbers and close to the beach. For fly rodders, mullet are easily mimicked with flies and they swim in the upper third of the water column usually leaving a V-shaped wake behind them. COLIN ARCHER

Right: Small box of Candies with bay anchovies, silversides, and sand eels. It's very important to be able to tie patterns that match the amazing size range of saltwater baits.

if you didn't succeed, often how the fly acts in the water will provide insight into how to fix your failures. Few flies work perfectly the first time out, and even good designs are never finished; they always evolve. Many flies fail initially but quickly rise again with a few little adjustments here and there. Is the keel strong enough? Does the material impart enough action? Does the silhouette look right? Is there too much flash or not enough? Does the fly fish in the part of the water column it was designed to? How well does it cast, and can it be cast accurately and effortlessly? Does the fly flutter too much? Can I cast it into the wind effectively? Does it foul excessively? Would some weight help? What, if anything, can I do to make it better?

One good example of simple refinements based on observation of a fly pattern in the water is my gradual move away from using long saddles and other feathers on my fleyes, such as Hollow Fleyes. I have learned through trial and error that long feathers that extend well past the bucktail tips look like seaweed or grass hanging off the back of the fly. Now, I make sure that the feathers or flash do not extend much past the tips of the bucktail.

Shape

Proper shape has always been paramount for me. When I view a fly from the side, I like to see nice flowing, natural lines that resemble the bait's overall shape. The lack of basic shape is often the first thing that comes up when I am asked to critique another tier's fly. To get them to think about proper shape, I generally ask them to trace their fly and then tell me what they see—it often doesn't resemble the form of any bait.

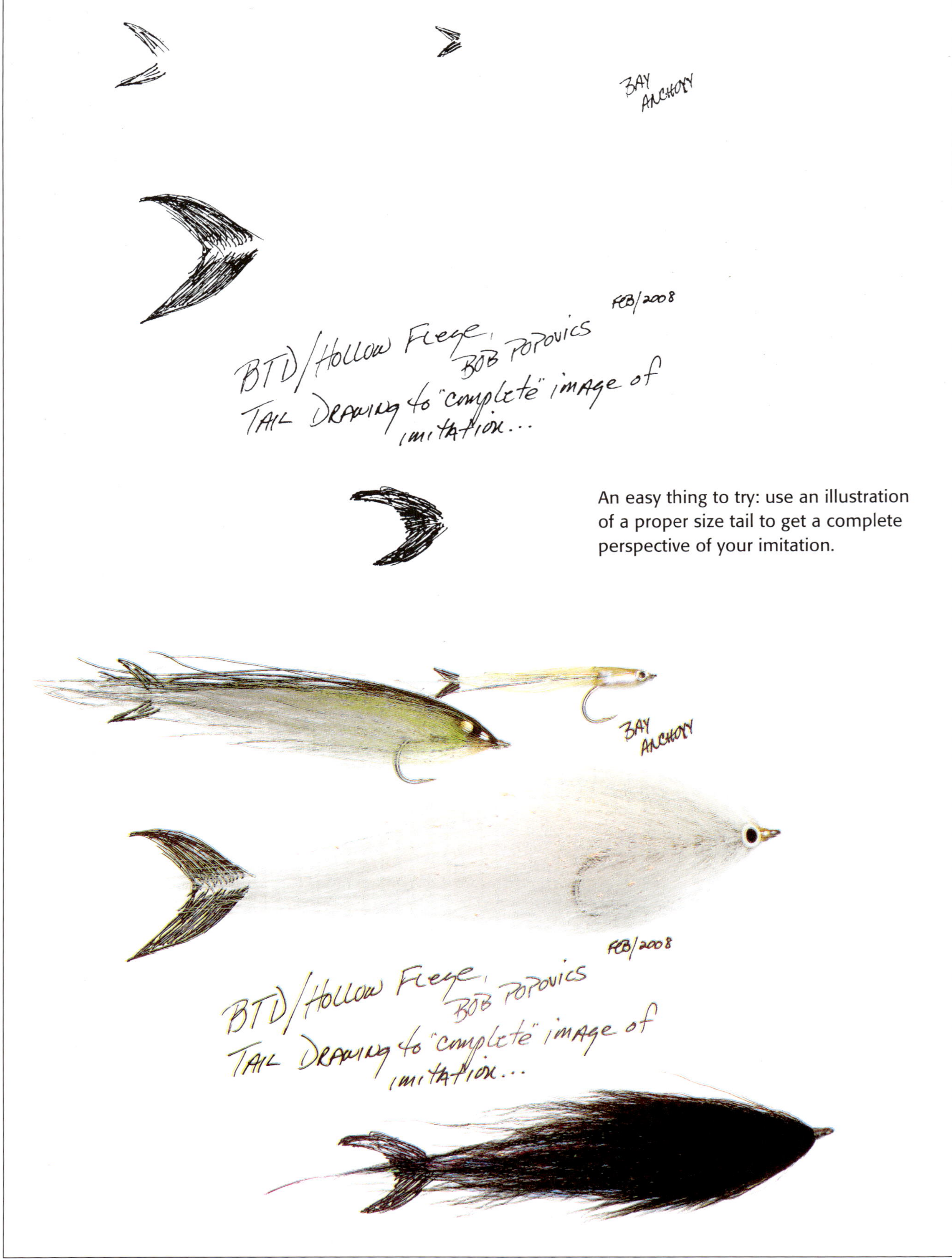

An easy thing to try: use an illustration of a proper size tail to get a complete perspective of your imitation.

To get my fleyes "in shape," I will trace the bait, add a tail and a hook, and use that as a form against which to complete my design. After I have an image of the bait and put a hook in there, I just fill in the spaces. The tracing helps me get the right image a little clearer in my mind. I am not a great drawer, but I can draw baitfish pretty well, because I spend so much time observing them. Interestingly, however, I cannot draw a tail, because I don't put tails in my fleyes. I guess you see what is important to you.

Tracing is a great way to get a handle on the basic two-dimensional shape. Another important basic two-dimensional shape consideration is that the fly has a taper from front to back. For the most part, no baitfish gets bigger past its shoulders, so the fly design needs to reflect that. I also like to create flies with flow that have no bulges or interruptions in the shape. It is also important that they have proper thread heads—no long thread heads that I call "beaks."

In addition to having the right profile, the fly must look right from all sides. The 3D made me focus on the simple subtleties of natural bait shape. All I needed to do was to incorporate these subtleties into the designs. A little bit more hair here and less there, and a more realistic and natural design took place. When I looked at the fly in the water, I noticed more action when I retrieved it. The 3D changed everything in my designs from that point on and has since influenced all of my fly designs, which is the main reason I begin the tying steps with it.

Lack of taper—whether it is a paintbrush-like clump of perfectly stacked fibers or a poorly conceived profile—takes the life right out of a well-designed fly. Taper is smooth and progressive, not erratic or out of sync. In the natural bait, good taper is extremely important to fish survival, contributing to a fish's ability to effectively swim for food and evade predators. To make flies with tapers that look natural and alive is not difficult. You just need to be aware of it, both in nature and your imitation, through good observation, and you must tie it into your fly.

Taper is not only important regarding overall shape, but also regarding movement, or action, in the water. The Bucktail Deceiver is a prime example because its electric action in the water is a result of both the taper of the individual fibers tips and the overall taper of the fly. On the slowest of retrieves, the entire fly still pulses in the water because of all the bucktail tips, and with faster strips, the back end kicks. This means the fly is always moving.

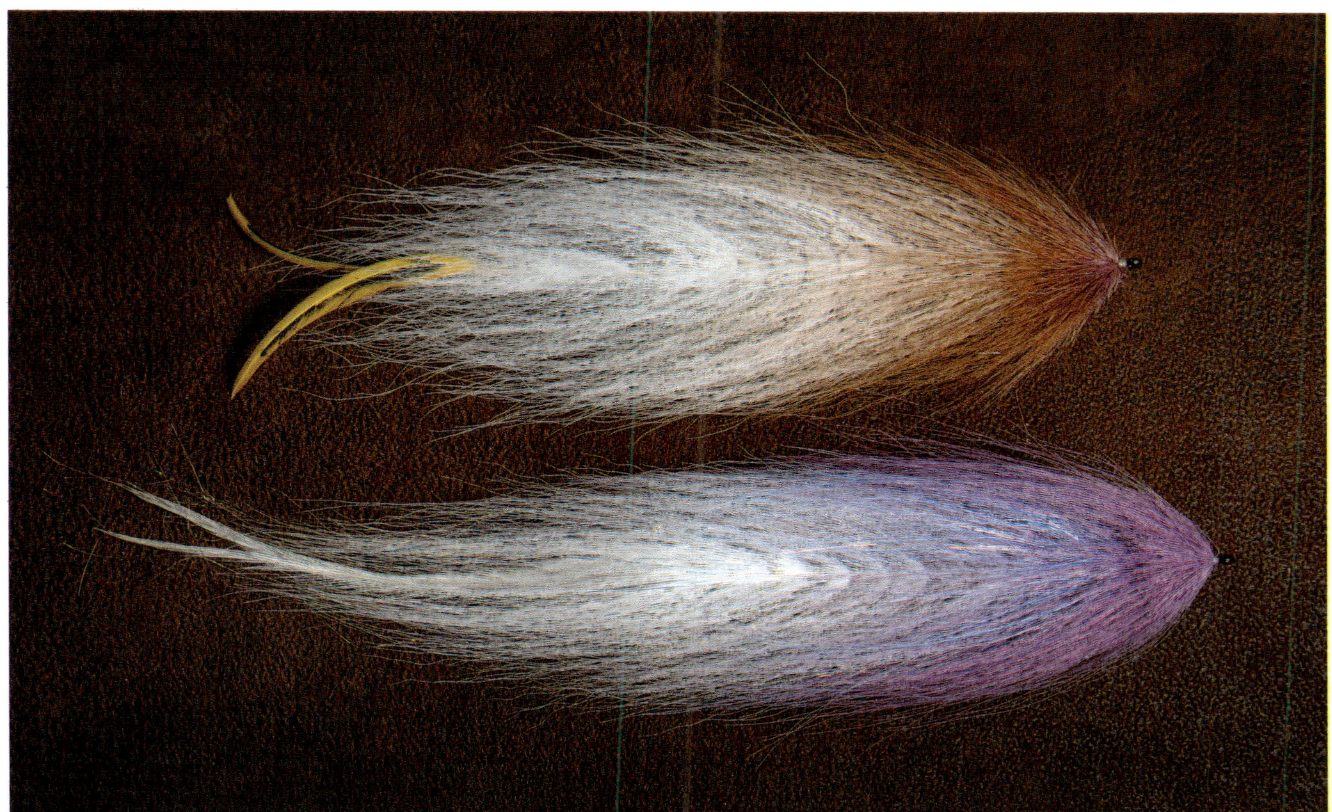

BULKhead Beasts. Even a huge fly can benefit from forward bulk to enhance its fish-catching action. The top fleye is a menhaden pattern tied with yellow feather tails on a monofilament extension. Menhaden have a forked tail with a prominent amount of yellow in it.

Body: Sparseness and Bulk

Over the years many tiers have asked me whether I prefer sparse or bulky flies, and I always reply that it is not an either/or proposition. Sparse, for me, is an obvious choice for smaller, translucent bait imitations. As the baits get larger, sparseness is less necessary because the baits become more opaque; however, I might opt to make larger flies sparse for ease of casting or to help them sink faster.

In general, I feel that using excessive amounts of material is a design flaw. I try to tie as sparsely as possible, while still retaining the effect I am aiming for, if only because subtracting unnecessary materials simplifies things. My Beast Fleye—which is a very large Hollow—has evolved over the years to become much sparser than the original versions. After observing the Beast in the water, I noticed that all the tips folded back over the preceding ones, which gave a relatively opaque appearance to a fairly sparse fly, so now I tie them sparse.

I'm not so sure that sparse flies have better action than bulky flies, which is something that people say, if only because I have noticed that heavily dressed patterns move well in the water, too. For me, the key to getting a fly to move in the water is to put bulk at the front of the pattern, which creates little currents that really move the fibers behind it. And if you look at many baits we imitate—bunker, squid, mullet, and more—only the last two-thirds of the body moves while the head is stationary. This principle of using bulk at the front to swim sparser fibers in the rear informs a lot of my fly design, especially for a fly like the BULKhead.

In addition to increasing action in the rear, forward bulk also holds the fly higher longer and can make a wake on top. The wake, or simply the water the fly pushes as it is being fished under the surface, creates vibrations that fish sense through their lateral lines—what Gary Borger calls the acoustic footprint. You can also add things like Pulse Discs or Banger heads to create even more disturbance.

Seeing the Future

When I sit down to tie a fly, I already have a vision of the bait that I want to imitate in my mind. The tying process

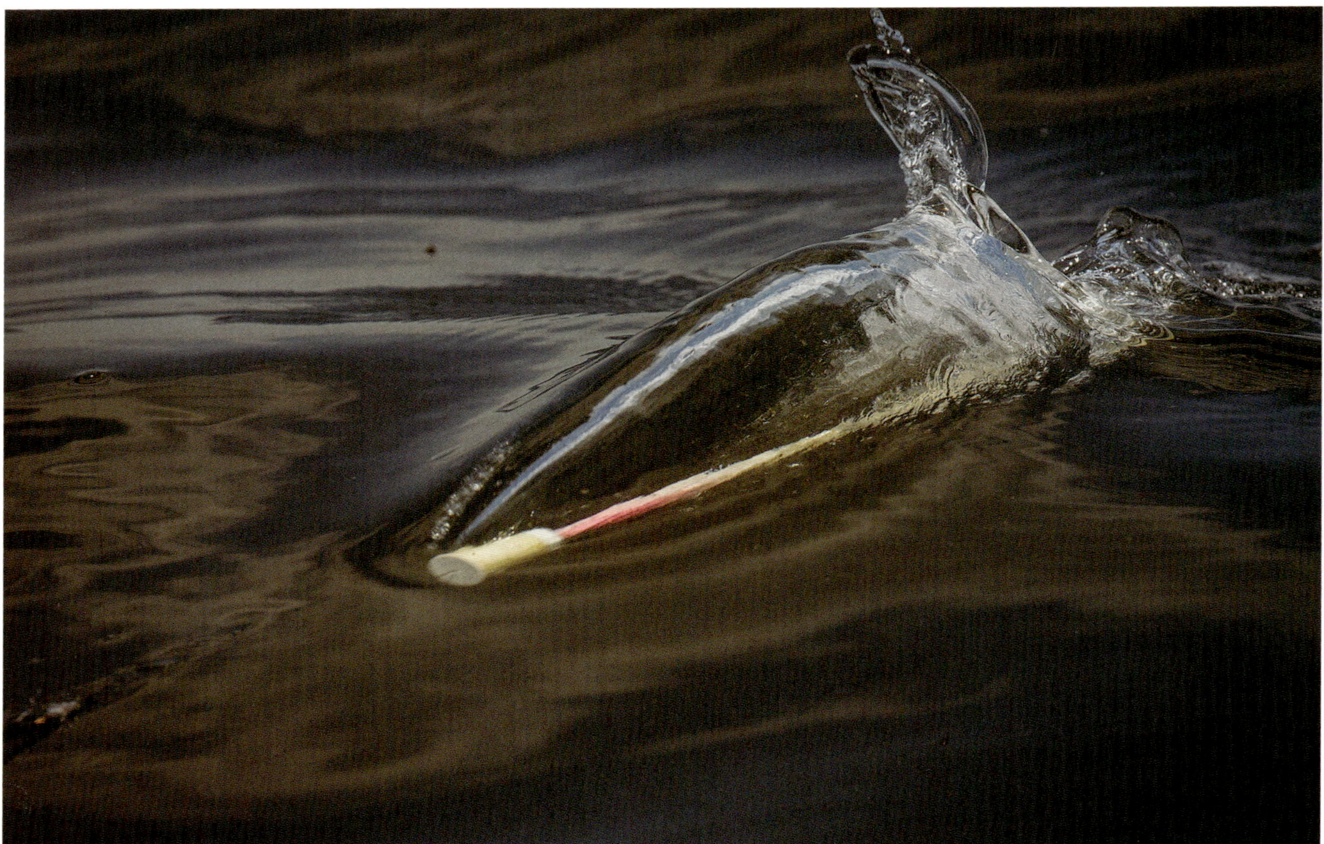

Adding a Banger head to a fly makes it plunge and swim, creating very dramatic noise and turbulence.

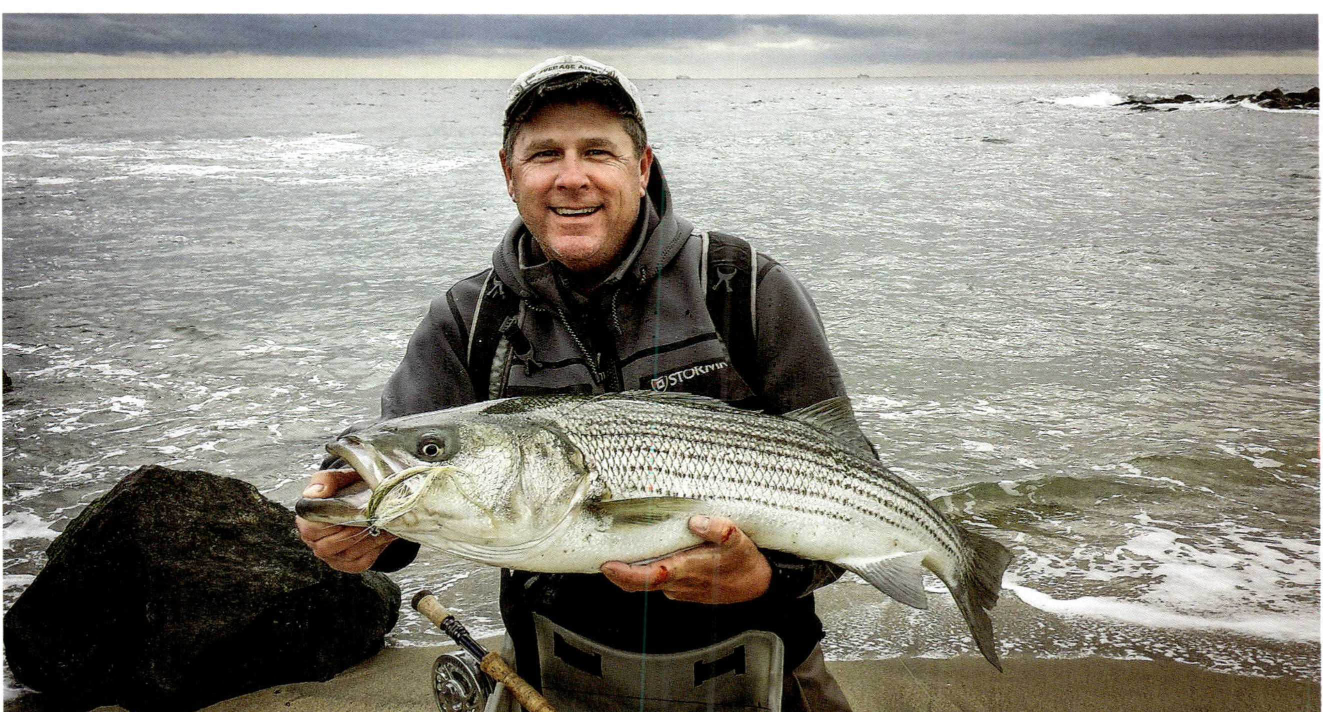

Anglers wait for years to be at the crossroads where bait, bass, and themselves meet at the same time. Colin Archer found a beach all to himself and caught several large bass that were in the wash along the Jersey Shore. COLIN ARCHER

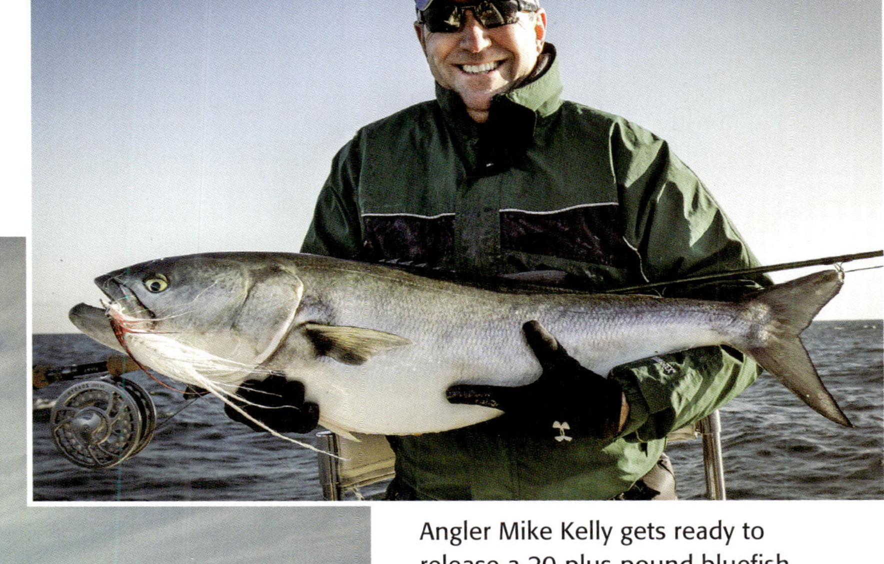

Angler Mike Kelly gets ready to release a 20-plus-pound bluefish taken on a Hollow Fleye. COLIN ARCHER

Left: This tuna was caught south of Martha's Vineyard by Rob Morrison. It took a Hollow Fleye. TOM RAPONE

becomes one of simply filling in the shape in my mind with the materials in my hand. This is not always easy because natural materials do not always want to behave, and if this is the case, then you must either switch gears or adapt to the material, which comes with experience. But the most important thing (which ties in with my previous comments about observation and importance of taper and multidimensionality in flies) is that having a vision for your flies ahead of time makes the process much easier.

As you work with, and respond to, the materials, you can also anticipate how they will respond and influence the final taper of the fly. How do you see the fly coming along? As you put that first bunch of material on, you can see how it reacts. You need to be able to respond to the materials. I've used bucktails with a wide range of characteristics and I've made beautiful Hollow Fleyes out of them, but some of them I have to get used to and understand in order to tie with them more consistently. And that came with time just like anything else. That's one of the reasons that tying with bucktail is so invigorating for me. Some forethought in material selection is also important and ultimately saves lots of time and frustration. When I find good bucktail for a certain fly, I will tie that fly, or save the bucktail for when I tie that particular pattern down the road.

Mimi Flies: Fly Dressing vs. Fly Designing

I am more of a fly designer than a fly dresser. For me, shape is the most important—that's the starting point and the backdrop on which everything evolves. I will add some simple flash and blend some colors, but in general, I am less concerned about fly recipes than overall shapes and designs. I prefer to provide the template and let the other fly tiers and fishermen who use the flies make them the way that they like.

These days, I like to make my fleyes as simple as possible and tie them to fish with. I like to minimize the tedious dressings and tie in just what's important to me. My fleyes are dressed casual—jeans and a T-shirt. I love to look at beautiful flies that are works of art, but as a fisherman first, I prefer to design basic, functional, well-thought-out templates, like a freshly cut Christmas tree

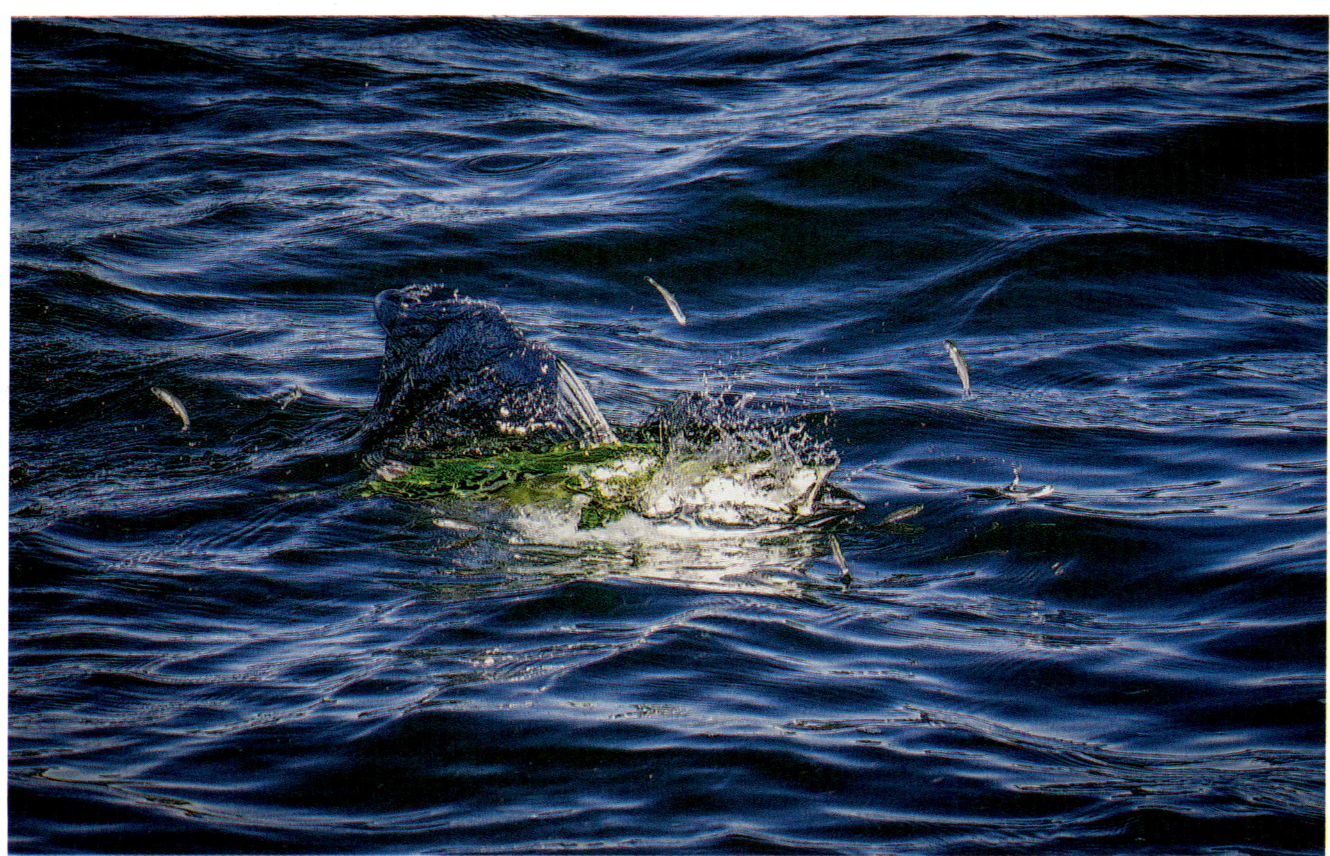

A speedy false albacore attacks bay anchovies (whitebait) off Montauk Point, New York. TOM LYNCH

A Look at Hooks

Choosing the proper hook to do the job in fly design is of utmost importance. To choose a hook simply because it's readily available or convenient without responsible consideration will, nine out of ten times, be insufficient. Mike Martinek once described it to me this way: "The hook's importance to the fly is like the proper hull to a ship. No matter what is in the ship, it's meaningless if it can't float and perform properly." Similarly, a fly will be less effective if the chosen hook doesn't tend to all aspects of the design—shank length, gape, and keel. A good saltwater hook must also be strong enough for your quarry, saltwater proof, and able to be sharpened.

Shank length: The shank is the "plot of land" on which to build your fly design. You tie on the shank, not the bend (usually) or the eye, so it needs to be long enough to accommodate the materials you intend to tie on it. For me, it is as simple as tying small flies on short shanks and longer and larger flies on longer shanks. Yet, many tiers squeeze their flies onto too short of an area, cramping the materials and making the tying more difficult or tedious than it has to be.

Long-shank hooks provide the necessary platform required for proper imitation and taper on a fly such as the Bucktail Deceiver. They also allow you to tie a significant amount of materials on the shank without closing the hook gape. Finally, you can tie on the back half of them to have a built-in bite guard for toothy critters such as bluefish.

Hook gape: What good is a beautiful imitation if the fly can't find the fish's mouth? As you put the materials on, you should always watch the gape (the distance from shank to hook point). If it gets closed up, the hookup percentage will decrease dramatically, as lots of material can block the hook point from finding a home. A long-shank hook has the extra shank length to move the forward tie-in point farther away from the gape so that you don't block it with materials.

Keel: The weight of the hook's bend and point (everything below the shank) is what allows the hook to track straight with the hook point down. Because of the excessive materials on big flies, you may need more weight below the hook shank to get a fly to track straight and not ride on its side during the retrieve. A properly keeled fly will dig into the current no matter the size and speed of a retrieve or current.

For larger flies, sometimes a simple fix is to go up one or two hook sizes to get more weight on the bottom. Another thing that I do is carry lead wire with me when I am fishing, and if I have a fly that is not keeling properly, I will wrap about an inch of wire at the bottom of the bend, just behind the barb.

You can also alter the keel by bending the shank (which relocates the bent portion of the hook to below the straight portion), altering the position of the wing, or weighting one side of the shank, such as with dumbbell eyes. In some cases, the fly might even keel better if you combine a couple of these tricks.

that tiers can adorn with whatever ornaments they please. On a fly like the Beast, or other large patterns, I consider the most important attributes to be silhouette and size. I don't dress them up much or feel the need to add eyes. Instead, I keep them pretty straightforward and find that the unadorned bucktail is perfect.

A running joke among some of my tying friends is that some of the garish flies that I see are just like Mimi Bobeck, the large lady from the late 1990s sitcom *The Drew Carey Show*. She wore so much makeup that in the first episode she wasn't hired for a cosmetics job. This is not an attack on other tiers, as much as a comment on my own evolution as a fly tier. Tiers go through stages, including preferences for different ways to tie, or different techniques or materials. And I am no different. In *Pop Fleyes*, on page 2, you can see Surf Candies tied with gaudy cheek feathers, and right above them an elaborate bunker that took all night to make. In Lefty Kreh's book *Saltwater Fly Patterns*, on the cover, the chartreuse Semper Fleye with painted cheeks and three-stage painted eyes is Mimi in full dress makeup! For the most part, I now prefer simple designs, a tendency that continues to evolve, even through this book where I no longer even like eyes on some of the bucktail designs that I originally tied for this project.

Now that I have stated my preference for simplicity, I will throw a curve. Fly tying is also a lot of fun and an extension of being on the water. I like to try different things when tying, and during those weathered-out days and nights when fishing is not possible, I find that fly fishing is not all that far away as I sit up in my fly-tying room and tie. It's no trouble to get a bit indulgent with a pattern—you never know where it will lead. I know that a simple bunch of proven patterns are going to do me just fine, but sometimes there isn't as much fun in that. The Feather Fleye is a good example of a fly that was a bit of an indulgence, yet it led to some interesting ideas for techniques and applications.

And sometimes you have to move beyond simplicity to make progress on a fly design. As I have mentioned, creating flies to me is problem solving. A fly that didn't last long or that fouled excessively were things that I couldn't stand back in my early days with the fly rod. The first fly I ever tied was just white bucktail with yellow bucktail over the top and peacock herl. Simple? Yes. Durable? No. Did it foul? Absolutely! The fly was simple without a doubt, but the design was flawed. To solve the problem I had to consider something more complicated. But the end result is worth the effort, if it works. The Surf Candy was my attempt at solving those problems. It sure was more complicated than that simple teaser fly, but it lasted far longer and didn't foul anymore. However, I didn't stop there because after observing the reaction of the epoxy and some materials (such as polar bear hair), I saw that realism was a possibility. Eyes, flash, tails, and gills were now a part of the whole. As it turned out, the tails were totally unnecessary and I just stopped putting them in—they were too complicated. But the eyes and flash and gills were simple to include. They are still in my Surf Candies today, although I have found an even easier and more efficient way to add them in with the Fleye Foils, which I feel is a major advancement. Do eyes and

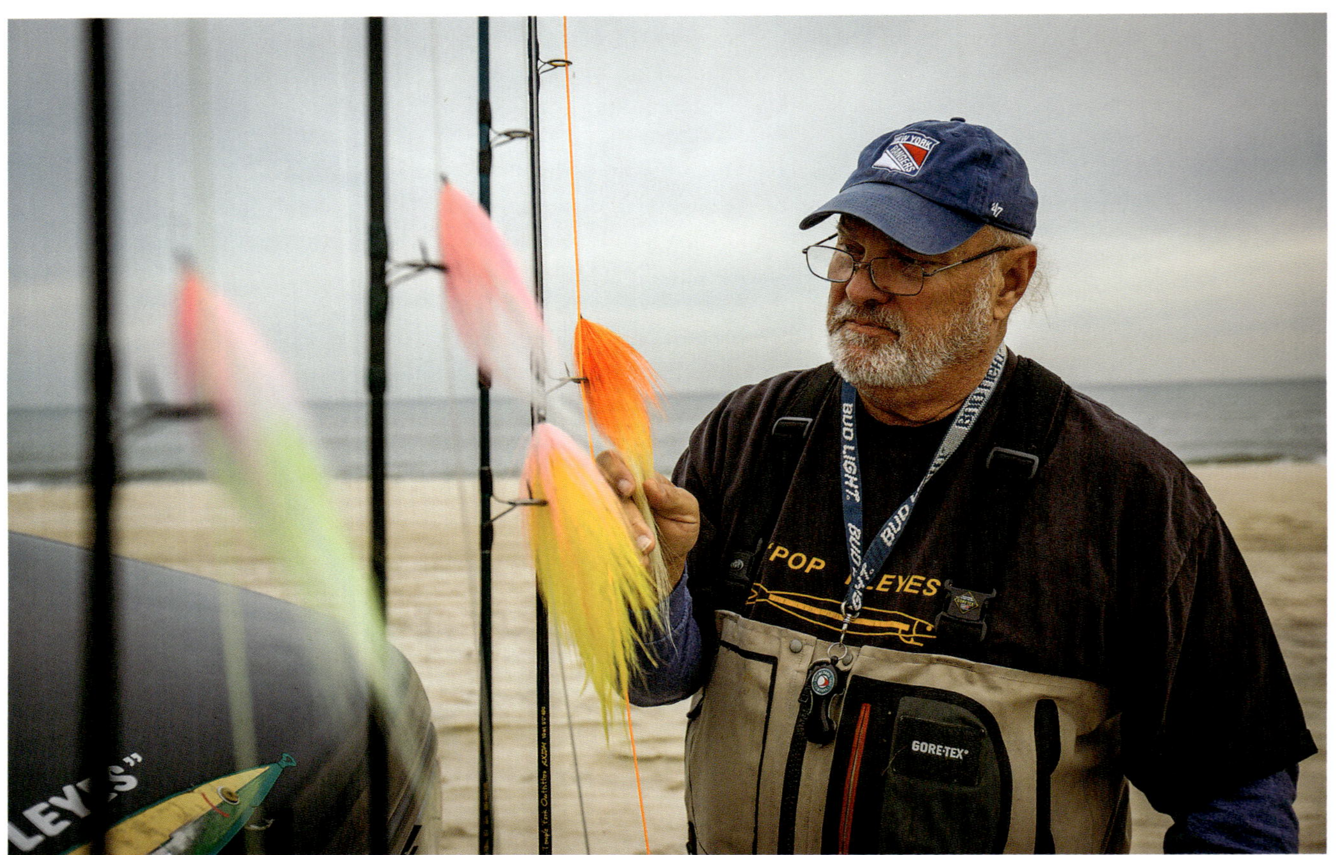

Bob Pop checks out his Beasts at Island Beach State Park, rigged and ready on the front of his 4x4 van for an on-the-water testing and evaluation session. The New York Rangers had just lost three games in a row, but they won that night. Could have been the hat. TOM LYNCH

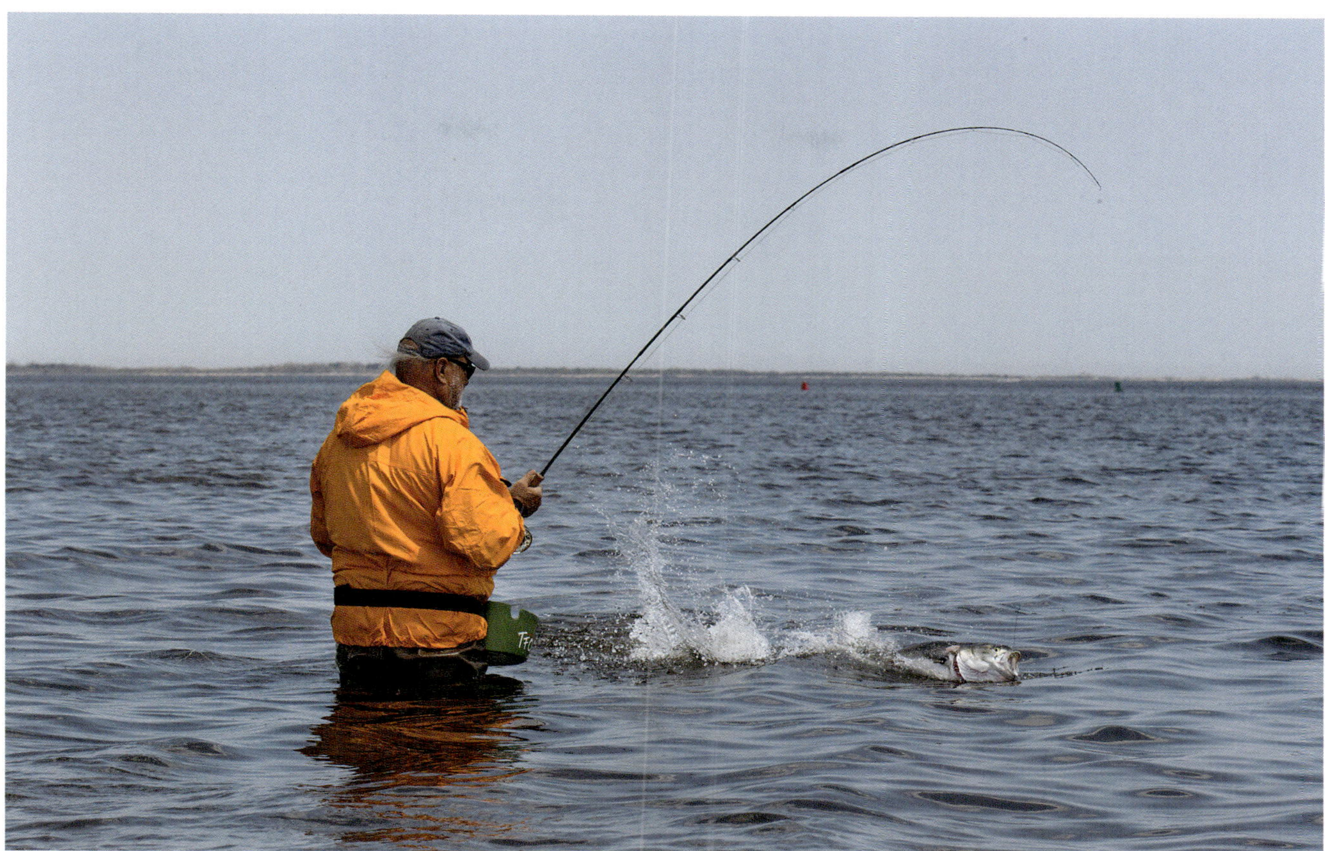

This bluefish jumped all over a Bucktail Deceiver fished on a wire leader. Artistic tying—tying for art's sake—does not interest me, though I am in no way criticizing those for whom it does. To me, tying flies is all about making something to go catch fish with. The easier and faster they are to tie, the longer the flies last, the less they foul, the easier they are to cast . . . those things are important in a fly. TOM LYNCH

flash make all that much difference? I don't know, but they are so easy to include that I say, "Why not?"

In the end, taper and shape—in the vise and in the water—combined with a fly that catches fish is my personal definition of perfection. I don't tie flies that look all alike, so machinelike consistency is not important to me. But when I have achieved what I have started out to do, I think that is as close to perfection as anything. When I have those rare moments, I chuckle at the end—and I am not the kind of guy who chuckles a lot. When I was tying, and retying, the prototypical Hollow Fleyes in my mind on a long car ride back from the Marlborough Fly Fishing Show, I was trying to work out all of the bugs and began to see an idea that would work, but I was also afraid that it would not. As soon as I got home, I went straight upstairs to my tying room and tried the technique, and it was exactly as I had imagined. After I saw that it would work, I went to bed because I was exhausted and then woke up and finished the fly in the morning. When I finished, I chuckled. So, when that happens—and it has with a few other patterns included in this book, too—I knew I am on to something real.

But the fly is only part of the complete picture. You have to fish it, and so the presentation—where you cast, how you retrieve, and how you rely on your own instincts, too—is more important than the fly, most of the time. You have to contribute more than just a fly to catch fish. You must contribute experience and instinct to do it successfully in all types of situations. When a fly doesn't seem to be working, I will change my presentation before I change my fly. Too often we give the fly too much credit when it works, and too much criticism when it doesn't. I believe in fine-tuning presentation first, then the fly. After that, the rest is up to instinct, and trusting that instinct is what separates great anglers from the others. Do you trust your instinct?

Chapter 6

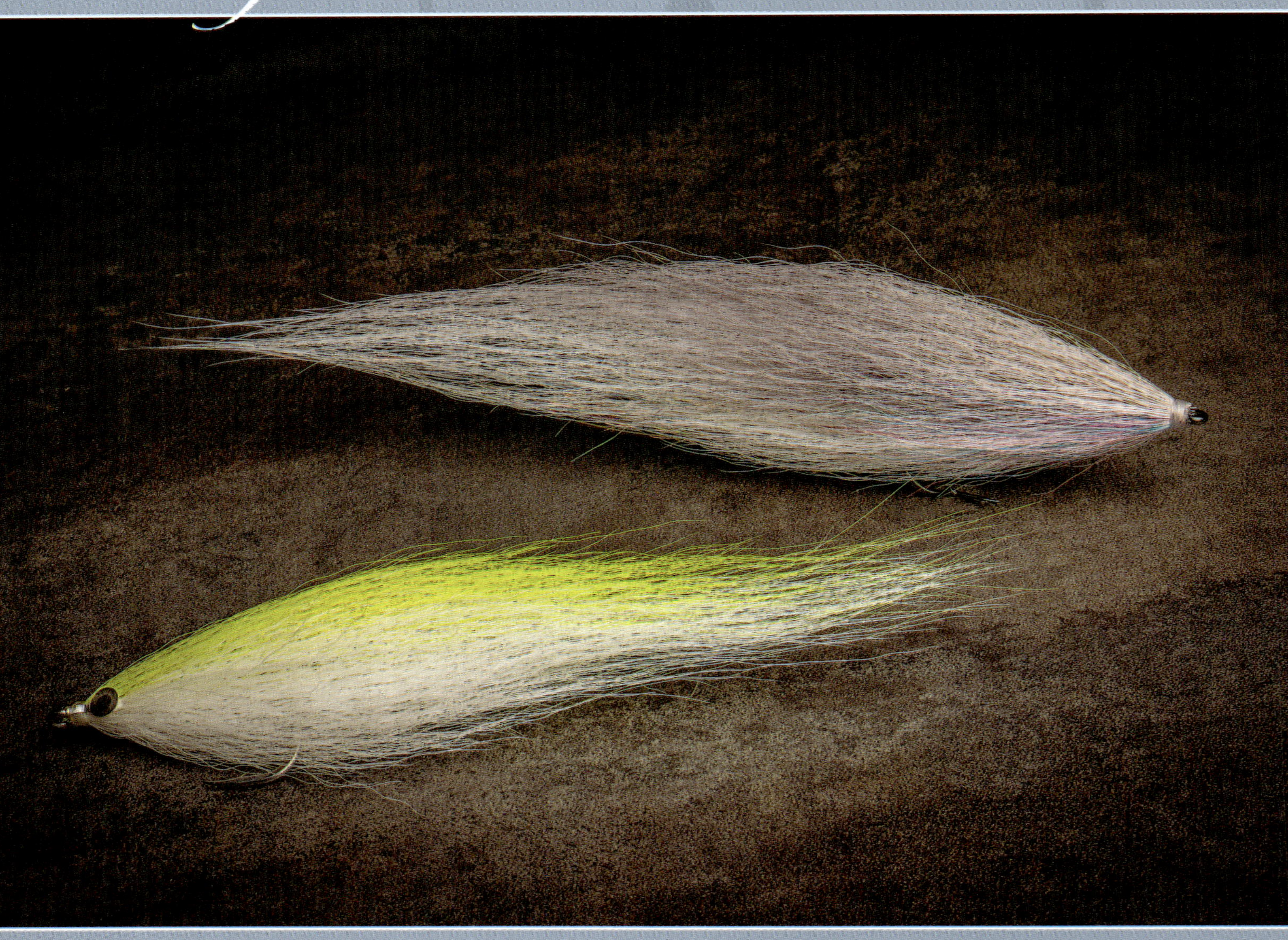

Lefty Kreh named the original synthetic version of this pattern the 3D as soon as he saw it. What I learned about tapering from the 3D was a major influence on my bucktail patterns such as the Bucktail Deceiver and Hollow Fleye, except that with the natural bucktail, I would have to create the taper with the natural material while I tied the fly, instead of trimming synthetics to shape.

3D Fleye

I've made almost as many casts with a net as I have with a fly rod, and I've been handling baitfish all of my life. Every day from September through November, I would net mullet commercially or for friends, and in the process of culling out all of the bycatch—anything from baby pompano to different shads, from mackerel to spearing—my hands would be in with the baits, feeling their shapes and subtle differences, the weight of their shoulders, their tapered bellies.

I can still remember taking a bunker fleye tied with Bozo Hair, putting it in my hand, and then comparing it to a live bunker. I wasn't satisfied. The imitation lacked body and depth; it was flat. This realization ultimately moved me to create a baitfish pattern with a more realistic shape. I wanted a fly that looked like a baitfish not just from the side, which is how most fly tiers create flies, but from every possible angle.

When I look back over the evolution of my fleyes, I can now say that the 3D was the father of the Bucktail Deceiver and Hollow Fleye, and that lessons learned from it have informed all of my designs since. I know that if I didn't do the 3D, the rest of the fleyes in this book would not exist. It was a point of maturity in my tying, an epiphany, that made me realize several important concepts. First, good imitations have multidimensional tapers, not just side profile. Second, if you want this taper, you must tie it in to the fly, and to create it, you must use fibers of progressively shorter lengths. Third, bulk in the front combined with a tapered tail contributes to a fly's action.

The 3D that we showed in *Pop Fleyes* was tied from synthetics, and that was how I first tied it before realizing that I could achieve better results with bucktail. I had tied a few 3Ds from bucktail before *Pop Fleyes*, but at that time it was still a fairly new technique for me. The 3D tied from synthetics required lashing all of the materials to the shank and then trimming away the excess to create the proper taper. Working with bucktail was almost the opposite: you had to tie the taper in with each step. Instead of trimming the fly at the end to get the shape I desired, I had to trim the fibers to length as I tied them in, leaving the tips untouched, which required a lot more precision and forethought than when tying with synthetics.

3Ds are a lot of work, and I've pretty much replaced them with Bucktail Deceivers and Hollow Fleyes. That's how my tying goes: it evolves. But the 3D represents an awakening for me, and tying it has really sharpened my sense of shape—every time I tie, I think in three dimensions.

3D Fleye

Hook:	#4/0 Gamakatsu SL12S or similar saltwater
Thread:	Fine monofilament
Body:	Chartreuse and white bucktail
Eyes:	Prism tab, silver with black pupil

TYING THE 3D FLEYE

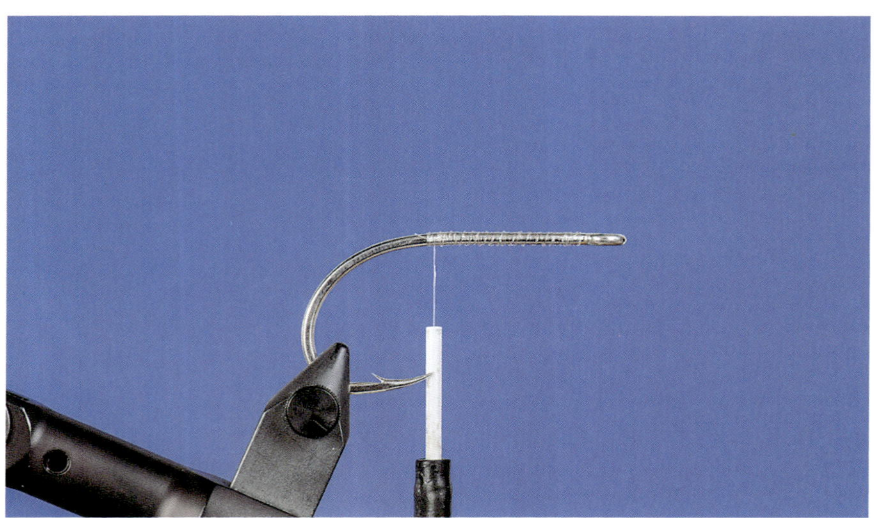

1. Place the hook in the vise and completely cover the shank with monofilament thread. By spiral wrapping the thread over an even base, you provide more surface area for the materials to grip. Choose a hook with a long enough shank so that you can evenly space the bucktail without running out of room.

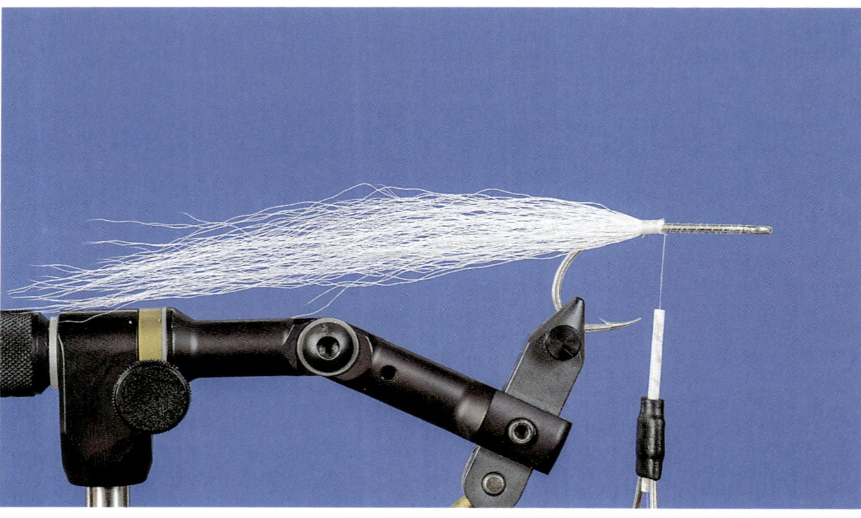

2. Select long, soft bucktail fibers from around the center portion of the tail and remove the shortest fibers. Cut the butts even so that in the next step you will be able to tie the next clump on top of the previous one. After you tie down the bucktail, distribute it 360 degrees around the hook shank as shown. Every time you tie in a bunch of bucktail, apply head cement to the butts before wrapping over them. Use your bodkin to free any fibers caught around the hook bend.

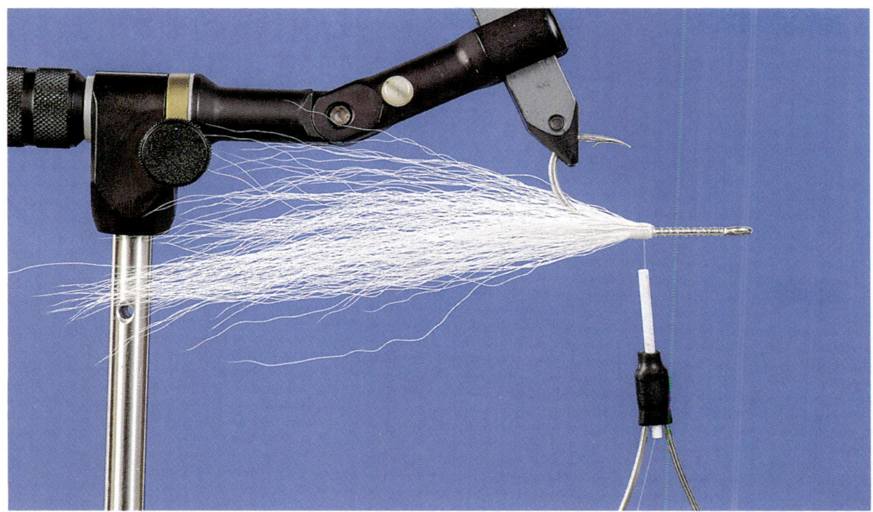

3. Turn the hook over, and tie in a slightly shorter length of bucktail that is also a little sparser than the previous clump to begin a taper at the belly. Here, I slightly shifted the fibers in my fingertips to increase the taper. Make sure the thread wraps are on top of the platform created by the tie-down area of the first clump. Do not distribute these fibers around the shank; instead, tie them down only on the underside of the hook shank.

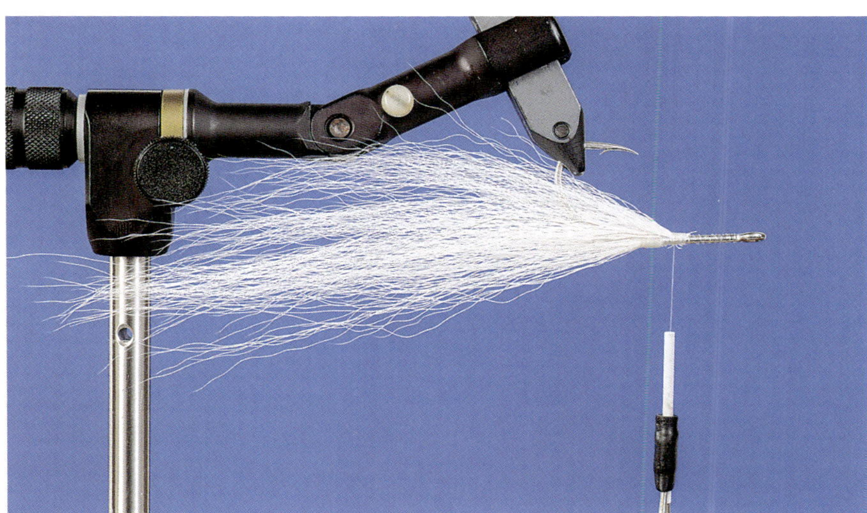

4. Wrap the thread forward (note the space between this tie and the previous one) and repeat the previous step to continue the taper of the belly. Be sure to keep the fibers on the underside of the hook shank. You want an approximately 45-degree angle, so be mindful of the space between the steps. If the bucktail butts up against the previous tie, you will have a steeper angle, which is undesirable. You should notice a taper developing on the underside by this time.

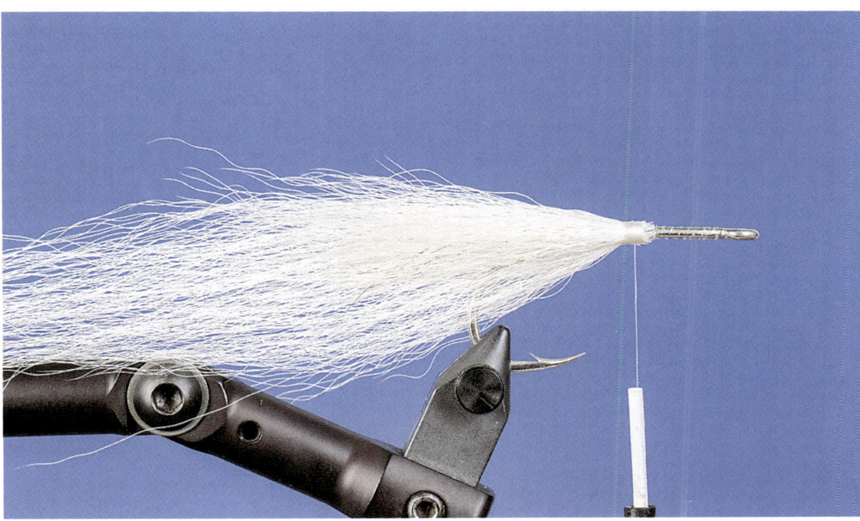

5. Turn the hook over, and make sure the thread is directly above the beginning of the previous step. Tie in short bucktail clumps that extend past the bend of the hook (half the length of the fly to this point) on each side to create width and fullness in the shoulder area.

(continued)

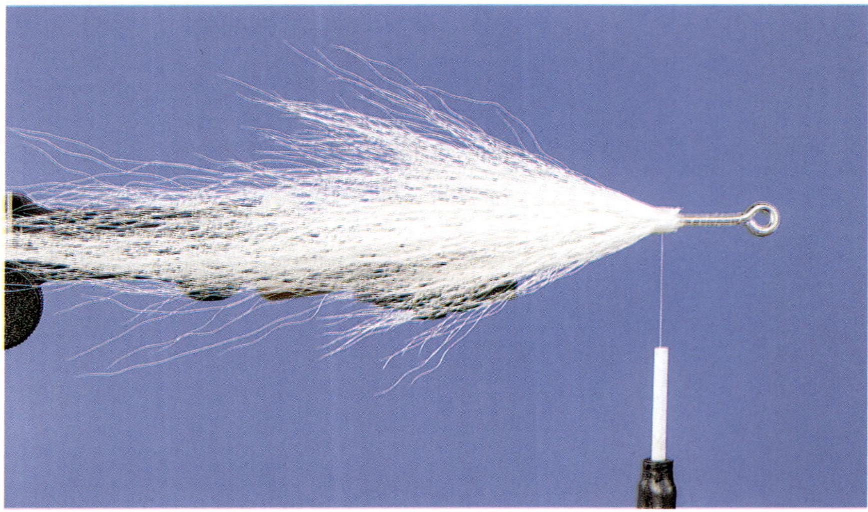

6. The top view here helps illustrate the tie-in point. Note the V that shows how the fibers are tied only on each side, not on the bottom or top. This thickness was lacking in flies that I tied before the 3D.

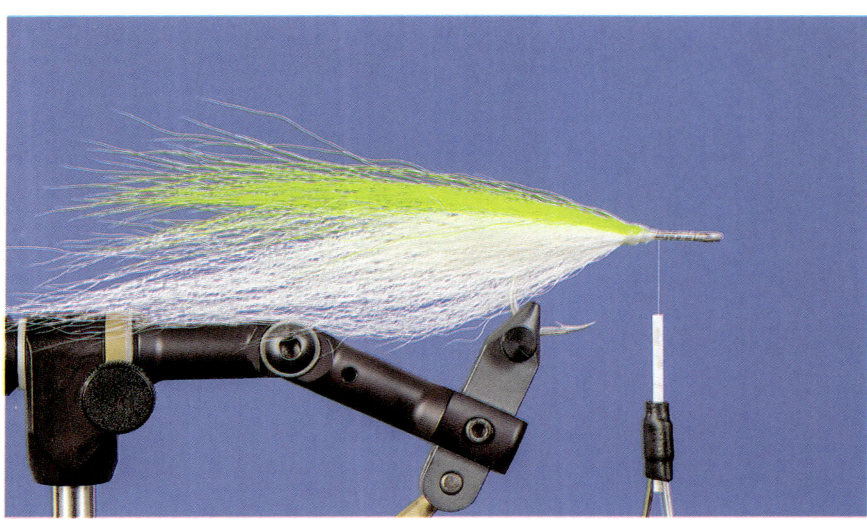

7. Tie down the top color of bucktail (chartreuse here) so that the butts align with the butts of the fibers that you used for the shoulders. When you select bucktail for the top color, choose fibers with similar characteristics to the previous fibers so that they blend well together and make the fly easier to tie. The fibers on top should be slightly shorter than the overall length of the fly. Create a smooth taper with the mono thread to the next tie-in point.

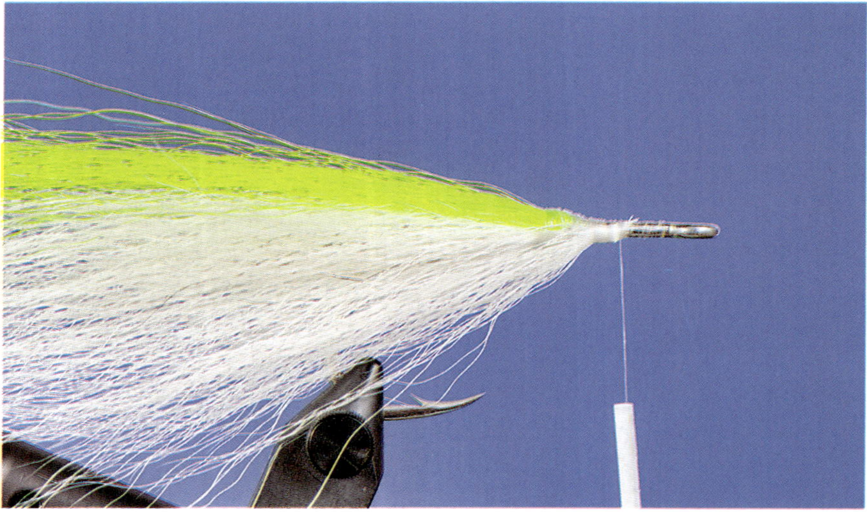

8. You can keep the hook upright or flip it over to tie in the next underbody section. Use half the amount of fibers that you used for the wing on top. Keep them directly below the shank, and don't allow them to roll up on the sides. If you overdress the underside, the fly may not hold its keel.

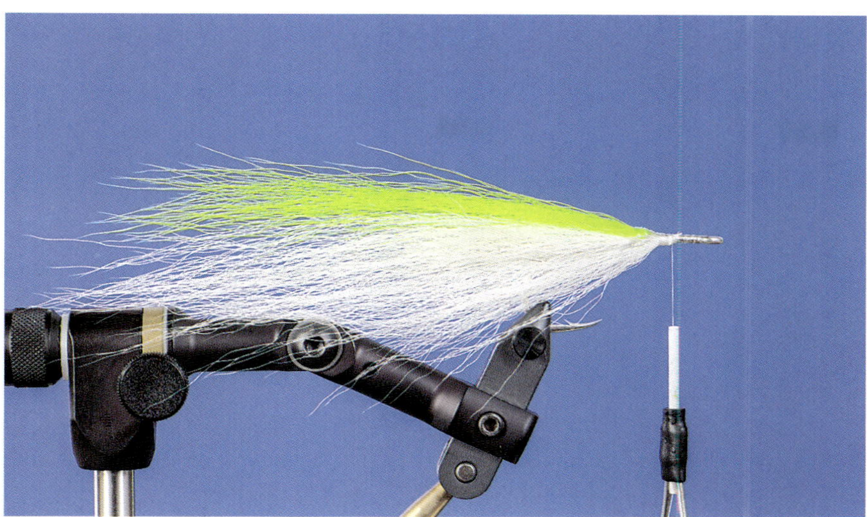

9. Note how the shape is developing underneath the fly. Since we are tying on a longer-shank hook, we have enough space to finish sculpting the taper.

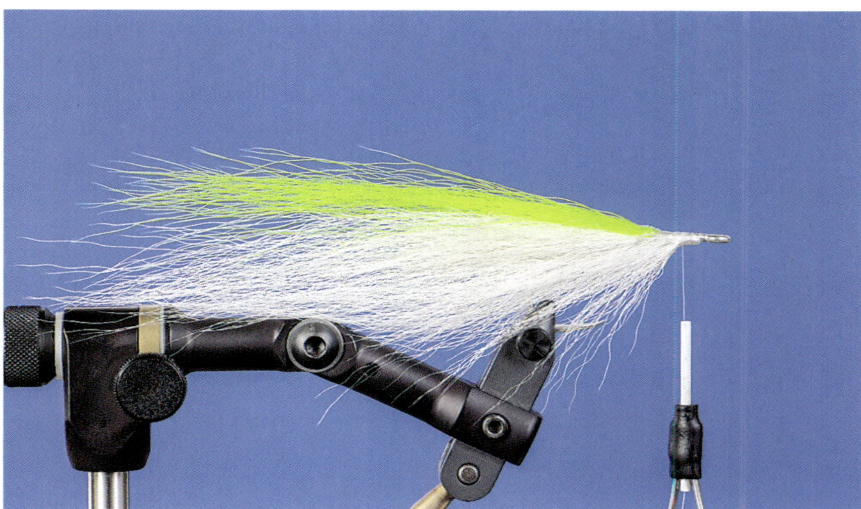

10. Tie in another section of bucktail on the underside. Use shorter fibers and flare them with thread pressure to create the belly.

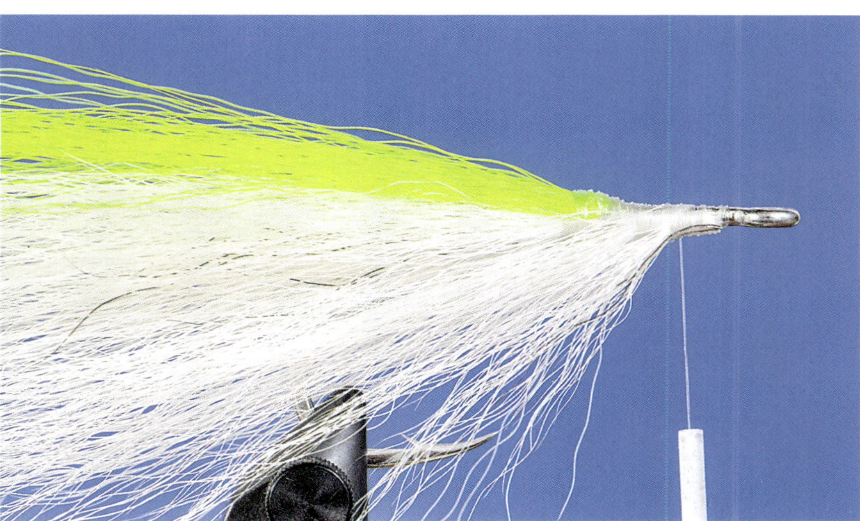

11. Remember to cut the butts straight so that you can work on top of the previous tie-in and to save space. When you flare the hair, the flat platform also ensures consistency and helps you control the angle—as if you are tying on a straight shank. This is critical. The thread is in the position to accept the cheeks.

(continued)

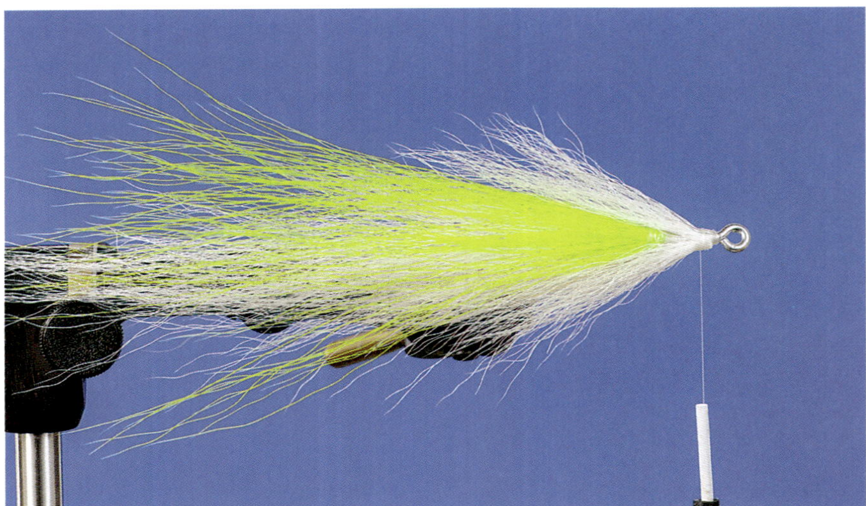

12. Make two more short ties on just the sides. Tie the inside bunch to the shank first, then attach another clump on the far side. Wrap over the butts of both, but not back so far so that they start to squeeze together.

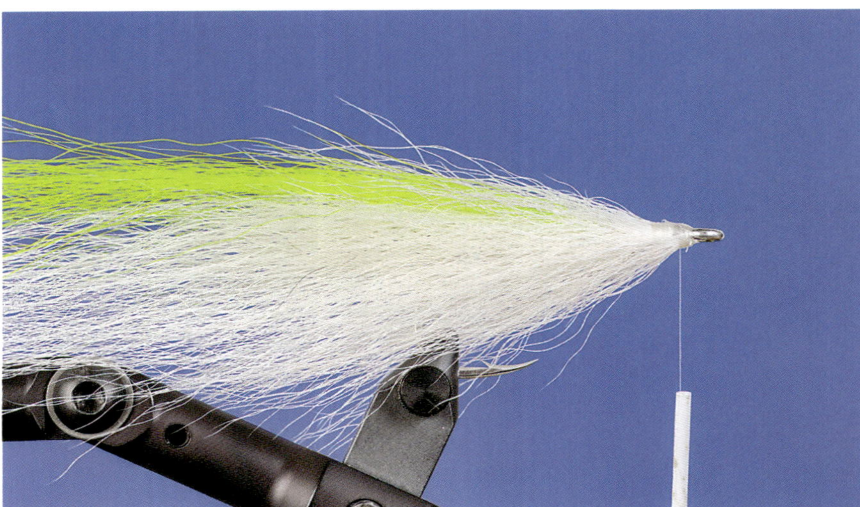

13. Tie in another bunch of bucktail fibers underneath the shank to complete the belly. At this point you want the thread close to the eye to prepare for the last bunch of fibers that you will tie in on top. Using a sparse amount of fibers here makes it easier to create a nice head on the fly.

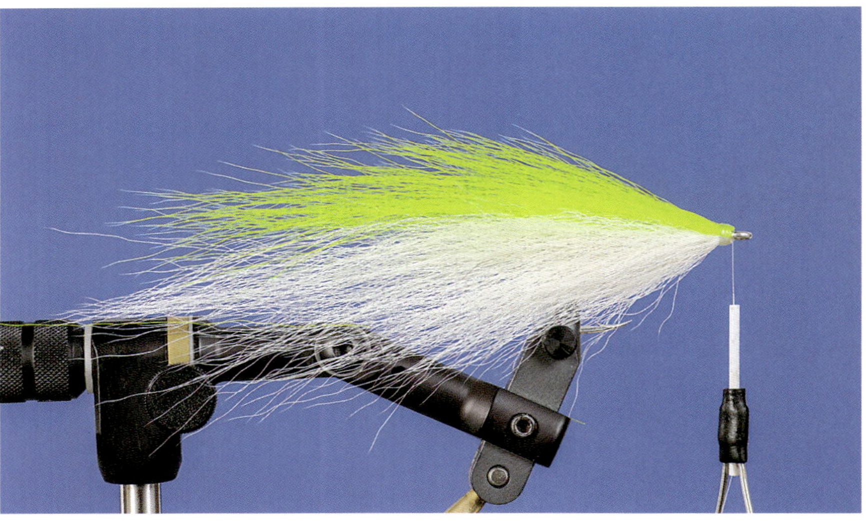

14. Add a short and somewhat heavy tie of bucktail. The bulk helps keel the fly, and also covers all the tie-in points on the underside. Once I select my bunch, I slide the butts with my fingertips about an inch to create uneven and tapered hairs. After tying the fibers in, I distribute them around the top half of the hook shank to fill in holes from tie-in areas on the underside.

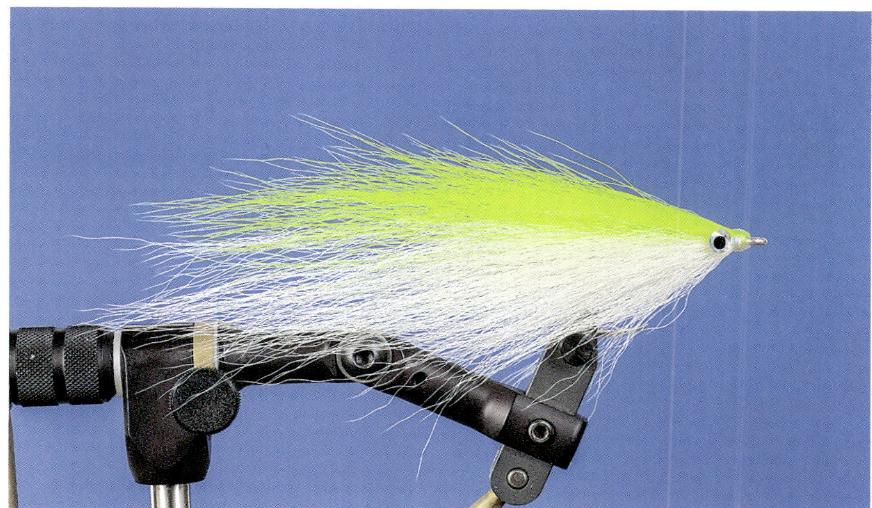

15. Select and tie on tab eyes if you like. They are completely optional. Whip-finish and trim the thread.

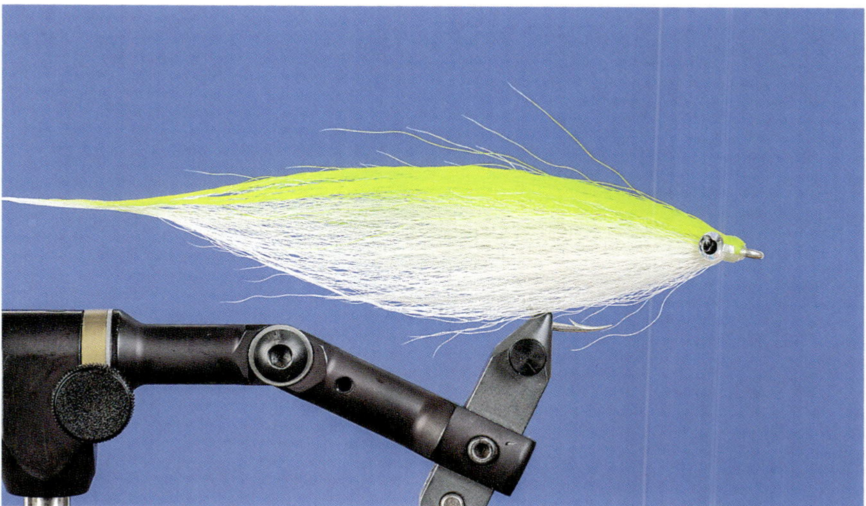

16. Wetting the fly will help take out the static and help the fibers assume their natural shape.

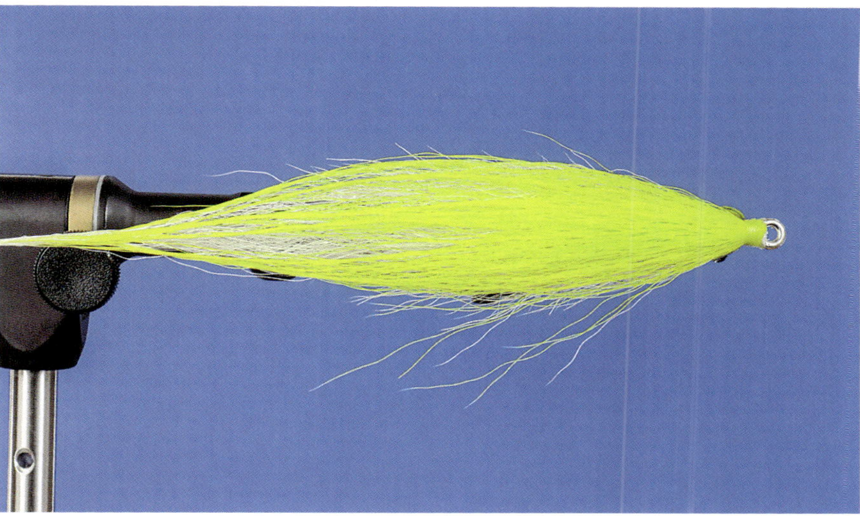

17. When you look at the fly from the top, notice the taper. The 3D is designed to look like a baitfish from every angle.

(continued)

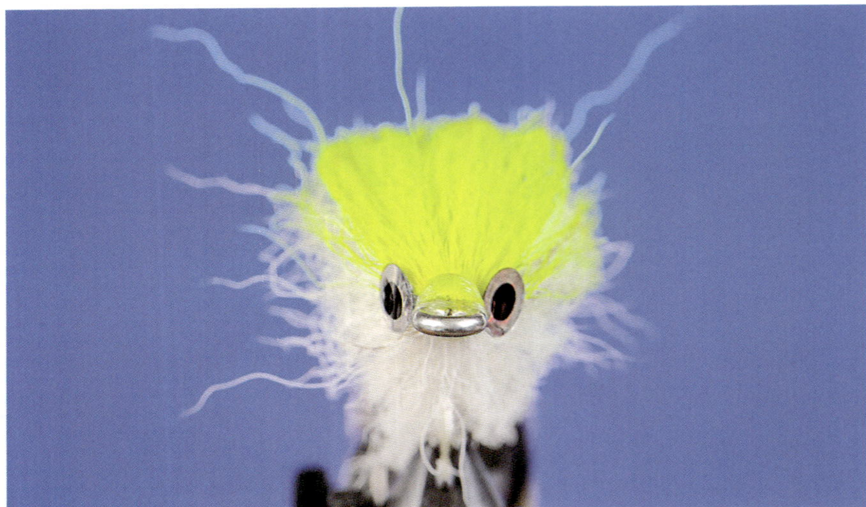

18. Notice from the front view the V-shaped, almost triangular, taper and how the finished fly has shoulders on the top that narrow in the belly. There are differences in the shape from every angle.

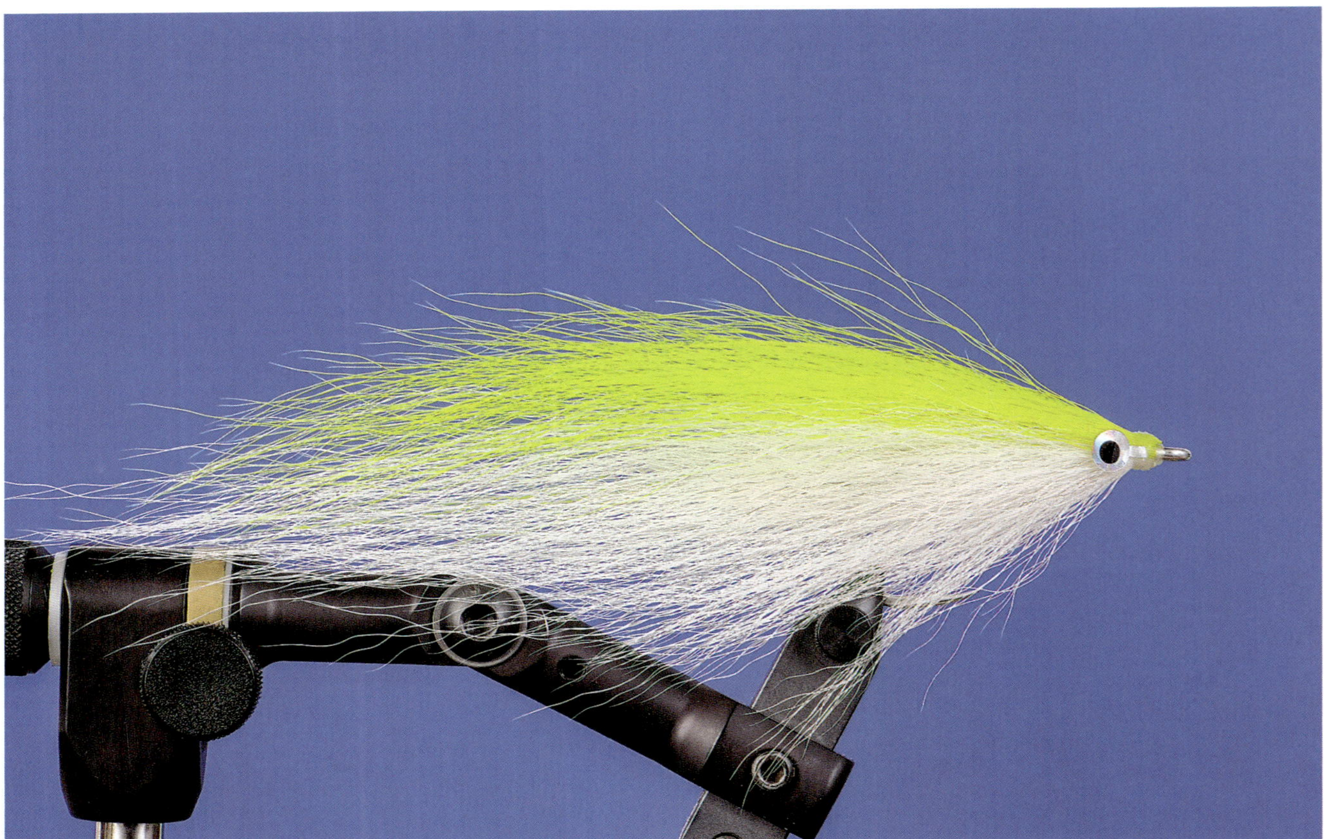

After the 3D Fleye has been wet and dried, it really starts to take shape.

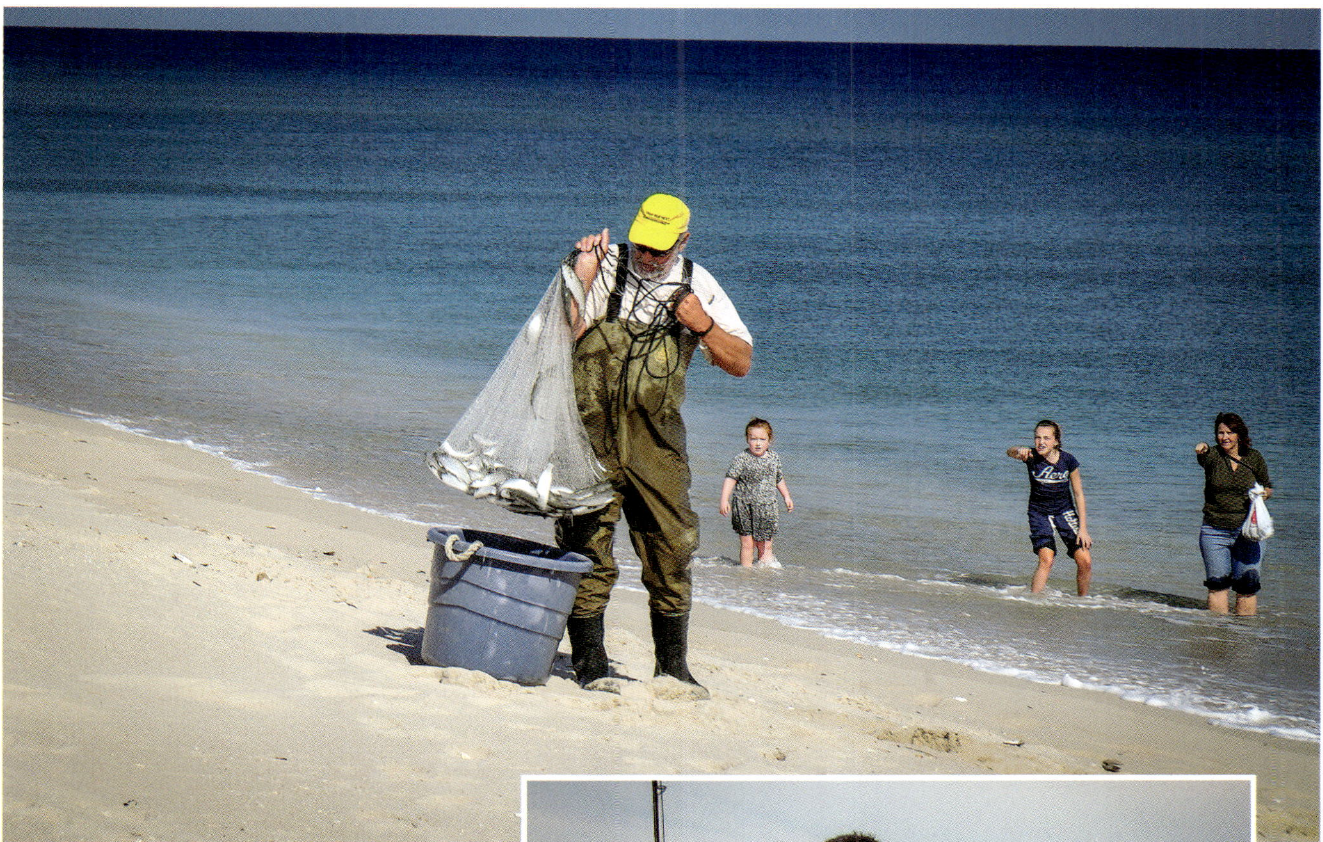

Capturing bait and feeling them in my hands has helped my fly design immensely. When you pick up a bait and put it in your hand, you feel the subtlest curves that will give you a much better idea of what you are trying to depict with your flies. Above, Lance Erwin gets ready to unload his haul of mullet as beachgoers look on.

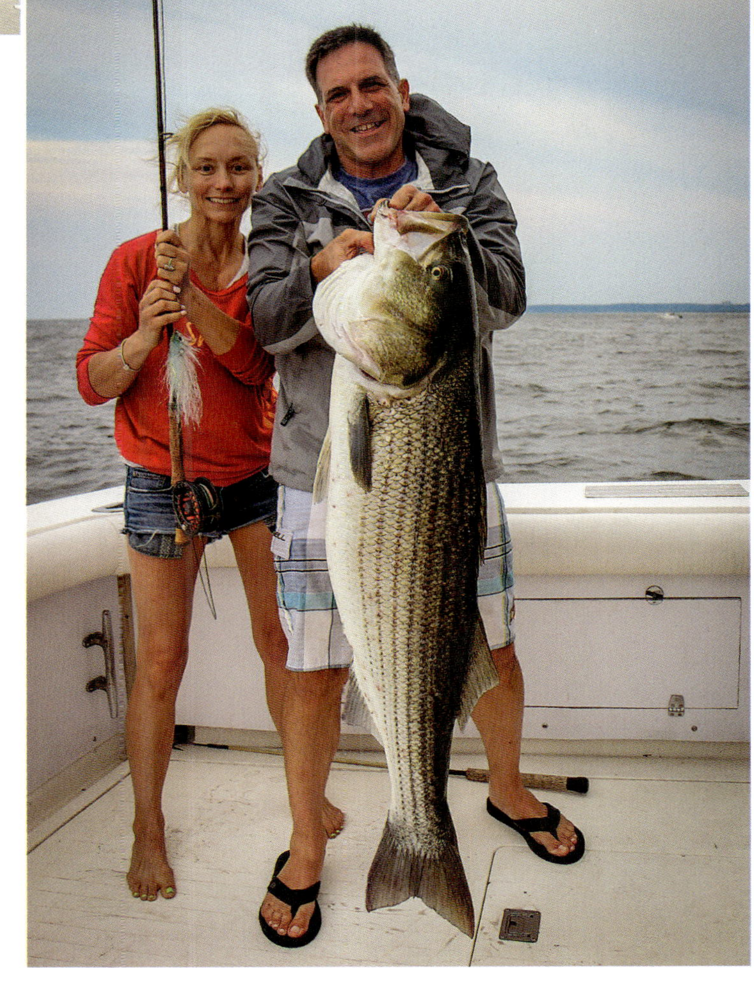

Right: Joe Mustari and Suzie Murphy with a striper estimated between 45 and 50 pounds (fish was released) caught on an 8-inch blue-and-white 3D Fleye on July 3, 2015. JOE MUSTARI

Chapter 7

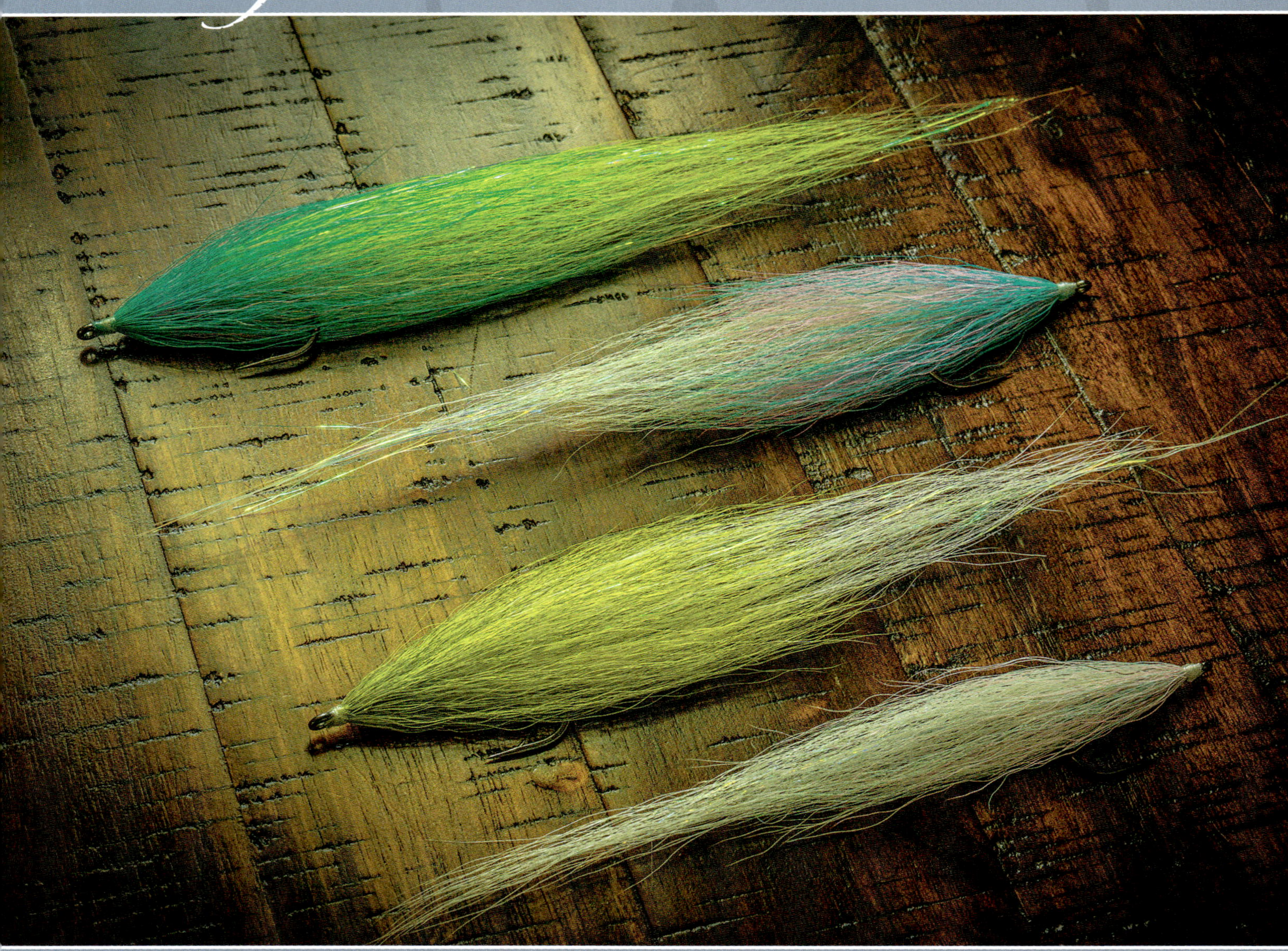

Various Bucktail Deceivers with subtly blended fibers.

Bucktail Deceiver

The Bucktail Deceiver, in its purest form, is tied only with bucktail, unlike the Lefty's Deceiver, which traditionally uses schlappen feathers for the tail. Formed from multiple ties of bucktail, often as many as eight, distributed around the hook shank to create the wing and collar, the Bucktail Deceiver's enticing movement in the water is the result of both the broad head and numerous tips of bucktail. You control the taper with each tie of bucktail, and by tying in progressively shorter lengths of fibers at each step, you expose more tips to the water, which in turn increases motion. The end result is a beautifully tapered fly that resembles many baitfish, imparts realistic movement, and has a lifelike shape. With its natural taper and silhouette, it captures the look of most saltwater baits, big or small, anywhere in the world.

Like the 3D, the Bucktail Deceiver began as a synthetic fly, tied with Kinky Fibre. I vividly recall tying them on the car ride up to Cape Cod. While Ed Jaworowski drove, I would lash the Kinky Fibre, bunch by bunch, to the shank (which I held in my hand), and then I would trim them into a brown paper bag on the floor. The flies were fast to tie because I wasn't concerned about shape while tying them—I would take care of that later. At the time, I was a huge fan of this technique because it was a fast, efficient way to get a realistic, beautiful shape with synthetics.

I always considered tying these flies with bucktail but was reluctant because I knew how labor-intensive it would be. Each tie would have to be precise to build the taper—I'd have to build the fly by adding materials, not taking material away. But, I eventually caved and tied one with bucktail anyway. Since then, I don't believe I ever made another synthetic one, not only because the results were so beautiful and organic, but also because they were extremely fun and satisfying to tie.

One of the synthetic version's greatest assets was that it was fast to tie, but I eventually streamlined the process with natural materials as well by tying in the fibers all at once and distributing them with my fingers, rather than the conventional way of tying a Lefty's Deceiver collar, which requires multiple ties of bucktail. Doing it all in one shot cut the amount of steps by half and made the design very practical.

In the water, the Bucktail Deceiver moved like no other fly that I had seen before. It looked like it was plugged into an electrical socket—everything turned on. Every little pulse of current or twitch of the rod made the fly move and pulse seductively. Currents moved around the collar and wiggled the tail side to side, just like a natural bait where the first two-thirds of the body is fairly stationary yet the last third moves. Yet even in the front of the fly, the tips never seemed to stop moving. I quickly learned that one of the keys to retrieving this fly was to let it breathe. Take your time on the retrieve and allow the water to move in and out and all around the bucktail tips. If you opt for a quicker retrieve, watch how the rear portion moves like a fish's tail as it swims through the water. At the end of your retrieve, you can shake your rod

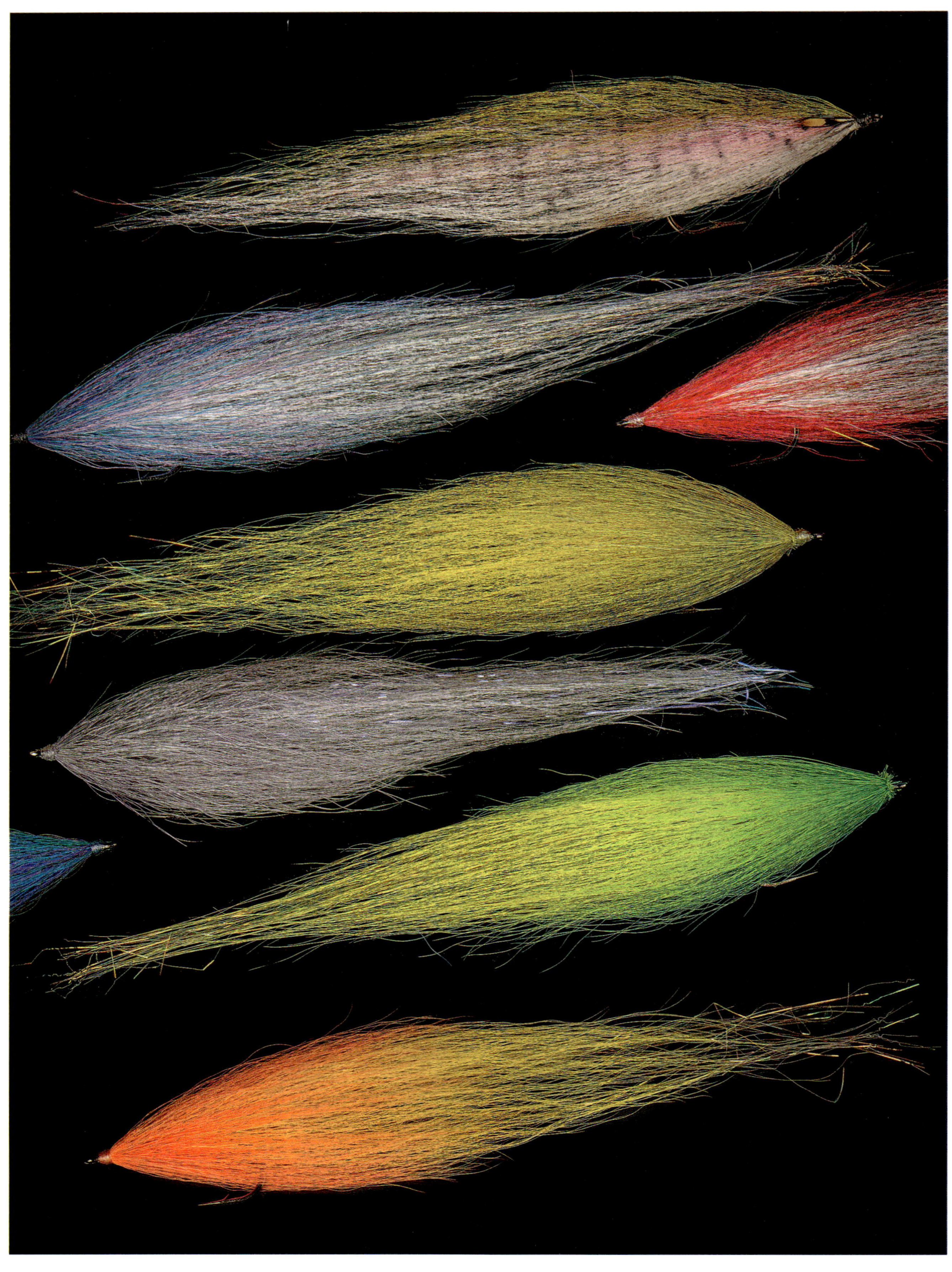

tip before bringing the fly out of the water to send movement down the line into the fibers. The fly goes wild.

Evolution of Design: Bucktail Deceiver Shapes

Like many of my fleyes, the Bucktail Deceiver is basically a template, a blank slate, that you can adorn as you please. Colors can, and do, run the gamut, and they are so influenced by local favorites that I am hesitant to give color recommendations. You can add flash, feathers, synthetics, eyes, and other elements to the basic design as you wish, but always maintain the general shape, the many tips that move, and the slightly bulkier collar that moves the sparser wing. These are fundamental design considerations that, when adhered to, create a fly that can go anywhere and catch fish!

More important than color and flash and other adornments, in my opinion, is how the bucktail is tied to the shank to influence fishing considerations such as profile and sink rate. The design of the Bucktail Deceiver has evolved over the years to suit various tying and fishing demands. The standard tie with fibers distributed evenly around the shank, 360 degrees, has a fairly universal three-dimensional profile that represents many common baits such as squids, mackerel, and mullet. We first showed that version in *Pop Fleyes*.

By squeezing the fibers from the side, you can add height and create imitations for taller, narrower baitfish such as bunker or herring. After tying in the fibers and distributing them 360 degrees around the shank, relax pressure on the thread, and squeeze the fibers from each side to force them above and below the shank. The loose fibers will always move away from finger pressure. Once the fibers are in the position that you like, tighten the thread. You can continue to relax the thread, reposition the fibers, and tighten them until you get the exact shape that you desire.

Instead of applying pressure from the side to get a high, thin profile, you can squeeze the top and bottom of the shank to flare the fibers horizontally and create "pontoons" on the sides. The end result will sink slowly and give a wide, realistic silhouette when a predatory fish views it from below and from the rear, which is how most fish see their prey before they eat. The technique for the flattened version is one of my personal favorites, especially for night fishing, where the "slow" motion of the fly through the retrieve is deadly for bass.

Another consideration when tying Bucktail Deceivers for night fishing is to make them as foul-proof as possible, because you can't see if the fly is fouled when it is in the water, and you don't want to be turning on your headlamp and checking it all the time. To create a foul-proof fly, I will use really short fibers for the collar, and choose fibers from the base of the tail, which not only flare more to achieve bulk and reduce fouling but also help hold the fly higher in the water.

A subtle variation is the triangular shape, which is flat on top with a V-shaped bottom. When you tie in clumps of bucktail, form a triangle with your fingers as you tighten the thread. Like the flattened method, this is another special-purpose shape for night fishing or for whenever I want a fly that sinks slower than the standard Bucktail Deceiver.

You can also combine these shapes, or variations of these shapes, into one fly. For instance, I sometimes combine the shapes for mullet, which have a flatter top section in the head and then a deeper belly. I also can use this shaping idea for shoulders around the hook bend and a narrower height and width in the front around the hook eye. Many baits are thicker in the middle of their bodies but get narrower in front.

Variations

In this chapter we are going to tie the standard Bucktail Deceiver and four variations that highlight or emphasize different techniques. The basic Bucktail Deceiver can serve as a blank canvas for your own designs. Make it your own, but consider the design concepts that are fundamental to the fly for the best fishing results.

The first variation is the squid, which is a simple Bucktail Deceiver that has a stick-on eye attached to a monofilament extension. The second and third variations illustrate narrow and wide profiles, respectively. The last variation is tied on a mono extension to create an extra-long Bucktail Deceiver. In this sequence we set up two vises to hold the monofilament, which is especially effective for thinner-diameter monofilament. The addition of a Banger head creates even more movement and commotion when the pattern is retrieved, and it is an excellent pattern for the fall mullet runs or whenever there are schools of large bait on the surface.

Previous page: The Bucktail Deceiver (BTD) can mimic a number of larger baits, including mullet, mackerel, bunker, herring, and squid. It is my go-to fly in the fall when larger baits are present. The BTD is quick and easy to tie; has a beautiful, natural taper; and the many tips of bucktail create an electric action in the water.

Fleye Shapes

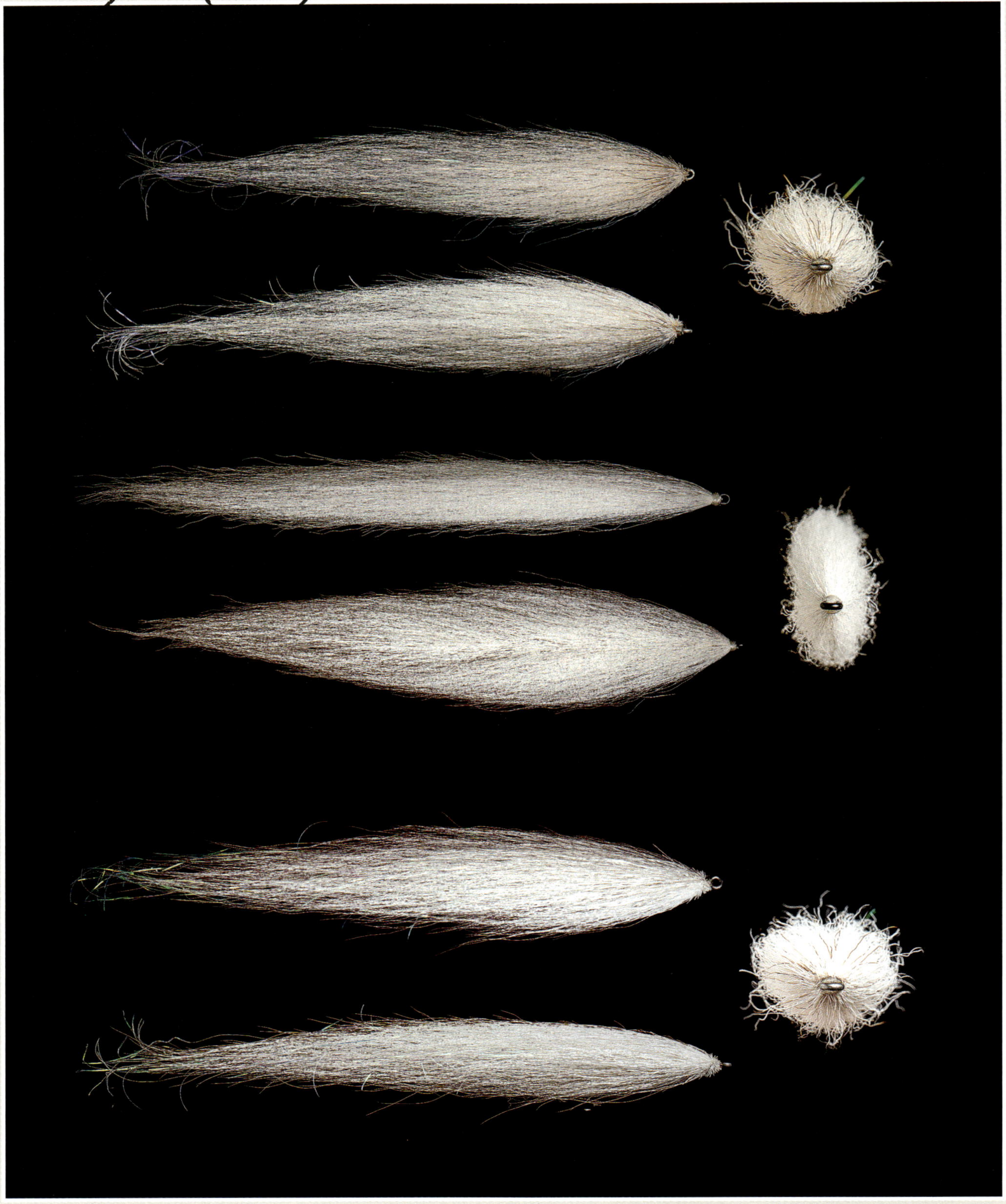

This composite image shows the front, side, and top views of the fundamental BTD shapes: round, narrow, and triangular.

Bucktail Deceiver

Hook:	#4/0 Tiemco 911S or similar long-shank saltwater
Thread:	Fine monofilament
Body:	Yellow bucktail
Collar:	Orange bucktail

TYING THE BUCKTAIL DECEIVER

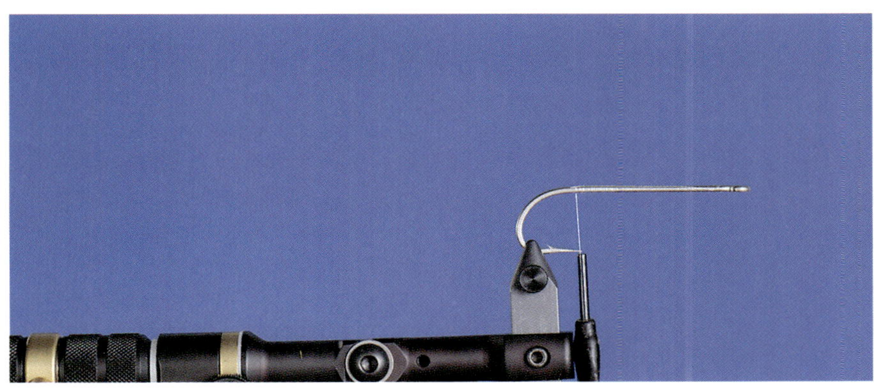

1. Insert the hook into the vise. Wrap monofilament thread over the entire hook shank, and bring the thread back to the bend. The #4/0 Tiemco 911S has ample space on the shank for the number of ties necessary to create the right taper. Coat the thread with head cement.

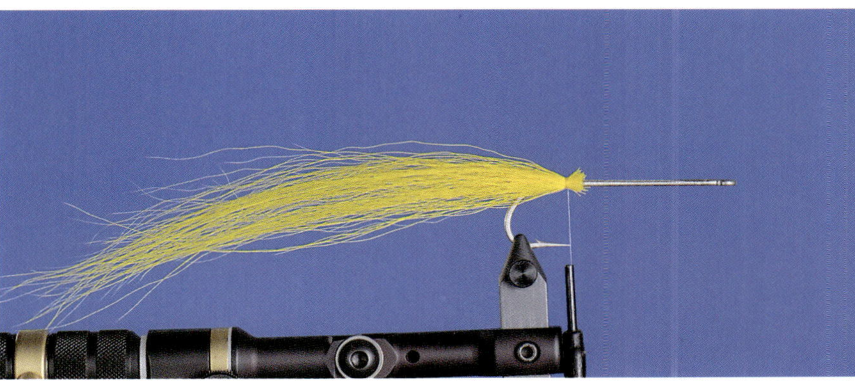

2. Select a sparse amount of bucktail and remove most of the short hairs. Clip the butts evenly and tie them in. The first tie of bucktail establishes the length, so you will need to select your longest fibers, but these are also the fibers that flare the most. Choosing a sparse amount and removing most of the shorter hairs allows you to manage them better. Refer to the steps on page 35 in the Techniques section for more detail on the method to distribute the fibers around the shank.

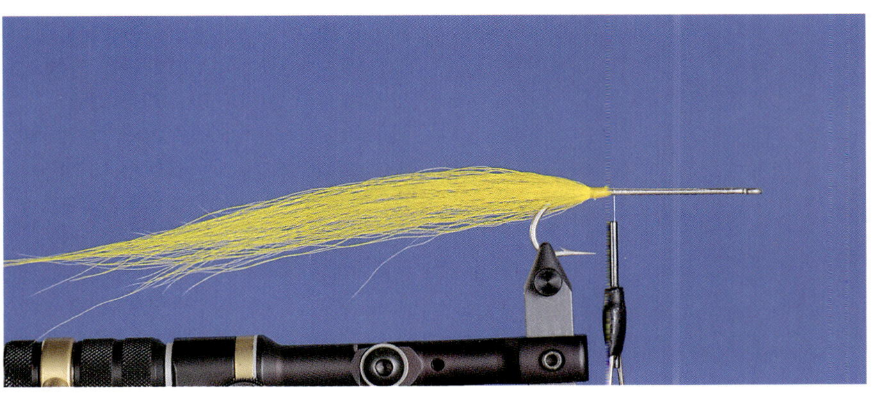

3. Before wrapping over the butts with the thread, coat them with head cement. Though I won't mention it every time, it is important to do this every time. Wrap to a point just in front of the tie-down area. At this time, I will often use a bodkin to make sure the fibers are straight and distributed around the shank, over the bend of the hook.

(continued)

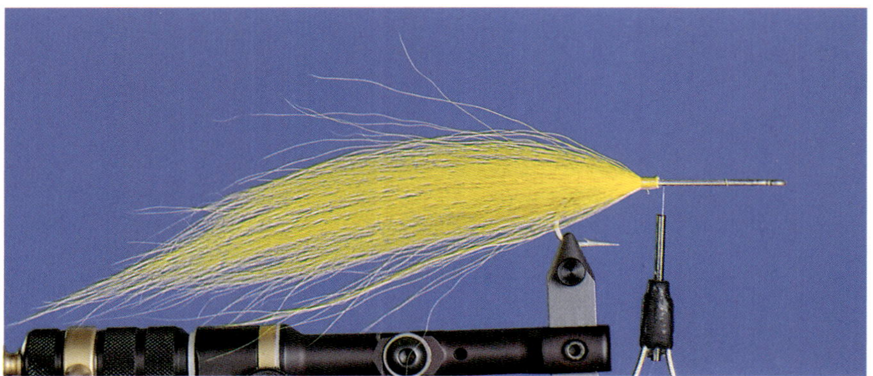

4. Tie in another clump with the same amount of fibers as the first, but make sure they are about 1/2 inch shorter than the previous step. Hairs of the same length that are spread apart evenly will ultimately create taper, but sometimes you'll have to trim the butts a bit as well, depending on how you visualize the taper. The taper should be gradual. Do not make it look like a staircase. Add head cement and tie down.

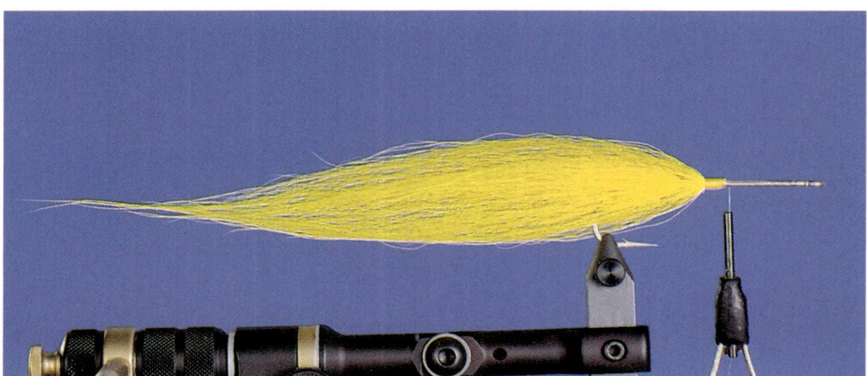

5. Here, I have moistened the fibers to get a better idea of form. I will do this frequently while tying to get a better idea of how the fly is progressing. Moving forward along the hook shank, tie in another clump of bucktail. Consider that you are advancing your thread approximately 1/4 inch each time. Because of this, you can use the same length fiber for each step, and it would be 1/4 inch shorter than the previous tie-in.

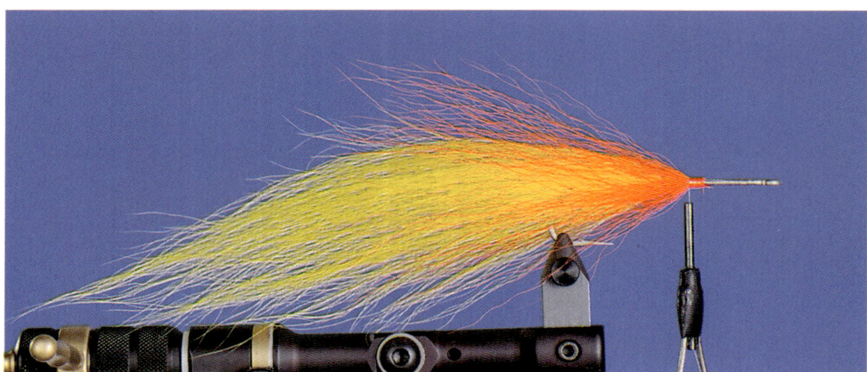

6. This is the point at which I would most often change color, if I wanted a two-toned fly. For the collar I like shorter and slightly wavier fibers to add more bulk.

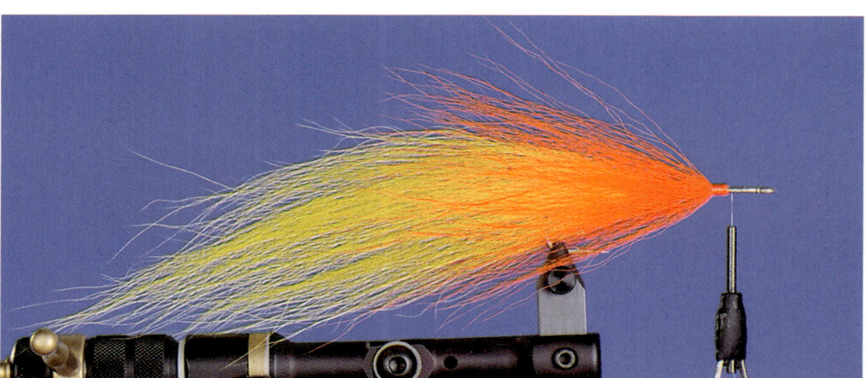

7. For the next tie, choose wavier fibers again to increase the bulk in the forward portion of the fly. This clump is more or less the same length as the previous one, perhaps a bit shorter. This is subtle, but I think worth mentioning. Sometimes when I get into the collar area, I want more height and bulk, which is achieved by using two sections the same length, spaced more closely together. Here, I am tying a little bit by the seat of my pants, based on my assessment of the material. Apply head cement and tie down the butts.

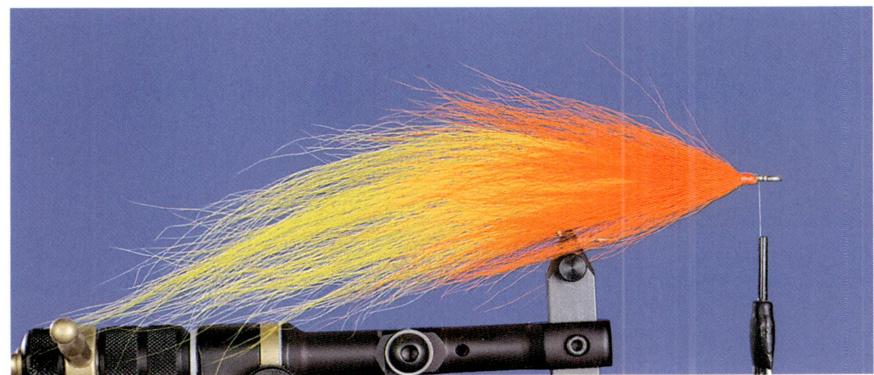

8. Tie down another clump of bucktail fibers. The increased bulk in the head (more fibers in each clump and closer spacing of the ties) will cause the fly to move more in the back end.

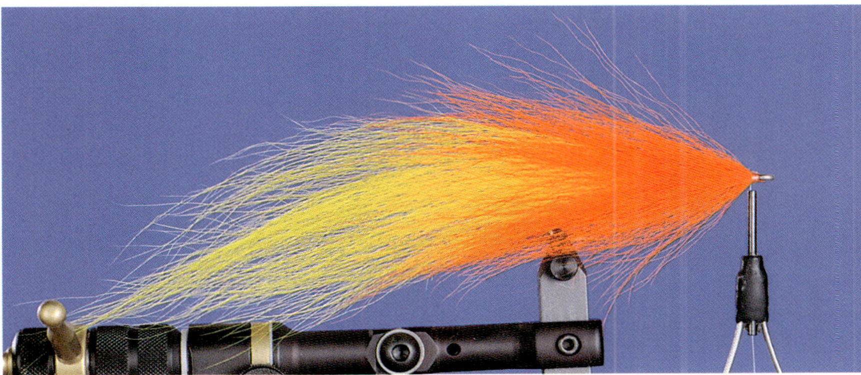

9. Apply the last bunch just at the hook eye. I like a short head, and the only way that you can get that is to clip the butt ends of the bucktail square before tying in the bunch. Sometimes when I am close to the hook eye, I will take the longest and shortest fibers out of the bundle so that I have a more consistently tapered bunch of fibers.

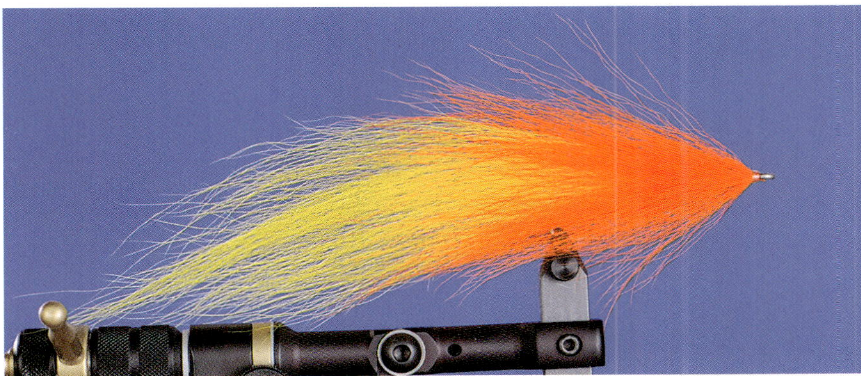

10. The finished Bucktail Deceiver.

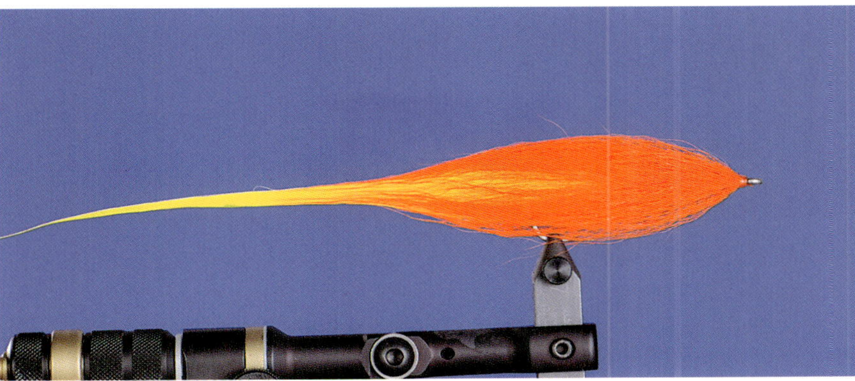

11. Completely wet the fly and let it dry.

(continued)

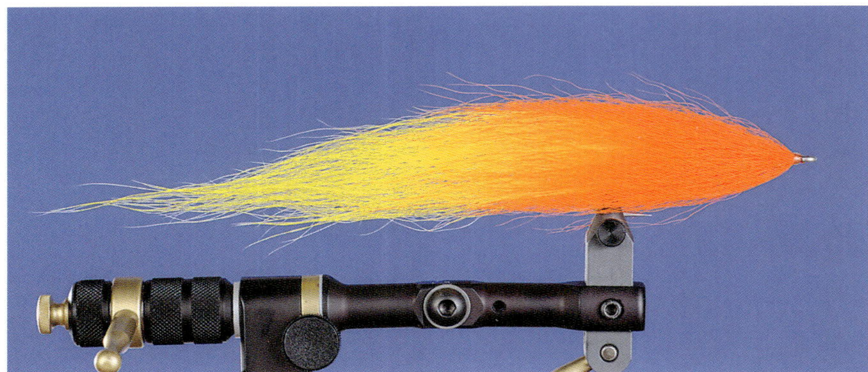

12. The Bucktail Deceiver template is extremely versatile and can be modified to create everything from superb flies for freshwater trout and bass to offshore species (with the addition of a Banger head). The shorter fibers in the front help create more turbulence in the water. The water pushing over and around the head and will tickle the sparser fibers in the wing, bringing the fly to life. The many exposed tips continually pulse in the water.

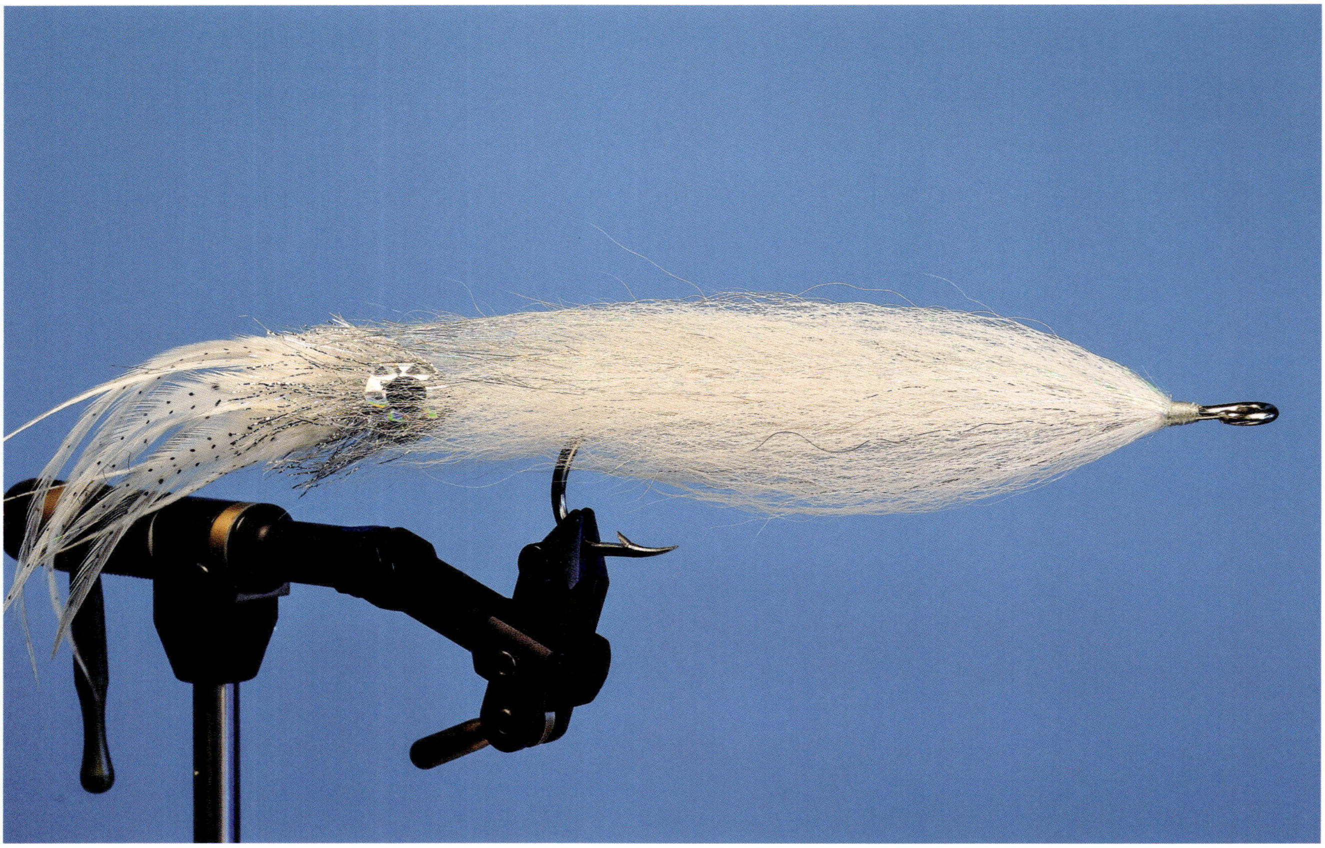

Achieving taper is sometimes complex, especially when a single fly has a combination of narrow, wide, flat, and full shapes such as this squid fleye, which incorporates both BTD and Hollow techniques to get the job done. Notice how the deep front tapers subtly to a narrow rear section; the top of the fleye is flat. Head and tentacles are tied on a mono extension with very short saddles, speckled with a marker.

Casting

You cannot buy a good cast or a mend or a soft, accurate presentation in the fly shop. To cast a fly with a fly line toward a target is the biggest part of fly fishing to me. Catching fish is the successful end to the game, but I often get satisfaction even without the catching.

Anyone can cast well. It simply takes time and practice. This learning is the most exciting and rewarding time in the evolution of a fly fisherman. Learn to cast well first before you find excuses about why you do not need to cast well. Distance is only one indicator of casting proficiency, and casting well is much more than that. It is dealing with a wide variety of conditions that often accompany fly fishing, fresh or salt. Wind, currents, waves, and obstructions are only some of the challenging obstacles we meet, and we need delicacy, finesse, endurance, efficiency, and the right flies to overcome those obstacles.

At times, fish will be blitzing at your feet or knocking at the side of the boat. However, there are more times that are difficult to handle, and only the better casters will be successful in these conditions. Open beaches have their own set of dynamics to throw at the fly fisherman such as wind, waves, outer bars, and upward-sloping beaches. These challenges favor good casters. If you can only cast 60 feet in optimum conditions, you will quickly be frustrated by windy days or distant edges or bigger flies. The better caster you are, the more conditions you will be able to endure, and as many surf fishermen know, the best days are often the nasty days.

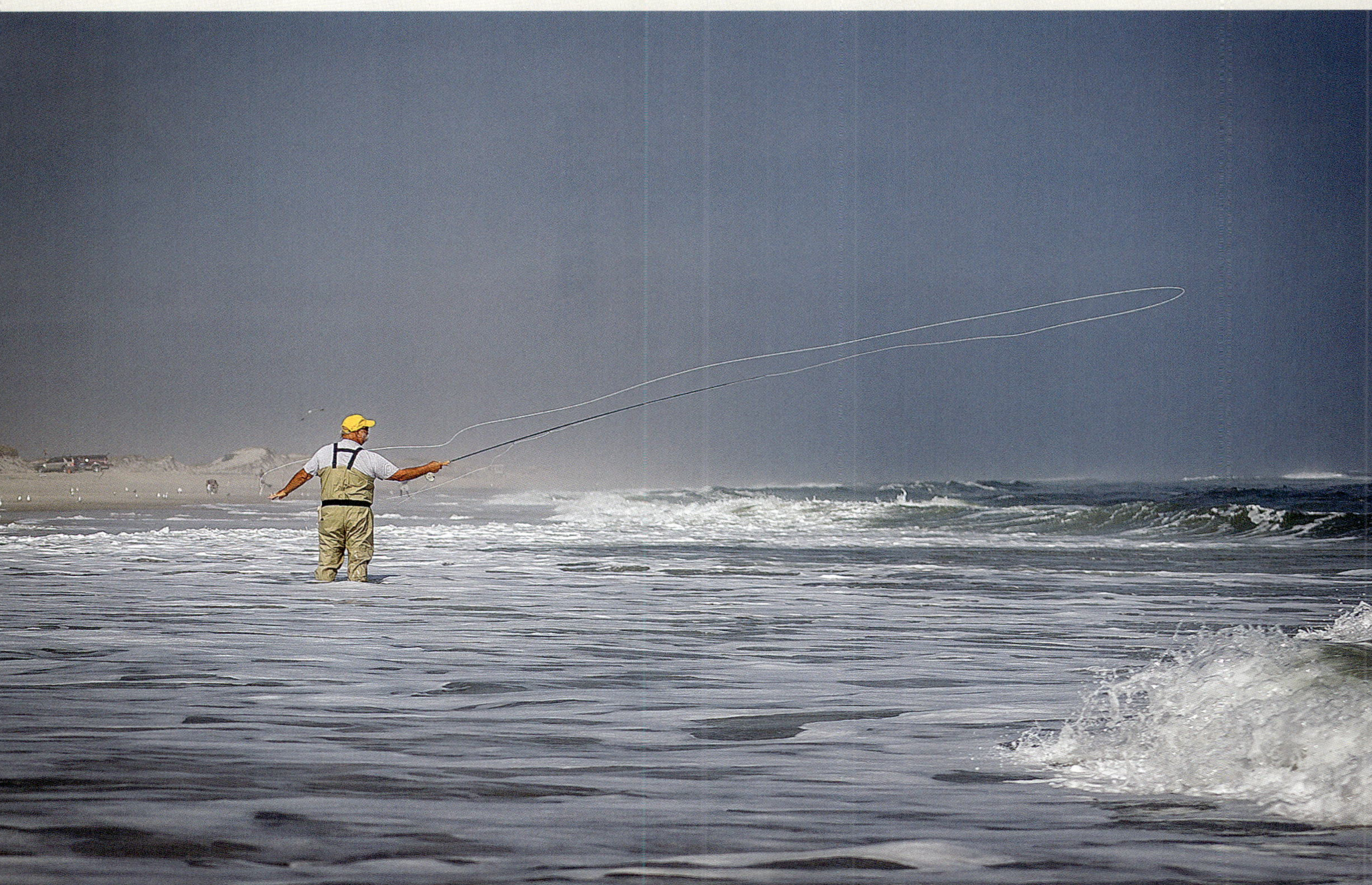

Presentation is a priority in my design process. A well-designed fly is durable, has good action, and can be cast with a fly rod. I continually try to refine and improve my patterns to make them perform better in the water. TOM LYNCH

Bucktail Deceiver Squid

Hook: #4/0 Tiemco 911S or similar long-shank saltwater
Thread: Fine monofilament
Eyes: Prism stick-on (large) attached to 30-pound-test mono straight
Body: Orange and pink bucktail

TYING THE BUCKTAIL DECEIVER SQUID

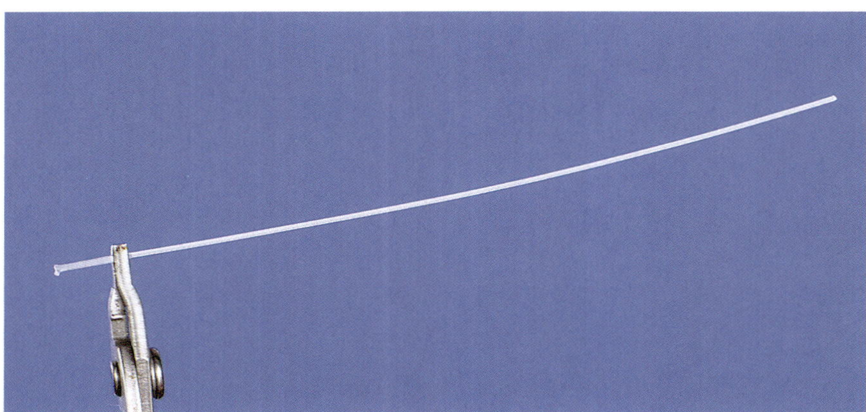

1. For this pattern we use straight, stiff, 30-pound-test monofilament to hold and properly position the stick-on eyes. Squeeze the mono with flat pliers so that you have a base on which to stick the eyes. The eyes have adhesive backs, but you can also add glue as an optional step.

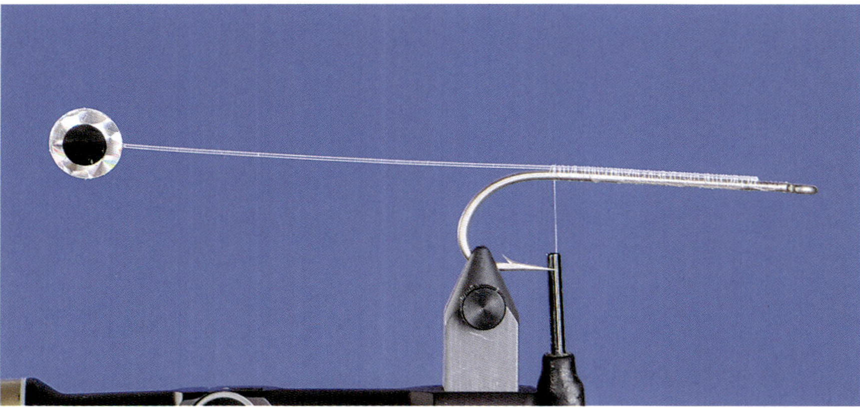

2. Cover the entire hook shank with monofilament thread, and tie the monofilament extension down at the hook bend, covering it with your thread and then coating it with cement.

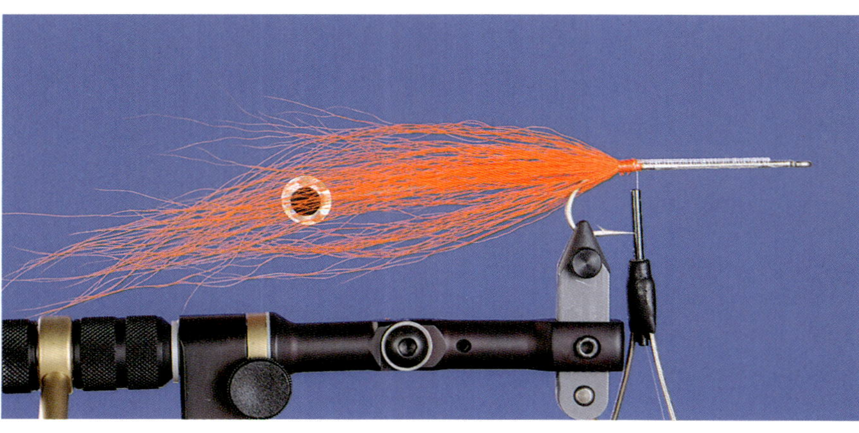

3. The first tie of bucktail is the same as with the Bucktail Deceiver. In addition to making sure that the fibers are completely distributed around the shank, you should make sure that they extend well past the eye. Apply glue to the butts and wrap over them with thread.

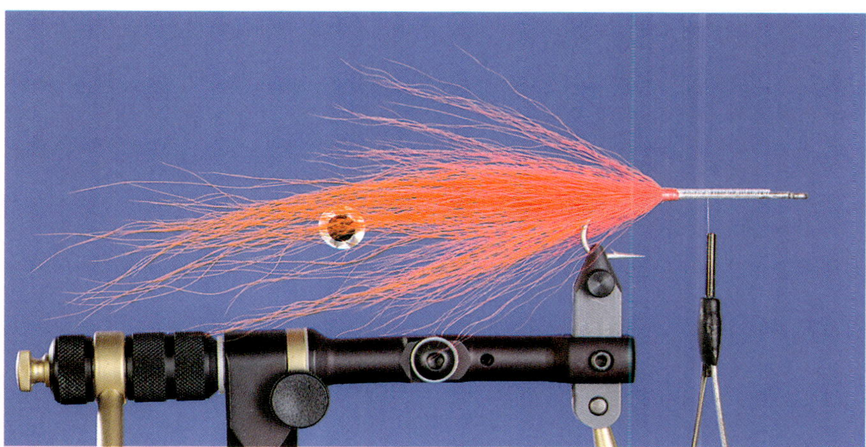

4. Continue tying in bunches of bucktail to complete the shape. The steps are exactly the same as with the Bucktail Deceiver. Remember, you are imitating a squid. Try to "see" the squid on the vise and fill the imagined outline with bucktail.

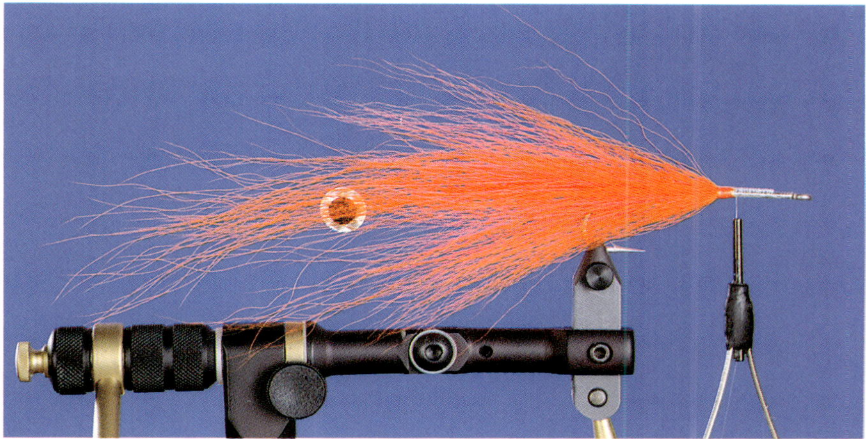

5. The mantle, head, and tentacles should join one another smoothly in a flowing sculpture. Do not leave any "steps."

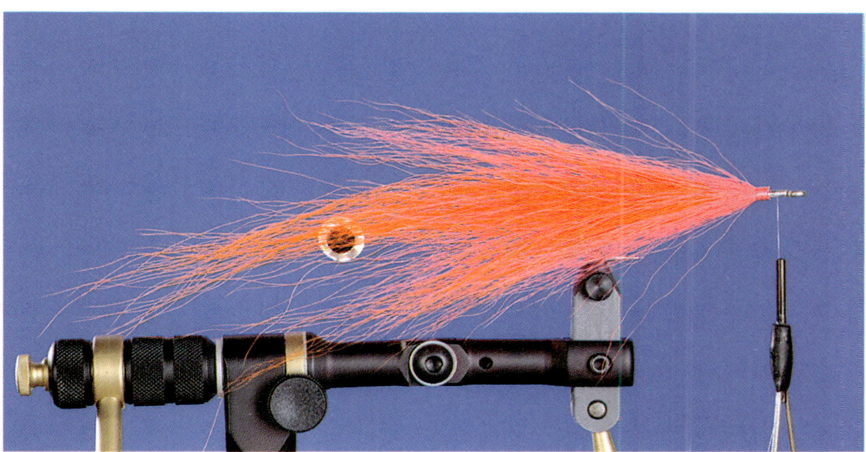

6. Once all ties are completed, you'll be able to see all the ends that will deliver great action from the front to the rear of the design.

(continued)

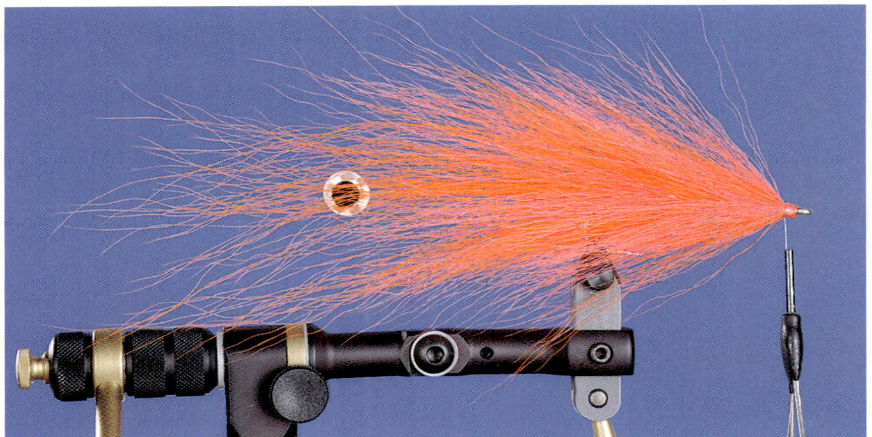

7. Completed Bucktail Deceiver Squid. Totally wet the fly and then let it dry.

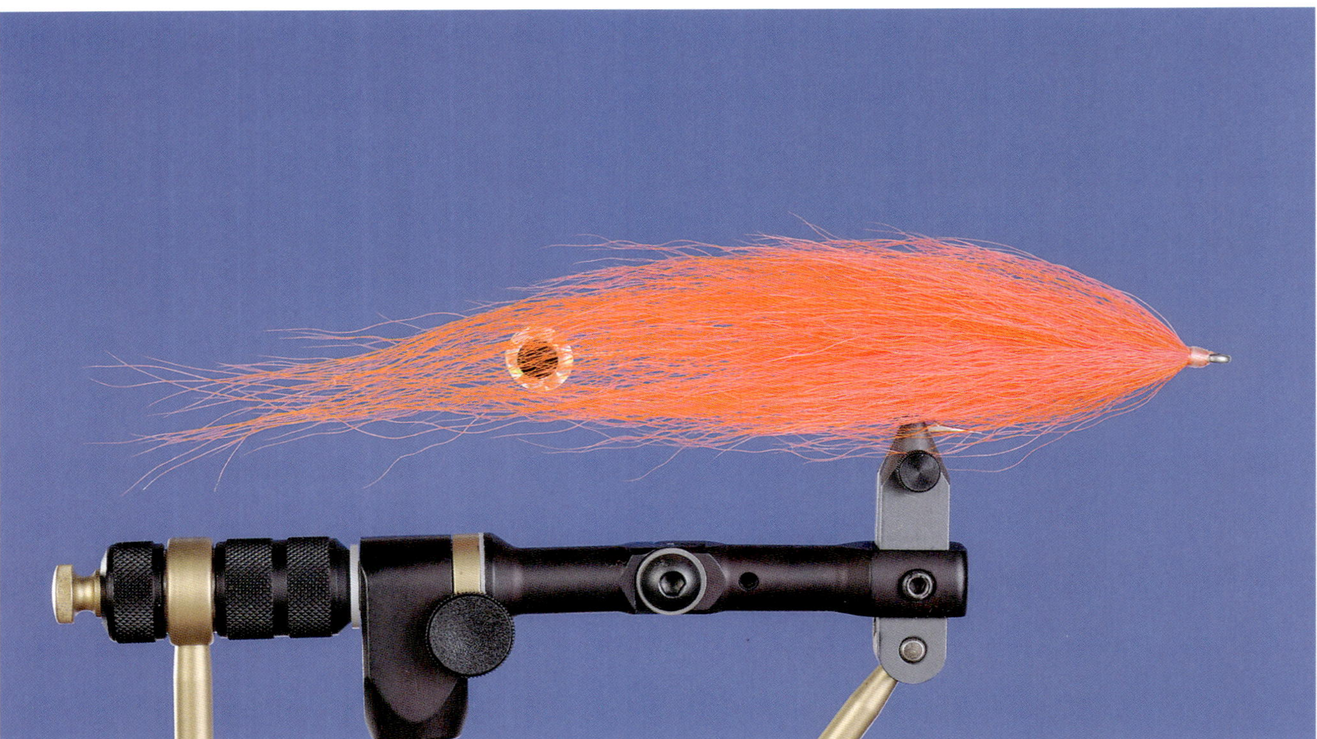

Squid are beautiful swimmers. Their sleek shape allows them to swim smoothly and effortlessly through the water. Visualize this while you tie the fly, and chances are good the final product will be better.

Bucktail Deceiver Herring

Hook:	Varivas 990S or similar short-shank saltwater
Thread:	Fine monofilament
Body:	White, chartreuse, pink, and blue bucktail
Eyes:	Jungle cock

TYING THE BUCKTAIL DECEIVER HERRING

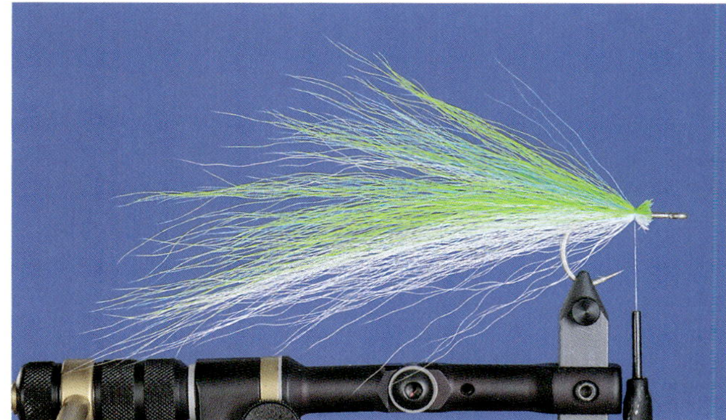

1. In this version of the Bucktail Deceiver, all of the steps are the same except for the way that you squeeze the fibers once you distribute them around the shank. Insert the hook into the vise. Attach the monofilament thread and wrap it to the hook bend. Prepare two colors of bucktail fibers and place them together neatly, with the darker color on top and lighter color below. After distributing them around the shank, squeeze the fibers tightly from each side toward the shank before tightening the thread. This creates a more narrow profile when viewed from the front.

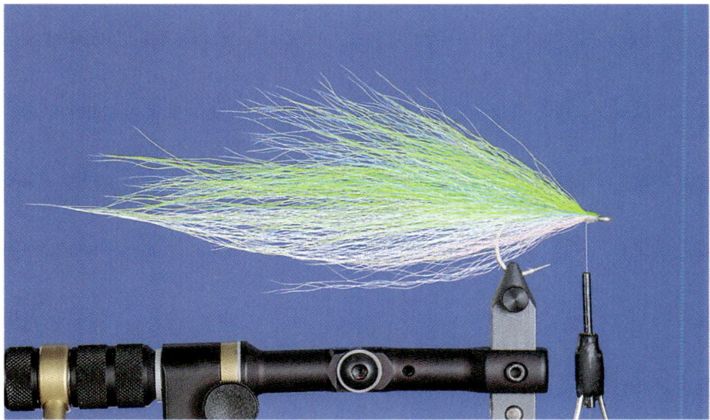

2. Repeat these steps and positioning of the bucktail going forward, paying attention to overall taper of the fly. Once at the hook eye, add a little belly color underneath. In this case I used pink.

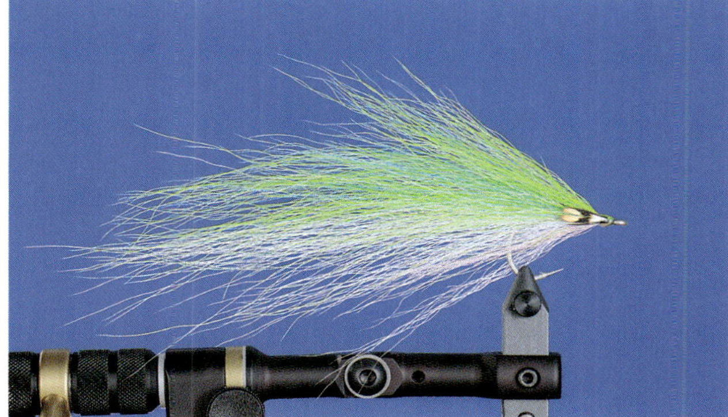

3. You can add eyes if you wish. Tab eyes or jungle cock eyes are good options. If you use jungle cock eyes, make sure that you capture some fibers when you tie down the feather. For more durability and to help prevent rolling of the feather, do not tie on a naked stem. Cementing the thread wraps at the head before tying in the jungle cock eyes can also be helpful.

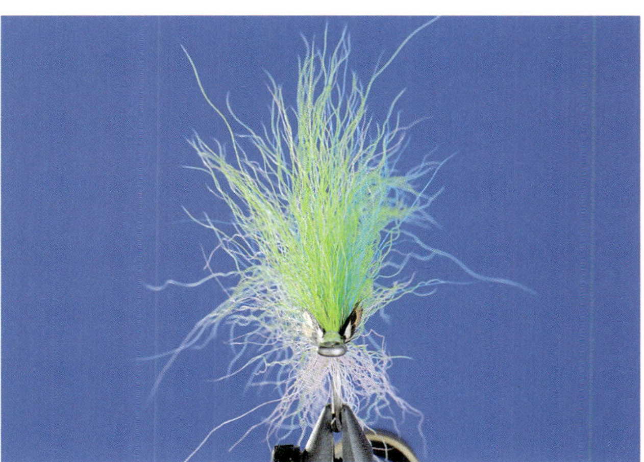

4. In just a few steps you have created a durable fly with taper and a broad profile.

Bucktail Deceiver (Wide)

Hook: Varivas 994S or similar long-shank saltwater
Thread: Fine monofilament
Body: White bucktail
Flash: Pearl Flashabou
Collar: Pink bucktail

TYING THE BUCKTAIL DECEIVER (WIDE)

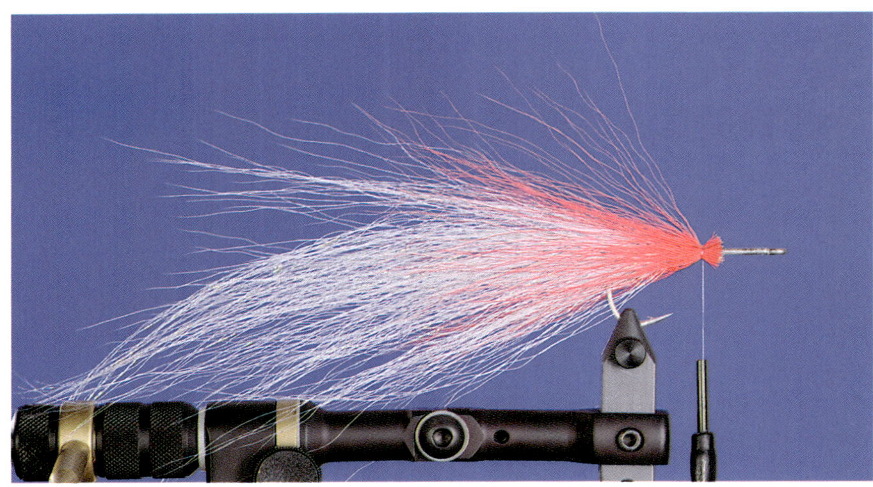

1. In this variation I am going to distribute the fibers around the shank as with the standard Bucktail Deceiver but create a flattened, wider collar by squeezing the fibers from the top and bottom when I tighten the thread. This splays the fibers out like pontoons. The rear portion of the fly is exactly the same as for the Bucktail Deceiver; the only difference is that you will add some flash and shape the collar differently. Pick fibers with a contrasting color for the collar that are slightly shorter than the fibers in the previous steps (the fiber lengths continue to get shorter as fly is tied), and tie them in as before, paying attention to the shape of the fly.

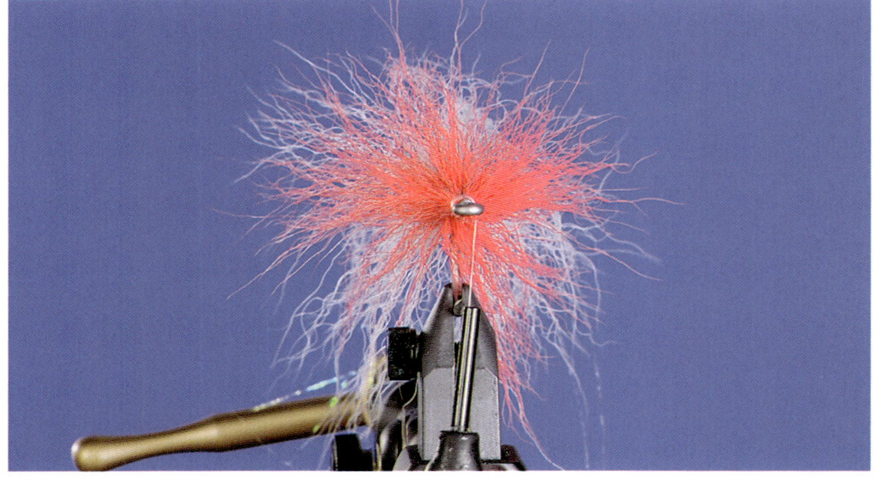

2. Note how the hairs are flaring to each side, creating a wider fly when viewed from the top down (or bottom up). After distributing the fibers around the hook, squeeze them hard on the top and bottom when tightening the thread.

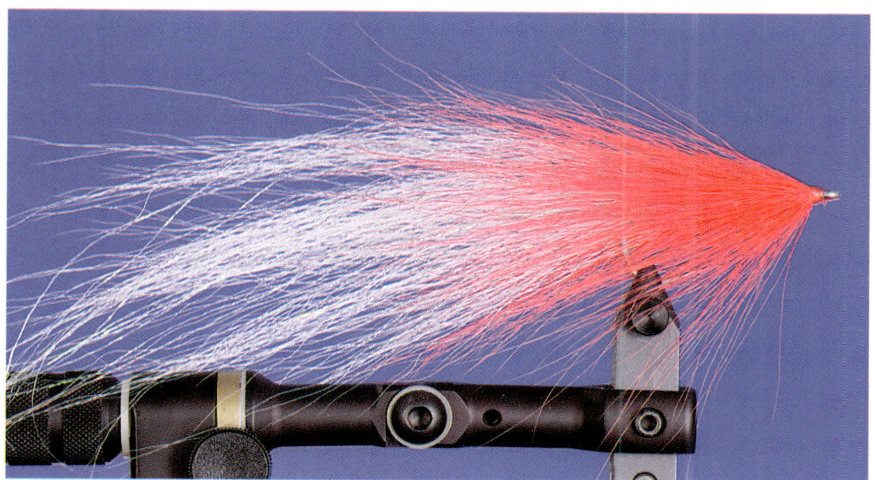

3. Continue building the fly, taking care to use shorter fibers once you are on the shank. If the fibers are too long, the fly can foul easier.

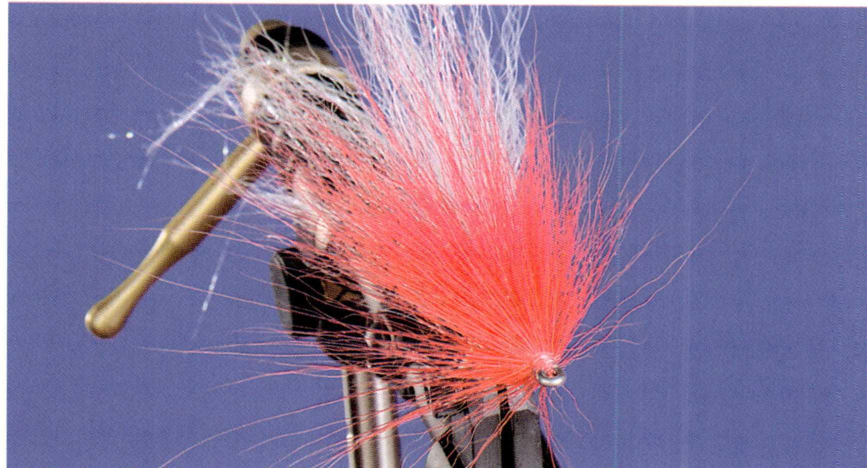

4. View from top front. The fibers in the collar splay out, which slows the fly's descent in the water.

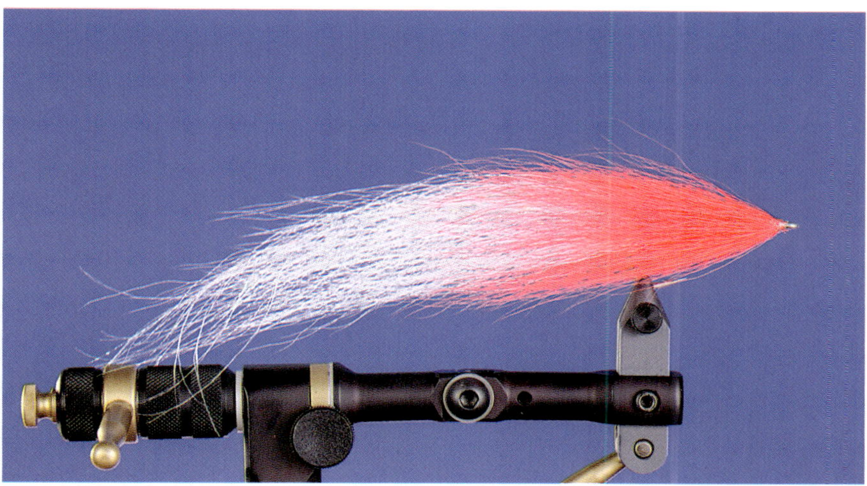

5. Totally wet the Bucktail Deceiver and allow it to completely dry before combing it out. In all black, this is the best nighttime fly that I know because it stays high in the water column longer.

Bucktail Deceiver (Extended)

Hook:	#4/0 Tiemco 911S or similar long-shank saltwater
Thread:	Fine monofilament
Extension:	30-pound-test mono
Body:	Long white and pink bucktail from the base of tail
Flash:	Pearlescent Flashabou
Head:	Full length closed-cell foam cylinder, sticky back prismatic tape, and extra large eyes

TYING THE BUCKTAIL DECEIVER (EXTENDED)

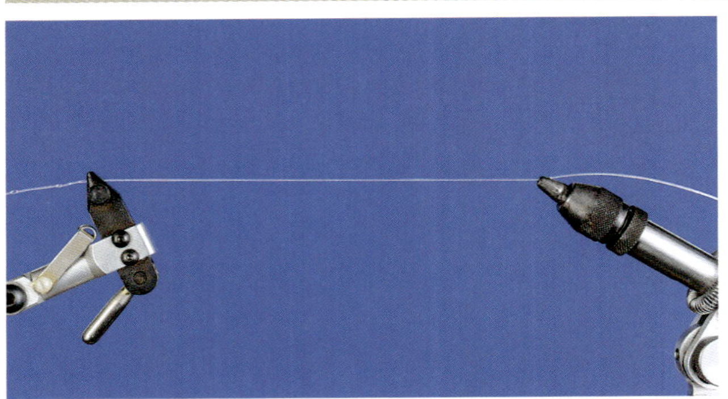

1. You can tie monofilament extensions using stiff monofilament straights as I do with the Beast (see page 147) or by stretching the mono between two vises as I do here. This is how I originally created monofilament extensions before I discovered the straights, and it is still a good way to go, depending on what materials you have on hand.

Begin by clamping the ends of the mono into two vises spread about 12 inches apart from jaw to jaw. For these pictures, the distance is closer than that, but you want to maintain 12 inches. Make sure the monofilament is stretched tight enough to sound like a guitar string when plucked.

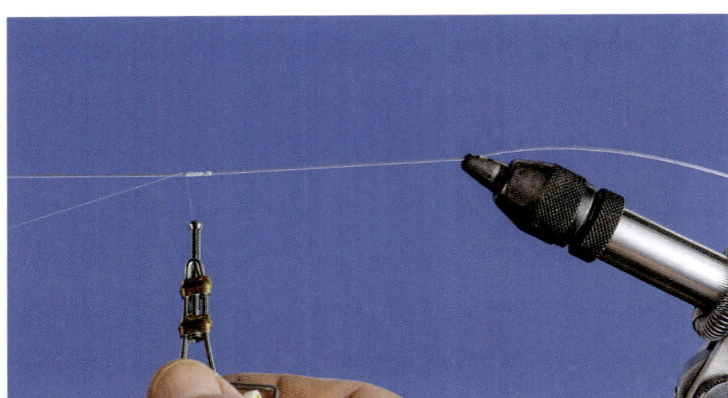

2. Increase the tension on the bobbin by removing one side of the spool from one of the legs of the bobbin and taking a few wraps of mono around the leg before returning the spool to its proper position. Attach the thread by hand to the mono extension, just as you would attach thread to a hook shank. You have to deliberately hand over the bobbin and thread to the other side of the mono, let it fall, and grab the bobbin again until it is secure enough to be spun without slipping.

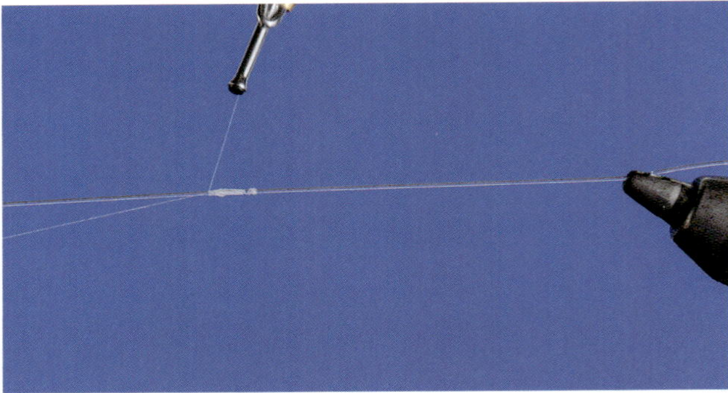

3. Once the thread is secure you can spin it around the mono straight and create a base very quickly.

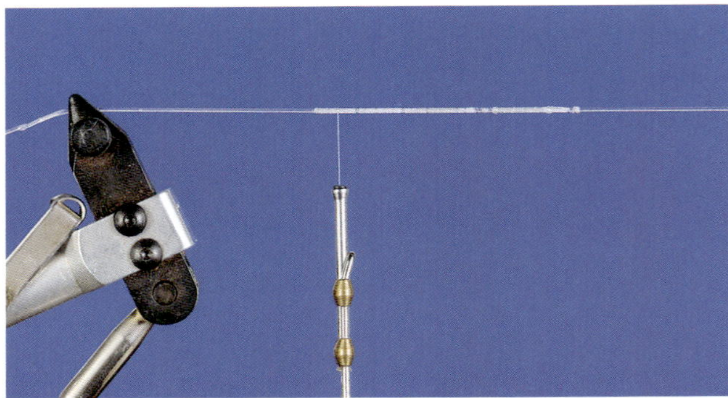

4. Wrap a complete base of monofilament thread over the mono extension so that the material adheres better. Note the location of the thread to accept the first bunch of bucktail fibers.

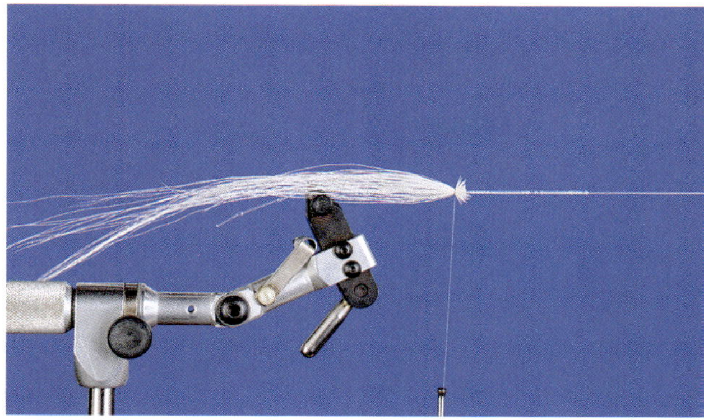

5. The first bunch of bucktail fibers establishes the fly's length, so select the longest fibers that you have. Remove as many of the short fibers as you can, and tie in a sparse amount to control flare. Distribute the fibers completely around the monofilament extension, and tie them down by holding the fibers tightly with your material hand and flipping the monofilament thread and bobbin straight up and over the mono, not at an angle. Hold the fibers with your material hand until you have secured them with the thread.

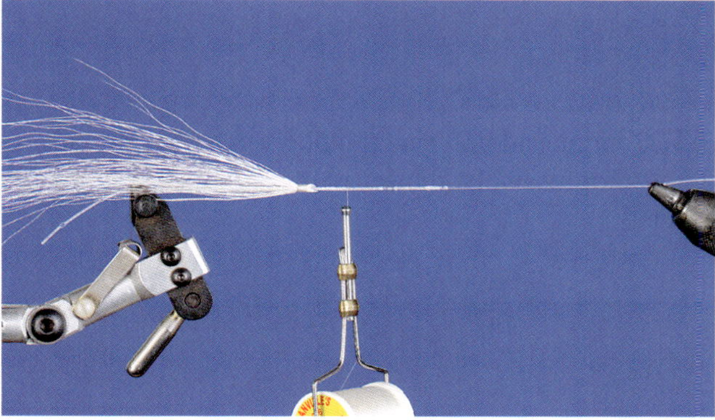

6. Coat the butts with head cement, and wrap over them to the next tie-down position. After tying in the second set of fibers, you can add some flash as I do here, but that is completely optional. Repeat, tying in slightly shorter bucktail fibers, and continue the taper. After you secure the fibers with thread wraps, advance the bobbin to the next tie-down position. You can add more flash if you wish. Remember that when you tie in the flash, you can get better distribution by giving yourself enough room to wrap back over the flash as you distribute it around the extension with your material hand.

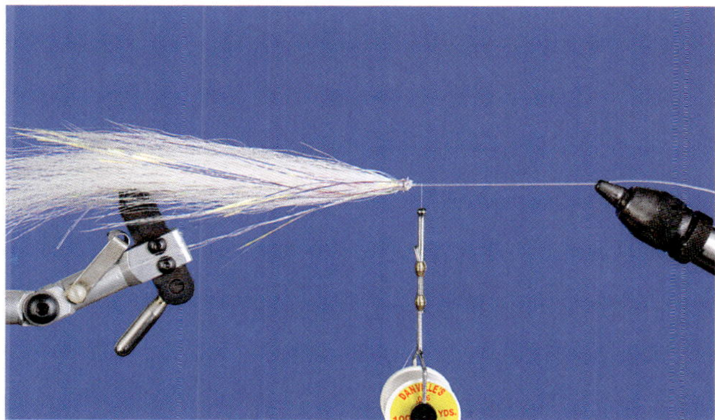

7. Tie in another clump of bucktail, again slightly shorter than the one preceding it. While the application of bucktail is repetitive, you must adjust the materials to maintain taper. Add some more flash, and tie off the thread. You want to make sure that you leave about two inches of bare extension to tie to the hook.

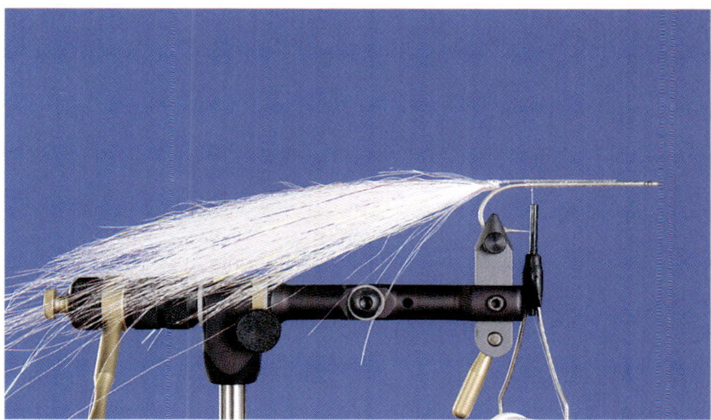

8. Insert the hook into the vise, attach monofilament thread, and completely cover the shank with thread. Tie the extension to the shank at the hook bend and wrap over it completely, ending with the thread at the hook bend. Add head cement (or a cyanoacrylate glue) to all exposed thread along the shank. After every application of bucktail, it's important to coat the butts with head cement. Since you spend so much time tying these and use your select bucktail, you want to make sure that they are as durable as possible.

(continued)

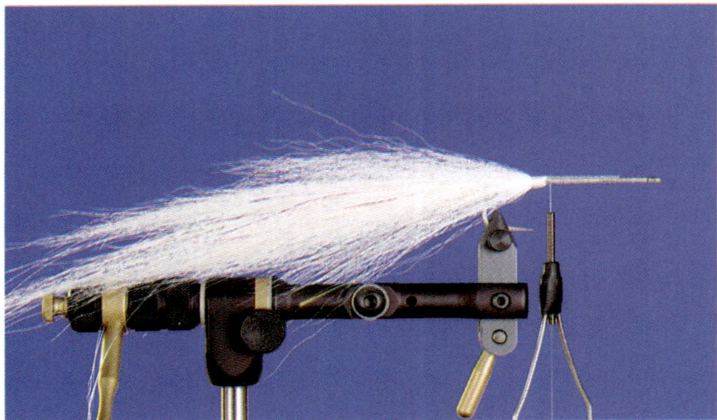

9. When you tie down the first clump of bucktail fibers and distribute them around the shank, make sure that they blend in with, and continue the taper of, the fibers on the extension.

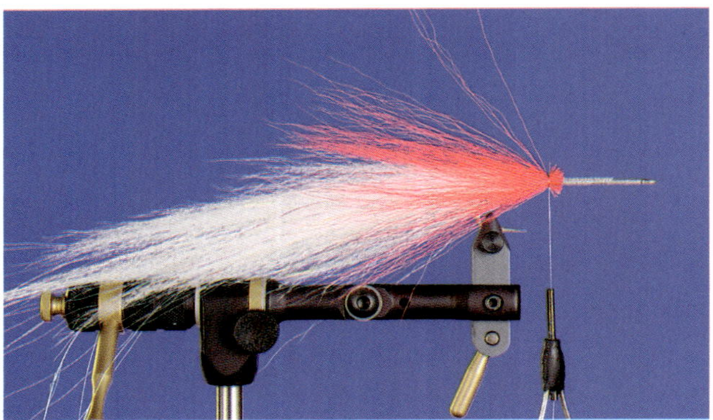

10. We are tying in contrasting-color hairs, although that is not necessary. When choosing the bucktail for the collar, I usually prefer wavy fibers that provide a fuller presence and a better overall look.

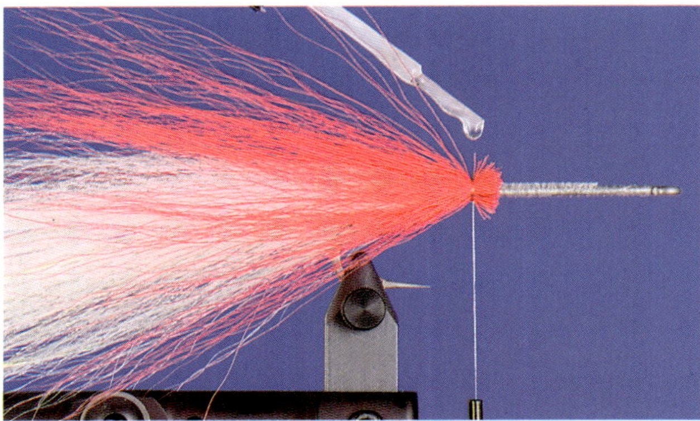

11. When the butts are flared, apply head cement to them before wrapping over them with thread.

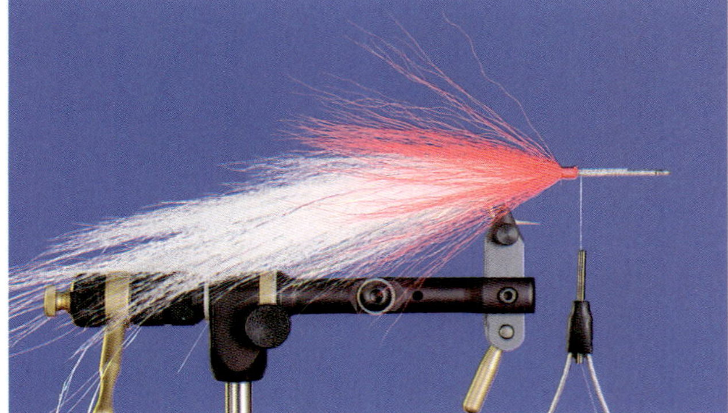

12. Wrap the thread over the butts after adding head cement to them.

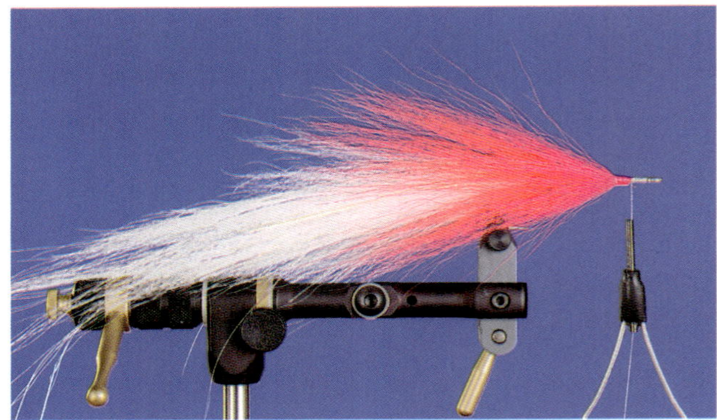

13. Continue adding bucktail fibers to build up the front, using progressively shorter hairs to maintain a smooth taper.

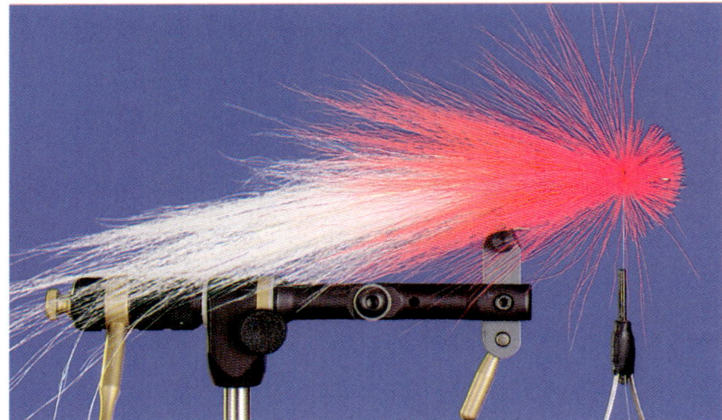

14. We are going to finish with a BULKhead on this fly, but you can also do a standard Bucktail Deceiver head as well. Using coarser fibers from near the base of a bucktail, choose fibers long enough to continue the taper of collar. As you tie in the fibers, flare them and make sure they are equally distributed around the shank. Refer to the BULKhead Technique on page 54 for more detail.

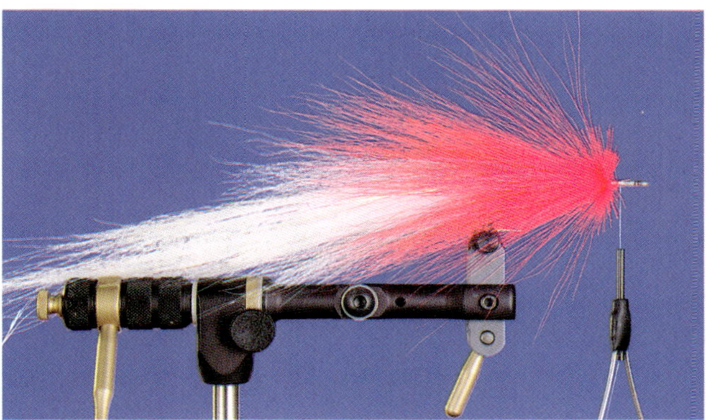

15. Cut the butt ends so that when they are pushed back, the uneven lengths will look more natural in the finished fly. Push the trimmed butts back with your pushing tool. Bring the thread in front of the butts, and advance it to the point shown to tie in the next clump.

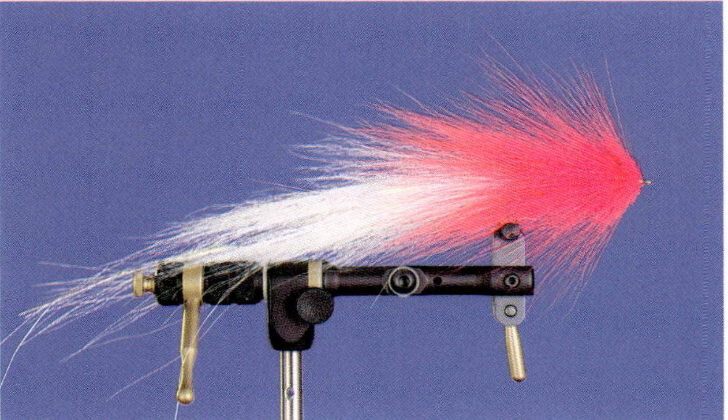

16. Repeat two more times to fill the rest of the shank and form a nice head. The finished fly should look like this before wetting and drying.

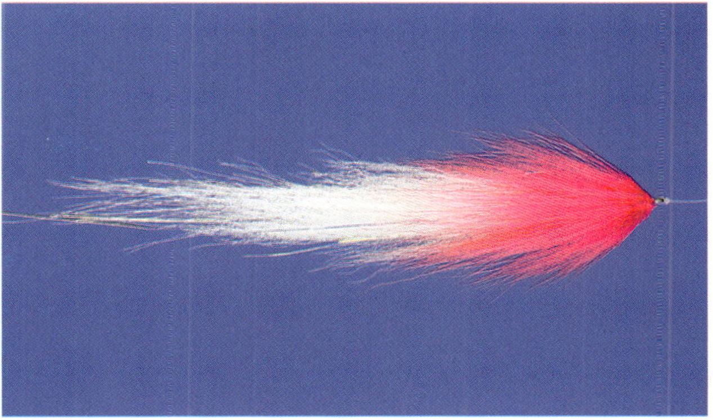

17. This fly will work great as is, but you can also create a Banger head for it. When fishing this fly with a Banger head, I use 12 inches of 60- to 80-pound-test monofilament for the bite tippet, connected to the main line with an Albright knot. Slip the Banger head onto the bite tippet.

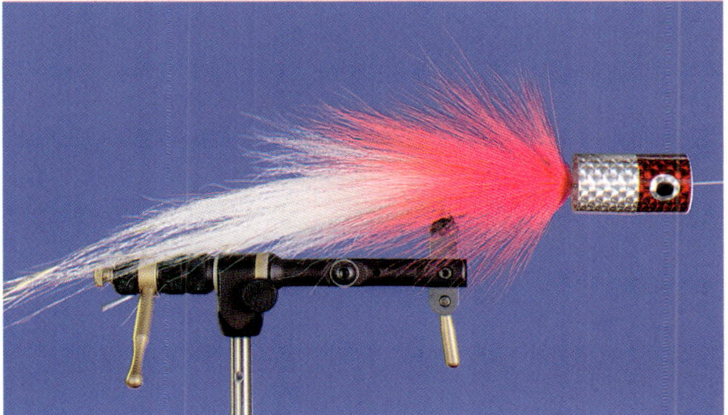

18. To create a Banger head, ream a center hole through an entire 1 1/2-inch-long Live Body foam cylinder with a heated bodkin or thin drill bit. Wrap prismatic tape around the cylinder, making sure to overlap it by at least 1/2 inch so that it is secure. Add a stick-on eye if you wish. The tape and eyes are optional and not having them on the fly doesn't seem to bother the fish. Keep in mind that you can fish the fly with the Banger head up close against the fly or well ahead of it on the shock tippet so that the fly dangles below the floating head.

Chapter 8

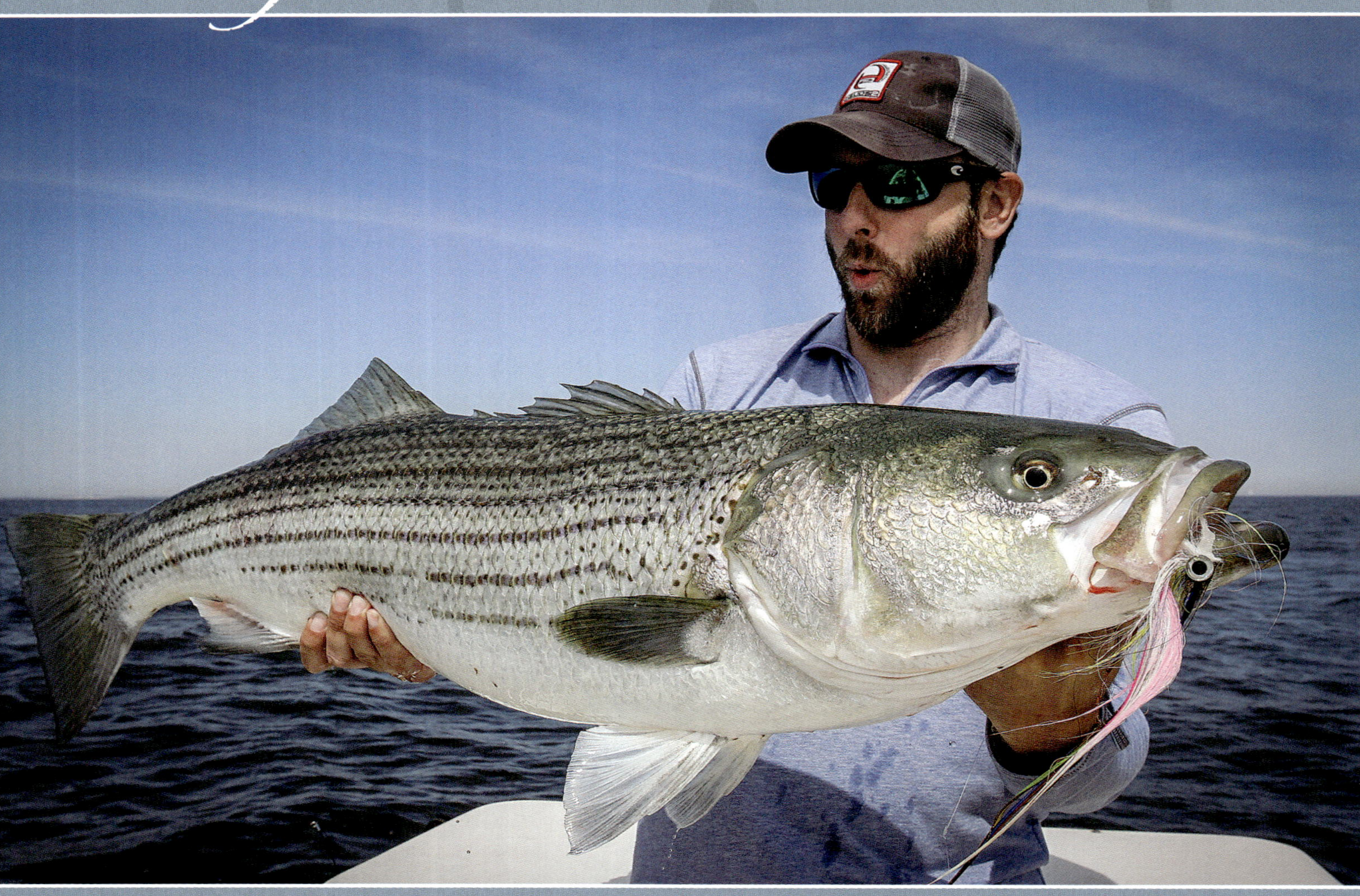

Andrew Hamilton holds a female striped bass that took a large articulated Hollow Fleye as the bass were on pods of bunker off the Jersey Shore. The Hollow Fleye technique to create big, broad bodies without bulk can be adapted to a wide variety of flies or combined with the other techniques shown in this book. COLIN ARCHER

Hollow Fleye

"You've got to take this to another level," Kenney Abrames said, smiling, as he walked toward my table at a fly-fishing show, pumping a red and white Bucktail Deceiver in the air. I had given him the fly shortly before, and now he was back.

"What do you mean by that?" I asked.

"Take it to another level," he repeated with a smile. And then he walked away.

Kenney, author of *Striper Moon* and *A Perfect Fish*, is an artistic fly tier who often talks in the abstract. Over the years, we have had many thought-provoking conversations about fly design, and while my tying style and general way of approaching fly tying was, and is, much different than his, I did appreciate his artistry and insights. I didn't quite know what he meant by taking it to another level, but I took it as encouragement to continue to explore the possibilities with the fly and its primary ingredient, bucktail.

As I drove the five hours home, I thought about what Kenney said. Though I don't know what he really meant by the comment, it was enough of a challenge to get me thinking about how to improve the Bucktail Deceiver, which was a revolutionary fly for me in its own right. I settled down into my mental fly-tying room and kept churning over ideas, which is something that I often do on long drives. Instead of having an obvious need to improve something, this challenge was like a force for me. I thought of the obvious—different flares, put feathers in it—but dismissed those as too easy and too simple. What could I do?

Ideas come from strange places, and I believe that if you pay attention to things going on around you, certain events or observations can reappear down the road as sources of inspiration for possible solutions to a particular problem. For instance, the two-handed-strip retrieve that I've come to use was directly inspired by watching a fisherman in Mexico. After launching his lure with a whirling overhead cast, I watched him retrieve it with his hands. He moved them violently apart from one another, strip after strip, giving his retrieve the speed he needed to fool the Sierra mackerel to strike. In this case, my mind wandered to Montauk, where I recalled anglers fishing with parachute jigs with trolling rods, and how they would sweep the rod back and forth to pull the fibers, which were tied at the front and extended out over the eye, open so that the jig would pulse in the water and give the illusion of size and life.

So as I started to think about how to get fullness without bulk, those jigs became a source of inspiration. It wasn't the answer, but it was a seed—the first step in the thought process. I had to think about how to achieve it in a fly form. The way that I tied the Bucktail Deceiver, and many of the previous saltwater flies, was that each step would be built on top of a previous step, and those steps in succession created the fly's bulk and shape. It occurred to me that devising a way of forcing the fibers directly up

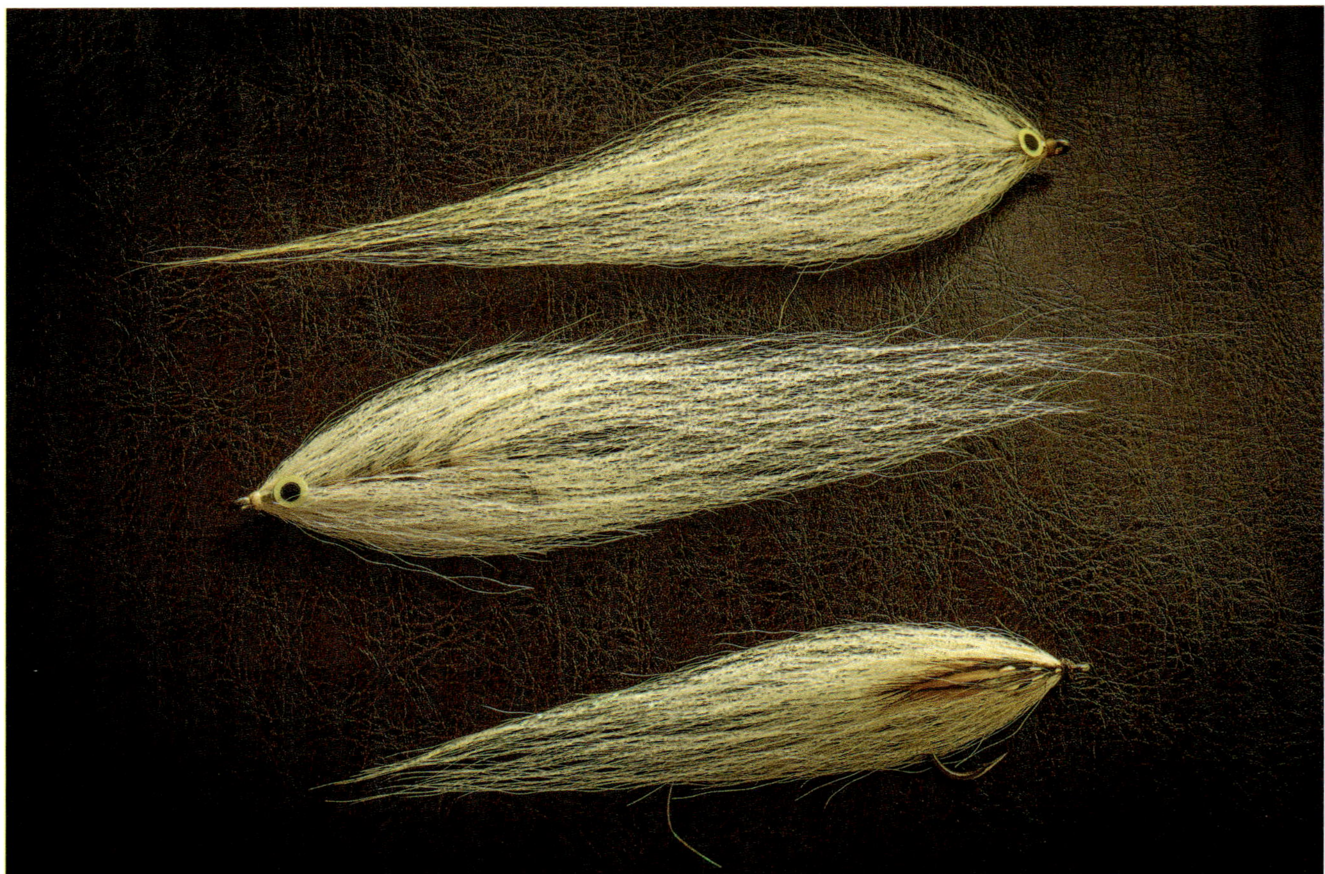

Early Hollows. From top to bottom you can see experimentations with different profiles, from wide to narrow, though these first Hollows were fairly conservative. When learning how to create the Hollow Fleye, I first needed to affirm that the technique was sound. It was, so I started at low angles then began to allow more and more flare.

and away from the hook shank when I tie it in would help me achieve immediate height, which would give me a lot more control because each tie is not dependent on the previous one for its shape. Just as the jigs had nylon fibers projecting out over the eye, which were swept back in a round parachute around the jig body when retrieved, I thought of tying in the bucktail in the opposite direction and pushing it back over the shank, using the thread to control the flare of the bunch, and then marrying each section of bucktail to the other to create taper. As I tied in my mind, looking for problems, snags, and anything that would get in the way of the process I was imagining, I could see the fly developing. I rehearsed the necessary steps over and over on the drive home.

I was tired from the show and the long drive, but I still went straight upstairs to my tying room, grabbed some bucktail, and tried the technique that I had worked through over and over. It played out exactly as I had envisioned it. After tying a few bunches of bucktail to the shank and experimenting with what would be the basic Hollow technique, I went to bed. The next day I got up, had my coffee, went upstairs, and started to assemble an entire fly.

The first versions had conservative tapers. I would just tie in the fibers and wrap back over them so that they would flare only a little more than a conventional Bucktail Deceiver. Later, I would increase the angle of the fibers coming off the shank by not tying down on them as much, and I could see the way for larger imitations. One of the biggest breakthroughs for me was realizing that since the fly was going to be pulled on the retrieve, all I had to do was take the fibers a little past perpendicular, cocked back toward the hook bend, and I was in the safe zone. This simple realization would give me confidence to allow the flies to stand tall at the vise and keep me from compressing the bucktail too much.

I was eager and a little nervous to see this fly in the water. But when that day did come, I was amazed at how beautiful the fly looked—it far exceeded what the Bucktail Deceiver did in the water. The Hollow breathed in the water as all the fibers moved, and the openness that allowed such freedom of movement prompted the name "Hollow Fleye." For me, the Hollow technique opened everything up, literally as well as figuratively. From then on, I could design large flies that had amazing action in the water, were reasonably easy to cast, and sank quickly.

When describing the Hollow technique, I use the term "reverse tying," but I want to make sure that beginning tiers, especially those coming over from trout fishing, don't confuse it with the reverse tying of Carrie Stevens, Keith Fulsher, and others. In those flies the bucktail is tied in so that the tips extend over the hook eye, but the thread remains behind the fibers and captures the bundle as the fibers are brought back, creating a bullet-type head. I do tie the fibers in a similar direction, but the key here is that I then bring the thread forward, through the pulled-back bucktail, and wrap back toward the hook point to adjust the angle at which the hair comes off the shank.

Variations

Though some tiers, such as Dave Skok, have mastered the technique for small flies, I typically reserve the Hollow technique for large, wide baits, such as bunker (6 to 12 inches), herring (6 to 8 inches), squid, perch, and butterfish, though I do tie some 4-inch Hollows for peanut bunker. To imitate extremely large baits, the Hollow technique is the best that I know of, and a supersized version of it called the Beast is my best tool when big-game hunting.

My favorite material to use with the Hollow style is bucktail, but you can also experiment with other natural materials such as polar bear hair or synthetics such as Kinky Fibre. The Hollow tie can also be used with other techniques for different effects or to accomplish a variety of different shapes. For instance, I often finish my Bucktail Deceivers with a Hollow tie to achieve a small, neat head. The more you play around with it, the more you will learn about it.

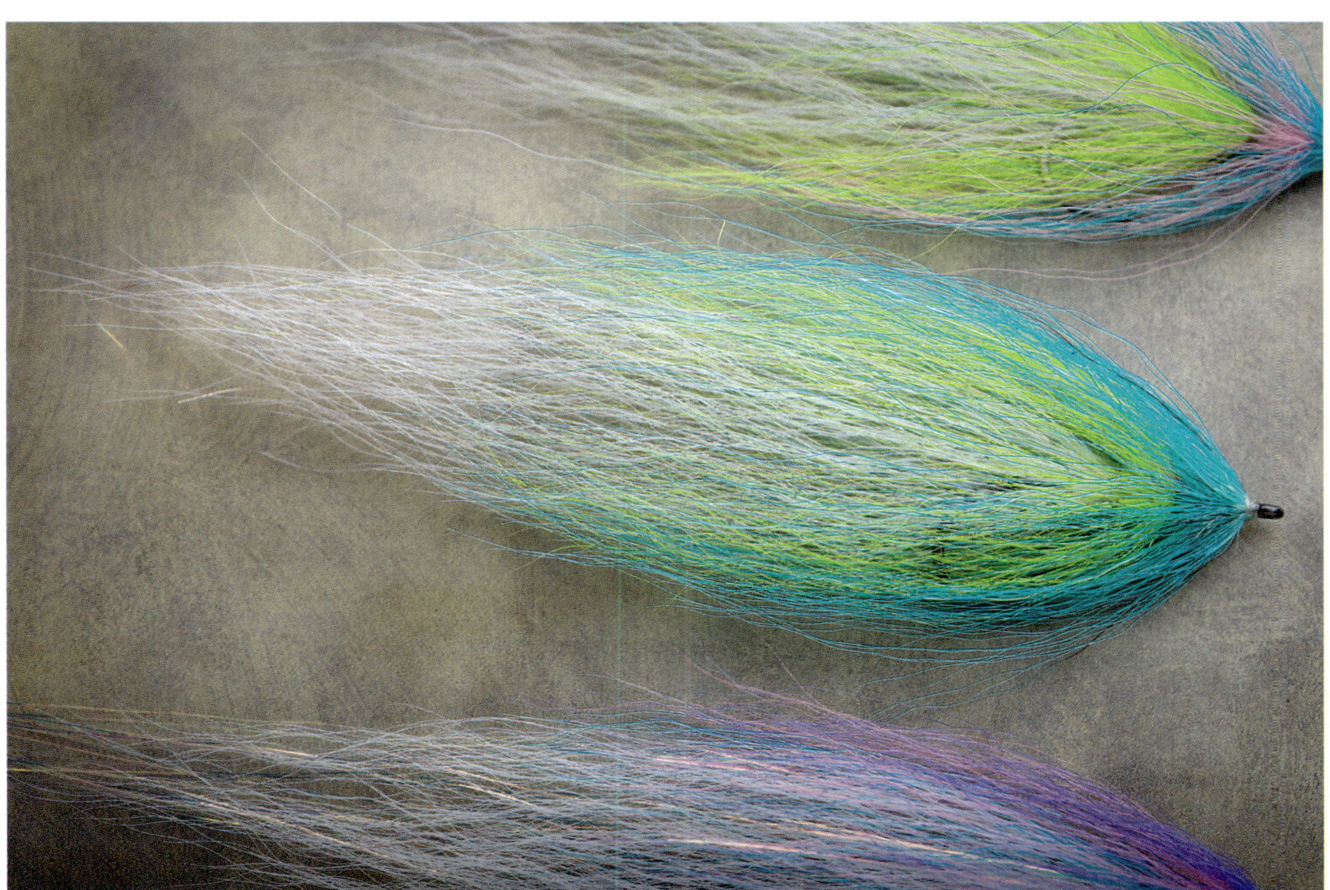

When tying Hollows, do not wrap over the hair too much. Many tiers wrap the thread back too far and push the fibers down too much. It's an easy fix technically, but many times a mental block is going on here too. Most tiers are so accustomed to seeing the bucktail a certain way that they are not satisfied to leave the fly alone.

Hollow Tying Tips

- Think about taper. You must make at least three ties on the hook shank to create a taper. The first tie should have the least angle, and then you should open up the angles with each successive tie. Remember, Hollow tying is a progression of steps that you gradually build higher if needed. The ties forward of the middle half of the fly need to be open (at greater angles) to achieve a fly with nice taper. If you take 1/4 inch off the butts before you tie them in, then move the thread forward 1/4 inch, you are going to automatically get shorter ties in each step (by about half an inch) as long as you work with fibers from the same area of the tail.
- Proper preparation. Preen out the shortest fibers, but tie with a bundle that has varying lengths. The short hairs in any given clump may have as many as four different lengths. Take only the shortest hairs out that don't contribute to the natural taper. I call these the first two layers. The third and fourth layers are the longest fibers, but there is still variation in the clump, which provides taper. Look at the fiber clumps closely and you will see two different lengths of fibers.
- Have faith in the finished fly. The fly looks strange with fibers sticking out wildly. But, that's what you may need to do. Allow it to be open when finished, and when you see it in the water, it'll make sense to you. Learning to tie a good Hollow took a certain amount of discipline to not wrap back over the fibers and maintain the angle. Often the best Hollows look wild in the vise. After you wet the fly for the first time and dry it, that will tame the fibers, and the fly will take its shape.
- Practice. Experiment with different types of bucktail and different amounts of fibers. The more you do, the better you'll get. Take your time and observe what is going on all the time. It's a different way to tie a fly, so you kind of have to learn all over again how the material reacts to what you do with it. With its many variables, the Hollow Fleye is the most difficult fly I have ever designed, but once you figure it out, you'll really enjoy tying it. It's creative tying, big time.

Because there is plenty of room in between each one of the ties, variations to the fly are endless. I frequently will add feathers and flash in those spaces and have also experimented with both weights and floats to get the fly to sink or suspend. One of my favorite ways of making a Hollow is adding spun deer hair in between the ties to create bulk in the collar section, which adds more density but does not detract from the overall shape and look of the fly. For this, I use deer hair from the base of the tail, and because it is shorter than the Hollow-tied fibers, it will only show up as an inner bulk concealed within the fly. When you hold it, you can feel the mass in the forward portion of the fly.

After the basic Hollow Fleye steps in this chapter, I demonstrate a High-Riding Hollow that uses short, blended, stiff-fiber bucktail to give forward bulk to the head. This is the forerunner of the BULKhead.

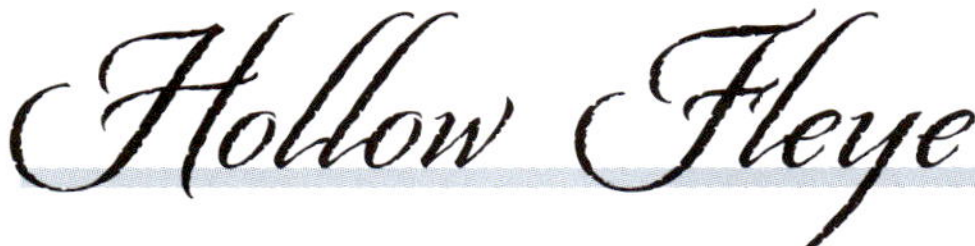

Hook:	Varivas 990S or similar short-shank saltwater
Thread:	Fine monofilament
Body:	Long white, chartreuse, and blue bucktail
Flash:	Saltwater Angel Hair

TYING THE HOLLOW FLEYE

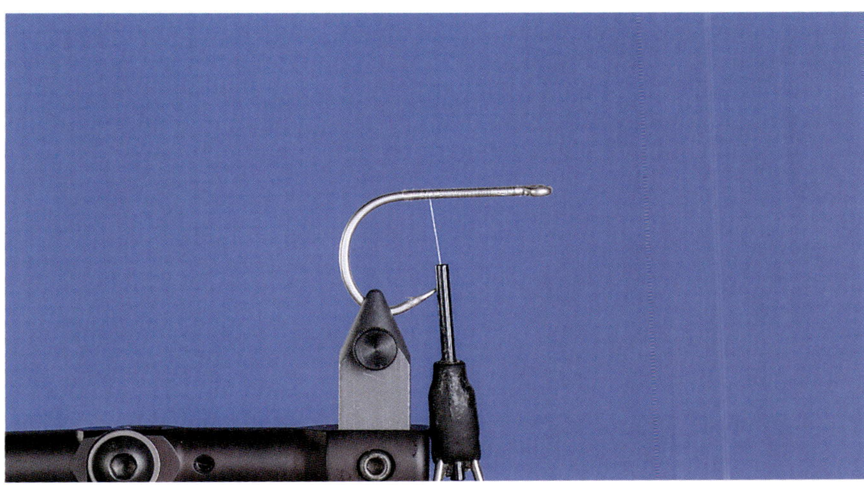

1. Insert the hook into the vise. Wrap a solid base of monofilament thread to the bend, and then wrap forward about 1/4 inch. The butt ends of the bucktail must rest against thread on the shank. This fly only has three ties—the minimum amount required for a taper—so you can work with a shorter shank hook than what you'd use for the Bucktail Deceiver.

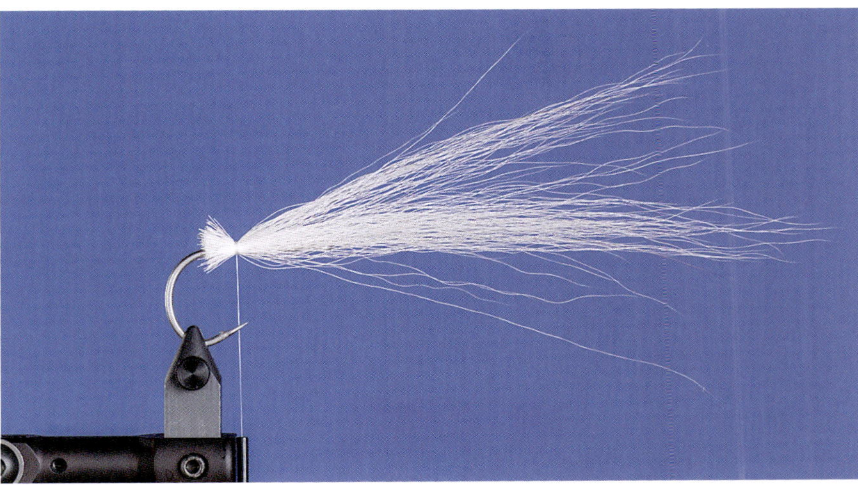

2. Select a fairly sparse bunch of fibers from the base of the bucktail. It's common for people to start out with too many fibers. You only want enough to suggest the shape and length. Ideally, you are looking for fine, soft hair with a bit of wave, but you can make do with any of your longer hair, except the coarsest, thickest fibers. After you preen out the shortest fibers and trim the butts, attach the bundle to the shank with the butts facing the hook bend. Be sure the fibers are equally distributed around the shank by holding the butts with the fingertips of your material hand while you tie them in. Tighten the thread to pull all the fibers into the shank equally. When you wrap your thread, be sure to come straight over and around the hook and not at an angle to the shank or the fibers will not flare equally.

(continued)

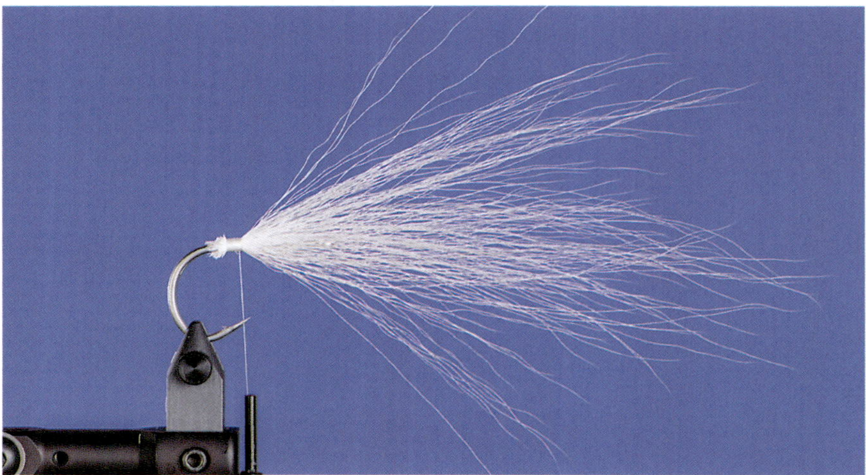

3. You can trim the butts to neaten them up. (I often skip this step.) After that, apply head cement and wrap over the butts, making sure the thread ends at the base of the collar, the transition point. Be careful with your thread as you negotiate the hook point.

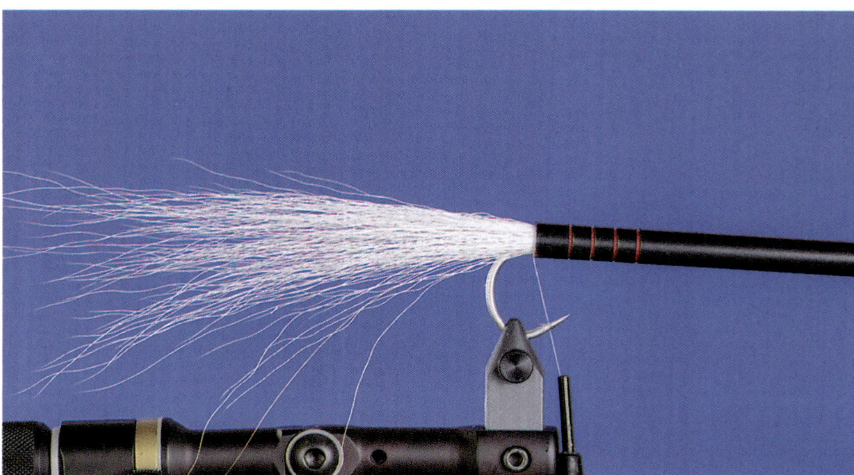

4. The next step is to move all the fibers rearward. While you can do this with your fingers alone, a pushing tool such as an empty pen cartridge helps push the fibers back far enough so that you can grab them easily with your fingers.

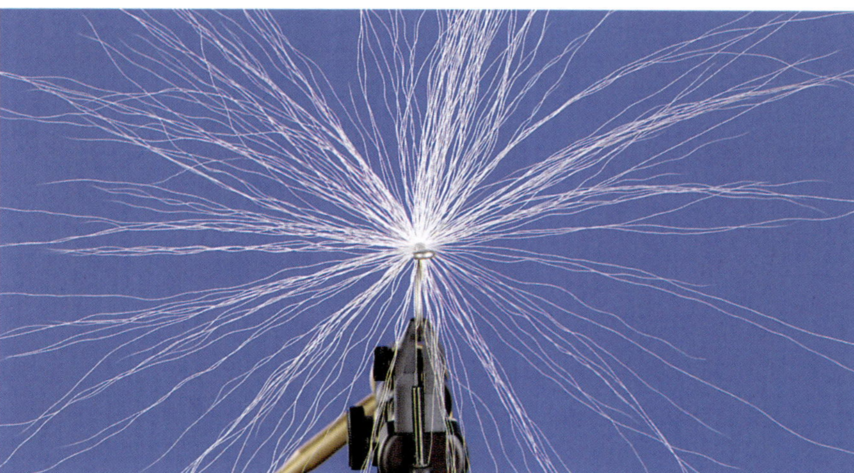

5. Try to evenly distribute hairs around the shank by slightly pulling fibers equally around the shank. That actually can move hairs at the base and make controlling flare with the thread easier.

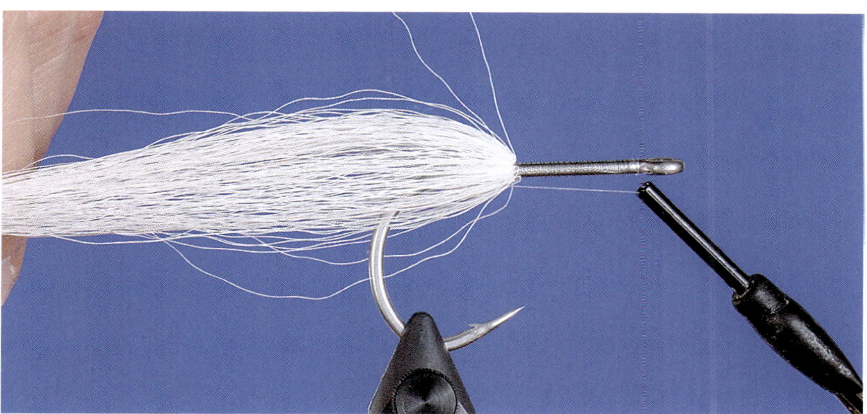

6. While holding the fibers in your material hand, bring the thread in front of them, making sure it is almost parallel to the hook shank.

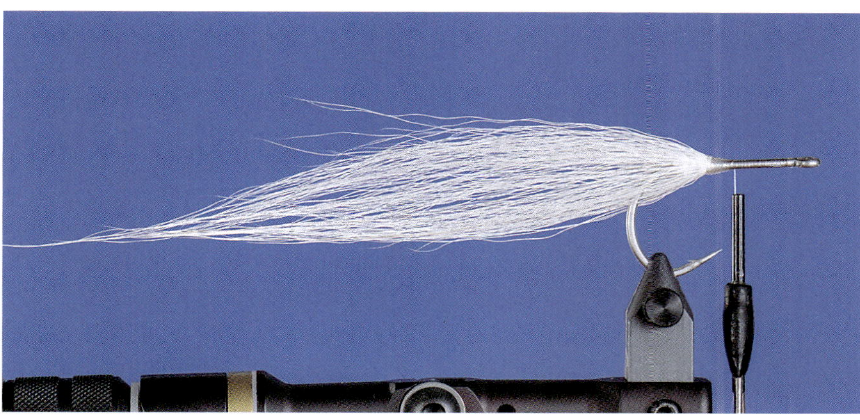

7. The first bunch of fibers should be at a low angle, which will require more thread wraps over their bases. You may need to wrap up, down, and then back up to create a stable ramp of thread, but remember to keep each wrap only one thread width.

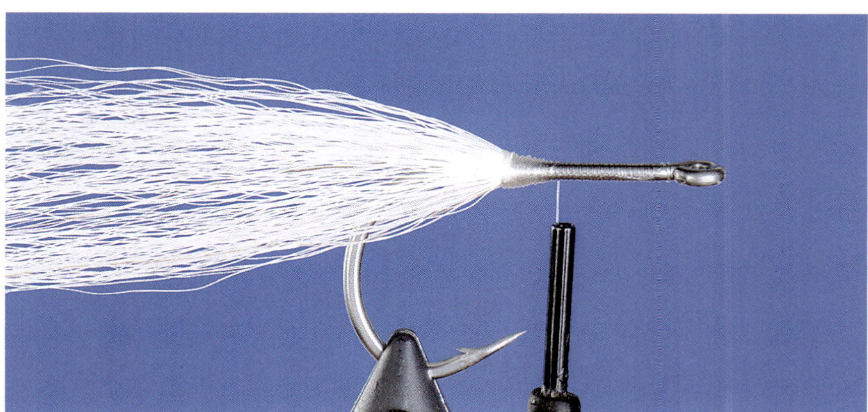

8. Note how wide the dam is to get the low angle and how it is built for stability. After you get the angle that you desire, wrap the tying thread forward about 1/4 inch for the next step. Add head cement after building the dam and in every other tie-in step from here on out.

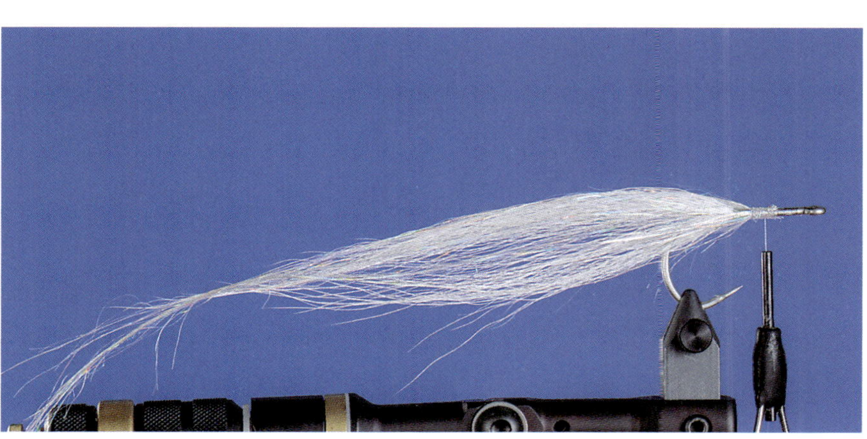

9. Because we are adding flash (here Saltwater Angel Hair) wrap another 1/4 inch so that you'll have room to wrap back over the flash before ending at the next tie-in step. Note the location of the thread for the middle section of bucktail. How far I choose to advance the thread is based on practice, experience, and the type of taper that I am trying to achieve on the amount of hook shank that I have to work with.

(continued)

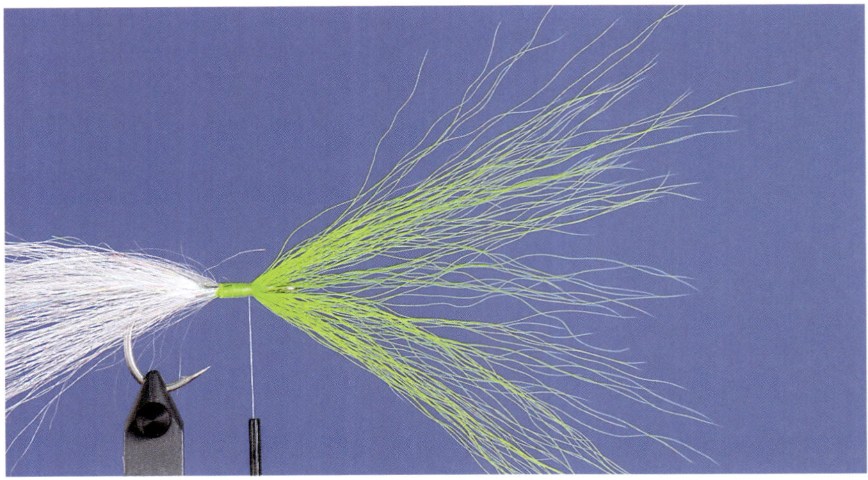

10. Tie in another bunch of fibers, and distribute them evenly around the shank. Make sure that you have trimmed the butts square and that they are not pushing against the previous clump and affecting its angle. Wrapping over the butts is not always critical, but if you don't, you must be careful that the butts don't catch the thread as you push the hair back so that you can pass the thread to the front of the fibers. Bring the thread back to the transition point. The length of these fibers, once folded back, will be about three-quarters the length of the white fibers in the first step.

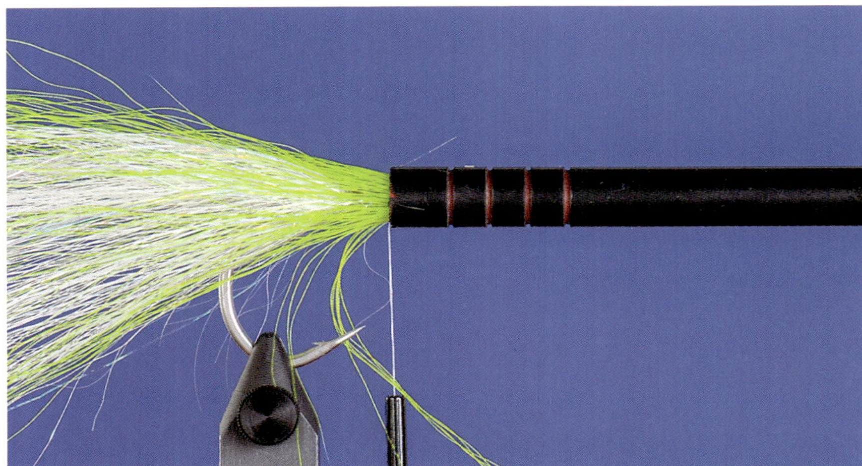

11. Push the fibers rearward with your tool. Rolling the pen cartridge around and back sometimes helps distribute the fibers better. The fibers must lie parallel to the shank and not be twisted.

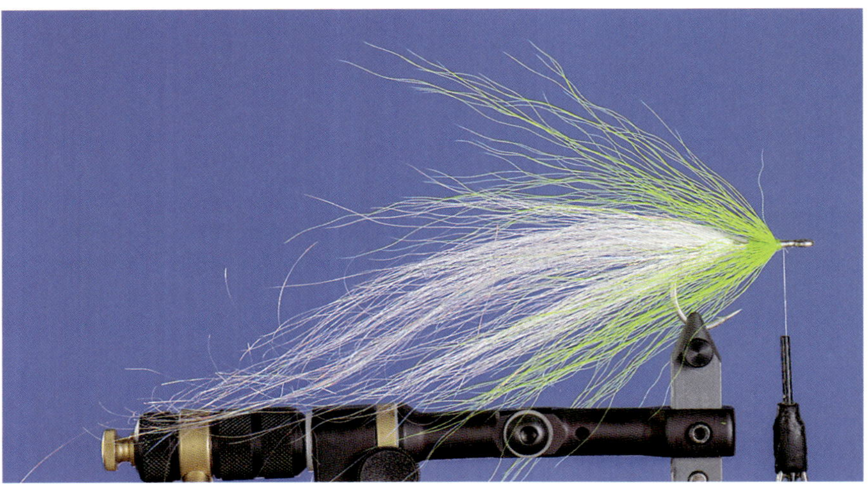

12. This angle is approximately 45 degrees and the first tie-in is about 25 degrees. You have complete control over the angle of the fibers. If you wrap too far and compress them too much, simply unwrap the thread to open up the angle.

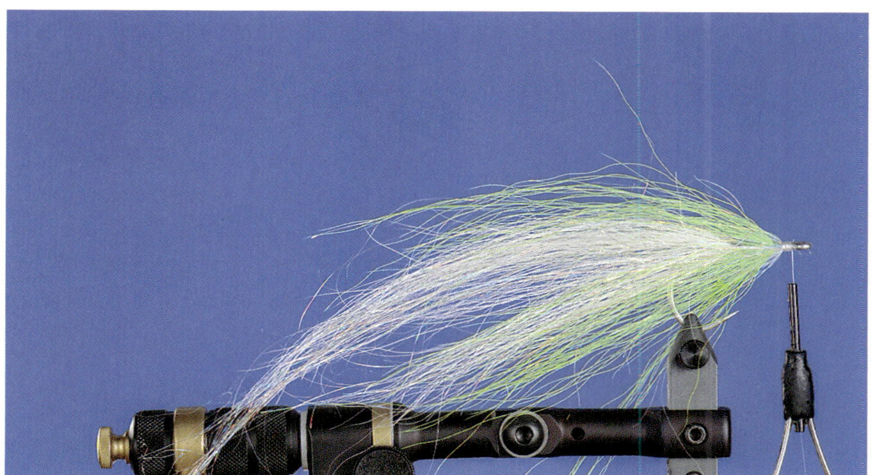

13. As I tie, I often moisten my fingertips and stroke the materials to remove the static and get a better picture of the finished shape. After you tie in the flash, bring the thread into position, up against the hook eye, for the final bunch of hair.

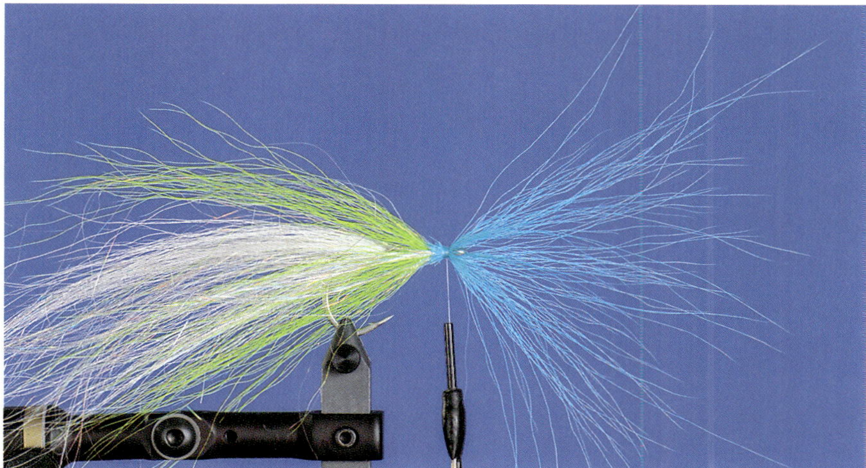

14. The last application of fibers is a little trickier because of the hook eye. I tie in the bucktail fibers right up against the hook eye, taking extra care that the fibers are evenly distributed around the shank before securing them. You might find it easier to tie the fibers on the near side of the hook shank instead of the top. The hook eye helps to separate the hairs evenly.

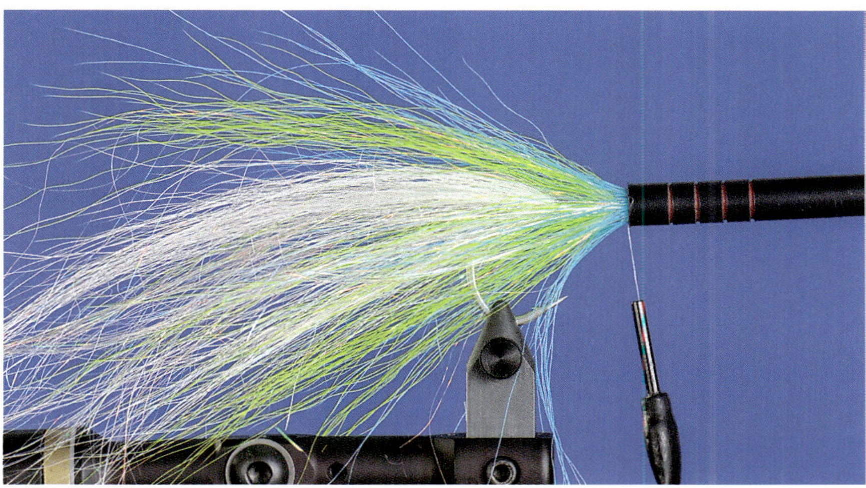

15. Push the fibers back with the pushing tool, grab the tips with your material hand, and bring the thread in front of the fibers. Wrap over the bases to get the angle that you desire.

(continued)

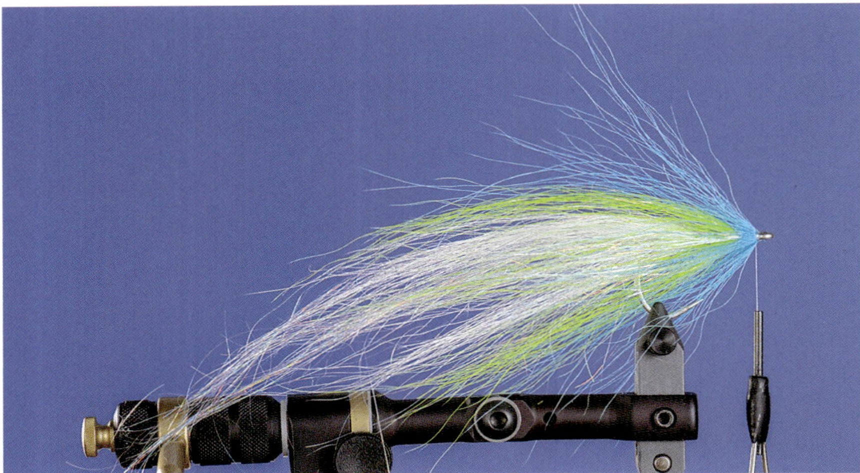

16. When the fibers are at the proper angle, tie off the fly. One of the reasons Hollow Fleyes look so pleasing in my opinion is because there's very little thread at the head. The material is secured completely at the butts, and the only visible thread is what is used to control the angle of the bucktail fibers. After you whip-finish, add head cement.

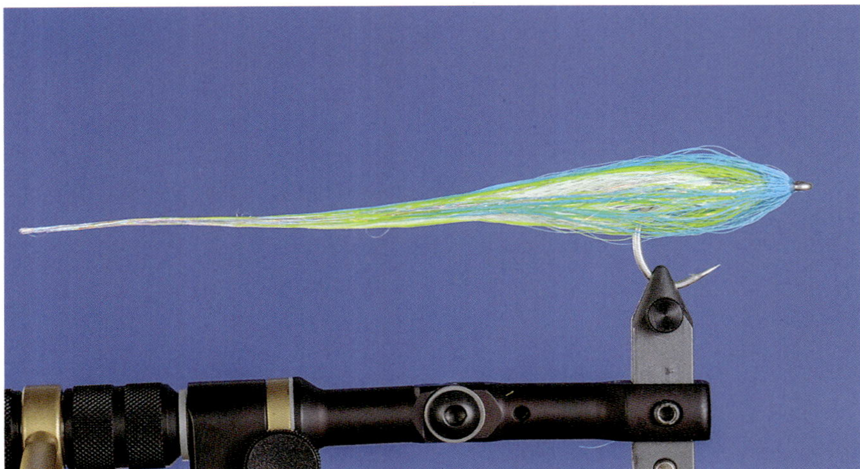

17. Before you wet it, this fly is going to look unruly. Most beginning tiers want to lay the fibers down. I have to remind them to leave the fly open and not try to tame it prematurely. After the fly has been wet and then dried, the tips will lie down and take on a beautiful curvature. Once this fly is dry completely, you can brush it with a comb.

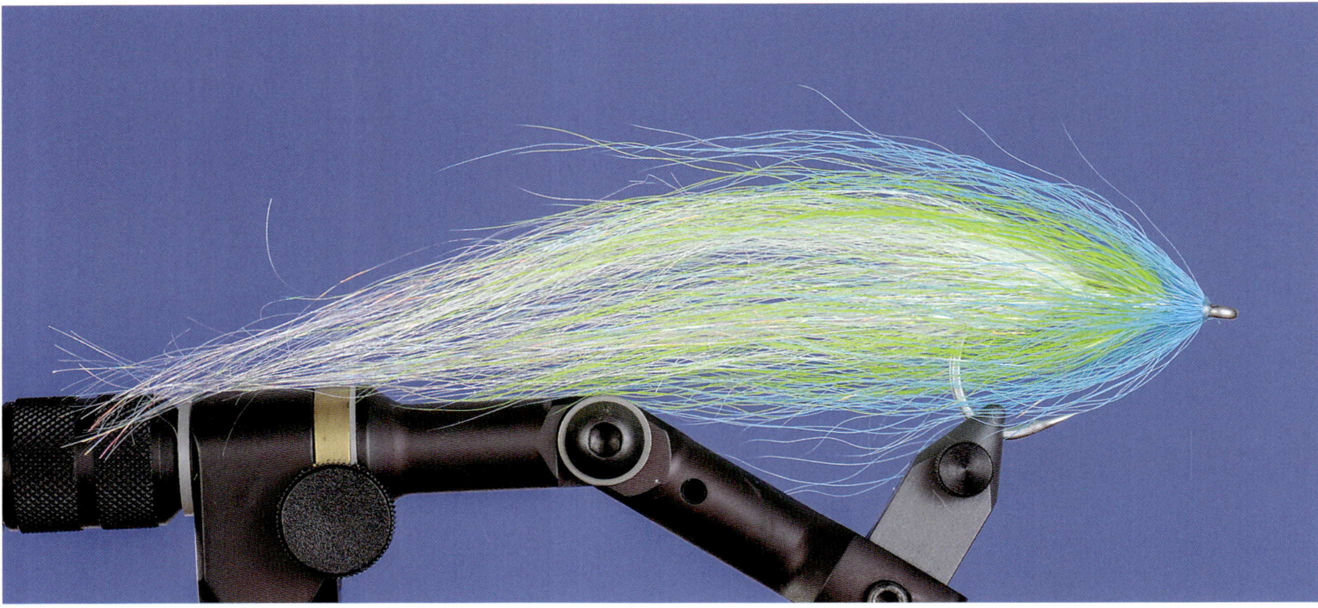

The fly is now dry and combed out. This is what the fly will look like in the water. Three basic lengths of bucktail: white is longest, chartreuse is three-quarters of that, and the blue is approximately three-quarters that of the chartreuse. On your flies, try to get a nice taper, with a roundness from the hook eye back.

TYING THE HIGH-RIDING HOLLOW

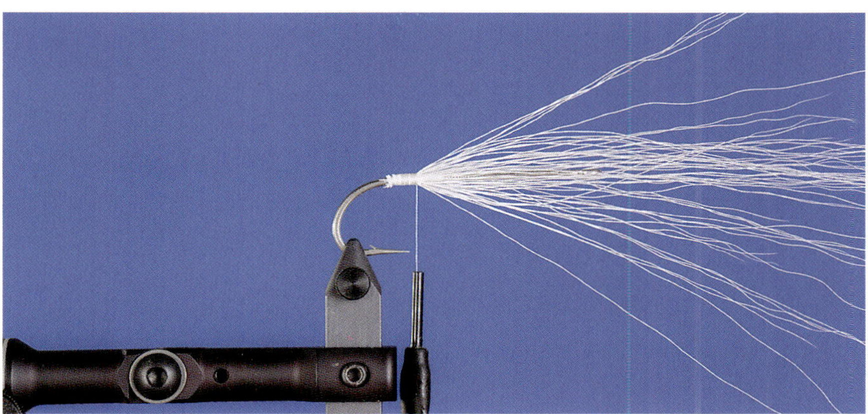

1. Insert a long-shank hook into the vise. This fly is going to require more applications of bucktail than the first one that we tied, so you need a longer platform. Wrap monofilament thread to the last third of the hook shank. Select your bucktail, remove the short hairs, and trim the butts evenly. Attach them with the tips forward and distribute the fibers equally around the shank. Wrap your thread to the transition point.

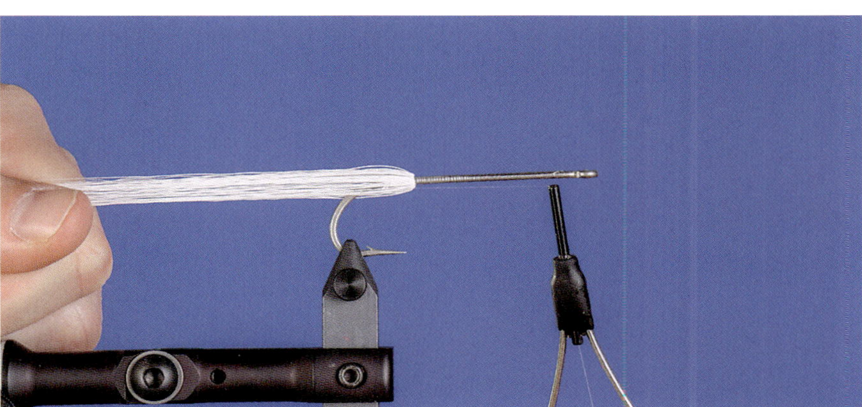

2. Push the hairs back with your tool, grab the tips with your material hand, and bring the thread in front of the fibers.

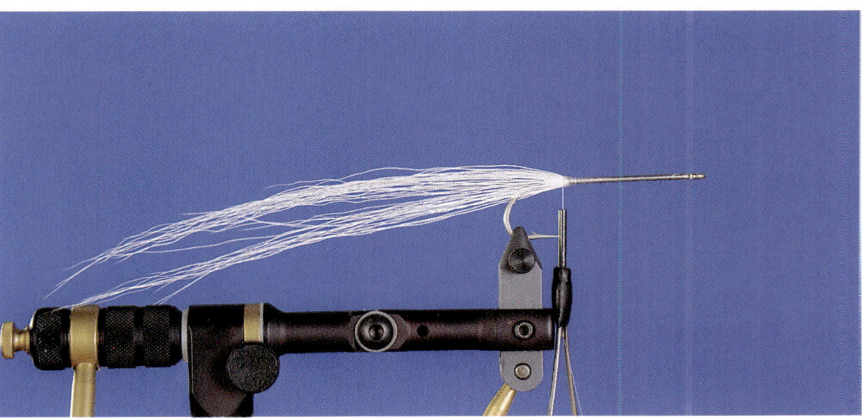

3. Since this is the first tie, keep the angle of the hair low and even with the hook shank.

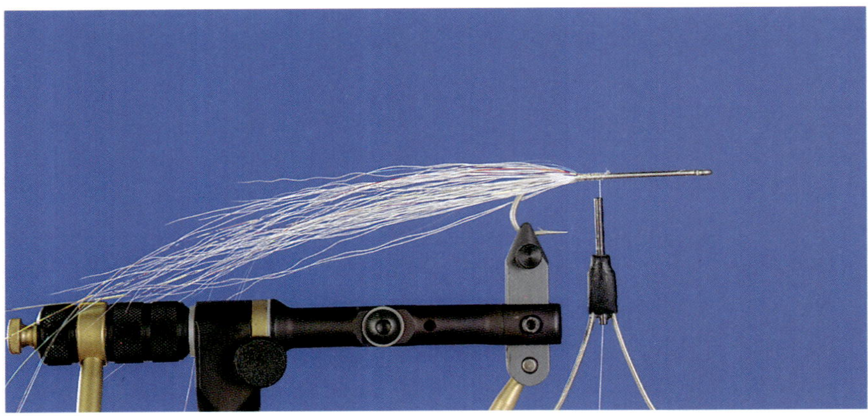

4. Apply some flash if you like and then wrap forward to the next tie-in point.

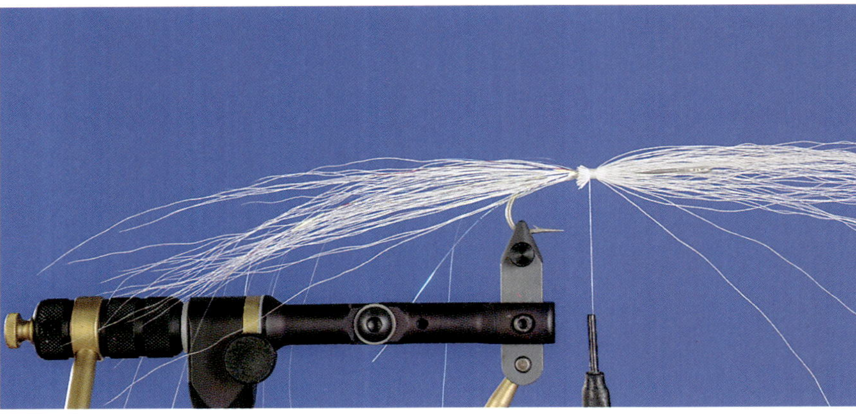

5. For the second application of bucktail, prepare the hair a little shorter than the first bundle of hair. Make sure you clean out the shortest fibers before you tie them in.

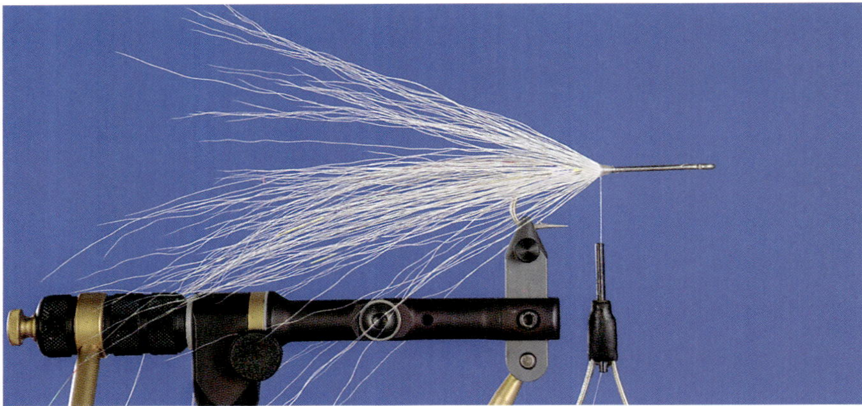

6. Push the hairs back and bring the thread in front of them. When you wrap back over the base of the fibers, make sure that you have an angle that is slightly higher than the previous tie. This begins the taper. If you like, tie in flash between each application of bucktail. Wrap the thread forward to the next tie-in point.

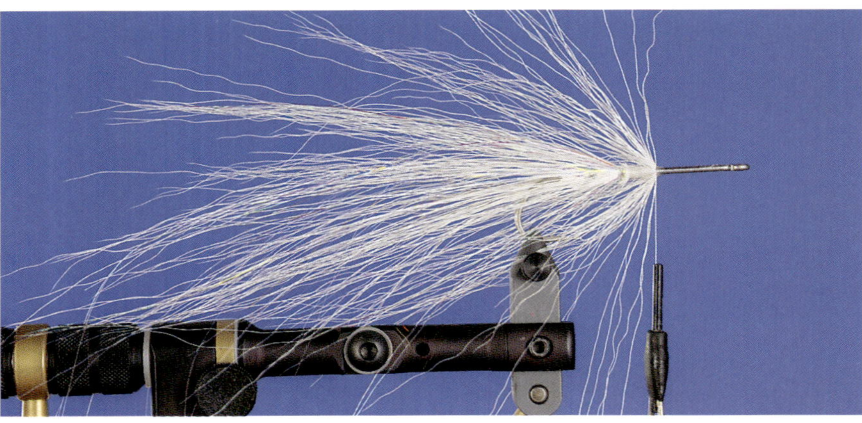

7. Tie in another bunch of hair, but keep a higher angle.

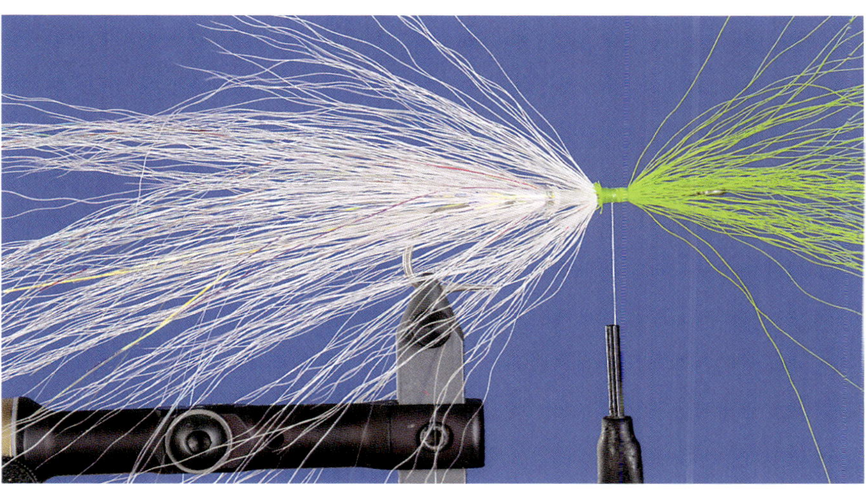

8. Now we are going to introduce another color. Remember to choose hairs that are slightly shorter than the previous hairs for taper and remove most short hairs before tying down the bunch. Tie down in reverse only at this time. The thread should be positioned in the center of the tie-down wraps for the next step. I am going to illustrate one way of using the space in between each of the Hollow ties.

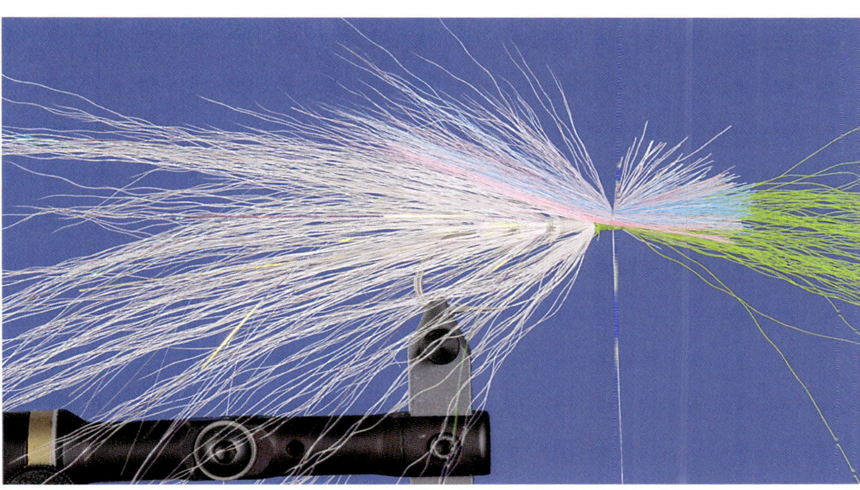

9. For the belly section, I blend light pink and light blue hairs using the technique shown on page 32. These hairs need to be shorter than the overall length of the chartreuse or collar hairs. These ties sit inside the main collar and provide subtle colors and create a little bulk in the forward portion of the fly. Tie down the prepared hairs in the space created by the reverse tie. Take a couple wraps of thread around the fibers and distribute them around the shank. Once they are in position, tighten the thread wraps and flare the fibers.

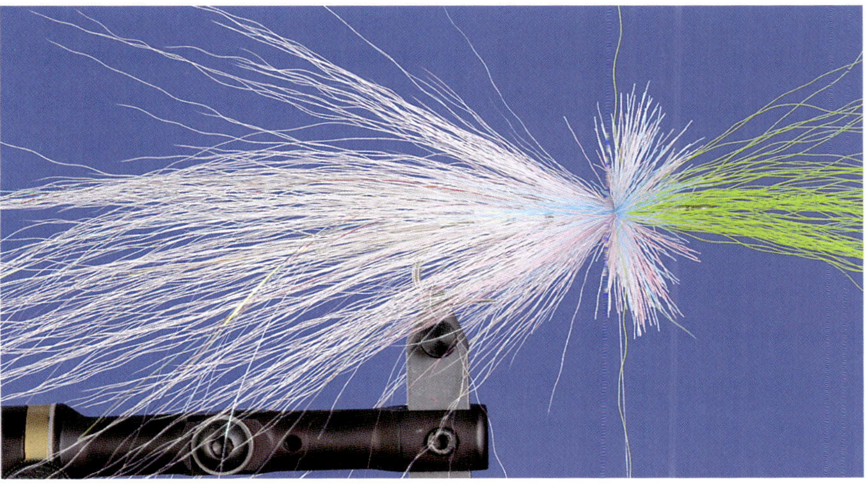

10. Make sure the fibers are distributed completely around the hook shank. Securely tie them down with a few tight wraps of thread and let the bobbin hang.

(continued)

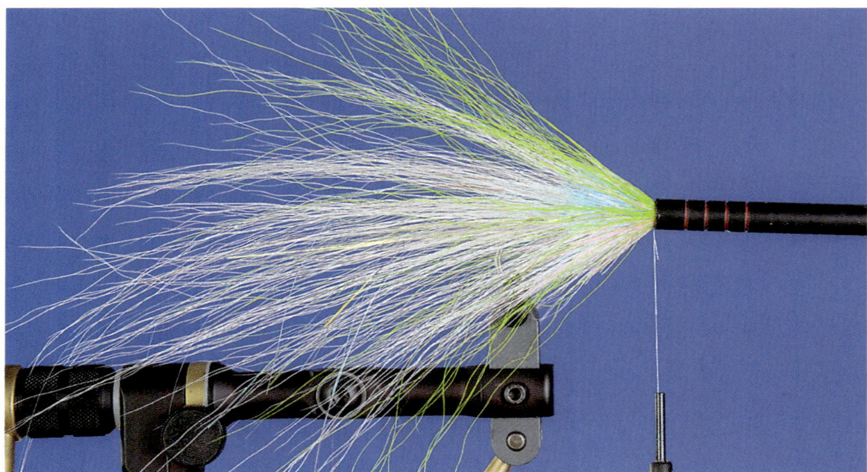

11. Push all the fibers back and bring the thread in front of them. Wrap back over their bases to control the fiber angle.

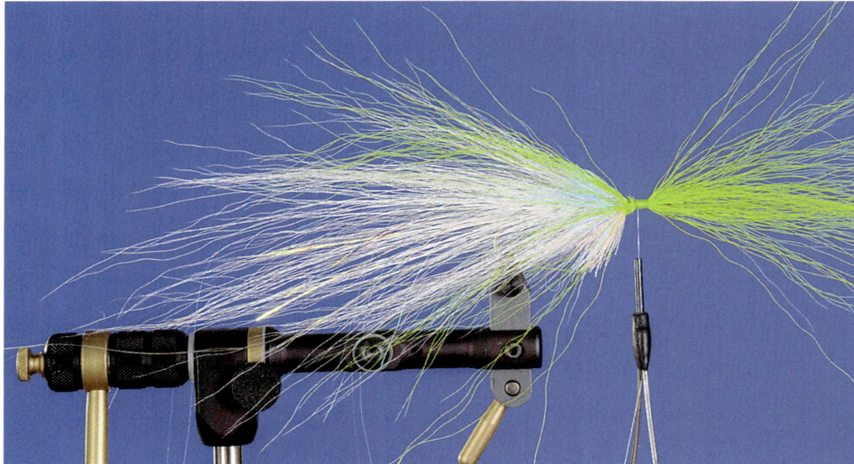

12. Move the thread forward to accept the next bunch of bucktail for the collar.

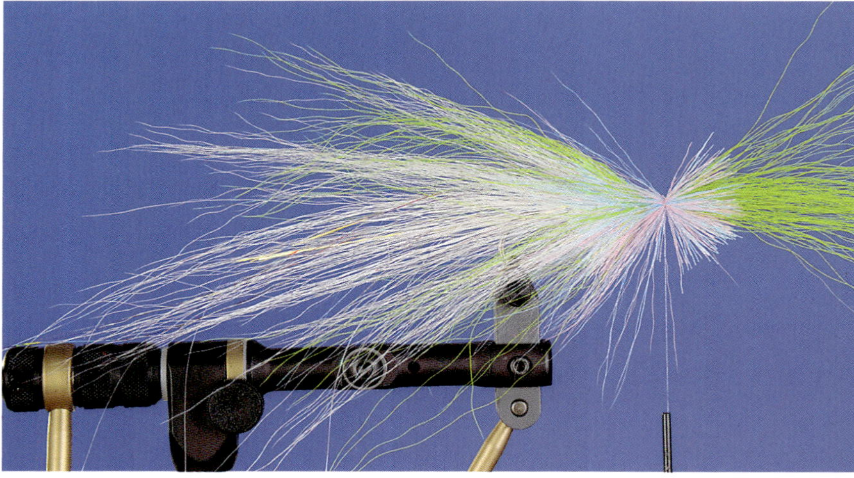

13. After you tie down the collar, tie in the multicolored belly hairs in the middle of the collar tie-down point and distribute them around the shank.

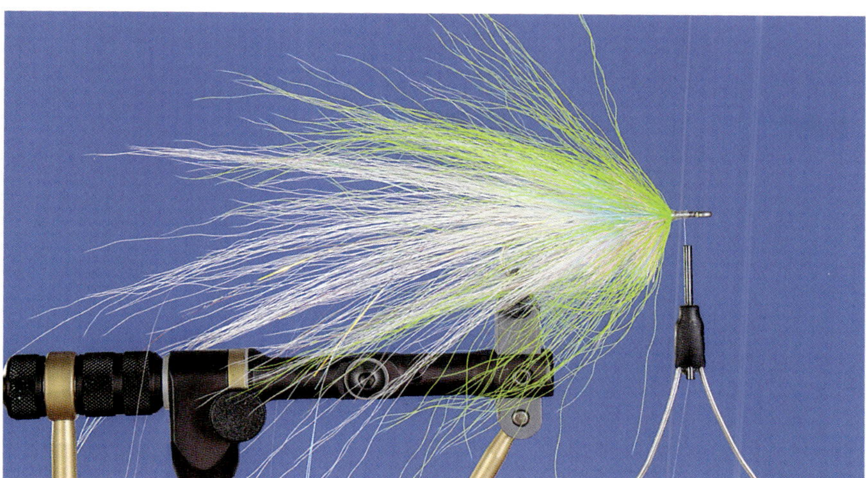

14. Push all the fibers back with your pushing tool, dam them up at the angle shown, and then wrap the thread forward to the next tie-in point.

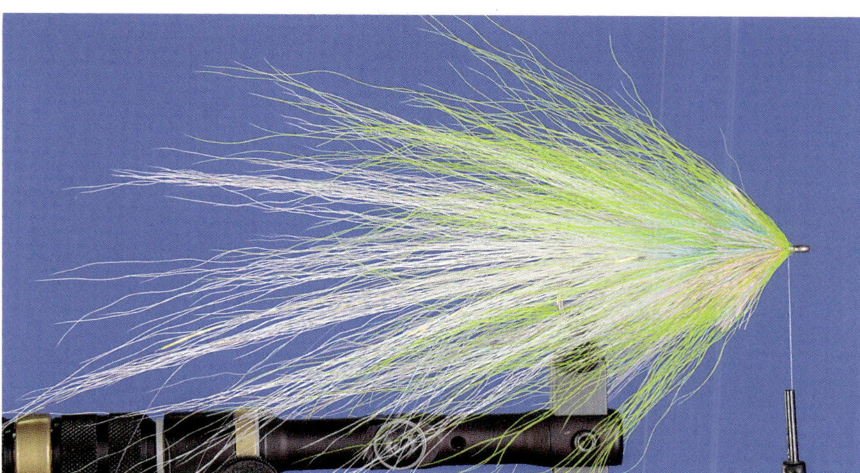

15. Tie in another section of collar, and then tie in the multicolored belly hairs in the middle of the collar tie-down point. Push all the fibers back with your pushing tool and then dam them up at the angle shown.

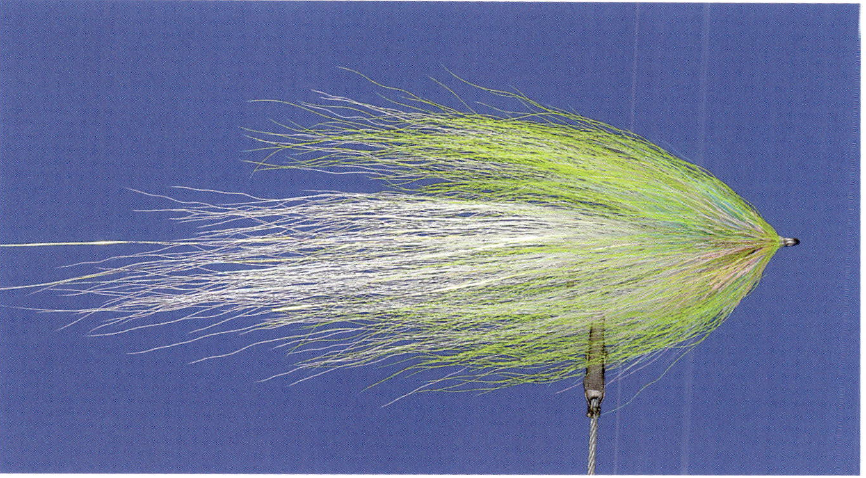

16. Note the taper of hairs and the fullness of the head section where the inner collar is within the main collar.

Hollow Fleyes

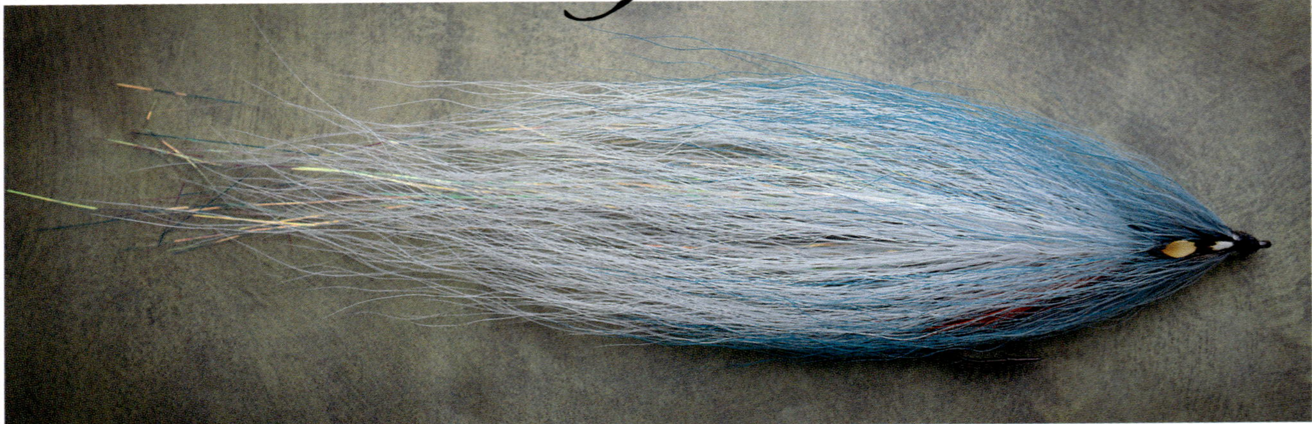

Very popular color of blue and white with jungle cock eyes and a little gill red feather in the right spot. Just a hint of Angel Hair Flash adds excitement.

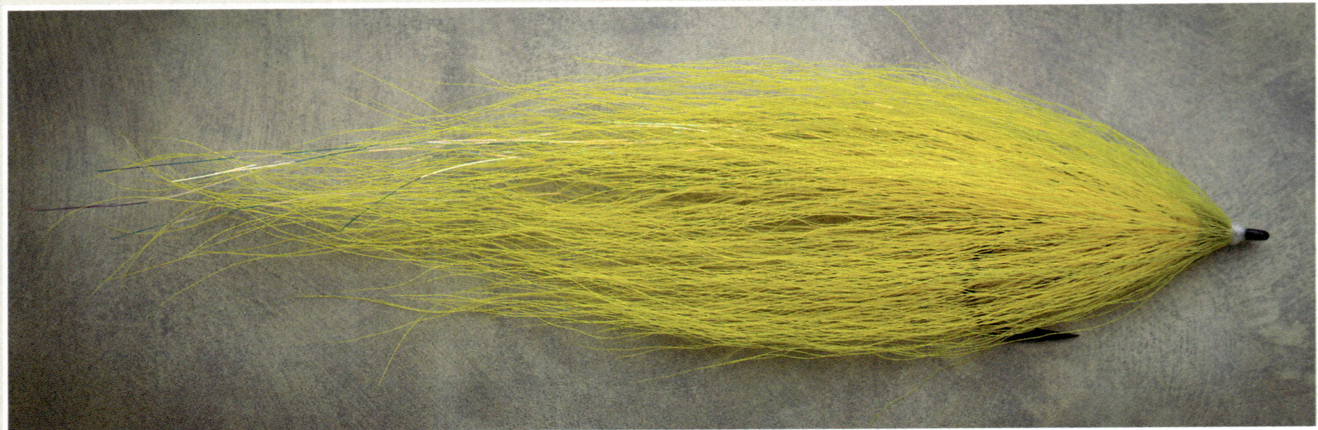

Large yellow Hollow. I like this color when fishing dirty water.

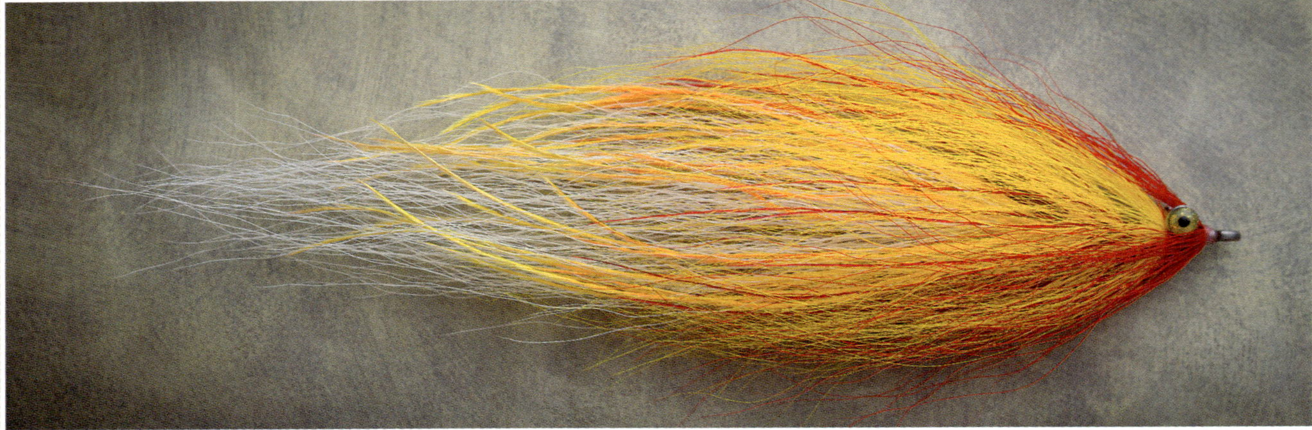

Huge Hollow with ostrich feathers added to increase movement. Lead dumbbell eyes are added for a little different retrieve motion. Often, having the weight so far forward on Hollow Fleyes is an asset to casting.

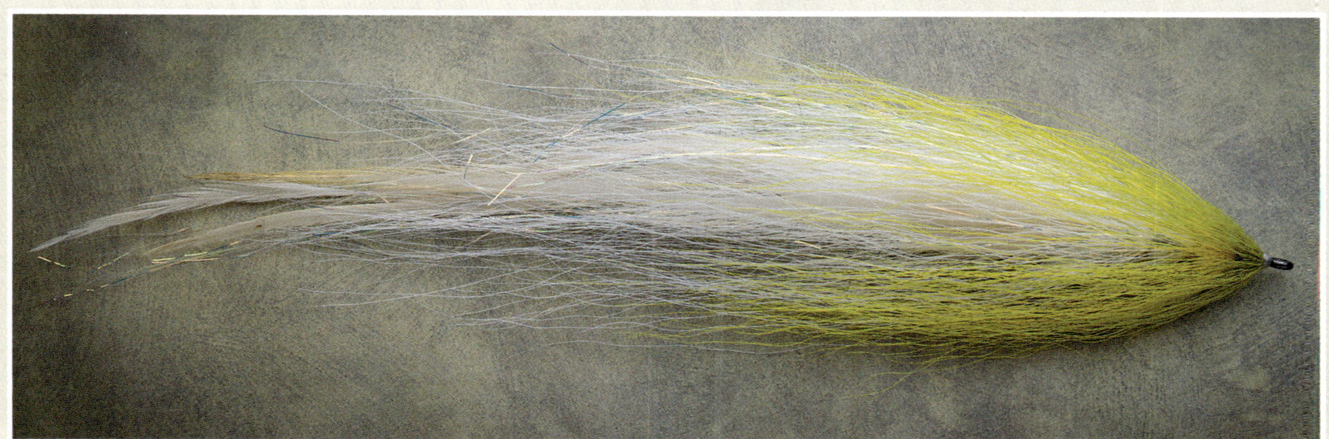

A narrower Hollow that sports a few long saddle hackles for added length and action.

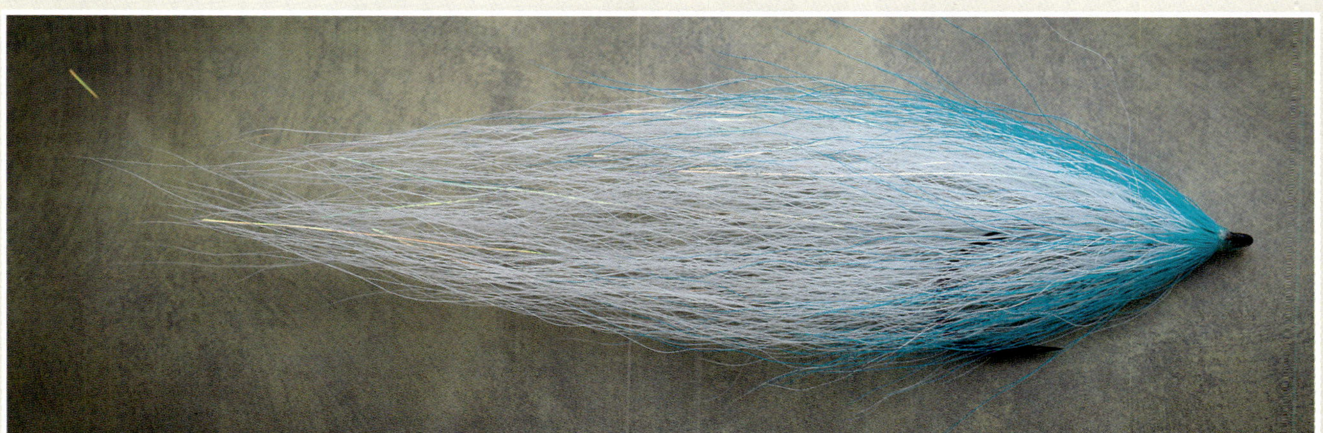

Offshore blue and white Hollow illustrates an open and full-volume fleye. No bulk materials—just the Hollow technique!

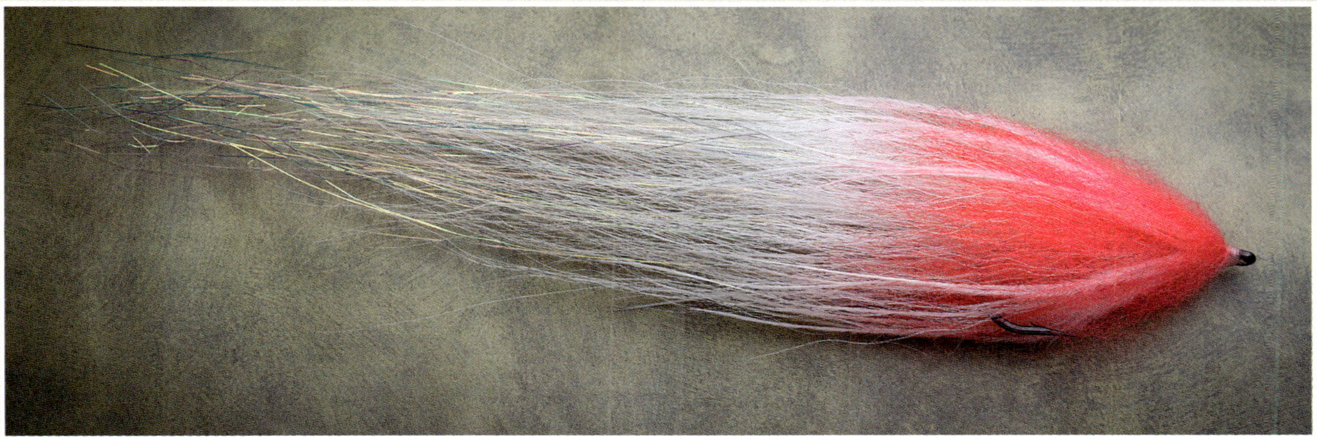

One of my favorites: a Hollow with gold pearl Angel Hair, bucktail, fleece, and ostrich collar. The fleece provides instant fullness to the head and pulls it all together smoothly.

Chapter 9

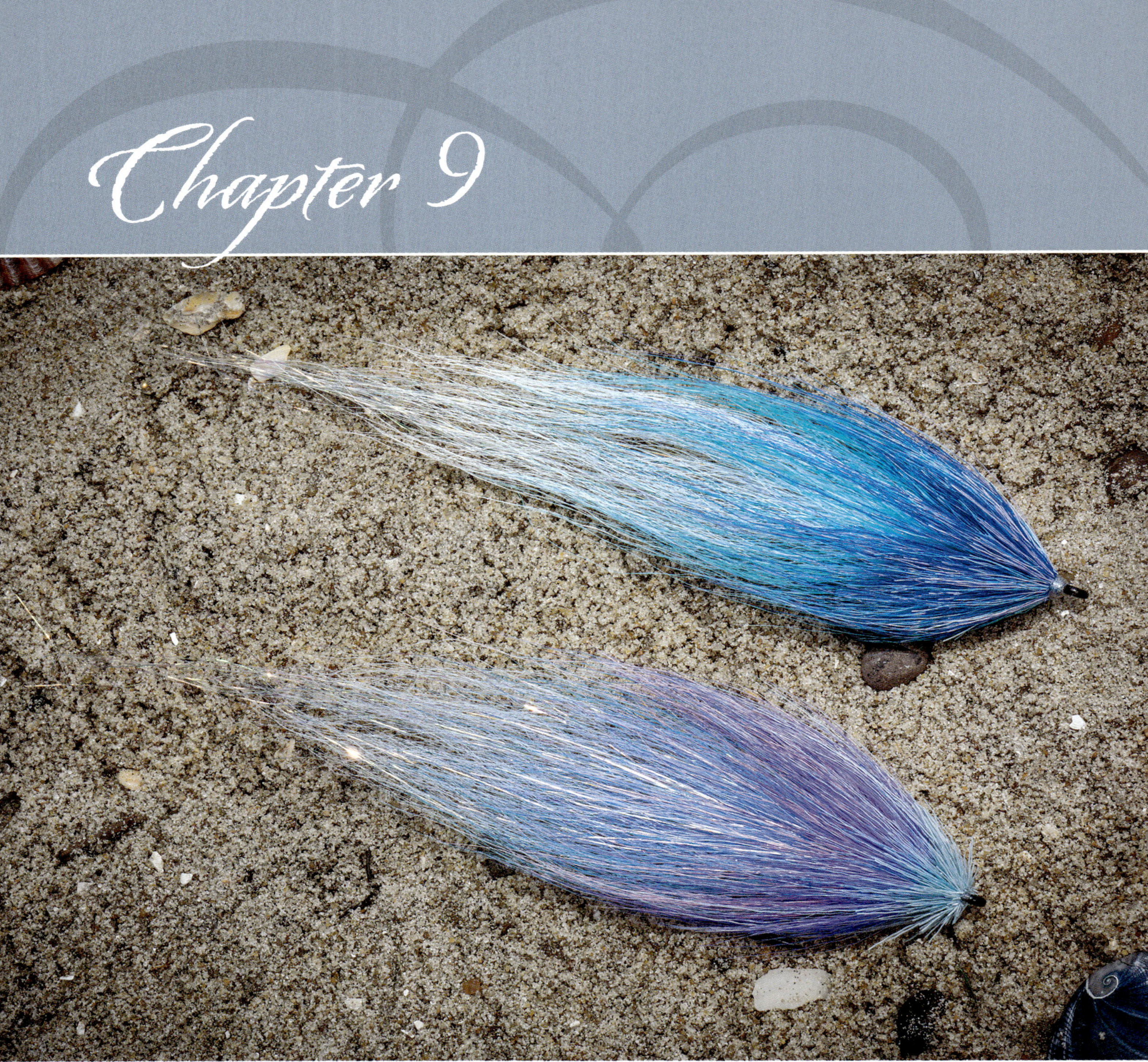

The BULKhead's taper mimics the natural lines of baitfish. Because the tapered ends of the spun deer hair head are left intact at each step, the bulk remains somewhat concealed underneath the longer fibers. The combination of the large head and the tapered tail creates an enticing action. One of the secrets of this fly is that if you try to be too perfect with it, the overall look of the pattern won't turn out right. You almost have to be sloppy and rough with your tying to make this fly look and fish right.

BULKhead Deceiver

The High-Riding Hollow from the last chapter demonstrates that when you add flared hair before bringing back the Hollow tie, you can achieve a wonderful veil of wispy bucktail over a more substantial tie that includes the butts of the bucktail fibers and shorter, tapered ends. By successively creating the front portion of the fly in this manner, I soon saw that I could create an inner bulk without interrupting the overall flow and taper of the fly.

From these results, the BULKhead Deceiver was born. The rear of the fly is tied more or less like a standard Bucktail Deceiver. As you come forward into the shoulders and head of the fly, you introduce slightly longer flared butts from the more hollow fibers at the base of the tail. The result, when it goes well, seamlessly integrates a flared deer hair head into the overall body taper and form of the Bucktail Deceiver. The trick of the fly is to maintain a smooth, uninterrupted profile from sparse tail to robust head that is aesthetically pleasing and natural looking while creating a head with enough presence to push water and kick the tail.

One of the great things about this fly is that it relies on the long fibers from the base of a bucktail with hollow butts—the fibers that most tiers discard. Sometimes this hair is cut off on commercial tails, but if not, you are in luck. The best fibers will flare easily and are still fine and soft enough to lie back and create the BULKhead. The perfect fibers are wider at the base of the fiber and hold the hollowness longer toward the tip.

When tying in the fibers, I do not spin them; instead, I just distribute them around the shank and then flare them, similar to what Bill Catherwood and Lou Tabory have done with their flies. Once the butts are flared and trimmed only slightly, you wrap back over their bases with a thread dam so that they lie back in a conical shape at approximately a 45-degree angle (angle depends on overall taper of head). The tips from the next tie will cover them so that you obtain a smooth, continuous taper on the outside of the fly. The loose flare (instead of the tightly spun and trimmed head typical of bass bugs) creates a bulky head that still pushes water and doesn't compact the butts so much that you have to spend excessive time trimming them. Part of the fly's visual appeal and fishiness is in its slightly unkempt appearance, and that is one of the secrets to tying a good one as well.

The technique of using flared butts to create bulk within a fly can be adapted in many ways, and it is still one of my favorite techniques for finishing a Hollow Fleye. And you don't always have to tie the butts in to the right. You can also tie in the fibers Hollow-style, with the tips to the right, to create a different effect. Place the butt ends toward the hook bend, then encircle the hairs with thread and pull tightly to the shank, flaring the butts to about 40 to 60 degrees. Secure the wraps in place, and

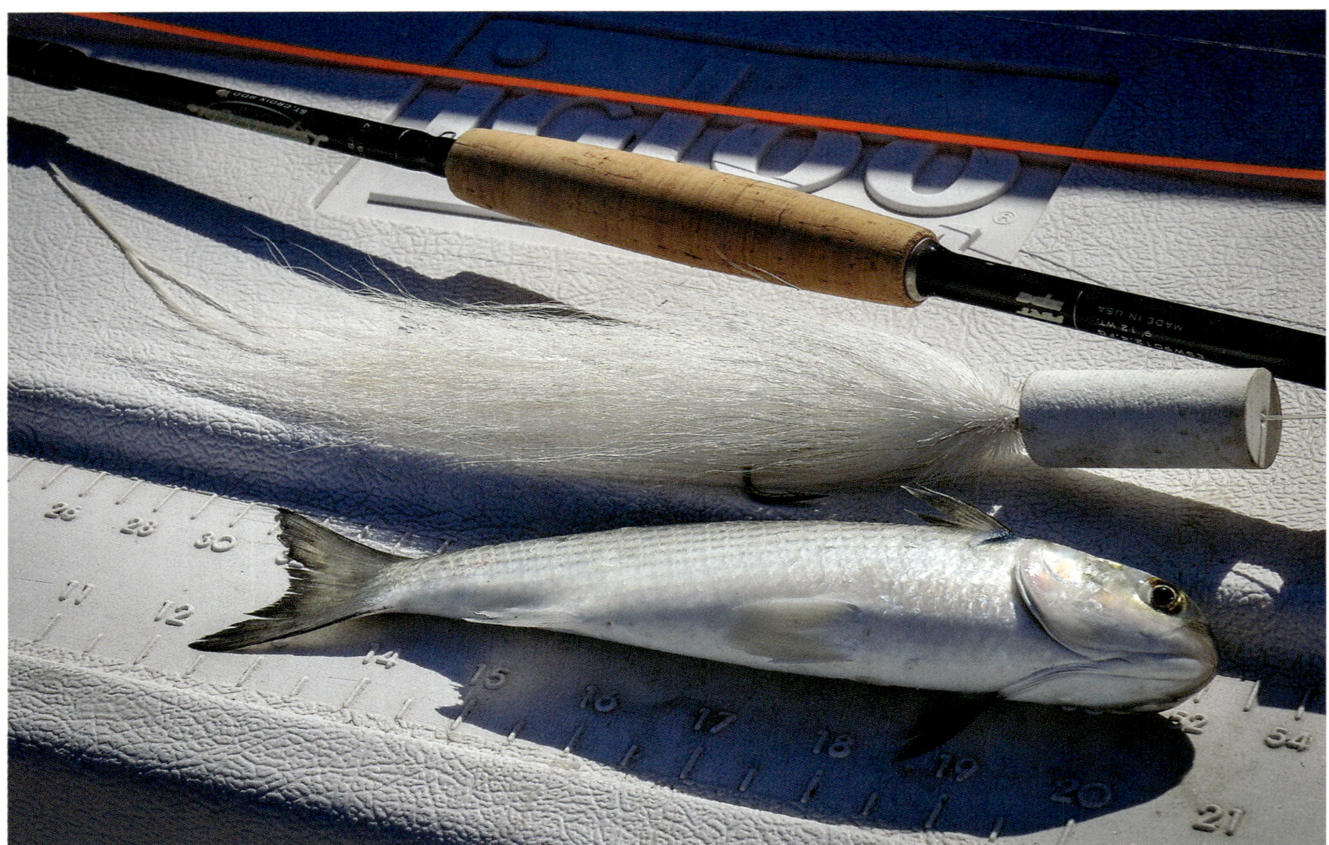

As a fly guy trying to get big fish from the beach, I will often go to a BULKhead and Banger setup. The Banger head creates all sorts of commotion, and the BULKhead (this one tied on a mono extension) just dances behind it. Try fishing this setup with either a steady swim retrieve or with an occasional "pop" or two. You can also move the Banger head forward on the leader to allow the fly to dangle enticingly below the surface.

then sneak the thread in front of the transition point. Pull the tips to the rear, and build the thread against the butt hairs. Some tiers may find this an easier method to create the BULK in the BULKhead Deceiver.

A good BULKhead is hard to predict, and the hair must dictate its use. If I get to the BULKhead portion of a BULKhead Deceiver and the hair doesn't react the way I need it to, then I will finish the fly as a regular Bucktail Deceiver. You have to listen to the material, and this fly, perhaps more than any other, requires instinctive, seat-of-your-pants tying. One nice BULKhead usually inspires a batch, because once I find the bucktail that is going to work nicely for the BULK portion, I get to tying them right then and there, or I at least save the tail in a bag marked "BULKhead." This is a fun fly to tie. When tied right, it looks even better than the best plug in a surf caster's bag.

BULKhead Deceiver (Mullet)

Hook:	Gamakatsu SL12S or similar
Thread:	Fine monofilament
Body:	White bucktail
Head:	Light blue and natural brown bucktail (coarse)

TYING THE BULKHEAD DECEIVER (MULLET)

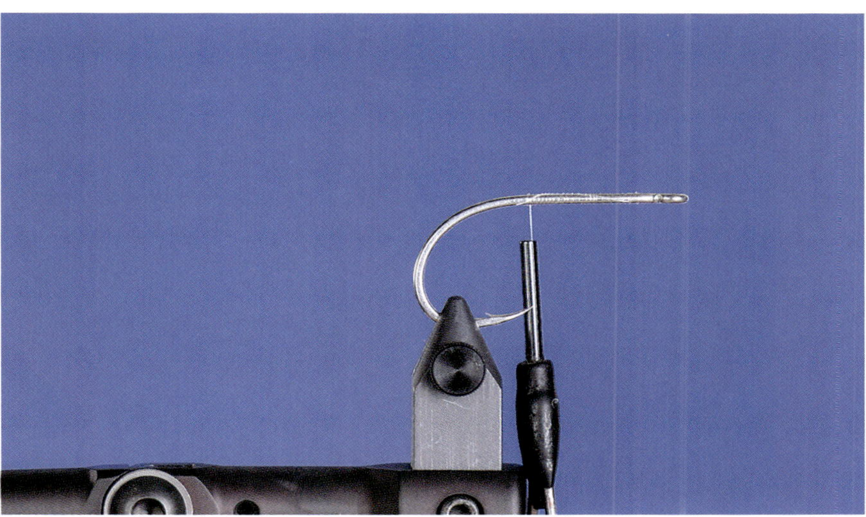

1. Insert the hook into the vise. Cover the entire shank with thread, and then bring the thread back to a point just before the bend so that you are tying only on the straight part of the shank.

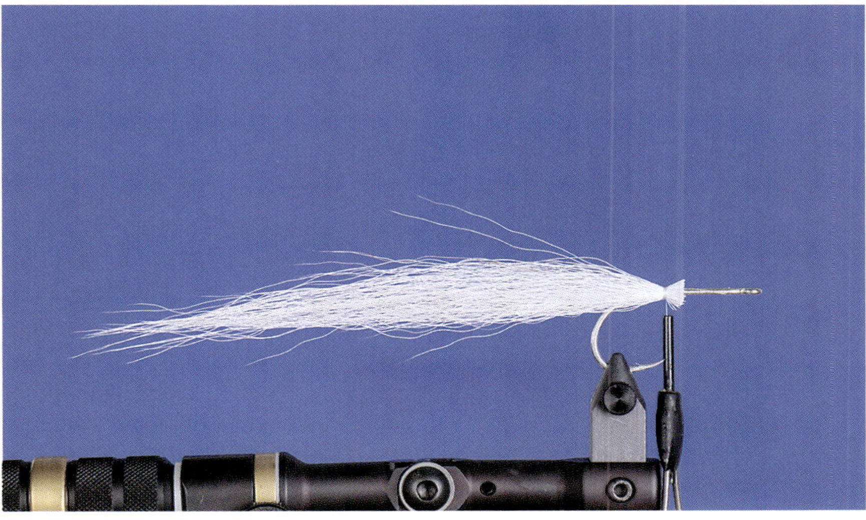

2. The rear portion of this fly is tied exactly like the Bucktail Deceiver. Prepare the bucktail by removing most of the short hairs, cutting the ends straight, and tying it in so that the fibers are distributed 360 degrees around the shank. Apply head cement before wrapping down over the butts.

(continued)

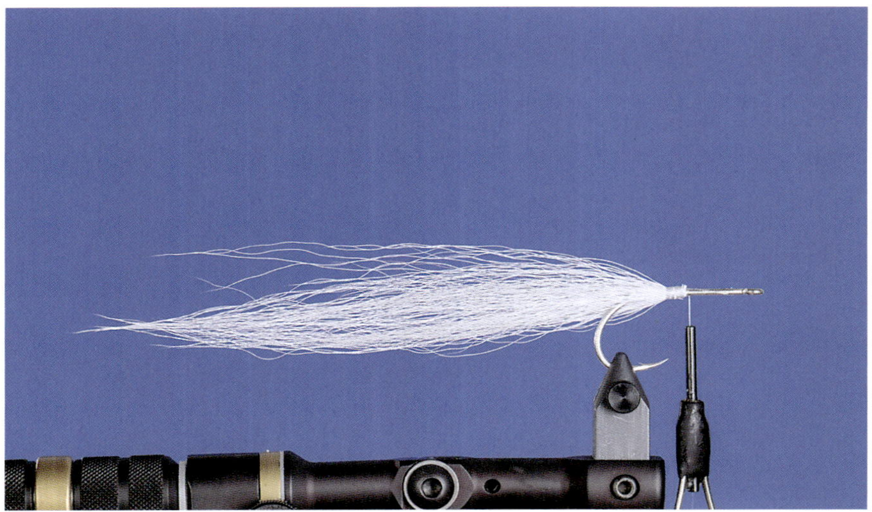

3. Wrap the thread over the butts to the next tie-in point. At this time, I will often use a bodkin to make sure the fibers are straight and distributed around the shank, over the bend of the hook.

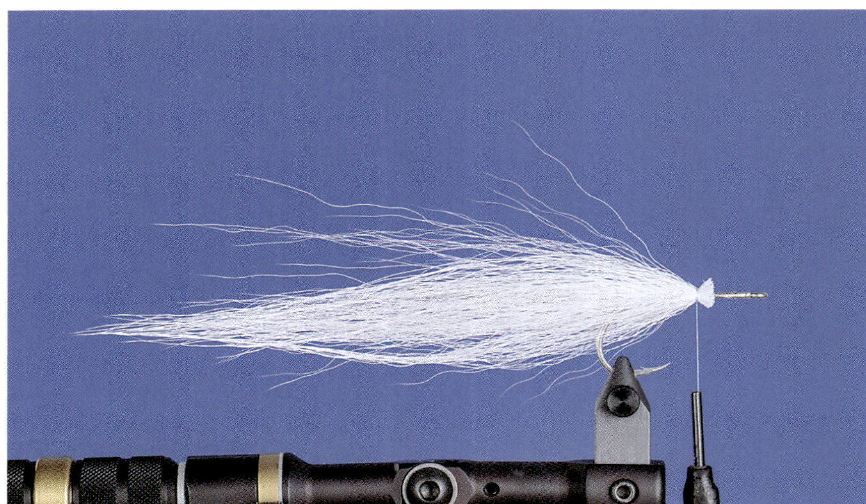

4. Tie in another bundle of fibers with approximately the same fiber count as the previous bundle. Distribute them evenly around the shank.

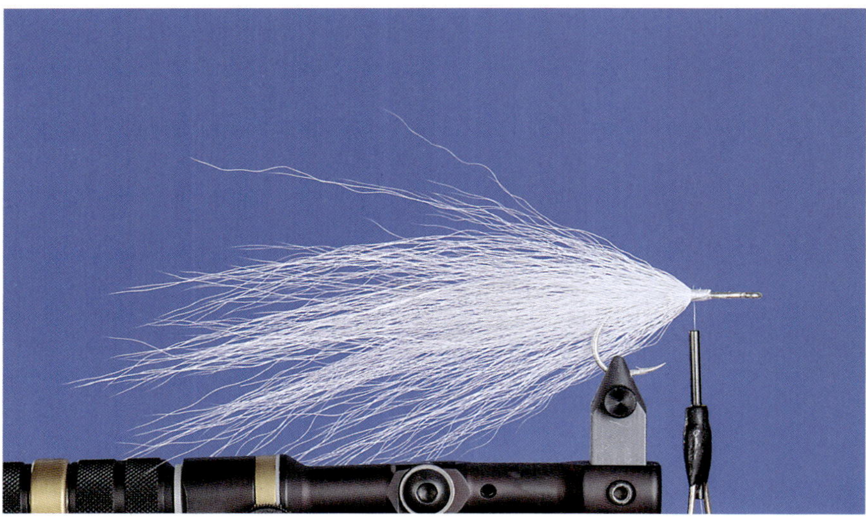

5. Make sure that you have a nice, uninterrupted taper in preparation for the front portion of the fly. The key to a good BULKhead is a smooth, continuous taper throughout, so try to maintain the flow of the fly. Note that the bobbin is positioned back toward the previous clump. You are going to tie the next step on top of this level base created by the thread and even butts.

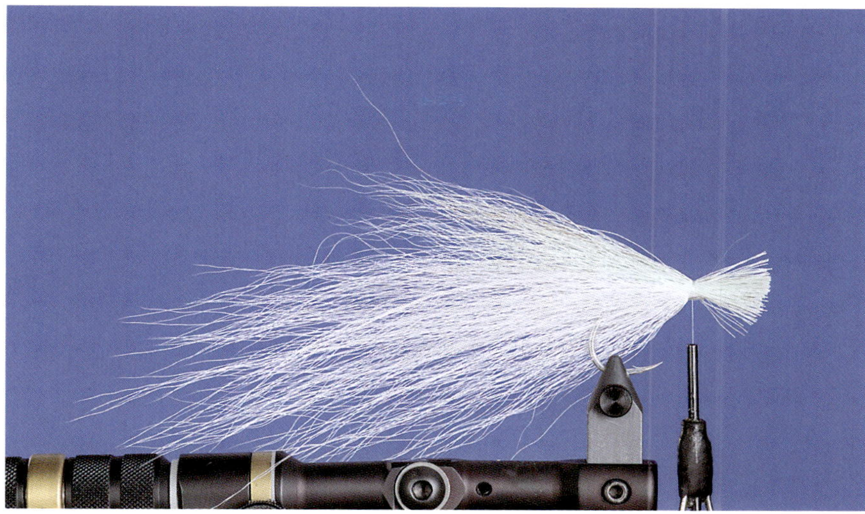

6. For the BULKhead collar, choose hairs from the base of the tail. Here we are using light blue and tan. If you use multiple colors, you can mix them or put them one on top of the other. The hair should be long enough to veil the wing and stiff enough to flare the butts to create a spun head. When you tie in the hair, the tips need to create a veil around the wing and the flared butts should be about 3/4 inch to 1 inch in length. This step shows bucktail controlled with three or four 360-degree wraps of thread around the fibers. The hairs have been maneuvered completely around the hook shank. The bobbin weight now holds the hairs in place.

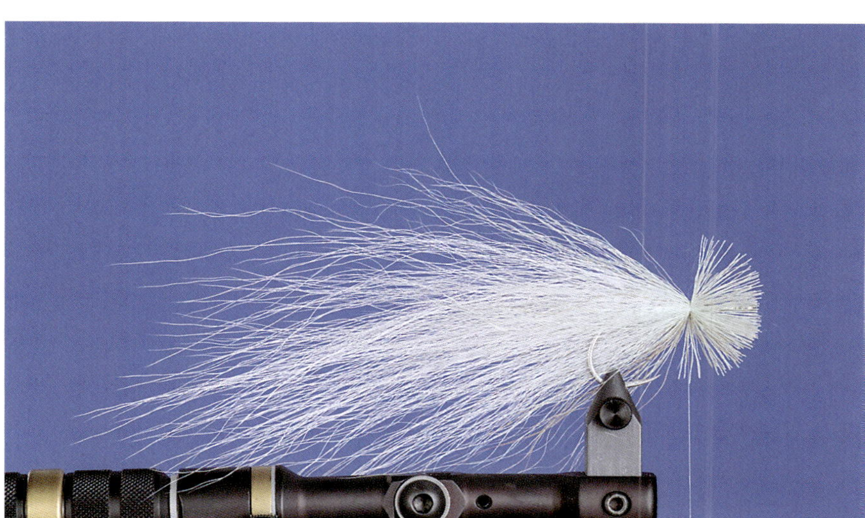

7. Pull the thread straight down, tightening all the fibers equally into the shank. Two more tight wraps will secure the hairs and flare the hollow fibers.

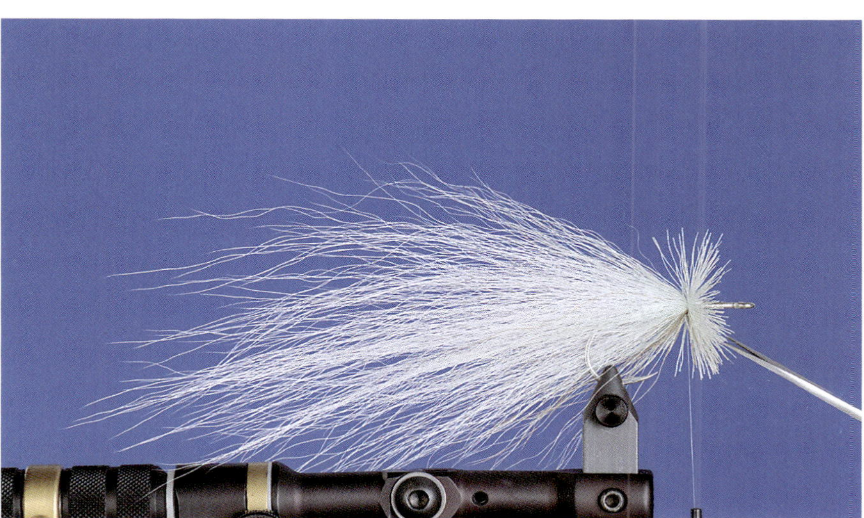

8. Trim the fibers closest to the hook shank to different lengths (not too much, no more than 1/8 inch) to get a head start on the taper, which will be more apparent when you push the fibers back. After trimming, push the fibers back with a pushing tool, move the thread in front of the butts, and wrap against their bases, forming a small thread dam and setting the angle of the fibers at approximately 45 to 60 degrees. Move the thread forward to the next tie-in point.

(continued)

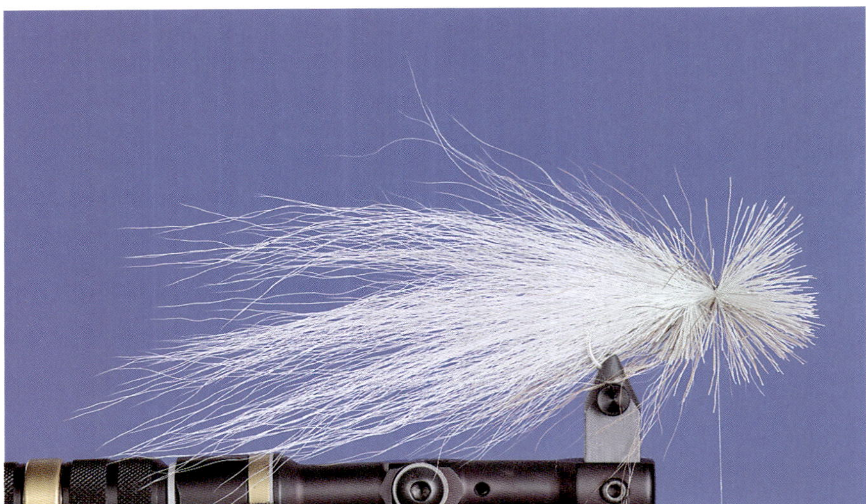

9. Continue to tie in bundles of hair until the hook shank is full, trimming the butts each time before you dam them up. Remember, do *not* cut the bucktail tips off at any time—they are important.

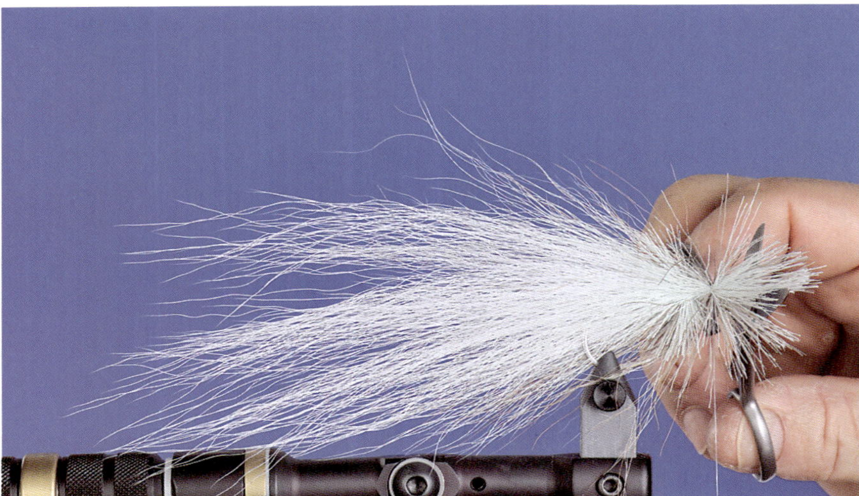

10. Once the fiber butts extend beyond the eye it is a lot easier to trim them. Here you can snip straight before pushing them back because there is no hook eye or shank in the way.

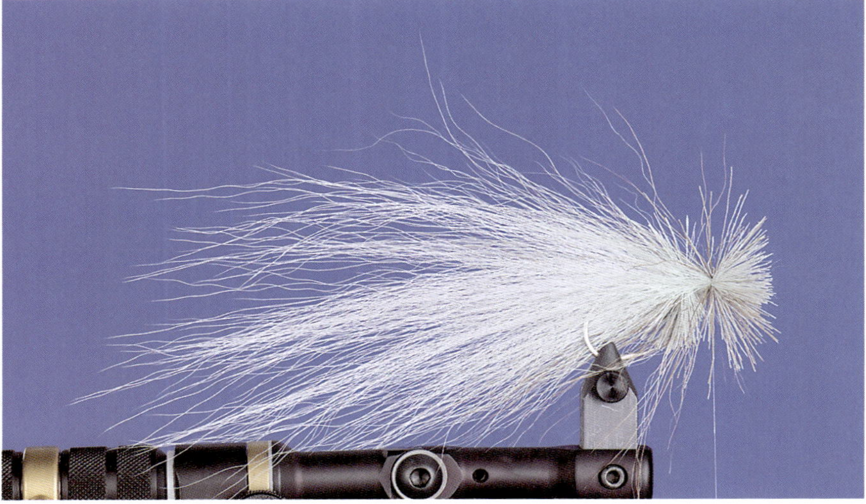

11. A simple straight cut will create enough taper when you push them back.

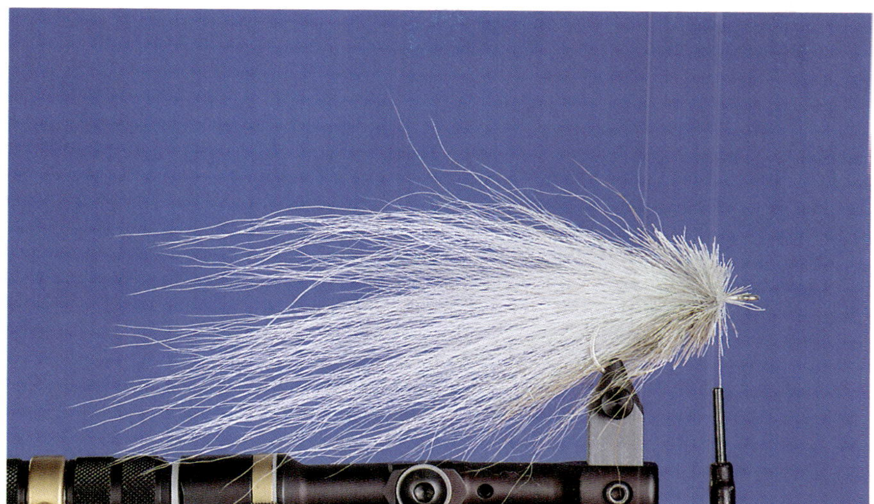

12. Move the thread forward. Sometimes I will use a comb or bodkin to separate any crisscrossed fibers. You want the fibers to be as free as possible so that you can see the shape of the fly as it is being tied.

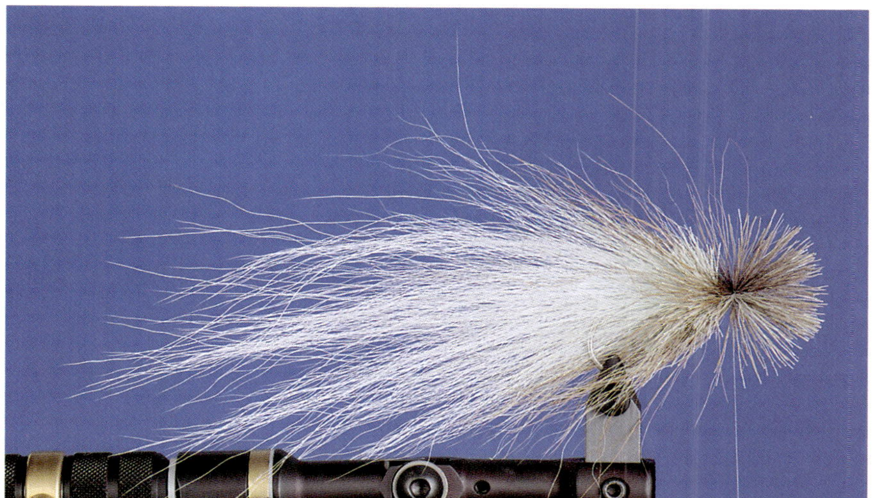

13. Apply the last collar of bucktail at the hook eye. Distribute the butts around the shank and flare them.

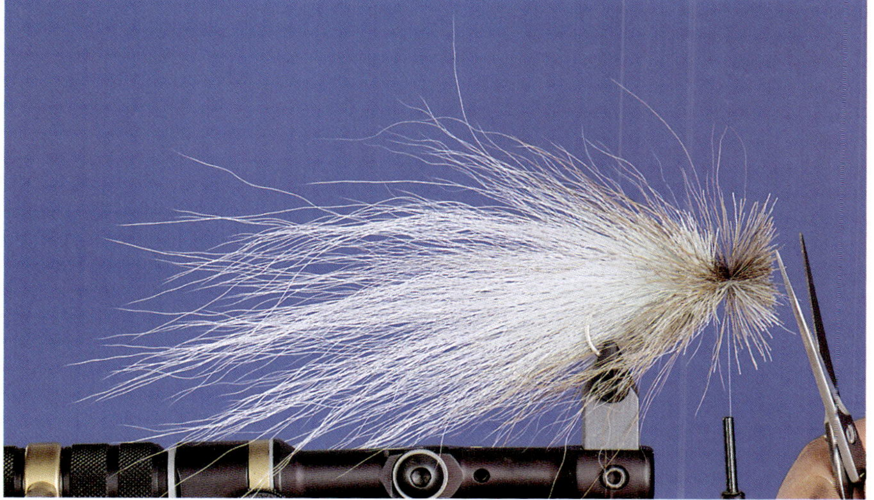

14. Trim the butts.

(continued)

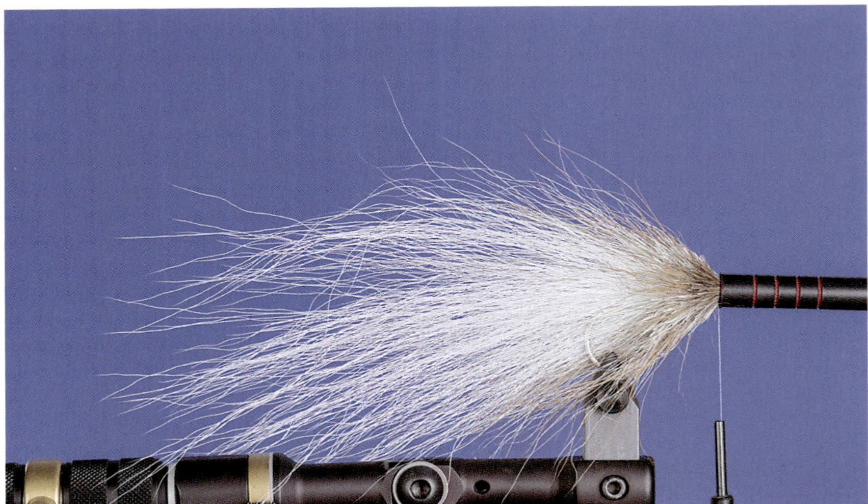

15. Push the fibers back with a pushing tool. I am using a hollow plastic tube from a ballpoint pen. Note the taper and the four distinct ties. If they weren't trimmed, they wouldn't look right.

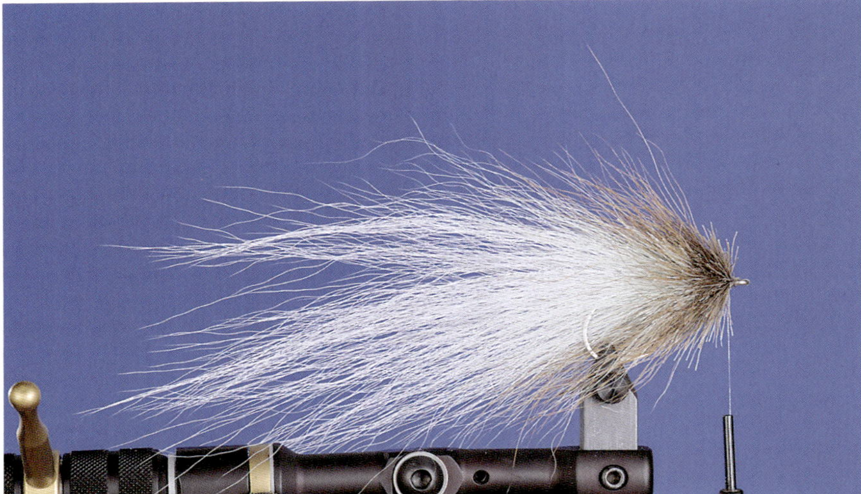

16. Move the thread in front of the butts, whip-finish, snip the thread, and add head cement.

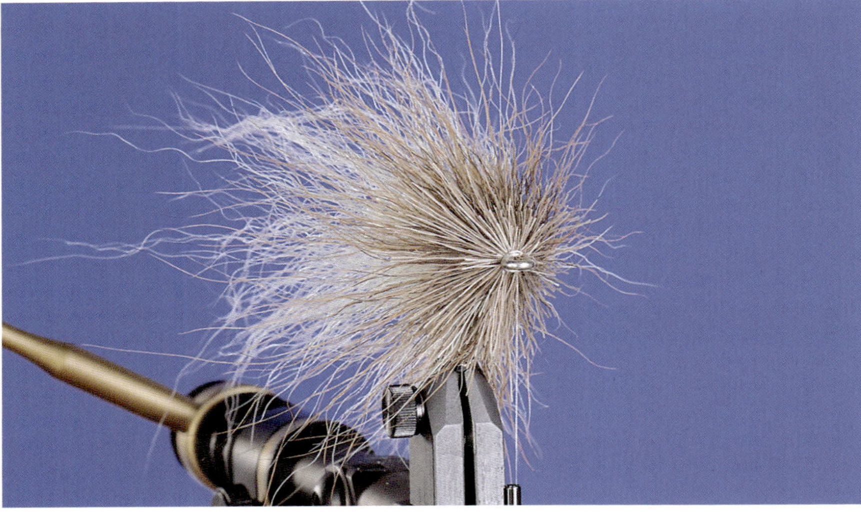

17. Front view. The irregular ends of the butts help the feathering of the taper.

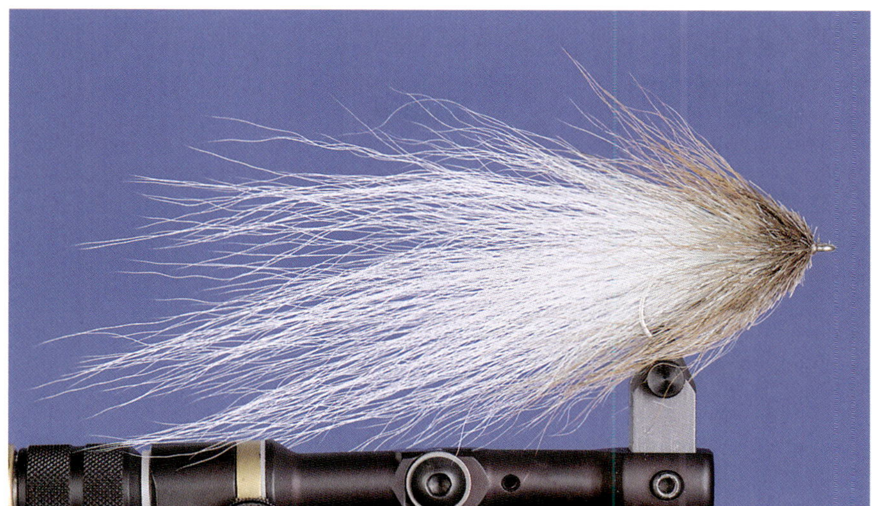

18. The BULKhead Deceiver is finished. One of the beautiful things about this fly is that it retains its taper from the bulky head to the tail, yet the bulk in the front of the fly is enough to move the tapered tail. By flaring the butts instead of spinning them you get a much more pleasing and seamless result.

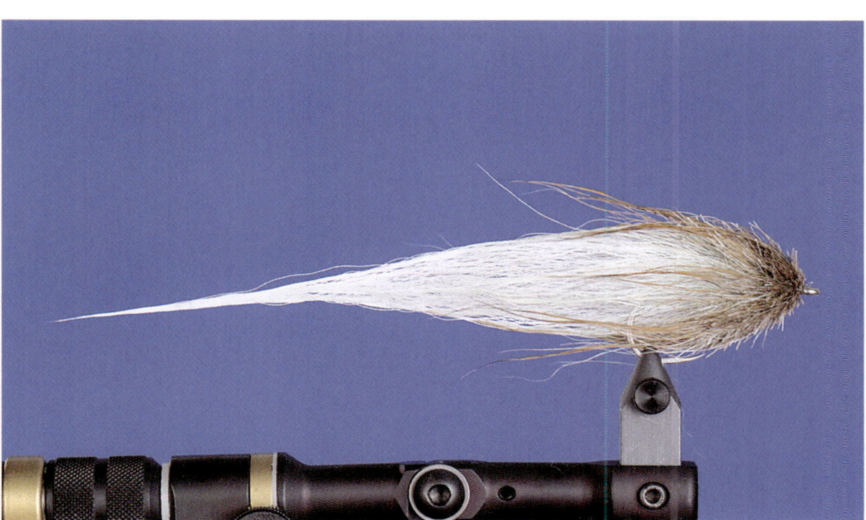

19. For the final trimming stage, wet the entire fly so that you can control the hairs and also see any butts that need to be trimmed easier. Grab the tapered tips, and hold them back so that the stiffer butt hairs stick up and you can trim them. For this fly I did not have to do a lot of trimming after it was tied, but I did snip a few of the longer butts in the head. Do not make it perfect—just a rough trim is best.

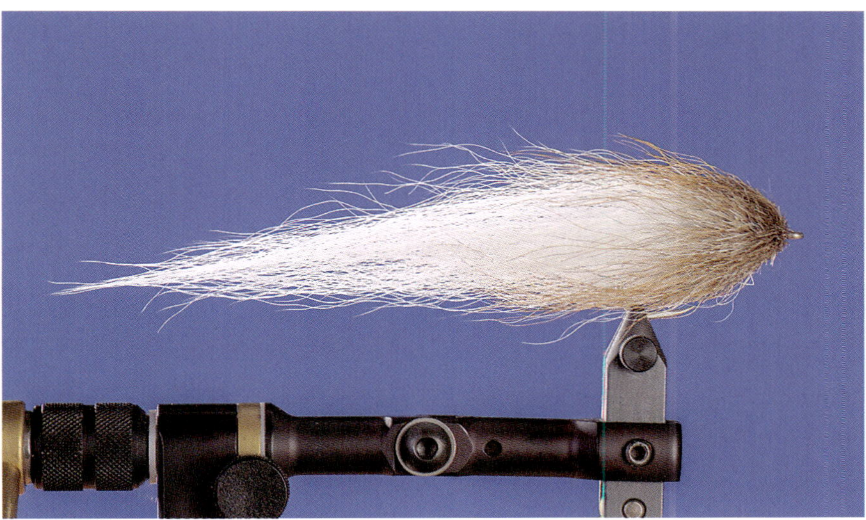

20. This fly is a simple example of a mullet shape. You can add ostrich herl, long saddles, and/or flash.

BULKheads

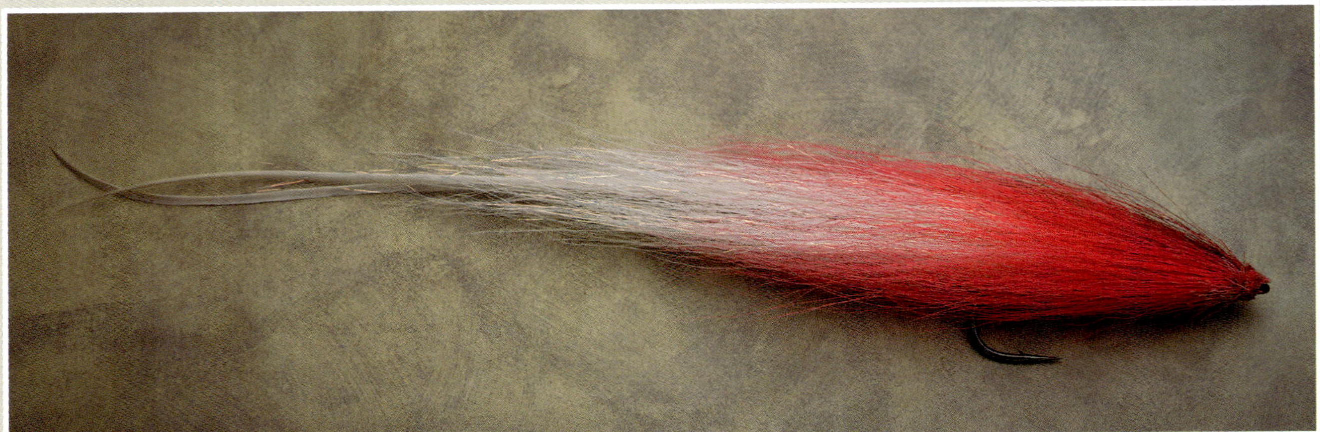

Red and white classic. Notice the head is flattened so that it stays high in the water column longer.

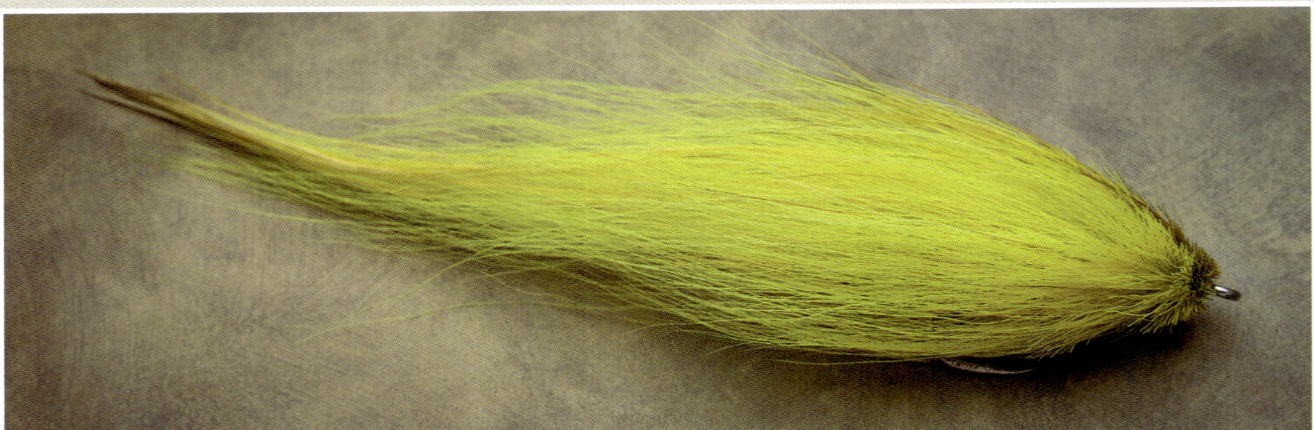

Triangular-shaped BULKhead sporting ostrich feathers surrounded by Hollow ties and three triangular BULK ties to finish. Uses a monofilament extension to help achieve awesome shape, action, and size.

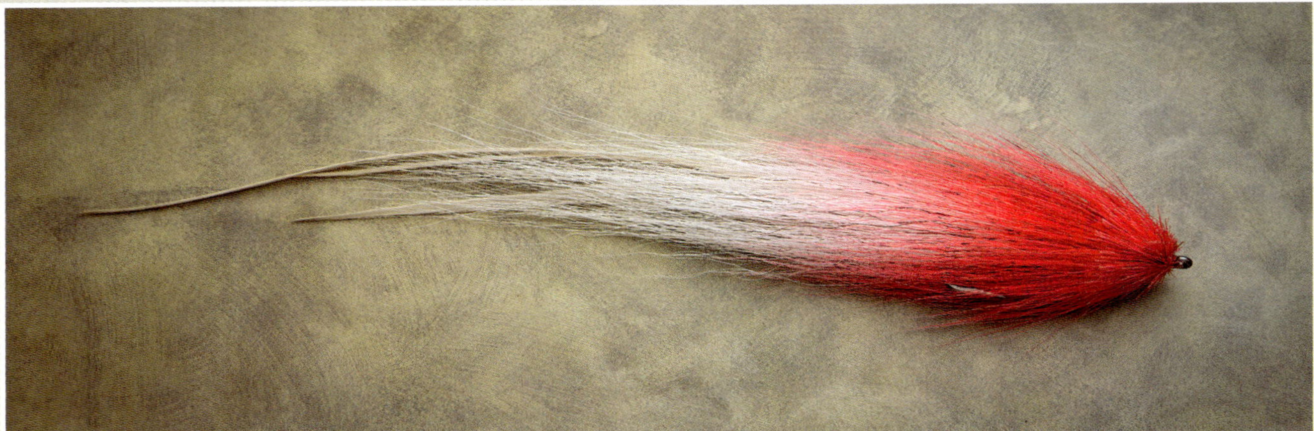

Another red/white classic but with a more rounded and broader forward bulk.

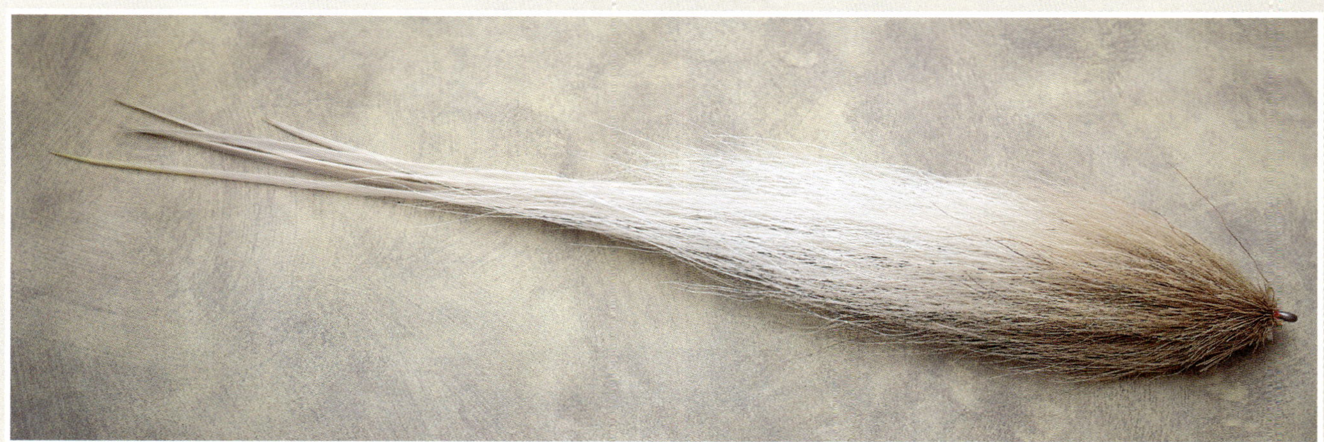

I love the smooth lines, from a rounded head to the slowly tapered body to the wispy feather tails, on this BULKhead.

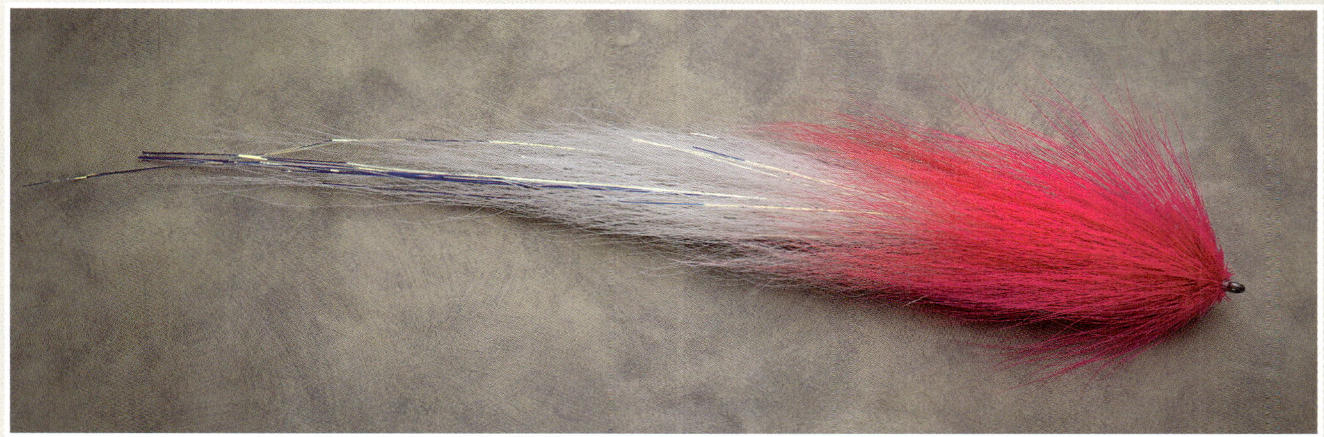

BULKhead tied on a monofilament extension with extra large head. It has great action.

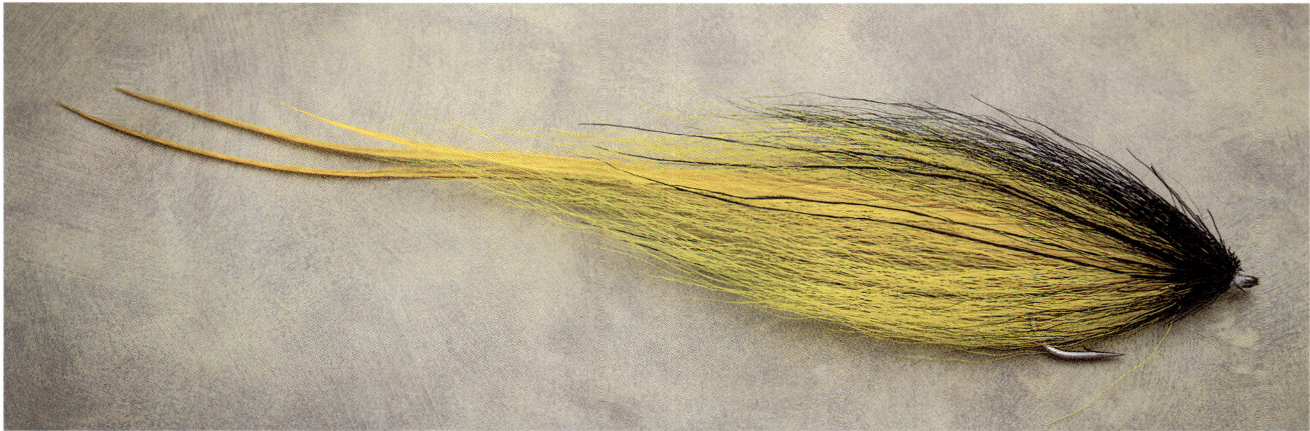

Yellow/black BULKhead. Yellow bucktail and feather tail accentuated with black ostrich and a BULKhead of black bucktail.

Chapter 10

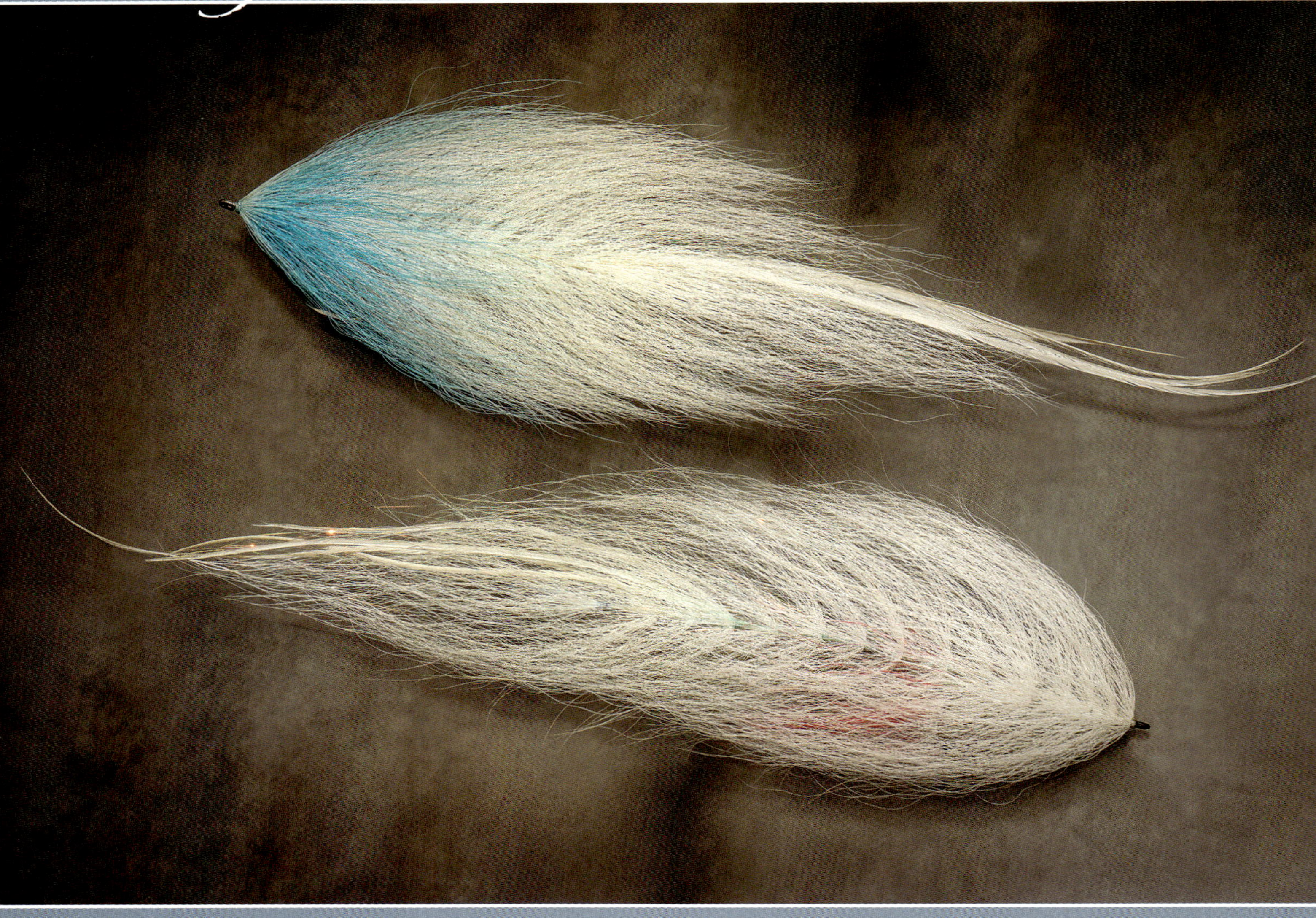

The Beast is an extreme Hollow Fleye designed to imitate large, mature baits such as menhaden, herring, shad, mackerel, and squid. It was born from my fascination with the challenge of tying very large flies that are fairly easy to cast and overcoming the limitations posed by traditional tying techniques. Using a monofilament extension allows you to create flies unrestricted by the hook size—up to 14 to 16 inches or more. The Hollow tying technique allows you to open the fly up to heights of 4 or 5 inches and thicknesses of 3 inches or more.

The Beast

"Jump in!" shouted Lance, as he approached my perch on the Barnegat North Jetty in his Mako. "You have to see the bunker outside the inlet!"

As he nosed the boat up against the rocks near a friendlier spot on the jetty, I jumped aboard (not before calling him crazy), and out to the inlet we went. Along the way, I quickly readied my rod with a large Bucktail Deceiver tied on a mono extension.

Sure enough, the bunker were all over the surface. But they were gigantic—larger than any I had ever seen before by about two inches in length and just much bigger overall. The fly on my line was simply not big enough—it looked like a simple bucktail alongside those horse bunker. We didn't find any bass in that school, but it didn't matter. Before Lance got me back to the jetty, my mind was calculating just how I might create a bigger fly. I had tied large fleyes before, such as the Spread Fleye, Cotton Candy, Shady Lady Squid, and the Big Mono Bunker. At one time they were considered big, but by today's standards they are not and they still wouldn't match the size of the baits that I saw that day. I decided to take my Hollow Fleye and tie it on a mono extension.

From this humbling experience, the Beast was born, and with it, I took big to another level—the first one that I tied was the size of a small bucktail. It was designed to be extra large in every way—length, height, and width—but also to have a dead-ringer shape throughout its length. The Beast was huge: 14 inches long, 4 inches high, and 2 inches thick. It included a BULKhead for more push and resistance in the water.

Now came the time to see how it looked in the water. I tied it on an 80-pound shock tippet and got it wet. From my stand on the 5th Avenue Pier in Seaside Park, I watched the new fleye swim with a natural, flowing movement through the water. The basic concept of forward bulk in front of a sparse, tapered wing did its magic. The currents sent rearward by the BULKhead gave the wing a wavy, realistic action. Its seductive rear movement seemed as natural as can be—not too much movement and not too little. No fly that I had tied before moved in quite this way. A few days later, while we were fishing together at Island Beach, Jonny King's jaw dropped when he saw it in the water and he christened it the Beast, based on its sheer size and the difficulty of casting it.

My first season fishing the Beast was memorable. I labored over it for quite some time, tweaking it until I was satisfied with the design. But I think it was well worth the effort. That year, people from all around reported to me about large fish they caught with the Beast or with large Hollow Fleyes. I even was lucky enough to land a striped bass in the surf that was over 25 pounds on it.

Still, the first version of the Beast was a little hard to cast, and that disappointed me. I figured it would be fine when used in special situations like from a boat, as a boat can maneuver closer to the baitball. Or when bunker schools would get tight enough to the beach to flop the Beast into the scrum. But I wanted to refine and improve it for other situations as well.

Inspired by the results of the fly in the water, I continued to refine the pattern. I started to tie with less material and increased the spacing between the ties so that the fly was lighter and easier to cast. The sparser use of materials also improved the way the fly swam in the water. Even though it is tied sparse, when the fly is pulled through the water, the tips overlap and create an overall density, an opaqueness, that is not immediately visible when the fly is in your hand or even at rest in the water. In other words, since each step overlaps the one preceding it, when you move the fly even 6 inches, all the fibers in the Beast that look almost skeletal and transparent, lay back slightly and overlap, creating a more solid silhouette that perfectly imitates larger baits. Another benefit of increasing the spacing between the ties was that the fly became much faster to tie.

The Beast is getting easier to tie as I refine it, and it is important to me that the fleyes I design can be tied by all levels of tiers. It has been, and hopefully will continue to be, simplified. I am still tweeking the Beast to this day, but as you'll see here, it's come a long way already. They are bigger, but sparser. They have more bulk in front and a lot less hairs in the back. They can be cast easily now with an 8-weight, and I hope now that it has earned its name not from how hard it is to cast, but because it is a true big fish catcher.

This fly's popularity has taken me a bit by surprise, but now, the Beast, and other large patterns tied with the Hollow style, have become important not only for saltwater anglers but also for muskie and northern pike fishermen, for whom large, easy-to-cast flies are a sort of Holy Grail.

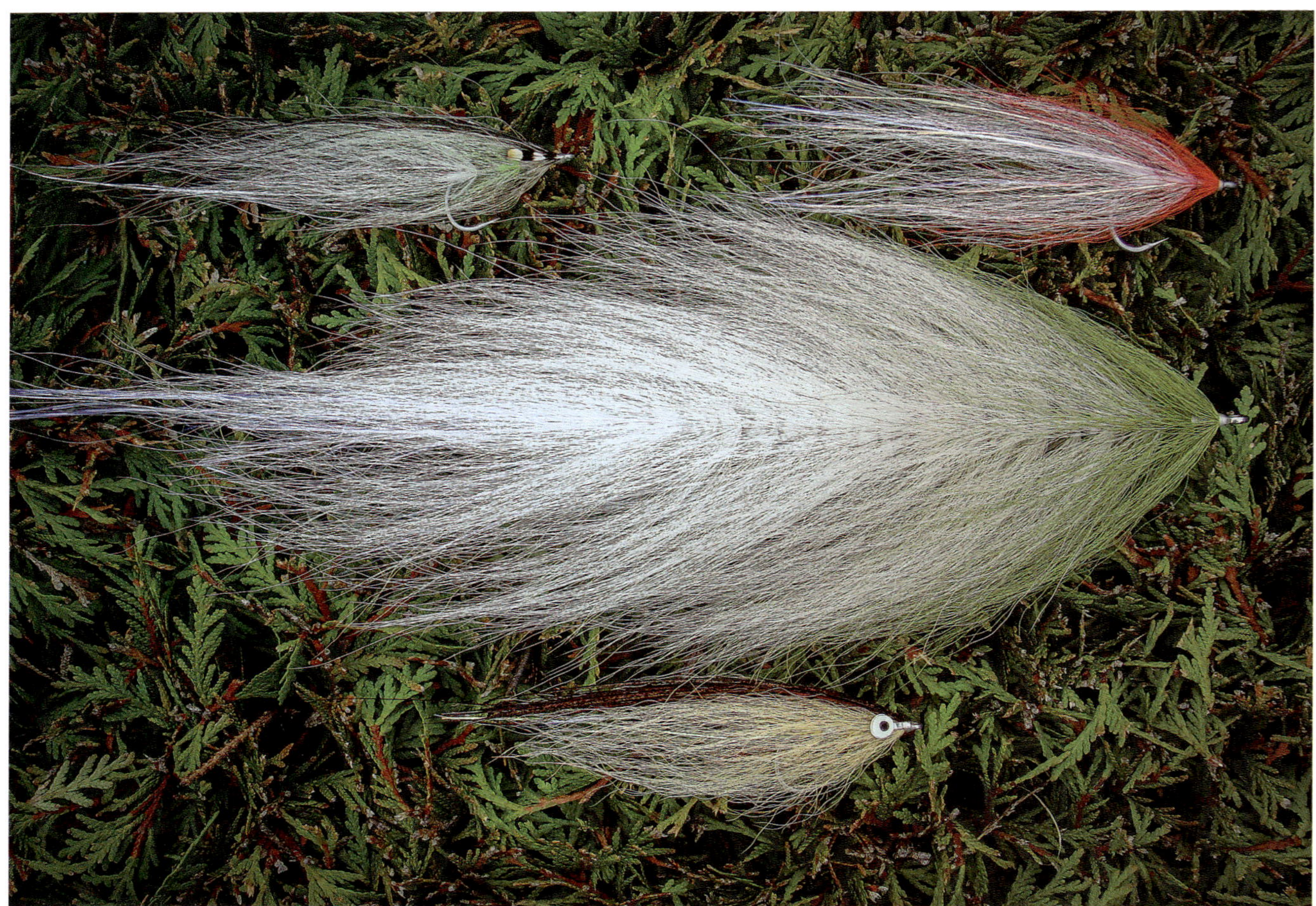

The original Beast surrounded by smaller Hollow Fleyes. The original Beast was massive—the same size as a small bucktail, precisely 14 x 6 x 2½ inches thick, and twenty-two ties (two regular and twenty Hollow-style). Though it was time consuming and a "Beast" to tie, it looked amazing in the water, which was enough inspiration for me to address the design shortcomings of its weight, the time it took to tie, and the challenge of creating a nice taper. The evolution continues, but it is currently lighter by at least half and streamlined tying techniques have made it easier to tie.

Beast Tying Tips

- In the steps below, I use a vise to hold the mono straight, and I think this is a good option for those who are new to this pattern. However, I typically tie the monofilament extension section without a vise, as I find it easier to spin the bobbin and manipulate the material by hand. If you try this, take a few wraps of thread around one leg of the bobbin so that you have a fair amount of tension on the spool. Spinning the bobbin around the mono straight in this manner is no different than the technique that you would use to whip a loop in the end of your fly line. If you do it this way, don't be afraid to use your vise as an extra hand when you are selecting bucktail for each step—I will often just rest the mono between partially opened jaws between each step. The tension from the bobbin wraps will hold all materials tight. No need for a half hitch.
- Another thing that I have started doing, especially when teaching this fly, is to use a Sharpie to mark the mono at even, 1/2-inch intervals. This seems to really help tiers maintain the discipline to space the tie downs evenly and also prevents them from adding too many ties, which creates unnecessary bulk. Even spacing not only looks right to my eye when tying this fly, but it also provides a built-in taper as long as the bucktail lengths are all similar. The 1/2-inch difference provides the perfect amount of taper.
- To achieve subtle nuances in shape, remember some of the lessons learned from the Bucktail Deceiver. On the Beast, I tend to squeeze each of the bucktail ties in the midsection of the fly (portion on the mono) so that they are taller than they are wide, and then at the collar I squeeze less so that it is rounded and completes the taper. Experiment and try to have a vision of the bait you want to imitate before tying it.
- If you don't have long enough bucktail fibers, don't be afraid to incorporate synthetics, especially for the tail portion of the fly. I tie many Beasts with Big Fly Fiber for the tails.
- To make your own straight lengths of mono, cut 60- to 80-pound-test sections about 12 inches long. Stuff them tight into a PVC pipe. Place the pipe into a pot of water and bring to a boil. Remove the pipe, place it in ice water, and let it cool.

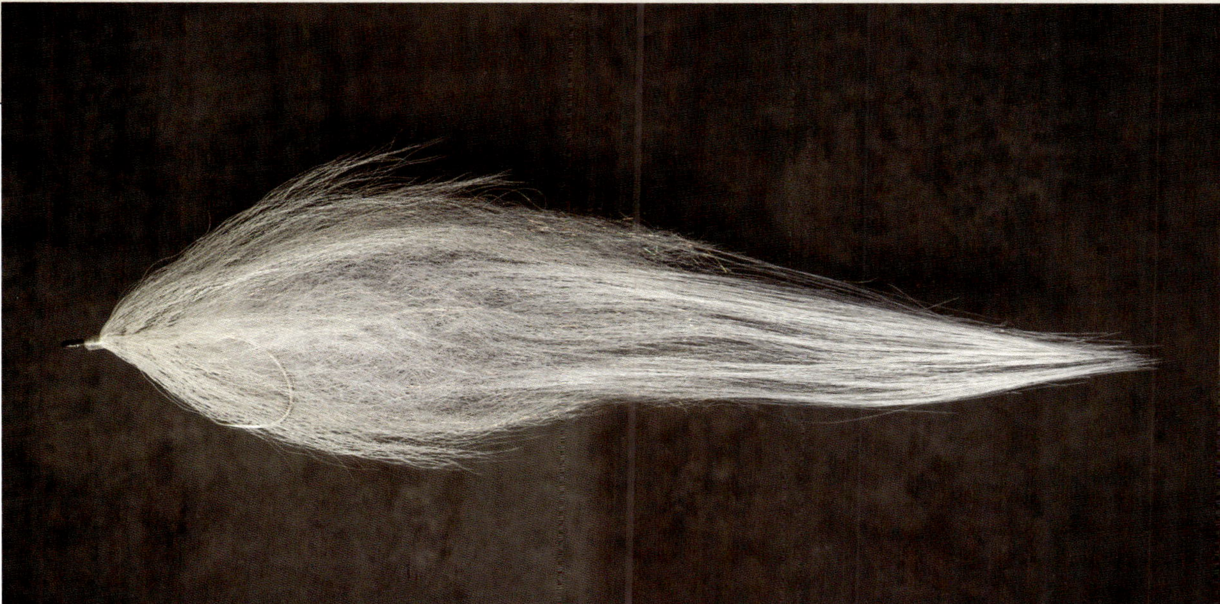

Here is a Beast that borrows the Big Fly Fiber that I used for the Cotton Candy in *Pop Fleyes*. Synthetics are readily available, shed water quickly, and move well in the water.

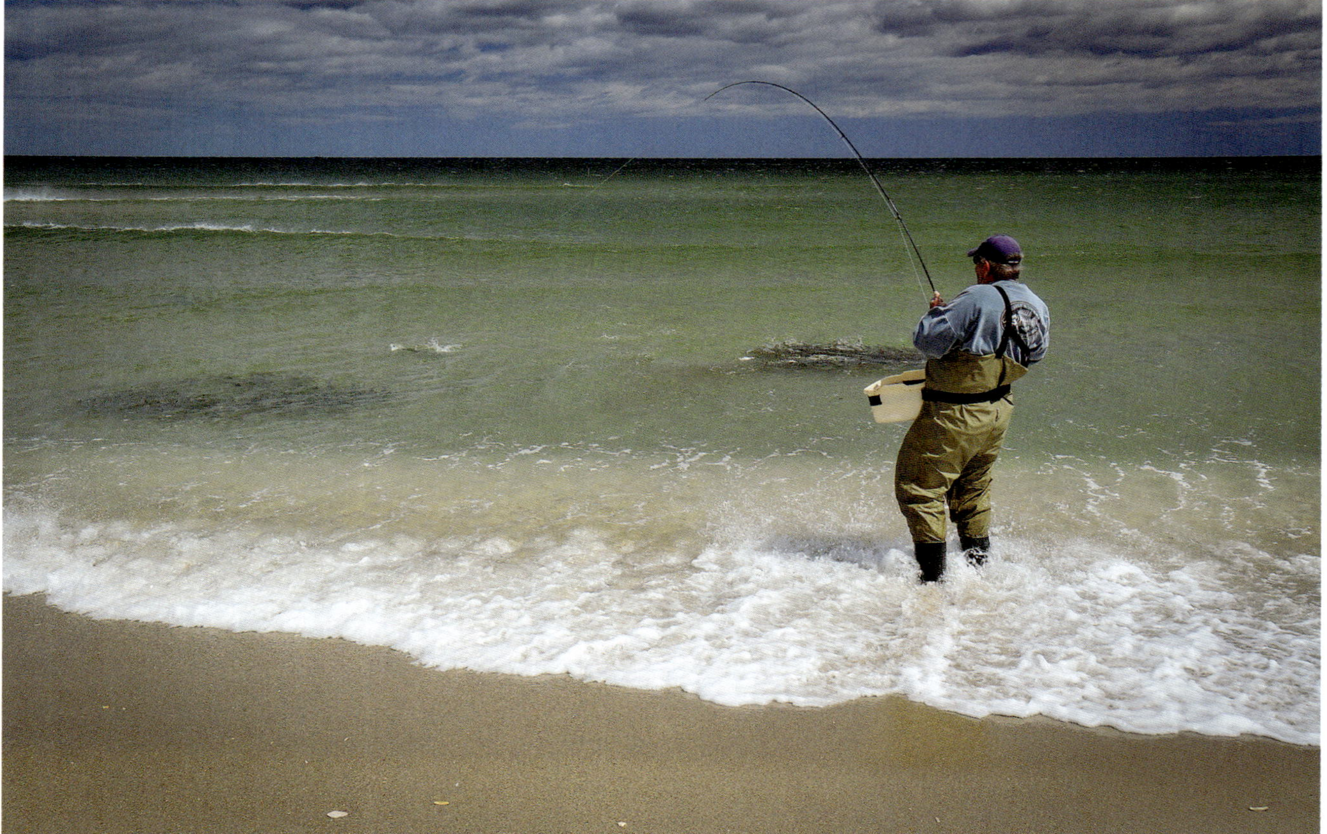

Lance Erwin hefts a large bluefish that attacked a Beast in the wash. Wild strikes on huge flies are the norm. It's not uncommon to see them hit the Beast from more than 10 feet away!

Designers such as Blane Chocklett have taken the basic concept of Hollow tying and are using multiple shanks instead of mono extensions to create flies for muskie with amazing movement in the water. Brad Bohen is popularizing the Hollow technique in his giant flies for pike and muskie throughout the Midwest. Some trout anglers fishing for behemoths on southern tailwaters are also using these techniques to create patterns that imitate 8- to 10-inch trout and suckers, among other things.

When casting the Beast and other large flies, I've found a few tips to be helpful. First, I don't go for distance. A lot of times with the big fish, from the beach or the jetty, everything is in close, and you don't have to cast that far. To move the larger fly, I go to heavier lines with a front-heavy taper or use sinking lines and shorten my leader. A heavy hook not only helps keel the fly and allow it to track straight on the retrieve, but the extra weight also helps carry the large fly through the air. Sometimes I'll even add lead wire wraps in the nose section to give the fly more weight. While it is important in all fly casting to keep slack out of your line, it is especially critical for large flies where there is no room for error.

The Beast

Hook:	#8/0 Partridge Universal Predator X (CS86X/SW)
Thread:	Fine monofilament
Extension:	60-pound-test mono straight
Tail:	Long, white bucktail and slender saddle hackles
Gills:	Red-tipped bucktail
Body:	Long, white bucktail
Flash:	Saltwater Angel Hair

TYING THE BEAST

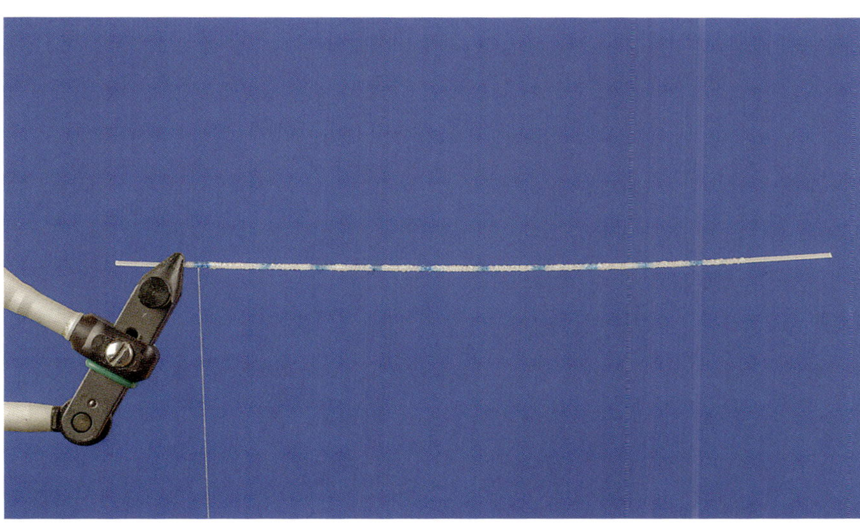

1. The advent of stiff, monofilament straights (available from tackle stores in 20-pount-test up to 100-pound-test) means that tiers no longer need two vises to hold the mono taut. Since the stiff mono can hold the bobbin without sagging, and the mono extensions are only about six inches at the most, you can tie on the mono almost as easily as you were tying on a hook shank. Prepare a 6- to 8-inch-long monofilament straight (60-pound-test) by covering it with monofilament thread. After you coat the wraps with head cement, mark the monofilament at 1/2-inch intervals with a marker.

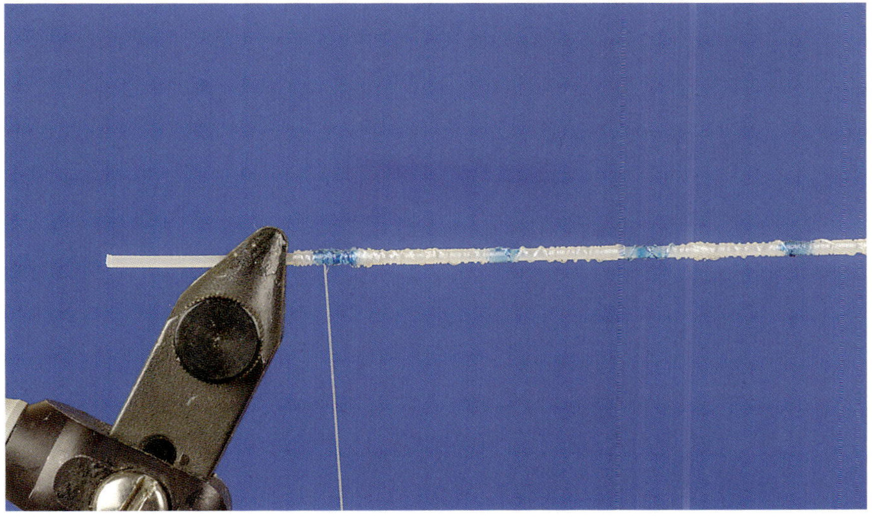

2. Whether you cover the entire straight at once, as I have done here, or you just cover it with thread as you tie, it is critical that you wrap a mono base to give the bucktail and other materials something to adhere to.

(continued)

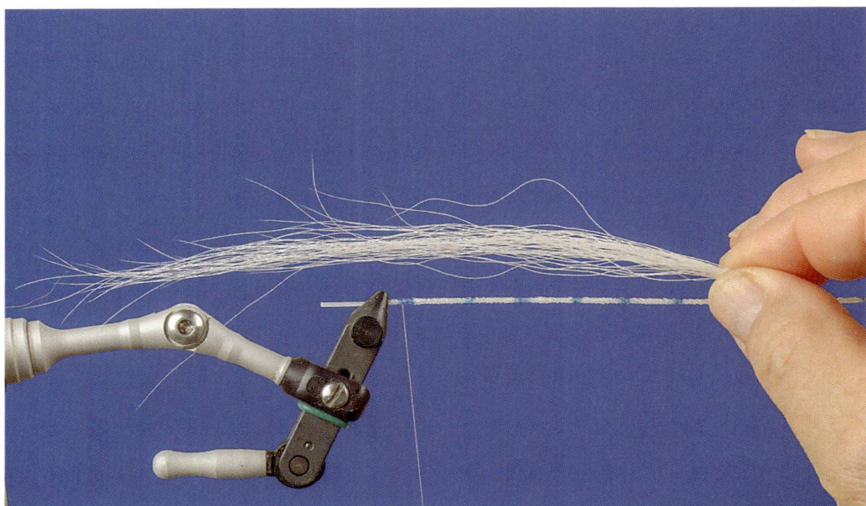

3. The first tie establishes the fly's overall length. This clump is tied in the same way that you would tie in the first bundle on a Bucktail Deceiver, not Hollow-style. Select a bunch of fibers about the thickness of a pencil.

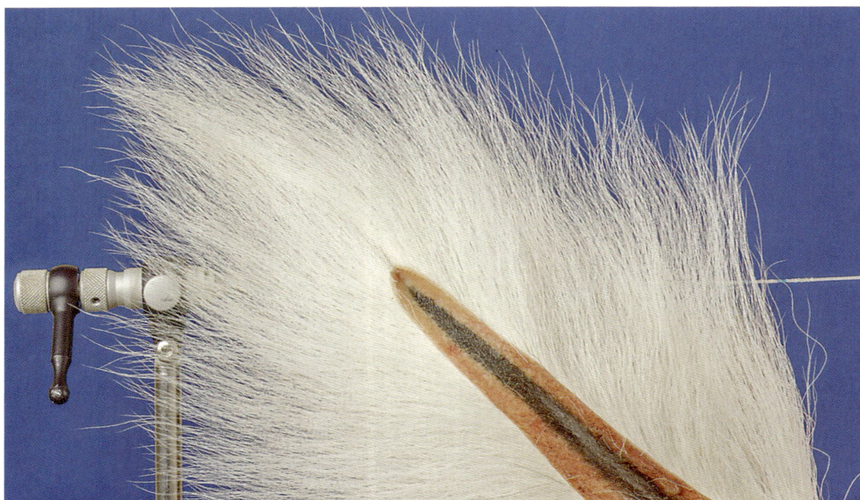

4. This is the tail from which I'll be selecting fibers. Hairs are long, thin, and fairly uniform, which should make it easier to capture the proper taper. Also, the finer hairs are much more manageable when tying hollows.

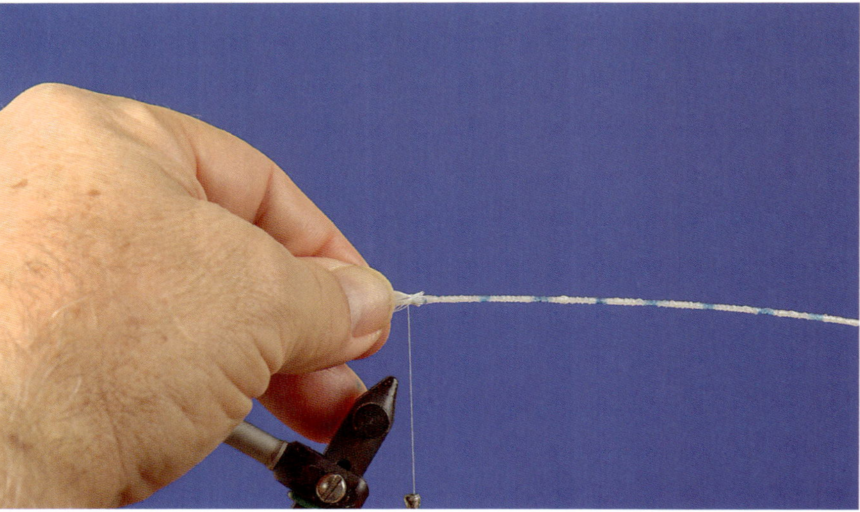

5. After you select the fibers, trim the butts square and tie them in.

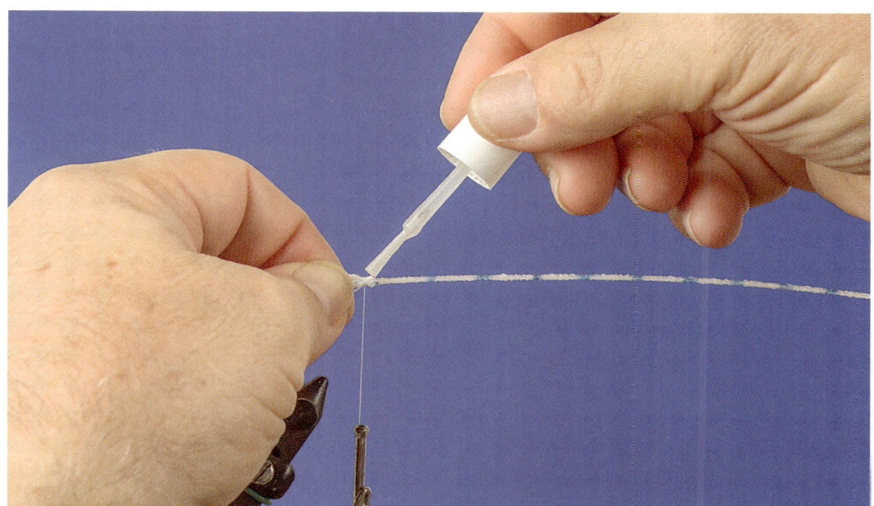

6. Coat the butts with head cement, and wrap over them with your mono thread. Do this with every bunch of bucktail that you tie in. With a fly like this that uses lots of premium hair and takes time to tie, you want to make sure it is as durable as possible.

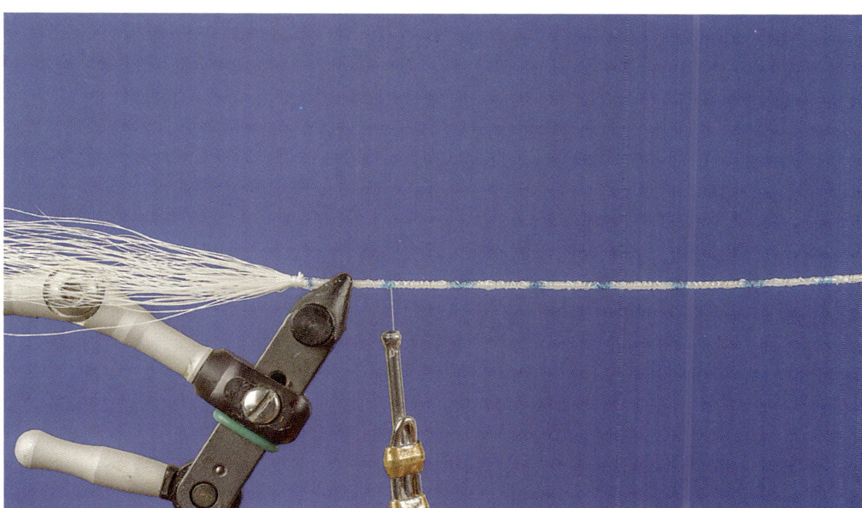

7. Reposition the mono extension in your vise. You'll have a few inches of tying area that extend out of the vise that are stiff enough to tie on before you must adjust it. Advance the thread to the next mark, where you will begin the first tie of bucktail in the Hollow style.

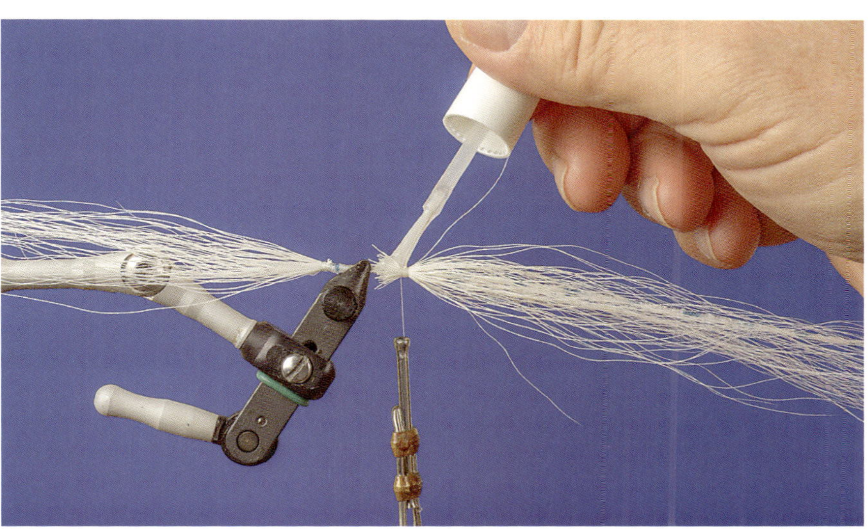

8. Select another bunch of fibers about a pencil-width thick, clip the butts, and tie them in so that they are distributed 360 degrees around the shank. The first clump of bucktail tied Hollow-style starts to create the taper, which is affected by the length of the bucktail and the final angle that you set with the thread dam. To get the right length, every step should come from the same area on the bucktail. Even lengths of bucktail fibers spaced at $^{1}/_{2}$-inch intervals should automatically create the desired taper. Add head cement to the butts.

(continued)

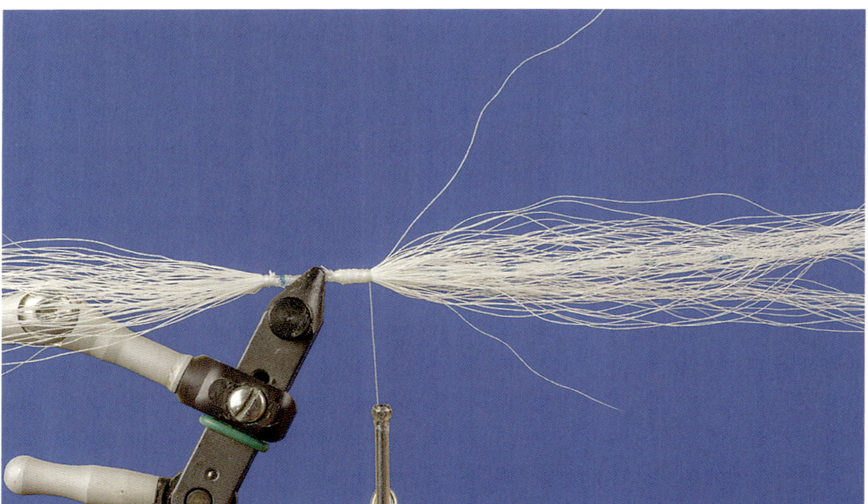

9. Wrap back over the butts, but do not go forward past the tie-in point.

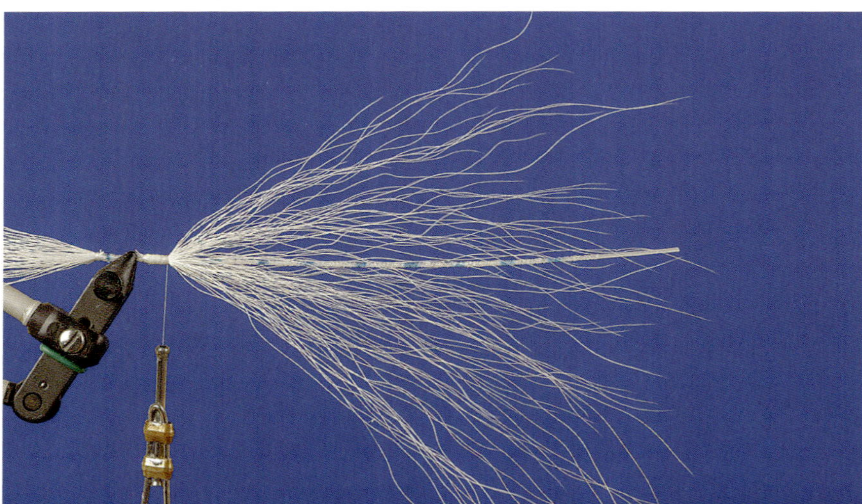

10. Preen the fibers to open them up and distribute them evenly around the monofilament.

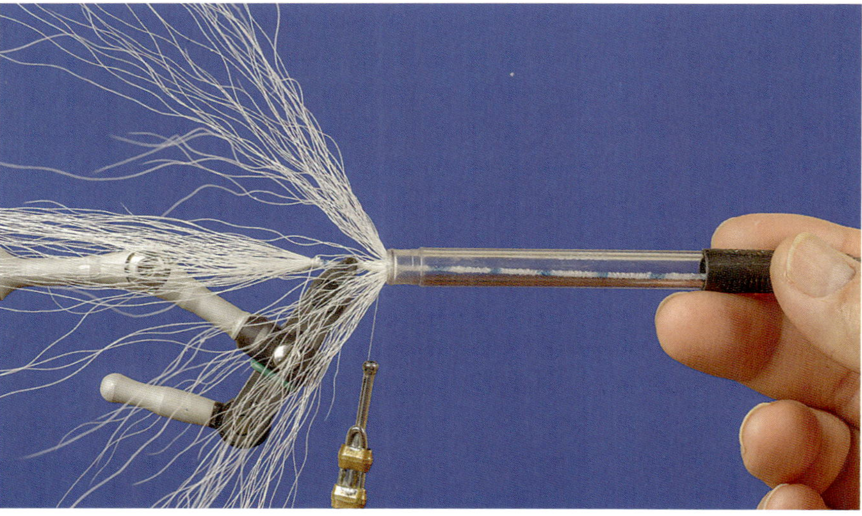

11. With your pushing tool, ease the fibers back so that you can grab them easily with your fingers.

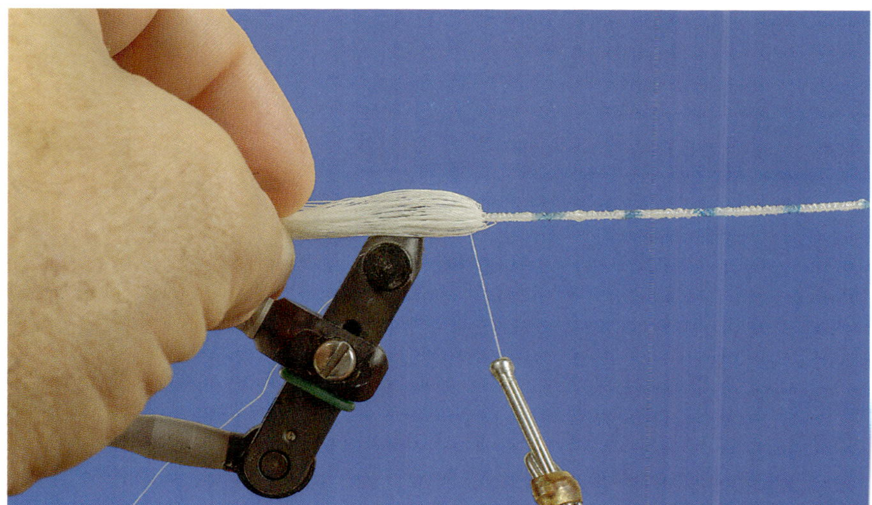

12. Grab the fibers with your left hand, and begin to move the thread forward to make the transition to the front of the fibers.

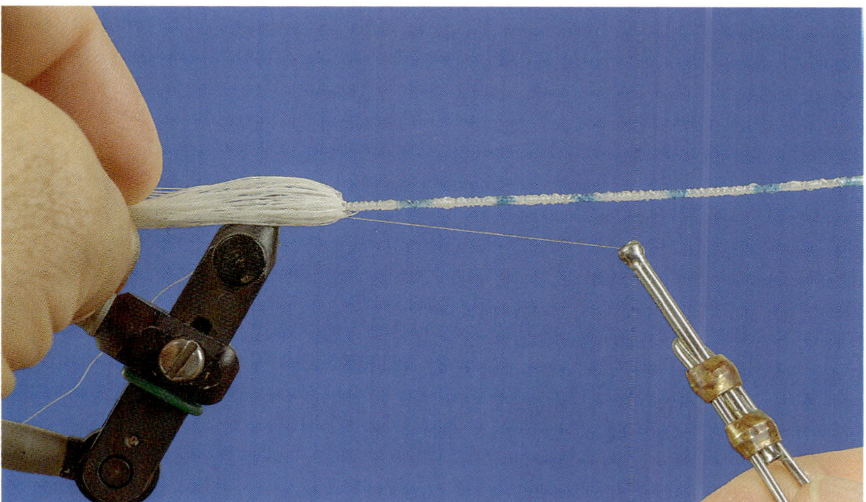

13. As with the Hollow Fleye, bring the thread almost parallel to the mono extension as you bring it through the bucktail and take a few wraps around the monofilament.

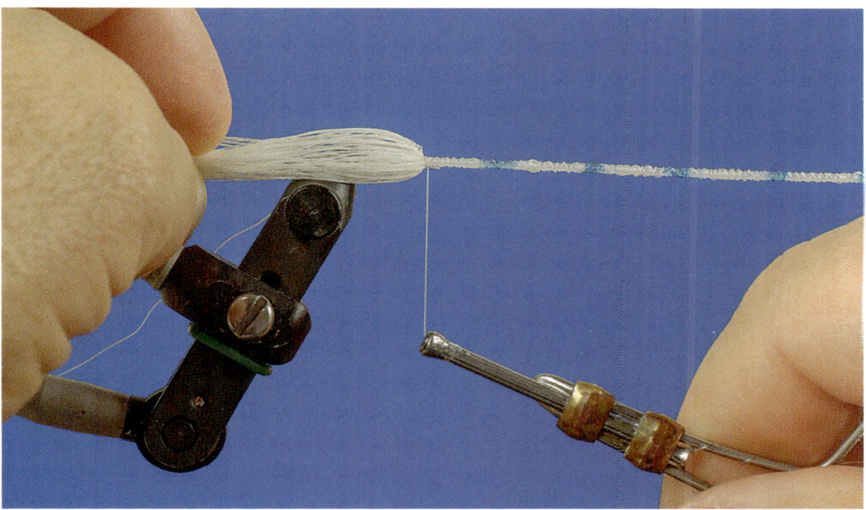

14. As you begin forming the dam that will wrap over the bottom of the hair and close the angle of the fibers, make sure that you wrap straight up and over the extension. You must not wrap at an angle or it will ruin the 360-degree distribution.

(continued)

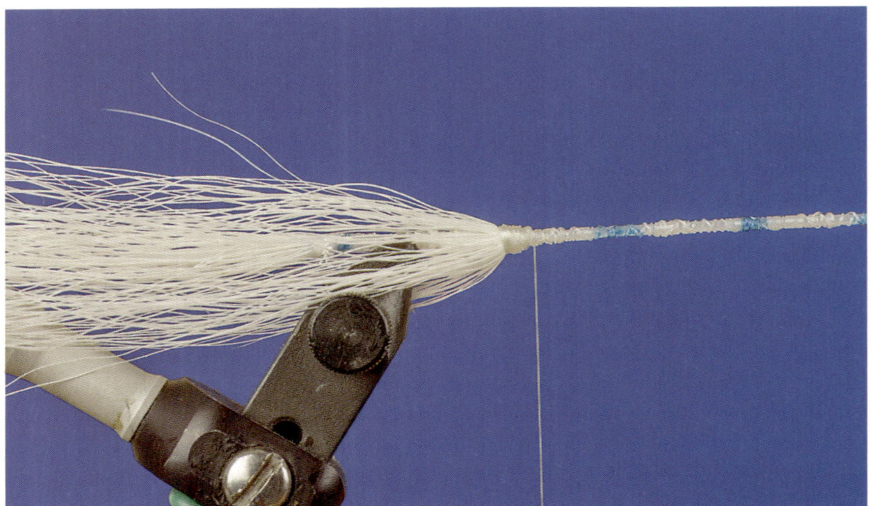

15. Wrap over the base of the fibers to achieve a fairly low angle, about 15 to 18 degrees. Length of fiber and angle both contribute to taper. In this step you want a slight angle, and then every subsequent tie-in should have a slightly larger angle (only a few degrees sometimes) than the preceding one.

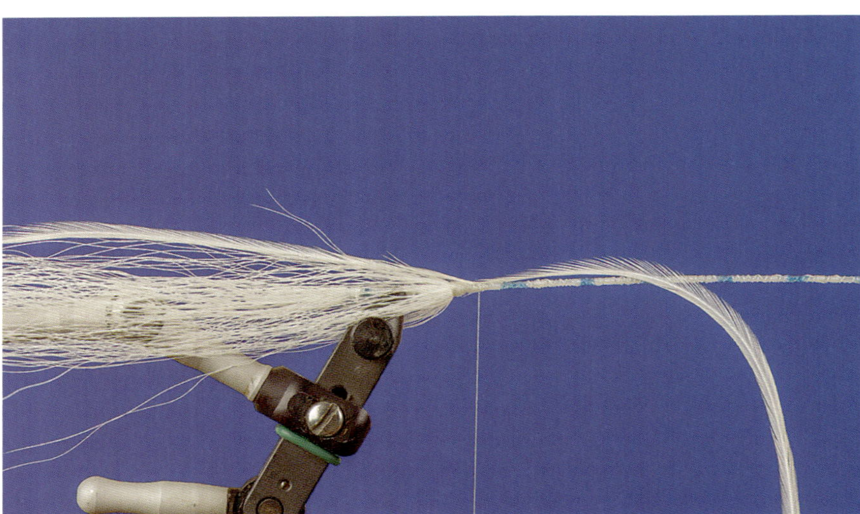

16. In between the ties of bucktail, you can add materials such as flash or skinny, long feathers if you like. Notice that the tie-down point of the feathers is almost exactly in between the 1/2-inch marks. You can tie down as many feathers as you like here, but I only use a few to enhance movement. More important is that the feathers do not extend too far past the tail of the fly—no more than 1/2 inch—or they look more like weeds.

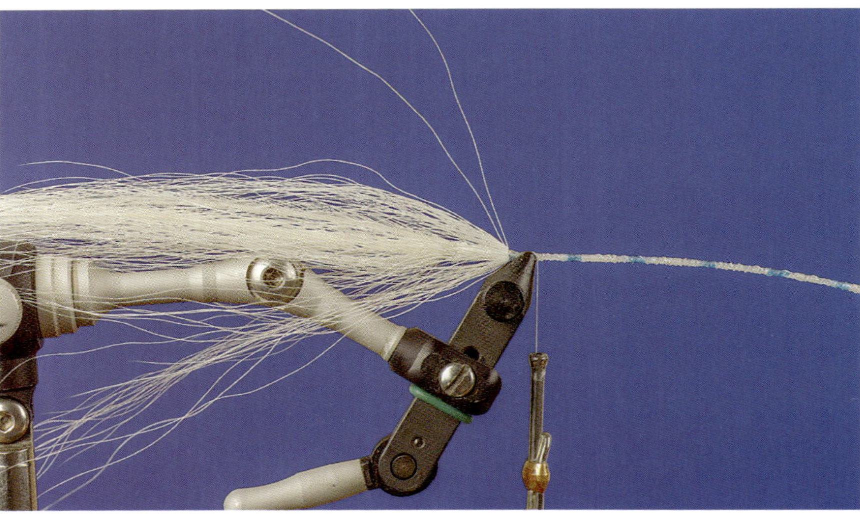

17. Tie in another section of bucktail and dam it up so that it is at a slightly greater angle. Then reposition the mono extension in the vise.

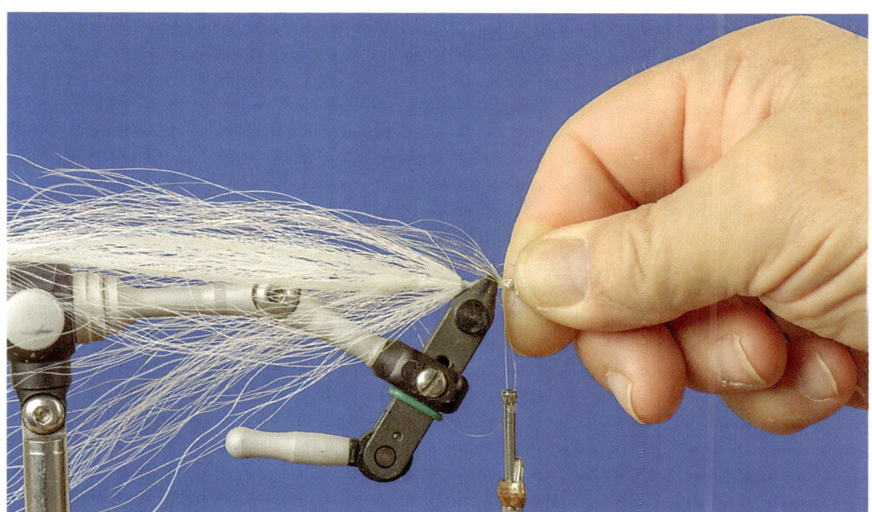

18. Adding flash is optional, but if you do choose to incorporate it into the fly you should tie it in between the marks. The flash that I am using here is Angel Hair. As with most flash, I like to tie it down in the middle and then fold it back, making sure to evenly distribute it around the shank. Once the flash is tied down, you can tie in another section of bucktail, this time at a slightly greater angle than the one preceding it.

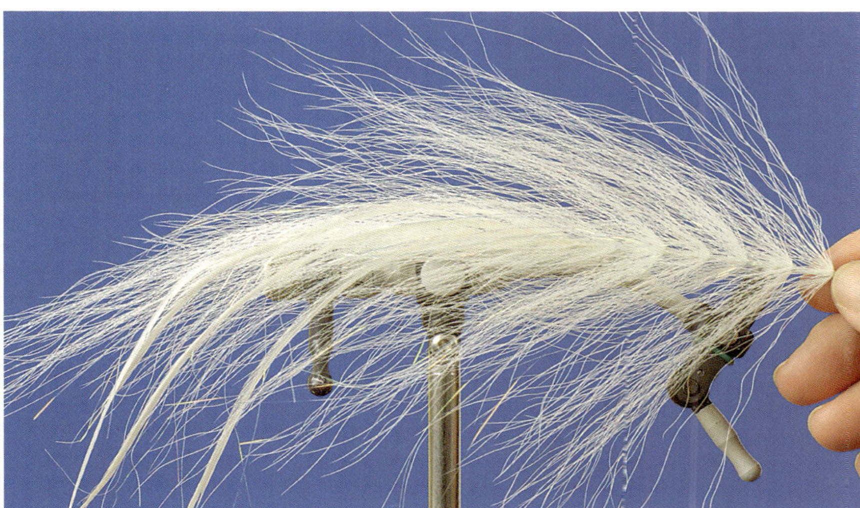

19. You can continue to tie in feathers or flash as you move forward, but the rest of the steps to finish the mono extension are the same. Whip-finish when you've reached the end of your tail assembly. This mono extension has eight total ties.

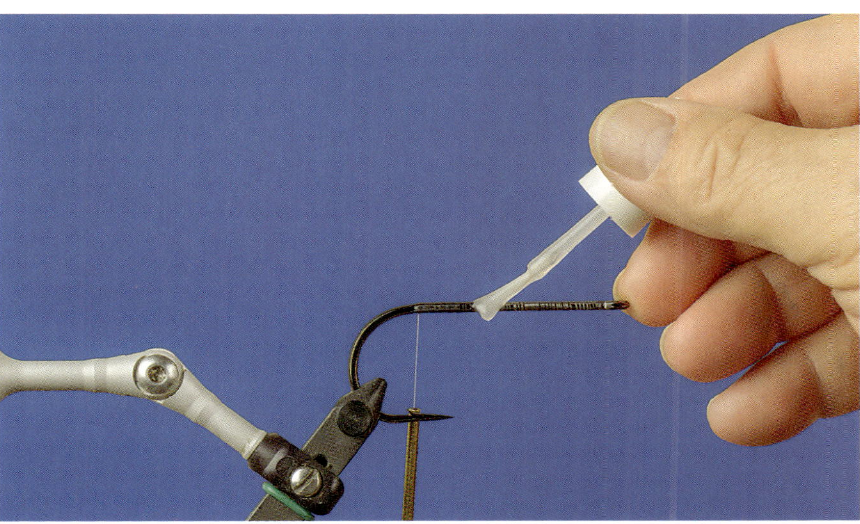

20. Insert the hook into the vise, wrap the shank with mono thread, and coat the wraps with head cement.

(continued)

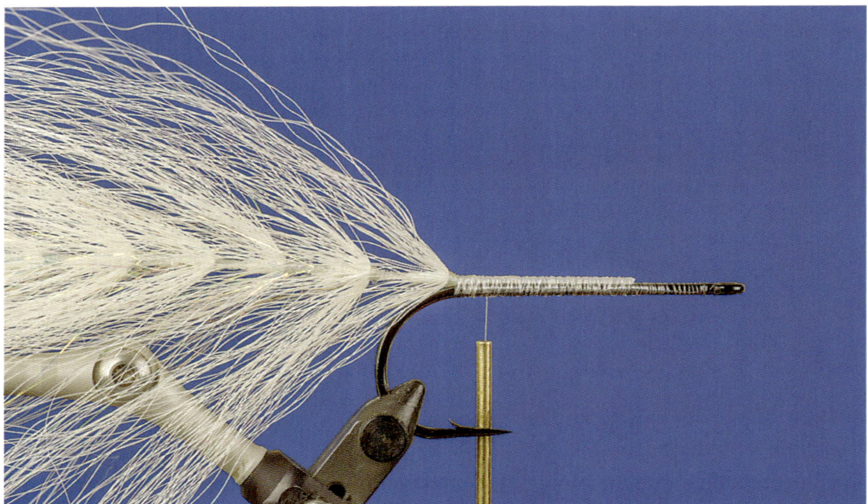

21. Flatten the end of the mono extension with pliers before tying it onto the hook shank and coating it with head cement. This makes a better bond to the shank than two round surfaces.

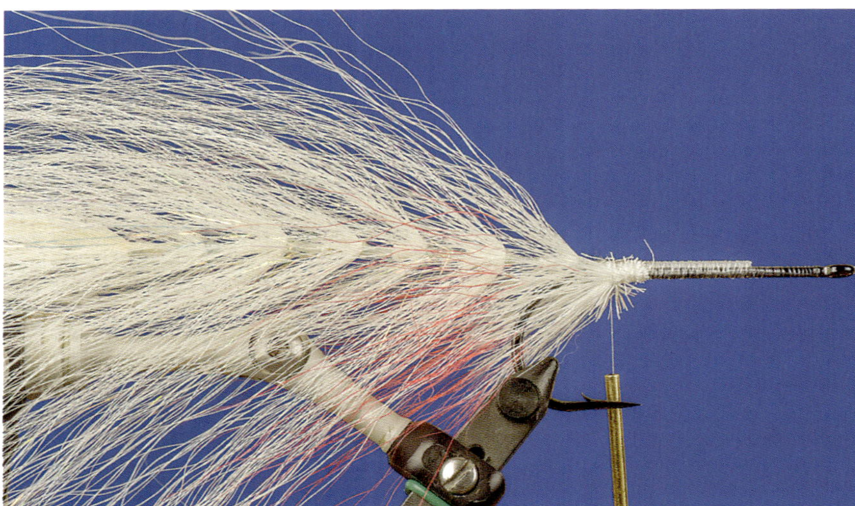

22. After tying in the extension, you can wrap the thread forward so that you are 1/2 inch from the last section of bucktail on the extension, or add feathers, flash, or other accents. Here we are tying in a small clump of red-tipped bucktail (just the tips are dyed) on the underside of the hook to provide the gentle illusion of gills. They are shorter than the other fibers. The red will be subtle in the finished fly, but fairly prominent when the fly is viewed from the rear.

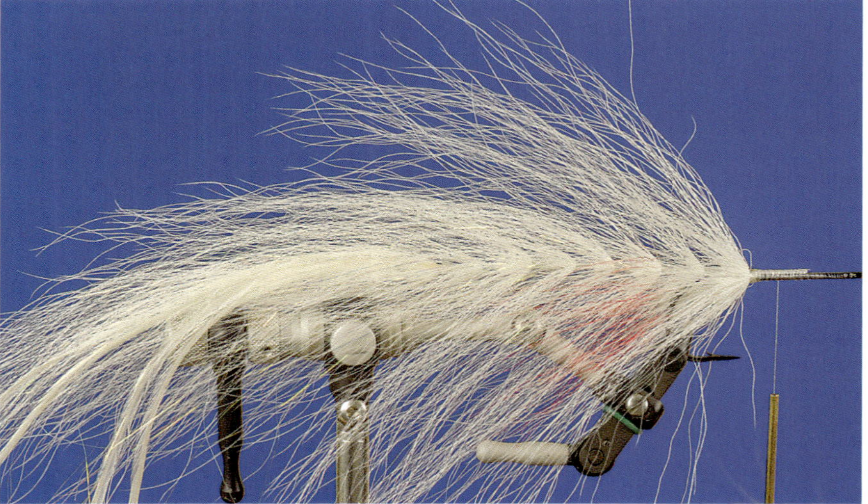

23. Advance your thread 1/4 inch to resume tying in the bucktail Hollow-style. This image shows two ties after the gills.

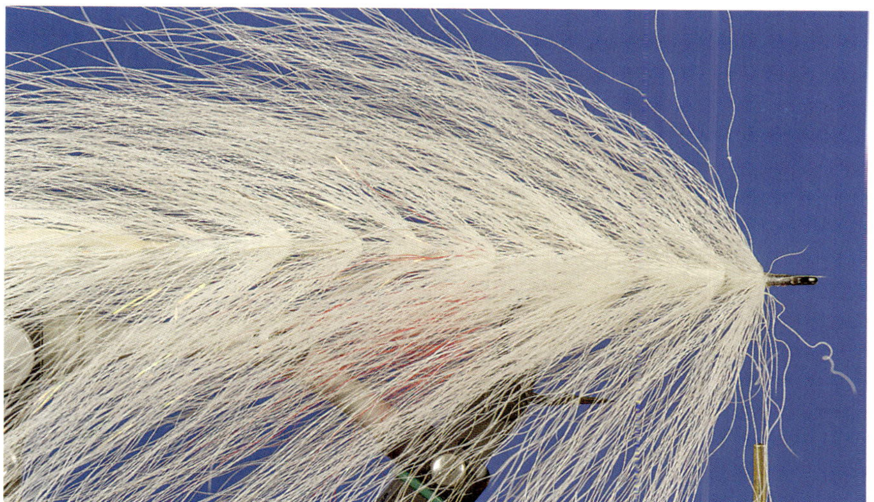

24. Continue tying in bucktail to complete the shank. Here are fourteen total ties for the fly. At times, I will reduce the space between the ties in the front of the fly for more bulk. Whip-finish.

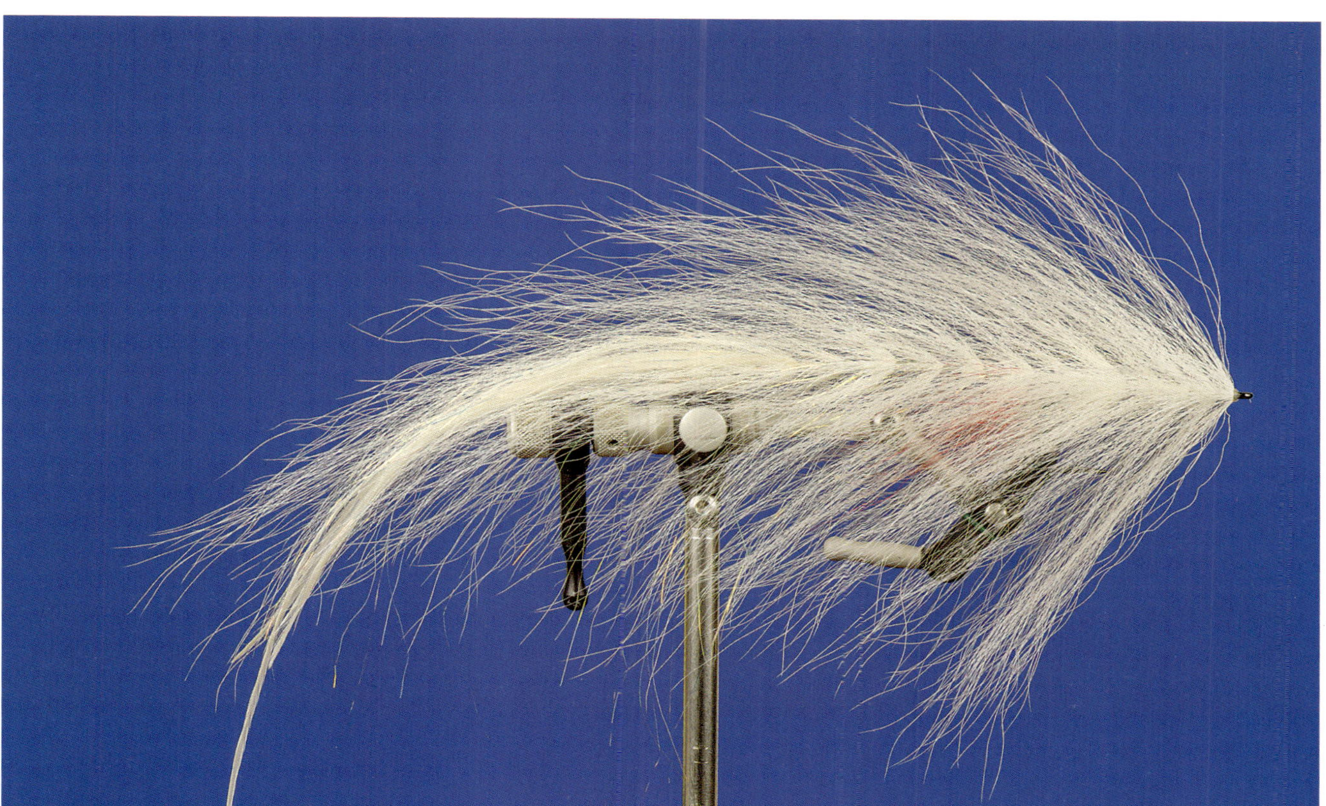

Note the slightly increasing angles of the bucktail on the finished fly. You must discipline yourself to leave the fly open as you tie it and let it be a little unruly—trust that the bucktail will lie back in the water. After you wet it, the fibers and tips will settle into a nice shape.

Chapter 11

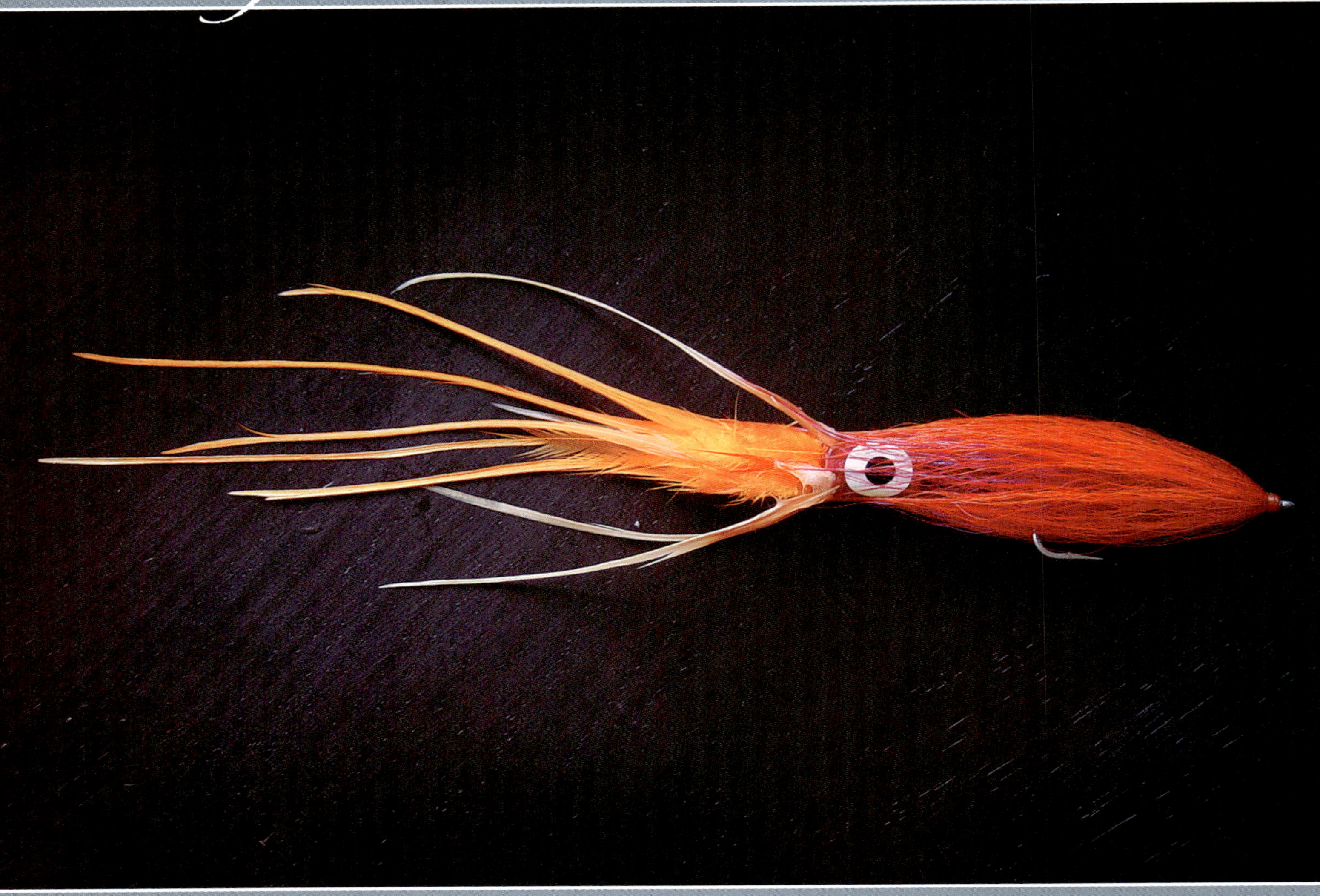

The finished version of the Rear Floating Squid, after working through several "crude" test models. Feathers protrude at a higher angle from around the outside of the foam cylinder to accent the action of the fly. The sleek body taper draws it all together.

Rear Floating Squid

Squid are found almost everywhere there is salt water (according to some sources, there are over 300 species), and they are favorites of all predator fish, from stripers to marlin. Intelligent and cunning creatures, squid are great swimmers with the ability to swim ahead or to the rear. The relatively short tentacles do not wiggle when the squid is swimming; they "point" their way either at the prey or away from predator.

Masters of camouflage, squid have special pigment cells in their skin that allow them to change colors to blend in with their surroundings, and they also change colors when threatened. Some species of squid can also glow, and have the ability to change both their color and the intensity of their light. Because of this, squid can be lots of different colors and shades and offer many creative possibilities for fly tiers.

More important than color, however, is the sleek fusiform shape and prominent eye. The oversize eyes of a squid draw immediate attention and are located well past the mantle. Another design consideration for good squid imitations is the proper proportion of the body, legs, and wings, and the full, robust figure. They are not skinny and pencil shaped.

The inspiration for the Rear Floating Squid came after watching squid in the rips in Martha's Vineyard during the annual spring squid run in June. They would come to the surface, or near the surface, and then all of a sudden disappear and then come out of the water 6 feet away. I have filmed them jumping out of the water as they were chased by marauding bass, only to be eaten when they returned. While a Bucktail Deceiver is still one of my favorite patterns for imitating large squid because it has that overall fusiform shape, I started to think about how to design a fly that would stay near the surface, yet be able to sink and dart under the water. It occurred to me that combining a buoyant popper head with a heavier hook might be a good solution and give the fly the action that I was looking for.

The result was the Rear Floating Squid, another pattern that is extremely fun to fish and has a distinctive action from the combination of a heavy hook that pulls the front of the fly down and the foam in the rear that wants to keep the fly near the surface. When you strip in line, the fly darts into the water and then settles back up to the surface. The pause and the rise really drives the fish crazy. I will vary the retrieve to include long, sweeping pulls (maybe two or three strips), then follow it with a momentary pause. Sometimes, to imitate the erratic swimming motion of a squid, I'll use a hand-over-hand retrieve with short pops to make it move about $2^1/_2$ to 3 feet in one strip, and then let it settle.

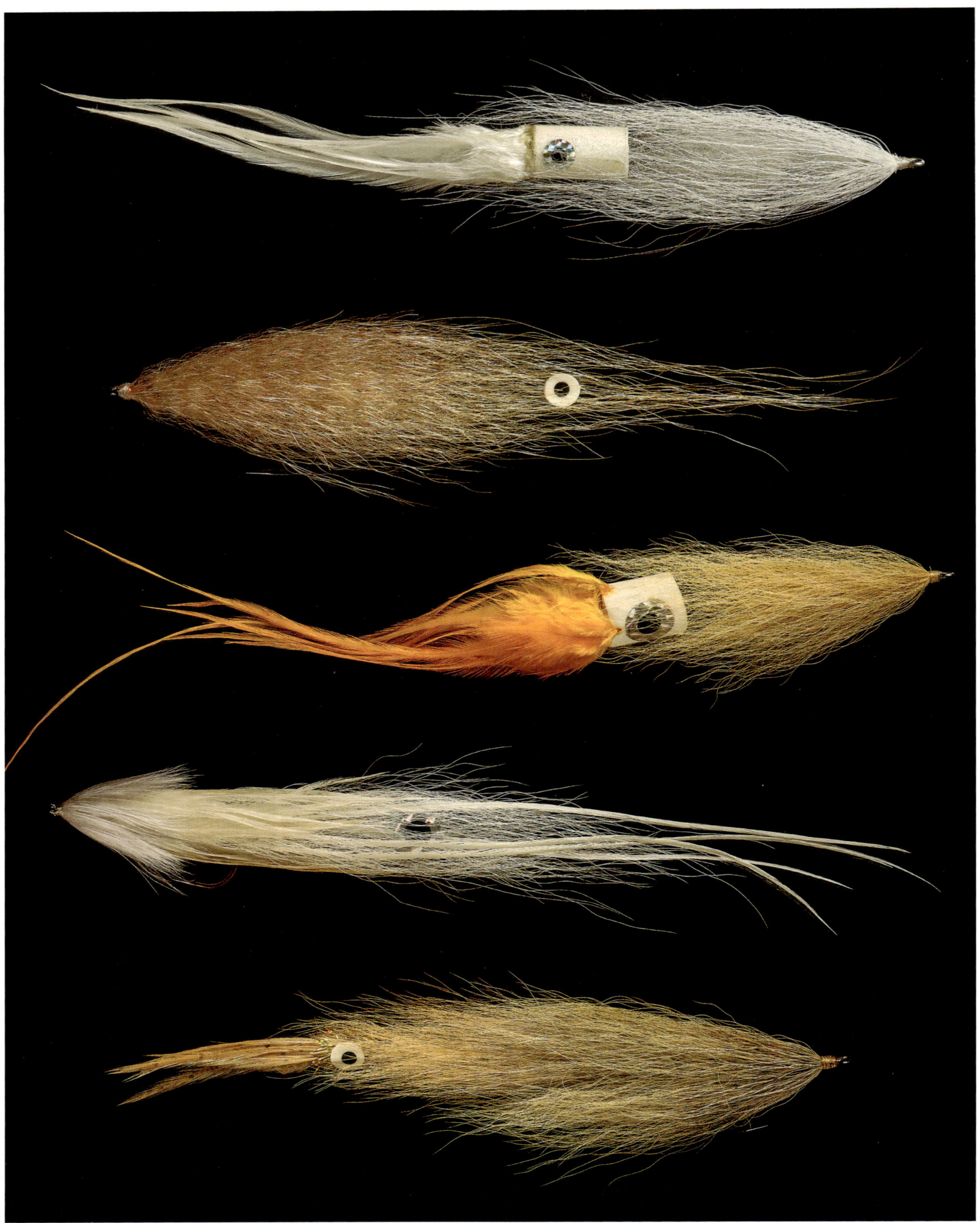

I have always been fascinated by squid, probably more so than any other bait. Nothing says "squid" better than a large eye toward the rear of a fly. A mono extension allows you to place the eye in the correct position, without being restricted by the length of the hook shank.

Rear Floating Squid

Hook:	Gamakatsu SL12S Big Game Saltwater
Thread:	Pink Gudebrod
Extension:	100-pound-test mono straight
Head:	Large Live Body foam cylinder, prismatic tape, and extra-large stick-on eyes
Tentacles:	Pink schlappen feathers
Body:	Orange bucktail over a core of pink fleece

TYING THE REAR FLOATING SQUID

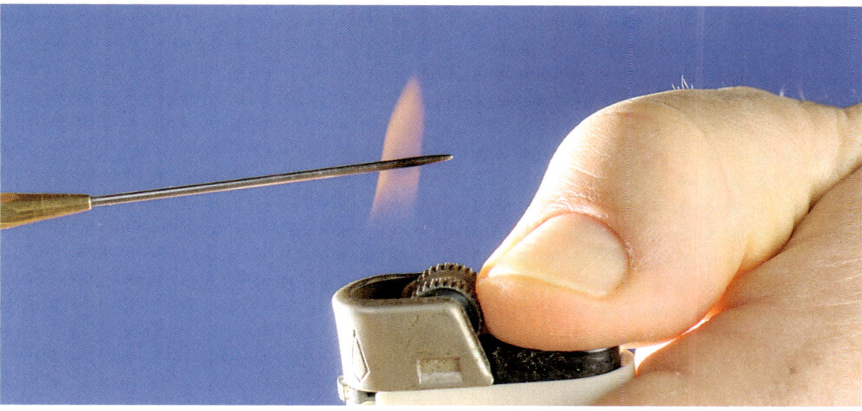

1. Heat the bodkin tip with a flame from a lighter or match.

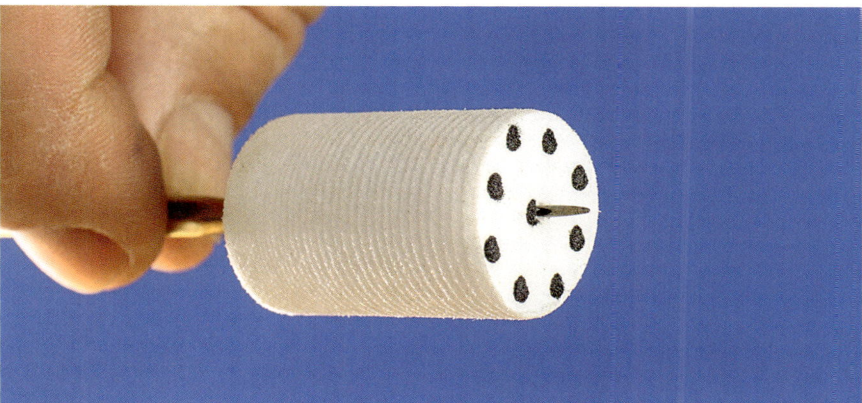

2. Mark holes on the Live Body foam cylinder (here $1^{1}/_{4}$ inch diameter) around the perimeter as a guide for the feather holes. Stick the heated bodkin through the center to create a hole for the monofilament straight.

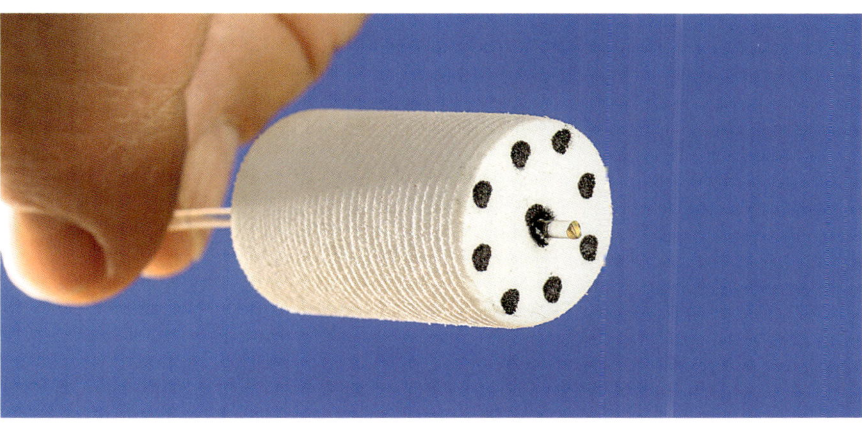

3. Insert the heavy mono (100-pound-test) through the center hole. You need to use monofilament that is stiff enough to hold the foam cylinder and still come straight off the hook shank when it is tied in.

(continued)

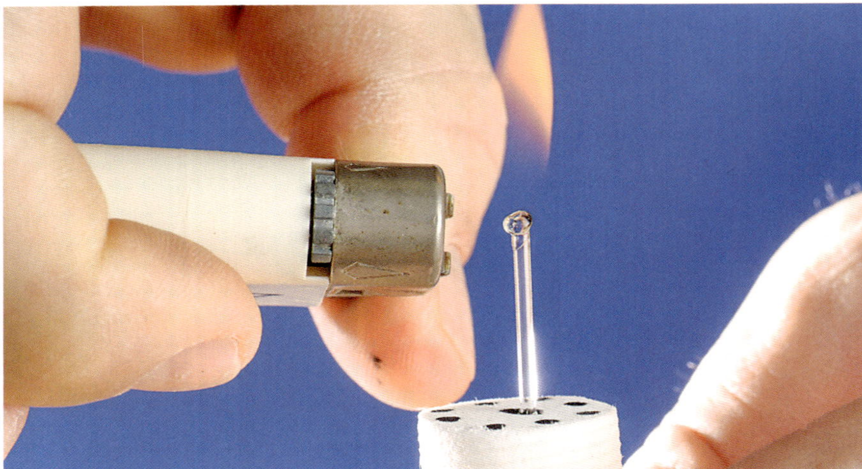

4. Light the end of the mono, and then blow it out after a sizeable ball has formed. Apply a bit of Krazy Glue to the shaft of the mono, and pull it down into the foam.

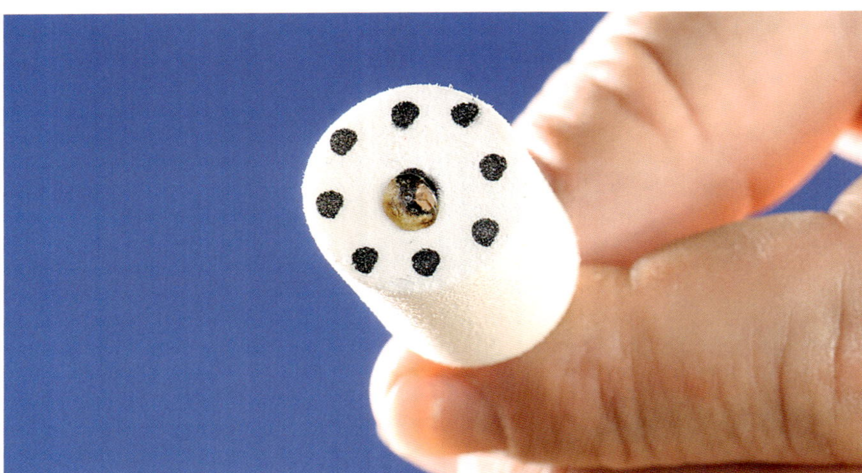

5. Wet your fingertip and smash the ball flat against the foam. Both the flattened mono and Krazy Glue ensure that the foam cylinder will stay in place, but you could probably simplify this step by just using Krazy Glue.

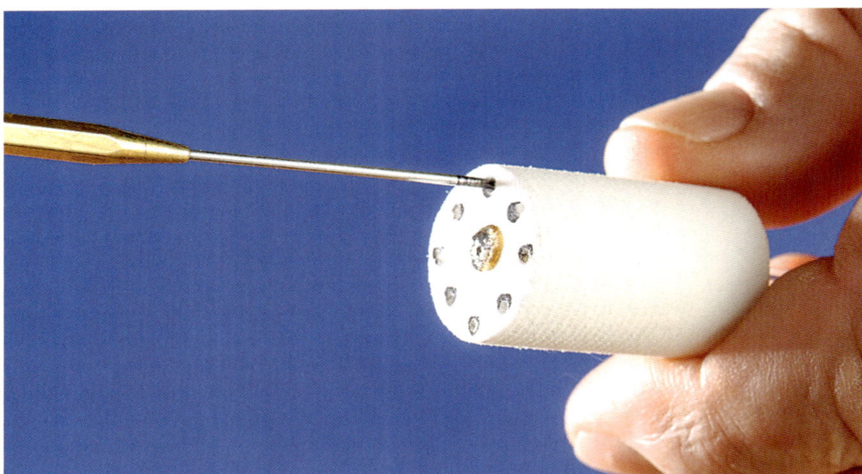

6. Heat your bodkin again, and create shallow, $^{1}/_{4}$-inch holes in the outside marks for feathers stems. As you insert the heated bodkin, roll it around a bit to make it easier to insert the feather.

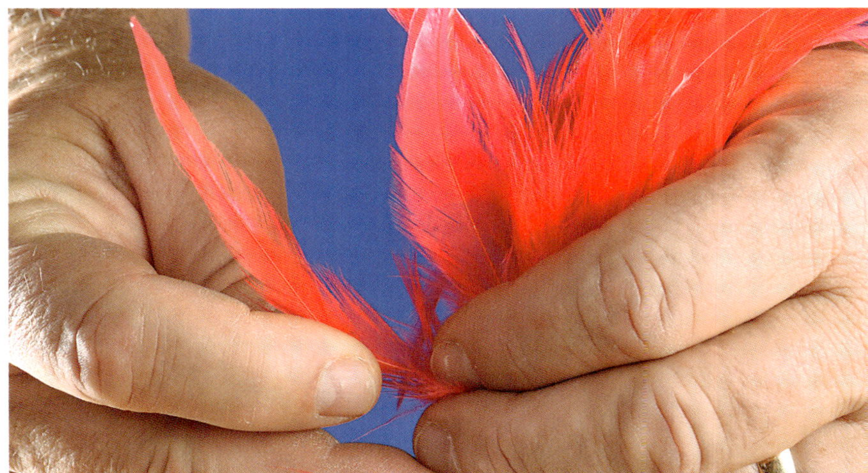

7. Saddle hackles with nice tapers and strong, durable stems are best for the rear tentacles.

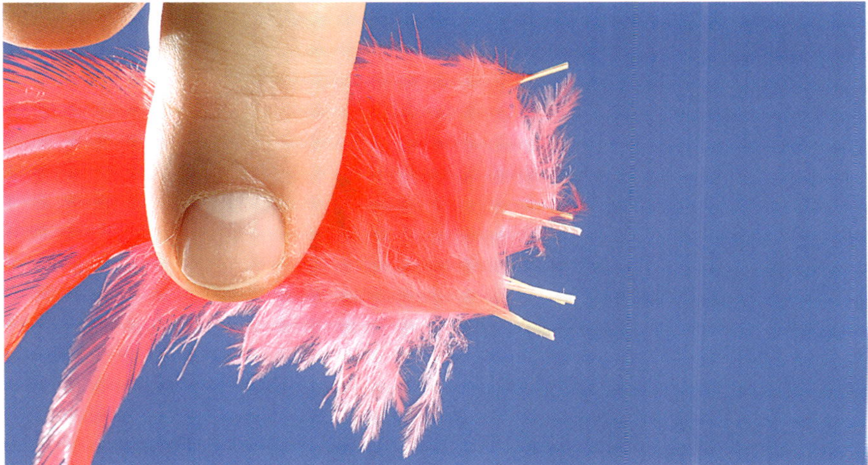

8. Prepare the feather by stripping about 1/8 inch of fluff to expose the stem, but keep another 1/8 inch of fluff so that the feathers seat into the holes and provide a nice transition from the wide foam cylinder to the feathers.

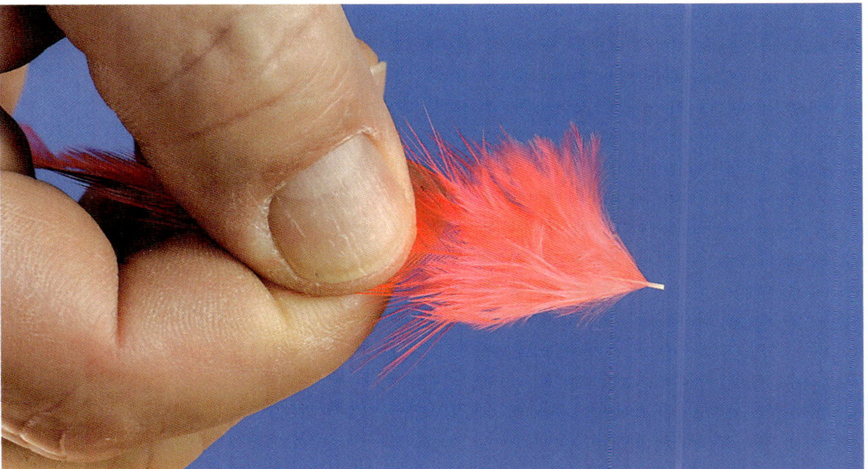

9. Trim all the stems to equal length.

(continued)

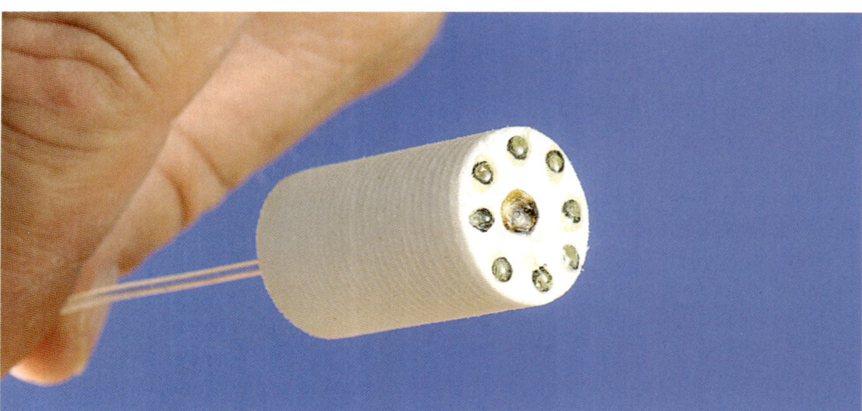

10. Mix a small batch of five-minute epoxy, which gives you more working time than Krazy Glue and doesn't require light like the light-cured acrylic. With a bodkin, place a dab of epoxy into each hole.

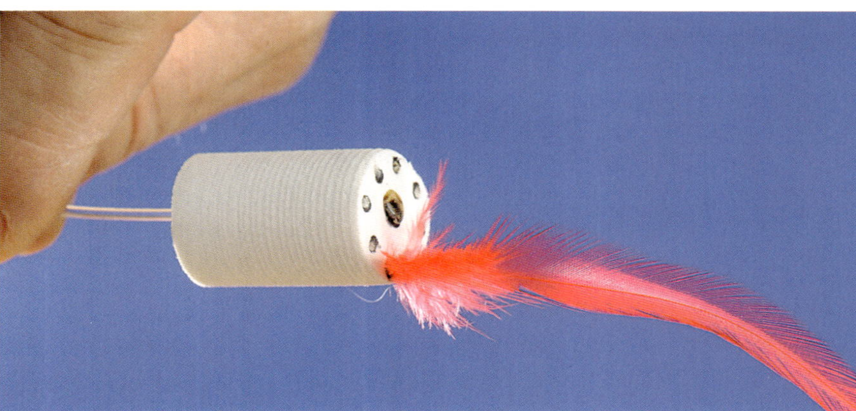

11. Insert feathers into all the holes. The dull side of the feathers should be on the inside.

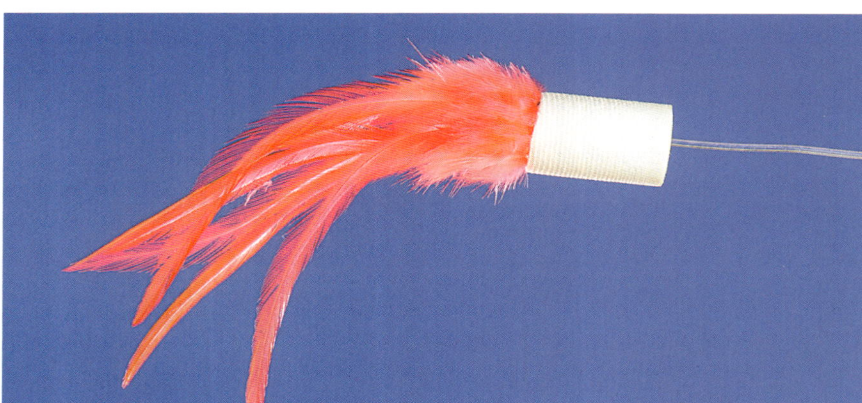

12. Notice how the fluff provides volume and a transition from the Live Body to the feather tips.

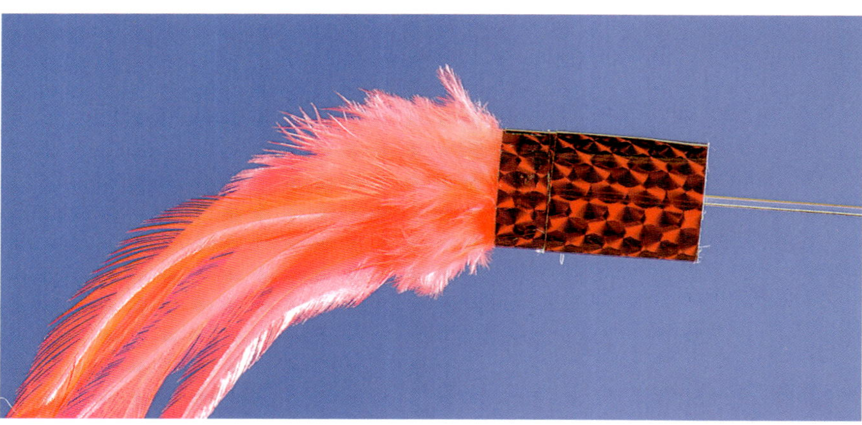

13. Apply prismatic tape to the Live Body. Be sure to overlap tape if necessary.

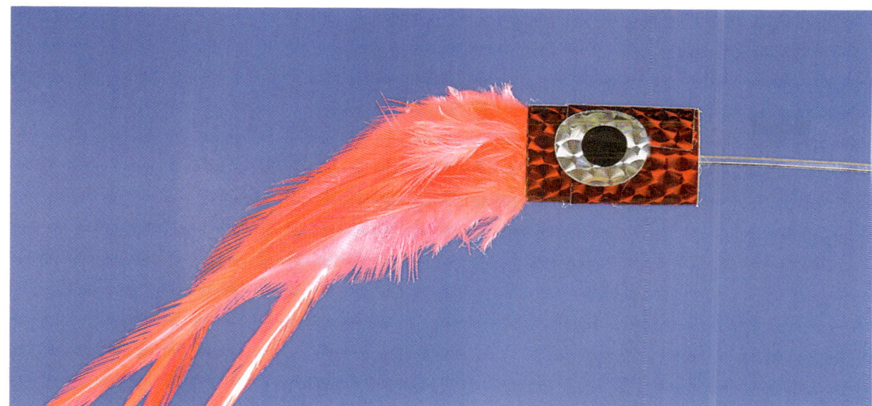

14. Attach extra large stick-on eyes over the prismatic tape. You can place a small drop of Krazy Glue under each eye for extra durability.

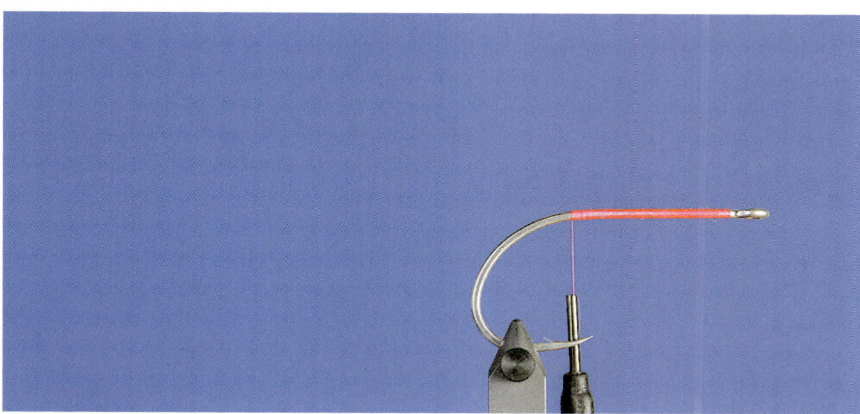

15. Attach the thread (here, Gudebrod A) to the shank and wrap a thread base over the shank to ensure that the mono assembly doesn't slip.

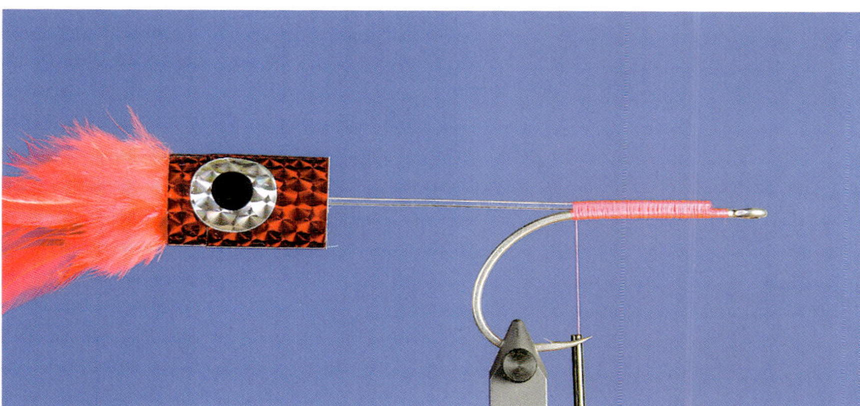

16. Tie on the mono assembly, and wrap along the entire shank to a point less than $^{1}/_{4}$ inch from the hook eye.

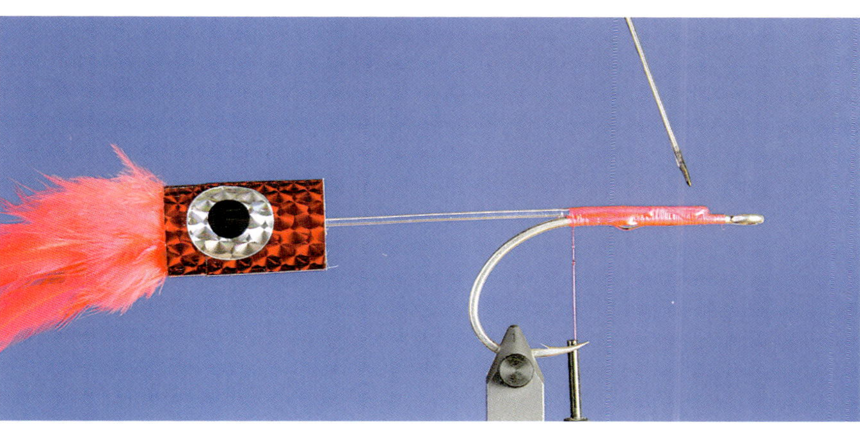

17. Apply head cement to the thread. The thread is now in the proper location to tie in your fleece or Estaz as filler.

(continued)

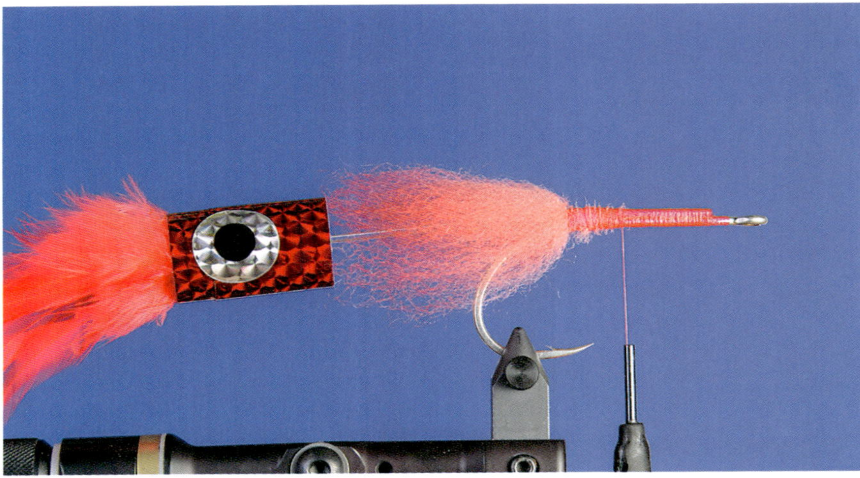

18. Prepare the fleece by first brushing the patch with a dog brush to remove tangles, and then cut a small tuft from the hide. Don't overdo the amount of fleece—it is just there to help open up the fibers a bit. Hold the fleece with your material hand while you tie it in so that it extends just past the hook bend and the tips reach the Banger head. Distribute it 360 degrees around the hook shank.

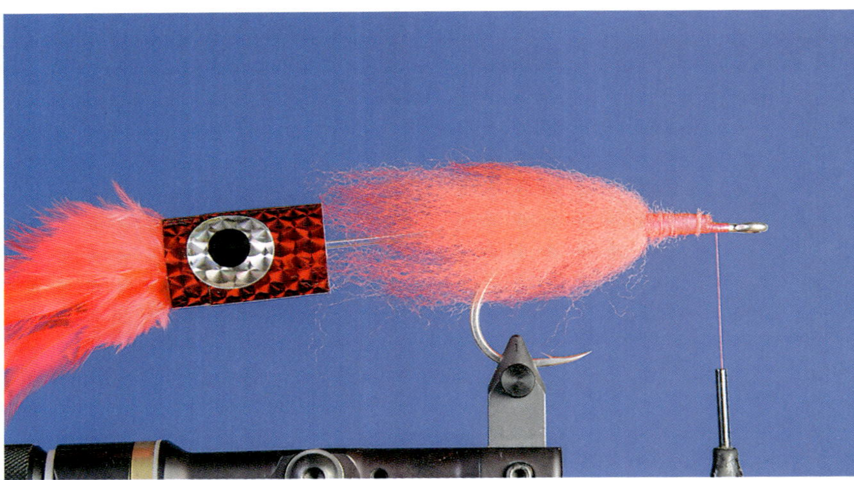

19. Attach another bunch of fleece and distribute it around the hook shank. The second tie of fleece should blend into the first. If you tie the fleece too far forward, it will interrupt the shape of the bucktail. You don't need a lot of fleece here; just two ties will suffice. You just want something to hold the bucktail open without ruining the shape of the squid, which has a longer snout.

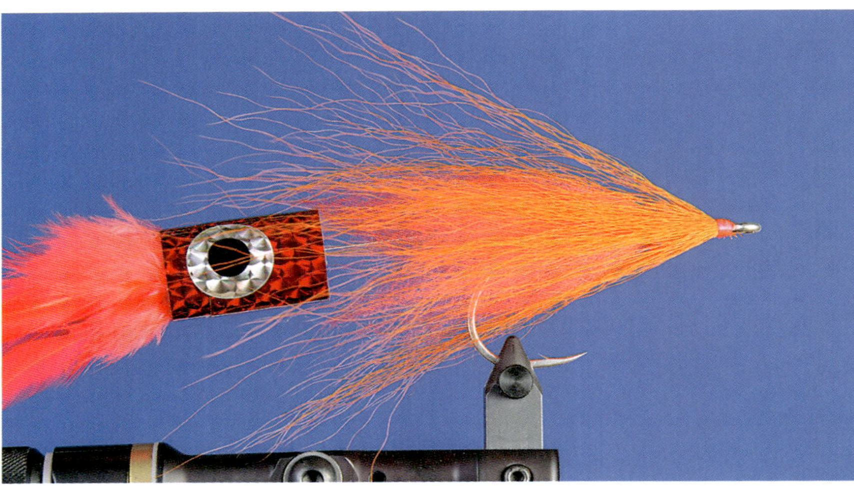

20. Tie in long bucktail to completely cover the fleece, and distribute it 360 degrees around hook shank, as you would for a Bucktail Deceiver. Notice the low angle that the bucktail comes off of the shank to imitate the profile of the squid. The fibers need to be long enough to get around the Banger head, at least halfway or to the end of the Banger head to provide continuity between the eye and the body, so that the eye looks like it is part of the fly. Whip-finish the thread.

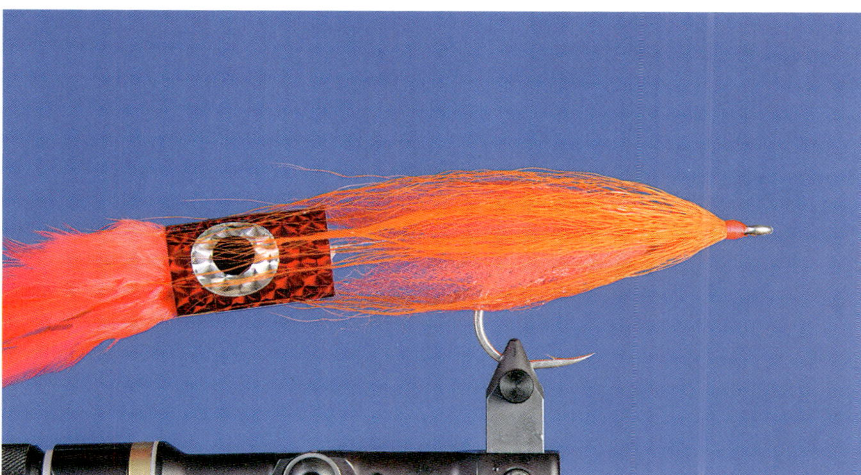

21. Wet the fly to control the fibers.

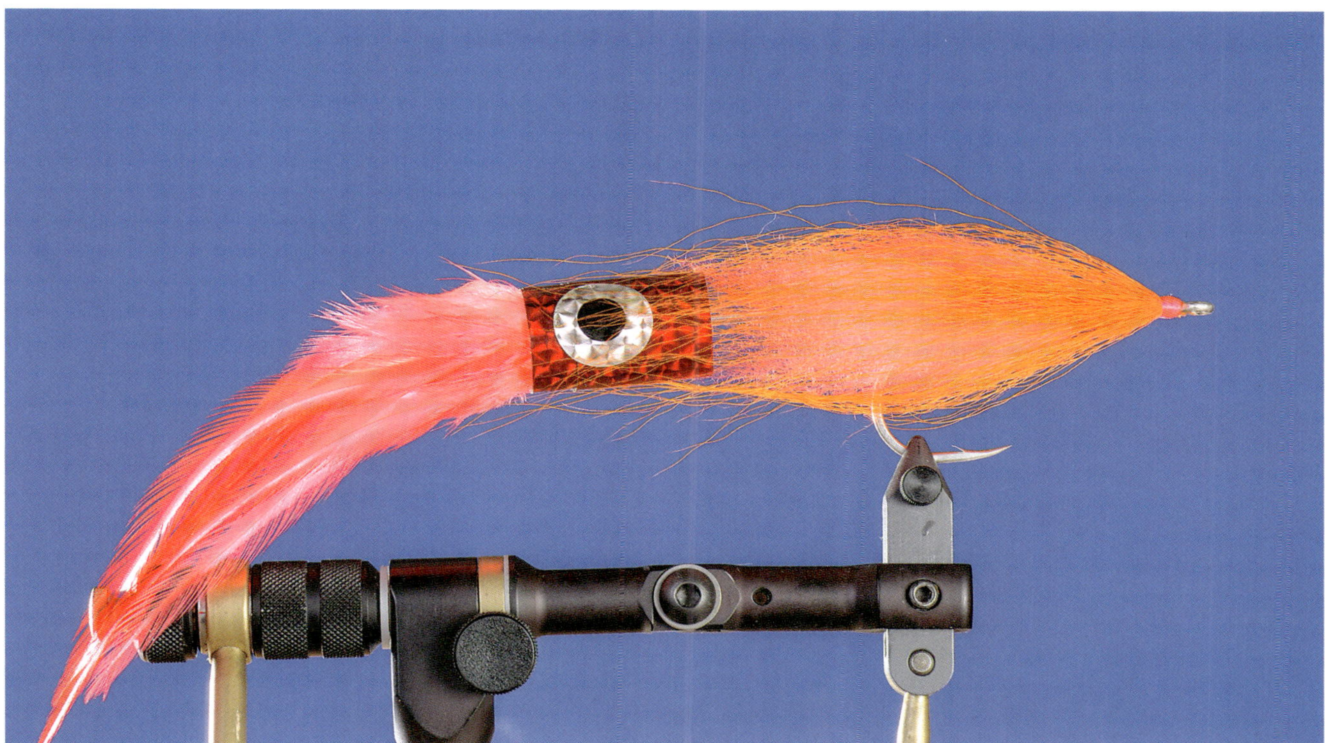

Try to visualize this fly in the water, resting with the hook pointing down and the Banger head suspended higher in the water. When you retrieve, the Rear Floating Squid will track down as it follows the line and leader, leaving a wake of bubbles from the Banger head, and then rise toward the surface.

Chapter 12

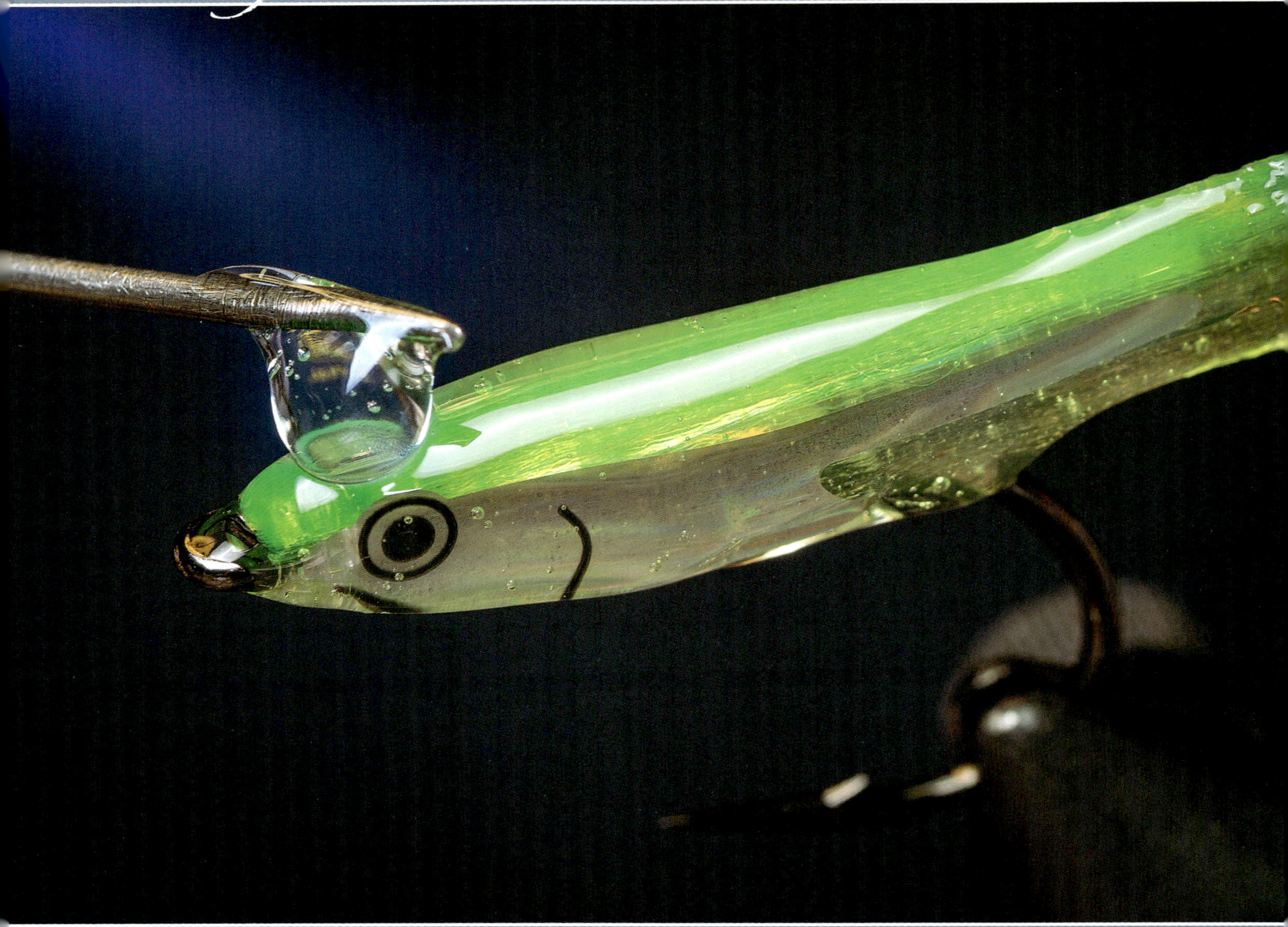

Adding one more coating of light-cured acrylic to a Surf Candy tied with a Fleye Foil. The new wave!

Light-Cured Acrylic Surf Candies

Epoxy has been used in fly tying for over thirty years, and discovering how to work with it to create effective baitfish imitations was a source of inspiration and creativity for me. But using epoxy as a fly-tying material was not without its problems. Everything had to be right; the mixing was critical, the application was messy and time-consuming, and controlling the dripping gel required extreme finesse. Then there was the unpleasant odor and yellowing to contend with. But epoxy flies looked and worked great and could stand up to abuse, so the hassles were worth it.

Seeing the Light

A couple of years ago, Dr. Ned Lunt, a dentist from San Antonio, Texas, introduced me to an epoxy alternative, which is actually a light-cured acrylic used in dentistry. Though I was skeptical at first, Ned came back East and showed me the potential of this material, which we later called Tuffleye.

After his quick demonstration, I could not wait to take a turn. As I worked with the material, I did everything exactly the same with the gel as I would with epoxy, and I was amazed. With epoxy, you first mix the resin and the hardener on a Post-it note and apply it to a fly with a bodkin. Then you create a shape and maintain it until the working time is over and the epoxy gets hard. With this new acrylic, there is no mixing—it comes straight from a syringe that I also use in place of a bodkin. Also, because you shape it and then instantly set it with the light, you have greater control with fewer steps and less waste. Over the next few months, I worked with Ned to fine-tune some things (such as using alcohol to remove the tackiness), and I have not used epoxy since—light-cured acrylics are not only easier and more convenient to use than epoxy, but they are also clearer and offer more flexibility for creative fly-tying applications.

Light-cured acrylics are much more expensive at the outset than epoxy; however, you have much less waste and you save a bunch of time, so for me the product is well worth the initial expense, especially since I believe the results are better. There's no mixing, no waste, no smell, no yellowing, no drying wheel, and no stress.

Core, Finish, Top Coat, and Flex

Because I prefer to use acrylics that are cured with a blue light over those cured with a UV light, I will discuss Tuffleye specifically, but other manufacturers have similar acrylics that you can use if you wish. Tuffleye comes in different viscosities: Core and Finish. It also comes in

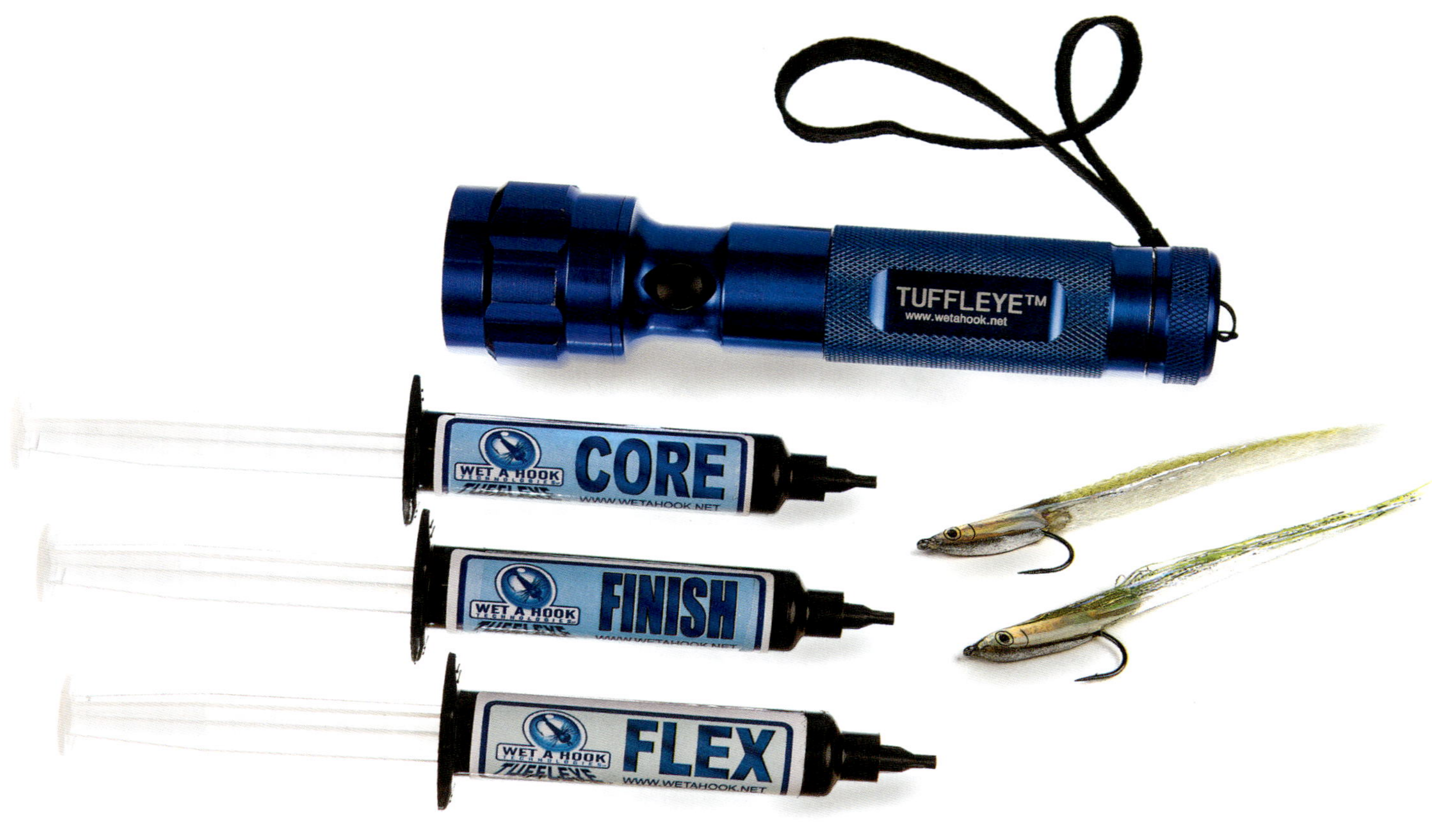

Flex, which is a different formulation altogether. Core is thicker and most like the consistency of epoxy. It is the easiest of the three to use because it stays in place without sagging or running (for a surprising length of time), can be adjusted over and over until you're satisfied with the shape, and quickly solidifies in seconds with the blue light. The Finish is thinner, moves quickly, and is excellent as a final coat to the Core. You can tie flies with the Finish, but I don't recommend it for beginners since it flows faster.

Core, Finish, and Flex have a tackiness after they are cured. This tacky surface is important because it allows subsequent coats to stick to one another and bond as one coat, not layers. If you are going to be using multiple coats, do not remove the tacky surface until that last coat. To remove the tackiness, simply wipe it with isopropyl rubbing alcohol and then apply Tuffleye Top Coat or Sally Hansen Hard As Nails.

Regardless of which product you use, you must penetrate the fibers thoroughly, and the type of fiber might influence your choice of acrylic. Sometimes, when tying small Surf Candies with Craft Fur, I will use the Finish because it saturates the fibers better. After you use the Finish to saturate the fibers, you can then add either Core or Finish to get a nice smooth and durable finish.

Flex has a similar viscosity to Core, but when cured, it feels like the bottom of a sneaker. It does not have a glassy feel, as Core and Finish do. I currently use it for both Surf Candies and Flex Fleyes. On a Surf Candy, I just like how it feels, though I'm not sure that it matters much to the fish. You should not use Core or Finish for Flex Fleyes, though. (For more on the Flex, see page 189.)

Acrylic Surf Candy

Hook: Varivas 990S or similar short-shank saltwater
Thread: Fine monofilament
Body: Olive and white Super Hair coated with Tuffleye Core
Flash: Pearl Saltwater Angel Hair
Eyes: Stick-on prismatic, silver with black pupil

TYING THE ACRYLIC SURF CANDY

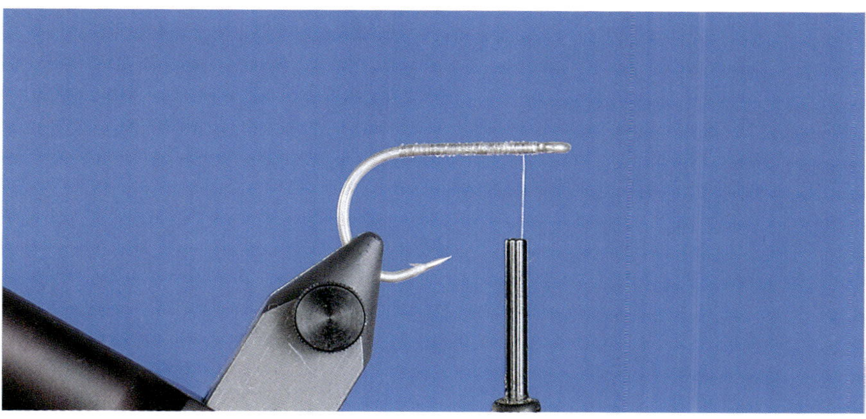

1. With hook in the vise, cover the entire shank with monofilament thread and bring it back to about 1/8 to 1/4 inch from the hook eye to begin the next step. The thread gives the light-cured acrylic something to bond to so that the materials are less likely to spin on the hook.

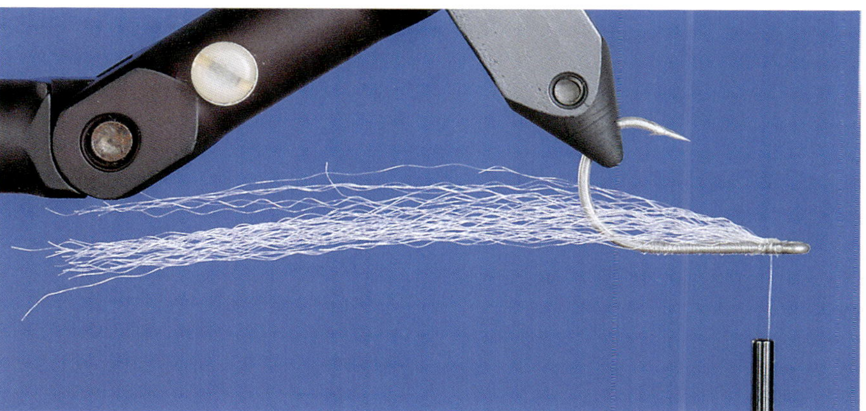

2. Rotate your vise or reposition the fly upside down, and tie in a light-colored wing on the underside of the hook shank. Keep the material sparse, and only use a few wraps to keep the thread bulk down.

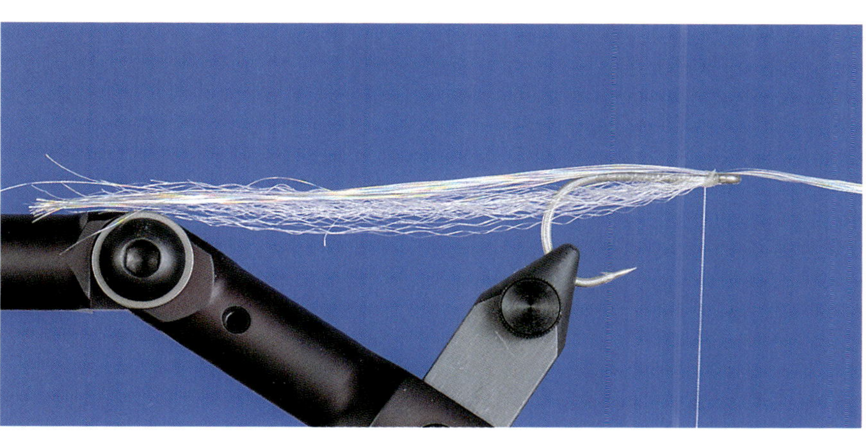

3. Rotate the vise or reposition the hook back to an upright position and tie in flash (pearl Angel Hair) in the middle of the bunch. Here I am using about 10 to 12 strands.

(continued)

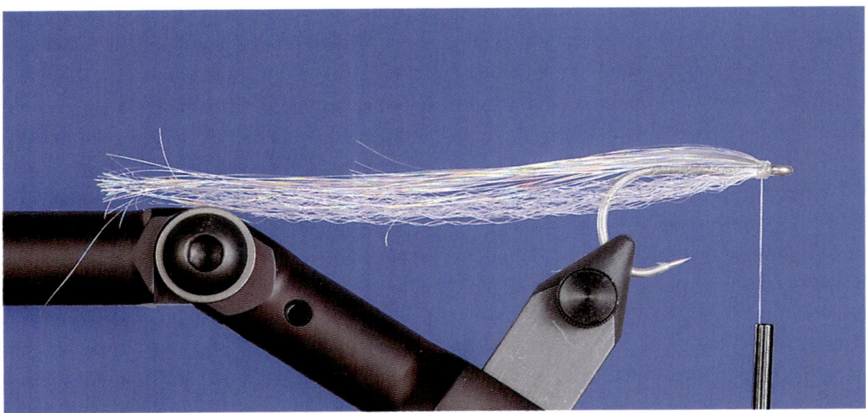

4. Fold the remaining flash hanging over the eye back over the rest of the bunch and wrap over it. After securing the flash, wrap the thread forward to receive the top color of fibers.

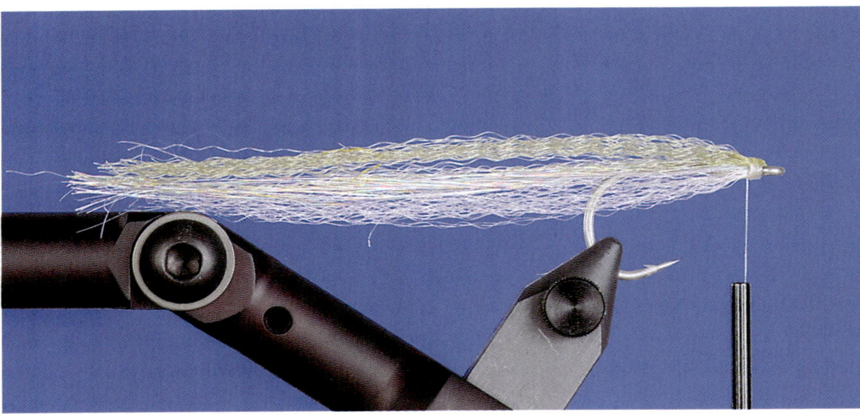

5. Tie the fibers directly on top of the previous ties. All the materials should be tied in at the same spot. Here we are using light olive for a silverside/spearing. Other good colors for spearing (aka silversides) are chartreuse over white, chartreuse and pink, and blue or gray over white. For bay anchovies, I like amber over white, or tan over white with or without some lavender, and chartreuse over white.

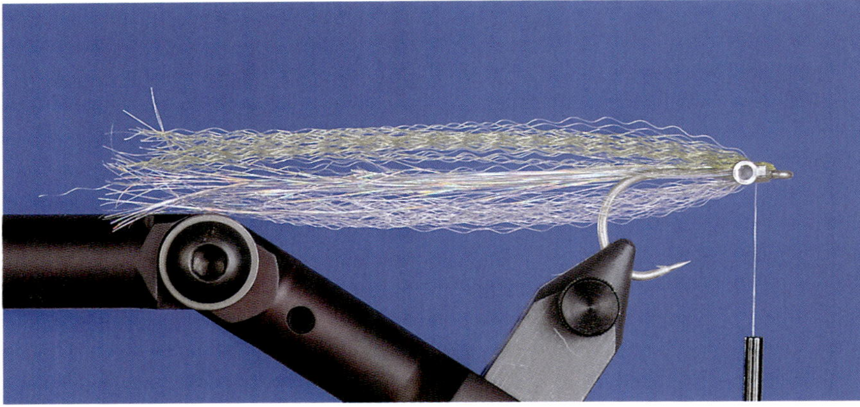

6. If using eyes with tabs, tie down the tab to the hook shank—one on each side. Cut the tab so that the eyes are fairly far forward to imitate the natural. If using stick-on eyes, place the eye on the head and wrap over it two or three times with the mono thread to hold it in place before you add the acrylic. Whip-finish, and you have completed the first phase, what I call the "blank." Sometimes I will tie a dozen blanks and then apply the Tuffleye all at once.

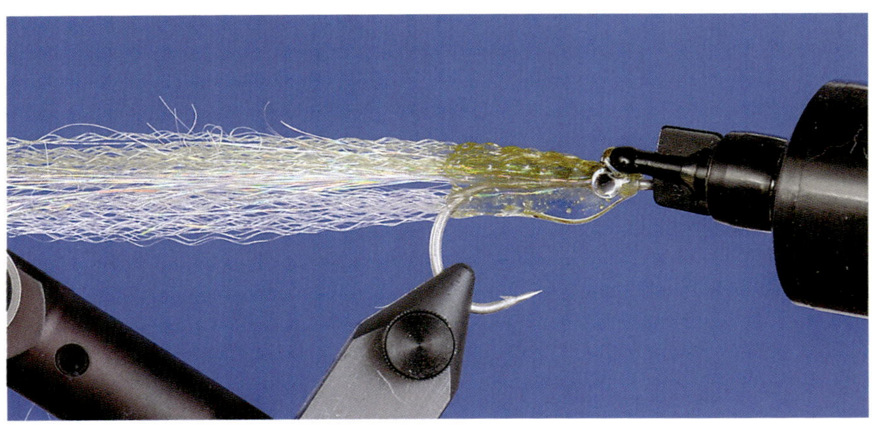

7. While holding all of the fibers firmly at the rear with your material hand, begin applying gel liberally from the hook eye to just behind hook bend. Press the gel into the fibers with the syringe tip to ensure complete saturation and fill all hollow areas. Once I apply the gel, I use the curved tip of the syringe or a bodkin (or both) to refine the shape.

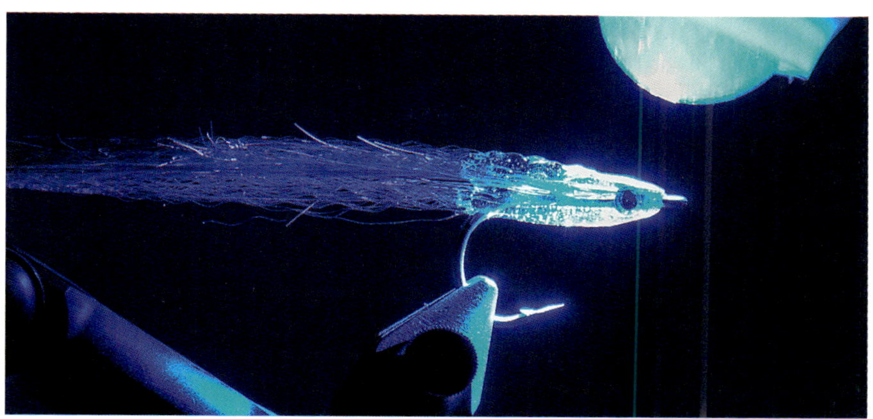

8. When I am happy with the shape and distribution of the gel, I go for the light. The gel will not set until you are ready. Here I am using the original light given to me by Ned. Keep the light close and move it slowly from front to back, and then repeat on all four sides. Note how close I am to the fly. When the acrylic on the fly is completely set, turn the light off.

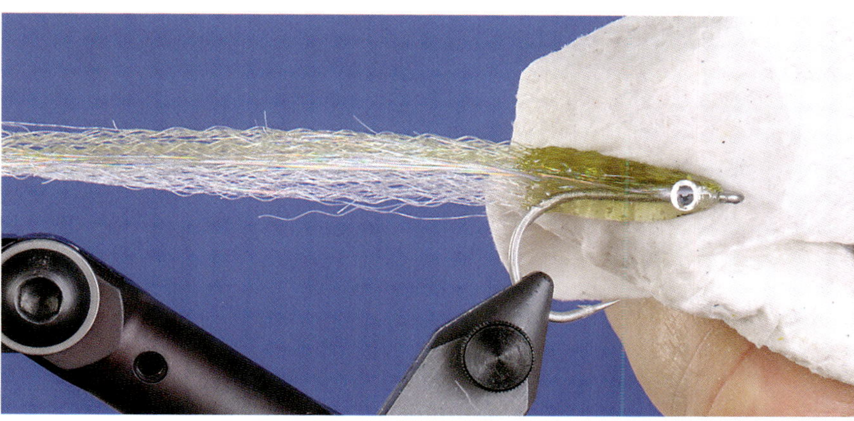

9. Wipe off the tacky residue with a paper towel and rubbing alcohol. This is a one-coat Surf Candy; if you add multiple coats, only wipe the last coat with alcohol. The tacky layer is what helps the layers bond.

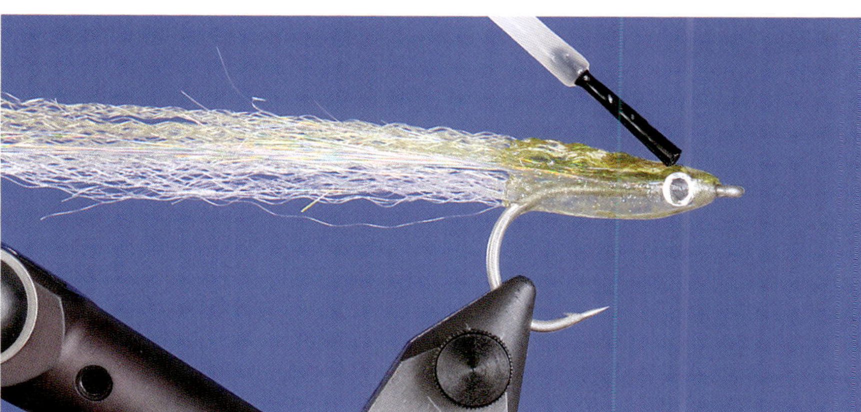

10. Apply clear nail polish or Top Coat to bring back the luster. This step is really more for the tier; once the fly enters the water, even if not treated with Top Coat, it shines.

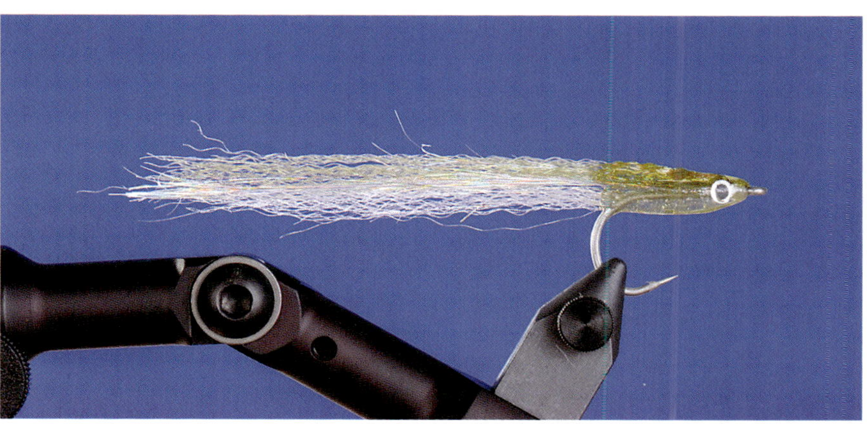

11. Now you are ready to trim the synthetic fibers to a nice, natural taper. The wing should always be thinner than the body on the shank.

(continued)

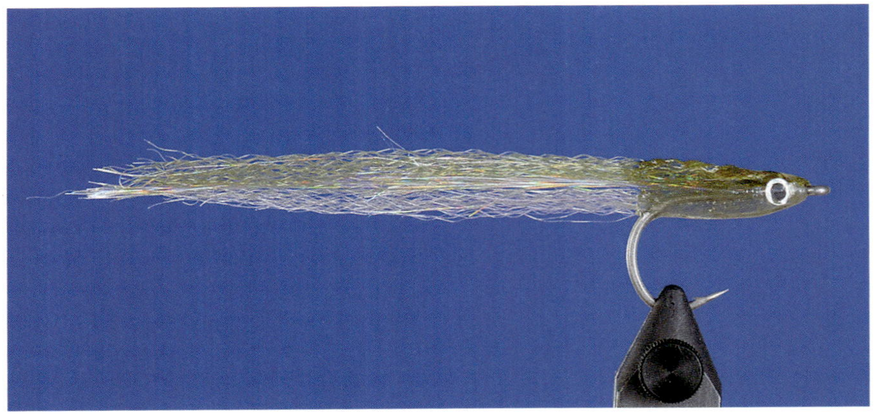

12. I did not paint the belly with silver paint on this fly to show how clear the acrylic is. One other virtue of the acrylic is that it gets clearer as the sunlight hits it, unlike epoxy, which yellows over time.

Surf Candy Variations

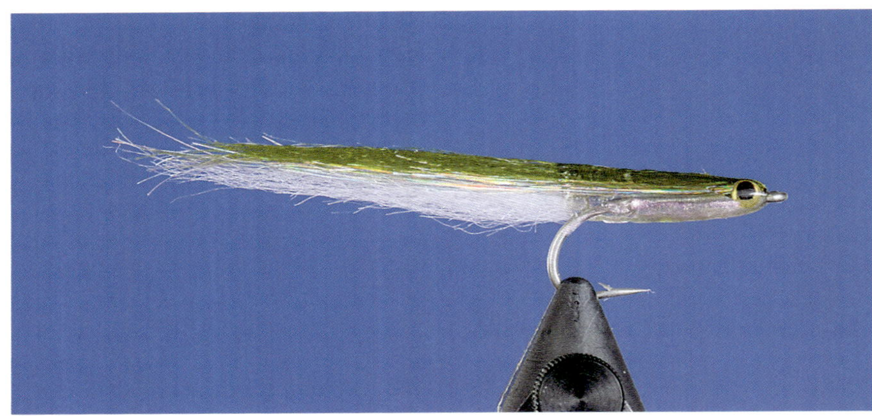

This is the Polar Fibre Surf Candy (for silverside). The fine, thin fibers add a little bit of movement to small flies. The belly is painted with chrome nail polish to imitate the belly sac of the natural, then coated with Tuffleye Top Coat or Hard As Nails. This is an example of a pattern tied with a stick-on eye, which is first held on with a few wraps of monofilament thread before coating with the acrylic.

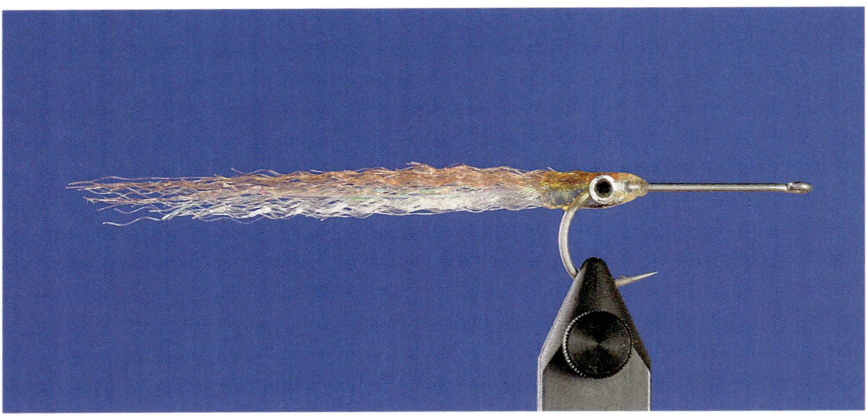

This pattern, tied with tan over white Super Hair, is an example of how you can use an exposed shank for a more durable fly for toothy fish, such as bluefish.

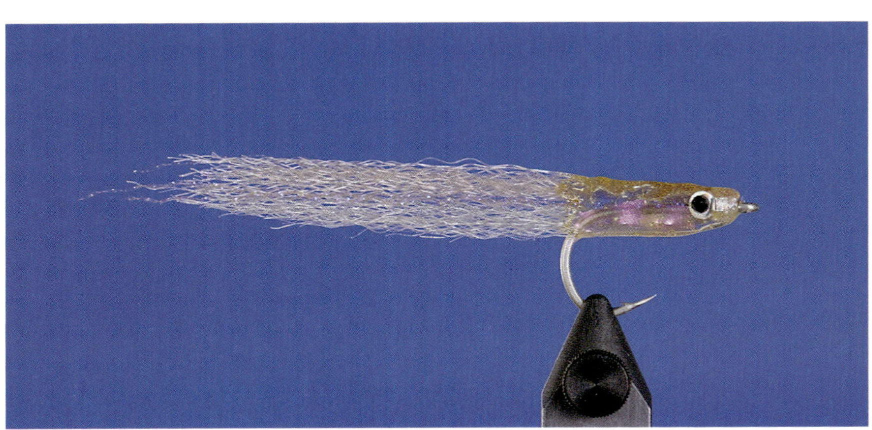

This bay anchovy Surf Candy is tied with Tuffleye Flex and has a subtle addition of pink pearl nail polish and a slight amount of pearl Krystal Flash.

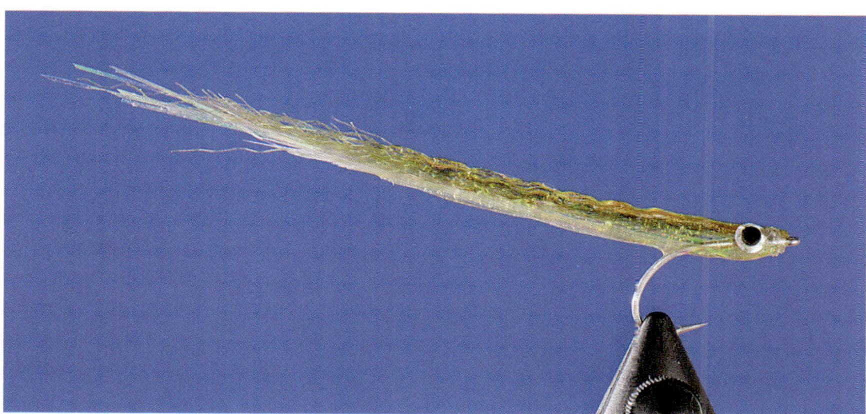

Light-cured acrylics make it easy to manipulate the body shape to get a thin profile. This sand eel–type fly is tied with Flex over olive and white Super Hair. In all black this is a great fly for Martha's Vineyard.

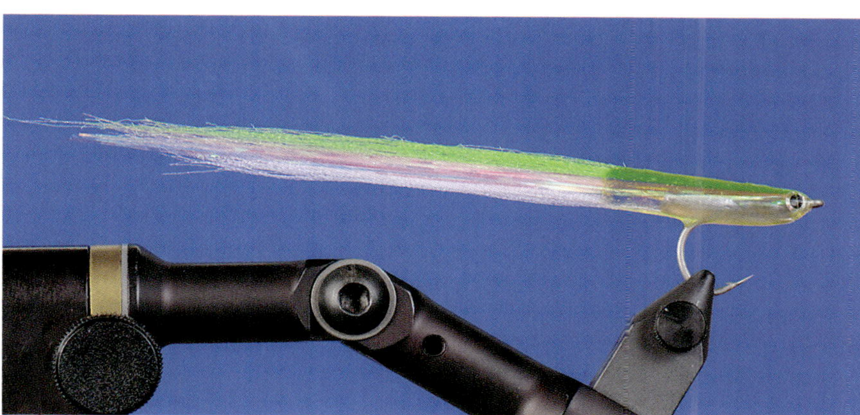

Here is a Surf Candy tied with chartreuse over white Fluoro Fibre. Fluoro Fibre is great to work with in combination with light-cured acrylics. Chrome nail polish extends from behind the eye all the way to the rear, and the acrylic extends well beyond the hook to prevent fouling. The tutti frutti color combination is a good option to use as a changeup.

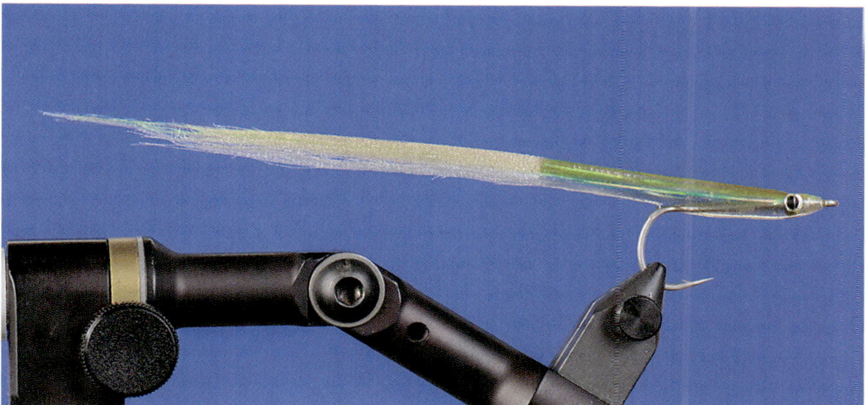

A sand eel Candy tied with tan over white Fluoro Fibre, coated with Flex.

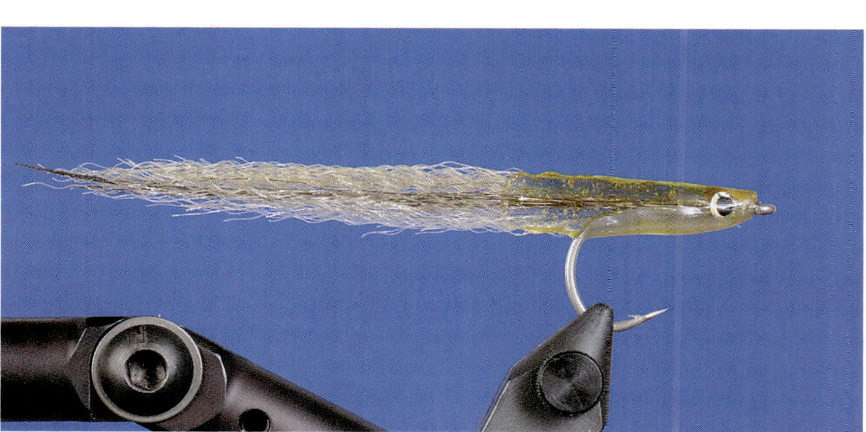

Attach the top fibers in a reverse style to achieve a prominent snout that more closely resembles a bay anchovy. This fly is tied with gold Angel Hair flash and tan over white Super Hair.

Chapter 13

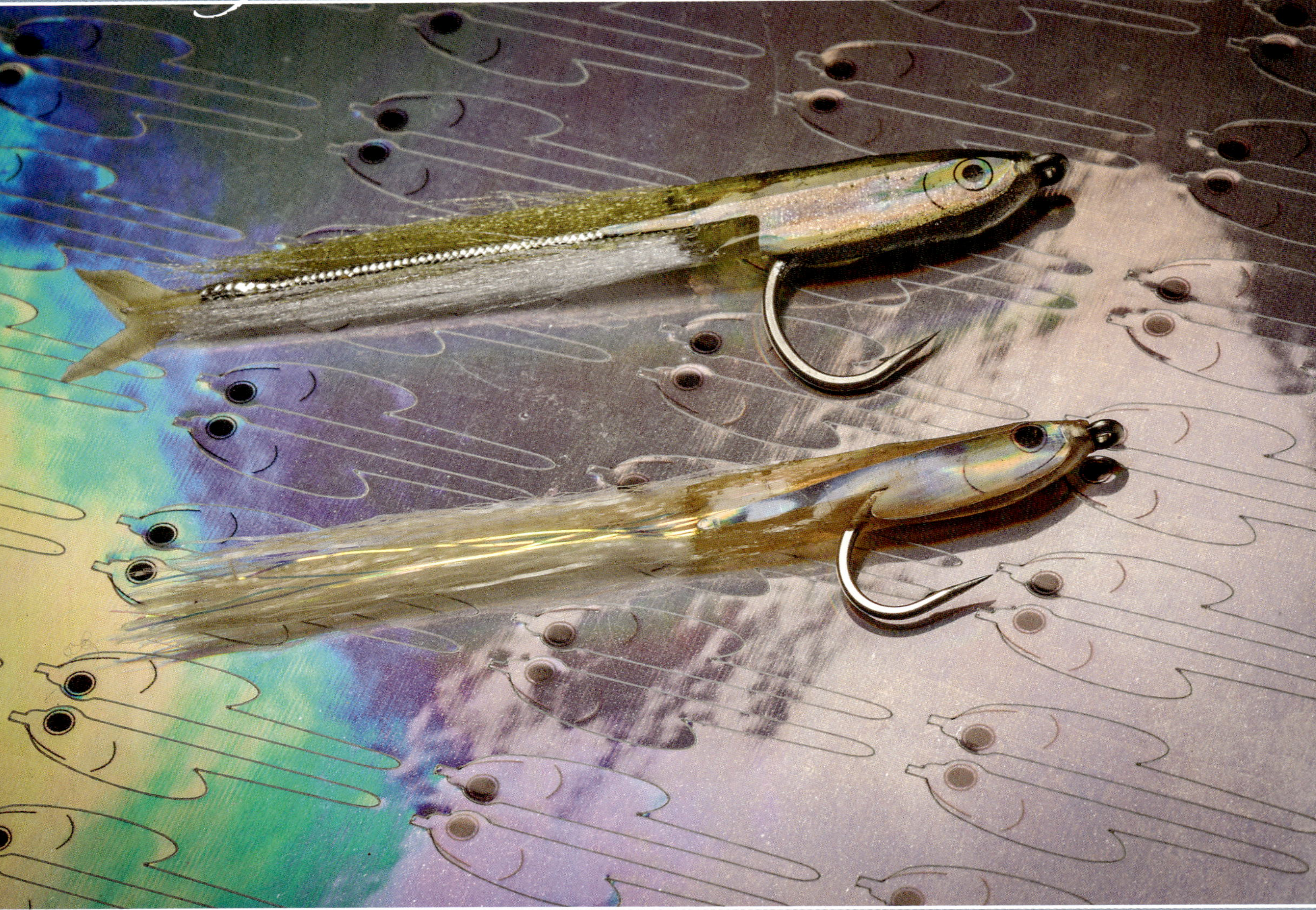

Fleye Foils come in different sizes and shapes and are now commercially available through fly shops (distributed by Wet A Fly Technologies in the United States). The fleye on the top is a Full Dress Acrylic Surf Candy (Silverside). This tail assembly is based on the one that I covered in *Pop Fleyes*, except in lieu of a feather, here I am using a latex tail, which was a prototype. I am sure manufacturers will eventually develop and produce prefab, realistic tails.

Fleye Foils

Surf Candies have always been one of my go-to patterns for small, translucent baits such as bay anchovies, silversides, and sand eels. The level of detail that I put into a fly is directly related to how translucent it is. On larger patterns, I don't feel the need to add a lot of specifics after achieving the right shape, but with smaller, more translucent baits, I believe it is important to tie in prominent eyes, lateral lines, and belly sacs. Though Surf Candies are fairly simple to make, this attention to detail nonetheless takes time. With Fleye Foils, I've been able to improve the Surf Candy by not only making it easier and faster to tie but also more imitative.

I had the basic idea for a premade shape for the Surf Candy for a long time and over the years had talked to some manufacturers about the idea, but it was always too expensive. A few winters ago, I met Ibrahim "Ibby" Mesinovic, a mechanical engineer and tier from Sweden, at one of the fly-fishing shows. He had some foils that had gels on them to simulate insect parts, and when he showed them to me, I knew he could make what I wanted. Because he was in Sweden and I was in New Jersey, I would draw what I wanted on a Post-it note, photograph it, and text or email the photo to him to fine-tune the different shapes and sizes.

The design of the foils offers several benefits. First, they have tabs in front that make attaching them to the shank easy. The length of the tabs can be trimmed to position the foil exactly where you want it. Second, each foil has two sides. Because they are not one solid piece that you fold over the back of the fly, you can reach the acrylic on the top and bottom of the fly with the light to cure it completely. You can also use these with epoxy.

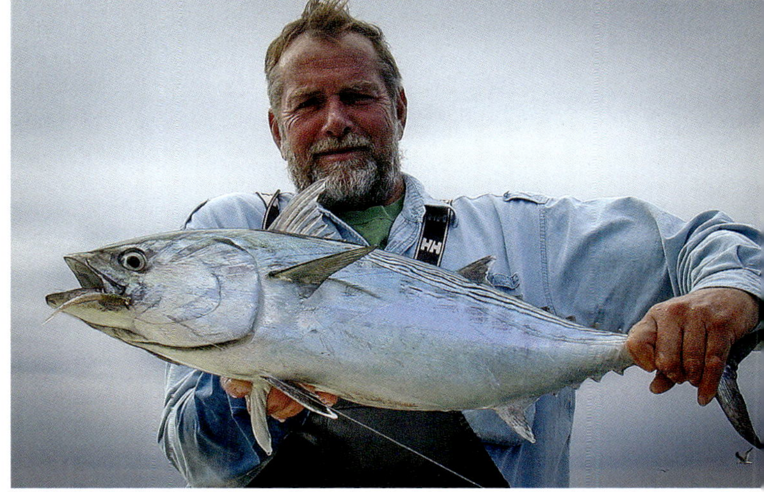

Lance Erwin lifts a brute of an albacore from Harkers Island, North Carolina. The fish took a Deep Candy, which incorporates durability and forward weight into one fly.

Perhaps the most exciting aspect of these foils is the quality of the imitation that you can achieve. Traditionally, it has been difficult to tie a thin fly with lots of flash in the belly, but with the Fleye Foils, you can achieve a wide, flat flash, almost like a mirror, that provides a bold, intermittent glint of light.

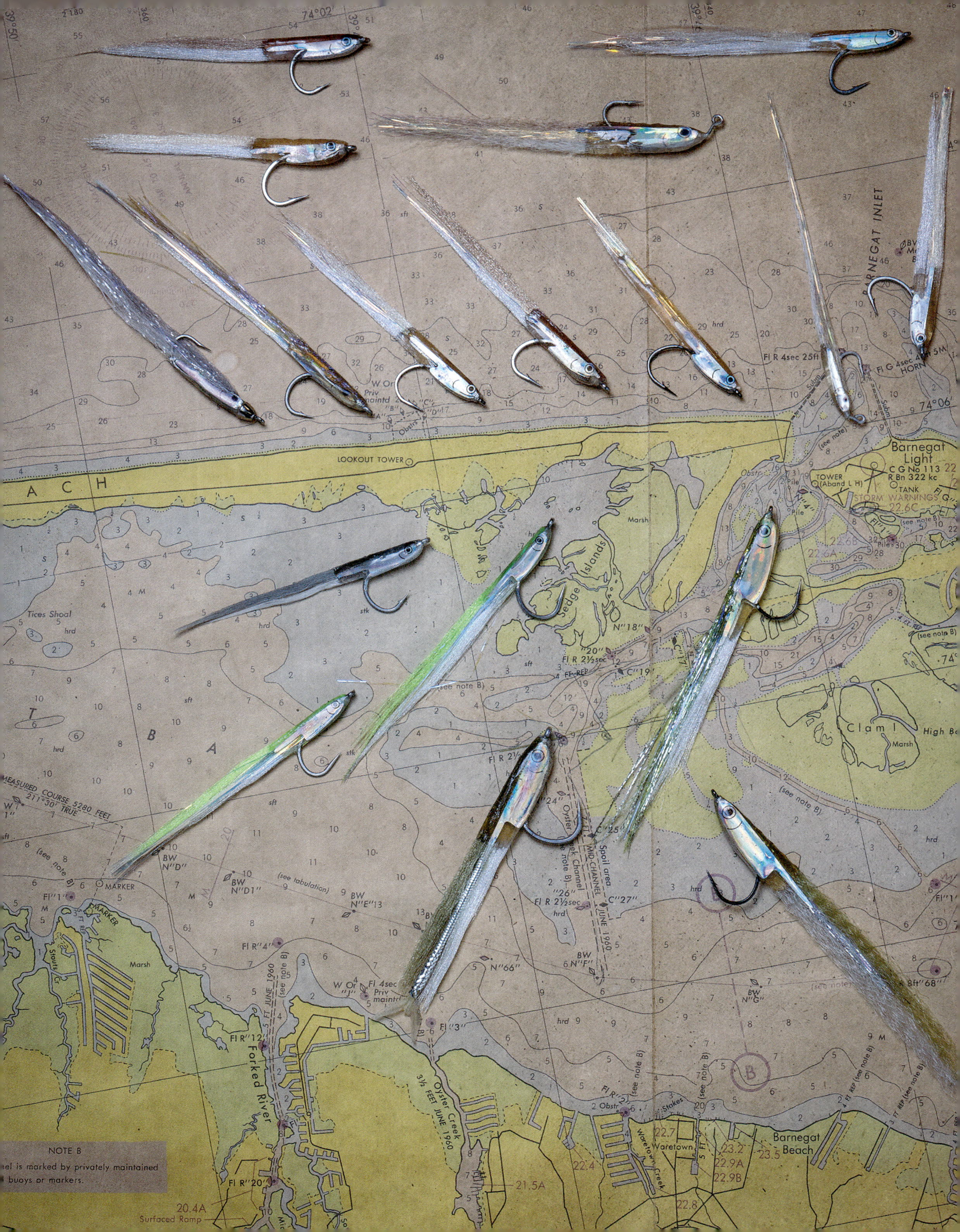

BARNEGAT INLET
LOOKOUT TOWER
Barnegat Light
Sedge Islands
Tices Shoal
Marsh
MEASURED COURSE 5280 FEET
Forked River
Oyster Creek
Waretown
Barnegat Beach
NOTE B
buoys or markers.
Surfaced Ramp

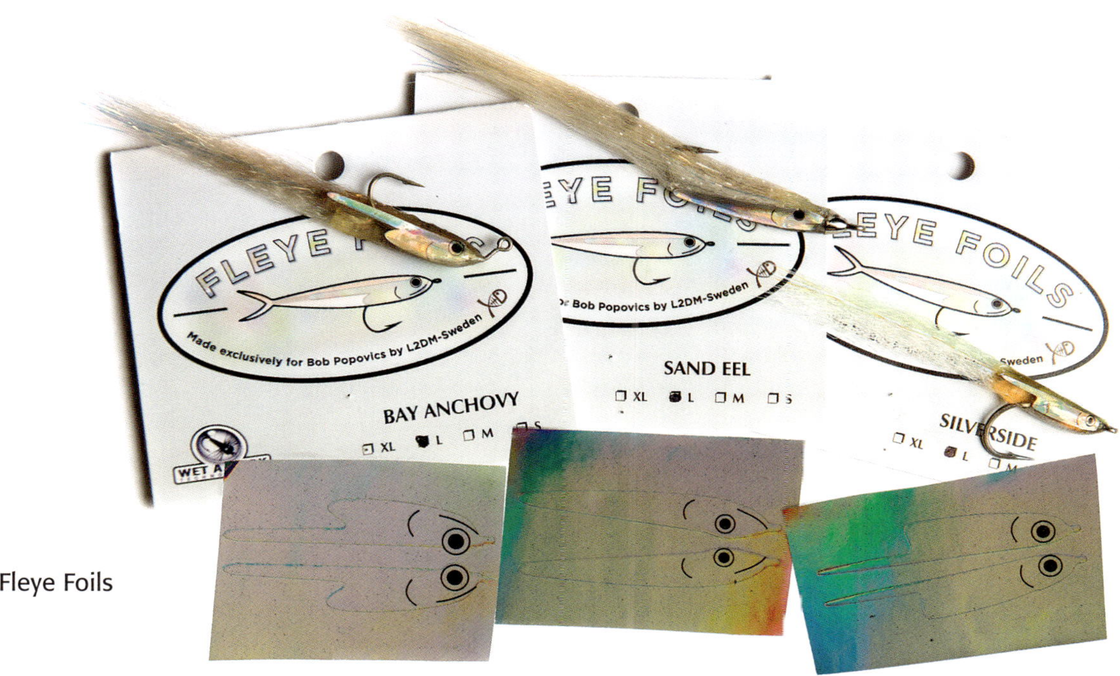

Fleye Foils

Fleye Foil Sizes

Silverside

Large, for hooks #2/0-4/0, bait lengths 3-4"
Medium, for hooks #1-1/0, bait lengths 3"
Small, for hooks #4-2, bait lengths 2-3"

Sand Eel

Extra large, for hooks #3/0-4/0, bait lengths 5-7"
Large, for hooks #1-1/0, bait lengths 4-5"
Medium, for hooks #2-1/0, bait lengths 3-4"
Small, for hooks #4-2, bait lengths 2-3"

Bay Anchovy

Extra large, for hooks #2/0-4/0, bait lengths 3-5"
Large, for hooks #1-1/0, bait lengths 2½-3"
Medium, for hooks #2-1, bait lengths 1½-2½"
Small, for hooks #6-2, bait lengths 1-2"

Squid Foils

Small squid are a common food for many offshore species. With Fleye Foils in a squid version, I was able to update the original Candy Squid that I showed in *Pop Fleyes*. Not only is this simple fly faster to tie, but it is more realistic. The Squid Foils are simply two sides of a squid-shaped skin body, with added specks to simulate a natural appearance and a round base at the rear to accept any eye that you choose. Like the other Foils, they have a tying tab in front to make it easy to tie them down. They are available in one size—in tan, clear, and pink.

Legs can be imitated simply by sparse bucktail, skinny feathers, or other premade leg materials. I keep it simple by tying in bucktail or synthetic fibers that extend from the hook eye to well past the bend, which serves as both the body and the legs. This keeps the same translucence throughout the squid, not lighter or darker in front or back.

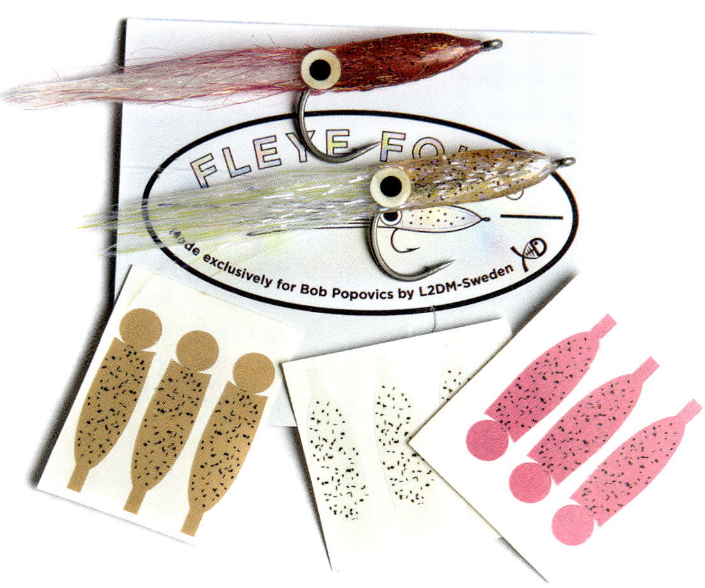

Squid Foils

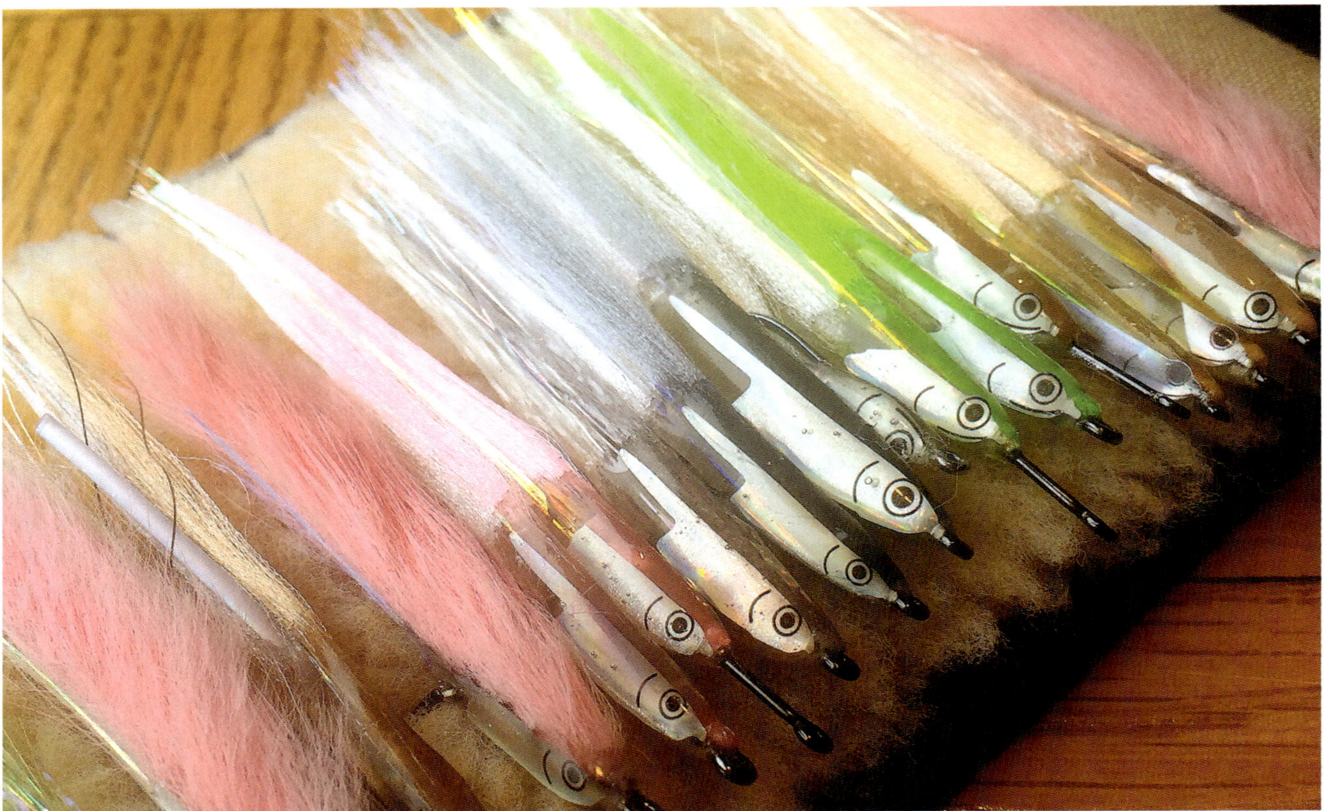

An assortment of Fleye Foil Candies, including some tied with rabbit.

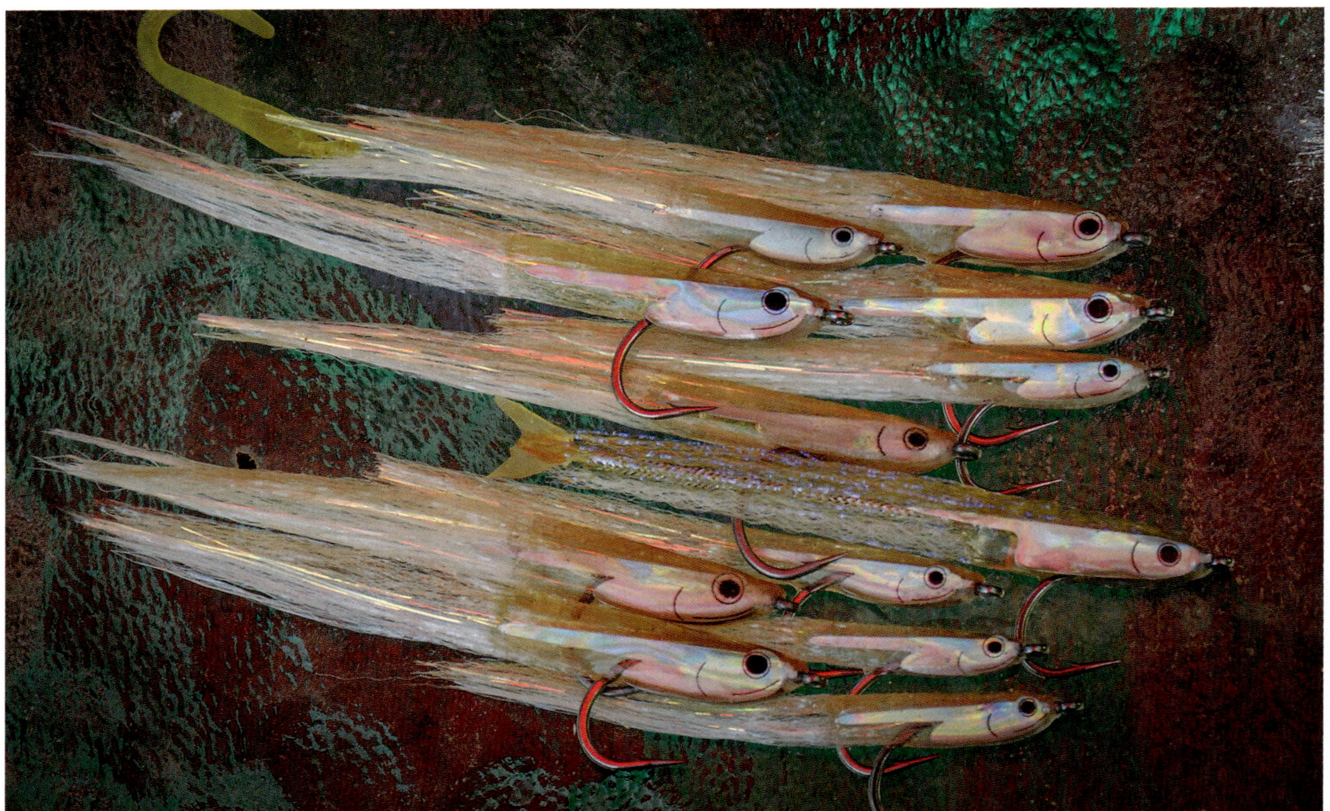

Early group shot of Fleye Foils, including some fleyes tied with latex tails.

Fleye Foil Bay Anchovy

Hook:	Short-shank saltwater
Thread:	Fine monofilament
Body:	Bay Anchovy Fleye Foil (small) coated with Tuffleye Flex, silver nail polish
Wing:	Fluoro Fibre
Flash:	Pearl Flashabou

FLEYE FOIL BAY ANCHOVY

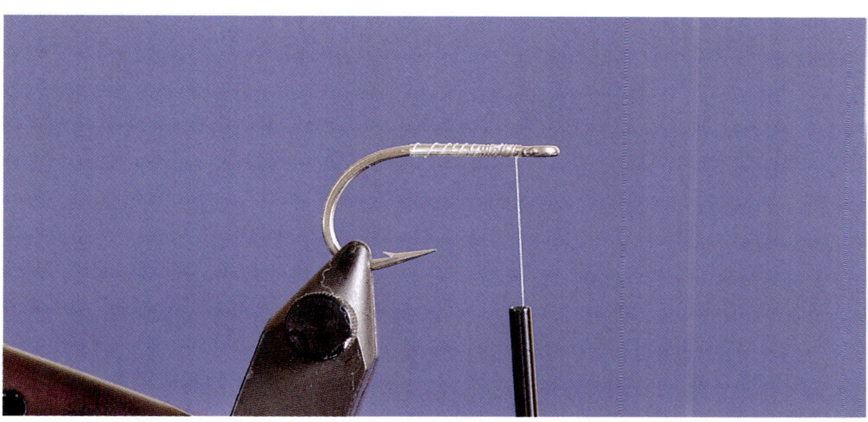

1. Insert the hook into the vise. Attach the monofilament thread to the hook shank just behind the hook eye, and wrap back over the shank and then forward again to cover it entirely. The thread gives the glue or acrylic something to grip to; without it, the finished fly could spin on the hook.

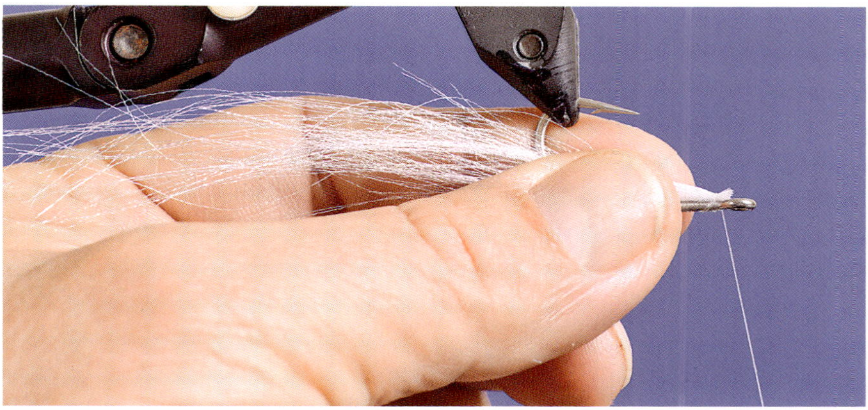

2. Rotate your vise to turn the hook upside down. Attach light-colored fibers (here I'm using Fluoro Fibre) just behind the hook eye and keep all the fibers on the underside. You don't need a lot of wraps to secure these fine fibers, so try to keep the head small. Every wrap from this point on should go toward the hook eye.

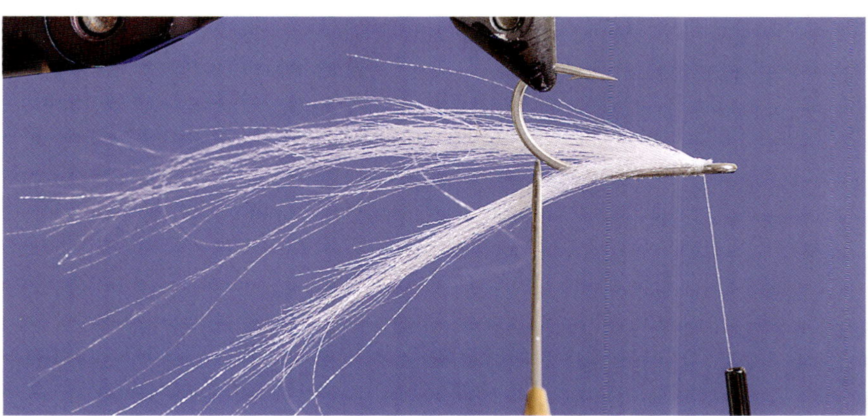

3. Using a bodkin, separate fibers equally to each side of hook so that the bottom of the fly is balanced before you put the gel on.

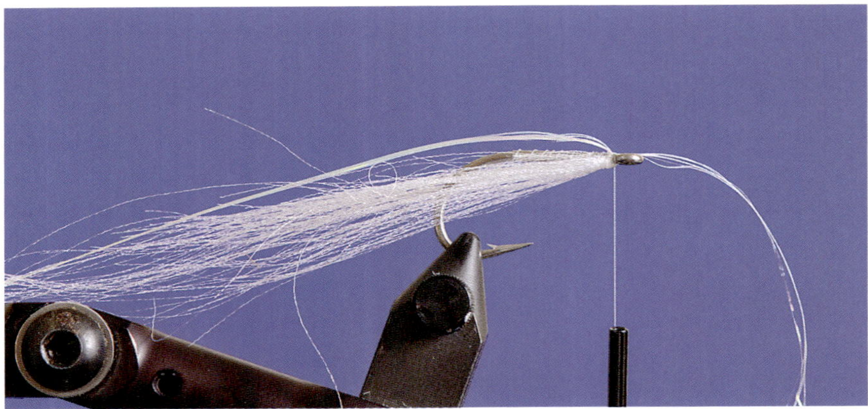

4. Turn the hook right side up. Separate a few fibers from a bundle of Flashabou, and tie them to the hook shank in the middle of the bunch. When Flashabou is backlit, it provides a prominent stripe; some of the other flashes don't.

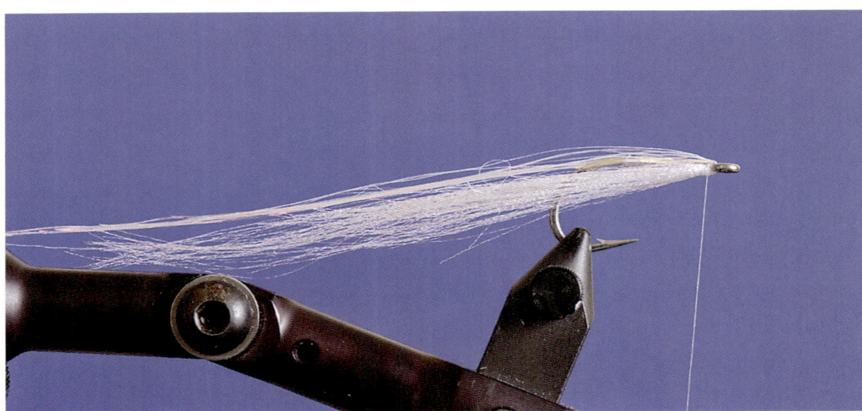

5. Fold the flash that is extending over the hook eye back over the fly, and take two or three tight wraps to secure it.

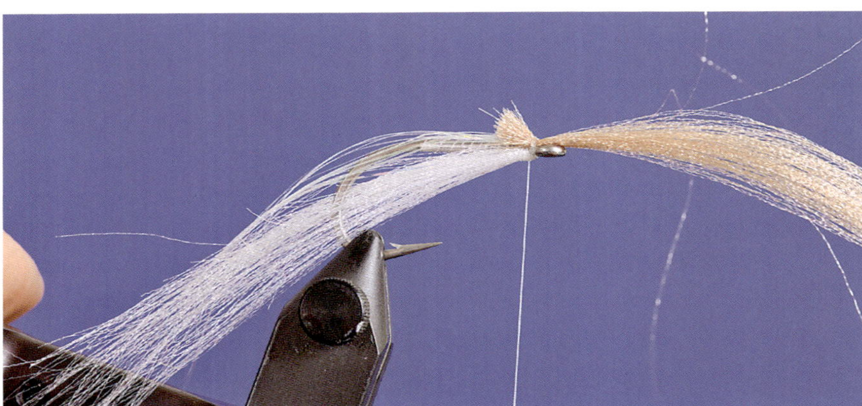

6. Bay anchovies have a prominent snout, so I tie in the fibers differently here. Tie in the top color in reverse, so that the fibers extend over the hook eye. Be sure to keep the fibers on the top for good color separation—this color will usually contrast with the bottom of the fly.

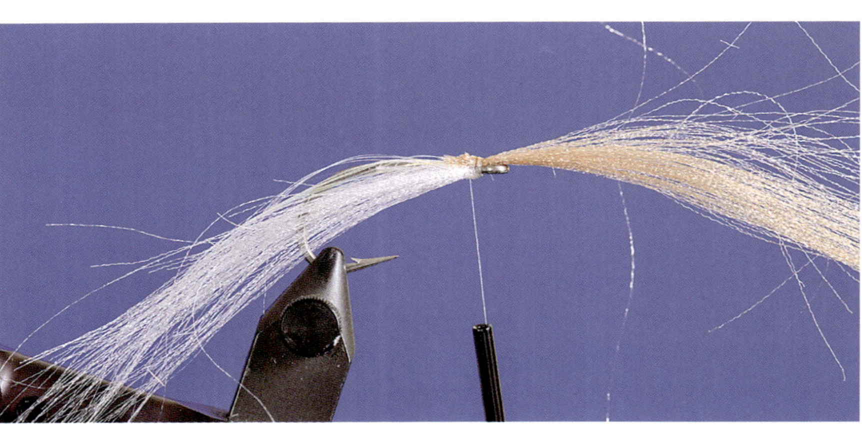

7. You can cut any excess fibers behind the tie-down area to neaten them up, or just leave them there. One interesting thing that I have noticed is that when I leave them there, the head area remains even darker when coated with acrylic, and it looks more natural, almost like the fish's skull.

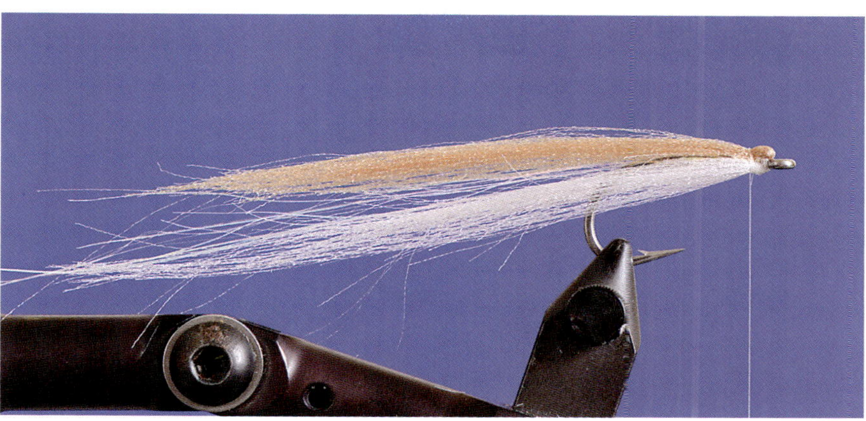

8. Pull back the top fibers and hold them in place with your material hand as you tie down the front with a few close wraps of thread. If you don't tie in reverse, the head will be too streamlined and won't look natural. Also, the flatter side makes a better platform for the foils.

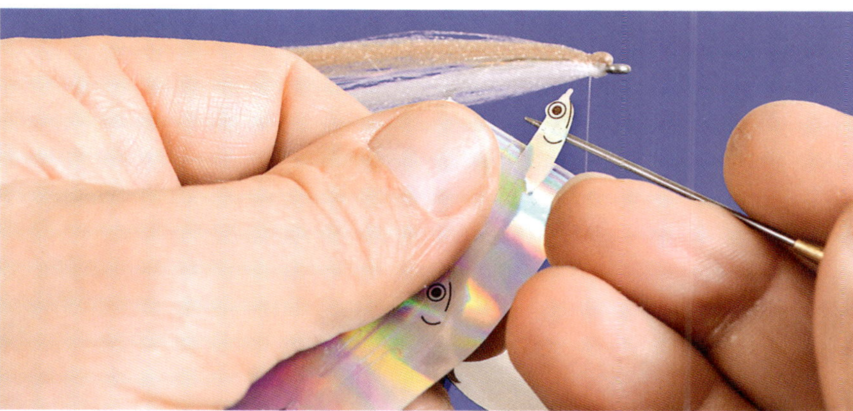

9. Peel one Bay Anchovy Fleye Foil side off the paper with a bodkin.

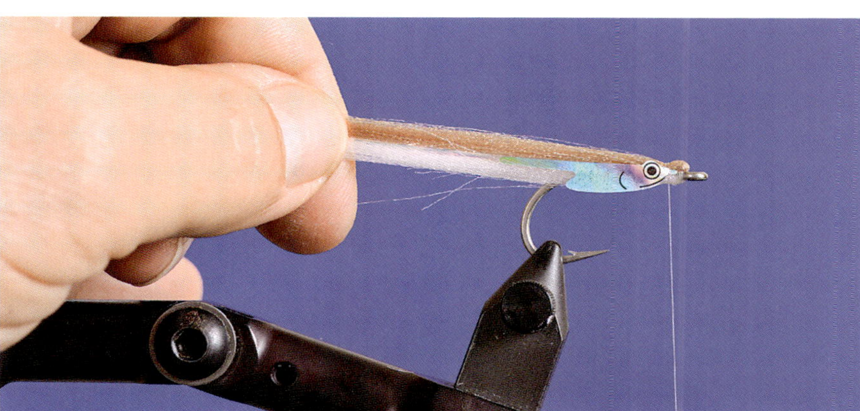

10. Place the foil against the side of the fly. Align the eye on the foil at the point shown on the left and secure it with two thread wraps over the tab. Repeat on both sides.

Tip: The stripe on the Fleye Foil should be centered directly between the top and bottom colors in the wing. Sometimes that causes trouble for the tier at this stage. After you whip-finish the fly, if you place a dollop of gel around the stripe area on the foil and then position it with your bodkin before setting it with the light, you can ensure its precise location while you complete the application of light-cured acrylic.

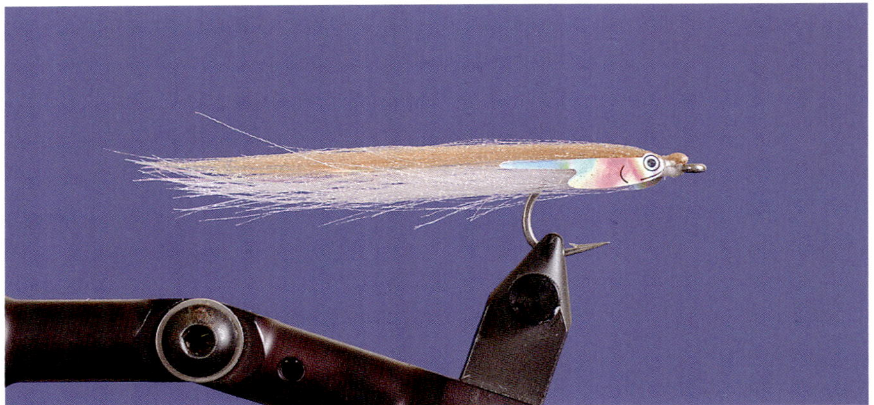

11. Whip-finish the thread. On this fly, I trimmed the bottom white fibers a bit, and tapered the top and bottom with scissors.

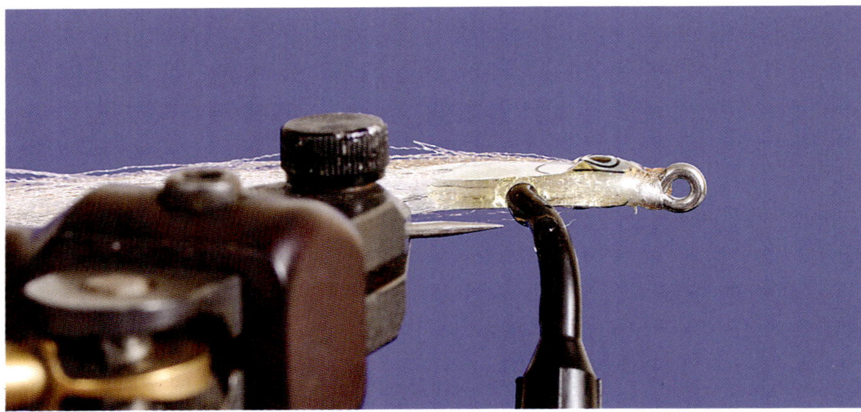

12. Begin applying the acrylic on the underside of the fly by dispensing gel between the sides of the foils so that the gel reaches through the fibers to the shank. Do not apply too much between the foils, either on the top or bottom, because too much gel can distort the sides. Apply the gel to just past the hook bend. Turn the fly over and do the same on top of the shank, and then coat the rest of the fly.

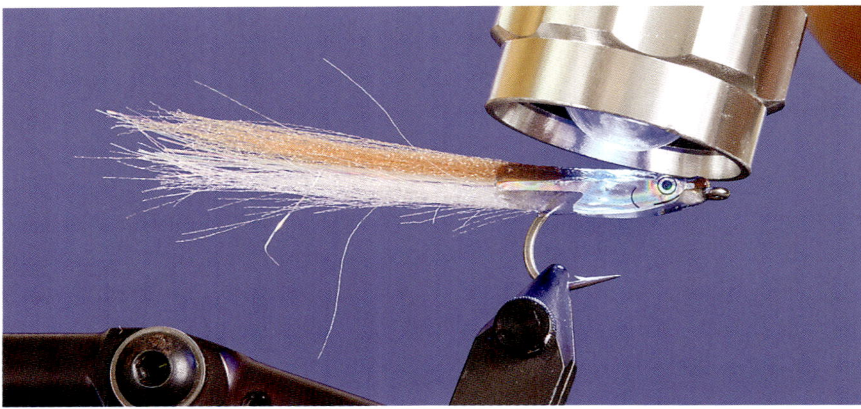

13. Set the gel with the light by placing it close to the gel, about $^1/_4$ inch, and move slowly front to back on the top, bottom, and both sides.

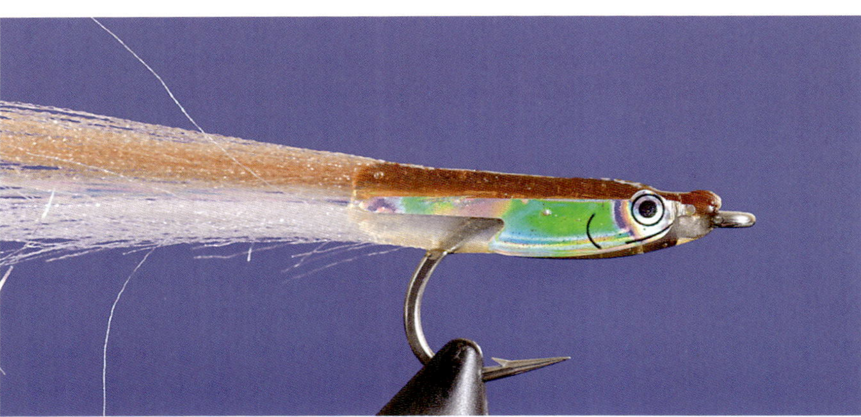

14. I often make Candies with one coat, but I will sometimes apply a second coat to fill in any low spots and to even everything out. Because of the small dip on the top of this fly, I will apply two coats. Do not wipe off the tacky layer just yet.

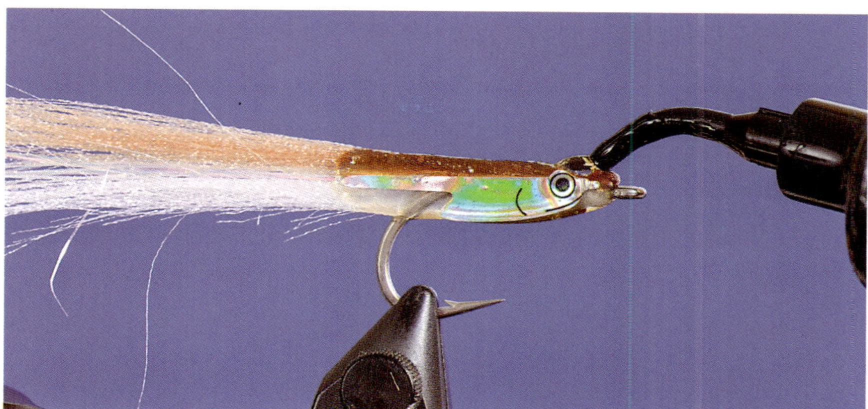

15. Apply a second coat to fill in the dip on top and smooth everything out.

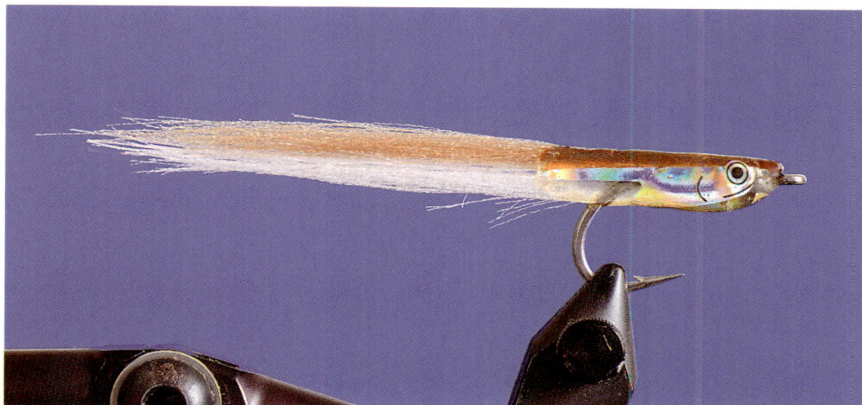

16. After you are done applying the second coat, set the acrylic with a blue light.

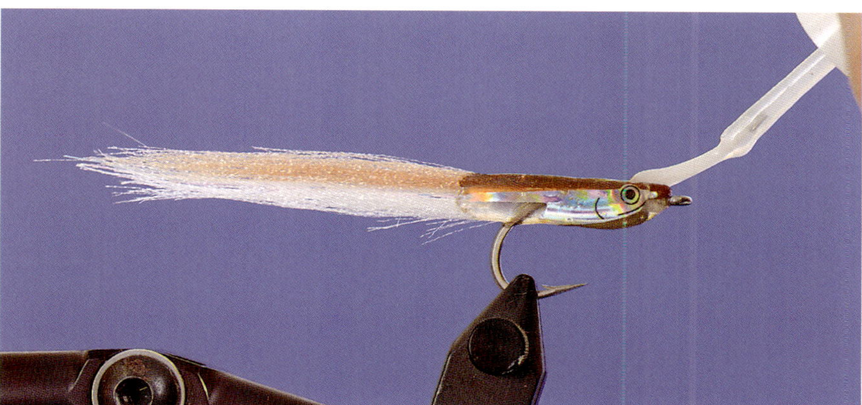

17. Wipe off the tacky layer with alcohol and a paper towel. Apply Top Coat for a clear, shiny finish.

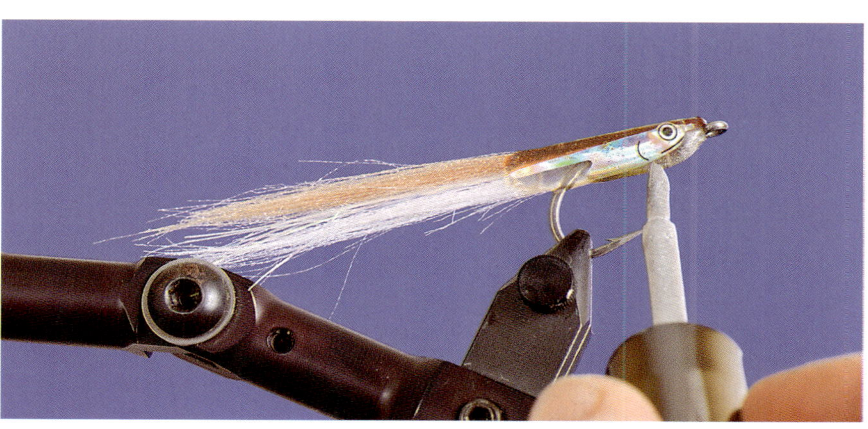

18. I'll often add some silver nail polish (silver flake) to the bottom of the fly after the Top Coat dries, but this is optional.

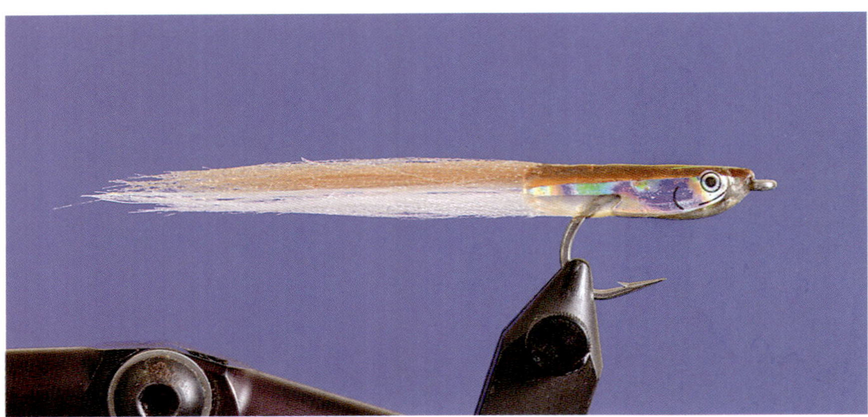

19. The finished Fleye Foil Bay Anchovy. Fleye Foils really simplify tying the fly, and they're fun. The foils give the fly a shiny belly, and quickly provide details such as eyes and gills with no hassle.

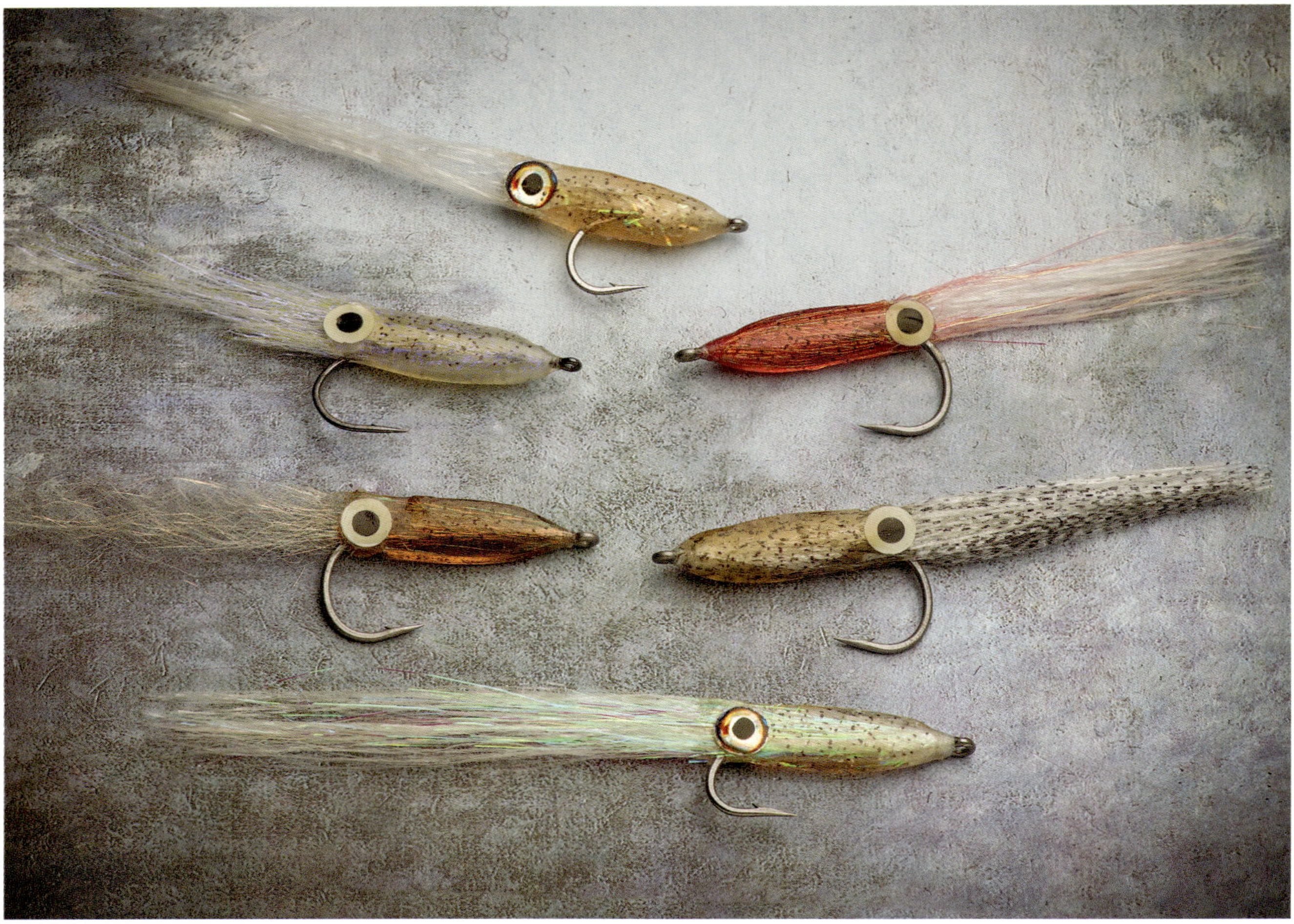

A variety of squid patterns in popular colors tied with Fleye Foils. They are very simple to construct with either Tuffleye Core or Flex.

Fleye Foil Squid

Hook:	#1/0-3/0 mid- to long-shank saltwater
Thread:	Fine monofilament
Body:	Steve Farrar Blend with Iceabou and Squid Fleye Foil coated with Tuffleye Flex
Eyes:	Prismatic stick-on, silver with black pupil

FLEYE FOIL SQUID

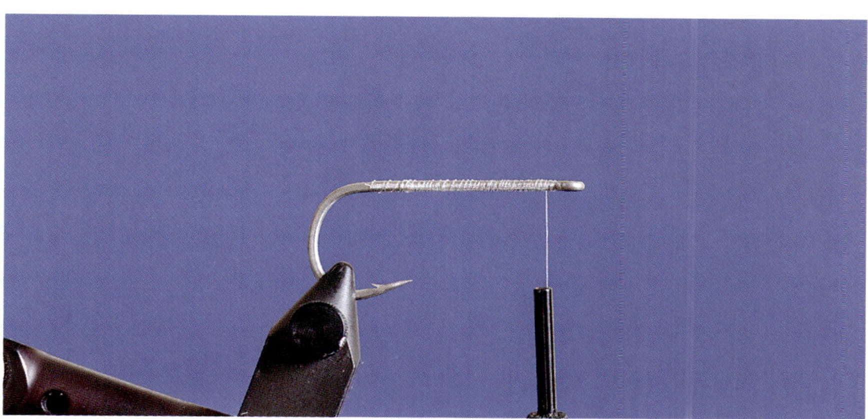

1. Insert the hook into the vise, attach monofilament thread, and cover the entire hook shank with it. Wrap the thread to a point just behind the hook eye.

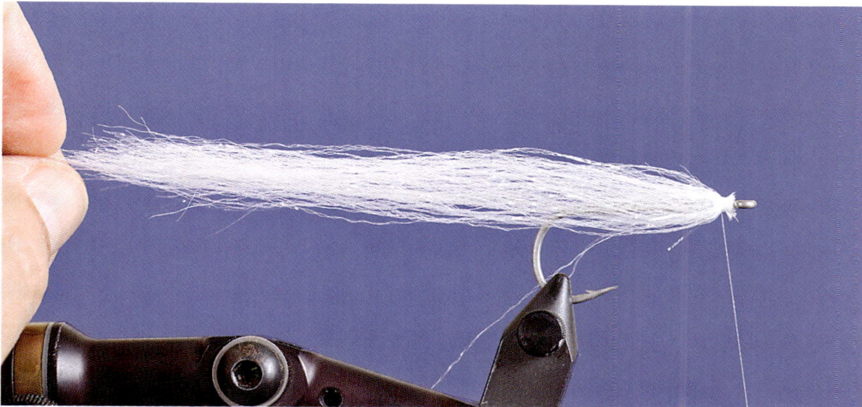

2. Attach the fibers behind the hook eye, and distribute them 360 degrees around the shank. You can use a wide range of materials. Here I'm using a Steve Farrar Blend with Iceabou flash in it.

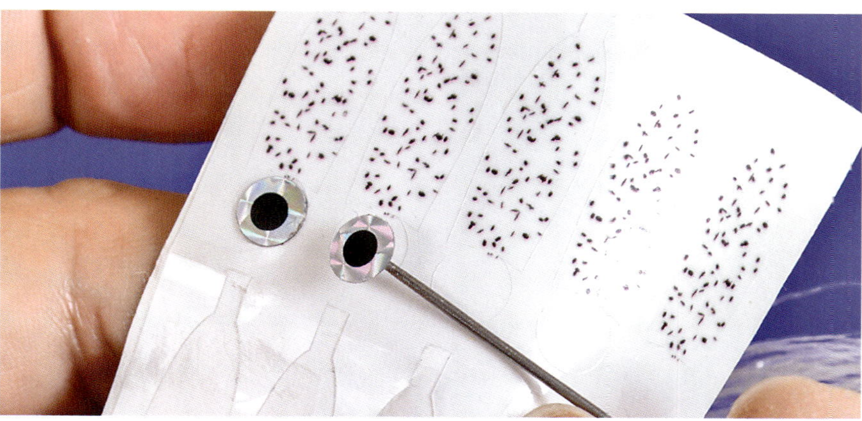

3. Squid Foils do not have eyes on them so that you can use eyes that you prefer. For this pattern, I'm using standard stick-on eyes, which I'll put in place with a bodkin.

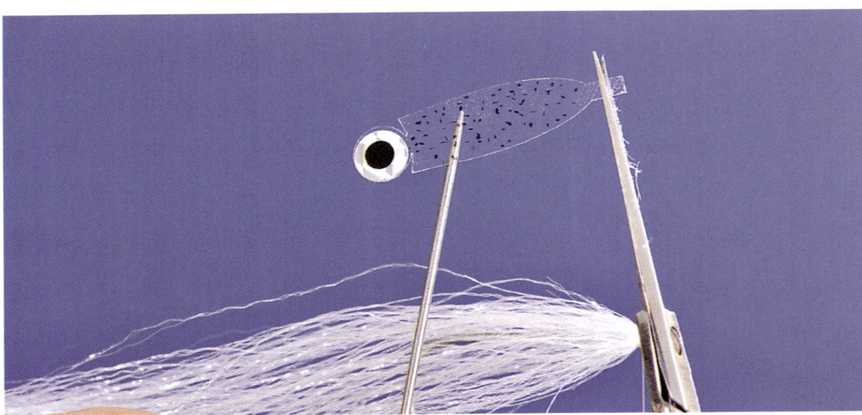

4. Trim the tying tab to length with scissors. In this case, you'd trim it in half.

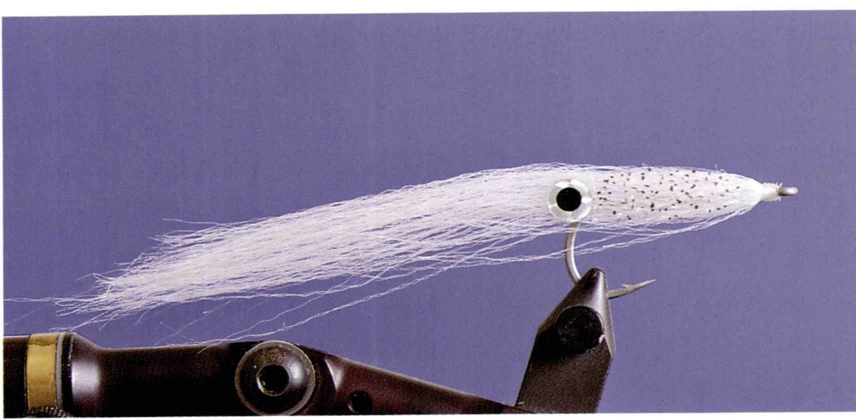

5. Attach a prepared Squid Foil to each side. Do this one side at a time and make sure that both sides are aligned and positioned so that the eyes are just behind the hook bend. Tie off with a whip-finish.

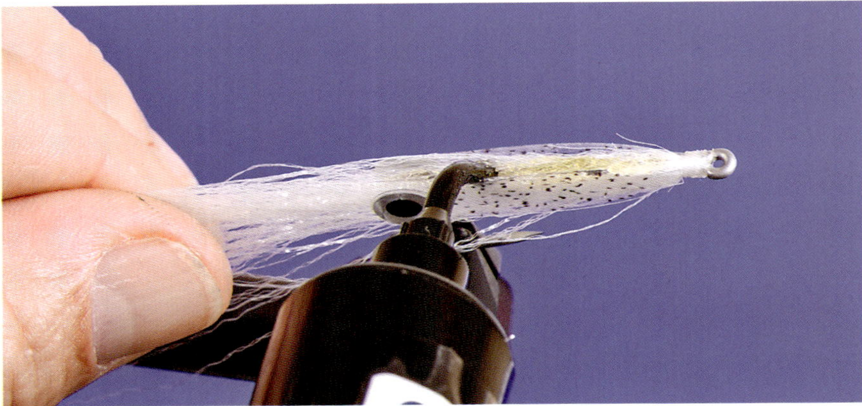

6. Apply gel to the top, ensuring that the gel completely penetrates through the fibers to the shank.

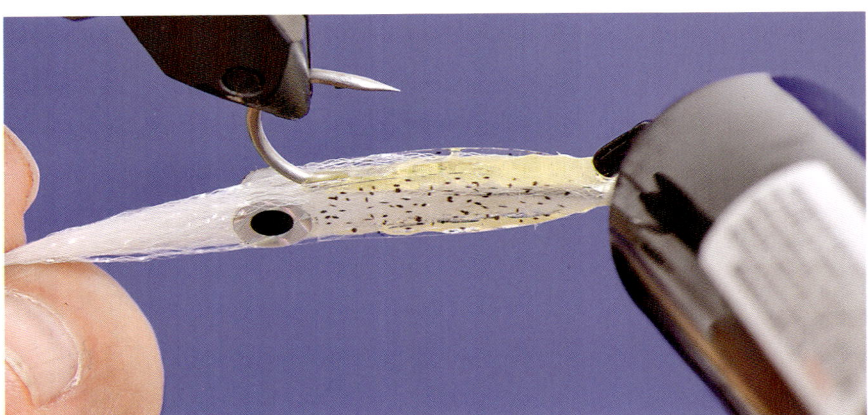

7. Apply gel to the bottom, making sure that it penetrates the fibers completely.

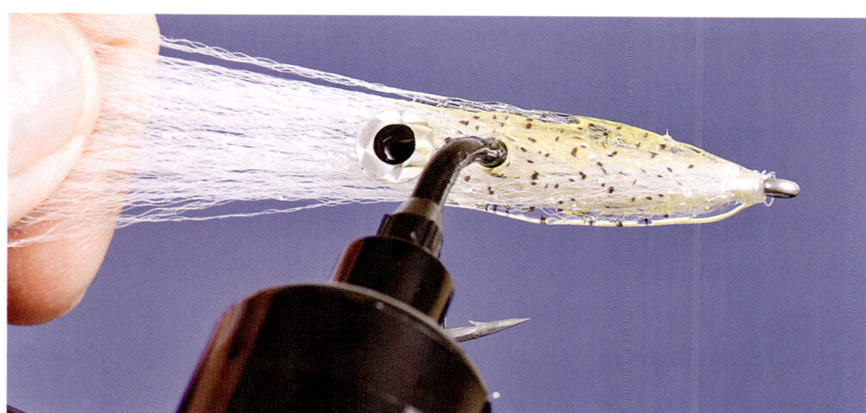

8. Apply gel to the sides. Do not overload the fly with gel; just a skim is best. Once you are happy with the shape, set it with the light.

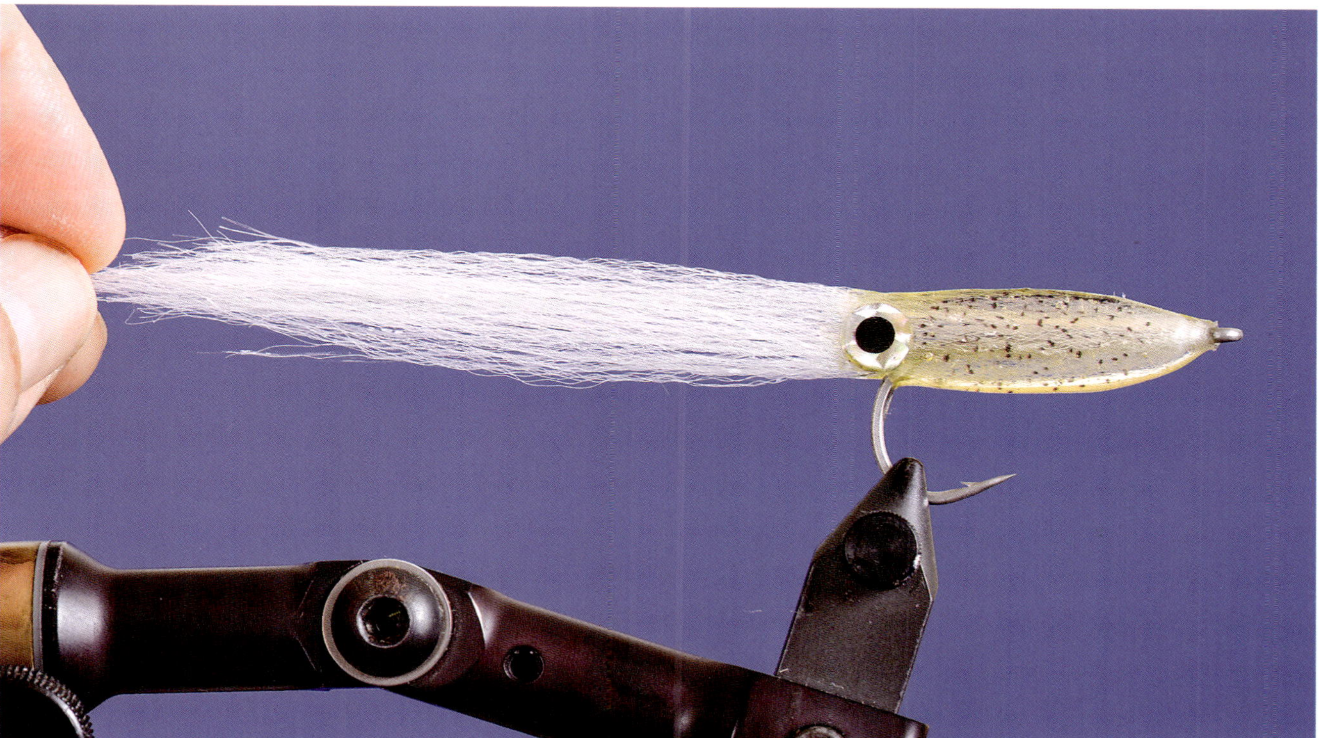

9. After you set the gel, wipe off the tacky layer with alcohol on a paper towel, and apply Top Coat.

Chapter 14

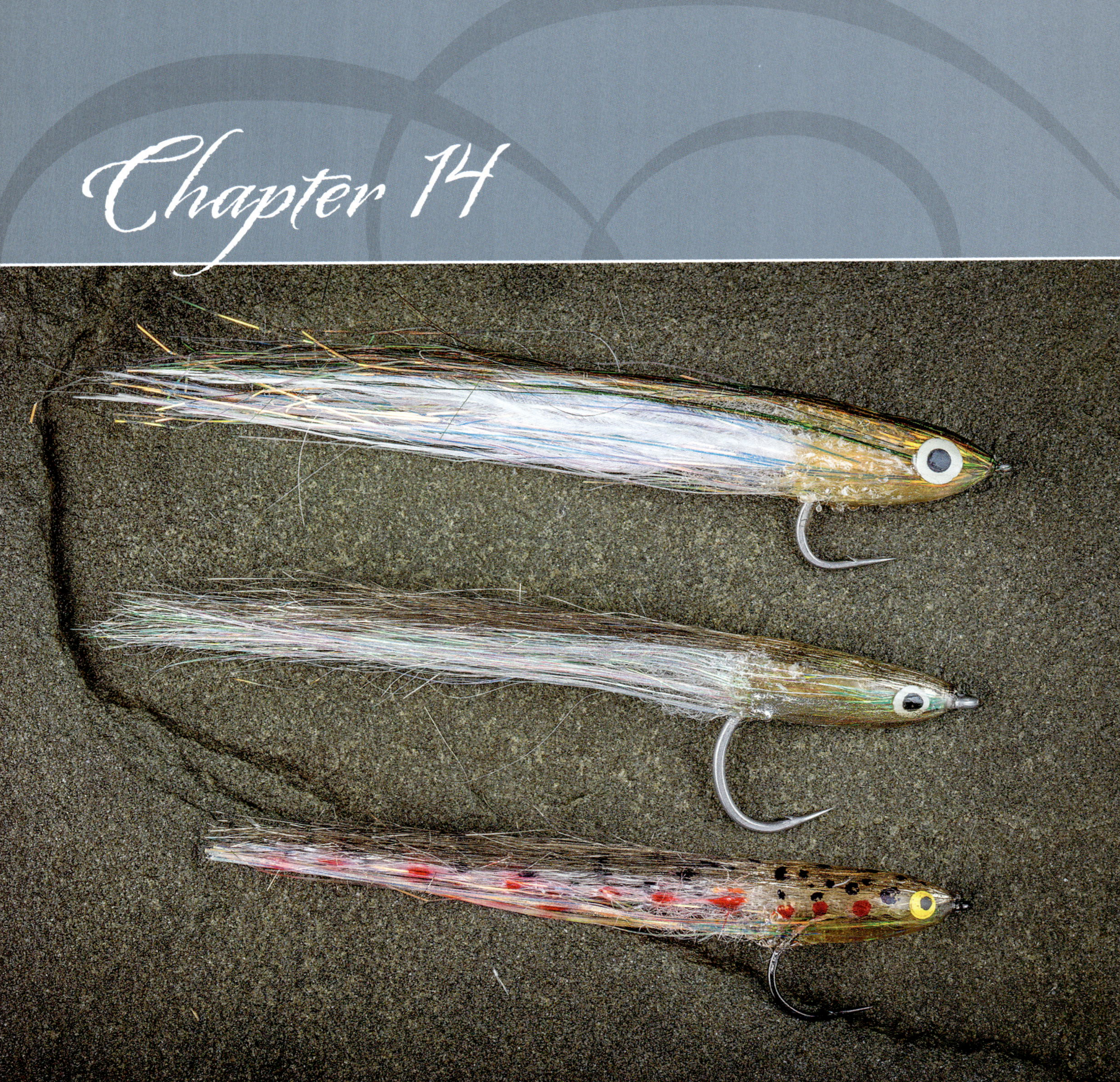

Flex Fleyes are light and easy to cast, they don't foul, and they have the look and feel of live bait. Flex Fleyes can range from silversides and squid to blacknose dace and small trout.

Flex Fleye

Siliclones and other Pop Fleye designs using silicone were big breakthroughs for my fly tying and fishing, and I included many of them in *Pop Fleyes*. Not only could you achieve realistic shapes by using silicone over fleece, but the flies had a distinct texture and action in the water, along with great durability. They would swim at the surface due to the natural buoyancy of the materials and the construction process, which traps air in the head of the fly, and during the retrieve they would dive and lift back to the surface, which drove fish wild. After the flies became waterlogged, they could either be fished deeper or squeezed out and fished near the surface again. Siliclones proved to be superb fish catchers around the country for everything from bluefish to smallmouth bass.

Siliclones were, and still are, effective designs, but like with all of my fleyes, I continued to try and find ways to make them easier and faster to tie. During the 1990s, I designed the Simple Clone, a much simplified version of the Siliclone. With the new fly, I no longer needed to tie on multiple layers of sheep fleece for the head and then precisely trim the fly to shape. Instead, I could tie in a simple fleece core 360 degrees around the hook shank, tie in a wing of bucktail 360 degrees around the fleece core like a veil, and then tie in one final veil of fleece over which I could form the head with a quick application of silicone. The result was a neat little fly for imitating mid-size bait, such as silversides, bay anchovies, mullet, and mackerel. Like the original Siliclone, the Simple Clone's inner core of soft fleece offered some tying advantages. The fly felt more natural than many other patterns, and it was also a lot faster and easier to tie. As an interesting side note, my first attempts at a Simple Clone had no inner core of fleece, which made it hard to keep the head from collapsing and the silicone from adhering to the hook shank. This forced me to use a bodkin to separate the silicone-coated materials from the hook shank. After dinner at the Timmermann's house on Long Island, New York, I took a short nap and woke up with the idea of tying in an inner core of fleece as the solution to the fly's "sticky" problem.

With the advent of Tuffleye Flex, the Simple Clone was refined once again, and the Flex Fleye was born. Unlike Tuffleye Core and Finish, Flex is soft and spongy when cured, similar to silicone. Like the other light-cured acrylic products, Flex stays clear, but it can give many flies a more natural feel.

Materials and Variations

As with the Simple Clone, the key to this fly is the soft fleece core that will ultimately provide the shell for the other materials coated with Flex. I look for fleece with a relatively soft texture and also make sure that I brush it out thoroughly before tying it in. After you tie it to the

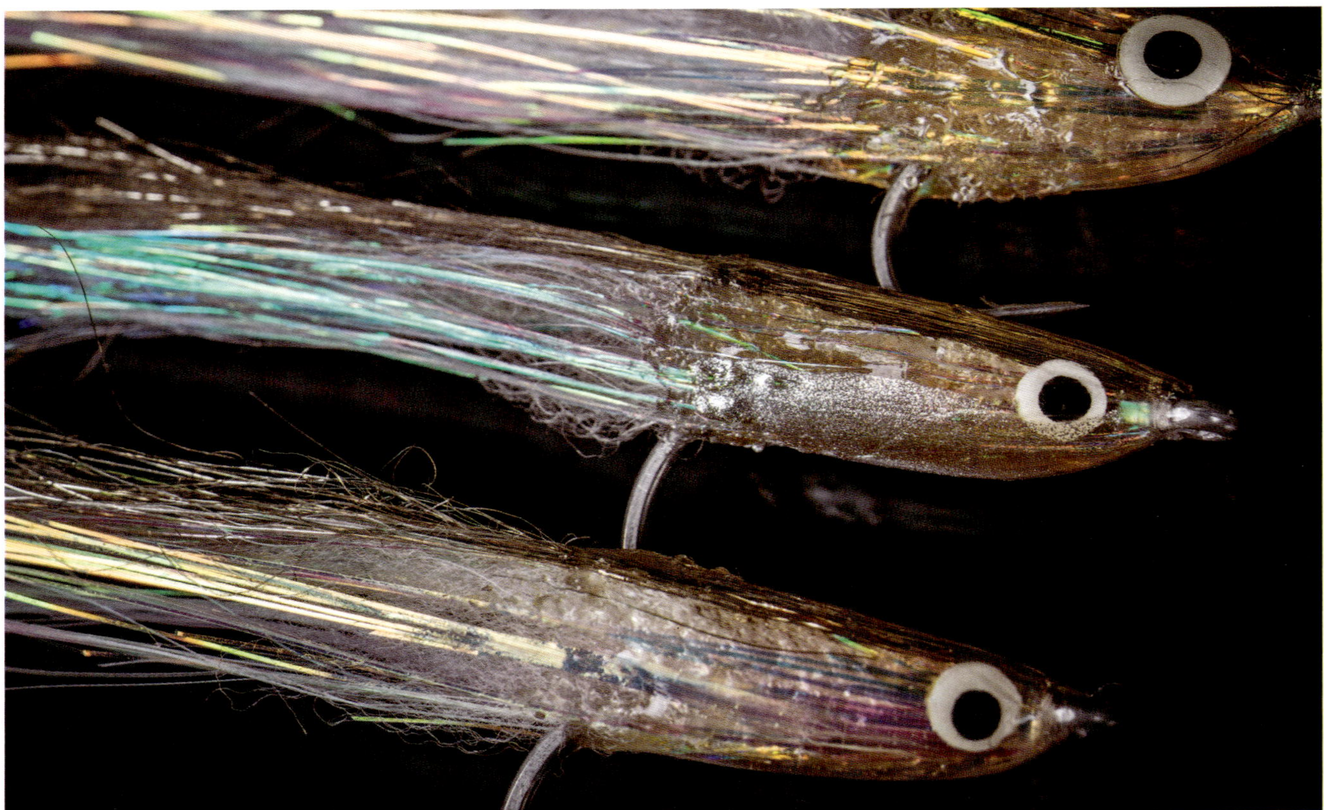

Fleece is an ideal core material, as it also releases any water quickly on the backcast, but you can experiment with any soft material that will provide a loose frame over which to pull the body materials. Any puffy natural or synthetic material such as Egg Yarn and wool will do. With proper technique you can even abandon the fleece core and simply use the butt ends of the wing material (tied in reverse) as a buffer for the Flex material around the hook shank.

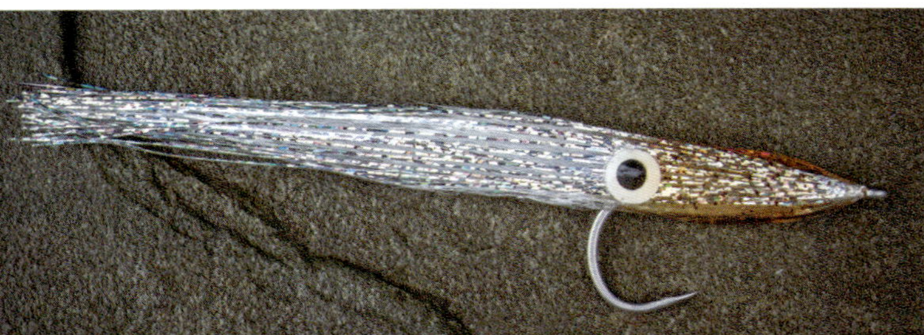

The Flex Fleye Squid is made using Tuffleye Flex, which makes the fly feel softer and more natural like the real thing.

shank, make sure that it completely surrounds the hook shank and that it is tangle-free. You can use your bodkin to pick out the fleece and ensure nice distribution. The fleece in this fly is not only a barrier, but it also impacts that overall shape of the finished fly.

You can tie the head and body of a Flex Fleye using many different materials, but my favorite ingredients are Steve Farrar's Flash Blend, Angel Hair, and feathers such as ostrich herl and saddle hackles, which easily accept the Flex gel and smooth out beautifully. Usually, one feather on each side of the fly does the trick to create a nice, clean appearance, but sometimes I will tie feathers on top of the fly, flat, and in staggered lengths. All you are looking for is a good balance of fibers to provide structure and flash to suit your tastes, so feel free to put your own spin on the Flex Fleye.

Once I found the mix of materials I liked for assembling the pattern, my next concern was durability. Saltwater flies are vulnerable to predators with sharp teeth and strong jaws. To improve the fly's durability, I wrap Body Braid around the shank to offer more bonding surface and add a heavier coat of Flex. No longer did the outside shell "float" freely around the shank—it was secured along the underside of the shank. This made a solid belly with the pillow of fleece above the shank while allowing a soft, cushiony body. Another subtle variation that you can try for sinking line applications is to apply the Flex on the top and sides with *none* on the bottom. This allows water to penetrate the fly right away, while keeping the same shape and most of the characteristics of the regular Flex Fleye.

Flex Fleye

Hook:	Varivus 990S or similar short-shank saltwater
Thread:	Fine monofilament
Buffer:	Sheep fleece
Body:	Steve Farrar Blend coated with Tuffleye Flex
Flash:	Saltwater Angel Hair
Eyes:	Glow-in-the-dark, stick-on

TYING THE FLEX FLEYE

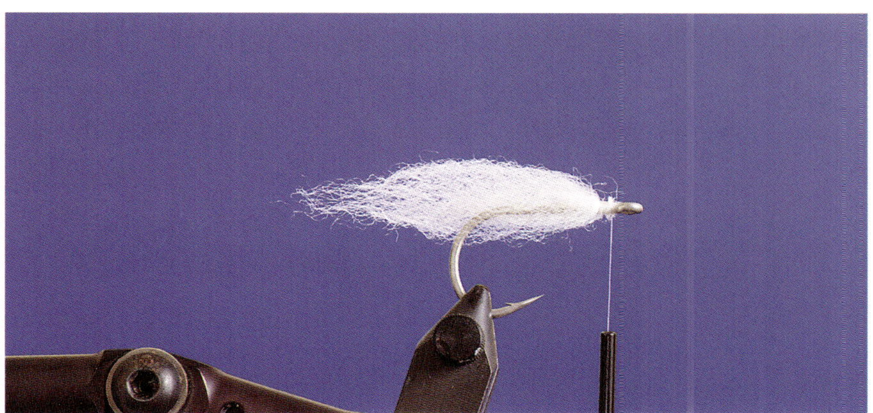

1. Insert the hook into the vise, attach the mono thread to the hook shank, and wrap a thread base over the shank, leaving the bobbin hanging at a point approximately one eye length behind the hook eye. Prepare the fleece by first brushing the patch with a dog brush to remove tangles and then cut a small tuft from the hide. Hold the fleece with your material hand while you tie it in. Aim for it to extend just past the hook bend and distribute it 360 degrees around the hook shank. Leave plenty of room for the wing materials.

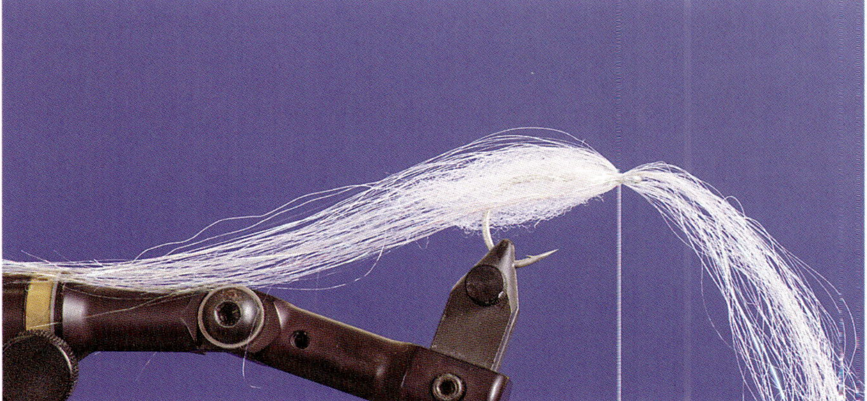

2. Pull off a section of flash material (in this case Steve Farrar Blend) that is at least twice as long as the fly you are tying, and tie it to the hook shank in the middle of the fibers with three or four wraps. Distribute the fibers equally around the shank with the technique shown on page 40 in the Techniques section.

(continued)

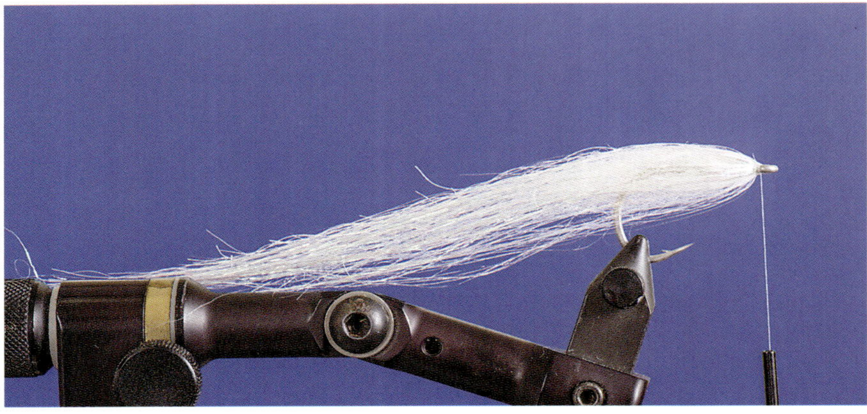

3. Pull back the remaining portion to cover the underside of the hook. Manipulate the material to ensure it is evenly distributed before tying it down.

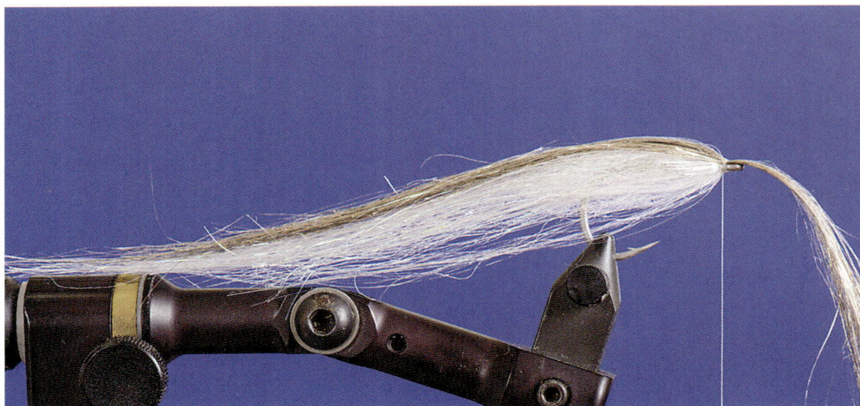

4. Tie in a contrasting color of Farrar Blend in the middle of the fibers.

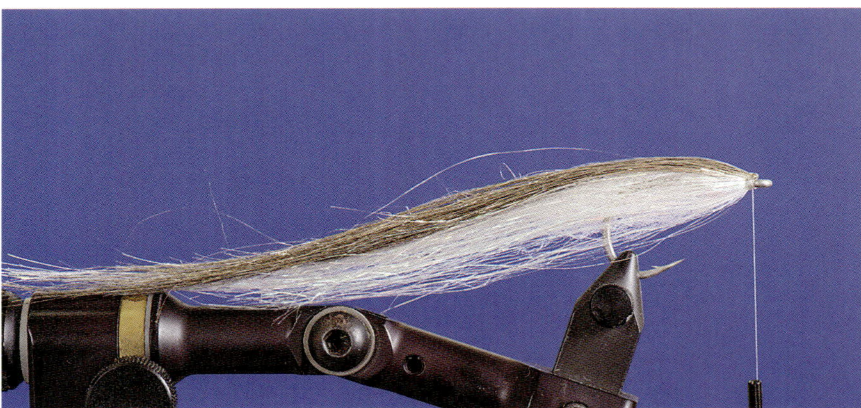

5. This time, keep all the fibers on top of the fly. Bring the fibers hanging over the hook eye to the rear, secure them, and whip-finish.

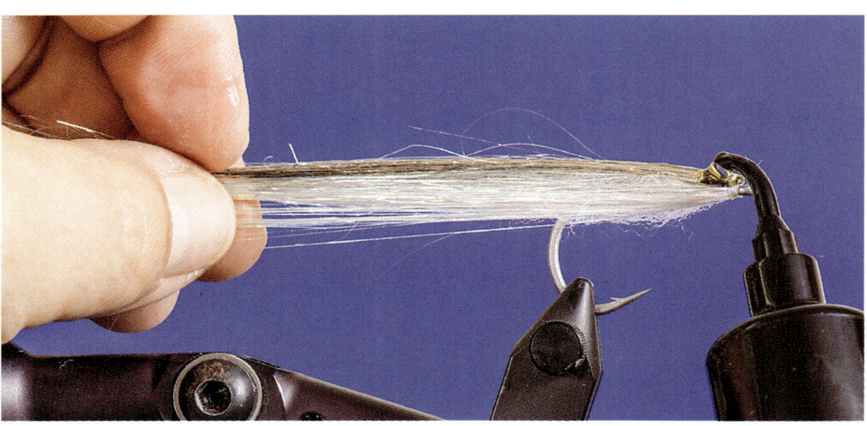

6. While holding the fibers with your material hand, begin adding tiny dollops of Tuffleye Flex around the fibers just behind hook eye, and then skim the Flex over the fibers with the syringe's curved tip. Always travel from the front to the rear of the fly so that you don't catch the shorter fibers. Do not press down on the fibers when you are applying the Flex. A gentle touch preserves the fullness of the fly.

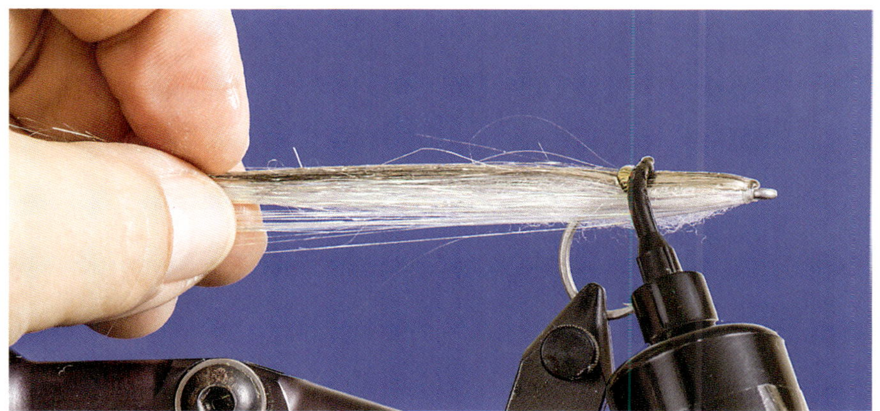

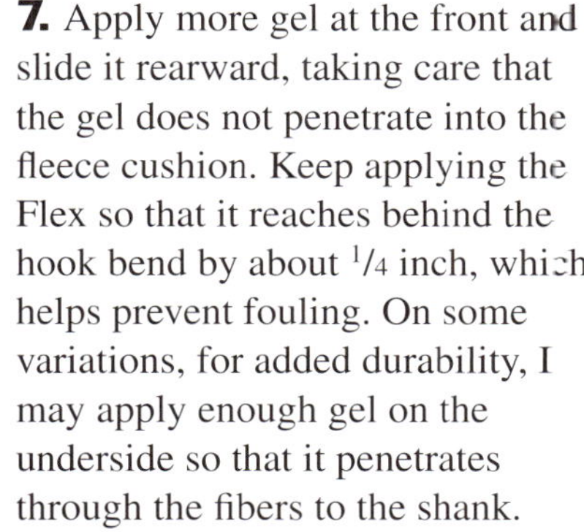

7. Apply more gel at the front and slide it rearward, taking care that the gel does not penetrate into the fleece cushion. Keep applying the Flex so that it reaches behind the hook bend by about 1/4 inch, which helps prevent fouling. On some variations, for added durability, I may apply enough gel on the underside so that it penetrates through the fibers to the shank.

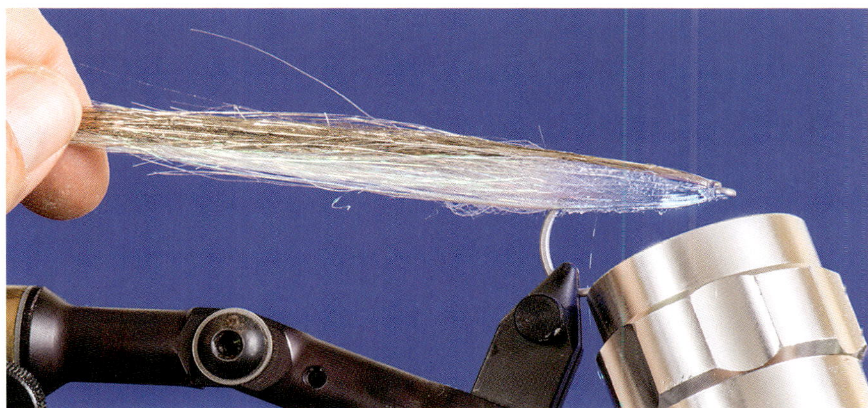

8. While pulling back on the fibers gently until you get the shape you desire, set the first coat of Flex with the blue light. At first, you might find it easier to do one side at a time because Flex cures in about half the time as the other formulations. Once cured, the coating will feel tacky. If you are going to add eyes, do not remove the tack just yet, as it will help the eyes stay in place. Clip and preen any unruly fibers.

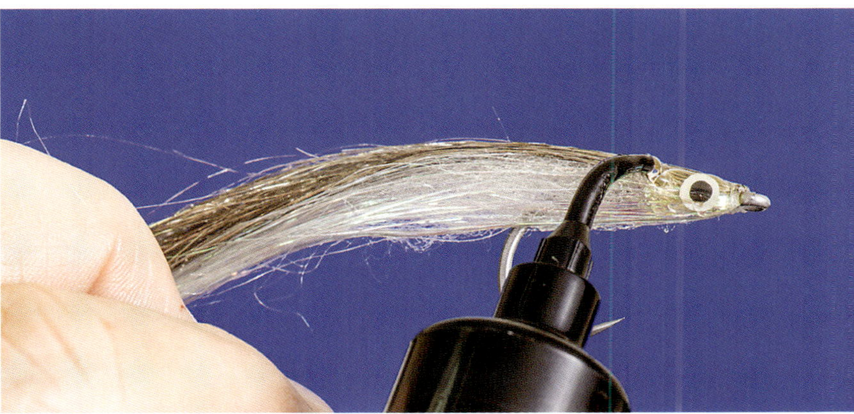

9. Add eyes if you wish. If you fold the eye while it is still attached to the backing, the crease will help it more easily conform to the Flex Fleye's shape. Remove it from the sheet with a bodkin and, while the eye is still on the bodkin, place it on one side. If the eyes do not stick where you place them, put a drop of Flex on each side of the head, and reposition the eyes.

The second coat is applied differently than the first coat. Rather than starting with a thick coat behind the hook eye and thinning the gel as you work toward the back of the head, apply an even coat of Flex over the entire first coat, using the applicator tip or bodkin. Allow the fly to set for a minute to allow the gel to level, and then cure the gel with the blue light. Then, apply more gel directly onto the eyes, top, and bottom around the hook eye. Once you have enough gel on the fly, then you can use your bodkin to distribute it. Like with epoxy, you need enough material to be able to gain control of it and sculpt it.

(continued)

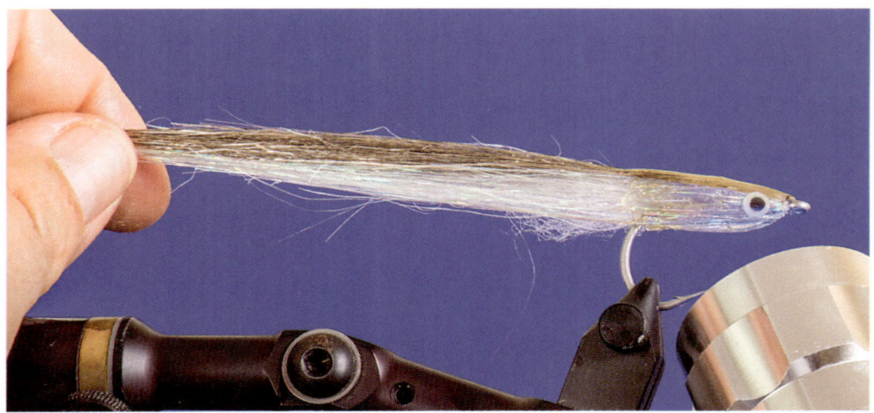

10. Set the gel once the body is smooth. Repeat on the other side. When you get better at it, you can do it all in one shot—apply the gel and set all sides.

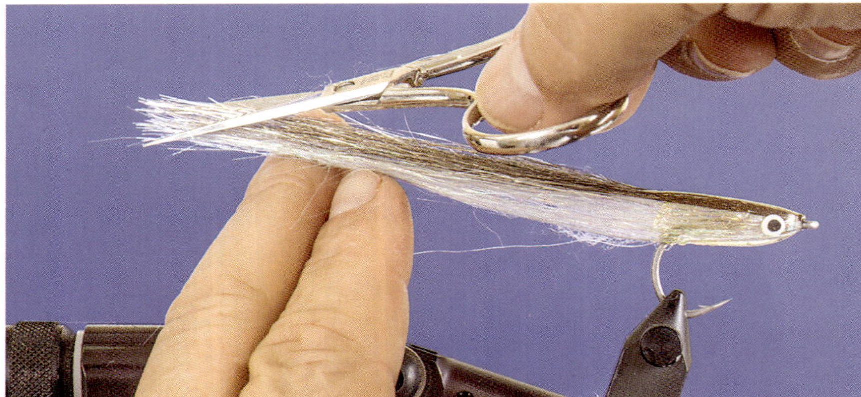

11. Trim the rear fibers at an angle. Stagger the cuts from at least a third of the way back.

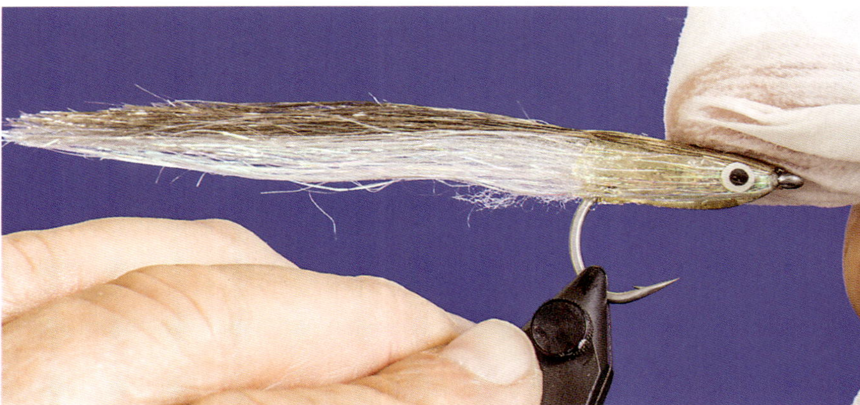

12. Wipe off the tacky layer from back toward the hook eye with alcohol and a paper towel. Don't wipe the tack onto the wing of the fly. The texture of the cured gel is more rubbery than the glasslike finish of the Core—it feels like sliding your finger across the bottom of a sneaker.

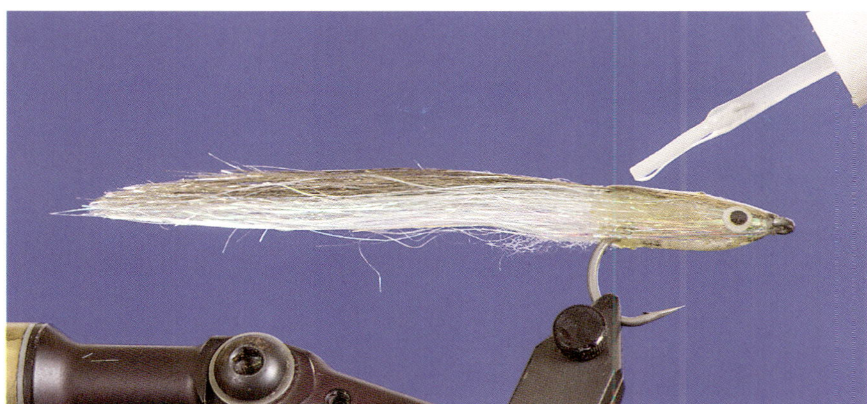

13. Apply one coat of Top Coat. I generally treat it twice with alcohol and leave it. You can use Hard As Nails as a slick and shiny coat, but I like the natural look best.

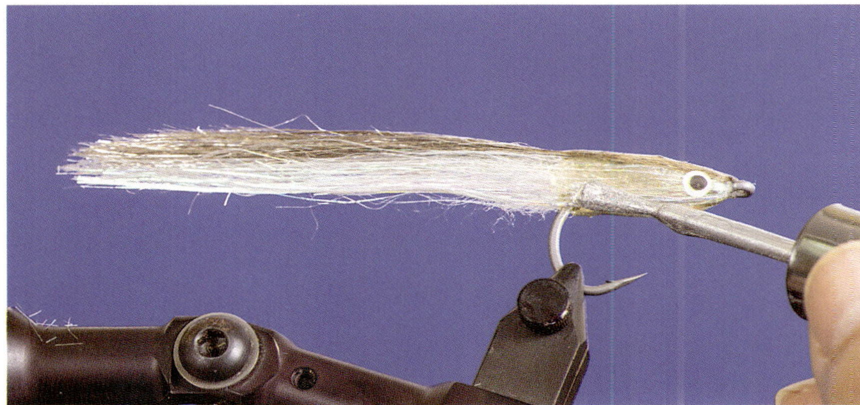

14. When the Flex has cured, you can coat the belly with silver nail polish (optional).

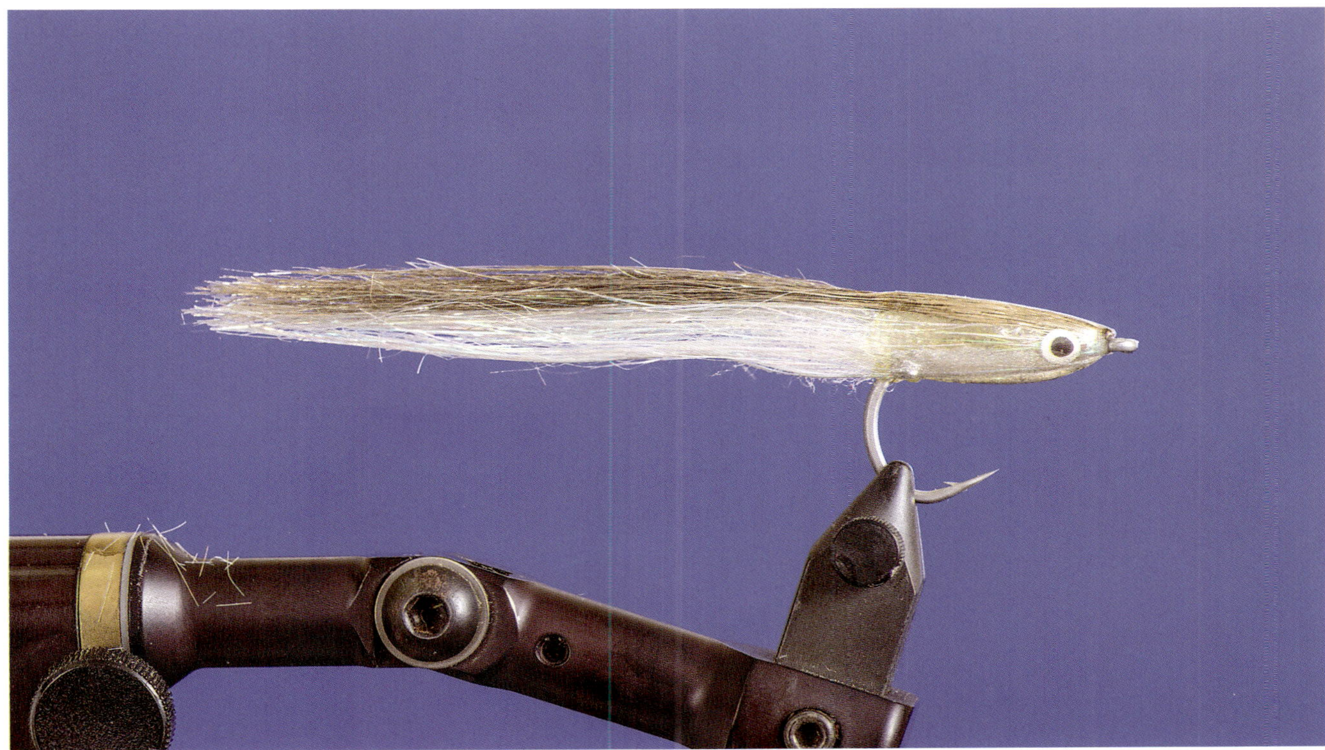

The finished Flex Fleye feels natural and is durable and shatterproof. I tie many of my Flex Fleyes using brightly colored materials, but I also make some with subdued colors and little flash.

Flex Fleyes

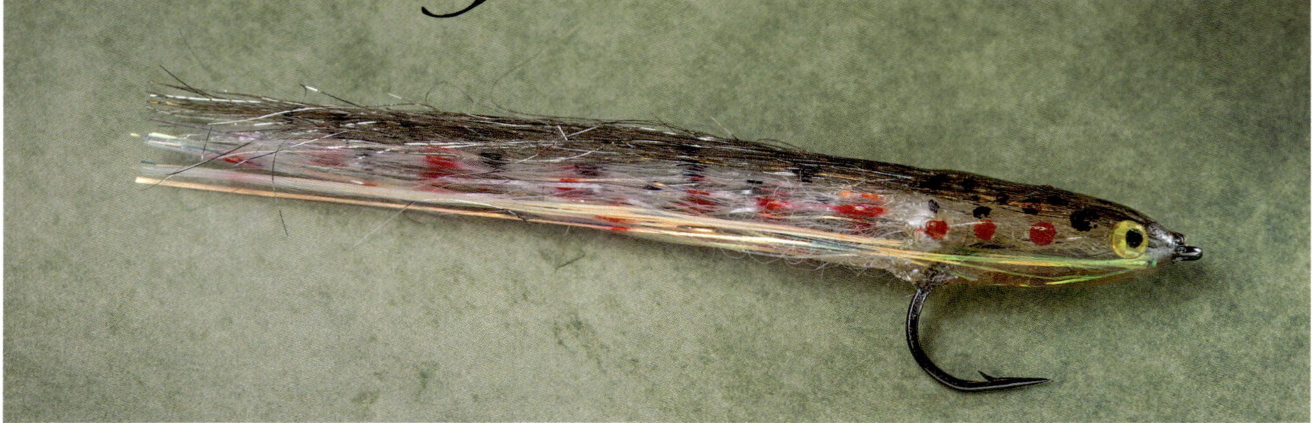

Flex Fleye adorned with red and black spots to imitate a brook trout.

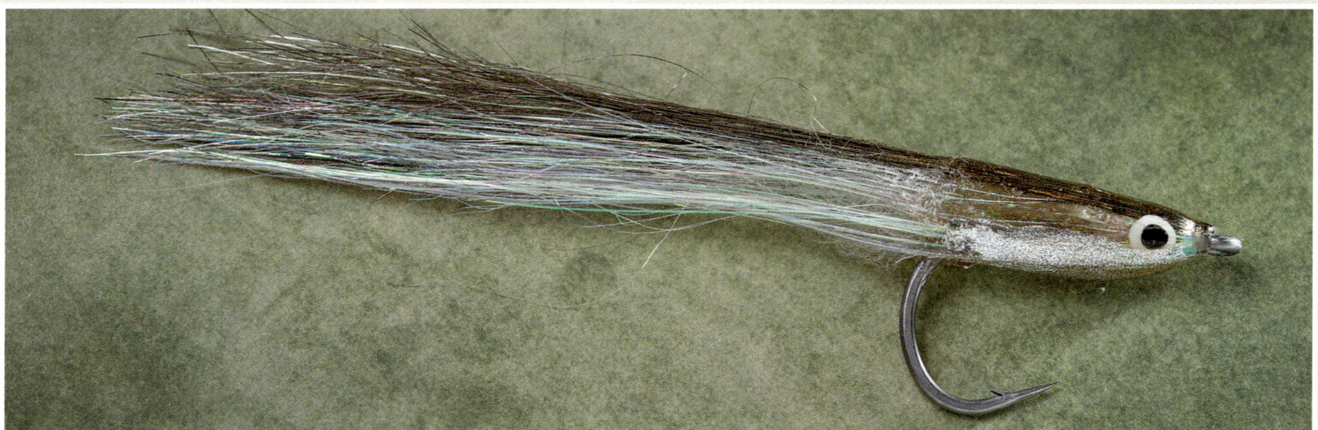

Flex Fleye designed to imitate a bay anchovy.

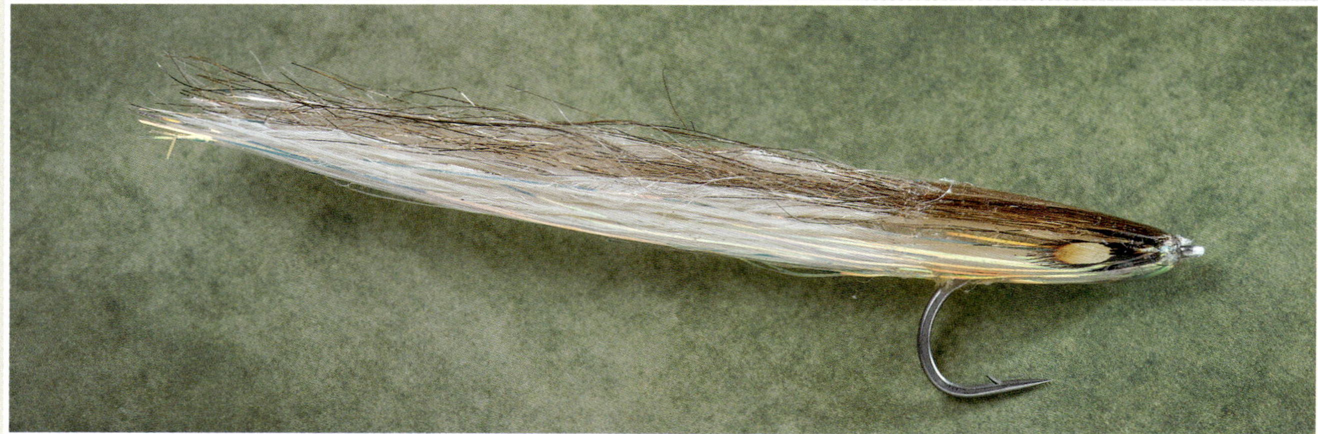

Flex can provide a durable, clear coating over fragile materials such as jungle cock.

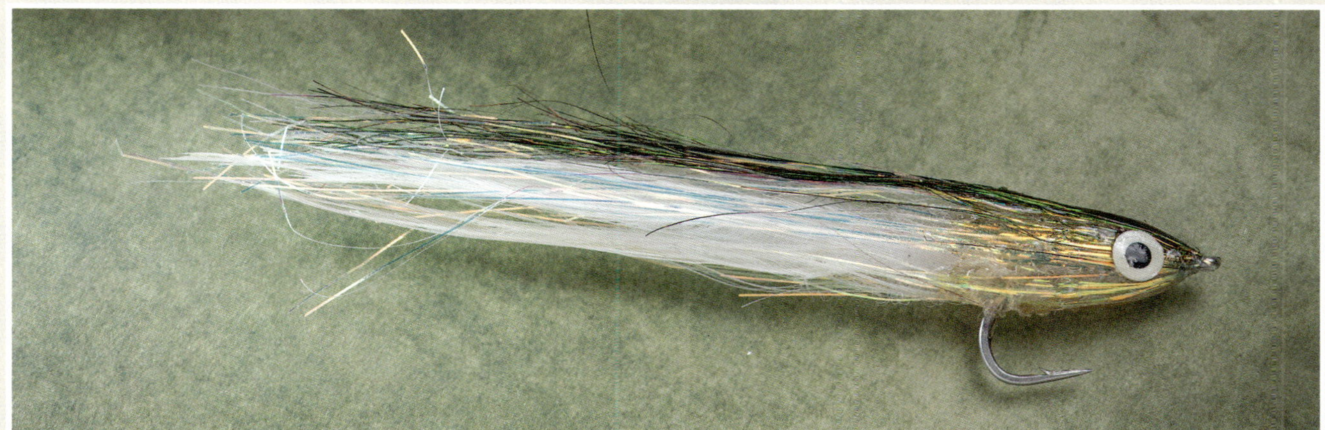

This wider profile Flex Fleye incorporating ostrich herl imitates a small bunker.

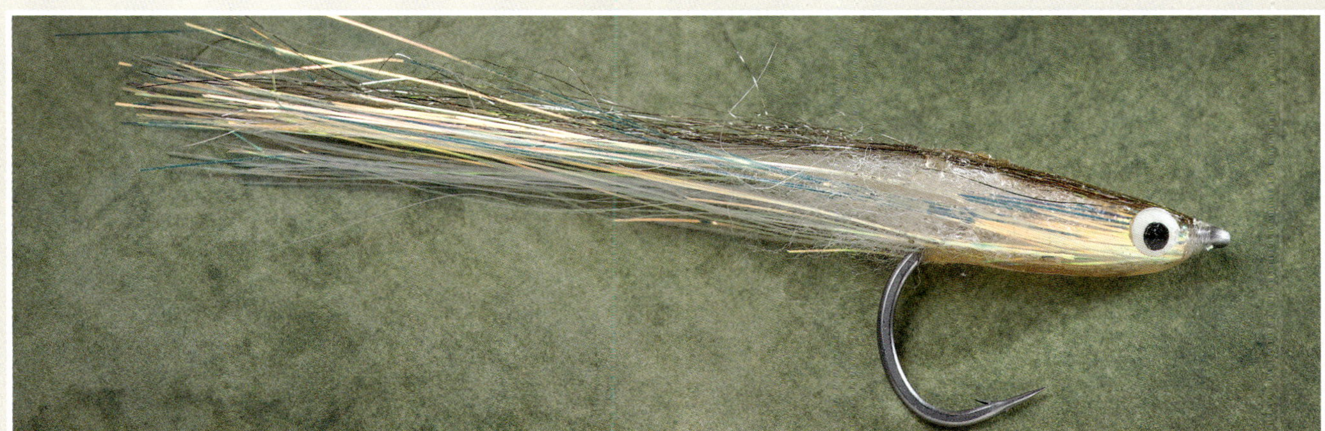

This bay anchovy pattern has a heavy gold pearl Angel Hair belly sac and glow-in-the-dark eyes.

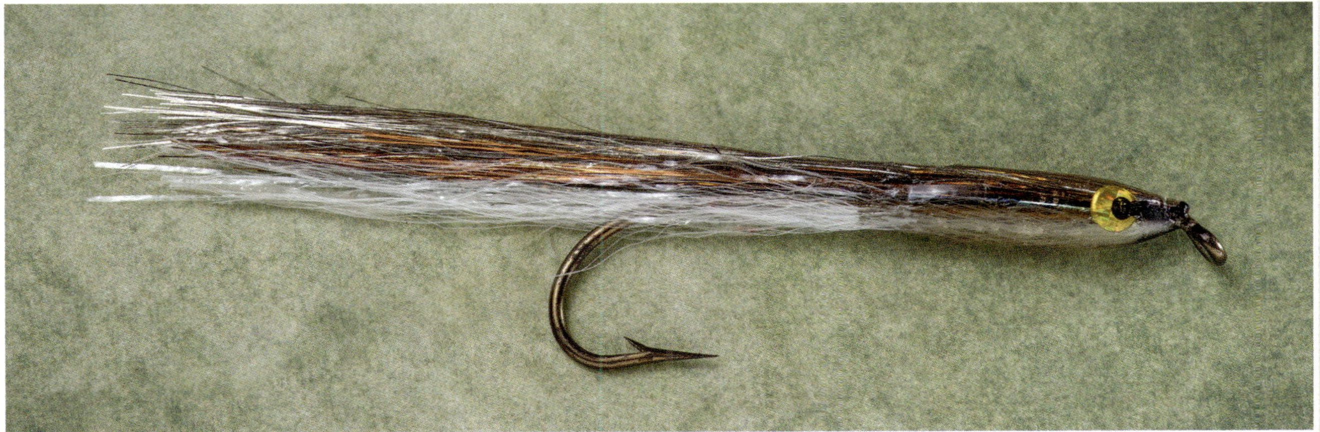

A freshwater blacknose dace.

Chapter 15

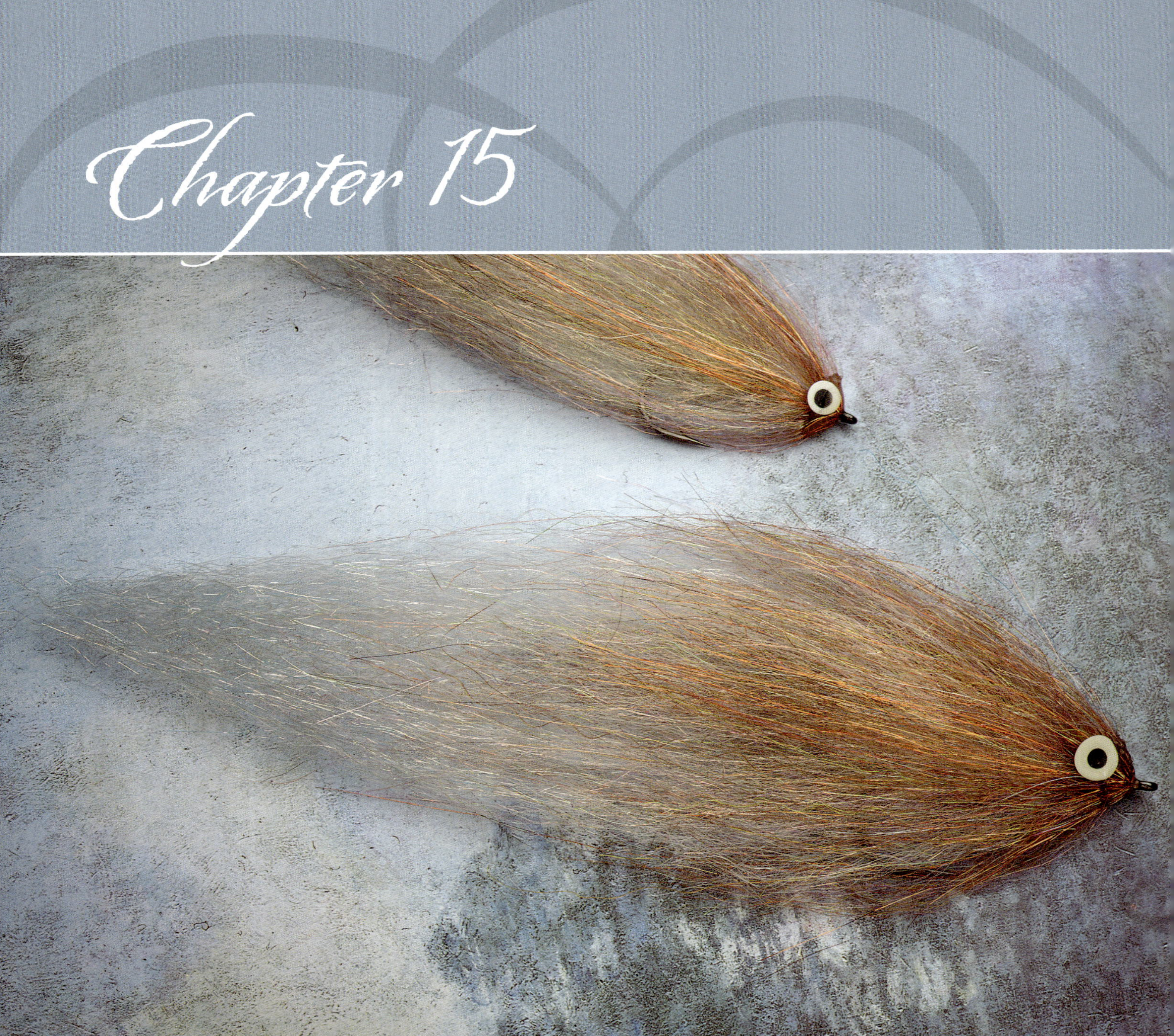

The Double Spread is a wide, light, extra-large pattern. The one above is built with two spreads along the shank and soft Farrar Blend fibers.

Double Spread

The first Spread Fleyes, using epoxy, were featured in *Pop Fleyes*. With proper timing, you could squeeze the epoxy at the head of the fly just before it hardened to create a thin but wide-profile fly. However, there was an element of chance to this technique: if I did it too late, it would not spread; if I did it too soon, it would stick to my fingers. The timing had to be perfect.

With Tuffleye, the process is a lot easier. Once you have all the acrylic distributed through the fibers, you can spread and pull the top fibers up and away to the desired angle and hit it with the light, and then do the bottom. By shaping the fly in stages like this, and not being concerned with the quick curing time of epoxy, you are in complete control. The Double Spread that we tie here has an inner spread that helps begin a wide profile on a large fly.

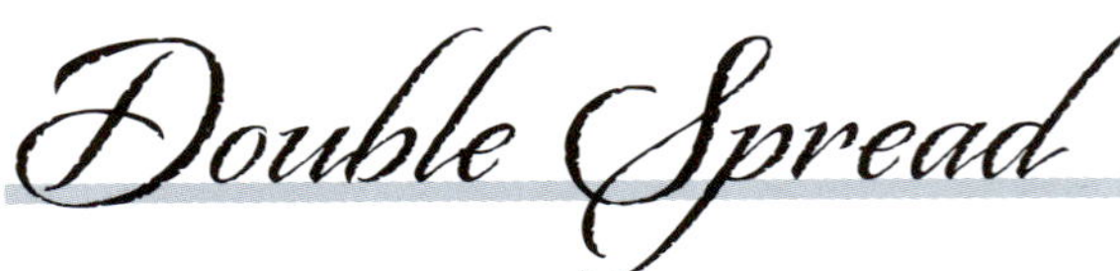

Hook:	Gamakatsu SL12S
Thread:	Fine monofilament
Body:	Steve Farrar Blend
Eyes:	Extra large stick-on

TYING THE DOUBLE SPREAD

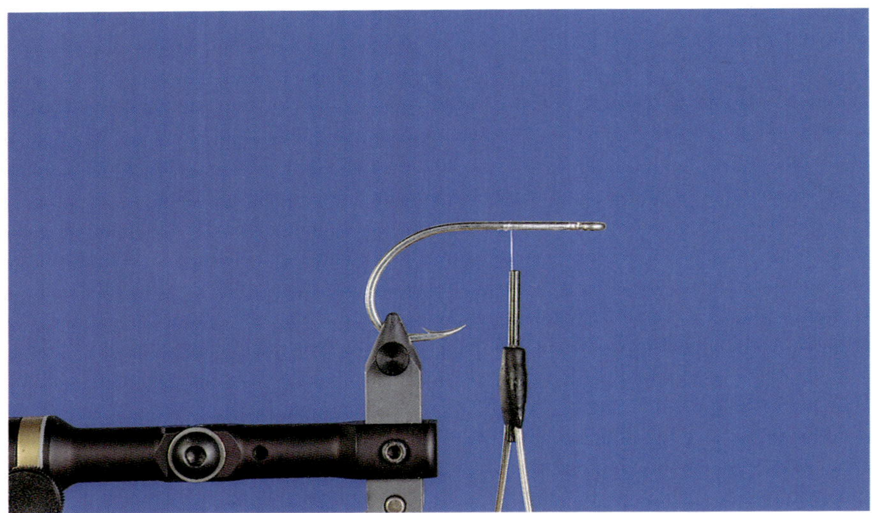

1. Insert the hook into the vise, attach the mono thread, and wrap a thread base to midshank.

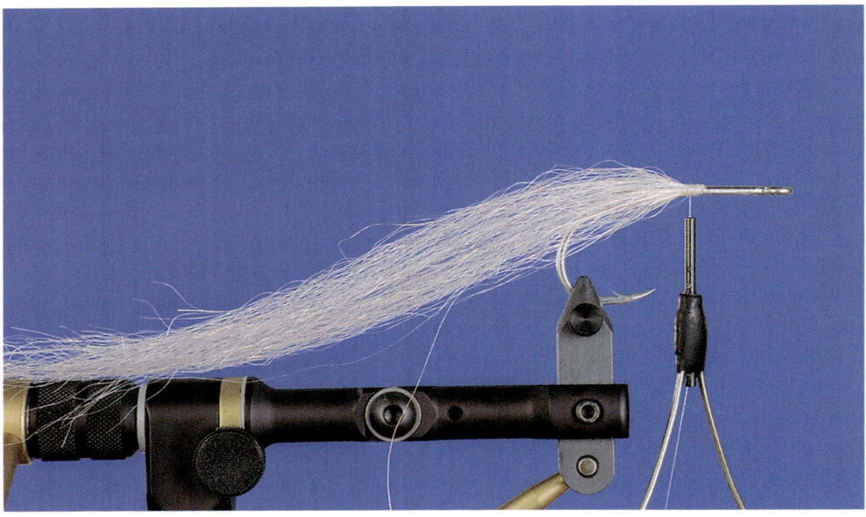

2. Tie in a bunch of Farrar Blend at the midpoint and secure it with several thread wraps.

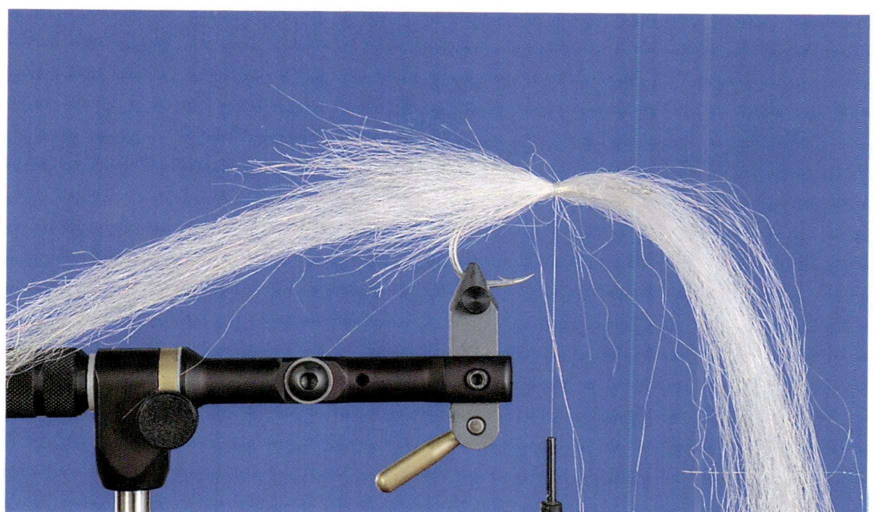

3. Reverse tie in another length of Farrar Blend, and leave about an inch or two to the left of the tie-down. The butts will help prop up the fibers when the fibers hanging over the eye are tied back.

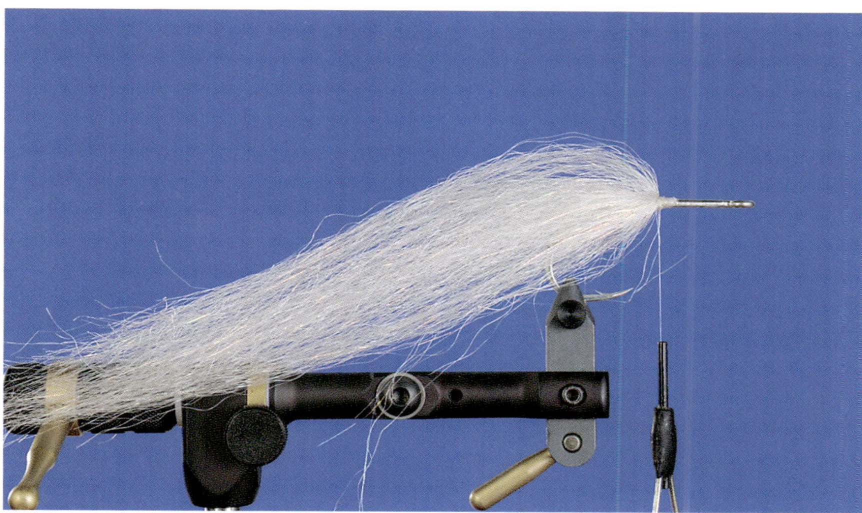

4. Pull back the remaining fibers, and spread them evenly above and below the hook shank. Return the thread to a point in front of the tie-down.

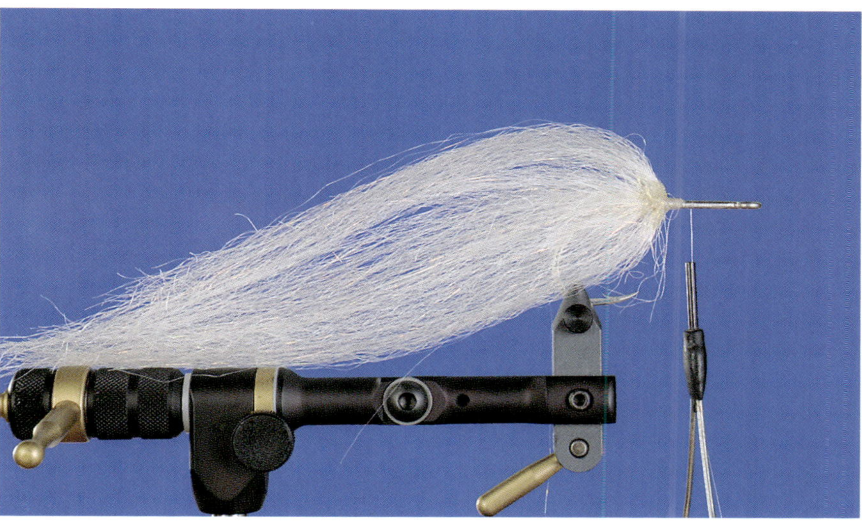

5. Apply light-cured acrylic to the bases of the fibers at the tie-down. Hold the fibers at a wide angle, and set them with the light to create height in the middle of the fly.

(continued)

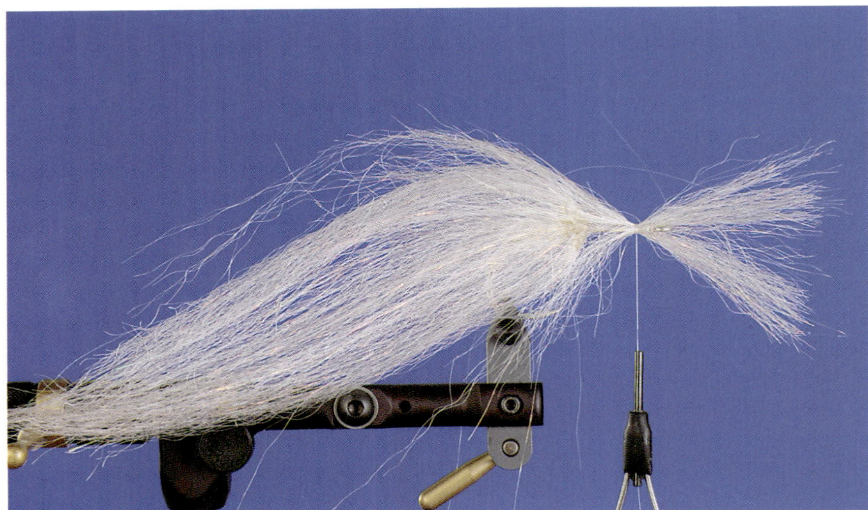

6. Cut a bunch of fibers about half the length of the first bunches that you tied in and attach them to the hook shank in the middle of the bunch. This is the added bulk you'll need for larger Spread Fleyes.

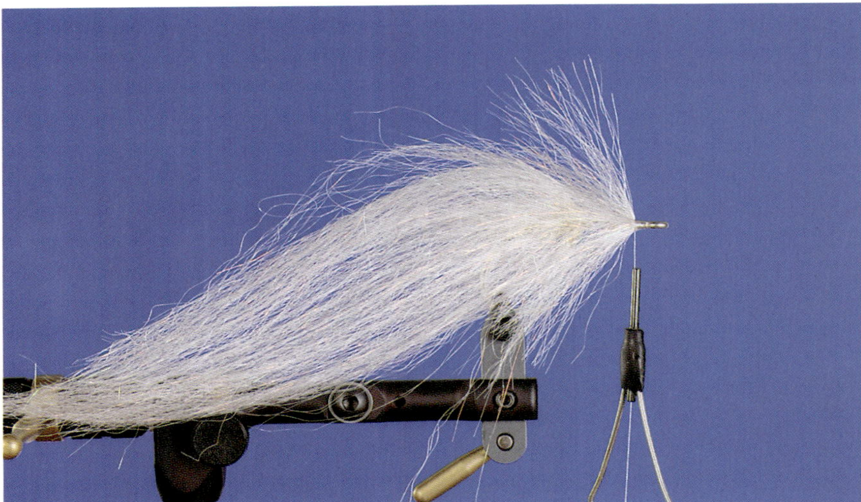

7. Fold back the fibers extending over the hook eye to add bulk.

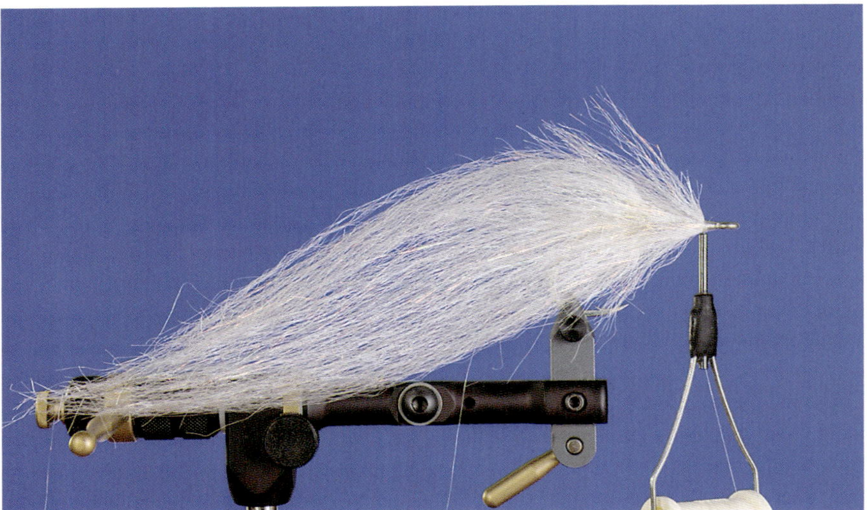

8. Tie the fibers back and dam them up with thread. Do not tie them down too low. Keep it high. Depending on the shank length of the hook I'm using, I might repeat these last two steps.

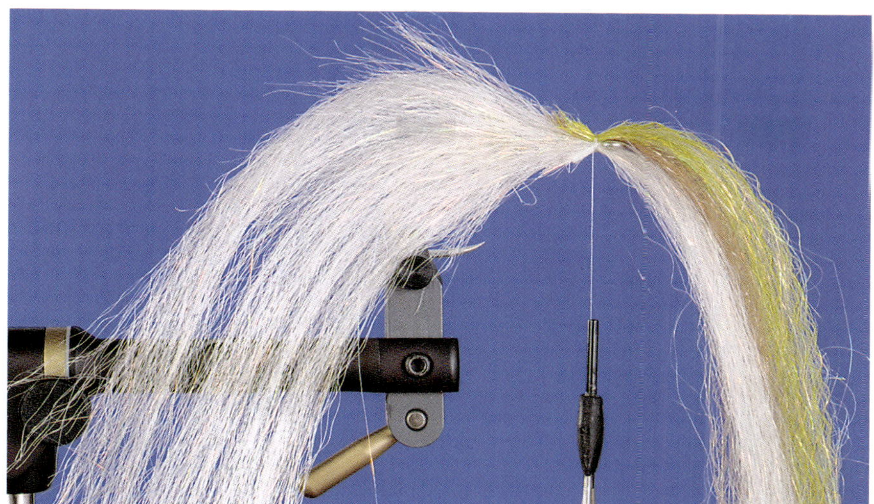

9. Select three colors of fibers that are as long as the full length of the fly. Here, I chose white for the bottom and shades of tan for above. Align them neatly on top of one another, and attach them to the shank all at once.

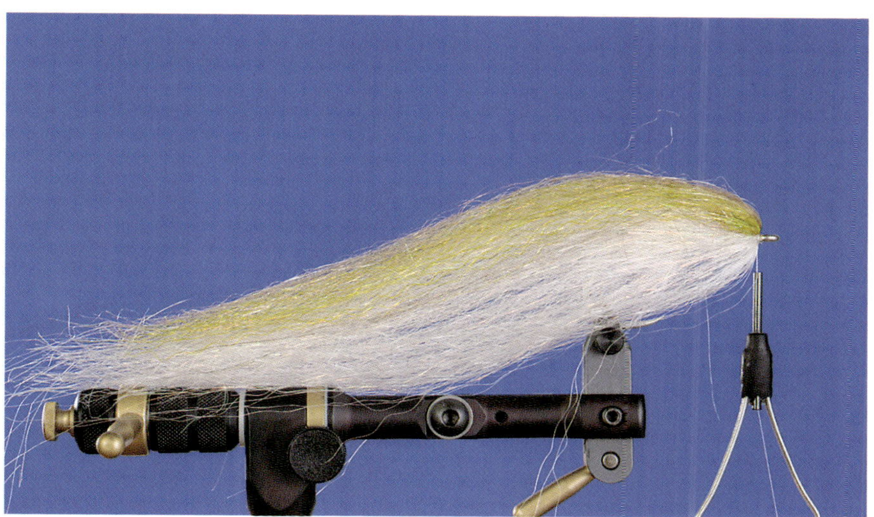

10. Pull the fibers hanging over the eye to the rear, and take a few loose wraps of thread over them. Push the clump down with your fingers until all of the white fibers are below the hook shank. Try to maintain a nice separation of colors. Tighten the thread and secure the fibers with a few more wraps. Bring the bobbin in front of the fibers, take a few more wraps against their bases, and whip-finish.

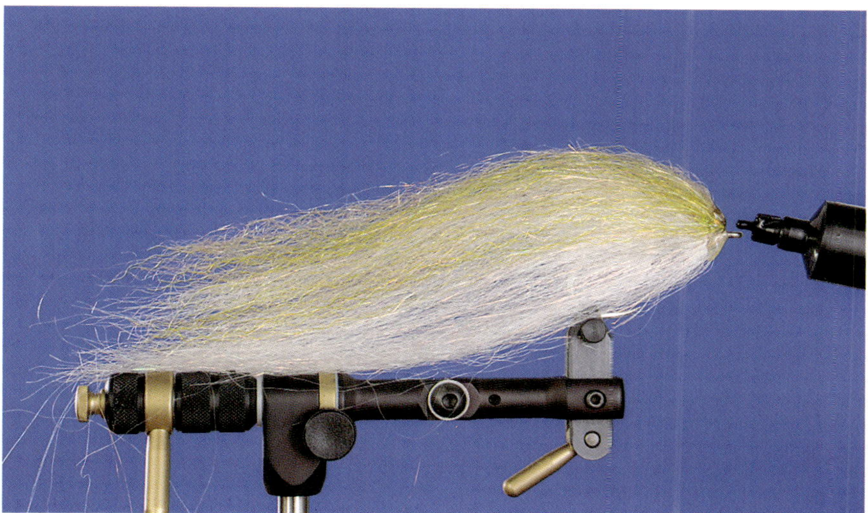

11. Apply gel just at the base of the fibers, closest to the hook shank. You only need a little bit to flare the fibers. Do not let the gel creep to the rear. Pull the fibers away from the shank with your fingers to create the profile you desire.

(continued)

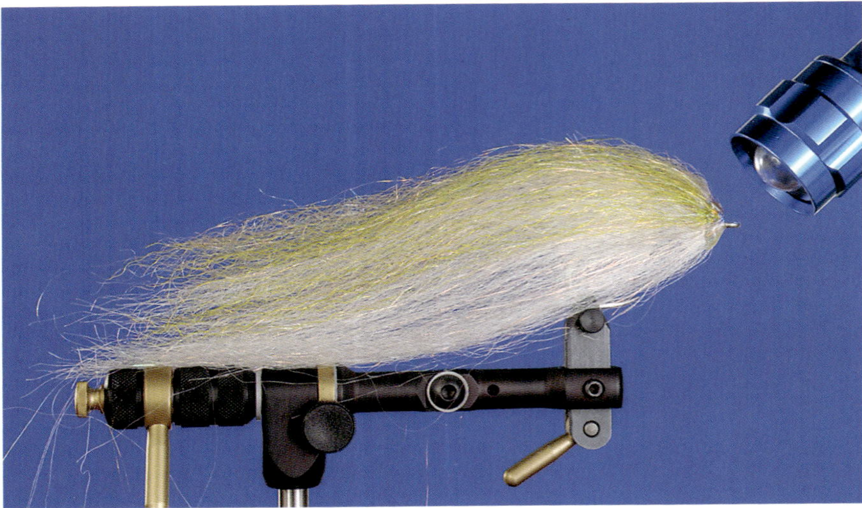

12. Continue to manipulate the flared fibers after the light-cured acrylic has been partially set, and once you have the final shape, you can set it completely with the light. You might find it easier to do this in two stages: first the top and then the bottom.

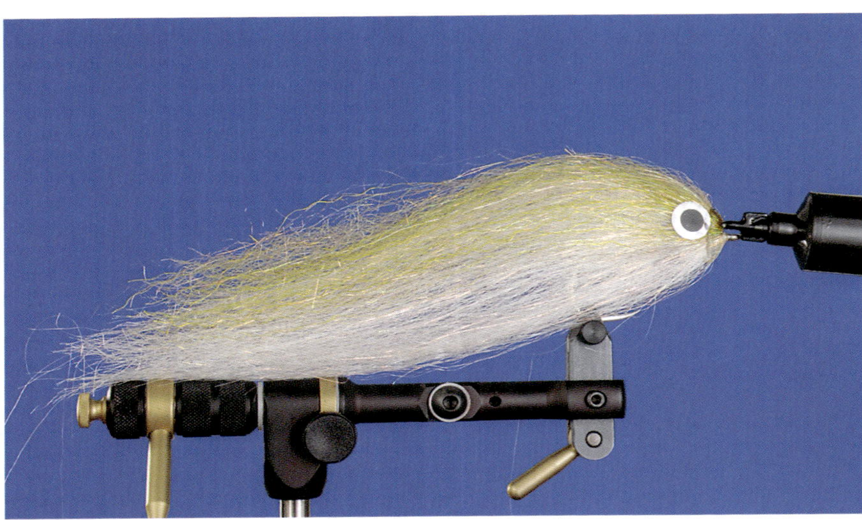

13. Place a stick-on eye on each side. Adding some gel on the edge of the eye helps it stay in place, or you can coat the entire eye if you wish. Hit it with the light.

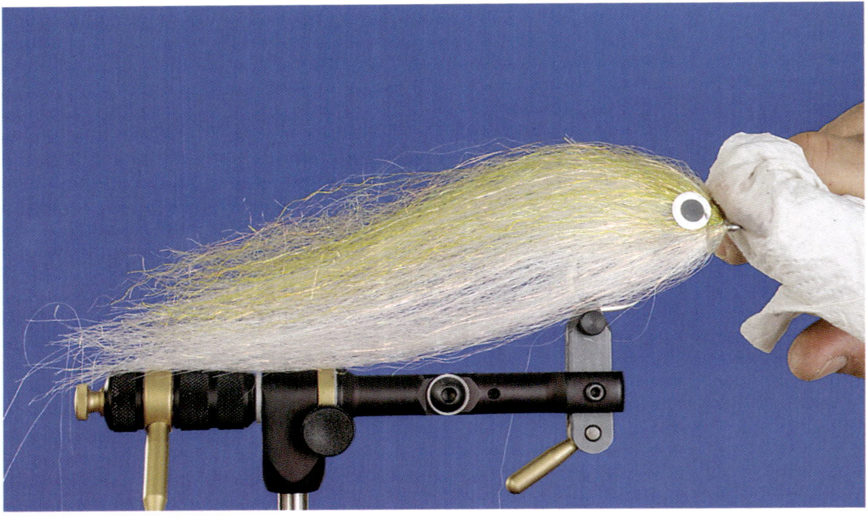

14. Wipe off the tacky layer with alcohol, and apply head cement to finish tying.

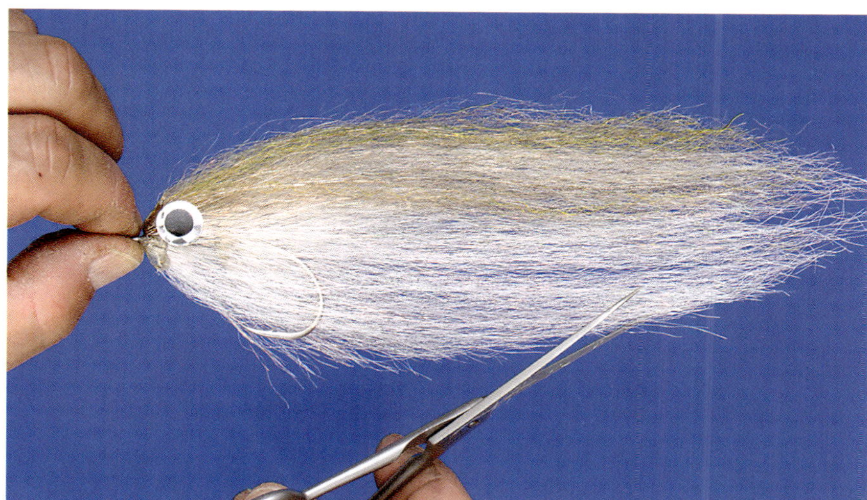

15. I like to take the fly out of the vise to get the final trim. Cut *with* the fibers and take off a few strands at a time. Go slow here. You want to try to get smooth lines from the hook eye to the end of the fly.

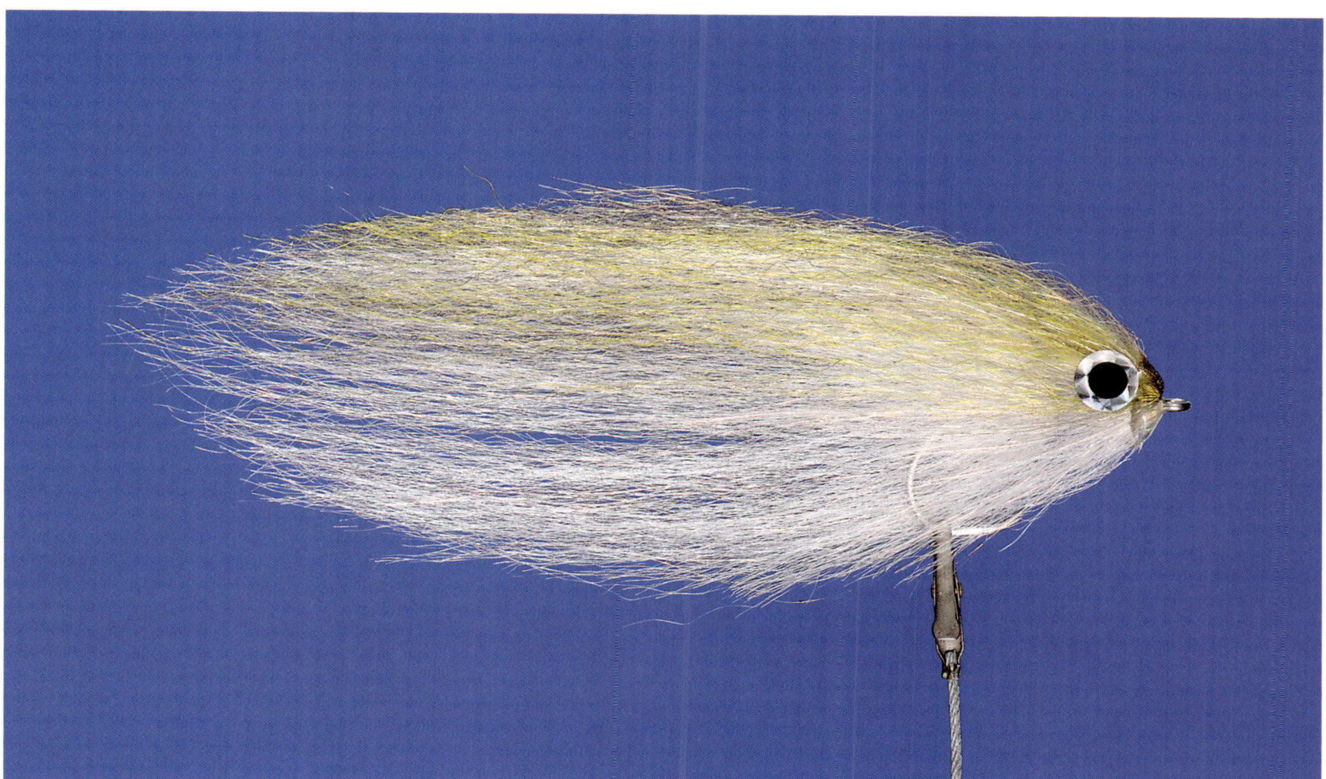

The Double Spread is effortless to cast. Its ultrathin design slices through the air. It also keels easily and won't roll on its side or spin in the current.

Chapter 16

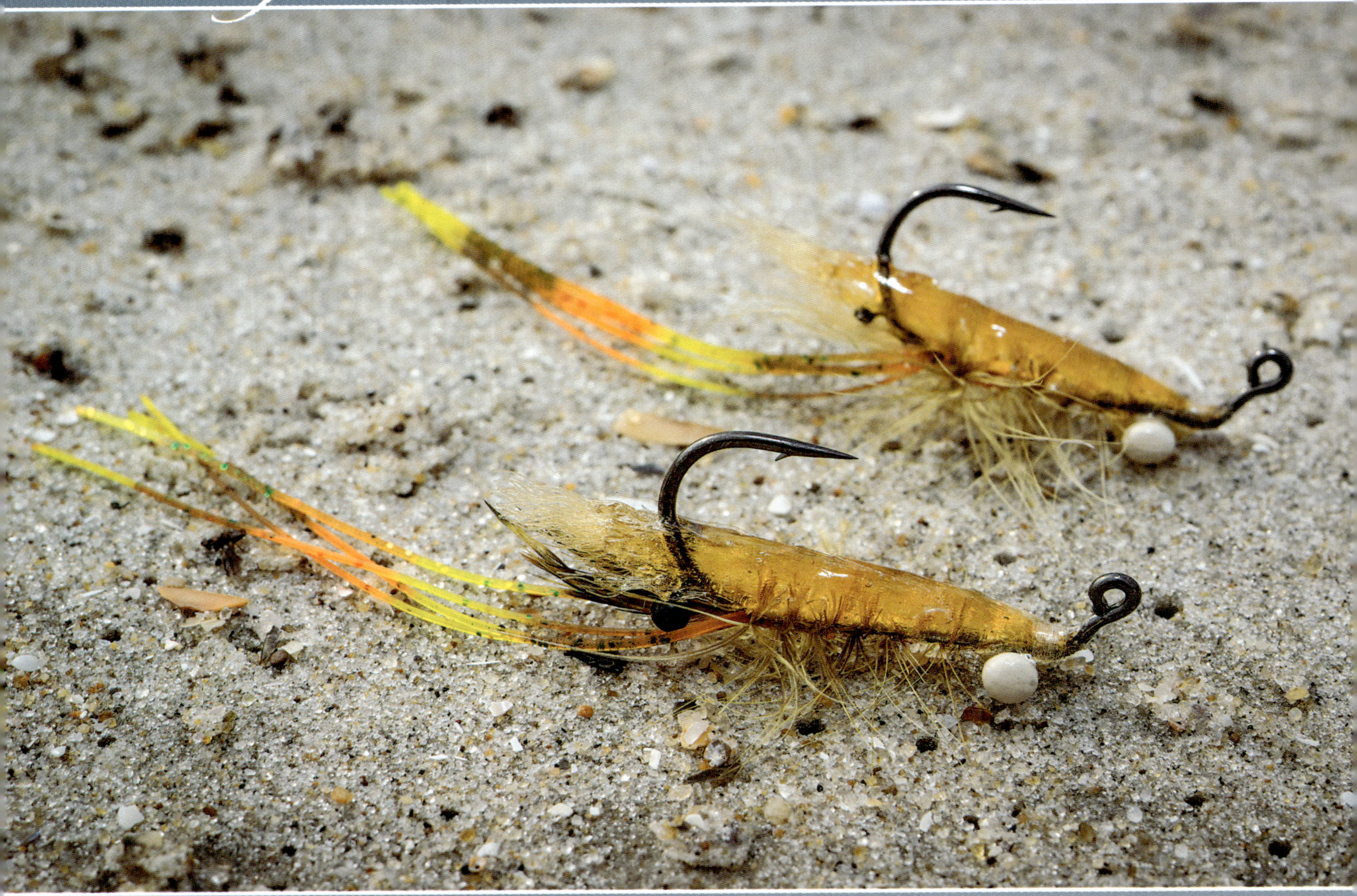

Tuffleye Sand Shrimp. Many kinds of materials can provide the right profile; however, the individual characteristics of different materials help fine-tune the design. In the case of the Sand Shrimp (above), it is the combination of dumbbell eyes, light-cured acrylic, and rubber legs.

Critters: Shrimp, Crabs, and Worms

It's often been argued that designing flies for saltwater species is not as challenging as designing flies for trout. Since I do not tie flies for or fish for trout very much, I cannot get into such a discussion. However, over the forty-five years I've lived "in the salt," I have made a few observations about saltwater flies and the challenges that a saltwater fly designer faces. The saltwater environment has such variety—from weather extremes to environments to species—that not only do patterns have to range from giant to small, they must also come in all different shapes. You are not simply creating different fish shapes, but also must imitate many different organisms, some of which live on the bottom of the ocean. Some of the most fun to design are what I call "critters"—crabs, shrimp, and worms. Predators seem to scrutinize imitations of these baits more than any other saltwater flies, possibly because the naturals are usually singled out before they are attacked.

Tuffleye Sand Shrimp

The Tuffleye Sand Shrimp is a simple, easy-to-tie, and realistic pattern for bonefish, weakfish, stripers, and other species that feed on small shrimp. It is a variation of the Ultra Shrimp, which I designed to fish outgoing estuary currents along the Northeast coast and to chum for stripers, weakfish, and fluke. The Ultra Shrimp design has been very successful for many types of anglers, and in many different fishing situations. Over time, the Ultra Shrimp has become popular for sight-fishing for everything from bass in the surf to bonefish in the Florida Keys. Many conventional fishermen use the Ultra Shrimp as a teaser when they bottom-fish for fluke. Because of the effectiveness of the basic design concept of the Ultra Shrimp, I simply modified it to better imitate the bottom dwelling sand shrimp by tying it on a jig hook with dumbbell eyes. Instead of epoxy, I use Tuffleye Flex or Tuffleye Core.

Tuffleye Sand Shrimp

Hook:	#1 Eagle Claw 413
Thread:	Fine monofilament
Weight:	Lead dumbbell, painted tan
Eyes:	Burnt mono
Flash:	Krystal Flash
Carapace:	Tan Super Hair coated with Tuffleye Flex
Legs:	Tan saddle hackle and orange-tipped rubber legs

TYING THE TUFFLEYE SAND SHRIMP (JIG)

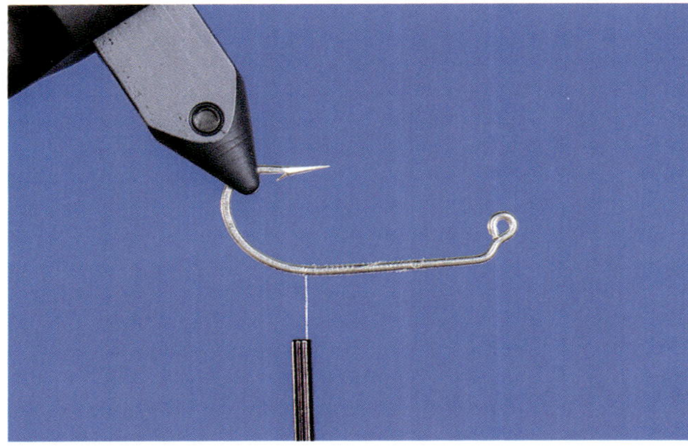

1. Insert the jig hook in the vise with the point up. Attach monofilament thread to the hook and cover the shank from the front to the rear of the hook, stopping just before the bend. Coat the thread with head cement.

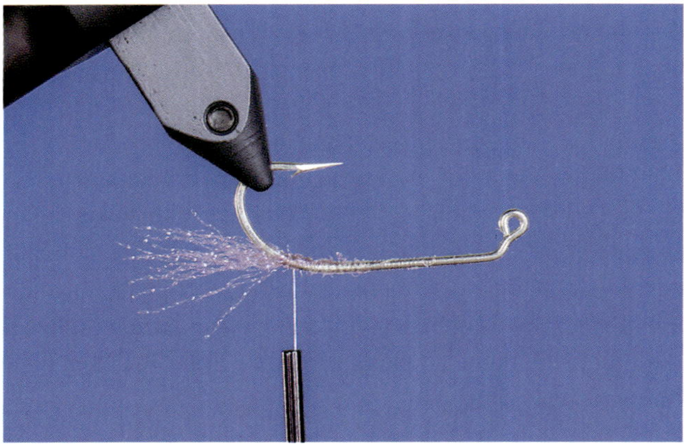

2. Attach a sparse amount of Krystal Flash about 1/2 inch long, and wrap over it slightly up the hook bend.

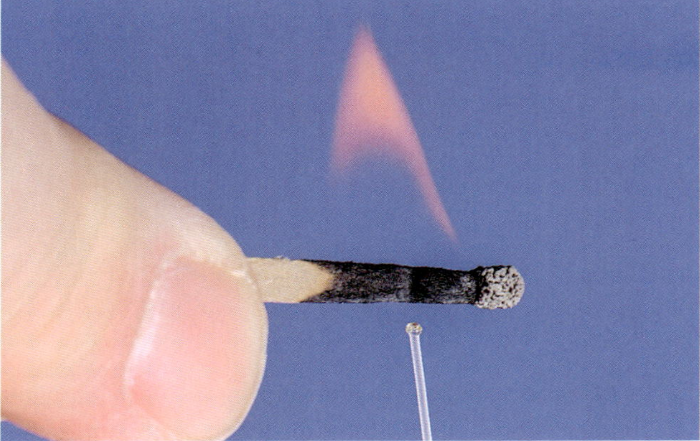

3. Prepare the mono eyes from 20-pound-test mono straights. Burn the tips until they form a ball, and then blow them out. I have found that monofilament creates a nice round ball, unlike fluorocarbon. Darken the mono eyes even more by coloring them with a black marker. If you plan on making a lot of shrimp, you might want to create a batch of eyes at one time.

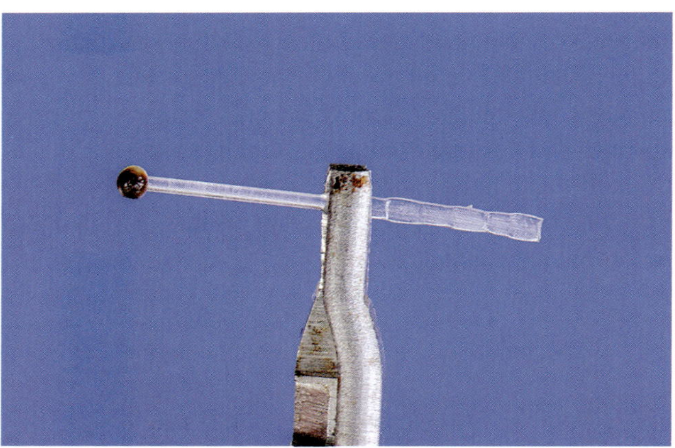

4. Flatten the mono with flat pliers so that it is easier to tie onto the hook shank.

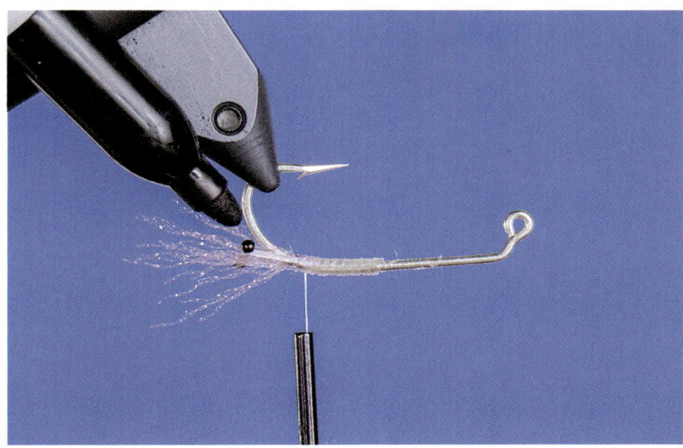

5. Tie in the prepared mono eyes, one on each side. The eyes should be up on the carapace of the fly, which means they need to be down on the hook bend. For me, the eyes are an essential feature of this fly.

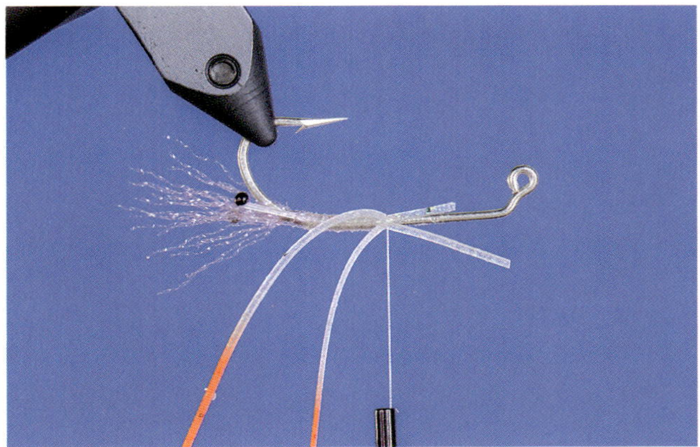

6. Wrap the thread forward to the middle part of the shank to attach the rubber legs, two on each side.

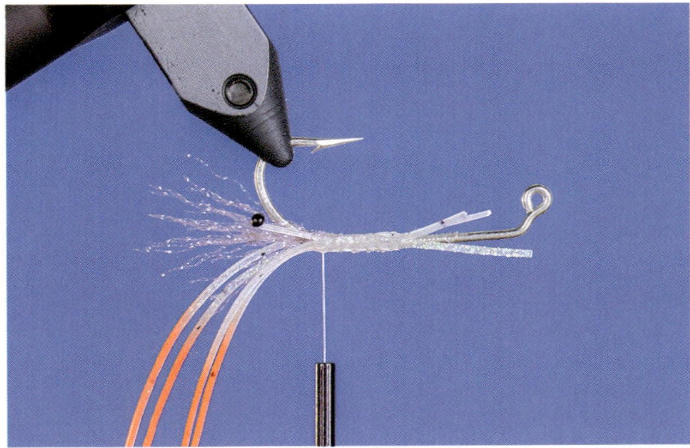

7. Wrap down the legs toward the hook bend to secure them.

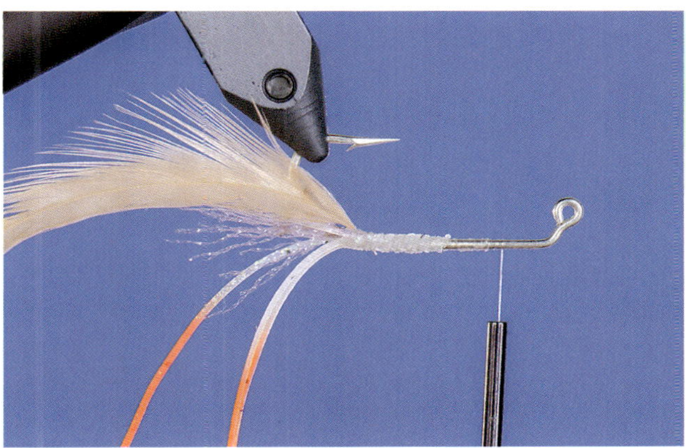

8. Trim the butts of the rubber legs flush and wrap over the legs once again with thread, finishing with the thread by the hook bend. Tie in a saddle hackle for the body legs, and move the thread forward about 1/4 inch in front of the hook eye. This is where you will tie off the feather.

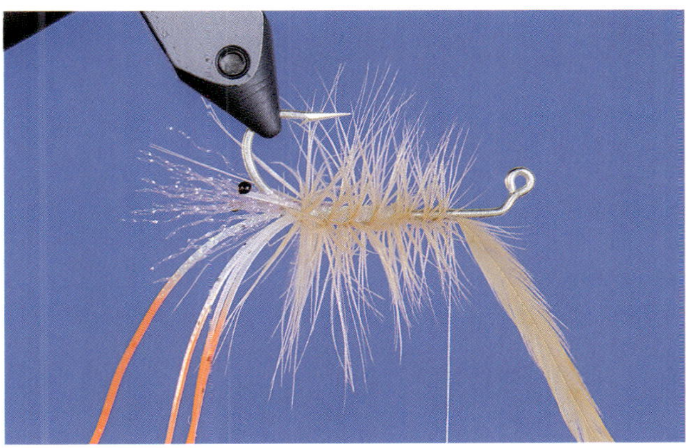

9. Palmer hackle the entire shank with an open spiral, except the last 1/4 inch.

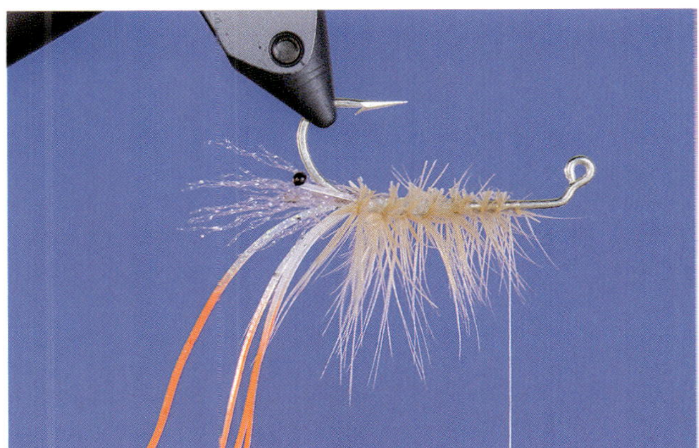

10. Tie down the hackle, trim the tip, and cover with thread. Trim the fibers on the inside of the hook.

(continued)

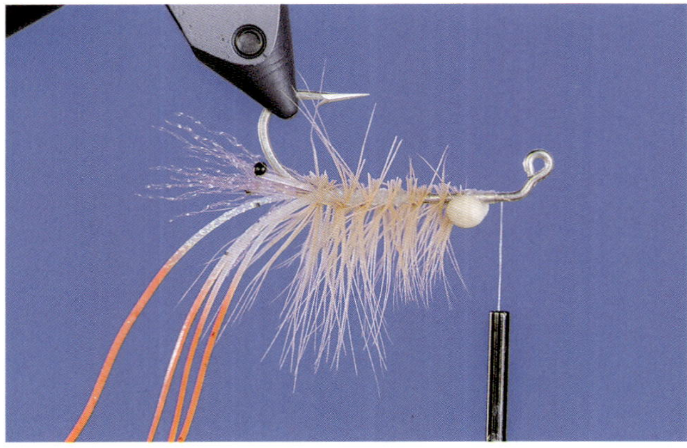

11. Attach lead eyes with figure-eight wraps adjacent to the hackle tie-down point. Apply head cement. If it is easier, you can turn the hook so that you are working on top of the hook shank.

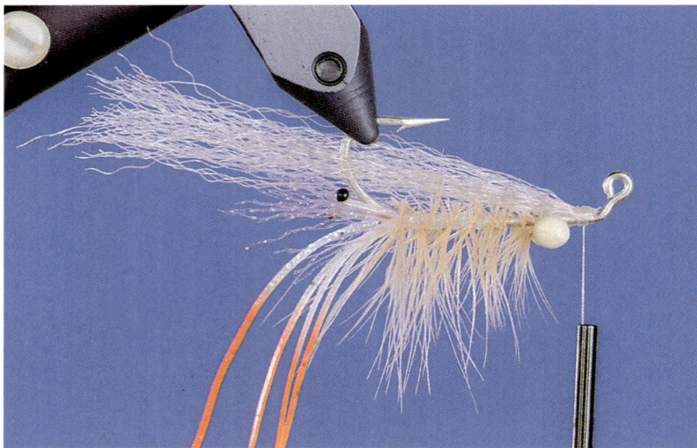

12. Tie down a fairly sparse carapace of Super Hair—about half a pencil width in thickness—in front of the lead eyes. Keep all fibers on the upper side of the hook shank.

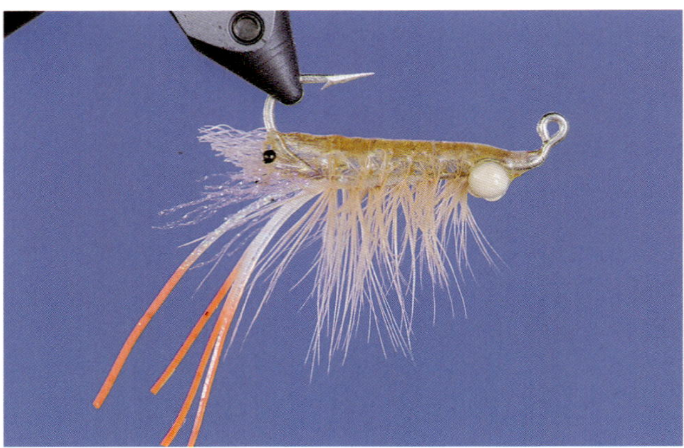

13. Apply Flex gel to the carapace as you hold the fibers firmly with your material hand. The carapace should be slightly angled up from the hook shank; don't put so much on that you start to close the hook gap. When you are happy with the distribution of acrylic, set it with the light, remove the tacky layer with a paper towel and rubbing alcohol, and add a final coat of Top Coat to finish the fly.

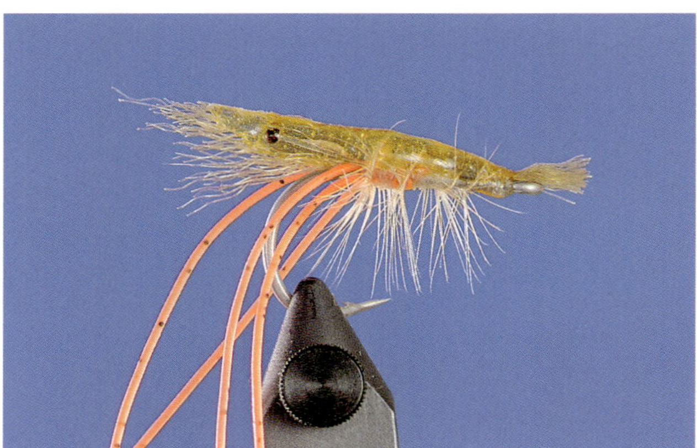

A basic Ultra Shrimp tied with Tuffleye Flex, sporting bright orange rubber legs. Orange can be a great color addition to many flats flies.

Jersey Long-Legged Crab

In July 2002, the water along the Jersey Shore was crystal clear. The stripers were in the shallows, looking for calico crabs. Until then, I had no need for a crab pattern, so I had to come up with one specifically for this situation, which was somewhat rare for New Jersey.

Because I had lots of sheep fleece available for other patterns that I tie, it seemed like a logical material to begin experimenting with for crab patterns. Fleece comes in many colors, is easy to control and shape, and it sinks. Through observing the naturals, what caught my eye was the movement of the legs and claws, so I knew I wanted to emphasize that and rubber legs seemed like a good choice. I started with fairly short legs, which were about the same length as the natural's appendages, but the fly didn't move the way I wanted. Tied in a lot longer, the legs moved a lot more, and that sense of life was what I was going for.

During that time when the stripers were feeding on crabs in the Jersey surf, and the water was clear enough to watch them, I soon discovered that if I moved the fly with short, 6- to 8-inch strips, the fish would get excited. Then, if I slowly crawled the crab fly away, with about a 1- to 3-foot strip, the fish would charge and take, and it was off to the races. The quick movement catches the fish's attention, and then the slow pull gets it to commit. The long legs are key to the effectiveness of the fly in my opinion, as they give the appearance of something alive. That summer, we caught lots of large fish while sight-fishing in the surf, some up to 25 pounds. In addition to stripers, this fly has worked well for cownose rays and even bluefish, fluke, sea robins, and lots of other kinds of fish that feed in the wash.

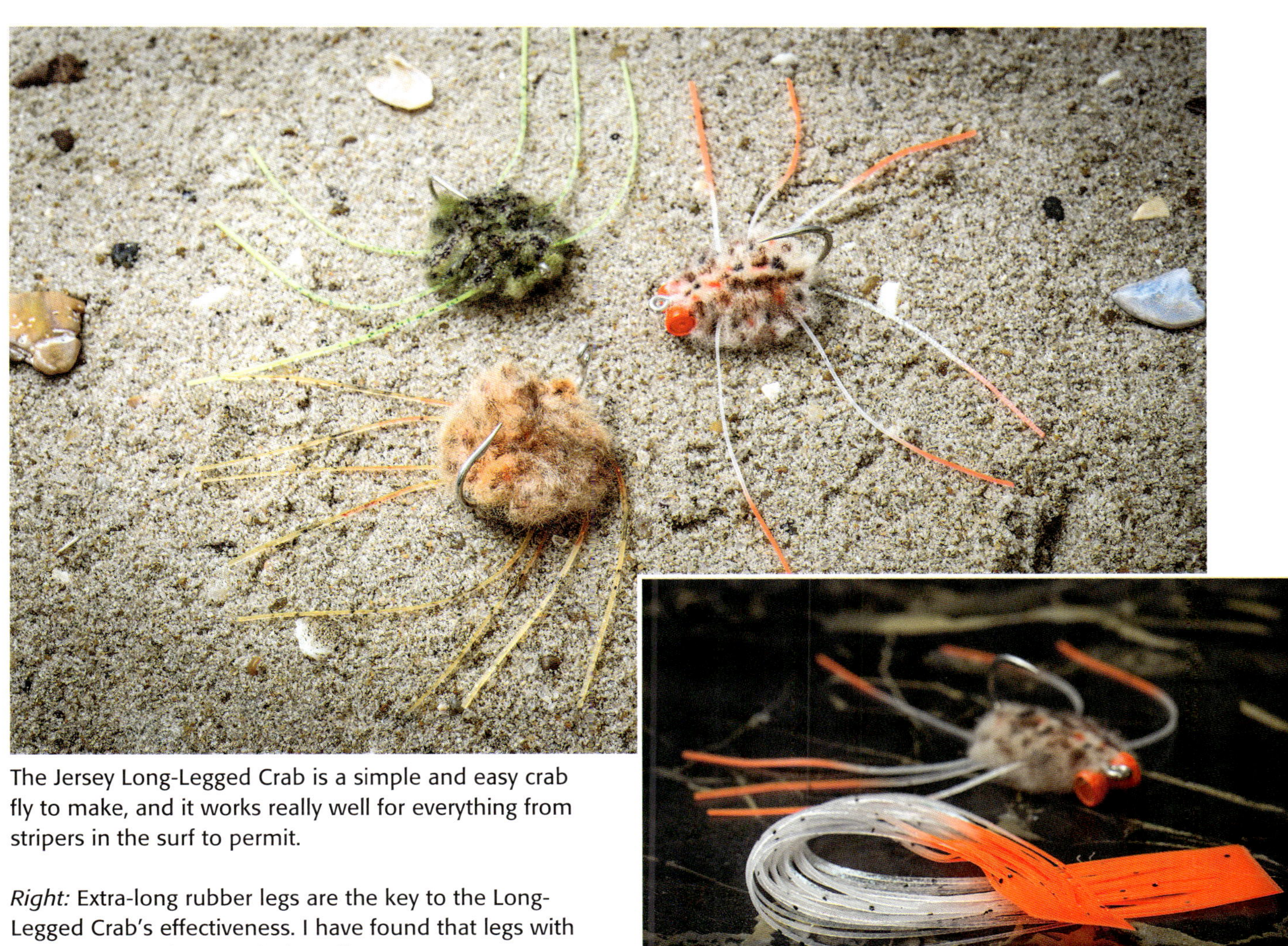

The Jersey Long-Legged Crab is a simple and easy crab fly to make, and it works really well for everything from stripers in the surf to permit.

Right: Extra-long rubber legs are the key to the Long-Legged Crab's effectiveness. I have found that legs with orange tips work particularly well.

Jersey Long-Legged Crab

Hook:	Eagle Claw 413 or similar jig-style
Thread:	Fine monofilament
Eyes:	Plastic dumbell
Legs:	Rubber
Body:	Sheep fleece coated with Tuffleye Flex

TYING THE JERSEY LONG-LEGGED CRAB

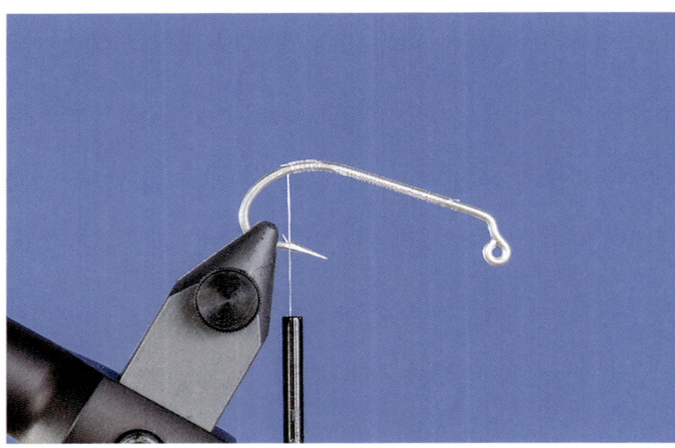

1. Place the hook in the vise with the shank angling downward a little to make it easier to wrap the thread on the shank and the bend.

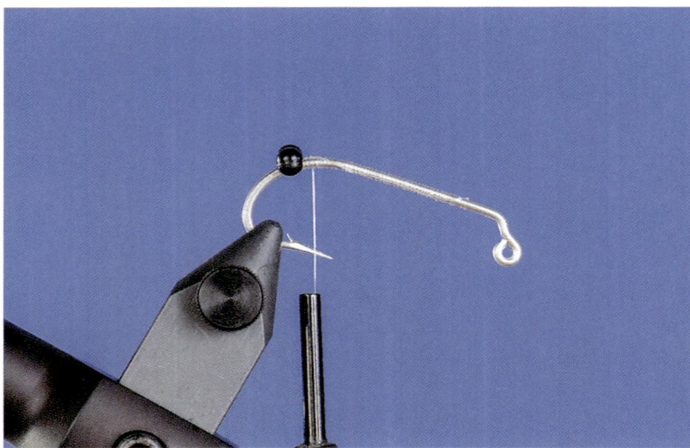

2. Tie on plastic dumbbell eyes with figure-eight wraps just past the hook bend on the underside. Coat them with head cement.

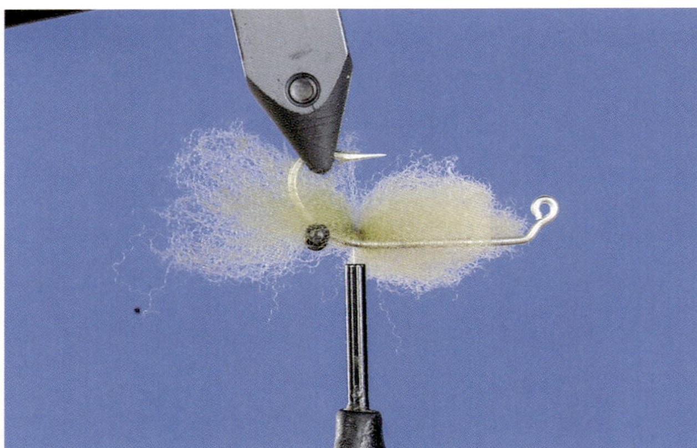

3. Turn the hook to a normal orientation, and wrap the thread to where the shank is straight. Prepare some fleece by first brushing the patch with a dog brush and then cut a clump from the hide about the thickness of a pencil. Do not trim the tips. Tie it down in the middle of the clump with the fiber tips facing to the rear. Keep all fibers on the inside of the shank to ensure that the hook rides point up in the water.

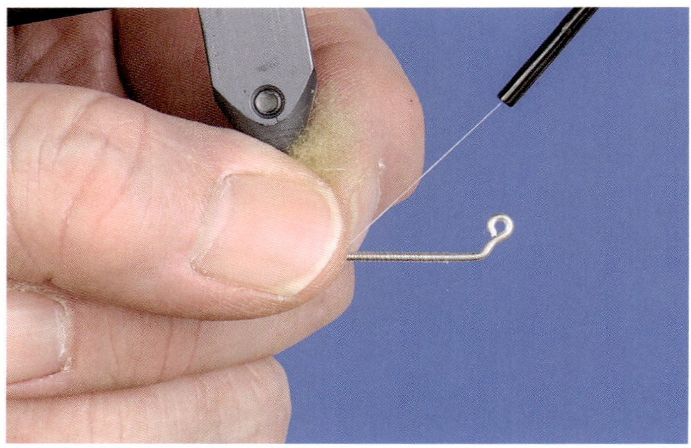

4. With your material hand, reach in and pull all the fibers back to isolate the thread. Bring the thread in front of the fleece tie-in point, and secure it with a few thread wraps.

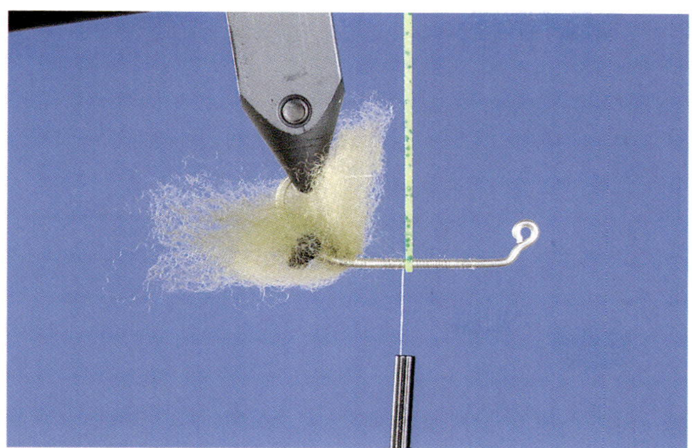

5. With the thread positioned about 1/4 inch from the base of the fleece, loop the rubber legs around the hook shank against the thread. The legs that you choose are up to you, but I like color combinations with pink or orange tips.

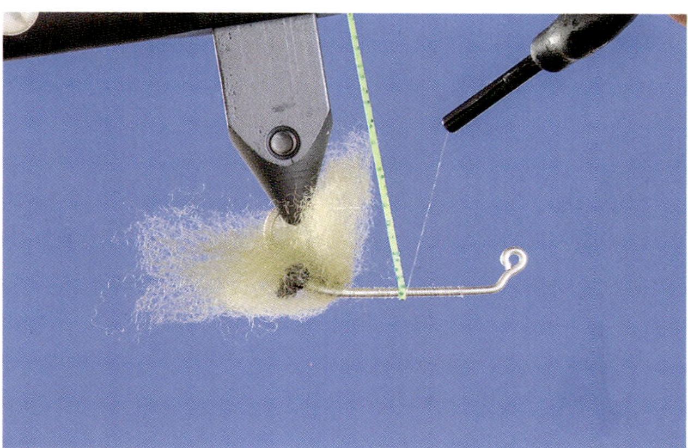

6. Wrap the thread over the doubled over legs, securing them to the shank.

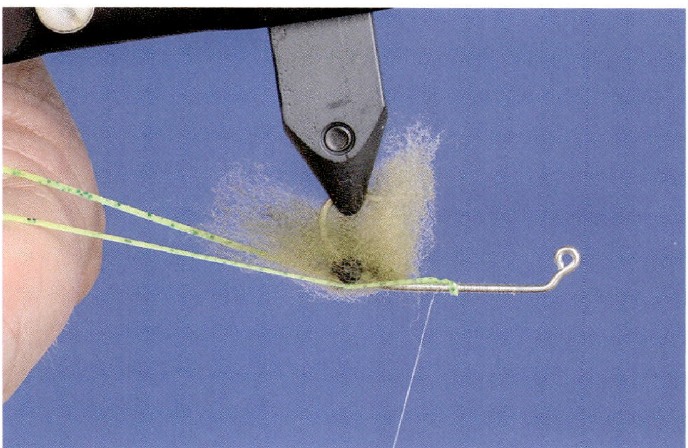

7. Separate the legs to each side of the hook shank. Hold them in position, and wrap back to the base of the fleece. This will keep the legs in the desired position, one to each side.

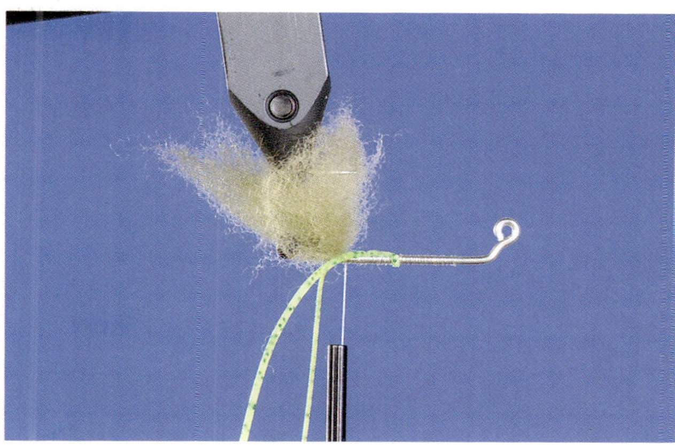

8. Make sure the legs are even on each side. If they're too long, you can always trim them back a bit, 1/4 inch at a time. Err on the side of caution because you can't undo your cuts.

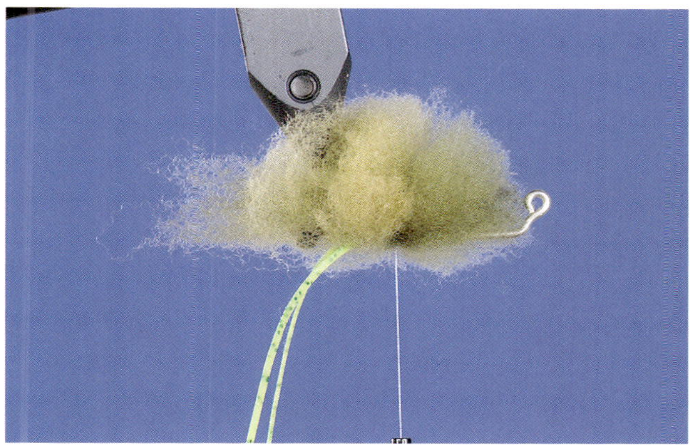

9. Bring the thread toward the front again 1/4 inch to tie in the next bunch of fleece. Prepare the fleece by cutting the tips off, leaving both ends cut square. Attach the fleece to the hook shank as before, being careful to keep the fibers on the inside of the shank.

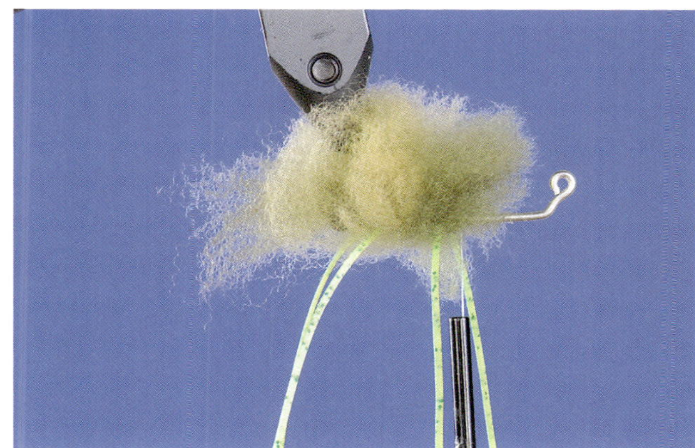

10. Pull back the fibers and bring the thread in front of the fleece tie-in point. Attach a second set of legs the same way that you did before.

(continued)

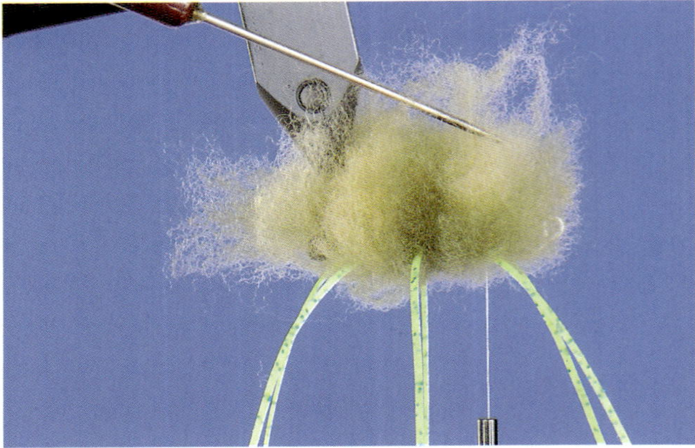

11. Tie in one more section of fleece and legs. At this point, free up any entangled fibers with a bodkin to get a good read on how the fleece fibers are lying and to make trimming in the future a lot easier.

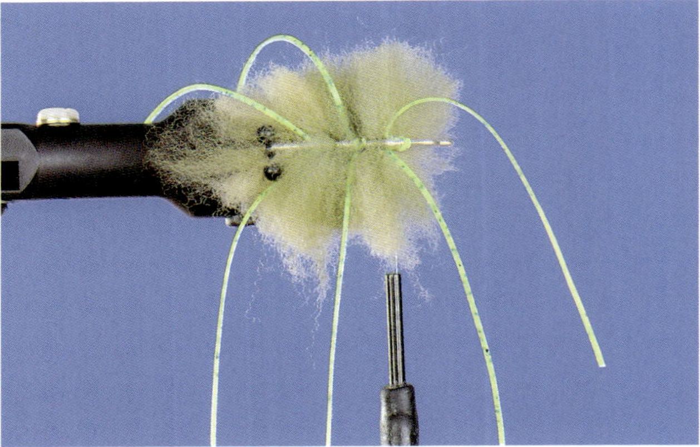

12. Take a good look at the underside of the hook shank to be sure that the fleece is located only on the inside of the hook shank. Cut away any fibers that are not in the proper position. Note here the distance between each tie of rubber legs.

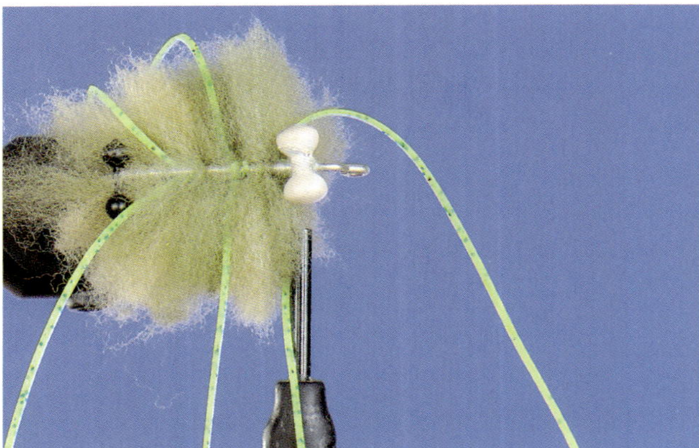

13. Tie in lead dumbbell eyes on the underside of the hook shank with figure-eight wraps. Position the thread in front of the eyes to tie down one last bunch of fleece.

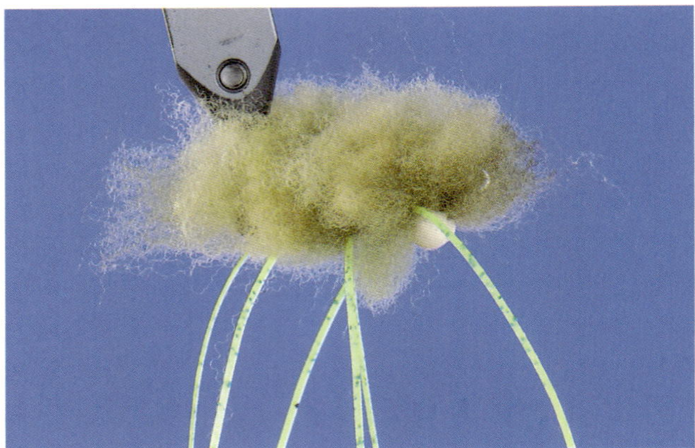

14. After tying it down, secure it with several wraps of thread. Cut off the thread. You are now ready to begin trimming the body.

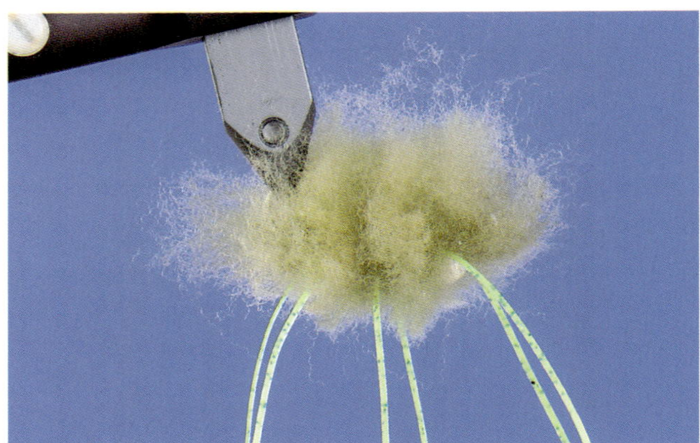

15. The body has to be "picked" with a bodkin once more before trimming it with your scissors. There is a crab in there; you just have to find it!

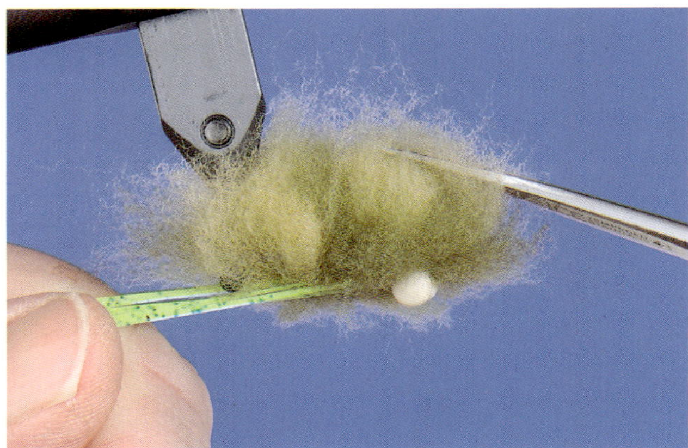

16. Holding the legs securely down and away from your scissors, start trimming with an angled cut from the top of the hook eye to just under the hook point.

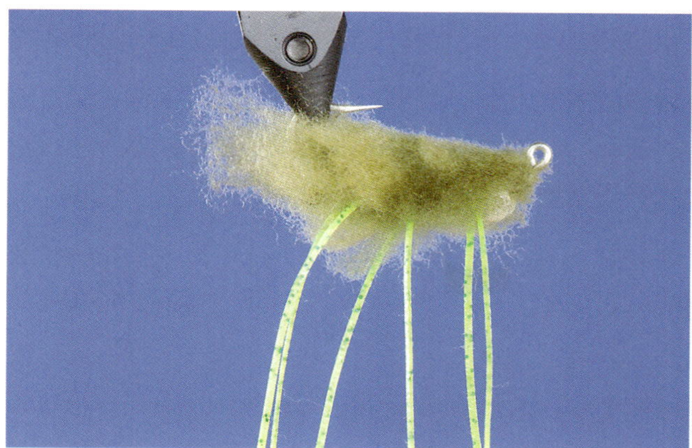

17. This is how the first cut should look. You want to remove the bulk in these first cuts and then do the fine trimming later.

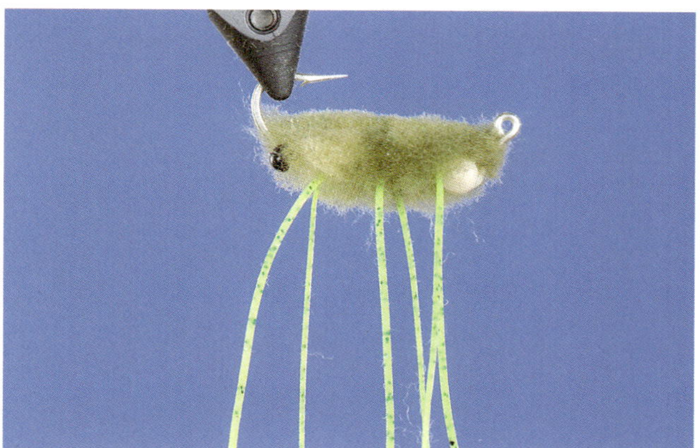

18. Continue trimming the fly to shape. It helps to look at it from all angles to get the proper shape.

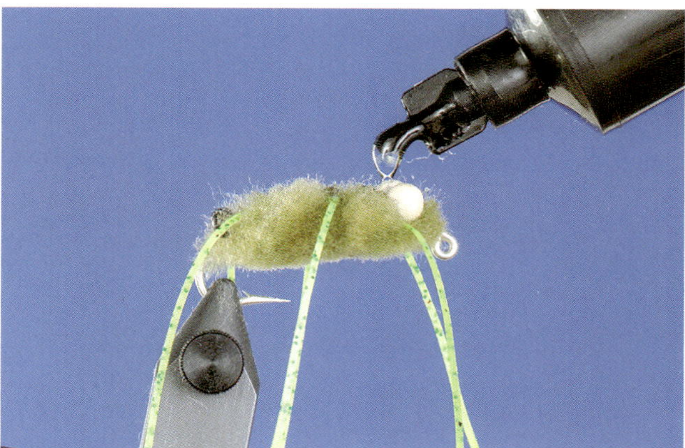

19. With the fly positioned so that the bottom is facing up, treat all the thread wraps with acrylic gel. This not only adds durability and realism to the fleece but it keeps the legs in position.

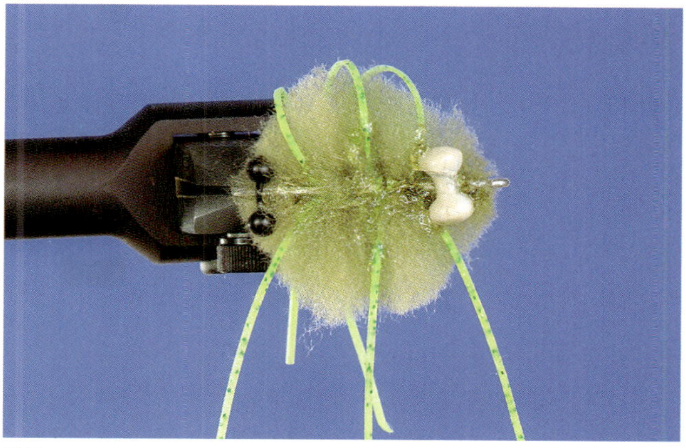

20. Here is a view of the underside of the fly with gel applied and hardened in place. You can see how the acrylic holds the legs in the proper position perpendicular to the shank. If you don't do this, the legs just sweep under the body of the fly and look strange and unnatural.

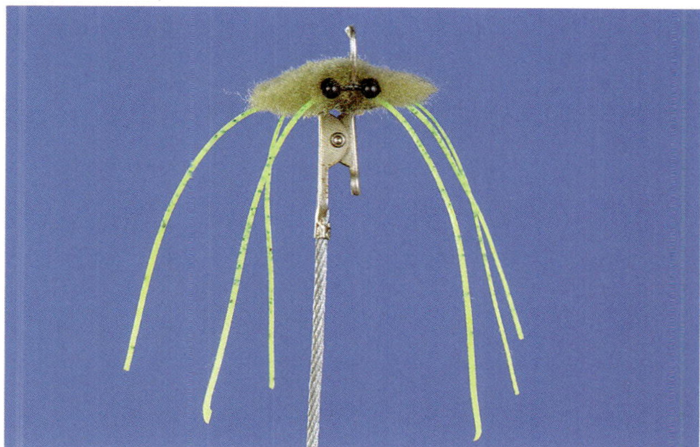

21. The finished Jersey Long-Legged Crab. From the front, you can see how the legs come out first before sweeping down. Underwater, they don't lie flat on the sand; they lift up, creating the illusion of a real crab with claws in a defensive posture.

Three-Feather Sand Flea

Sand fleas (aka sand crabs or mole crabs) are a plentiful bait along our coasts. They burrow into the sand, but they are often unearthed with the currents in the wash. When this happens, they bounce and tumble along until they can right themselves and find cover in the sand again. Sand fleas are not strong swimmers. Before they can burrow back into the sand, they are at the mercy of the surf currents and frequent predators that feed in the wash.

My intent with the Three-Feather Sand Flea was to capture the overall shape of these baits and suggest the subtle markings and coloration. The feathered collar breathes in the water, and the short rubber legs bring additional movement.

I fish this fly by casting up into the surf zone and allowing it to sweep down into the wash zone (the first step into the water from the beach that is slightly deeper). This area is the best fishing spot in the entire surf area because everything is at the mercy of the currents in there. Most of the time, I will be able to spot the fish and watch its reaction to the fly.

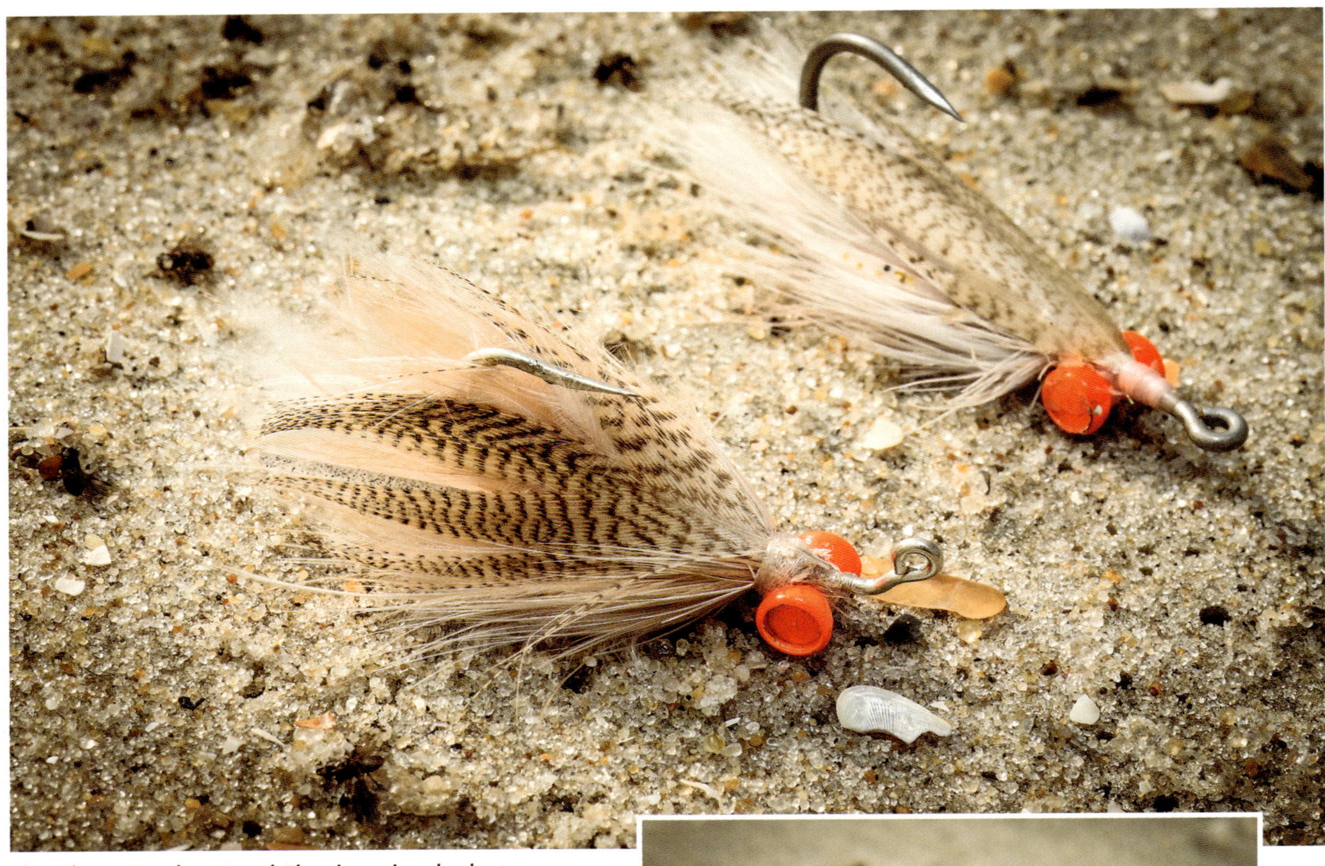

The Three-Feather Sand Flea is a simple, but effective pattern. When you fish it, allow it to tumble in the wash like the naturals.

Right: Sand fleas (female shown) roll around in the surf all day and are a major food source for stripers.

Three-Feather Sand Flea

Hook:	Eagle Claw 413 or similar jig-style
Thread:	Fine monofilament
Eyes:	Orange dumbbell
Body:	White (or gray), tan, and light pink saddle hackles
Carapace:	Wood duck (or dyed mallard) feather
Legs:	Clear rubber

TYING THE THREE-FEATHER SAND FLEA

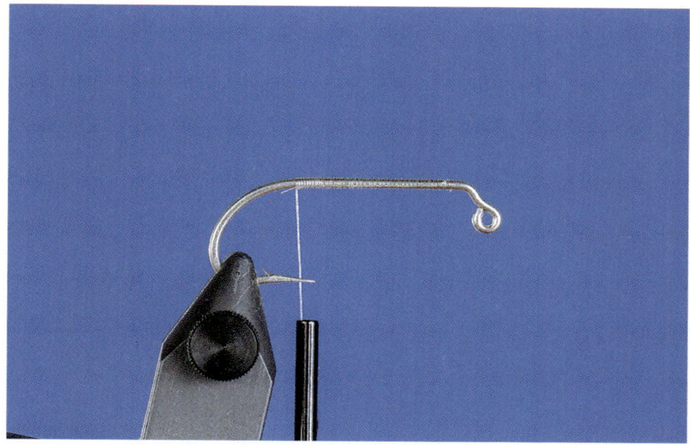

1. Place the hook into the vise with the bottom of the shank facing up. Attach the thread and wrap it back to a point just before the hook bend. Cover the thread wraps with head cement.

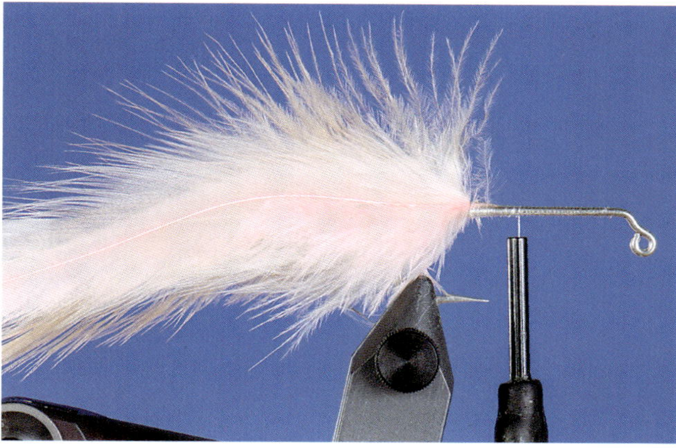

2. Choose three webby feathers with similar characteristics—one white, one light pink, and one light tan. Gray is another terrific color to use instead of white. Remove the fluff, exposing the stem, and align the three feathers together in your hand—color order doesn't matter. Tie down all three feathers at the bend with the concave sides down.

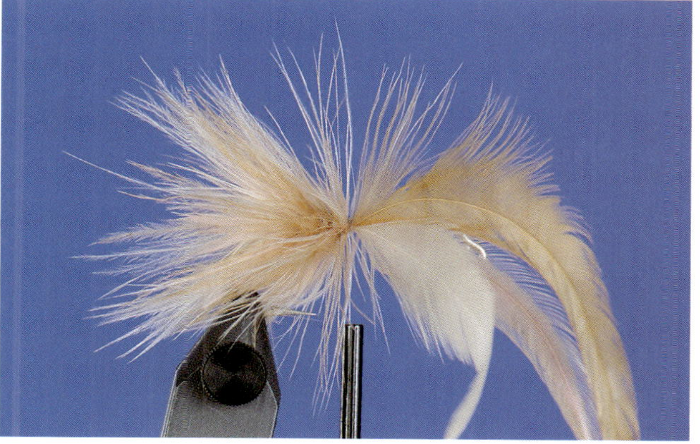

3. Palmer wrap all three at the same time to get a blend of colors. Palmer only the web portion of the feathers—about three wraps. Tie down and secure. You will repeat this step three times.

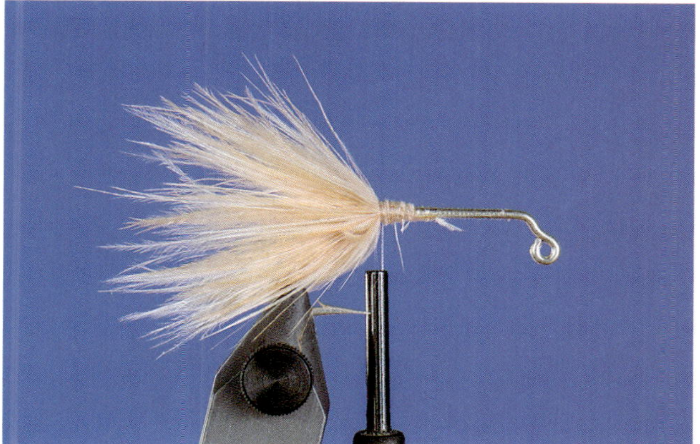

4. Cut off the saddles and wrap back over them to push them back slightly.

(continued)

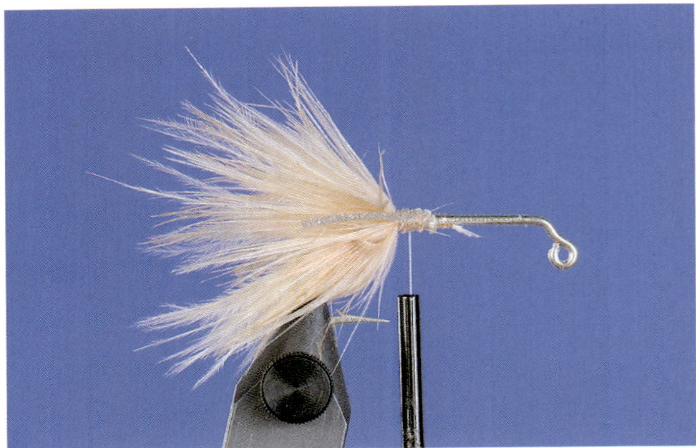

5. Tie in one leg on each side, and make them only slightly longer than the length of the fibers. Legs on sand fleas are short and barely noticeable, but it's better to err on the long side because you can always cut them later. Tie in the legs by looping them around the thread under the hook shank and wrapping back over them, as you did with the Jersey Long-Legged Crab.

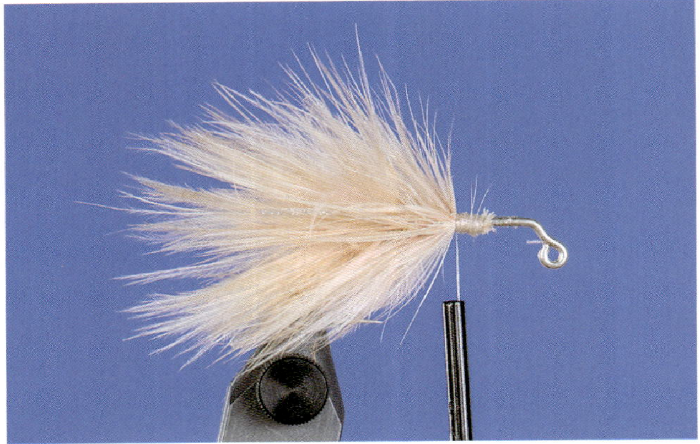

6. Tie down another three feathers, and wrap the thread forward so that it is out of the way. Palmer the feathers as you did before, tie them down, and trim the stems.

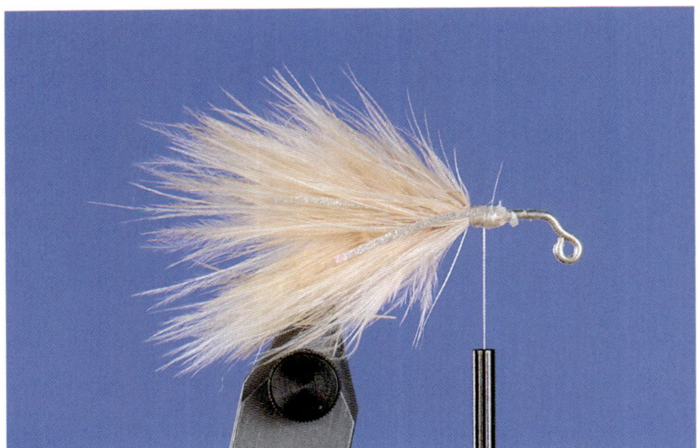

7. Attach the second set of short rubber legs.

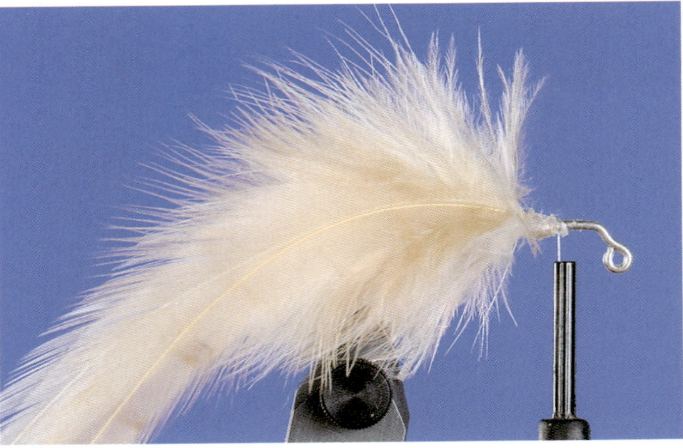

8. Tie in the last set of feathers, but do not palmer them yet. Wrap the thread forward to the point shown.

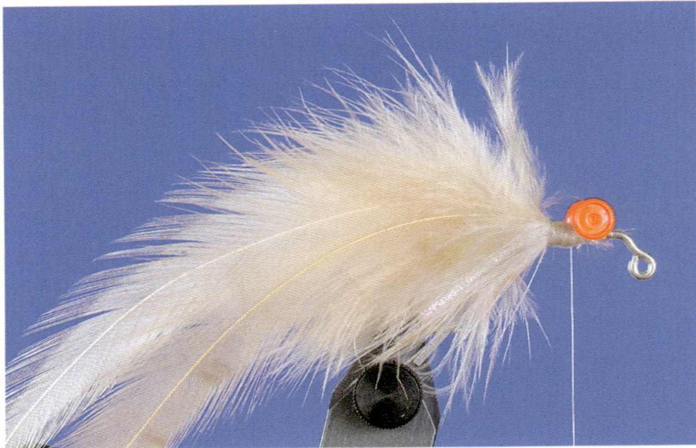

9. Tie down the lead dumbbell eyes with figure-eight wraps 1/8 inch behind the bend in the jig hook and coat them with head cement.

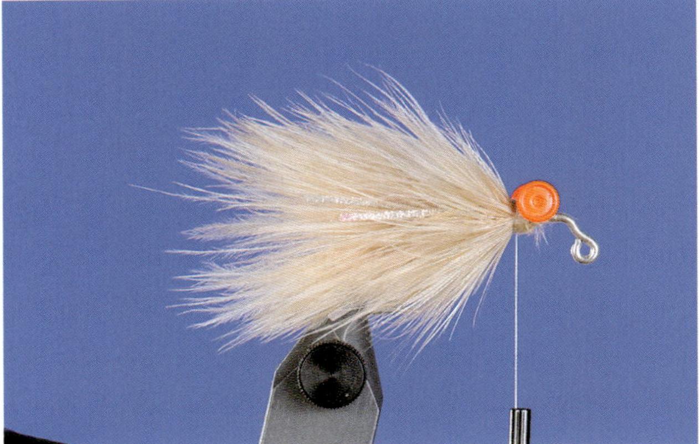

10. Palmer the feathers forward to fill in the gap at the base of the lead eyes and secure them. Trim the excess feather stems.

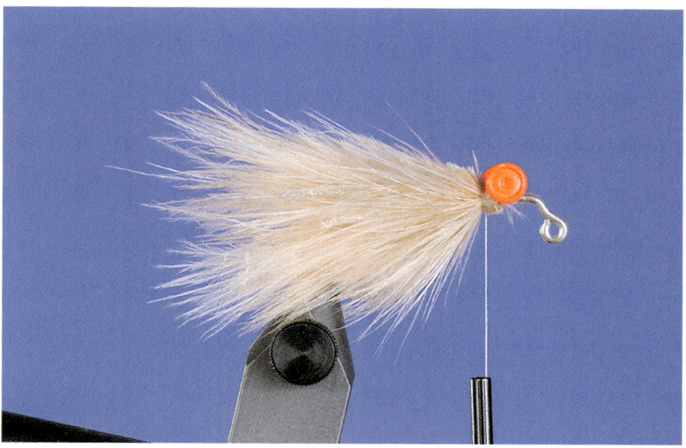

11. Trim the fibers on the bottom flat, but don't trim all the way to the hook shank. I always trim from the hook eye to the bend.

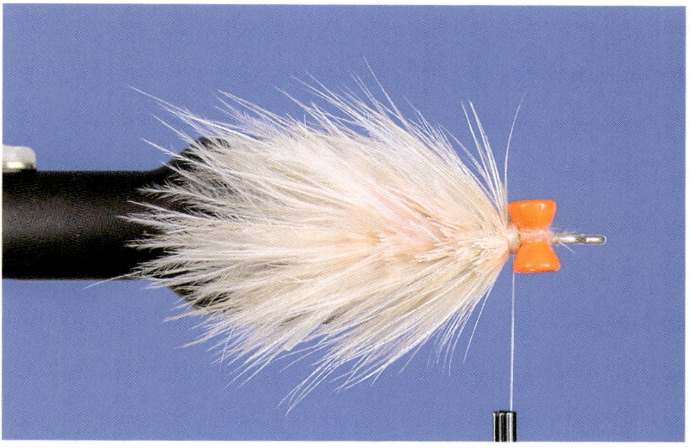

12. This is how the bottom should look after it has been trimmed.

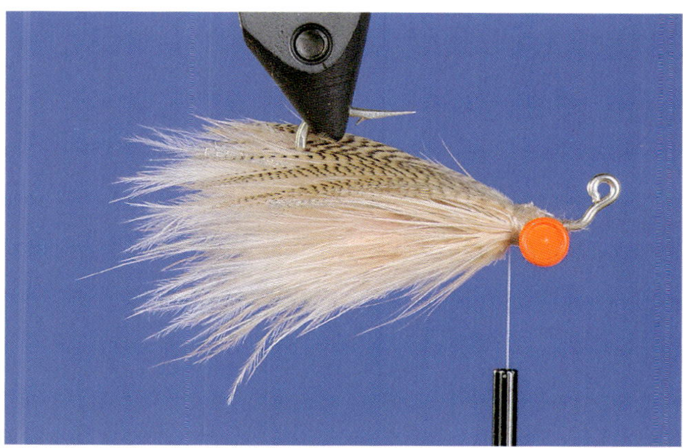

13. Tie in a prepared duck feather on top to imitate the speckled shell. Select a feather that covers the entire back of the fly and not just the middle. Whip-finish once again and add head cement to the wraps.

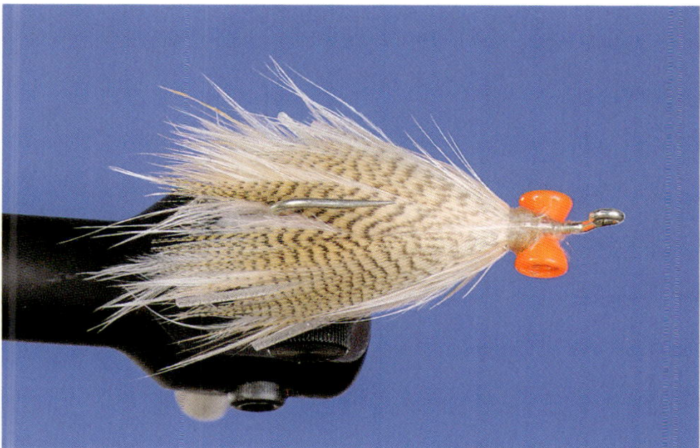

14. The finished Three-Feathered Sand Flea. The subtle pink hue combined with a mottled back suggest the natural.

Worm Fleye

Several seasons ago, Dave Skok sent me some Ezee Bug Yarn from Umpqua Feather Merchants, suggesting I try it for making a crab fly or possibly a shrimp pattern. This three-strand yarn comes in a wide range of colors, and though it looked interesting, I was not happy with the short lengths of the fibers for those types of patterns.

After spending more time looking at the material, I wondered about its possibilities for a worm pattern. I soon discovered that by picking out more of the fibers along the side of the yarn, I could create the look I wanted. A long bead of Tuffleye Flex down the middle finished it off.

I tied it to the back of a hook with no concern other than fouling. I realized I could just tie the worms first, and then tie them onto hooks later. I could make them in a couple of variations this way. I could use a spun deer hair head and a short piece of Worm Fleye, or tie on a hook with a triangular Live Body head, or I could "go long" by tying it onto a hook with lead eyes, which makes a nice sandworm imitation to entice bass on the Northeast flats.

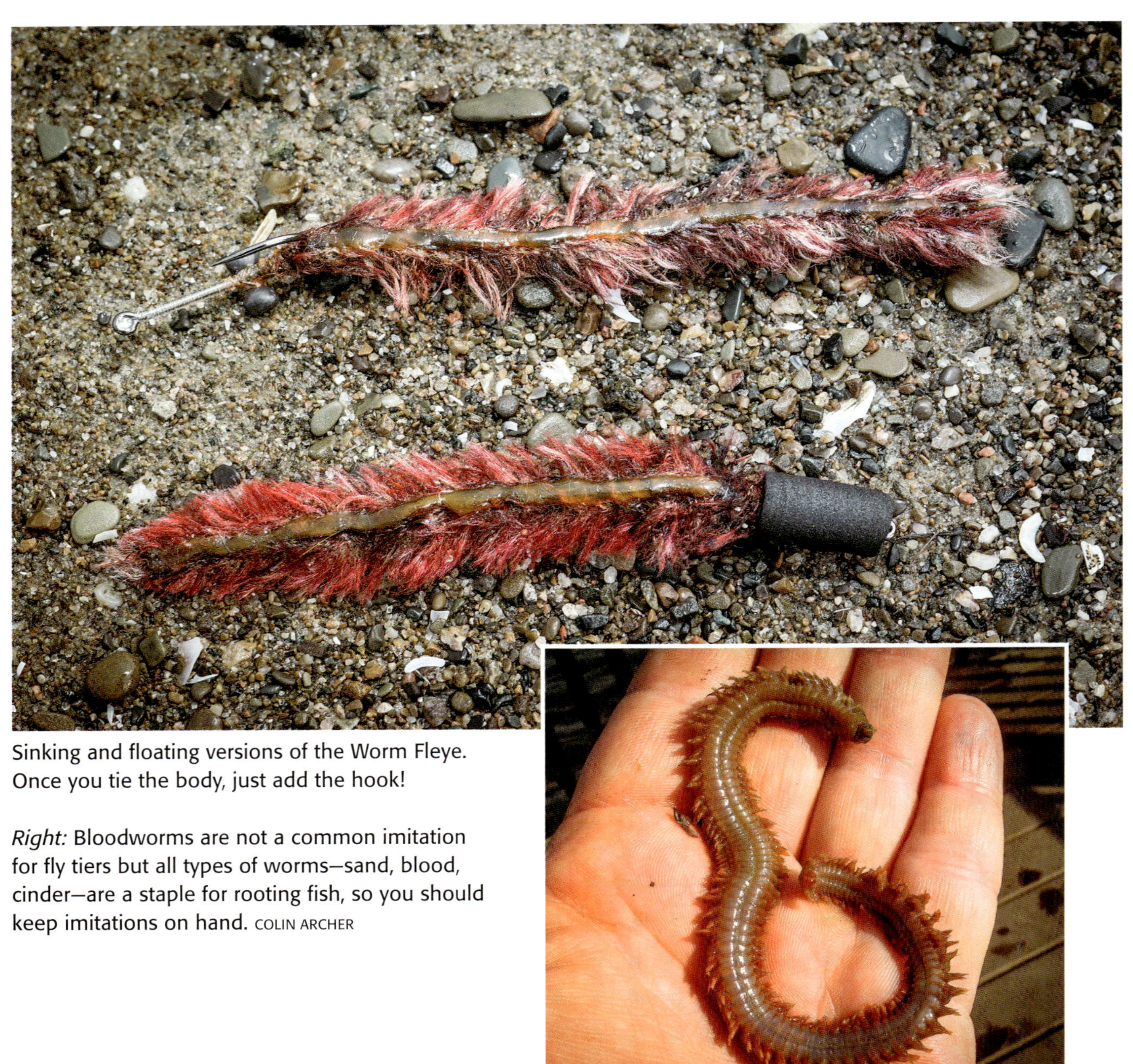

Sinking and floating versions of the Worm Fleye. Once you tie the body, just add the hook!

Right: Bloodworms are not a common imitation for fly tiers but all types of worms—sand, blood, cinder—are a staple for rooting fish, so you should keep imitations on hand. COLIN ARCHER

TYING THE WORM FLEYE

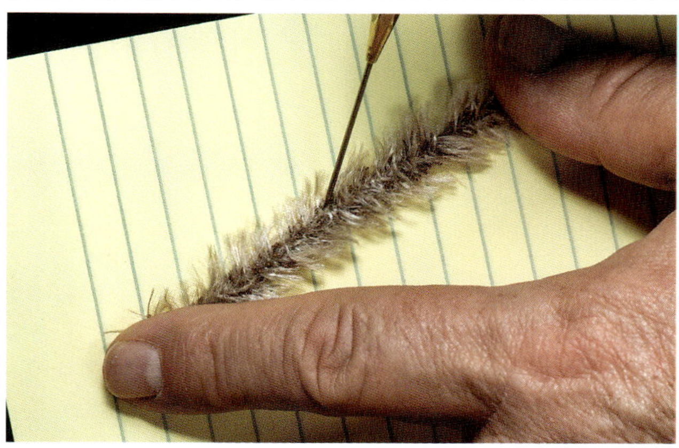

1. Cut the Ezee Bug Yarn into 4- to 6-inch lengths. Lay it onto a Post-it notepad or other surface and pick the fibers out as shown.

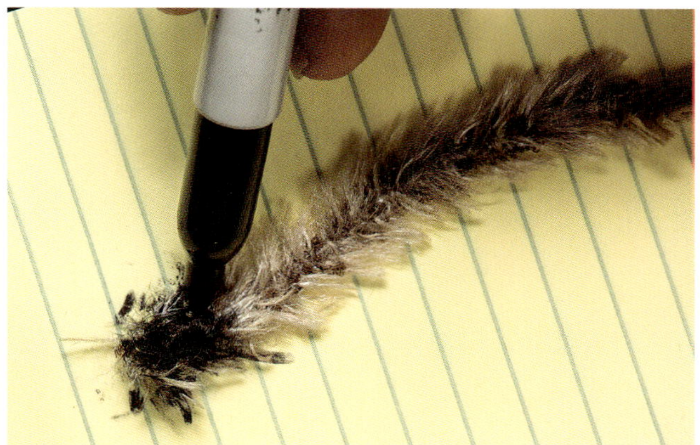

2. Color the first 1/2 inch of the yarn with a black Sharpie. Flip the yarn over and do the same on the other side.

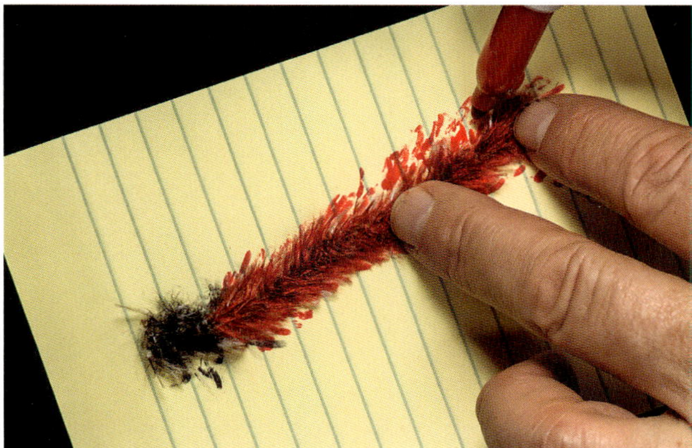

3. Color both sides of the rest of the yarn with a red Sharpie.

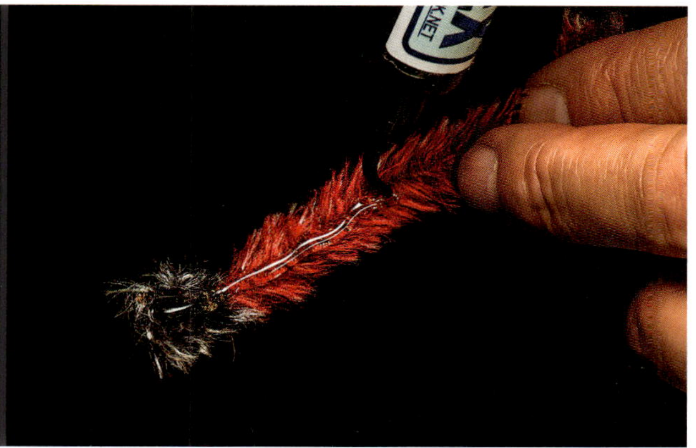

4. While laying the yarn flat, apply a long bead of Tuffl-eye Flex gel down the center from end to end. Stay in the middle. Do this on both the front and the back sides of the material.

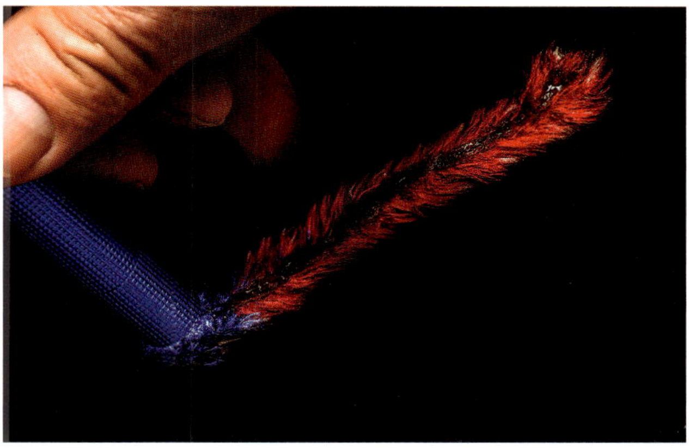

5. Set the gel with a blue light (here I am using a small pen light, which is ideal for travel). Remove any tack with rubbing alcohol and apply Top Coat. That's it! You can tie this basic Worm Fleye on to the hook in several different ways for both floating and sinking flies.

PART III

Evolution of Fleye Design

INFLUENCES & ADVANCES

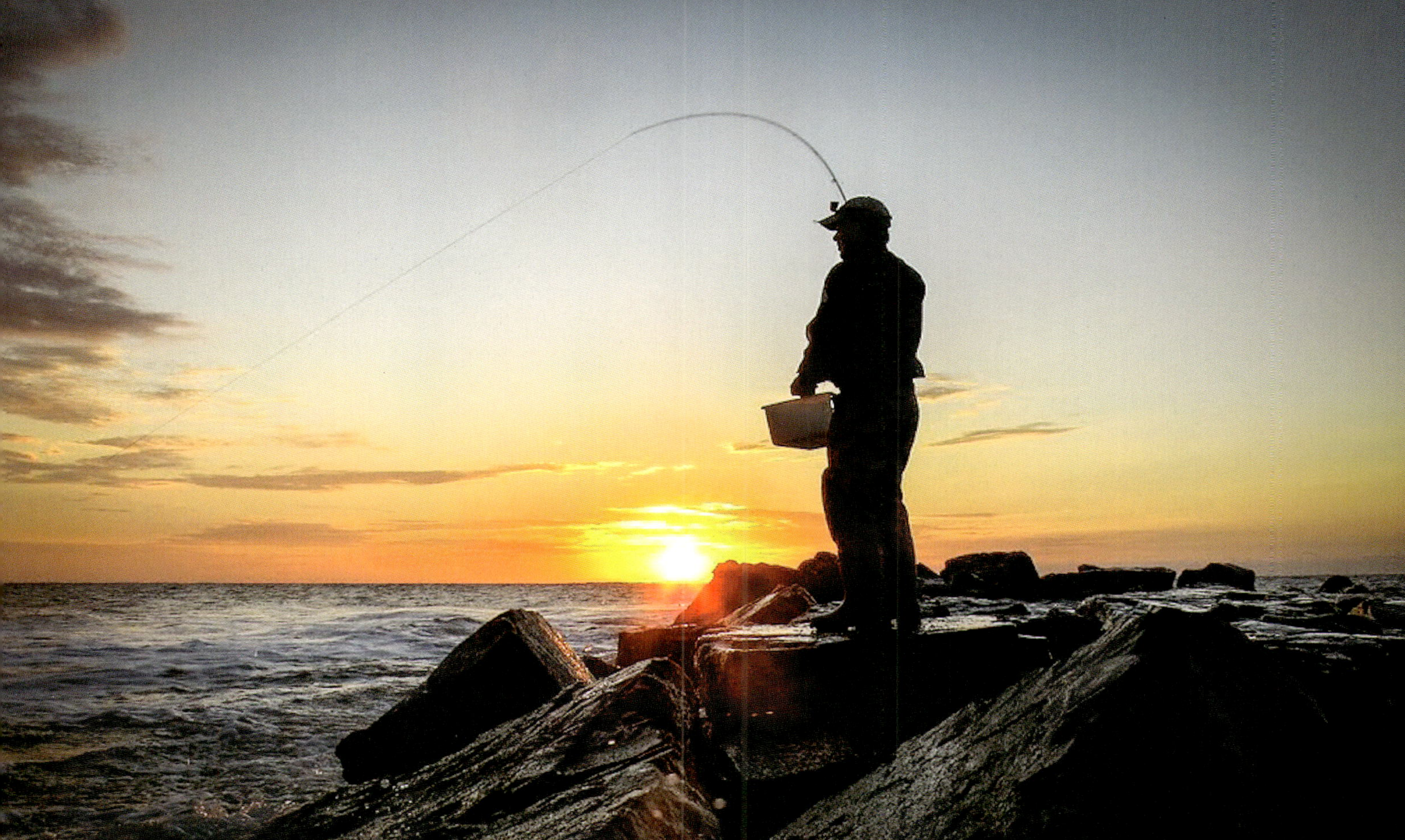

Rich Racioppi hooked up on a fly rod bass. Sloping rocks in the groin can provide a ramp to land fish and return them quickly back into the water. COLIN ARCHER

Chapter 17

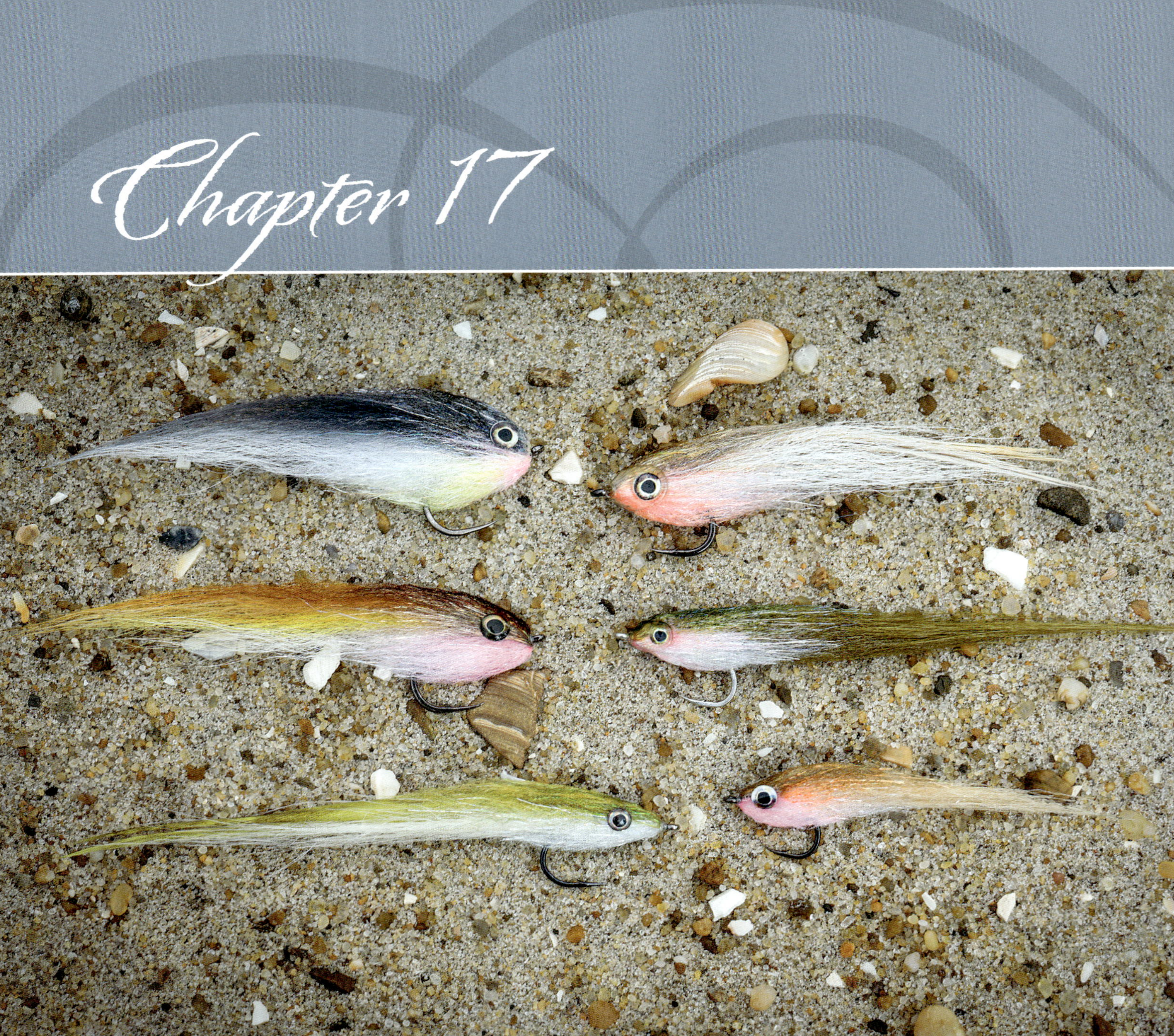

The Hoo Fly style is adaptable to almost any baitfish profile, from wide-bodied bunker and shad to smaller anchovies and spearing. Just brush the Laser Dub head into the desired shape and fix the profile with a coating of Liquid Fusion. From top to bottom: Shad Hoo Fly, Bunker Hoo Fly, Sand Eel Hoo Fly (left column); Bunker Hoo Fly, Silversides Hoo Fly, Bay Anchovy Hoo Fly.

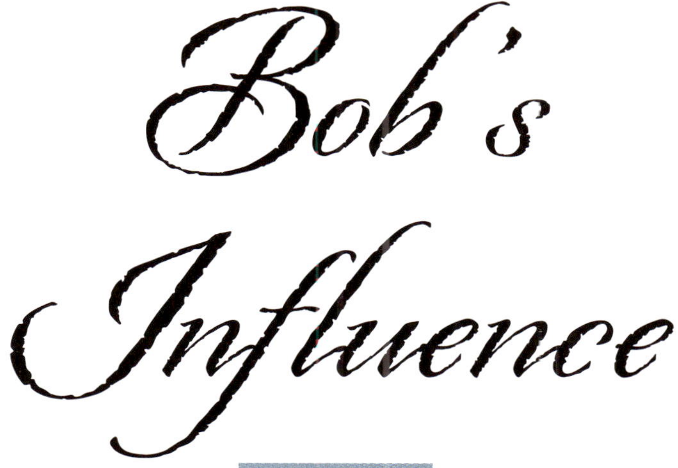

Bob's Influence

Jonny King

Influence and inspiration are subtle things. I know from my own life as a jazz musician how other musicians and composers can change the way I approach music in both conscious and unconscious ways. The same is true for tying flies. Sometimes the inspiration is direct and literal—we recreate what our heroes have contributed. With a little confidence, we may progress to adopting a technique or a trick we learned from them into our own patterns and styles, tailored to our own experiences and requirements. And finally, the influence may be less a conscious decision and more a broad philosophy about our chosen avocation. Both during the twenty-five years I've admired his fleyes and during the more recent years when he's become my close friend and tutor, I've felt Bob's influence in all these ways.

At the literal level, I've been tying Bob's patterns from my first transition from trout and bass flies to saltwater flies more than twenty-five years ago. I remember in particular seeing those first Surf Candies in an article and marveling at how they looked more like a spearing—a bait I encountered regularly on the beaches north of Boston—than any fly I'd ever seen. The pattern was simple, accessible to a transitioning tier, and so realistic and effective I was stunned. I still tie and use lots of Bob's patterns today, ranging from his old staples, like Surf Candies and Jiggies, to his more recent contributions, like the Hollow Fleye and Bucktail Deceiver.

But in copying and using those patterns, we've all learned the more important lesson of the techniques they teach. The Hollow Fleye method, a new way of creating a wide-bodied baitfish with open collars of bucktail, applies to all kinds of patterns, from bunker imitations to poppers and squid patterns. Again, it's devilishly simple—just tying the bucktail in the "wrong way" and posting it backward around the shank—but it solves a problem and creates an option that no prior fly ever offered us, and you can see its influence on every beach and all over the Internet. There are lots of other examples: Bob's "squeeze and release" method of attaching bucktail 360 degrees around the hook shank, and the ingenious Spread Fleye method of creating a tall but thin profile with a small application of epoxy (or more recently Tuffleye) are two of my favorites.

Beyond the actual techniques, Bob's discussion and understanding of the mechanics of fly design have invaded my own tying. He can explain why broad shoulders on a mullet imitation help suspend the fly in the water column, or how critical a hook's weight and dimensions are to how a fly swims. He stresses how a bulky head followed by a long wispy tail—best illustrated by his BULKhead Deceiver—creates current lines that make the tail kick like a real baitfish. These mechanics are basic physical principles, built into lots of fly patterns. But Bob has crystallized them for me and for others, and helped us understand them in ways that let us implement them in our own patterns.

And yet more compelling than all these patterns and techniques is Bob's power of observation and gentle

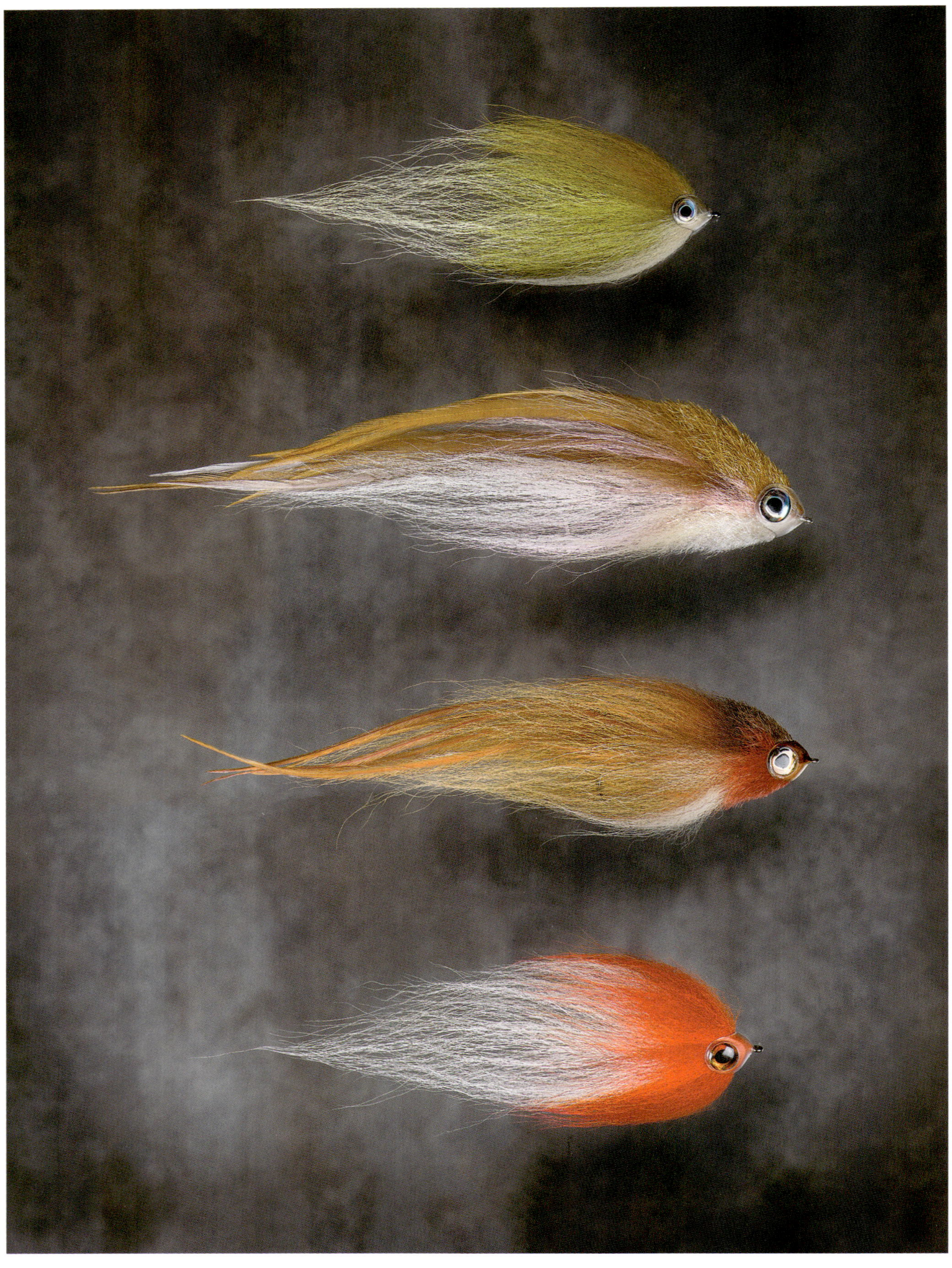

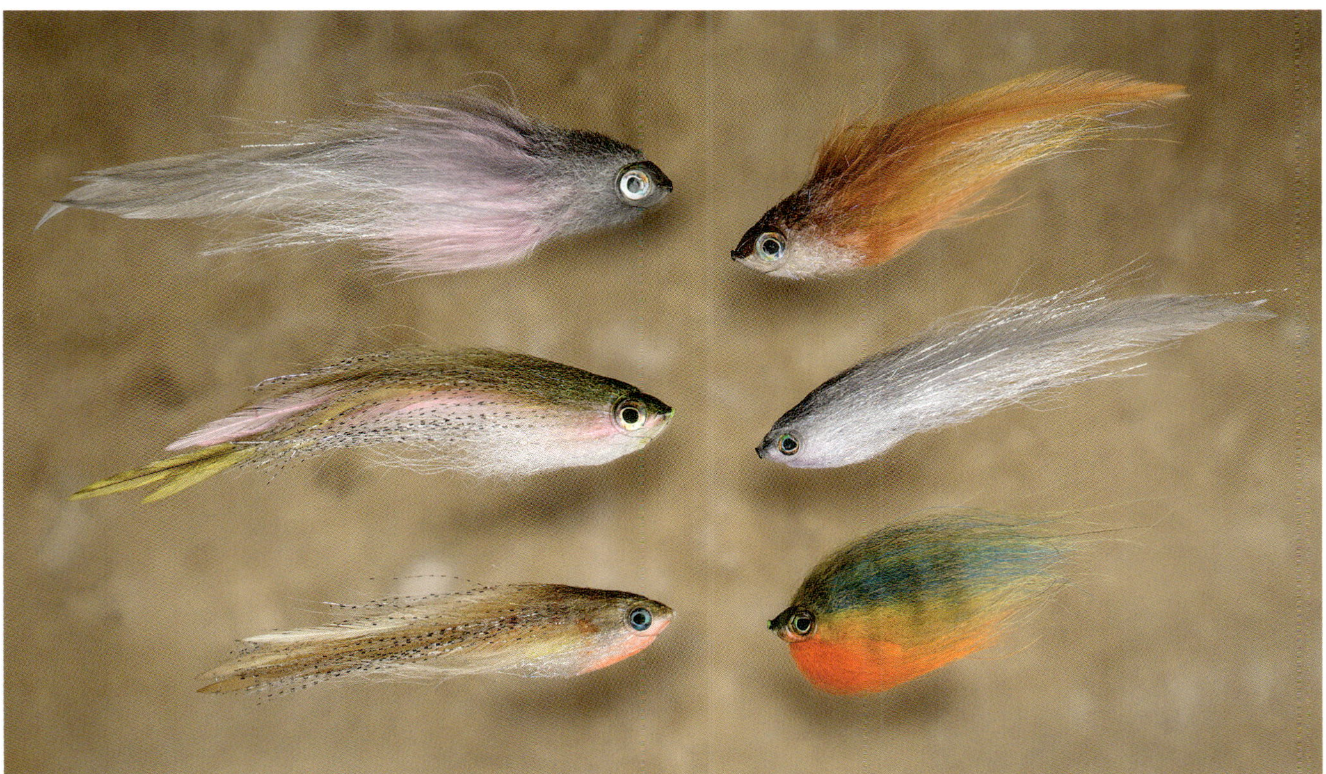

Tube flies offer real functional advantages for baitfish patterns. With a system like the Pro Sportfisher components, you can weight the fly at different points along its length, tie the fly to ride hook point up to make it weedless, and use any of a number of heads to reverse the materials back on themselves Hollow-Fleye-style. From top to bottom: Mullet Kinky Muddler tube, Rainbow Trout Hoo Fly tube, Brown Trout Hoo Fly tube (left column); Sucker Kinky Muddler tube, Finger Mullet Hoo Fly tube, and Bluegill Fox Hollow Fly tube.

nudging for us to be more observant on the water. With his slides and stockpile of photos and videos, he'll get you to see that a bunker is not a symmetrical oval, but that it has a gently sloping back and a deep, V-shaped belly, and it wiggles in its tail area most. He'll show you that a slender sand eel on the flats is different, because its belly is opaque, but its back is translucent—the opposite of a spearing. As Bob likes to point out, the transition from the darker back of a baitfish to its lighter belly isn't stark, because "things don't stick out like a sore thumb" in nature. I know Bob has studied these things scrupulously for decades, because I've seen his endless stock of videos that illustrate what most of us just ignore. His patterns capture that essence of the profile and movement of real baits in simple and essential ways, and they encourage us to scrutinize what we see a little more closely and objectively.

But maybe more important than all these other contributions and influences is his philosophy about the legacy of sharing and camaraderie of fly fishing and fly tying. When I first tentatively approached Bob at the end of a long weekend at a consumer trade show, he greeted me warmly and pawed attentively through my box of patterns, admiring what I'd done well, and, later, suggesting areas for improvement. Mine was probably the ten-thousandth box of patterns foisted on him that day. There was no sense of ego or inaccessibility, but rather an openness to anyone of any experience or skill level who wanted to talk tying or fishing. I've seen him approach every fan or fellow enthusiast the same way.

Previous page: The Hollow Fleye style of reversing bucktail makes a great wide-profile body for any baitfish, whether for pike or stripers. The middle flies pictured have Hollow bodies with heads tied Kinky Muddler style on an articulated shank. The top and bottom flies are Hollow Fleyes with a front collar of fox fur reversed with a Pro Sportfisher Soft Head. From top to bottom, Bunker Hollow Fleye veiled with Fox Fur, Articulated Bunker Kinky Muddler Hollow Fleye hybrid, Articulated Pike Kinky Muddler/Hollow Fleye hybrid, Pike Attractor Hollow Fleye veiled with Fox Fur.

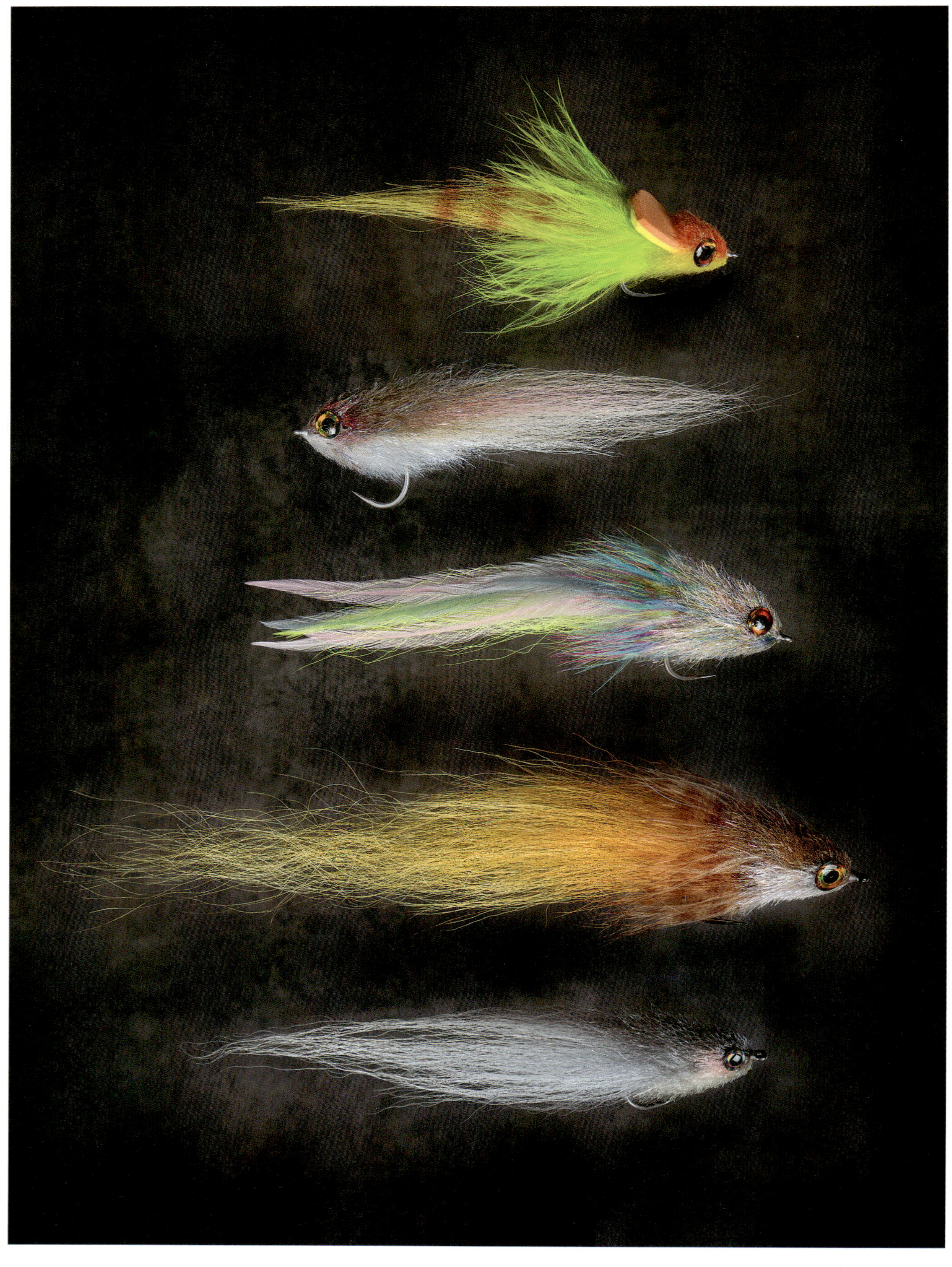

His philosophy is to share and encourage and show you that you too can do it.

And when, with his encouragement, I started to publish articles and tie publicly at the various trade shows and exhibitions, Bob admonished me that those more public displays were "not about you" or "showing off your skills," but about teaching others and proving to them that they too can enter this sport and create their own designs. It turns out that saltwater tying's greatest expert and innovator is also its most democratic, accessible, and inclusive advocate. It is that philosophy of collaboration and sharing that is Bob's greatest influence, both on me and on the general fly-fishing community.

Baitfish: Profiles in Three Dimensions

How do you imitate a baitfish? Each has its own dimensions—shape and profile, taper and heft—that mark the species and identify it to predators. Historically, even some of the greatest streamer flies were unlikely replicas of real fish food. The venerable Mickey Finn and Black-Nosed Dace, like many traditionally styled streamers, sport "wings" of bucktail, but baitfish don't have wings or backs that swim independently from their bodies. The mighty Muddler Minnow looks nothing like its namesake; its bulky head is separated from the body and wing by a valley that appears nowhere on a sculpin. The first streamer I ever encountered that reflected the shape of a real baitfish was Lefty's Deceiver, with its 360-degree collar of bucktail. Catching my first striper on a blue and white Deceiver in the 1980s began a quest for that perfect profile.

Bob's fleyes have dimension like no others. When Bob and I took one of his original "Beast" Hollow Fleyes for a swim at Island Beach State Park, it was the first fly I'd ever seen that captured the real presence and motion of an adult bunker; everything else I'd seen looked lifeless and anemic. A dark purple Bucktail Deceiver kicking around the back of Bob's van was equally startling. It actually lay in my hand with the heft and profile of a real baitfish, with the bucktail applied to give it broad shoulders and a thinly tapered tail akin to a real mullet.

A number of Bob's multidimensional fleyes have been particularly influential on me. In messing with Bob's 3D style of tying a number of years ago, I over-trimmed some Kinky Fibre, only to learn that the effect was akin to spun deer hair. Knowing I'd seen a similar effect elsewhere, I flipped through *Pop Fleyes* and found my reference—a little squid 3D Fleye with Super Hair producing the same rounded, fuzzy effect. As I played with the results, I refined the technique to apply the synthetic hair in a series of V-shaped ties on the top and bottom of the shank, straddling the shank on both sides, and then trimmed the fibers to shape. That method, unlike the typical Hi-Tie, distributes material both up and down and side to side, creating the kind of three-dimensionality I'd learned from Bob's patterns. Better yet, because the hair isn't really "spun" perpendicular to the hook shank like deer hair, but rather layered back on itself at a 45-degree angle, it blends seamlessly with the tail to create an uninterrupted baitfish profile and smooth transition from head to tail.

True to another of the design principles Bob and I had discussed, I also knew that I needed a soft, tapered tail to complete the baitfish profile and exploit the benefits of the dense synthetic at the front of the fly. Combining the "spun" Kinky Fibre head with a tail of bucktail, feathers, or even simple Craft Fur or fox fur, resulted in a fly that swims just like a baitfish. Water washing over the 3D head as it swims through current is diverted into all kinds of minicurrents and turbulence that make the tail materials wiggle and kick just like a real baitfish. A simple Bucktail Deceiver with the densely packed synthetic head is one of my favorite variations for a midsize imitation, while a Hollow Fleye version works great for deep-bodied baits.

I call the fly a "Kinky Muddler" because it has the bulky head of a Muddler made out of Kinky Fibre. It lends itself equally to a fat-headed mullet, a tall-but-thin bunker, a snaky eel, or any of a number of shapes and profiles used in backcountry, freshwater, or attractor patterns. The Kinky Muddler has taken stripers, blues, and albies in the Northeast; tarpon, snook, and redfish in the tropics; and golden dorado, trout, bass, peacocks, and pike in fresh water.

The Siliclone was yet another of Bob's innovations in creating a three-dimensional fly. The mullet version pictured head-on in the original *Pop Fleyes* fascinated me both for its uncanny resemblance to the real article

Previous page: The Kinky Muddler head technique works for all styles of baitfish. The top warmwater fly uses a collar of foam that makes the fly float and dive. The second and last flies are tied to imitate the profiles and colors of a bunker and mullet. And the third and fourth are attractor patterns that could work for stripers, roosterfish, pike, or virtually any other predator. From top to bottom: Kinky Muddler Diver, Bunker Kinky Muddler, Rainbow Kinky Muddler, Pike Kinky Muddler, and Mullet Kinky Muddler.

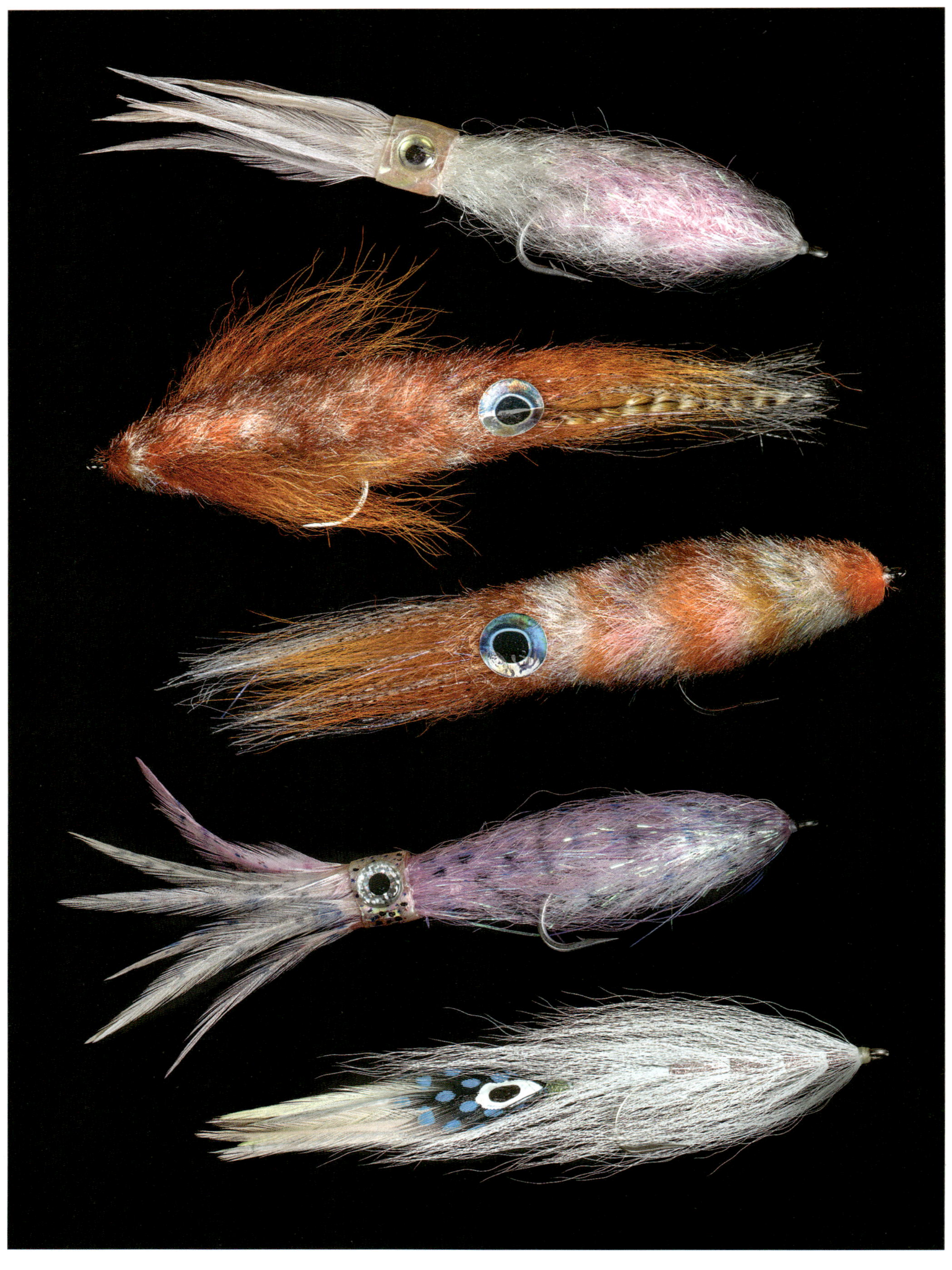

and for its unorthodox combination of trimmed fleece and flexible silicone coating. I've found flies with coated heads, inspired by the Siliclone, to be some of the simplest and most efficient ways to create a convincing baitfish profile. I've coated everything from fox fur and bucktail to synthetic hair, with glues of all kinds, but my favorite variation is called the Hoo Fly. It has been my most effective small baitfish fly over the past five years, yielding plenty of good-size stripers and albies.

The Hoo Fly uses a chopped synthetic yarn called Senyo's Laser Dub covered with a thin and flexible skim coat of Liquid Fusion, a urethane glue. The key is to tie in the Laser Dub with V-ties, as described above, and then comb it carefully to align the fibers before fixing its shape with Liquid Fusion. Instead of trimming, you effectively paint the soft Laser Dub into the desired profile by brushing its surface with the Liquid Fusion. It easily conforms to any profile you coax out of it. The coated head veils the tail material—usually Craft Fur, bucktail, or feathers—and becomes wonderfully translucent when it hits the water.

If the Kinky Muddler is my primary big bait imitation, the Hoo Fly is my small fly staple, best suited to bay anchovies, sand eels, spearing, finger mullet, baby bunker, butterfish, and freshwater minnows and juvenile trout and bass. Ultimately, both flies descend directly from Pop Fleyes. They represent my effort to use all Bob has taught me about profile, fly mechanics, and material choice in creating my own flies and solutions for the situations I encounter on the water.

Squid

Shortly after I met him, I presumptuously sent Bob some photos of squid patterns I had been tinkering with, and his response ignited years of correspondence about squid, both real and artificial. We started with the living creatures themselves—their anatomy, manner of movement, and kaleidoscopic coloration. So many squid patterns bear the wrong proportions, with excessively long tentacles and a too-short body or mantle. Squid also move freely backward and forward, but as Bob again pointed out, they will jet with their mantle forward when fleeing from a hungry striper, and it is primarily their tentacles that move and squirm, with the body remaining fairly rigid. After years of dialogue, Bob even sent me a National Geographic VHS about squid—we share that level of obsession.

My first squid flies (and still among my favorites) drew directly from Bob's patterns, with the head and tail assembly of saddles and eyes on an extension of heavy mono or narrow tubing off the hook shank. Bob's various bucktail techniques make for effective but very different bodies. A Hollow Fleye squid is open and translucent, and sinks quickly, whereas a Bucktail or BULKhead Deceiver version is denser and hovers higher in the water column. My favorite eyes for these all-natural squid are cheeks of Guinea feathers marked with fabric paint. You can see those eyes from 70 feet away!

Bob's Rear Floating Squid provided the impetus for a different style of cephalopod imitation. One of the least realistic attributes of most squid patterns is the means by which the head, eyes, and tentacles are all pinned to a single tie-in point, sandwiching the tentacles unnaturally. On a real squid, the head is a broad cylinder, with the eyes set wide apart and the tentacles distributed around a semicircle. The only technique I've ever seen for copying that layout appears on a few of Bob's patterns, such as his offshore Bangers or Rear Floating Squid, where saddles are glued around the circumference of a foam cylinder.

Adapting that template for a sinking fly, I attach saddles around a ring of flexible adhesive sheeting, like Sili Skin or Crystal Skin, and then slide the ring onto the end of a body of synthetic hair tied Hollow-style. In between collars of the synthetic, I wrap any of the flashy hackle materials, such as Palmer Chenille, Estaz, or Polar Chenille, to give the mantle an interior glow like Bob's "inner flash" technique. The Emergent Sparkle Squid (named after Gary LaFontaine's famous Emergent Sparkle Pupa) has a translucent "bubble" of a body trailed by a cylindrical head with open, flowing tentacles.

More recently, I've adapted the Kinky Muddler method to squid bodies, yielding a denser overall construction but the same widely spread eyes and free-flowing tentacles, usually of fox fur. My squid flies, like the baitfish imitations, are always evolving based on experience on the water, inspiration from Bob and others, and new materials. I figure that if Bob can still tweak, perfect, and refine his already stellar designs after so many years, the rest of us should do the same.

Previous page: The key to any squid fly is combining the right proportions with movement in the right place. You need a cylindrical body for about $^2/_3$ the length of the fly, followed by a prominent eye and mobile tentacles. These principles govern whatever style you tie; here synthetic and natural materials are combined in each fly for optimum profile and movement. From top to bottom: Emergent Sparkle Squid, Winged Kinky Muddler Squid, Kinky Muddler Squid, Emergent Sparkle Squid, and Hollow Fleye Squid.

Chapter 18

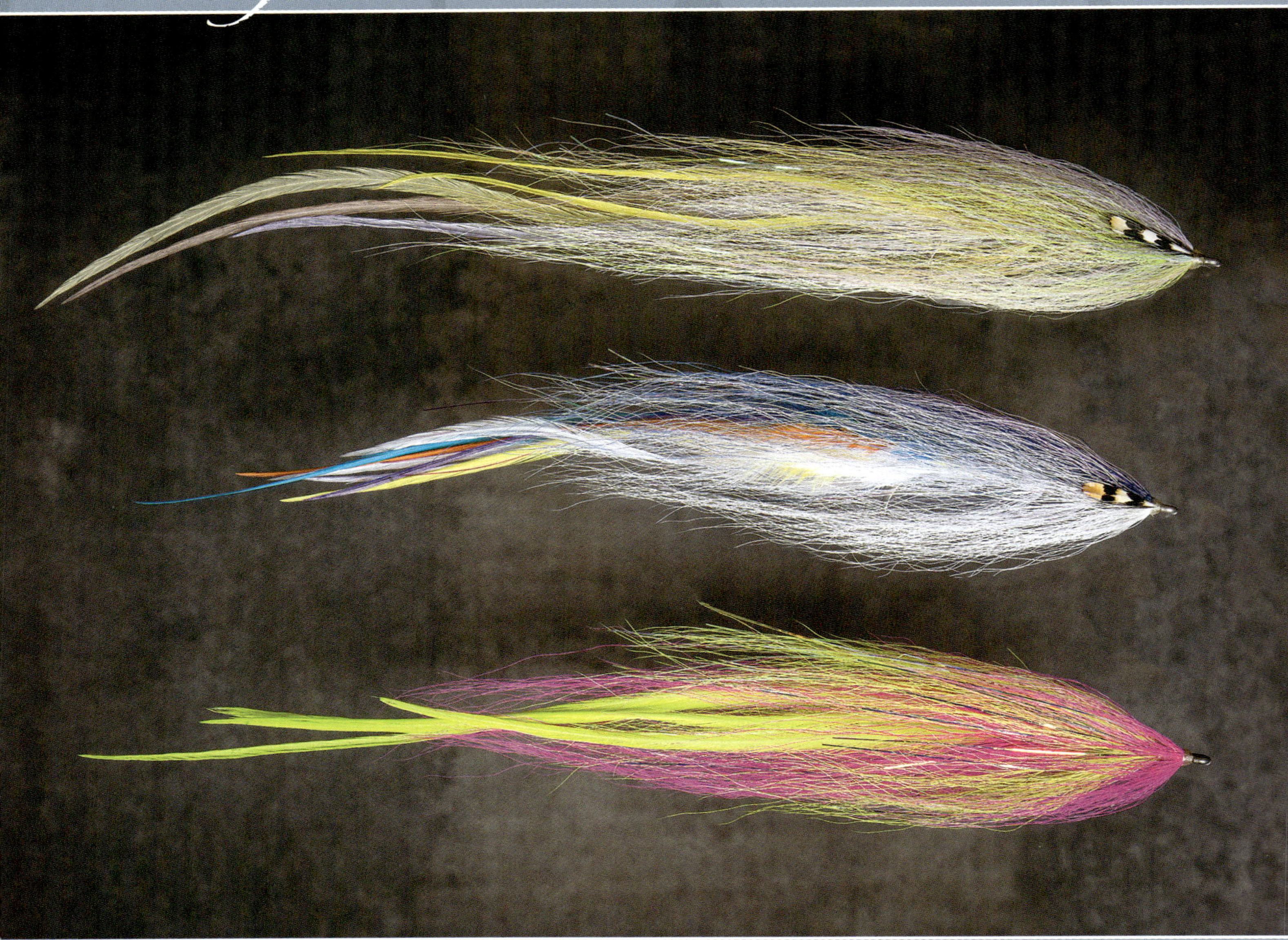

Three very early (2002–2003) Hollow Semper Fleyes. "I didn't have extremely long bucktail then," says Farrar. "So I would compensate by using longer hackle. Combining Popovics's Semper and Hollow techniques gave me the proper profile and symmetry."

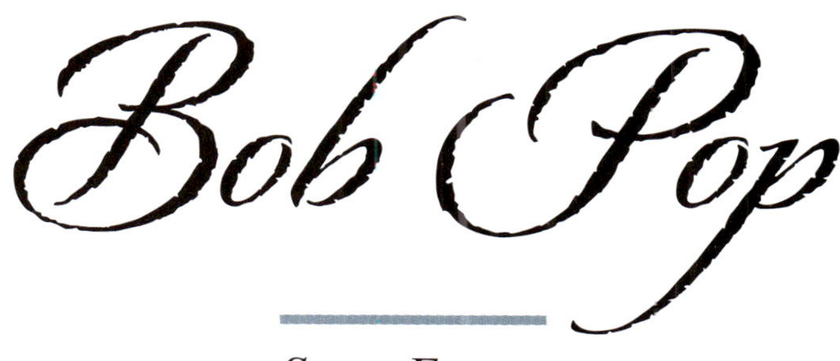

Bob Pop

Steve Farrar

Lefty calls Bob the most innovative fly tier he's ever known. I call Bob friend, mentor, and master fly innovator. All who know Bob agree that he has special talent when it comes to fly tying, fly design, and sharing and educating. His techniques are well thought out, with simplicity and durability always at the forefront. Bob's fleye design has only one goal—to catch fish. Bob is one of the best at combining observation, technique, and critical analysis to achieve the overall look and movement of a given baitfish.

I first met Bob after joining the Atlantic Saltwater Flyrodders (www.aswf.info) in 1999. As time passed, I started to pick up additional techniques from Bob and apply them to my fly tying. They were like adding new precision tools to a toolbox, each one with a specific purpose to be selected and used at the opportune time either alone or in combination with other tools. Over time, as we exchanged ideas on tying, our friendship grew. My earliest published work had tremendous influence from Bob's techniques and designs. I am thankful for that friendship and for Bob's critical thinking, which just makes tying better and better.

Patterns

My favorite technique of Bob's is the Hollow tie. It's effective in a long list of patterns. It can be tied sparse, bulky, open, closed, with naturals, with synthetics, long, short, and so on and so on. The technique is difficult to master but leads to an incredible range of material or hair control. I use it predominantly in two applications: first, in the Hollow Semper Fleye (a combination of two of Bob's fleyes) and second, as a concluding tie in any fly where I want total beak elimination in a symmetrically round or oval head. It enables me to craft a head where the only thread visible is a few wraps at the hook eye—visually pleasing while providing a realistic profile.

Spearing, Bay Anchovy, and Sand Eel

We've always had a reasonable number of spearing in our local waters. Their numbers appear to be sufficient and rather constant as a norm—a good bait to replicate and count on as forage for predators. Since spearing run in schools of varying size, you could tie just one size and be certain it would match at least some of a given school, as long as the fly wasn't radically small or large.

Bay anchovies and sand eels on the other hand have undergone a more dramatic variation in their numbers. Not more than ten years ago, the numbers of these baits that you could see from the beach seemed almost nonexistent except for certain times of the year. Since then, their numbers seemed to increase each year. Now they appear in greater numbers and for longer periods when I can count on them as a readily available food source.

Both appear in juvenile and fully mature sizes, traveling in schools of like-size fish. The bottom line is they've been added to my fly arsenal on a more regular basis. The two patterns I rely on most for these imitations are my Sili Skin and MV Baitfish versions. Both are easy to craft, don't foul, and use synthetics and perhaps a single hackle on some. In particular, I like to use a blend of Angel Hair and Unique Hair or Super Hair. The Sili Skin versions make use of Sili Skin (invented by Blane Chocklett and Harrison Steeves) and EZ Body or a similar braid.

Mullet

Of all the baits I enjoy observing in the surf, mullet are my favorite. Although present in our estuaries and bays in spring and summer, it's in the fall during the September full and new moons when they school up and move to the ocean. This is the start of their migration south in groups of several hundred, typically within a fly cast of the beach. Once these baitfish are discovered by bluefish and striped bass, a highly visual game of cat and mouse begins. Mullet typically range in size from the length of a finger (hence the term "finger mullet") to almost a foot. For these patterns, I use Simple-Simple Clones (a variation of Popovics's Simple Clone fleye), a modified Hi-Tie with more hi-ties on the side to achieve thickness, or a version of the MV Baitfish, again with more hi-ties on the side. All are tied with a synthetic blend of Slinky Fibre and Angel Hair, sold as Steve Farrar Flash Blend from Fishient Group.

You can make a synthetic-based mullet more buoyant by injecting thinned Plasti Dip in many random areas from the hook eye to just behind the hook bend. This also beefs up the durability of the pattern and helps to further prevent fouling.

Peanut Bunker

The peanut bunker was almost nonexistent along New Jersey beaches in the fall of 2008—in sharp contrast to years prior. But when the peanuts are present during the run, they are one of my favorite fish to imitate. I tie them varying in size from 3 to 6 inches in length. I also use varying tying methods to replicate them. The version I use most often is the simple Hi-Tie using a blend of Slinky Fibre and Angel Hair. When using a full-length

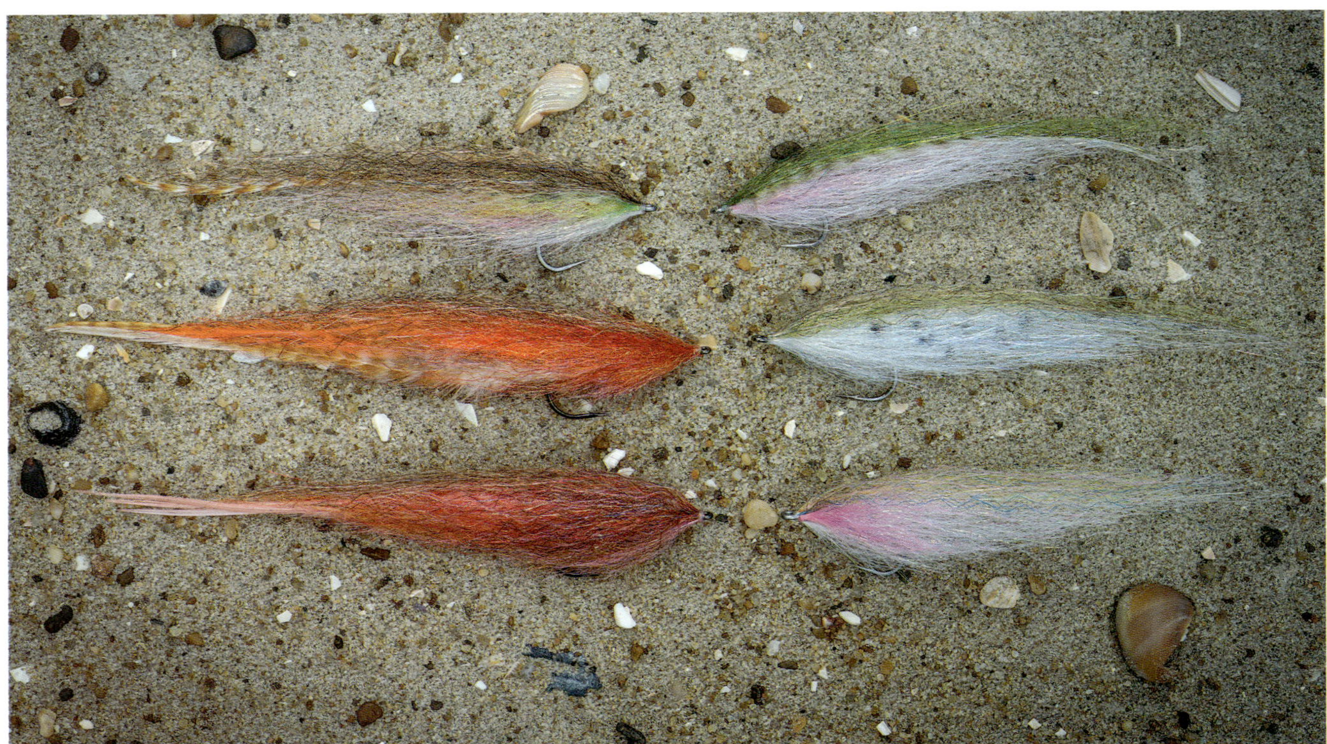

A selection of flies tied MV Baitfish–style using Steve Farrar's SF Flash Blend and natural hackle. From top to bottom, column one imitates a generic baitfish and two variations for squid. Column two imitates generic baitfish, peanut bunker, and mullet. These flies are quick to tie, nonfouling, and durable. I have observed no advantage to adding eyes fishing my local waters.

blended mixture, these will be in the 5- to 6-inch range with size 6 molded epoxy eyes secured in place with Plasti Dip. All the thread wraps are beneath the eyes and also encased in Plasti Dip. It makes for an extremely durable and lifelike pattern. I'll comb and retrim a fly after using it several times. One tip on fishing this fly: when you can't seem to get a hit, especially when the bait is thick, try casting into the middle of the bait and, without stripping, just let the fly sink and flutter to the bottom perhaps with nothing more than a seductive twitch. I've had several occurrences where stripers will take the fly either as it's on its way down or even on the bottom.

Blending Flash with Synthetic Material

Whether it be naturals or synthetics, using good quality material in your fly tying will make a significant difference. Using materials of similar length and thickness, especially when using different materials, can add to the look of a fly. Over the years, I've found blending flash with synthetics gives a more natural and appealing look to many patterns as opposed to layering flash between synthetic ties. However, blending synthetic with flash at each tying step can become tedious and time-consuming at best. I've found that blending larger quantities ahead of time and storing the blend in a way that's easy to use can make tying more enjoyable and certainly speed it up. I refer to this process as "flash blending," and I make use of it for several types of material. Again, an important key is to blend material and flash of similar length and thickness.

The one I use most is a blend of Angel Hair and Slinky Fibre. The Slinky Fibre is consistent in thickness. However, the Angel Hair can be too thin and brittle in some colors, so I don't use those. In the past, I would tie certain flies with Angel Hair alone, but the flash would easily tear and durability suffered. It was also too difficult to achieve any level of bulk or thickness in the pattern. Blending the Slinky Fibre with Angel Hair adds tremendous durability, and the distributed flash provides a distinct look. Varying the ratio of flash to fiber is up to personal preference. I use a blending ratio of up to three packs of flash to one pack of Slinky Fibre but more commonly one to one and even less if I'm tying flies where I want the flash to be more subtle.

Although I use Slinky Fibre and Angel Hair most, there are other blended versions I've used in my tying. The key is to make sure you blend flash and fiber of a similar length and thickness. I use Unique Hair or Super Hair blended with Angel Hair for many of my thin-profile bait patterns that imitate spearing, bay anchovy, and sand eels. For the largest patterns, I'll blend a thicker and longer flash like Dave Skok's Mega Mushy with Yak Hair or Bozo Hair. The combinations are many and, again, up to personal preference, but the technique remains the same.

Whether you've blended it yourself or purchased it, the blend should be loose in a plastic sleeve with the ends feathered. This feathering is important, as it provides a more natural look when tied into a fly. The feathering is a natural side effect of the blending process, resulting in the ends having a random-length appearance.

When tying the blend into a pattern, I'll make a few wraps to secure it, then fold the length in my hand over what's on the hook shank. I always want the piece folded over to be either longer or shorter (depending on the pattern). If I need the piece folded over to be trimmed, I'll do that trimming while it's still being held, and I'll make sure to trim it at an angle front to back. On a pattern such as the MV Baitfish, tying the fibers in at their midpoint and then folding and trimming them in this manner allows each tie to create volume and support subsequent ties. The amount of material used for each tie will determine profile and bulk. Additional side, top, and bottom tie-in points may be used approaching the eye to create bulk such as in a mullet pattern. Finally the securing glue (I use thinned Plasti Dip) is injected liberally along the shank and then randomly inside the pattern from the eye to behind the bend.

For patterns that are more vertical in profile, like peanut bunker, the lengths are tied mostly at the top and bottom with few or none tied to the sides of the shank. For patterns where I want a round or oval profile (when looking head-on at the fly), I tie more lengths on the sides of the shank.

When I want either the width or height of a pattern to be exaggerated, I make sure each tie is as close as possible to the previous one so that it flares, or kicks out, more than normal. I also make sure I use as few wraps as possible on the folded-over portion, and I make sure those wraps are at the very end of the fold.

In any pattern, long lengths of material on the outer profile will tend to foul more than those inside. One way I deal with this is to build the length of a pattern closer to the inside of the pattern—that is, to tie the longer lengths in first, then to tie in shorter and shorter lengths as the pattern progresses toward the hook eye. Another option is to use a material with greater stiffness or to create that stiffness with glue, epoxy, or heavy mono when you want longer materials on the outside profile of the fly.

BLENDING TECHNIQUE

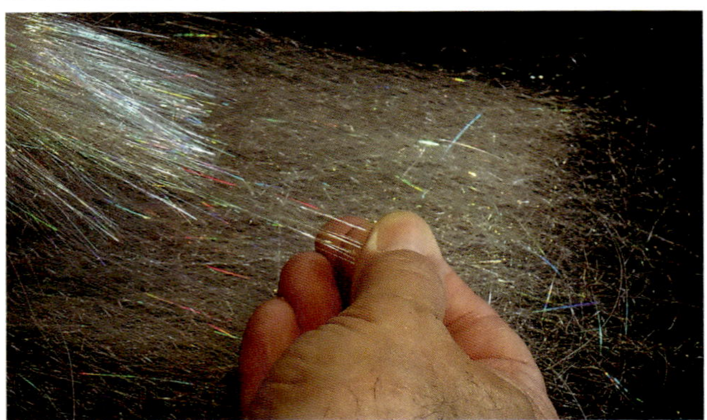

1. For this blend we will use a 1:1 ratio of one pack of Angel Hair to one pack of Slinky Fibre. The blend is up to you. Cut the Slinky Fibre away from the tie, and then cut to the same length as the Angel Hair. Strip a thin layer of Slinky Fibre onto your work area, and then strip a thin layer of Angel Hair on top of it.

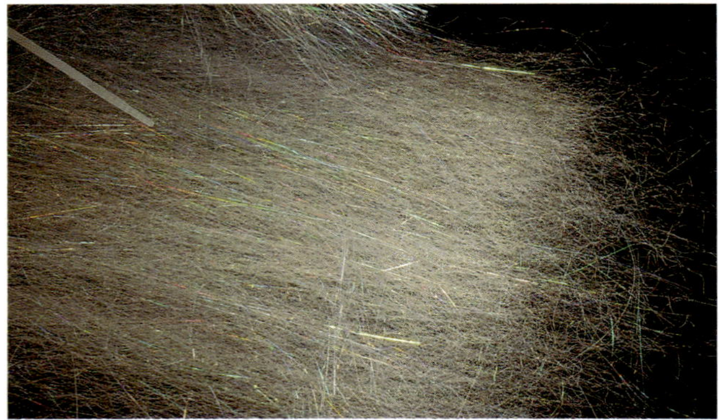

2. Continue alternating layers until the Slinky Fibre and Angel Hair is used up. Thin layers produce better results.

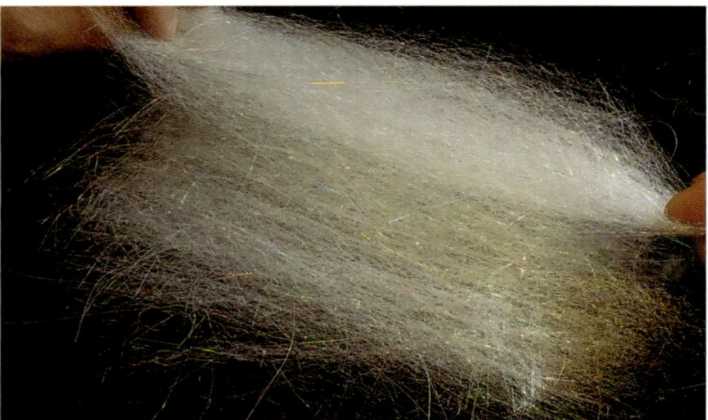

3. Roll up the resulting blend. Hold it in one hand while stripping it back onto the work surface with the other a little at a time. Continue this process until the two materials look like one.

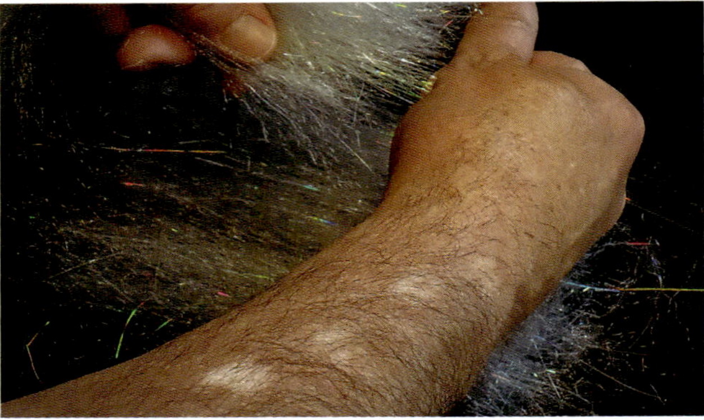

4. Strip thin layers of the resulting blend onto your work area. The thinner the layers that are created in step 1, the fewer times you'll have to repeat the blending process.

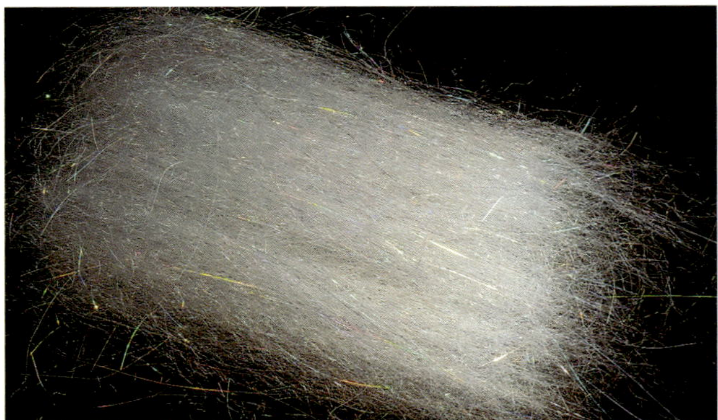

5. Repeat until thoroughly blended.

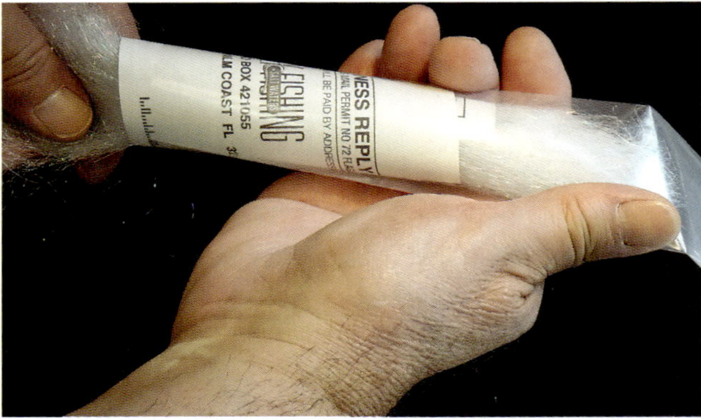

6. Get a postcard from one of your magazines. Roll the postcard around the blend and use it as a funnel to slide it into a large plastic sleeve.

Blended packets (yours and that sold prepackaged by Just Add H2O) store conveniently in a clear plastic utility container, such as the Plano 3700 plastic storage box. When using the blend, I strongly advise leaving it in the sleeve and just tapping so about an inch is hanging out. It's then easy to pull out just enough for one tying step.

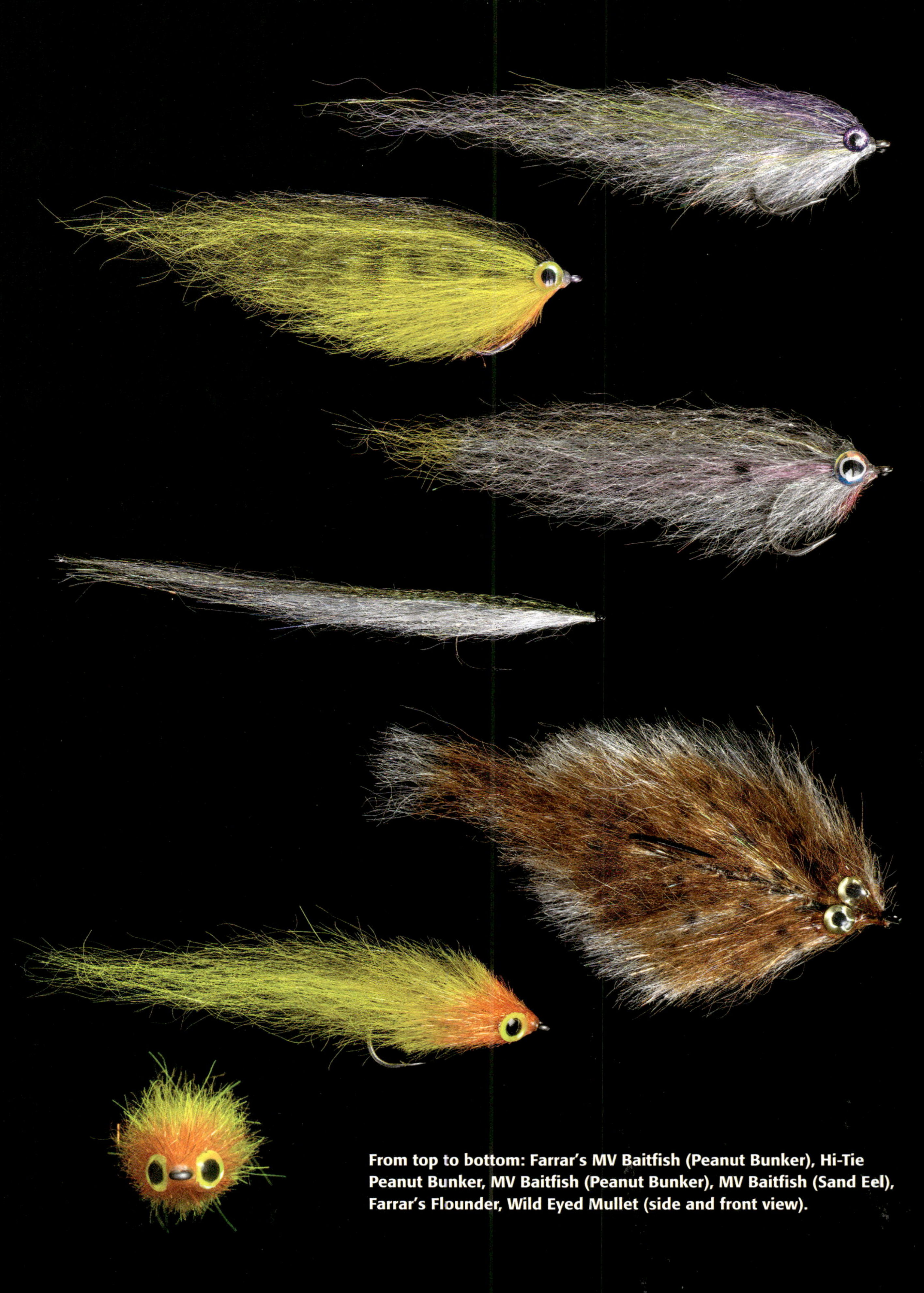

From top to bottom: Farrar's MV Baitfish (Peanut Bunker), Hi-Tie Peanut Bunker, MV Baitfish (Peanut Bunker), MV Baitfish (Sand Eel), Farrar's Flounder, Wild Eyed Mullet (side and front view).

Chapter 19

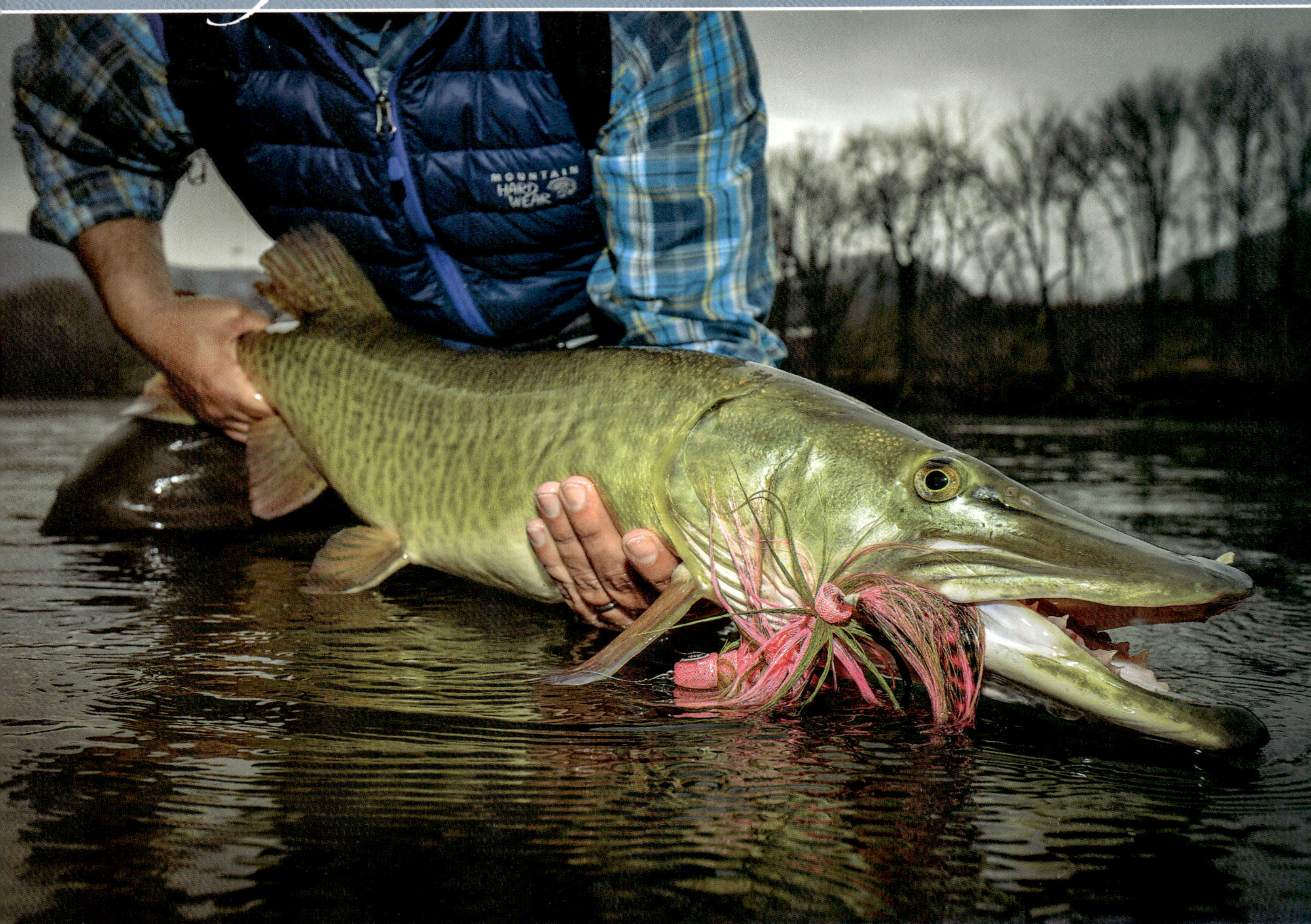

This James River, Virginia, muskie took a T-Bone, which borrows heavily from the Popovics style of tying bucktail in reverse to create bulk. Using his techniques and applying them to different design ideas has truly revolutionized muskie fishing on the fly.

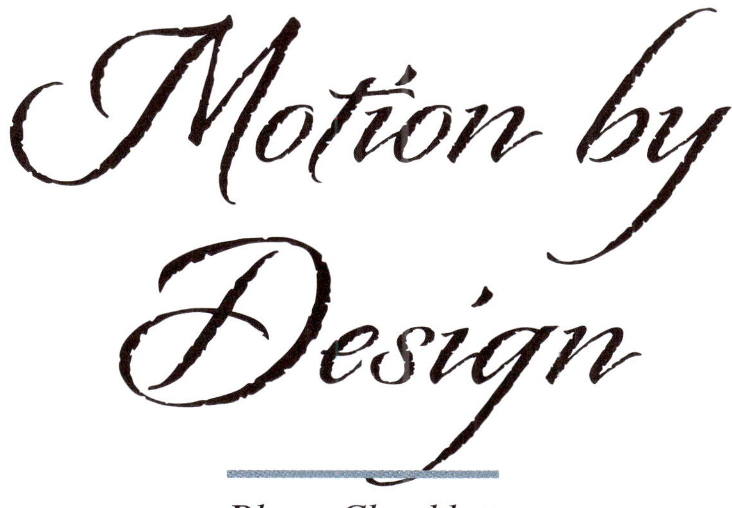

Motion by Design

Blane Chocklett

Two of Bob's greatest gifts to fly tiers and fishermen have been his Hollow and BULKhead styles of tying. These techniques of reversing bucktail to give the illusion of mass without adding bulk or weight have, in my opinion, changed the pursuit of large predatory fish with a fly forever and have helped carve my success in the pursuit of muskie on the fly.

Muskie are some of the hardest fish to catch on any type of rod and reel. Muskie are attracted to underwater vibrations and do a lot of hunting based on feel before they pick up the prey by sight. Adding the reversed bucktail technique helped give my flies more of a presence underwater by adding mass and pushing more water.

Another key factor in getting muskie to attack flies is a side-to-side motion. By this, I mean that predatory fish with teeth, such as muskie, are programmed to attack their prey by grabbing them. The teeth help them hold on to a prey item as well as slice and maim it. One of the best ways for muskie to grab their prey is from the side, and a fly that constantly turns in the water will show its side profile to predatory muskie. In my opinion, this causes a natural trigger that muskie can't easily turn off.

My T-Bone fly has these key characteristics built into it. The T-Bone has a series of linked shanks, called articulated fish spines, and spreaders that prop up the bucktail for the illusion of mass. The head on the fly can either be Bob's BULKhead or a head made out of Flex Cord. Either way the head needs to have mass to push water. The head design causes water to be deflected out from the body causing the fibers behind to swim. This chain reaction helps add in the side-to-side motion, which is accentuated by the articulated shanks.

The Flex Cord spreader dams are my version of Bob's reverse style. I spin the bucktail in front of the spreaders, and then work forward and add another spreader. The way I make the dams is by taking a 1 1/2" x 1/4" Flex Cord and burning both ends. Then, I slide one end over the shank or hook. After that, I reverse the entire cord over itself. I push it forward again, and tie the other end directly over the end I tied in previously. Finally, I push the cord back over itself, hiding the thread wraps from the fishes' teeth and creating a cone shape for the bucktail to rest against.

Using this technique moving forward on the fly allows you to change the angle of the bucktail by adjusting how far back the next Flex Cord dam pushes back over the hair. The more the cord pushes back over the hair, the lower the profile; the less the cord touches the hair, the more the hair will stand up. Working forward on the fly adding spreaders and shanks causes the fly to be articulated. It also helps in the T-Bone's swimming action, which is where the fly gets its name from.

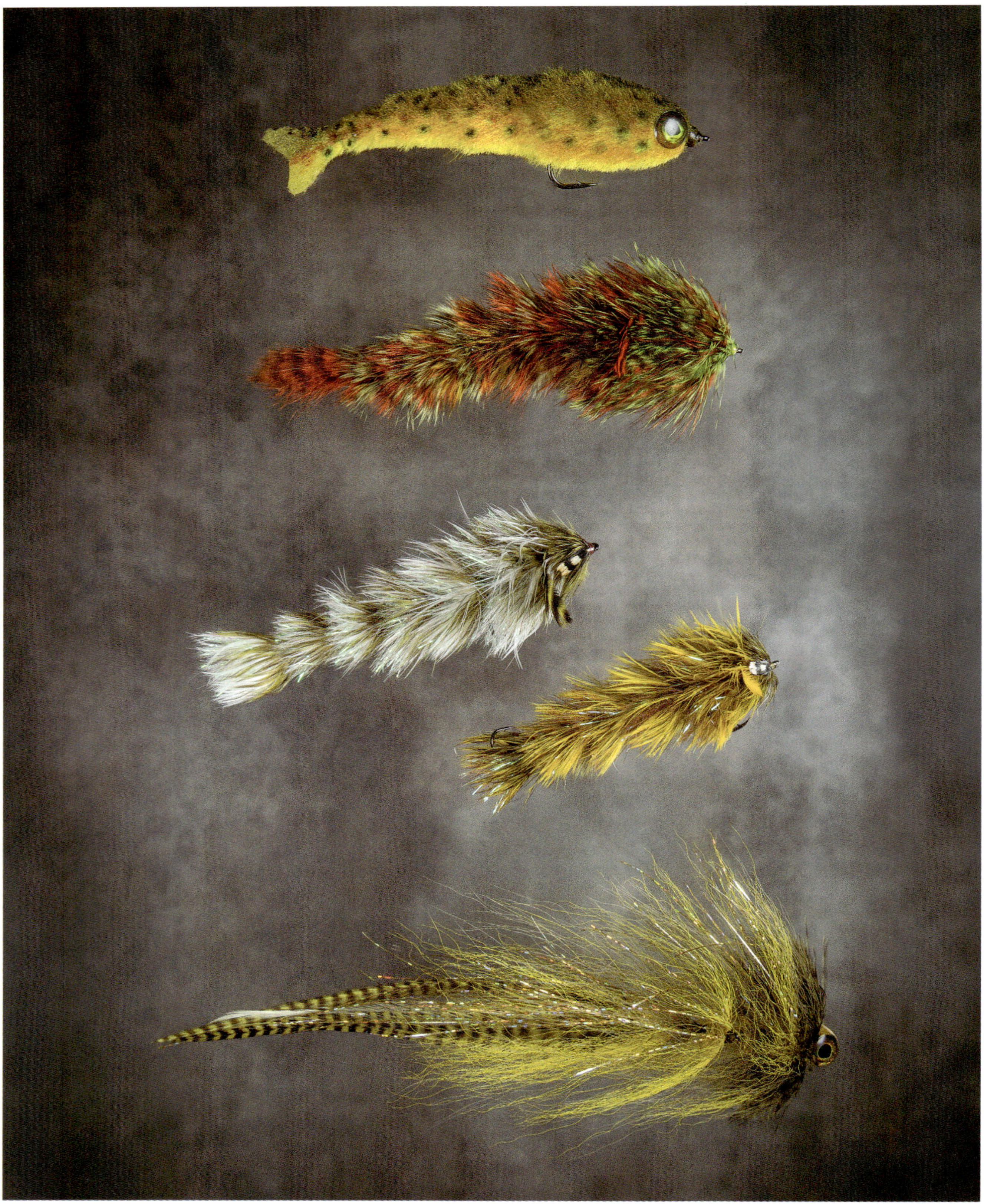

The Feathered Game Changer is more of a technique than a specific pattern. You can tie this fly in many sizes, shapes, and color schemes to catch a wide variety of fish. To date, the Feathered Game Changer has taken trout in both fresh and salt water, snook, tarpon, both large- and smallmouth bass, and stripers to name a few. From top to bottom: Brown Trout Game Changer, Feathered Game Changers (Fire Tiger, Rainbow, Baby Brown), and a Baby T-Bone.

Feathered Game Changer

One of many things I've learned from Bob over the course of my tying career is that a new pattern usually evolves from a problem. This problem could be lack of movement, shape, size, durability, or weight. The Feathered Game Changer is a prime example of a pattern evolving and changing due to a need based on several of those components.

I developed the Game Changer series of flies after thinking long and hard about how fish swim. First, a fish is powered by its muscles. Second, they move and change direction with their fins, aided by their muscles. Third, and most important, all of their movement starts with the spine and the independently moving vertebrae. Stripping fly line provides the "muscle," and I knew I could place and manipulate material to fill the role of fins. But, I was stumped on the spine.

While articulated flies have been around for years, I was looking for something that would be faster and easier than tying on broken hook shanks. To really get what I wanted I needed a series of short connections of wire (vertebrae) to form a flexible backbone for my fly. Eventually I developed exactly what I needed with Flymen Fishing Company, and flies such as the T-Bone and original Game Changer (tied with synthetic fibers) were born.

The Feathered Game Changer came to be after a trip down in Arkansas on the White River. I'd noticed that a new variation of the Game Changer tied out of bucktail that I was fishing didn't sink quickly and was hard to cast. When I got home, I called Bob, we discussed the problem, and he told me to try feathers as a substitute for deer hair. This was based on his use of feathers in his Semper Fleye design. This palmered feather technique was exactly what I needed to solve my pattern's problem.

Taking Bob's advice, I sat down and created the Feathered Game Changer, using a series of connected metal shanks and palmered hen saddle and schlappen. The results of this new concept have paid huge dividends for me on the water since its inception. When designing the T-Bone and original Game Changers, I knew that it was critical to have a head on the fly that resisted water because the water needed something to push against to create a side-to-side swimming action. However, the webby feathers also create a barrier for water to push against that helps aid in the swimming action of this fly. Adding the feathers to the pattern also keeps the fly light for easier casting. This alone solved several problems I had with the original Game Changer and the bucktail version.

Since tying the first Feathered Game Changer, I have refined it more to save time on the vise. I now add palmer chenille and only use half as many feathers. Doing this saves material and tying time. To achieve the desired profile, I use the natural alignment of feathers on the hen saddle skin to achieve the desired taper. The feathers on the skins are smaller in length and width down at the base. If you choose the feathers at the base of the skin and work up toward the top of the skin, you can create a natural taper without having to cut any of the feathers.

Tying Notes

Original Game Changer (Brown Trout)

Form the tail with yellow Chocklett's Body Wrap (by Hareline) and Clear Cure Goo (CCG) Flex. Apply the Flex and smear it through the entire tail, creating a fan shape, and then cure it with the light. Trim the tail into a V shape after the fly is complete. In this fly, I use the 10-millimeter Fish-Spine (by Flymen) for the tail and first part of the body, then a 15-, 20-, and 25-millimeter, respectively. The last connection to the hook is 20- to 30-pound Berkley Nylon Coated Wire secured to the hook midshank. I then wrap back down the shank to the hook bend, slide the eye of the 25-millimeter shank through the wire, and fold the wire back over the top of the shank. The opening of the wire to the shank should only be the size of the eye of the 25-millimeter shank. Secure the remaining wire to the hook shank by wrapping forward to the hook eye.

As you tie in each section of the body, trim the yellow Chocklett's Body Wrap to size and at a slight upward angle, continuing to move forward from the tail to the head of the fly. The hook on this fly is a size 1/0 Gamakatsu B10S. The eyes are CCG Chameleon (size depends on fly size). Add a dab of CCG Flex to each side of the head, and then add the eyes. Next, cure the glue through the eyes with the CCG light. Then add a light coat of CCG Flex over and in front of the eyes. Cure with the light, add another coat of CCG Hydro, and then cure again.

Fire Tiger Feathered Game Changer

The tail is two grizzly orange Chickabou saddles (Metz) tied in at their butts on each side of a 10-millimeter shank. Follow that with one orange hen saddle (chosen from the base of the skin) tied in by the tip and wrapped

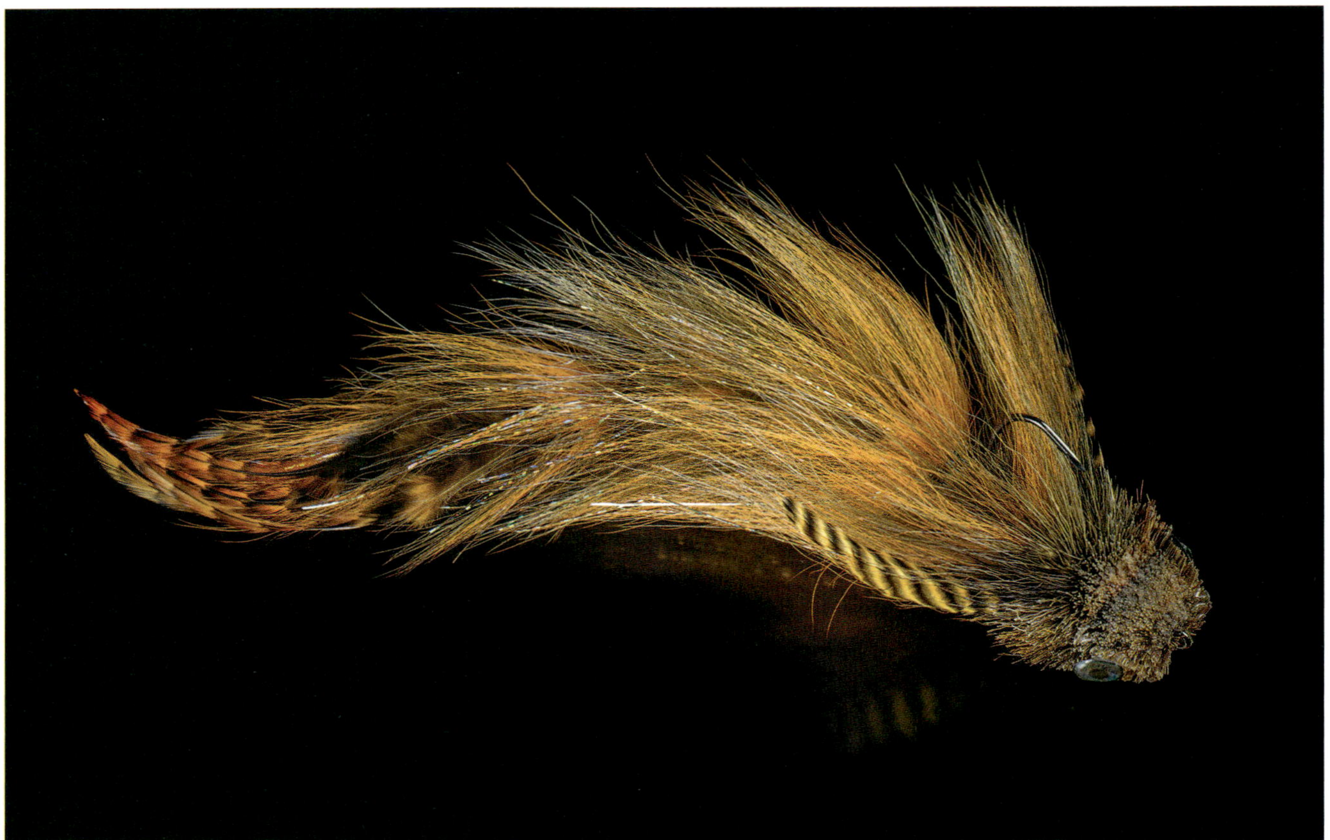

Bucktail Game Changer with a Tommy Lynch–style Drunk and Disorderly head. This fly, tied on a jig hook, has a remarkable action in the water.

forward in tight turns, and then a chartreuse hen saddle feather tied the same way.

The body consists of five 15-millimeter Fish-Spines. Each shank will have alternating Metz Magnum Hen Saddles tied in by the tips and wrapped forward. I select feathers from the base of the saddle and then move up the rows toward the top, choosing the appropriate feather for each spine. This tapering of feathers provides a perfect baitfish profile. I use as many hen saddles as needed to cover the shank, but each fly usually requires two to four per shank. The tighter you wrap the feathers on the head, the denser the forward portion of the fly, and the better movement it will have. The pectoral fins are two grizzly orange Magnum Hen Saddles taken from the bottom third of the skin. Tie the feathers in by the butts, concave side out, giving a good profile to the fly and adding to the swimming motion.

Rainbow Trout Feathered Game Changer

This fly is tied on four 15-millimeter shanks; the tail hook is size 6 Owner Mosquito. To form the tail, take three wraps of large pearl Cactus Hackle (by Hareline) and large Magnum Hen Saddle wrapped in by the tips side by side. Then pinch the material together, flatten the sides, and fan the flash and feathers out to form a fish tail shape. Once you are happy with the shape, apply CCG Hydro at the base of the materials and cure with the CCG light. Next, wrap a grizzly olive hen saddle feather from the bottom/base of the skin in front of the tail.

The body is large pearl Cactus Hackle (three turns), and white and olive hen saddles tied in by the tips and wrapped side by side, moving forward up the shanks. As with the other Feathered Game Changers, start with feathers from the base of the skin and work your way up as you tie the fly. The pectoral fins are two olive Magnum Hen Saddles; eyes (optional) are grade B or C jungle cock.

Baby Brown Feathered Game Changer

This fly is tied the same way as the rainbow trout version, but with medium rootbeer Palmer Chenille and yellow and olive grizzly Magnum Hen Saddle selected from the middle of the skin. After forming the tail, tie in an olive grizzly Magnum Hen Saddle by the tips. The underbody on this fly is three 15-millimeter Fish-Spines.

Baby T-Bone (Brown Trout)

The tail on this pattern is a combination of spun yellow bucktail, prismatic gold Flashabou, and two yellow hackles about 3 to 5 inches long from a Metz Magnum Saddle. After you tie these in, tie in yellow and then olive bucktail, Hollow Fleye–style.

On the middle body, which is tied on a 15-millimeter Fish-Spine, I tie in a 1/8-by-1 1/4-inch Chocklett's Body Tubing and reverse it to form a spreader for the yellow bucktail spun around the tubing.

The head is tied on a 25-millimeter Fish-Spine with a 1/8-inch Body Tubing cut to 1 1/4 inches to form a spreader for the olive bucktail. After an application of prismatic gold Flashabou, tie in one more section of tubing and yellow bucktail, followed by one olive schlappen feather tied in and wrapped to form a collar. Lastly, add a 1/4-by-3-inch section of Body Tubing reverse tied to form the head. Add eyes with CCG Flex, and then coat the head with CCG Thick, followed by a top coat of CCG Hydro.

Another head coating favorite of mine is mother-of-pearl Sili Skin. Simply cut a strip of Sili Skin, and wrap it around the head, starting on the underside and folding up. Trim the excess material. The Sili Skin will stick to the Body Tubing. Then cut a strip about 1/4- to 1/2-inch wide and a little longer than the length of the head. Cover the seam and trim the front flush with the eye of the shank.

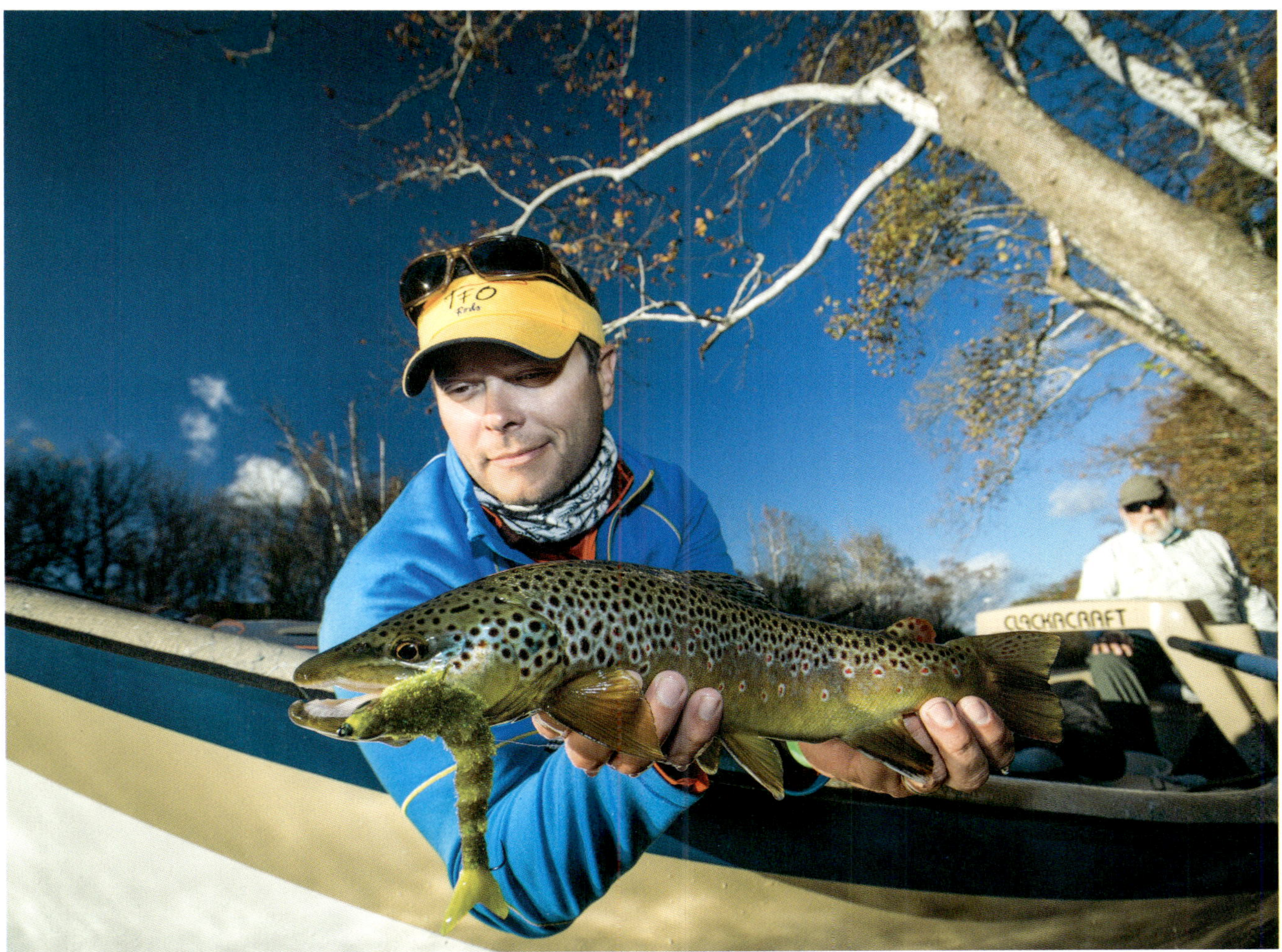

The Game Changer design has changed the way that I fish for large trout. In many ways, large browns act similarly to muskie.

Chapter 20

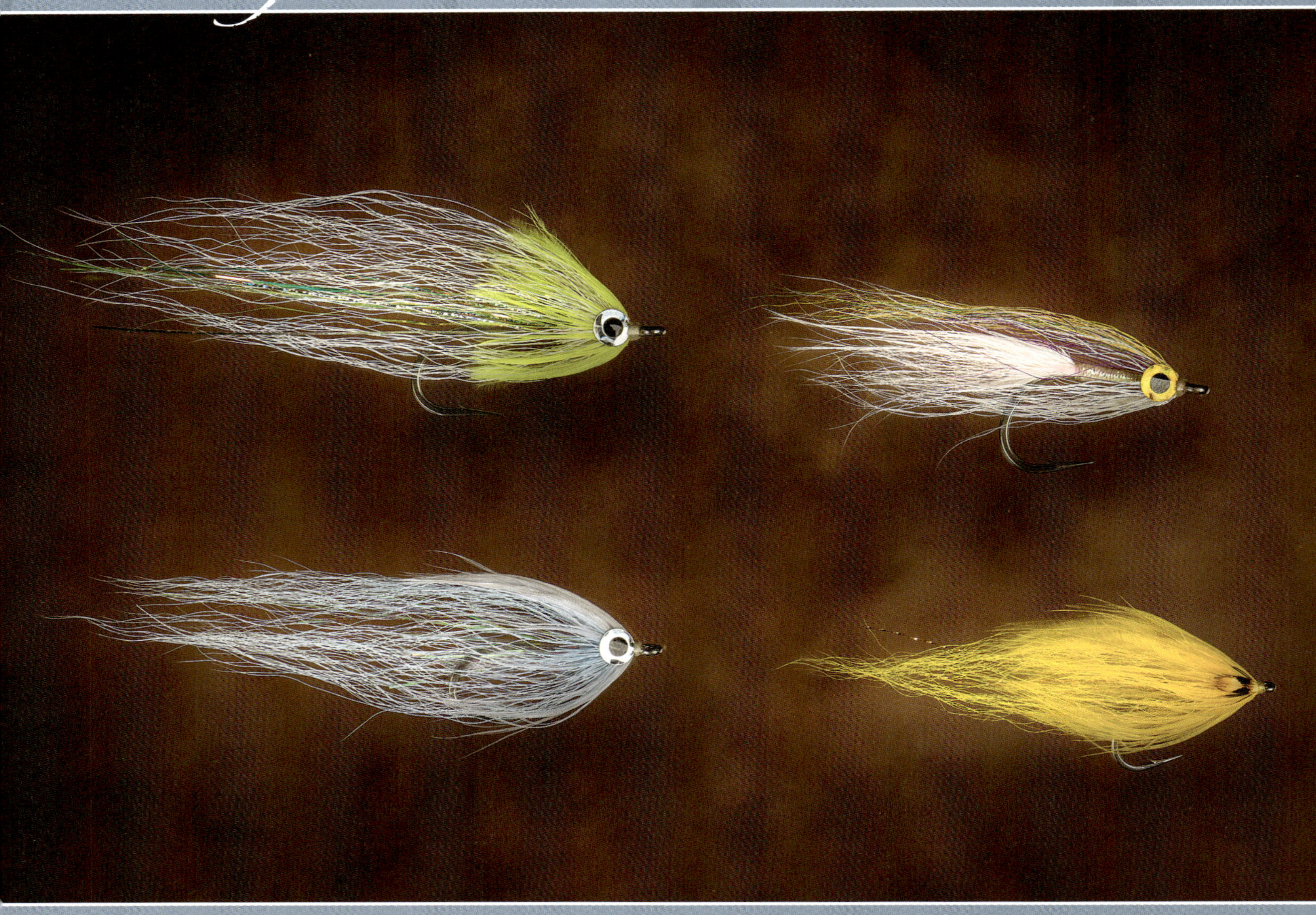

The Hollow style of tying can be adapted to small flies, as well. Above, a selection of Hollow Peanuts.

Pop's Indispensables

Dave Skok

Perhaps you've fished for trout with a fly and have heard of Tup's Indispensable? The "Tup's" is an early twentieth-century dry fly created by R. S. Austin that is still popular today. It was G. E. M. Skues, the father of modern nymph fishing, who exalted the pattern and dubbed it "Tup's Indispensable." "Tup's" was considered an absolute must-have for any fly fisher plying the waters of Britain's chalkstreams for picky trout. As a progressive angler and tier, Skues was a proponent of the then-heretical notion of fishing flies under the water and in a constant rivalry with his dogmatic contemporary, Frederic Halford, who accepted dry-fly fishing as the only suitable method of targeting trout. The reason I bring up all this ancient fly-fishing history is that, in my mind, Bob Popovics is both a modern day Austin for creating such iconic patterns and a modern day Skues who has never been afraid to break new fly-tying (and fly-fishing) ground. And, while it's impressive that R. S. Austin created the Tup's Indispensable, it's also impressive that Bob has come up with at least a dozen patterns that have shattered the conventional "rules" of fly tying. From epoxy to silicone to acrylic resin, Bob has set new standards for fly realism, durability, and fishability. As for Skues, I would love to have seen his heather tweed and pasty face alight in blue while torching another 'Poxyback Pheasant Tail Nymph. Ha!

My introduction to the incredibly fertile mind of Bob Popovics came late in the winter of 1990 when my copy of *American Angler* showed up. Surf Candies were featured on the cover and in a truly enlightening article by Ed Jaworowski. I was sixteen and my mind, like the minds of many other tiers, was completely blown. I thought to myself, "Those look *exactly* like silversides!" My hand was not nearly as deft as Bob's, so I ended up with epoxy on my tools, my table, my fingers, and just about everything else within a yard of my vise—real "fun" for anyone who is familiar with the terrible stink and burn of five-minute epoxy curing on human skin! After a while, I got better at handling the epoxy and learned to love Candies. The false albacore wholeheartedly agreed. A sizable raised dollop of brown epoxy is still there on that old magazine page. It's left a mark that has rippled through all the other pages of that issue, just like Bob's techniques have throughout the global fly-tying community.

Bob has produced numerous tying innovations. The extended body of the Shady Lady Squid, the "no power tools needed" Bob's Banger, and the nearly indestructible Siliclone and Flex Fleyes that look so good you want to fillet them and fry them in butter when you're done hitting them with the light. The list goes on and on. The impacts of his innovations are just about everywhere you

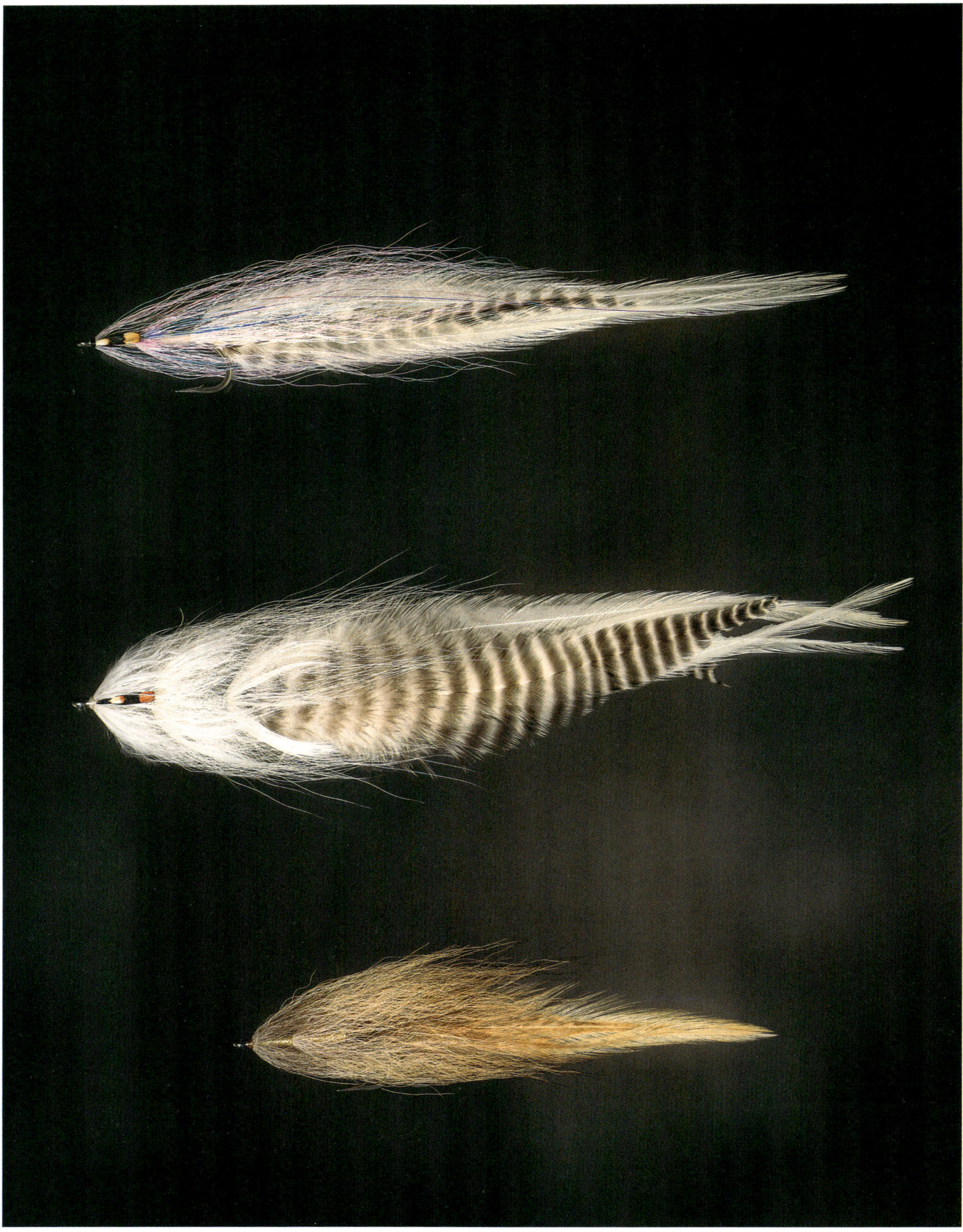

My favorite Popovics pattern is the Hollow Fleye. Many of my Hollow Deceivers have multiple collars of bucktail and saddle hackle or schlappen tails.

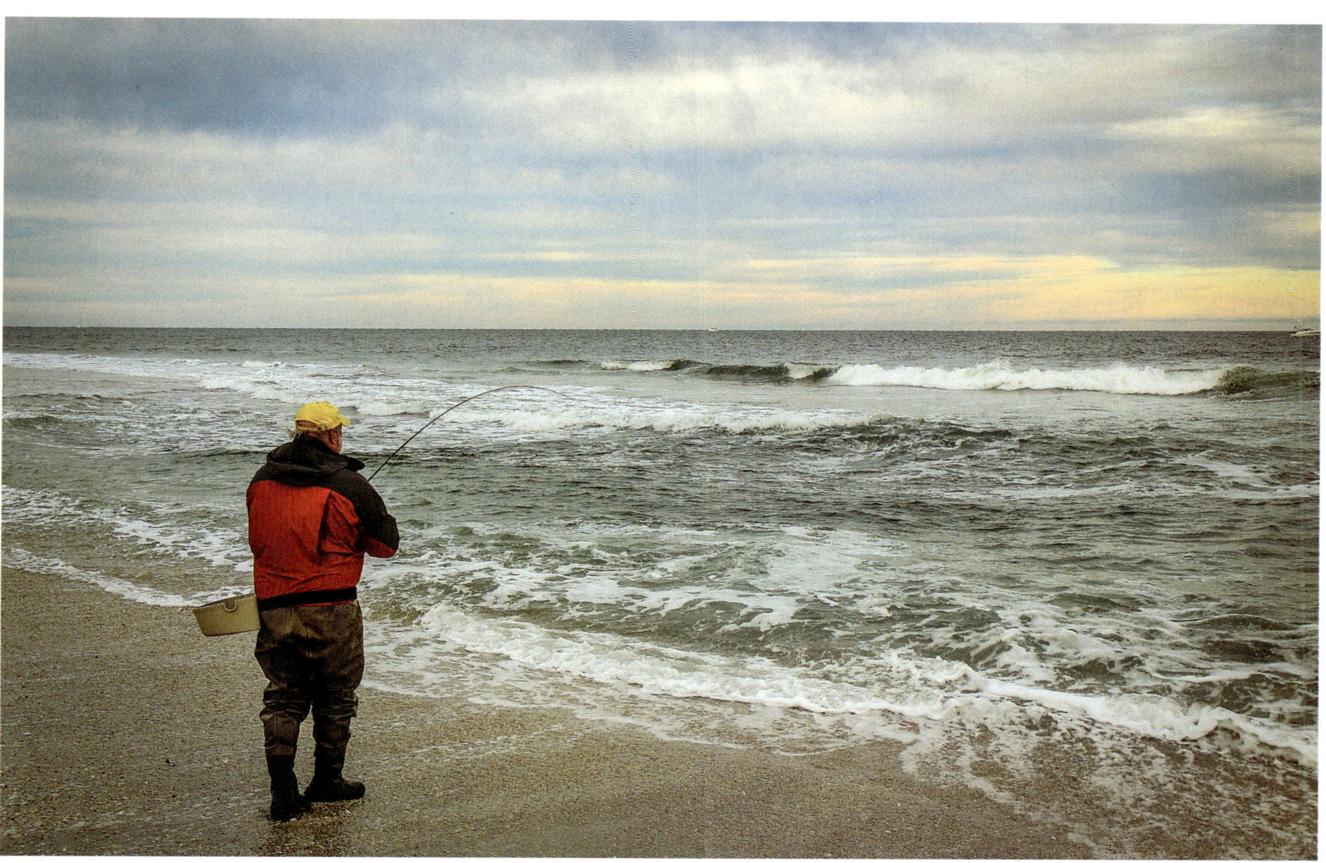

Bob Popovics plays a fish at Island Beach State Park, in Seaside Park, New Jersey. It's a perfect overcast day with whitewater at the Jersey Shore beaches with stripers at every edge. Late fall season means sand eels in tight.

look. The Mushmouth, the Albie Whore, and twenty-first-century muskellunge flies are all direct descendants of Pop Fleyes. Open any fly catalog and you'll see more Surf Candy and 3D Fleye knockoffs than you can count.

My favorite Popovics pattern is the Hollow Fleye. I like it best on a 3/0 or 4/0 hook with three collars of bucktail, a saddle hackle or schlappen tail, and just a hint of flash. I fish it from May to November. It's a perfect imitation of both river and sea herring and many other herring-like baitfish. It's so deadly that I'm not sure I would want to go striped bass fishing without it.

If you haven't already, perhaps someday you'll run into Bob. You might see him rolling down the beach in his custom four-wheel-drive van. Or maybe you'll find him sailing effortless loops over the outer bar and its rolling green and white waves. If you're lucky, you might even run into him while he's saddled up at the counter of Betty and Nick's Bait and Tackle for a double shot of pork roll, egg, and cheese on a fresh Portuguese roll. Either way, please take a moment to thank him for his inventive contributions to the world of fly tying.

Chapter 21

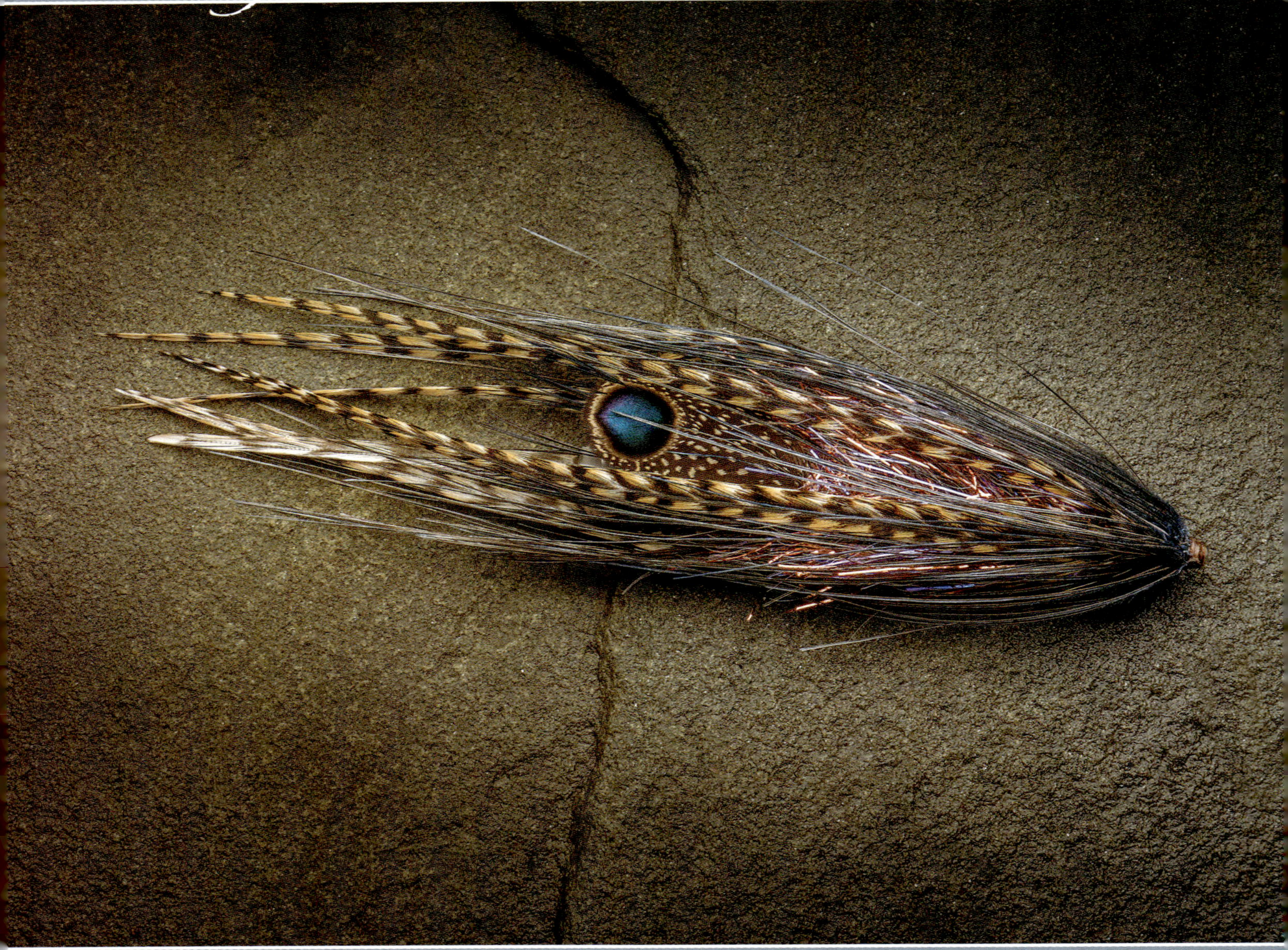

I started tying tubes for anglers fishing for steelhead and thought that tubes also would translate well to saltwater patterns, though you can also tie this fly on a long-shank hook. The rhea and cree hackle tied Semper style at the head of the Natural Squid Tube (above) create a 3D effect and have amazing movement in the water. The eye assembly is olive polar bear hair with peacock pheasant eyes. Reinforce the eyes with Scotch tape on the back and then coat the face of the eye with Flexament.

Squimpish Flies

David Nelson

The patterns and techniques that Bob Popovics has shared over the years have stood the test of time, not just in the East but worldwide. In my opinion, the most influential aspect of Bob's contributions to this sport and art are in the realm of sharing and caring. Bob seems to get an inordinate amount of pleasure in sharing his ideas with you and then encouraging you to make them your own. I can hear him now as I write this: "Listen, David, I just like to put the idea out there, share it with someone like you, and then see how you tweak it . . . how it progresses through your tying, how you make it develop, and how you make it your own."

One lesson, of many, that stands out for me is the first time that I saw Bob trace a fly on paper. I was at the Fly Fishing Show in Somerset, New Jersey, looking over someone's shoulder as Bob traced the outline of his fly on paper, removed the fly, and then drew in eyes and tail. Presto. A perfect fish silhouette. After the show, I went home and did the same thing to some of my flies. I could see that they were pretty good, but not quite right yet, and over the years I have come to do this for all my fly patterns, whether squids, shrimps, or baitfish. Sometimes, I photograph the fly and completely remove the color so that I only see the shape. Seeing the negative space of the fly makes the process more complete in my opinion, as it allows you to imagine how materials will interact with each other, which helps develop shape and taper in your flies—water and hydraulics are the only missing ingredients.

Because of the importance of flow and taper, I prefer to use natural materials in general. They have taper, unlike synthetics that you must cut to shape. When they absorb water, materials such as bucktail, peacock herl, and chicken and pheasant feathers flow, blend, and interact with one another—they become one yet remain separate components.

This interaction of materials is an important part of my fly construction. It starts with the front of the fly, where a good strong mass allows water to swim over the back and bottom of the fly and kick and flutter the fibers in the rear. I first saw this large mass in front of the fly in Bob's Cotton Candy Fleye, and when I asked him about it, he explained to me that it is the tips of the material that really move and flutter (and that to have currents moving over these tips, there needs to be a large mass ahead of the material). As a result I try to build shape and taper by tying in materials at different points so that the tips of the fibers are moving throughout the fly.

This leads to another important design consideration—a wispy tail and purposeful sparseness in the rear of my flies, which can be achieved with bucktail fibers or saddle feathers or peacock herl or fur. Bob has filmed baitfish extensively underwater, and he once explained to me that when viewed underwater, the back ends of baitfish disappear or fade out, as if they were ghosts. There are a lot of variables above and under the water and differences among the baits, of course, and though there is a lot that we will never know, I don't think that you can go wrong with basics such as silhouette and movement in a fly.

The Natural Squid Tube reflects some design concepts gleaned from Bob—proper eye placement and tying techniques from the Semper Fleye. Toward the end of a past Fly Fishing Show in Somerset, New Jersey, Bob picked up a squid fly that I had tied with a pair of jungle cock nails for eyes. He told me that he liked using natural materials for the eye, but that I should reconsider where I placed them. In the pattern that he was holding, I had tied them in at the start of the hook bend, but he pointed out that just

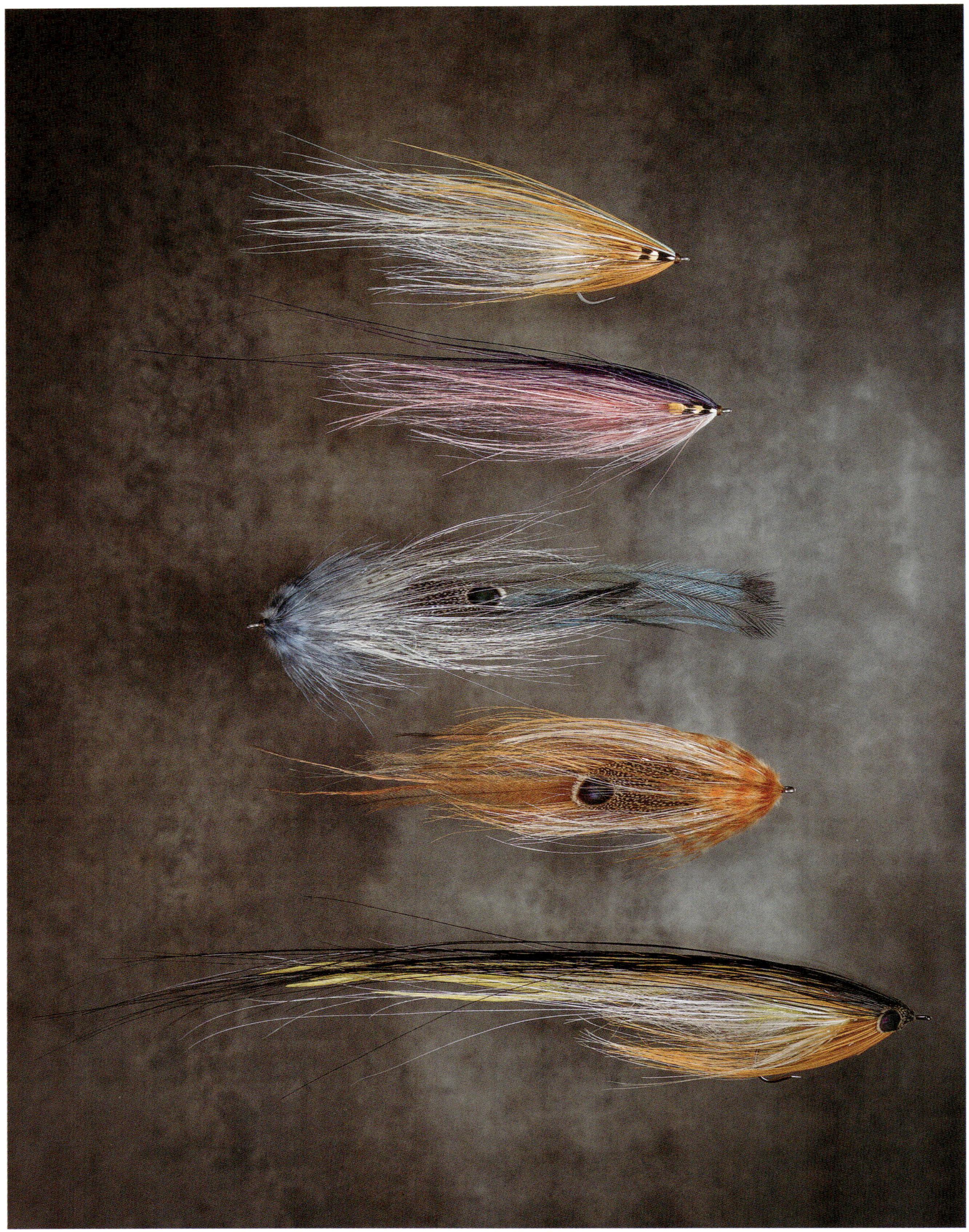

From top to bottom: Peacock Streamer, Albino Peacock Big Eye Squid, and Peacock-Eyed Fat Back Streamer.

moving the eyes back from the head by 1 inch didn't really make a contrast for fish looking for triggers—squid eyes are far in the rear. He asked if there a way to make a fly with a natural eye but get that eye farther back.

So the wheels turned, and I looked through some materials and saw the long peacock pheasant eyes, which had a long stem that when tied in would position the eyes perfectly. You can increase the durability of this beautiful feather by covering the back of it with a strip of Scotch tape and then brushing some flexible cement across the face of the feather eye.

As soon as I discovered it, the Semper tie quickly became my preferred method for constructing rear portions of baitfish and squid. A Semper tie is where slender to wide saddle feathers are tied 360 degrees around the hook shank as the tail (as opposed to just on top and flat like a flat wing or praying hands on either side like a Deceiver). After one tying session, I looked at the finished flies that I had tied and wondered, "Why not apply a Semper tie at the head of the fly?" When combined with a supporting collar of bucktail or a few turns of the actual feathers as a collar, it creates a 3D effect in the front of the fly.

Peacock-Eyed Fat Back Streamer

Hook: #4/0-4 Ad Sweir Pike
Tail: Natural polar bear clump and olive saddle hackle
Rear Body: Olive Palmer Chenille
First Collar: Albino peacock eye feather
Front Body: Silver Body Braid
Second Collar: Albino peacock dyed orange
Wing: Dyed black stripped peacock herl
Eye: Peacock pheasant "eye" feather, backed with Scotch tape and front coated with Flexament

Notes: This fly shows how Bob's ideas and techniques really get inside you. Instead of bucktail tied Hollow style, I use albino peacock eyes wound as hackle collars. This idea carried forward into other baitfish and squid patterns shown here.

The teardrop shape of this fly is an homage to the Fat Back/Temple Dog–style flies of Scandinavia. The dropped bend pike hook keels the fly perfectly. I designed this fly to be fished near the surface with a floating line for freshwater predators such as largemouth and smallmouth bass on the reservoirs in my area as well as muskie on the lower Delaware River.

Peacock Streamer

Hook: #2/0 Varivas or #2/0 Sakuma 410
Tail: White polar bear and 15 to 20 pieces of white albino peacock herl stripped from a tail feather
Rear Body: Pearl Body Braid
First Collar: Albino peacock eye feather dyed pink, tied in at tip, folded, and wound 2 turns
Front Body: Silver/pearl Palmer Chenille
Second Collar: Natural white albino peacock eye feather
Wing: Claret dyed peacock herl
Eyes: Jungle cock

Notes: This is a generic-shaped baitfish pattern for small Atlantic herring, Pacific sardines, or similar baits. Rear collar should be longer than front collar but shorter than tail. Changing the length of materials can yield different shapes. With a longer front collar, you will achieve a fatter profile, as the rear collar would now be a hoop inside the front (similar to the Peacock-Eyed Fat Back). The extra half turn of the eye feather should be tied off on top of the fly to help with proper keeling during the retrieve. This fly fishes well on a sinking line and should be thoroughly soaked prior to fishing for best action.

Albino Peacock Big Eye Squid

Hook: #2/0 Tiemco 911S
Tail: Polar bear clump surrounded by dyed-blue emu feathers tied Semper style
Eyes: Peacock pheasant tail eye feathers
Body: Silver Palmer Chenille
First and Second Collar: Albino peacock eye feather and natural Amherst pheasant fibers spread around as accents
Head: Barred marabou, color to match

Notes: Peacock pheasant eyes are reinforced for durability as in the other patterns. The marabou over the albino peacock eye feather in the front collar pulses with life. You can also substitute saddles for the emu. This fly is great on a sinking line when fishing the rips when squid are prevalent (think Watch Hill in June).

Chapter 22

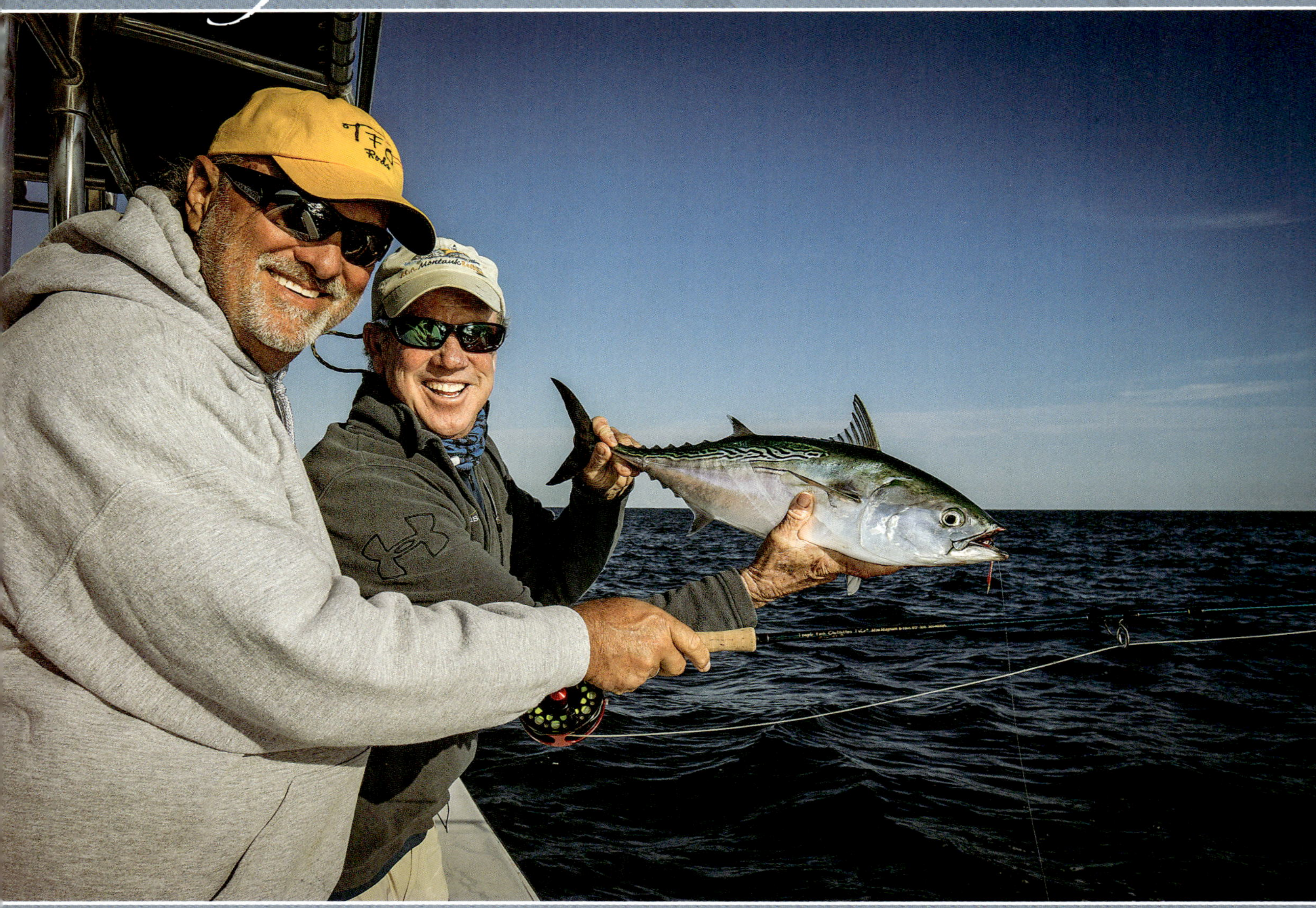

Bob Popovics and Capt. Paul Dixon with a false albacore caught off Montauk, New York, September 2015. The albie bite was phenomenal that day, with marauding packs of 5- to 8-pound fish gorging on whitebait (bay anchovies). TOM LYNCH

Innovator Extraordinaire

Paul Dixon

One of my first excursions fishing in salt water was in the early 1970s. It was my second year in college, and my friends and I were going to Cabo San Lucas in Baja, Mexico, for spring break. For me, it wasn't just about girls and partying. Even though that was foremost on my mind, I had ulterior motives. I was also dying to catch a roosterfish on a fly.

I grew up in Newport Beach, California, where my dentist had a mounted roosterfish on the wall in his office. Every time I got my teeth cleaned, he would regale me with his tale of catching the huge, comb-backed fish. I had endured years of mouth probing by dreaming about catching my own monster rooster. Having learned to fly-fish in Idaho the summer before our college trip, I was determined to master the salt water with a fly rod. Baja and the roosterfish seemed to present the perfect opportunity to realize my dream.

Our first night in Cabo, we trolled the bars for babes, with nothing to show for it the next day except throbbing heads. I spent the days flailing the beaches for the wily roosters. Oh, yes, I found them; they were there. But like the girls at night, they just wouldn't take the bait. They would sniff, nip occasionally, and follow the fly to my rod tip, but they would not hit.

I hobbled through the next decade of fly fishing using store-bought flies and learning to tie a few of my own with only a fair rate of success. In those days there just wasn't a large selection of saltwater flies to choose from. There were the Joe Brooks Blonde, Lefty's Deceiver, the Clouser Minnow, and few others, but it wasn't till I heard and read about Bob Popovics that things started to change for me. Bob was using methods and material to create baitfish imitations that boggled my mind. This guy had taken fly tying to a whole new level, and I wanted to be part of it. I was hooked on Pop Fleyes!

I finally got to meet Bob Popovics in the late '80s when I ran the Orvis booth at the Somerset Fly Fishing Show in New Jersey. Bob was whipping up his creations and drawing a small crowd of admirers, myself included. This was before the explosive growth of saltwater fly fishing. Now when you see Bob tying at a show, there are hordes of admirers, waiting eagerly to ask him about Bob's Banger, Shady Lady Squid, Ultra Shrimp, Surf Candy, or a dozen of Bob's other patterns. Bob Popovics is arguably the most innovative saltwater fly tier in the world today.

I began fishing and shooting video with Bob in the early '90s, which was about the same time I started my own fly shop and guiding service on the East End of Long Island. Since then, Bob and I have spent countless days on boats in Gardiners Bay, Montauk, Florida, and the Bahamas. In all those areas, Bob would always be problem solving. What is the bait? How does it swim? What material can I use to imitate it? He was always curious, always inquiring. At night, Bob would sit at the bench and produce the creations he'd been visualizing all day. Sometimes they worked, and sometimes it was back to the drawing board. But, inevitably, by the next time I saw Bob, he'd have some kind of new creation that blew my mind. Problem solved!

One day in June, while sight-fishing for stripers in Gardiners Bay, fellow fly fisherman Nick Curcione, Bob, and I were forced off the water by a strong northwest wind. Bob decided to use the downtime to test his newest creation—the Pop Lips—in the swimming pool at my house. While Nick and I observed the fly's action from underwater, Bob's job was to cast the Pop Lips and trim the silicone lip of the fly to maximize its action. Two hours later, Bob had the fly swimming perfectly. Nick and I were waterlogged, but a fly was born.

Over the years I have spent thousands of days guiding fly fishermen up and down the East Coast. Like most guides, I believe what's in my fly box to be critical to my success. There may be twenty different types of flies in the box, but I probably only use a handful throughout the season. Of that handful of flies, more than 80 percent are Pop Fleyes. Yes, I still use Clousers and Deceivers. They are great flies, but when I'm trying to "match the hatch," as they say, Bob has a fly to mimic almost any size, shape, or form of baitfish.

When I'm fishing the herring run in Montauk in late fall, I use Bob's Spread Fleye. It gives the perfect profile of the herring, is durable, and is easy to tie. If I'm fishing for big bass in the rocks and rips using sinking lines, I'll often use a Deerhair Deceiver. When you fish it real slow for the old cows, the Deerhair Deceiver pulsates and breathes. It just cries out, "Help me!"

I do a fair amount of teasing of bluefish and bass in the summer. I will tie on a Bob's Banger for my client and have him stand ready to cast. I will throw a hookless plug and tease the fish into casting range of the Banger. I like the Banger because its flat head creates tremendous commotion, and the fish will come to it instantly when the teaser is pulled.

Often in the spring, while I'm poling the flats in Gardiners Bay, we'll see stripers following sea robins. The sea robin, an orange, ugly little critter, is rooting along the bottom and will spook grass shrimp. The shrimp will bolt to the surface trying to escape the robin, and the bass will race forward to inhale the shrimp before the slower

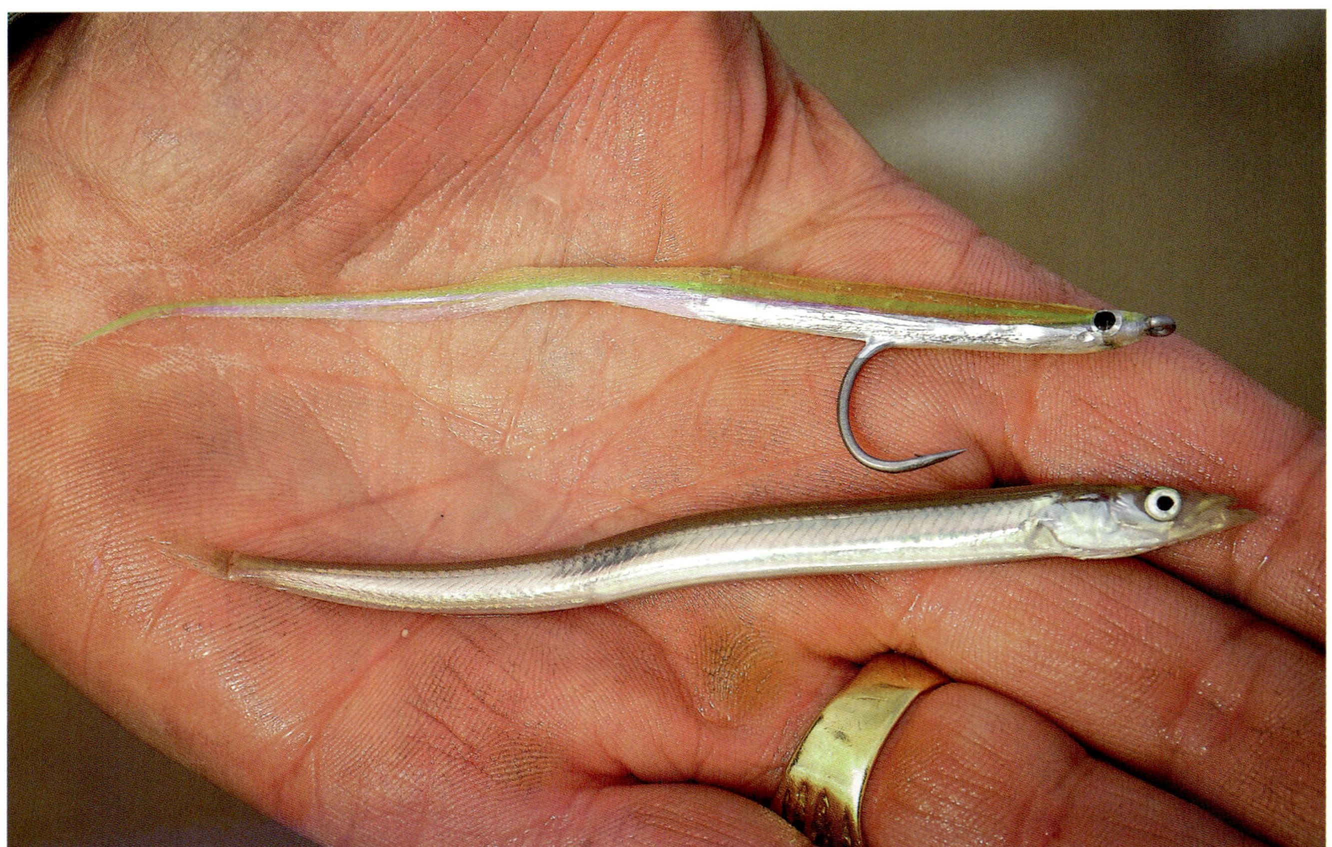

Sand Eel Surf Candy. Not only does the fly imitate the natural sand eel, it is tied on a strong hook and the elongated body ensures that it won't foul.

sea robin. When I see a bass following a robin, I quickly tie on one of Bob's Ultra Shrimp, and then it's game over for that bass. The striper will pound that Ultra Shrimp before the sea robin knows what happened—which is lucky for the robin, not so lucky for the bass.

So, as you can see, I tie and use a lot of Bob's fly patterns, but none as much as the Surf Candy. The Surf Candy gives such a realistic representation of a variety of small baits, depending on how you tie it. Most baits in the spring on the flats in Gardiners (such as sand eels) and in Montauk in the fall (such as bay anchovy) are small. I usually tie my epoxies with different-colored Polar Fibre. Polar Fibre breathes and looks realistic even when fished slow.

The Surf Candy, or epoxy fly, was developed by Bob in the early '70s to create a durable fly to withstand toothy bluefish. By adding synthetic material and epoxy to a hook, Bob helped revolutionize the sport of saltwater fly fishing. That bit of epoxy and material created a translucent baitfish imitation that fooled even the most wary gamefish. Nowhere is this truer than when fishing for false albacore. The Surf Candy erases the frustration of fishing for albies that we used to encounter in the old days, when fly refusals were the norm. The albies just hammer the thing! Whether it's Bob Clouser adding lead eyes to a hook or Bob Popovics adding epoxy, it doesn't matter. It all starts with the creator.

A few years back I began experimenting with different flies when I was fishing the flats for stripers. I had been having trouble later in the season with finicky fish refusing the fly. The norm up until that point had been to use intermediate lines and sinking flies. In the early days of sight-fishing for striped bass, I had tried floating lines and surface flies with no success. Most stripers could not be enticed to the surface, and the few that could refused the offering. So for years we used what worked, until one day it didn't.

They say necessity is the mother of invention. After a morning of ripping out what little hair I had left on my head due to fly refusals, I jumped down off the poling platform and started digging through my fly box. We could see schools of sand eels, but the bass didn't seem to even care about them. Still, nothing else was working. I tied on a small Surf Candy that looked about as close to a sand eel as you can get. I told my client to lead the next striper by a few feet so the fish could get a chance to see the fly over its head, as they tend to hug the bottom. That fish rocketed off the bottom and whacked that Candy. It was a eureka moment.

I now use a skinny Candy and floating line in almost all of my sight-fishing for stripers. I attribute my earlier failure with flies to the fact that they were impressionistic rather than realistic looking. That is why Bob's fleyes work so well in many conditions. If you hold one of Popovics's fleyes next to actual bait in your hand, it's easy to see why they catch fish. They look like fish.

It's been many years since that college trip to Baja and my uneventful quest, for women and roosterfish, but I can honestly say that I have had more success on both counts through the years. For the latter, I can definitely thank Bob Popovics. If it weren't for his innovation and tireless dedication to the art of fly tying, fly fishing would be a far more frustrating endeavor. Come to think of it, Bob's flies may have helped me indirectly with women as well. The fly that acts right, looks right, and is dressed right is sure to catch fish. That's a lesson I wish I'd known before I got to Baja.

About the Contributors

Nick Curcione

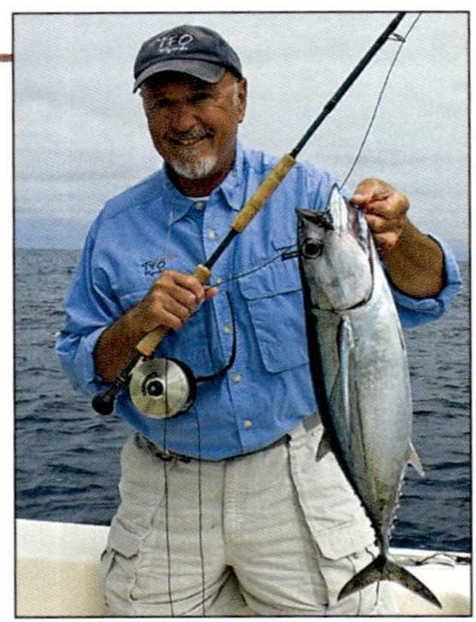
JOHN LOO

In addition to his former 35-year career as a university professor, Nick is an internationally recognized outdoor writer, instructor, lecturer, and tackle consultant with a lifetime of angling experience. He has been on the sportfishing-show circuit for more than 40 years. His writing credits are extensive, with numerous articles in local, national, and international publications, and he has authored three fly-fishing books. In 2011 he received the FFF Silver King Award for his contributions to saltwater fly fishing.

Ed Jaworowski

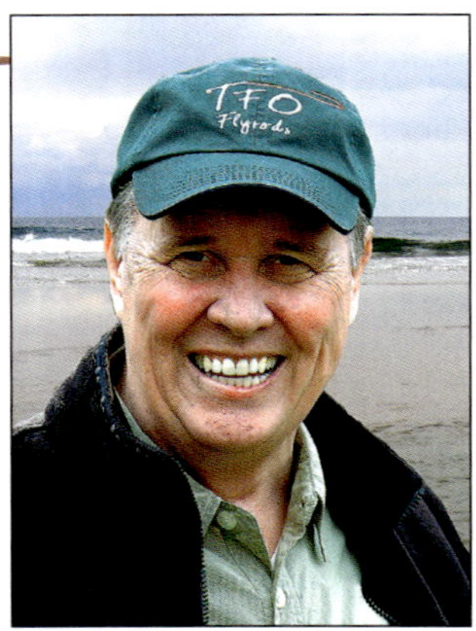
LEFTY KREH

Ed Jaworowski is an internationally known fly-casting coach, writer, photographer, speaker, and tackle consultant. He and Bob Popovics have been close friends and angling companions for more than 40 years. They collaborated on the first book about Bob's flies, *Pop Fleyes*.

Richard King

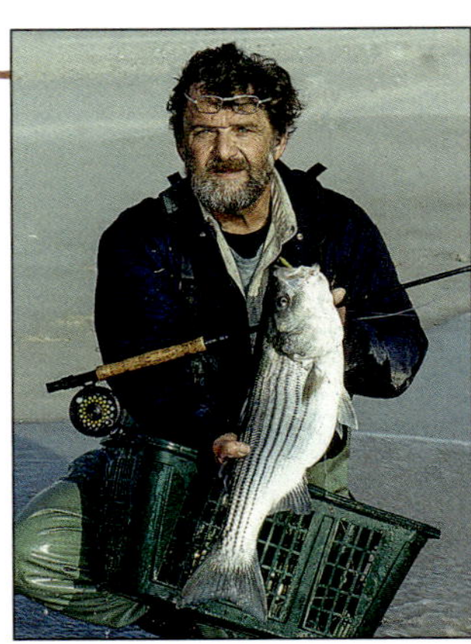
RON RODGERS

Richard King has had a lifelong obsession with fishing and the natural environment, particularly New Jersey's Barnegat Bay Estuary. Being introduced to saltwater fly rodding by Elwood "Cap" Colvin, its founder, in 1970 opened his mind not only to fly rodding, but to one of the most productive ecosystems in the world. Richard has since photographed thousands of organisms, from grasses, algae, invertebrates, and forage fish to herons, blues, stripers and weakfish. He is determined to photograph and study the full range of wildlife—including small and underappreciated species at the base of the ecosystem that allow larger, more popular species to exist—in order to give a true image of a wonderful place you won't see on a map. His website is www.richardkingwildlifephotography.com.

Steve Farrar

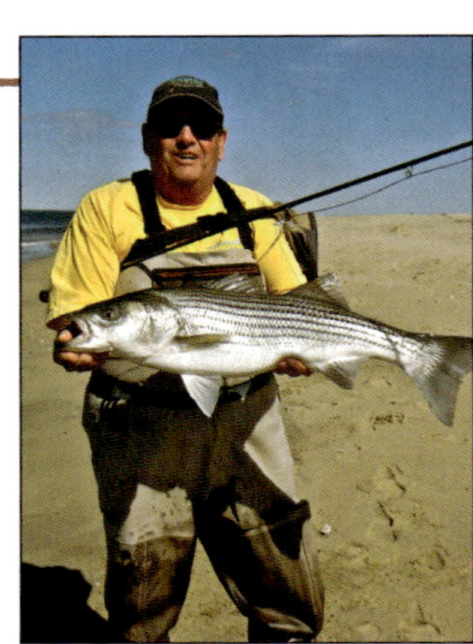
GERARD FABIANO

Born and raised in New Jersey, Steve Farrar started fly fishing and tying in the early '90s. He joined the Atlantic Saltwater Fly Rodders in 1992, where he first met Bob Popovics. Steve has developed a variety of blends using synthetic fibers and flash, including the popular Steve Farrar's SF Blend, which is distributed worldwide by Fishient.

Jonny King

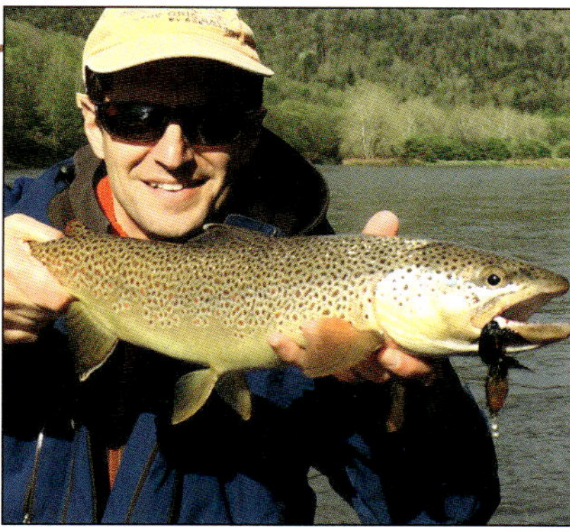

BEN RINKER

Jonny King is a lifelong fly fisherman and tier from New York City. He taught himself to tie as a young boy reading Poul Jorgenson's instructional books and has developed successful patterns for virtually all fresh and saltwater species. His flies, commercially available through Orvis, have claimed a number of world records. Jonny has written numerous articles for *Fly Fishing in Salt Waters* and *Fly Fisherman*, and his flies are regularly featured in *American Angler*, *Fly Tyer*, and many other U.S. and international magazines.

Blane Chocklett

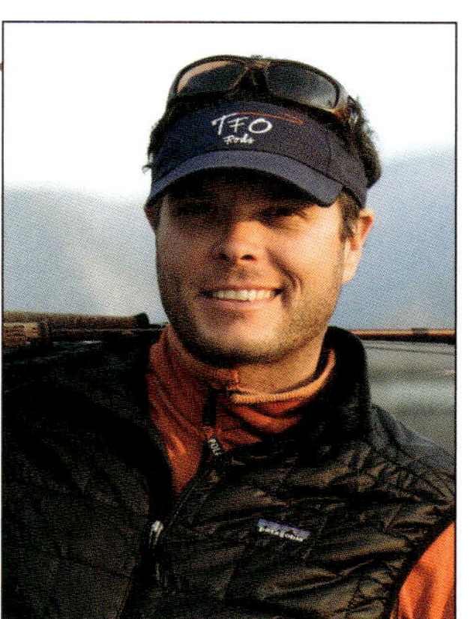

JACK HANRAHAN

Blane Chocklett is a full-time guide and fly designer specializing in musky, bass, trout, and stripers. He is an Umpqua Feather Merchants signature tier, on the TFO rod design team, and has been featured in publications such as *Fly Fisherman* and shows such as Larry Dahlberg's *The Hunt for Big Fish*.

Dave Skok

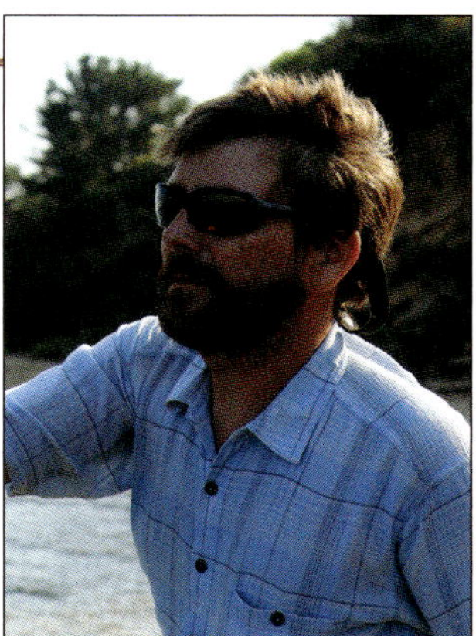

VAN MILENKOVICH

Dave Skok is a Boston-based fly tier and photographer who has been learning from Bob Popovics since he was a teenager in Connecticut.

David Nelson

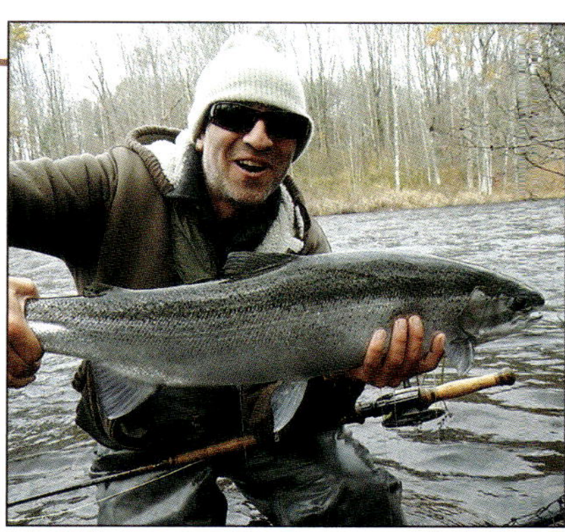

PATRICK ROSS

David Nelson is a fly fisherman and tier who lives near Kensico Reservoir in White Plains, New York. His grandmother instilled in him a love for the outdoors at a young age, and he enjoys fishing for stripers, trout, albies, and steelhead throughout the year, as well as sight-fishing for carp.

Paul Dixon

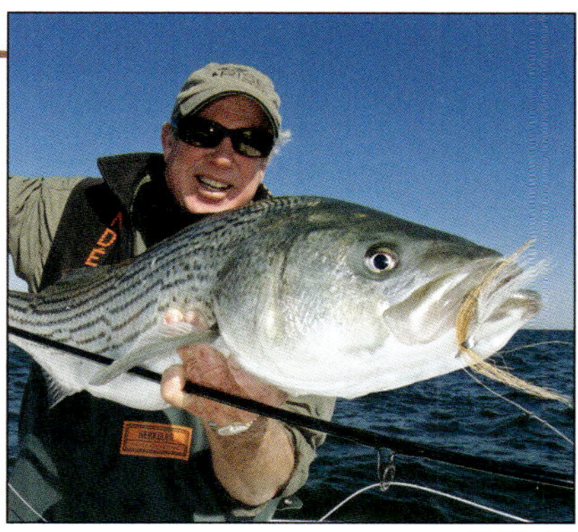

PAT FORD

Paul Dixon is a fly-fishing guide in Montauk, New York, who pioneered the sport of sight-fishing for striped bass on the waters of Eastern Long Island. He has been guiding in those waters for over twenty years and spends the winters in the Florida Keys guiding for bonefish, permit, and tarpon. Paul has traveled the world fly-fishing in the Seychelles, Belize, Bahamas, Mexico, British Columbia, and across the United States. He has also been featured on several ESPN fishing shows such as *Guide House: Montauk*, *Spanish Fly*, and *Walker's Cay Chronicles*.

Index

Page numbers in italics indicate photographs.